Orthopaedic and Sports
physical
therapy

Mosby's Physical Therapy Series

Orthopaedic and Sports Physical Therapy, ed. 2
edited by **James A. Gould III, M.S., P.T.**

Cardiopulmonary Physical Therapy, ed. 2
edited by **Scot Irwin, M.S., P.T. and Jan Stephen Tecklin, M.S., L.P.T.**

Neurological Rehabilitation, ed. 2
edited by **Darcy Ann Umphred, Ph.D., R.P.T.**

Orthopaedic and Sports
physical
therapy

Edited by

James A. Gould III, M.S., P.T.
Associate Professor of Physical Therapy
Department of Physical Therapy
University of Wisconsin-La Crosse
Editor, Journal of Orthopaedic and
  Sports Physical Therapy
Co-editor, Orthopaedic Physical Therapy Practice
La Crosse, Wisconsin

Second edition

with 703 illustrations

The C. V. Mosby Company

ST. LOUIS • BALTIMORE • PHILADELPHIA • TORONTO • 1990

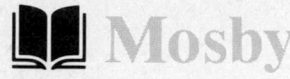

Editor: Richard Weimer
Developmental Editor: Kathryn H. Falk
Assistant Editor: Ellen Baker Geisel
Production Editor: Cynthia A. Miller
Design: Liz Fett

Second Edition

The C.V. Mosby Company
11830 Westline Industrial Drive, St. Louis, Missouri 63146

Library of Congress Cataloging-in-Publication Data
Orthopaedic and sports physical therapy/edited by James A. Gould
    III.—2nd ed.
        p.   cm.
    Includes bibliographical references.
    ISBN 0-8016-2908-X
    1. Physical therapy.   2. Orthopedics.   3. Sports medicine.
  I. Gould, James A.
    [DNLM: 1. Orthopedics.   2. Physical Therapy.   3. Sports Medicine.
  WB 460 077]
  RD736.P47078   1990
  615.8′2—dc20
  DNLM/DLC
  for Library of Congress   89-12910
                                                              CIP

C/MV/MV   9 8 7 6 5 4 3 2 1

Contributors

Tzvi Barak, Ph.D., P.T.

Adjunct Instructor, Downstate Medical Center, Physical Therapy Program, State University of New York, Brooklyn, New York; Adjunct Instructor, Touro College, Huntington, New York; Private Practice, East Side Orthopaedic and Sports Physical Therapy, New York, New York.

Richard W. Bowling, M.S., P.T.

Assistant Professor, School of Health Related Professions, University of Pittsburgh; Private Practice, President, Forest Hills Orthopaedic and Sports Physical Therapy, Pittsburgh; Pennsylvania.

Ronald Steven Brocato, B.S., P.T.

Private Practice, Rehab Pine, Richmond, Virginia.

Carl DeRosa, M.S., P.T.

Associate Professor and Chairman, Physical Therapy Program, Northern Arizona University, Flagstaff, Arizona.

John S. Eggart, M.S., P.T., A.T.C.

Chief Physical Therapist, Student Health Center, University of Wisconsin-La Crosse, La Crosse, Wisconsin.

Mark H. Friedman, D.D.S.

Private Practice, Mount Vernon, New York.

James A. Gould III, M.S., P.T.

Associate Professor of Physical Therapy, Department of Physical Therapy, University of Wisconsin-La Crosse; Editor, Journal of Orthopaedic and Sports Physical Therapy; Co-editor, Orthopaedic Physical Therapy Practice, La Crosse, Wisconsin.

Ivan A. Gradisar, Jr., M.D.

Professor of Orthopaedics, Northeastern Ohio Universities, College of Medicine, Rootstown, Ohio.

John W. Halbach, M.S., P.T., A.T.C.

Director of Sports Medicine, Orthopaedic and Sports Physical Therapy, La Crosse, Wisconsin; Clinical Affiliate, Department of Physical Therapy, Indiana Central University, University of Wisconsin-La Crosse, Marquette University, and University of Miami, Florida.

Dennis L. Hart, P.T., Ph.D.

President, Assessment Centers Technology, Arlington, Virginia.

Dixie L. Hettinga, B.S., P.T.

Director of Physical Therapy, Department of Physical Therapy, Wausau Hospital Center, Wausau, Wisconsin.

Gary C. Hunt, M.A., P.T.

Department of Physical Therapy, Medical Center for Federal Prisoners, Springfield, Missouri.

Gregory W. Kaumeyer, M.S., P.T., A.T.C.

Co-Director, Physical Therapy and Sports Injury Rehabilitation Ltd; Private Practice, Hazel Crest, Illinois.

James S. Keene, M.D.

Associate Professor, Team Orthopedic Surgeon, University of Wisconsin Athletic Teams; Section of Sports Medicine, Division of Orthopedic Surgery, University of Wisconsin Hospitals and Clinics, Madison, Wisconsin.

Glenda L. Key, P.T.

Physical Therapist, President and Founder, Key Functional Assessments, Inc., Minneapolis, Minnesota.

Donald T. Kirkendall, Ph.D.

Associate Professor, Department of Health, Physical Education, Recreation and Dance, Illinois State University, Normal, Illinois.

David Leigh, M.I., Ph.D.

Head Athletic Trainer, Marquette University, Department of Athletics, Milwaukee, Wisconsin.

Barney F. LeVeau, Ph.D., P.T.

Professor and Chairman, Southwestern Allied Health Sciences School, Department of Physical Therapy, The University of Texas Southwestern Medical Center, Dallas, Texas.

Terry R. Malone, Ed.D., P.T., A.T.C.

Executive Director of Sports Medicine, Associate Professor of Physical Therapy, Assistant Professor of Surgery, Duke University, Durham, North Carolina.

Robert E. Mangine, M.Ed., P.T., A.T.C.

Administrative Director of Rehabilitation, Cincinnati Sports Medicine and Orthopaedic Center, Cincinnati, Ohio.

Thomas G. McPoil, Jr., Ph.D., P.T., A.T.C.

Assistant Professor, Department of Physical Therapy, Northern Arizona University, Flagstaff, Arizona.

James Allen Porterfield, M.A., P.T., A.T.C.

Faculty Member, Graduate Curriculum, Department of Physical Therapy, Cleveland State University, Cleveland, Ohio and Ohio State University, Columbus, Ohio; Owner, Crystal Clinic Rehabilitation and Health Center, Akron, Ohio.

Cheryl L. Riegger, P.T., Sc.D.

Assistant Professor of Physical Therapy, Division of Physical Therapy, University of North Carolina, Chapel Hill, North Carolina.

Paul A. Rockar, Jr., M.D., P.T.

Adjunct Assistant Professor, School of Health Related Professions, University of Pittsburgh; Private Practice, Forest Hills Orthopaedic and Sports Physical Therapy, Pittsburgh, Pennsylvania.

Elaine R. Rosen, M.S., P.T.

Associate Professor, Program in Physical Therapy, School of Health Sciences, Hunter College of The City University of New York, New York, New York; Private Practice, Queens Physical Therapy Associates, Forest Hills, New York.

Mark J. Rowinski, Ph.D., P.T.

Director, Physical Therapy Program, University of Rhode Island, Kingston, Rhode Island.

Barbara Sanders, M.S., P.T.

Director and Assistant Professor, Physical Therapy, Southwest Texas State University, San Marcos, Texas.

Michael Sanders, Ed.D.

Assistant Track Coach, Men's Intercollegiate Athletics, University of Texas, Austin, Texas.

A. Joseph Santiesteban, Ph.D., P.T.

Associate Professor, Physical Therapy Program, Indiana University, Indianapolis, Indiana.

Christine E. Saudek, M.S., P.T.

Managing Editor, Journal of Orthopaedics and Sports Physical Therapy; Co-editor, Orthopaedic Physical Therapy Practice, La Crosse, Wisconsin.

H. Duane Saunders, M.S., P.T.

Physical Therapist, Saunders Therapy Center, Edina, Minnesota.

Roslyn Sofer, P.T.

Clinical Instructor, Program in Physical Therapy, Downstate Medical Center, State University of New York, Brooklyn, New York and Touro College School of Physical Therapy, Huntington, New York; Private Practice, Community Physical Therapy, Middle Village, New York.

Robert T. Tank, M.A., P.T., A.T.C.

Adjunct Faculty, Department of Physical Therapy, University of Evansville; Director, Department of Sports Medicine and Rehabilitation, Orthopaedic Associates, Inc., Evansville, Indiana.

Greg Vergamini, M.S., P.T., A.T.C., S.C.S.

Sports Medicine Coordinator, St. Mary's Medical Center, Duluth, Minnesota.

Carolyn Thaxton Wadsworth, M.S., P.T.

Lecturer, Physical Therapy Program, University of Iowa, Iowa City, Iowa.

Lynn A. Wallace, M.S., P.T., A.T.C.

Director, Ohio Physical Therapy and Sports Medicine; Consulting Athletic Trainer, Case Western Reserve University and Lake Erie College, Cleveland, Ohio.

Joseph Weisberg, Ph.D., P.T.

Associate Professor, Department of Physical Therapy, Downstate Medical Center, State University of New York, Brooklyn, New York.

Michael Zito, M.S., P.T.

Associate Professor, Department of Allied Health, University of Connecticut, Storrs, Connecticut.

To my wife Deborah and daughter Kimberly
who have guided me and reinforced my
endeavors through their love and support.

JAG

PREFACE

Physical therapy is in the midst of a tremendous revolution in practice and philosophy. Established in the early 1900s by a group of physical education persons called to work with polio epidemic victims, the profession has evolved to the point where recognition of clinical specialists is beginning. The clinical specialists in orthopaedics and sports are just now being certified. The growth in the number of orthopaedic and sports specialists will lead to greater recognition of physical therapy as a vital component of the health team at a time when the health care team concept is in turmoil. The team concept is being questioned because of alteration of the medical model. The historical medical model regarded the physicians as the "commander of the ship" or the captain of the health care team.

Presently the medical model is shifting to a shared leadership concept, a transition that is difficult because shared leadership requires trust and respect. The health care team members have all received their education and training in relative isolation from each other and it will take a great cooperative effort to balance the team leadership in the health care team of the future. Physical therapy's role in the health care team is yet to be fully establshed. Therefore specialized physical therapists who can take command of aspects of the health care team will ensure a vital role for physical therapy in the future.

It is for the training of the orthopaedic and sports specialists that the individual chapter authors of this text have updated their respective chapters.

As we work toward increased independence of health care practitioners with increased responsibility, the information contained in these chapters shall be of even greater value to the practicing physical therapist.

James A. Gould III

CONTENTS

Part One

Basic sciences: Musculoskeletal System

Chapter 1

MECHANICAL PROPERTIES OF BONE

Cheryl L. Riegger

Bone is a living tissue that provides support and structure to the body. Through attachments to bone, the muscular system initiates and sustains movement, which allows us to carry out the activities of daily living. When most professionals study bone, it is the dead, dehydrated, brittle bone found in skeletal models. What we must remember is

I would like to thank Dr. Christopher Ruff, for guidance in the development of this paper, and my mentor, Dr. Whitney Powers.

that bone is a dynamically adaptable material that continually undergoes subtle remodeling. This fact is the key to understanding the mechanical properties and behavior of bone.[66] There are seven categories of bone:[66,78]

1. Long bones are tubular—usually longer than they are wide—with a shaft or body and convex or concave articular ends. The shaft usually contains a hollow center, the medullary cavity. Examples of long bones are the femur and humerus.
2. Short bones are generally small and cuboidal. Of their six surfaces, four or fewer are articular and two or more serve as attachment sites for tendons and ligaments or entry sites for blood vessels. Examples of short bones include the carpal and tarsal bones.
3. Flat bones consist of two plates of compact bone, with cancellous bone and marrow located between the plates. The skull, sternum, and scapula are examples.
4. Irregular bones, such as facial bones and vertebrae, are usually composed of various nonuniform shapes.
5. Pneumatic bones contain air cells or sinuses with a cortical shell of bone surrounding the air spaces. The mastoid portion of the temporal bone is a pneumatic bone.
6. The round or oval sesamoid bones are located within tendons. They not only protect the tendon but also increase the mechanical advantage of the muscle involved by increasing the angle of application at the muscle attachment site. Examples of sesamoid bones are the patella and the bones connected to the flexor pollicis brevis and flexor hallucis brevis.
7. Accessory or supernumerary bones develop when an

extra ossification center appears in, or a usually oc-curring ossification center fails to fuse with, the main part of the bone.

The main functions of bones are to provide support for the body, to facilitate joint movement, to produce red blood cells (including some lymphocytes, granulocytic white blood cells, and platelets), to protect various body structures and organs, and to store calcium, phosphorus, and magnesium salts.

MECHANICAL PROPERTIES OF MATERIALS

External forces acting on tissues, as well as other struc-tures, can be defined in mechanical terms. Such forces cause internal reactions within a structure, which can be expressed in many forms: load, deformation, stress (σ) or load/unit area, and strain (ϵ), or the percentage of defor-mation occurring within a structure. Units of measure for force, deformation, stress, and strain are listed in Table 1-1. Types of stresses and strains are listed in Table 1-2.

Equal and opposite distracting external loads, which tend to pull a structure apart, cause tension. The structure elongates, and tensile stress and strain result. Maximal tensile stress occurs on a plane perpendicular to the ap-plied load; that is, if stresses were assessed on a plane other than a perpendicular one, a reduced tensile stress would occur (Fig. 1-1).

External crushing loads equally applied on opposite sur-faces of a structure produce compression and tend to shorten and widen a structure, resulting in compressive stress and strain. Maximal compressive stress also occurs on a plane perpendicular to the applied load. These stresses represent resistance to crushing loads (Fig. 1-2).

Shear stresses occur when equal but not directly oppo-

Table 1-1. Units of measure for expressing forces on bone

Force	Deformation	Stress	Strain
	Millimeter	Pounds per square inch (psi)	Percentage change in length
Pound	Centimeter	Pascal (Pa)*	Angular defor-mation in radians
Newton (N)†	Inch	Megapascal (MPa) (equals 1 million Pa or N/m²) Gigapascal (GPa) (equals 1 billion Pa or N/m²)	

*A pascal is 1 n/m² and is the pressure produced by the force of 1N ap-plied uniformly over an area of 1m.²

†A Newton is $\dfrac{1 \text{kg m}}{\text{sec}^2}$ and is the force that, when applied to a mass of 1 kg, gives an acceleration of 1m/sec.²

Table 1-2. Types of stresses and strains

Reaction	Symbol	Method of determination
Tensile stress	Tσ	Tensile force/unit area
Tensile strain	Tϵ	Increase in length/original length
Compressive stress	Cσ	Compressive force/unit area
Compressive strain	Cϵ	Decrease in length/original length
Shear stress	$\tau\sigma$	Shear force/unit area
Shear strain	$\tau\epsilon$	Angular deformation

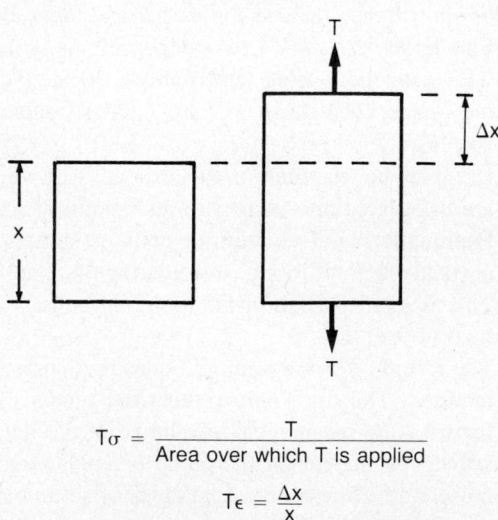

$$T\sigma = \frac{T}{\text{Area over which T is applied}}$$

$$T\epsilon = \frac{\Delta x}{x}$$

Fig. 1-1. Tensile stress and strain.

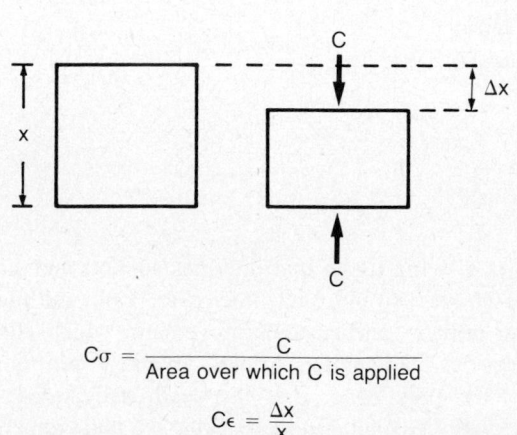

$$C\sigma = \frac{C}{\text{Area over which C is applied}}$$

$$C\epsilon = \frac{\Delta x}{x}$$

Fig. 1-2. Compressive stress and strain.

site loads are applied to opposing surfaces or structures. Normal shear strain is a linear deformation that occurs as molecules move past each other (Fig. 1-3). Shear stresses and strains result when both tensile and compressive loads are applied to a structure. At any point within the structure, tension and compression are maximal in two orthogonal planes and these maxima are called the *principal stresses*. At the same point, the shear stress and strain are zero in the direction of the principal stresses and maximal in a plane at a 45-degree angle to the principal stresses (Fig. 1-4). Angular shear strain results when shear stresses and strains are caused by tensile or compressive stresses (Fig. 1-5).

The strength of a material—as defined by the area under the load-deformation curve (energy storage)[41] or by the ultimate failure point—and its stiffness—as defined by the load/deformation ratio or slope in the curve in the region of elastic deformation—can easily be studied by drawing a load-deformation curve for that material. However, for comparison of different materials, it is necessary to standardize loads as loads per unit area and deformations as deformations per unit length or percentage of deformation. The result is a stress-strain curve.[41] Many important measurements can be determined directly from this curve[14,41,84] (Fig. 1-6). The measurements that can be determined include the following:

1. *Strength*. The area under the load-deformation curve or the stress-strain curve area defined by the ultimate failure point or ultimate stress or strain.[1]
2. *Yield point*. That point *(Y)* at which the material no longer reacts elastically; that is, some deformation is maintained after the release of the load.
3. *Ultimate failure point*. That point *(U)* where ultimate failure occurs.
4. *Stiffness (modulus of elasticity, Young's modulus, E)*. The slope of the elastic portion of the stress-strain curve for tensile or compressive loads, σ/ϵ.

For an elastic material or a material loaded within an elastic range, stress and strain are linearly related such that stress equals E × strain (Hooke's law).

5. *Shear modulus of elasticity*. The slope of the elastic portion of the stress-strain curve for shear loads or, sometimes, the slope in the initial portion of the torque-angular deformation curve, τ/ϵ.
6. *Ultimate stress*. A ratio that can be expressed as load at failure over the initial area of the cross section of the material that equals the stress at the point of failure or the stress at the point of failure.
7. *Ultimate strain*. The strain at the point of failure.

Materials are either ductile or brittle or a combination of the two, depending on the amount of deformation they can withstand before failure.[41] A ductile material deforms a great deal before failure and therefore has a long plastic region. A brittle material has no plastic region, deforming very little before failure. At the time of failure, the two ends of the brittle material can be fitted together to conform to the original shape of the material.

Loading systems produce bending if two force pairs act at opposite ends of a structure (four-point bending), or three forces cause bending (three-point bending), or if an already bowed structure is loaded axially[29,41] (Fig. 1-7). In any case, the original structure has one element, the neutral axis, that does not change in length. However, on bending, the convex portion of the structure is subject to tensile stresses and is elongated, whereas the concave portion is subject to compressive stresses and is shortened. Since a structure may be asymmetrical, the tensile and compressive stresses may not be equal. Tensile and compressive stresses are maximal at the furthest distance from the neutral axis and are proportional to the square of that distance. Shear stress is greatest at the neutral axis (Fig. 1-8).

The bending produced in a structure is called the *bending moment*, or the tendency for a load to move a structure clockwise or counterclockwise around a fixed point. The bending moment is determined around a point or axis by multiplying the load times the perpendicular distance from the action line of the load to the axis, that is, bending moment M = force × distance[111] (Fig. 1-9). In static equilibrium, the sum of the forces in any direction equals zero ($\Sigma F = 0$), and the sum of the moments around any point also equals zero ($\Sigma M = 0$) for any coordinate system.

If accelerations are involved, the inertial resistance to such movements must be calculated. In a linear sense, force = mass × acceleration describes the relationship of a linear force (F) and a resultant linear acceleration (a). The inertial resistance of an object rotating around a point is determined by the object's mass and the object's weight distribution. For example, a pendulum with a heavy mass distant from the point of rotation will resist changes in motion more than a pendulum of uniform weight. The mo-

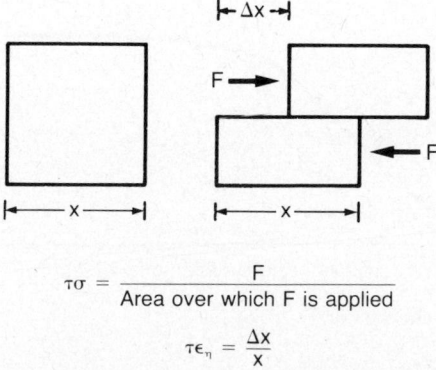

$$\tau\sigma = \frac{F}{\text{Area over which F is applied}}$$

$$\tau\epsilon_\eta = \frac{\Delta x}{x}$$

Fig. 1-3. Shear stress and strain.

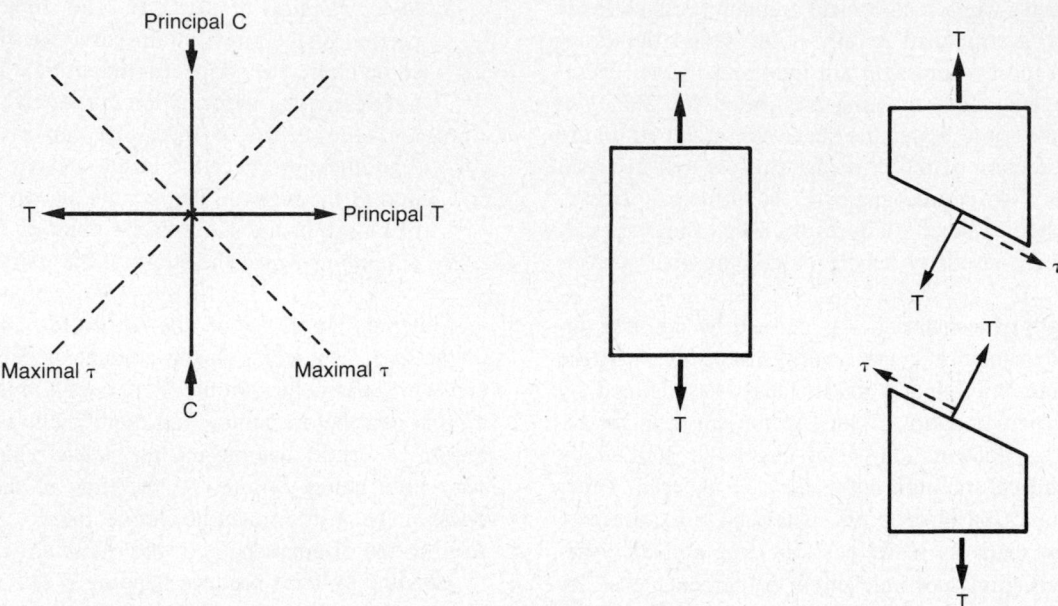

Fig. 1-4. Maximal shear occurs in a plane 45 degrees to the planes of principal tensile and compressive stress.

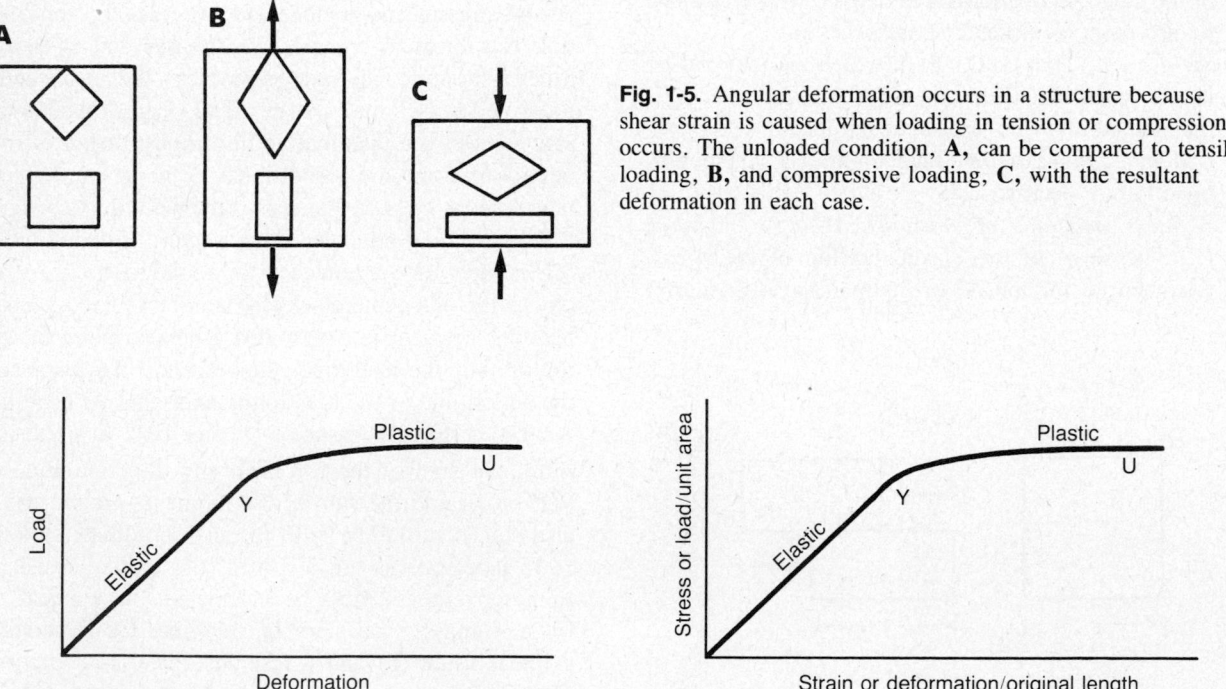

Fig. 1-5. Angular deformation occurs in a structure because shear strain is caused when loading in tension or compression occurs. The unloaded condition, **A,** can be compared to tensile loading, **B,** and compressive loading, **C,** with the resultant deformation in each case.

Fig. 1-6. Load-deformation and stress-strain curves.

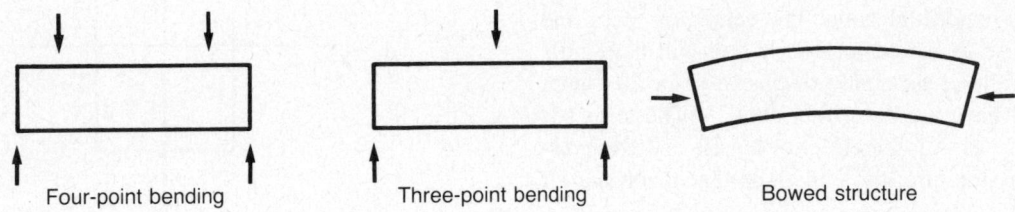

Four-point bending   Three-point bending   Bowed structure

Fig. 1-7. Four-point bending, three-point bending, and axial loading of a bowed structure.

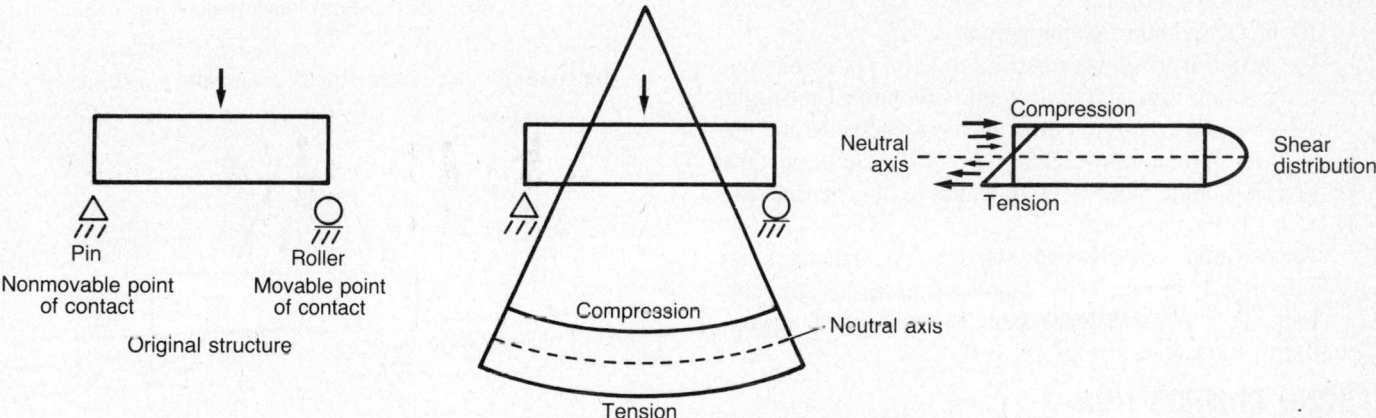

Fig. 1-8. Bending results in tensile, compressive, and shear stresses and strains.

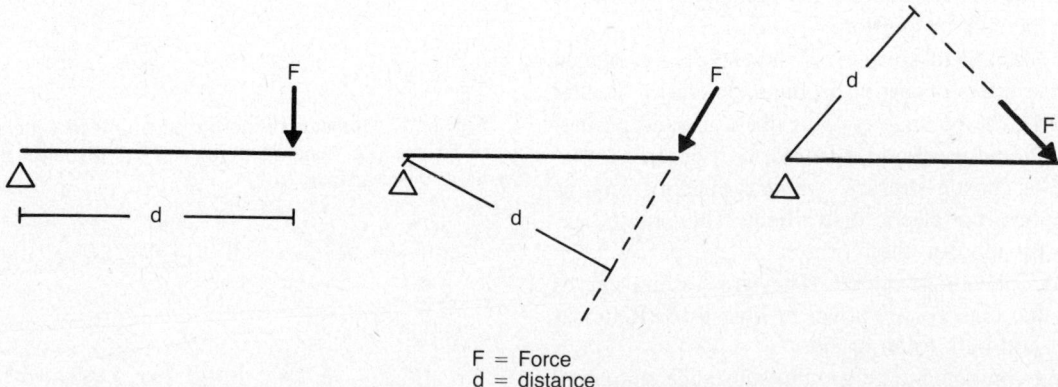

F = Force
d = distance

Fig. 1-9. Bending moment = (load) force × distance, which is the perpendicular distance from the action line of the force to the axis.

ment of inertia, or I (the second moment of the area), is a constant for a material of specific shape and indicates the ability of the segment to resist angular movement. The value I is determined about the point of rotation by summing each mass times the square of its distance from that point (Fig. 1-10). The equations show that I will be minimal when rotation occurs about the center of mass and mass that is close to the center of rotation will have little effect on I. It follows that mass displaced from the center of rotation will have a great effect on I.[111] The term I is used in conjunction with the effect of tensile and compressive loads on a structure; the equations that incorporate I are seen in Fig. 1-11.

The polar moment of inertia (J) indicates resistance to changes of angular movement resulting from torsional (twisting) loads. J is determined by the equation $J = \int r^2 dA$, where dA is each small mass of the material and r is the distance of that mass to the center of rotation (0) (Fig. 1-12). For a cylinder, as shown in Fig. 1-12, 0 is the center of the cylinder, or the neutral axis.

The result of torsion loads (Fig. 1-13, *A*) is shear stress over the entire cross section of the structure. The magnitude of the shear stress is directly proportional to the distance from the neutral axis (Fig. 1-13, *B*) and is maximal on planes parallel and perpendicular to the neutral axis (Fig. 1-13, *C*).

Tensile and compressive stresses on structures are shown visually in Fig. 1-14. The net stresses for structures undergoing combined loads can be determined algebraically, as illustrated in Fig. 1-15.

BONE COMPOSITION

Bone is classified as a connective tissue, as are cartilage, ligaments, tendons, and fascia. The connective tissues have three parts—a fiber component, a ground substance with a tissue fluid component, and a cellular component. The first two components form the extracellular matrix and make up the bulk of the connective tissue, as compared to the cellular portion.

The fiber component consists of three types—collagen or large-course fibers occurring in bundles; elastin smaller fibers; and small branching reticular fibers located primarily in lymphoid and myeloid (bone marrow) organs. Collagen fibers resist tensile stresses, whereas elastin fibers, as the name implies, are elastic or resilient. They can be extended and still recover their original shape easily when the stretching force is removed. The stress-strain curves for collagen and elastin are shown in Fig. 1-16. Reticular fibers merely add bulk to an organ.

The second component is a ground substance composed of amorphous glycosaminoglycans (GAGs, formerly known as mucopolysaccharides), the constituents of which are protein-sugar combinations (proteoglycans, glycoproteins, chondroitin sulfate, and keratan sulfate) and hyaluronic acid (Fig. 1-17).

This ground substance–tissue fluid component helps

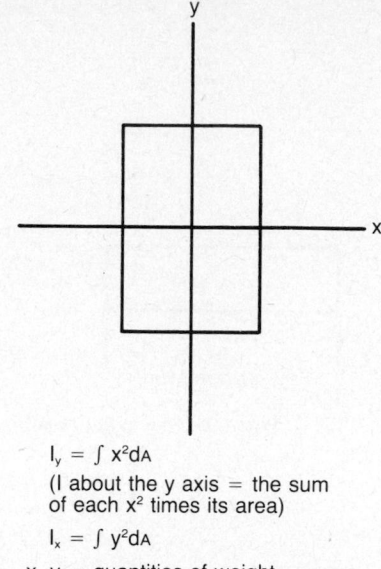

$I_y = \int x^2 dA$
(I about the y axis = the sum of each x^2 times its area)

$I_x = \int y^2 dA$

x, y = quantities of weight
dA = the distance of each weight from the axis

Fig. 1-10. Moments of inertia (I) around the y and x axes.

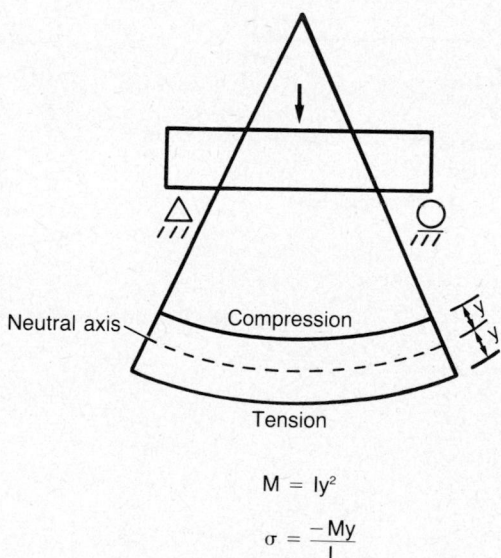

$M = Iy^2$

$\sigma = \dfrac{-My}{I}$

Fig. 1-11. Moments of inertia: equations that incorporate moment of inertia *(I)*, bending moment *(M)*, distance from the neutral axis *(y)*, and stress *(σ)*.

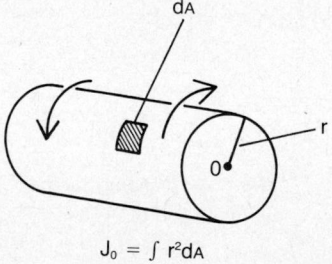

$J_0 = \int r^2 dA$

Fig. 1-12. Polar moment of inertia *(J)*, or the resistance of a structure to torsion loads, is calculated by $J_0 = \int r^2 dA$.

SHEAR STRESSES

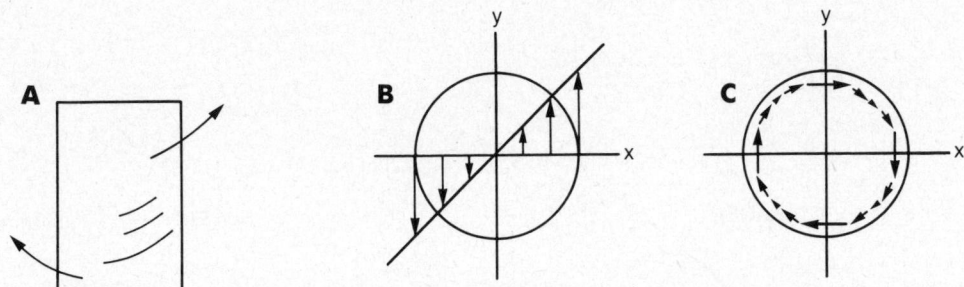

Fig. 1-13. A, The result of a torsion load is shear stress over the entire surface of the structure. **B,** The magnitude of the shear stress is directly proportional to the distance from the neutral axis. **C,** Shear stress is maximal on planes parallel and perpendicular to the neutral axis *(C)*.

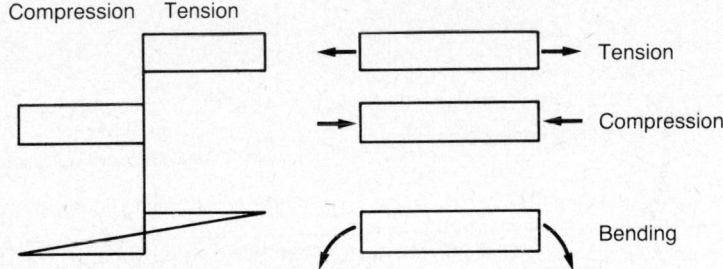

Fig. 1-14. Visualization of tensile and compressive stresses.

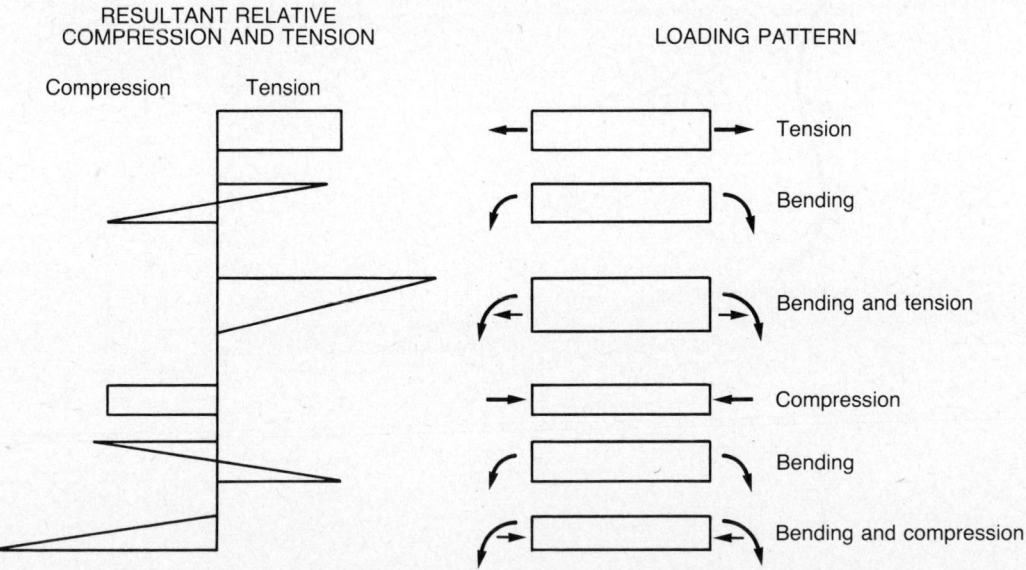

Fig. 1-15. Net stresses resulting from combined loading.

Fig. 1-16. Stress-strain curves of collagen and elastin.

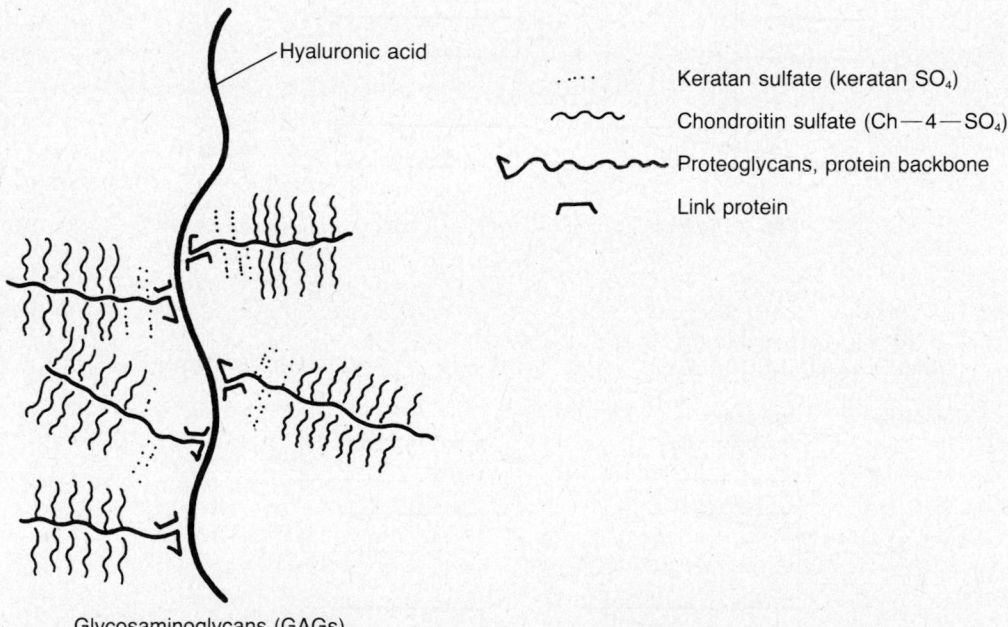

Fig. 1-17. Structure of glycosaminoglycans.

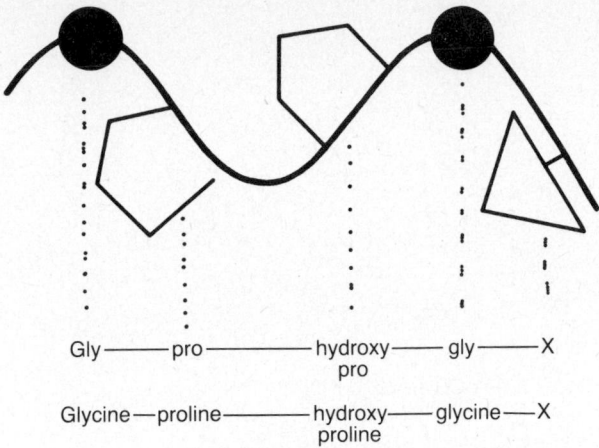

Gly —— pro —————— hydroxy —— gly —— X
                        pro

Glycine — proline ———————— hydroxy —— glycine — X
                              proline

Fig. 1-18. Amino acid sequence of collagen.

maintain tissue water and electrolyte balance, controls the diameter growth of collagen fibrils,[69] forms linkages with collagen fibers,[69] decreases friction between fibers, resists tissue compression, and helps transmit tensile loads between collagen fibers by filling in the spaces.

The third component of connective tissue is the cellular component. It contains fibroblasts and fibrocytes, from which fibers are produced, as well as cells that are tissue specific.

Mechanical properties of the different connective tissues can be determined by the percentages and contents of the three components and direction of fibers.

Bone consists of a collagenous fiber component, a ground substance of mostly calcium phosphate ($Ca^{++}P$)—which is reordered to form hydroxyapatite, GAGs, and hyaluronic acid—and a cellular component of osteoblasts, osteocytes, osteoclasts, and osteoprogenitor cells. Bone is unique in that it has both an inorganic mineral component, mainly hydroxyapatite, and an organic component, mainly collagen.[84] Since the properties of bone differ significantly from the properties of either of its original components, bone is called a *composite material*.[66] Bone has been viewed as a two-phase material[106] in which the hydroxyapatite crystals are considered the high-modulus, or stiff, portion and collagen is the low-modulus portion. Wall, Chatterji, and Jeffrey[106] state, however, that an accurate representation of bone requires a three-phase model—mineral, organic, and fluid.

Approximately 40% of bone tissue is organic and consists not only of collagen but also GAGs and lipids.[66] Collagen has the general amino acid sequence, glycine-proline-X, and contains another amino acid, hydroxyproline (Fig. 1-18). In humans collagen alone contains hydroxyproline. Collagen exists in a greater relative amount in bone than in any other tissue, and bone collagen has the shortest half-life.[11] These facts suggest that detection of hydroxyproline in urine, for example, may yield valuable

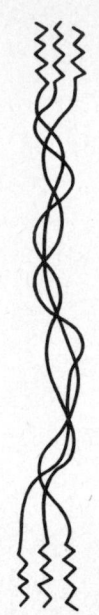

Fig. 1-19. Triple alpha helical chains forming tropocollagen.

information about bone deposition and resorption in different states of growth, adaptation to exercise, and disease. Collagen originates from a precursor, tropocollagen, and has a triple alpha-helix formation[84] (Fig. 1-19). The stability of collagen is increased during maturation via crosslinkages formed between alpha-helices and various intramolecular and intermolecular bonds, including those of water, with the polar groups in the collagen backbone (Fig. 1-20).

When fibroblasts are placed in tension and stretched as a result of muscle traction forces at a tubercle or because of bending that caused tension on one side of a bone, they elongate and align to lines of tensile stress. Collagenous fibrils then appear along these lines to counteract the stress.[108] Water is attracted to and fills the intervening spaces between collagen fibrils, allowing the fibrils to develop even more of a parallel arrangement, thus increasing their structural stability. This parallel alignment allows collagen to resist tensile loads. However, since collagen does not have equal mechanical properties when loaded in different directions, it is termed *anisotropic* (Fig. 1-21). The ground substance portion of the organic phase of bone acts as a glue, lubricant, and shock absorber.[84]

The hydroxyapatite crystals of the inorganic or mineral phase of bone, composed of calcium and phosphorus, are slender rods 200 to 400 Å (angstrom = 10^{-10} m) long by 15 Å thick and are located between and within the collagen fibrils.[84,88] Other mineral ions are citrate, carbonate, fluoride, and hydroxyl ions.[84] The mineral phase gives stiffness (two thirds that of steel), rigidity, and hardness to bone.[56]

New bone is formed of osteoblasts that mature to become osteocytes; bone is resorbed by osteoclasts. Osteo-

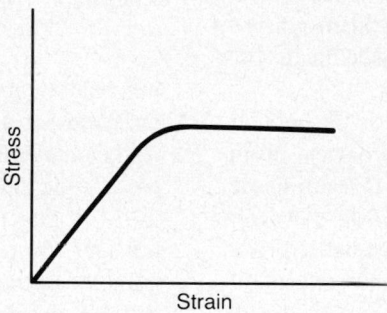

Fig. 1-20. The main collagen cross-link in bone is dehydrodihydroxylysinonorleucine.

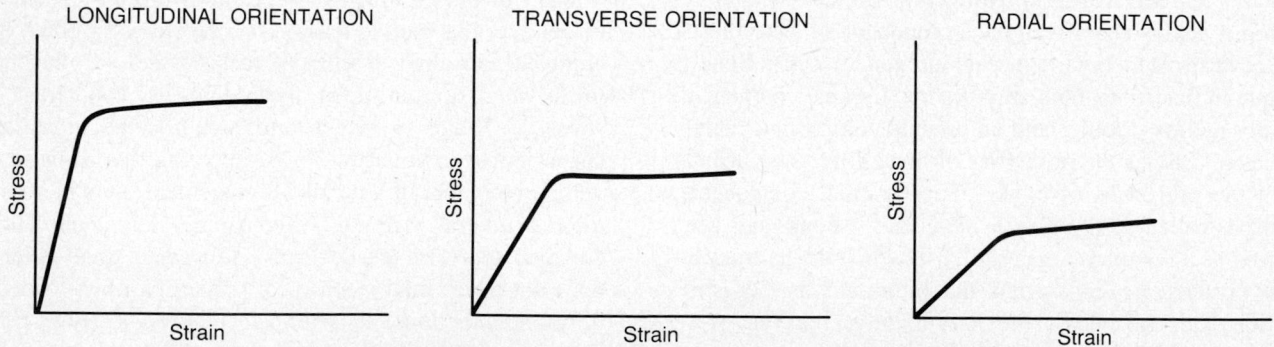

Fig. 1-21. *Top,* An isotropic material has a similar stress-strain curve independent of the direction of loading. *Bottom,* Different stress-strain curves result if nonisotropic material is loaded in different directions.

blasts synthesize enzymes that modify collagen fibrils and GAGS to produce osteoid or bone matrix.[88] Lysosomal, neutral pH phosphatase activity is unique to differentiated skeletal cells (i.e., osteoblasts, osteocytes, and osteoclasts) and to cartilage cells. A major difference between osteoblasts and osteoclasts is the tremendous quantity of lysosomal enzymes produced in the Golgi apparatus around the cell nucleus in osteoclasts.[88] Since osteoblastic activity causes bone formation and osteoclastic activity causes bone decomposition, a greater osteoclastic than osteoblastic activity will result in osteoporosis. Osteoprogenitor cells are located in the endosteum (inside) and periosteum (outside) of bone. Also, since there is no periosteum at attachment sites for ligaments and tendons, where articular cartilage is found in sesamoid bones, or at the subcapsular area of the femoral neck and on the talus, there is a lack of osteoprogenitor activity at these sites.

BONE GROWTH

Bone can develop in two ways, either by endochondral (enchondral) bone growth, which produces an intermediate cartilaginous model of the bone, or by intramembranous bone growth, in which bone is formed directly without a cartilaginous model.[10,28,30,63] The skull, sternum, and part of the clavicle are formed intramembranously, whereas the other bones are formed by endochondral bone growth. As one of the connective tissues, bone is derived from embryonic mesoderm, which is called *mesenchyme*. Mesoderm is one of the three embryonic germ layers, the other two being ectoderm and endoderm (entoderm). Bone of the skull and jaw, formed from the branchial arches (embryological tissue of the throat) is mesectodermal (mesoderm and ectoderm) in origin. Mesenchyme also differentiates into other connective tissues, such as tendon, ligament, cartilage, and blood, and a nonconnective tissue, muscle. Mesoderm forms lateral, intermediate, and medial (somite, paraxial) portions. Fig. 1-22 shows the three portions of mesoderm and their skeletal derivatives.

Endochondral bone growth

The relative time schedule for the development of bone by endochondral growth[28,78,79,107] is as follows:

Prenatal period

Week 3 (after fertilization). Mesenchymal cells begin migration from the intraembryonic mesoderm to specific locations.

Week 4. The migrated mesenchymal cells aggregate and condensation occurs. Somites are formed from the paraxial mesenchymal cell aggregations. The somites consist of (1) a ventromedial portion, the sclerotome, which is the precursor for bone, cartilage, and ligament within the axial and a small part of the appendicular skeleton; and (2) a dorsolateral portion, the dermomyotome, from which the dermis of the skin and skeletal muscle will form, again for the axial skeleton plus a small portion of the appendicular skeleton.

The sclerotome migrates in three directions—ventromedially to surround the notochord and form the intervertebral disk, dorsolaterally to cover the neural tube forming the vertebral arch, and ventrolaterally toward the body wall to form the costal processes (future ribs) on the thoracic vertebrae and portions of the transverse processes on other vertebrae (Fig. 1-23).

Week 5. Mesenchymal models of future bones have

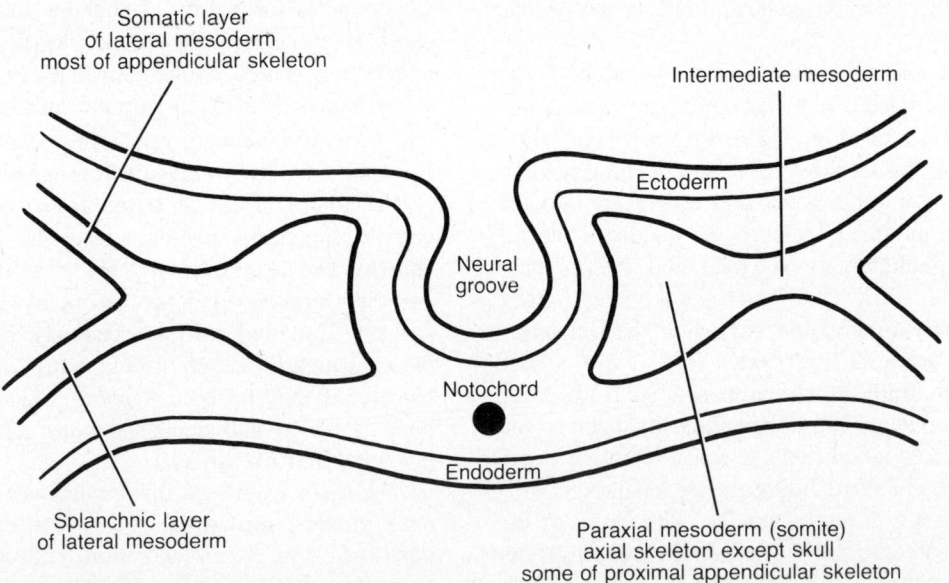

Fig. 1-22. Paraxial, intermediate, and lateral portions of intraembryonic mesoderm and their skeletal derivatives.

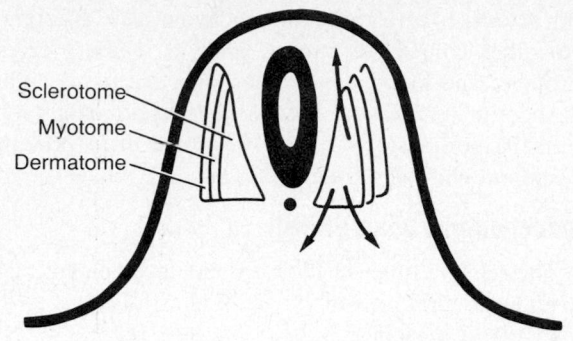

Sclerotome
Myotome
Dermatome

Fig. 1-23. Migration of cells from the sclerotome includes cells migrating ventromedially, dorsolaterally, and ventrolaterally.

now formed, with the upper extremity models at a slightly later stage of development than those of the lower extremities. The carpal bones have formed in the hand, but metacarpal bones and phalanges have not yet appeared.

Week 6. Mesenchymal cells further differentiate into chondroblasts, resulting in cells that form cartilaginous models of future bones. Hyaline cartilage forms these bone models. Growth occurs by cell division in the middle of the cartilage (interstitial growth) and by proliferation and differentiation of new chondroblasts at the periphery of a cartilaginous mass (appositional growth). The deep part of the perichondrium contains cells capable of forming new chondroblasts, which can secrete ground substance and eventually become mature chondrocytes. Cartilaginous models occur in the hand for carpals, metacarpals, and proximal phalanges only (Fig. 1-24). Joint capsules of the shoulder and elbow are not present.

Embryological cartilage forms by the condensation of undifferentiated mesenchymal cells into centers of chondrification. In the vertebral column, five chondrification centers appear in each mesenchymal vertebra, two in the centrum, two in the vertebral arch, and one in the pedicle (Fig. 1-25).

Week 7. Three primary centers of ossification (bone) appear in the vertebrae, one in the anterior centrum and one in each pedicle area (Fig. 1-26). Primary ossification in cartilaginous models of the long bones of the limbs occurs as early as the seventh week and continues until the fourth intrauterine month. Cartilaginous models of the future hand bones include the proximal and middle phalanges.

Week 8. Primary ossification begins in the diaphyses (shafts) of the future long limb bones (Fig. 1-27). Chondrocytes located centrally in the diaphyseal shaft hypertrophy, become vacuolated, and accumulate glycogen in the vacuoles. These cells die, perhaps because of toxins or lysosomes in the matrix surrounding the degenerating cartilage cells, and create a central cavity. The walls of the spaces or primary areolae that are left by the dead cells become calcified cartilage as calcium phosphate is deposited.

The cartilaginous bone model, except at the articular surfaces, is enclosed in a dense, irregular connective tissue

covering called the *perichondrium*. The deepest part of the perichondrium of the diaphysis contains osteogenic stem (osteoprogenitor) cells that differentiate into osteoblasts, which lay down a layer of young fenestrated bone (bony collar) at the middiaphyseal area. As the bony collar forms, the connective tissue covering of the bone model is called the *periosteum* instead of perichondrium. Blood vessels invade the bony collar first and then the central cavity, bringing osteoprogenitor and hematopoietic (blood-forming) stem cells to the interior (Fig. 1-28). As the blood vessels proliferate longitudinally in both directions, the invasion of vascular connective tissue stimulates further cartilaginous hypertrophy and degeneration, leaving calcified cartilage (bone mineral) at the ends of the bone. The bone mineral is a complex calcium phosphate similar to hydroxyapatite $[Ca_{10}(PO_4)_6 OH_2]$ and contains also calcium carbonate $(CaCO_3)$, citrate, fluoride, Mg^{++}, and Na^+. The hydroxyapatite crystals become intimately related to the collagen fibers that have been carried in by the vascular connective tissue. Trabecular (primary spongiosa, spongy marrow, woven-fibered, cancellous, and interwoven) bone is formed as osteoblasts attach to the calcified cartilage spicules, break them down, and replace them with bony spicules, which then attach to other spicules (Fig. 1-29). Some osteoblasts become surrounded by the matrix and sit within lacunae, remaining connected to other cells by canaliculi. These cells are now called *osteocytes*.

Vascular connective tissue from the deep periosteum carries osteoclasts as well as osteoblasts through the collar and into the central cavity. Walls of the primary areolae are then eroded to form secondary areolae (medullary spaces). Calcified cartilage becomes covered with osteoblasts, which lay down osteoid matrix and develop into osteocytes if they become trapped in lacunae. Subperiosteal bone is added and endosteal bone removed to form the primitive marrow cavity.

The main events of this eighth week include cartilaginous growth, formation of a central cavity via cartilaginous hypertrophy, degeneration, and calcification; formation of a bony collar; vascular invasion; cartilaginous changes toward the ends of the bone; and replacement of calcified cartilage spicules by bony spicules.

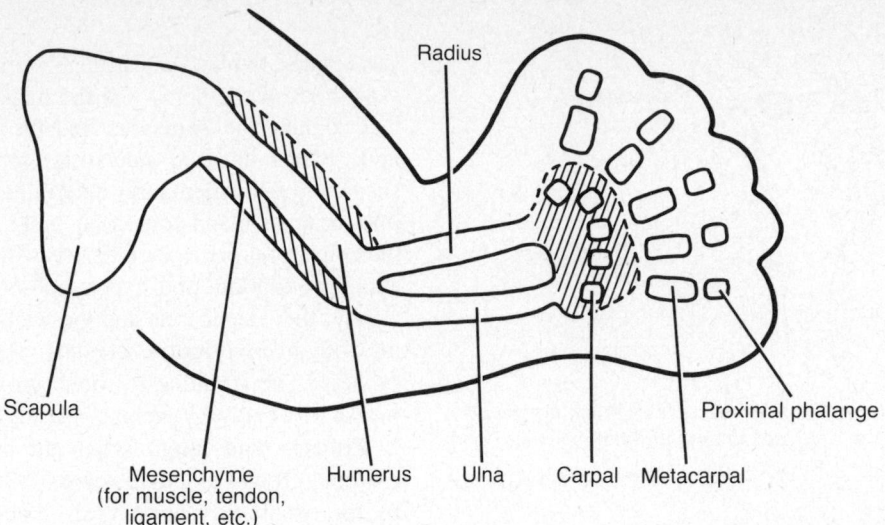

Fig. 1-24. The cartilaginous model of the hand bones includes metacarpals and proximal phalanges at 6 weeks of embryological development.

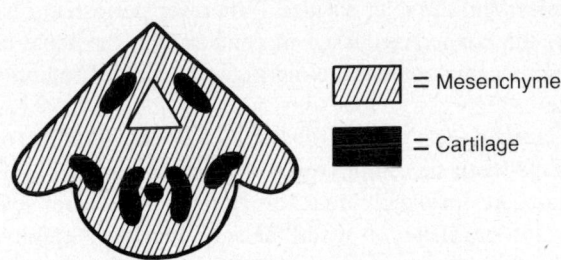

Fig. 1-25. Five chondrification centers in the vertebra at 6 weeks of embryological development.

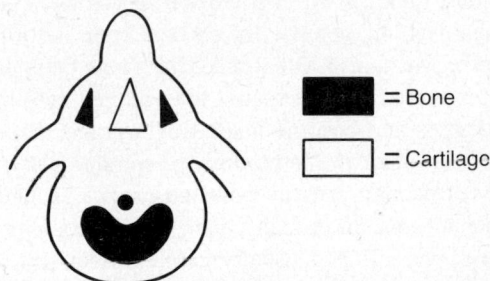

Fig. 1-26. Three primary centers of ossification in the vertebra at 7 weeks of embryological development.

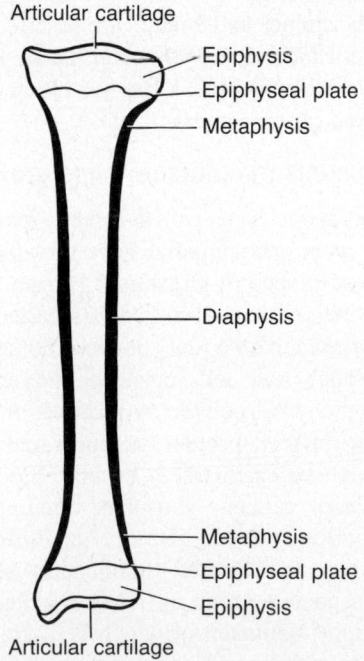

Fig. 1-27. The portions of a long bone.

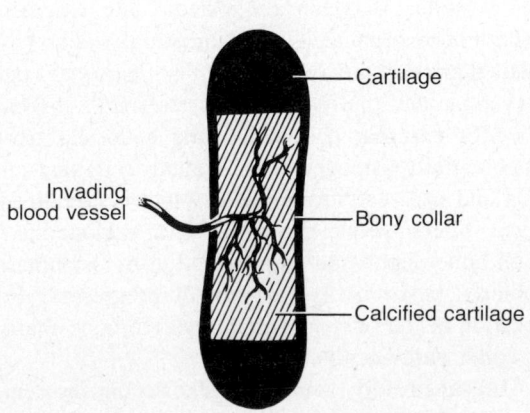

Fig. 1-28. Blood vessel invasion of bone.

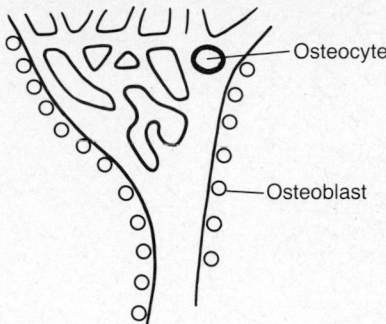

Fig. 1-29. Trabecular bone forms as osteoblasts break down calcified cartilage spicules and replace them with bony spicules.

Week 12 and after. Cartilage cells in the remainder of the bone model continue to grow by appositional and interstitial growth. Within the model, areas of reserve, proliferative, mature, and hypertrophic cartilage can be seen. As cancellous bone is formed, space develops around the bony spicules. As compact or cortical bone is formed, the trabeculae thicken and the space between them narrows. Collagen fibers from the matrix are secreted onto the walls of the spaces and become increasingly organized as parallel bundles, either in longitudinal or spiraled patterns. The osteocytes occupy roughly concentric rows around a central channel, the haversian canal, which contains nerves and blood vessels and usually capillaries or postcapillary venules, but only occasionally an arteriole.[9, 10]

The haversian canal system forms the bone's nutritional source. The longitudinally coursing haversian canals are interconnected by transversely and obliquely running Volkmann's canals (Fig. 1-30). These canals are unnecessary in cancellous bone, since nutrition can occur there by diffusion. Haversian systems that are not fully developed but exist as sequential rows of osteocytes are called *primary osteons,* or *atypical haversian systems.* These systems are eventually eroded and replaced by osteons characterized by layers of osteoid matrix around the osteocyte. These are then called *secondary (lamellar) osteons* or *haversian systems.* Between the osteons are fragments of lamellar bone, organized into interstitial systems. There are also sharp demarcations, called *cement lines,* between the haversian and the interstitial systems (Fig. 1-31).

The fibrovascular periosteum and endosteal tissue remain potentially osteogenic and contain cells that undergo mitosis and can secrete new matrix that is combined with collagen fibers. Bone modeling and remodeling occur through bone deposition and resorption by osteoblasts and osteoblasts, respectively, as growth progresses. Primary ossification centers extend throughout the bone shafts. The bony collar continues to thicken.

Postnatal period (years 1 to 2). Secondary centers of ossification begin to form, with vascular invasion of the epiphyses, which proceeds as previously described. Epiphyseal plates, or plates of cartilage, remain between the epiphyses (ends of the bone) and the metaphyses (areas of bone that connect the epiphyses and the diaphyses). Cartilaginous plates undergo interstitial growth, with the plate shape and cell orientation determined mostly by principal lines of tension and compression. Zones of cartilage within the epiphyseal plates include areas of cell reserve, proliferation, maturation, and hypertrophy. After the cells hypertrophy, they degenerate and the walls of the empty lacunae fill with hydroxyapatite crystals. Bones lengthen by this process. The stimulus for bone growth in length is compression, usually by weight bearing.

Puberty and later. When the epiphyseal plates have ossified, growth in length ceases. Most bones have ossified by the twentieth year. Not all bones have two secondary centers of ossification. Hyaline cartilage, devoid of nerves and blood vessels, remains on the articular surfaces of bone. Therefore, periosteum is absent from the articular bone surfaces, as well as from the attachment sites of tendons and ligaments, sesamoid bone surfaces (such as the patella), and the talar surface. Wherever periosteum is absent, the connective tissue in contact with the bone lacks the osteogenic potential to aid in the healing of fractures in the area.

Cartilaginous growth plates can occur at areas other than between the epiphyses and metaphyses of long limb bones. At localized areas of attachment where several muscles originate or insert closely together, epiphyseal plates will be found. Since muscle contraction causes a traction or tensile loading that stimulates bone growth at these areas, these epiphyseal plates are called *traction epiphyses,* or *apophyses.* A traction epiphysis is found at the greater trochanter of the femur, where many hip muscles, which mainly abduct and rotate, are inserted. Bones that ossify by endochondral growth are listed in Table 1-3. Included in the table are the locations of the primary and secondary ossification centers.

Intramembranous (membrane) bone growth

Intramembranous bone growth[28] takes place earlier and more rapidly than endochondral bone growth. It occurs in the bones most in need of protection. During the formation of the flat bones of the skull (frontal, parietal, temporal, and parts of the mandible and sphenoid bones), condensations of mesenchymal cells occur in proximity to blood vessels. Mesenchymal cells in some areas of the body begin to produce a mucoprotein (organic) matrix called *osteoid,* in which collagen fibers become embedded. Inorganic crystals of calcium phosphate accumulate around, inside, and on the collagen fibers. This results in a mineralization of the osteoid matrix (ossification). From the calcium and phosphate a group of minerals called *apatites* are formed, the most abundant of which is hydroxyapatite.

In the intramembranous growth areas, mesenchymal cells differentiate into osteoblasts, which secrete osteoid.

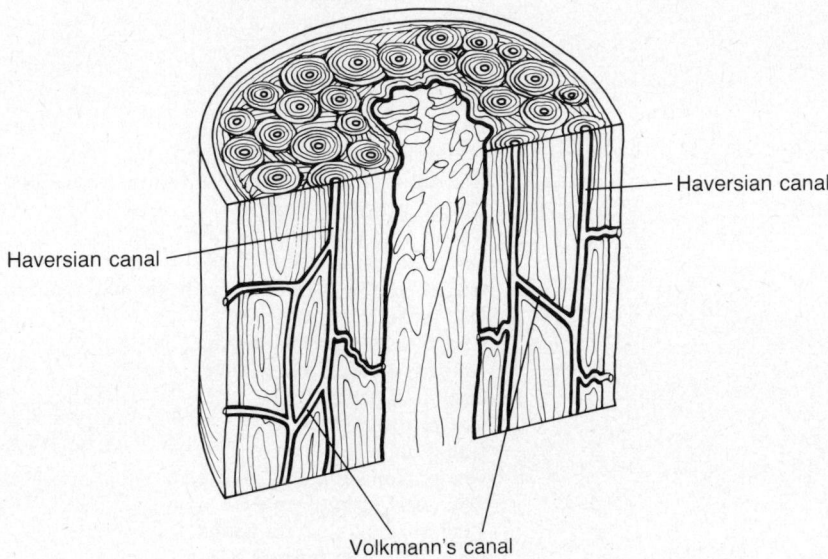

Fig. 1-30. Interconnection of haversian and Volkmann's canals.

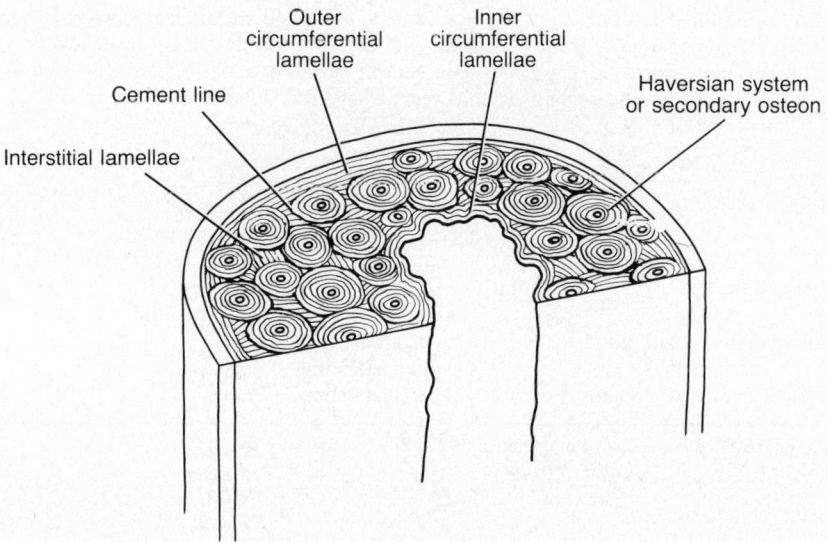

Fig. 1-31. Secondary bone with lamellar (secondary) osteons or haversian systems, interstitial lamellae, and circumferential lamellae with demarcating cement lines.

Table 1-3. Primary and secondary centers of ossification

Bone	Primary center	Secondary centers
Humerus	Shaft	One proximal epiphyseal plate Apophysis at greater tubercle Apophysis at lesser tubercle One distal epiphyseal plate
Radius	Shaft	One proximal plate One distal plate
Ulna	Shaft	One proximal plate One distal plate
Metacarpals	Center	One proximal plate for thumb One distal plate for digits 2 to 5
Phalanges (hand)	Body	One proximal plate (begins to form in years 3 or 4)
Vertebrae	Centrum	One at spinous process One at each transverse process One at superior edge of body One at inferior edge of body, beginning at puberty
Femur	Shaft	One proximal plate Apophysis at greater trochanter Apophysis at lesser trochanter One distal plate
Tibia	Shaft	One proximal plate One distal plate
Fibula	Shaft	One proximal plate One distal plate
Metatarsals	Center	One proximal plate for hallux One distal plate for toes 2 to 5
Phalanges (feet)	Body	One proximal plate (fused by years 11 or 12)
Clavicle	Growth is intramembranous in center and endochondral at ends.	
Scapula	Body	Two at coracoid process Two at acromion One each at medial border, inferior angle, and lower rim of glenoid cavity
Sternum	Manubrium ossifies from one, two, or three centers—first and second sternebrae (one of four sections from which sternum develops) usually from one center and third and fourth usually from two centers. These centers appear in fifth intrauterine month. Union between centers occurs at about puberty for third and fourth sternebrae, 25 years of age for first and second, and 40 years of age for xiphoid process.	
Ribs	Rib 1 (shaft)	One at head One at tubercle
	Ribs 2 to 10 (angle of rib)	One at head One at articular part of tubercle One at nonarticular part of tubercle
	Ribs 11 and 12 (shaft and head)	
Pelvis	Ilium (above greater sciatic notch)	Two at iliac crest One at acetabulum
	Ischium body (month 4)	One at acetabulum
	Pubis superior ramus (months 4 or 5)	One at acetabulum

Modified from Tachdyian MO: Pediatric orthopaedics, Philadelphia, 1972, WB Saunders Co.

The osteoid quickly becomes mineralized and osteoblasts embedded in it become osteocytes. Extensions from these osteocytes emerge and contact other cellular extensions via pathways called *canaliculi*, which carry ions and nutrients. The space around the nucleus of the osteocyte is called the *lacuna* and is formed by the removal of osteoid.

Spicules of bone form and unite with other spicules or trabeculae to form a meshwork of primary cancellous bone. A layer of osteoblasts forms deep to the superficial dense sheath of connective tissue and becomes the cam-

bium layer of the periosteum.[31] These osteoblasts deposit subperiosteal layers of bone called *lamellae*.

Near the time of birth the primary cancellous bone becomes compact in some locations. This involves a thickening of trabeculae by the addition of concentric lamellae around osteocytes and trabecular rearrangement into haversian systems or secondary osteons. The bony trabeculae in the relatively large marrow spaces are called *primary osteons*. Eventually the original marrow space becomes only a small tubular pathway, a central osteonal or haversian canal, which contains a single capillary and nerve fiber. The haversian system is composed of four to twenty (usually six or less) concentric lamellae. The canal is about 50 μm in diameter and the concentric lamellae are 3 to 7 μm thick. With formation of many secondary osteons, the cancellous bone becomes compact bone. Where trabecular bone remains, trabecular growth ceases and vascular tissue differentiates into hematopoietic tissue. Therefore, compact bone forms the outer portions of the intramembranous bone growth areas, surrounding marrow cavities called *diploë*, which are located centrally and directly surrounded by cancellous bone. When the bone reaches its eventual size, the osteoblasts revert to resting osteoprogenitor cells. Bone modeling and remodeling occur by the same mechanism of osteoblastic-osteoclastic activity.

The secondary osteons in the compact bone usually course along the length of the bone. Cement lines, which are highly mineralized and devoid of collagen fibers, clearly mark the outer limit of each secondary osteon. The communication system among the haversian canals and between the canals and the periosteum is by the transverse and obliquely coursing Volkmann's canals.

All bones have an outer shell of cortical or compact bone and an inner mass of trabecular bone, except where the latter is replaced by the medullary cavity or an air space.[78,79] Cancellous bone gradually becomes cortical as the outer surface of the bone is approached.[31,84] In long bones the epiphyseal and metaphyseal areas are mostly trabecular, whereas the diaphyses are mostly compact bone. Cortical bone is distinguished from cancellous bone by the amount of mineralized tissue per total bone tissue volume. Measures of mineralized tissue include bone porosity (percentage of nonmineralized tissue), apparent density (mineral tissue/total bone tissue volume), and ash density (ash weight/total bone tissue volume).[20] Ash weight is a measure of the mineralized portion of bone. Advanced densitometric techniques have made the accurate measurement of bone density and skeletal loss possible.[50]

Cortical bone is 5% to 30% porous; that is, 5% to 30% of the tissue is nonmineralized, whereas cancellous bone is 30% to 90% porous.[41] Interestingly, the term cancellous is derived from *cancelli,* the Italian word for the open lattice screens behind which Roman judges sat. Spongy bone is a three-dimensional lattice or meshwork of bony spicules (trabeculae or rods) and thin plates (lamellae).[57,98] The term *trabeculae* is used here to indicate only the rod portion of cancellous bone, but it is often used loosely to indicate all elements of cancellous bone. Human cancellous bone may be of many types, varying in a composition as follows[97]:

1) rods only (deeper parts of the ends and walls of the marrow cavities in the shafts or long bones)
2) rods and plates
   a) large plates with rods (as in the pubis and lateral angle of the scapula)

b) thick rods with irregularly shaped plates (the calcaneous)
   c) plates crossed by rods (the epiphyseal bone close to some articular surfaces or adjacent to some articular surfaces—the patella or bodies of upper cervical vertebrae)
3) plates only (as in the ends of the tibia)

The rod structure may be more conductive to providing support along the medullary canals, whereas the plate structure gives more support near articular surfaces. Since the plate structure exists at the tibial plateau area, which is subject to high shear stresses, this type of structure would appear to offer strength to resist shear stresses as well.[97]

MECHANICAL PROPERTIES OF BONE
Stresses causing and resulting from bone shape

The loads placed on a bone can be viewed as having a similar effect as loads placed on a simple beam. Bone has an elastic deformation range and a yielding point that delineates the deformation range from a nonelastic or plastic range.[13,41] Bone is not entirely linearly elastic in the initial portion of its stress-strain curve but curves slightly.[41] Therefore, bone is subject to nonrecoverable deformation ("creep," or plastic flow) but can yield under stress and recover from deformation within a range (elastic range of the stress-strain curve). However, bone does not exhibit large recoverable deformations when significant energy loss or hysteresis occurs during loading and unloading.[5] Bone is neither ductile nor brittle but a combination of the two,[41] with the mineral phase being more brittle and the organic (collagenous) phase being more ductile. Since bone demonstrates time-dependent characteristics (changes in mechanical properties with altered rates and duration of load applications), it is considered a viscoelastic material.[22,37,57]

Tensile loads on a bone cause tensile stress and strain. A bone is strengthened in tension if the collagen fibrils (one fiber being composed of many fibrils) are aligned parallel to the tensile load.[87] With use of the scanning electron microscope, it is possible to identify the spatial orientation of the collagen fibrils in bone. The concentric rings in the osteons of cortical bone contain collagen fibrils that are arranged in parallel for each layer or lamella. However, the collagen fibrils in consecutive layers do not course in the same direction. Several investigators have described fibril directions in consecutive layers as alternating in a longitudinal and then circumferential (in reference to the haversian canal) pattern[107] or in a longitudinal, then circumferential, then oblique pattern, with most periosteal collagen fibrils oriented in the direction of the bone axis and additional fibrils interconnecting with the concentric lamellae.[56,66] Osteons with a predominately longitudinal or predominately oblique direction of collagen fibrils or a mixture were also observed.[40]

Bone organization with layers of collagen fibrils coursing in different directions would allow bone to be strengthened by tension[63] in several planes, since deformation from tensile loads is resisted when the load is applied parallel to the fiber direction. More and more layers of bone (an increased cross-sectional area) lead to increased bone strength and stiffness as well. At bony attachment sites, collagen fibrils often become oriented parallel to a large tensile (muscular, ligamentous, or tendinous) stress. The primary orientation of the collagen fibrils in the tibial tuberosity is shown in Fig. 1-32. The fibrils have been aligned for the most part parallel to the pull of the patellar ligament.[97] The maximal tensile stress from any of these sources is located on a plane perpendicular to the tensile load (Fig. 1-33). Therefore, an increase in cross-sectional area will increase bone strength and stiffness in tension, as long as the tensile loads are applied axially (i.e., not as bending loads).

In periosteal, endosteal, and trabecular bone, most of the collagen fibers are oriented in the direction of the bone axis or along the axis of the trabeculae, indicating their function in resisting tensile or compressive stresses.[66] The hydroxyapatite crystals exist as rods and plates oriented with their long axes parallel to the local direction of the collagen fibrils.[56]

Similar to tensile loads, compressive loads on bone cause compressive stress and strain, with maximal compression occurring along a perpendicular plane to the applied load (Fig. 1-34). An increase in the cross-sectional area of bone increases the strength and stiffness of axially compressed bone. Vertebrae and inferior femoral neck regions receive the greatest compression loads.

Shear stress and strain occur with both tensile and compressive loads. Marked shear loads occur in cancellous bone. A specific anatomical area that receives great shear loads is the tibial plateau area.

Bending loads cause tension, compression, and shear stresses and strains. Increasing the moment of inertia of a bone in a particular direction by increasing the amount of bone or displacing the bone farther from the axis will increase the resistance of bone to bending in that direction. An example of axial loading is the load placed on the bent femur during weight bearing if the vertical component of the ground reaction force is used in the calculation. Fig. 1-35 shows that the bending moment caused by the vertical component equals the force times the perpendicular distance ($M = F \times d$) from the action line of the force to the neutral axis.

Torsion loads caused by twisting result in large shear stresses over the entire surface of the bone, with maximal shear occurring on planes that are perpendicular and parallel to the applied loads and with maximal tension and compression occurring on diagonal planes. Increasing the polar moment of inertia of a bone in any one direction will increase the resistance of the bone to torsion (twisting).

Usually there are combined loads on bone. Many com-

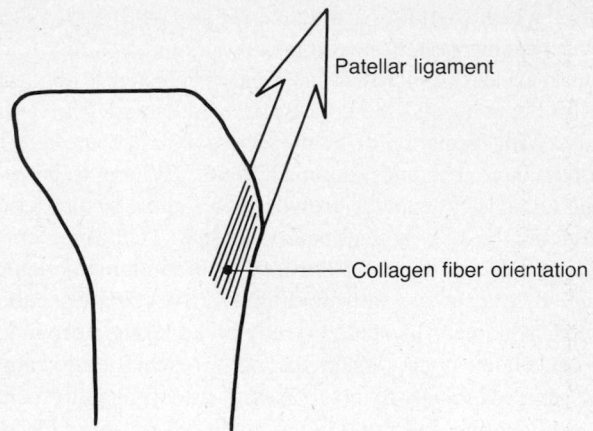

Fig. 1-32. Alignment of collagen fibrils parallel to the pull of the patellar ligament.

binations serve useful functions in decreasing the net effect of a particular load. For example, the femoral neck sustains large compressive loads inferiorly and large tensile loads superiorly as a result of bending loads during weight bearing. However, the hip abductors, particularly the gluteus medius, are active during weight bearing, causing a compressive load superiorly on the femoral neck, which produces a marked decrease of tensile loading on the superior neck (Fig. 1-36). Since bone is weak in tension, this is of great benefit to the integrity of the femoral neck.

Bone is a living material, and although metabolically expensive to produce, it can be modeled (development of the initial shape) and remodeled (ongoing alterations of the shape with aging or after a fracture). (This is in obvious and striking contrast to the analogy of bone as a simple beam.) The approximate shape of bone is genetically determined, evidenced by protuberances, although underdeveloped, and bendings in newborns' bones.[71,81] However, much of the detailed form of bone is produced by stresses and strains caused by weight bearing, tendinous, muscular, and ligamentous loads.[43,80] The long weight-bearing bones resemble slightly curved beams, so that bending stresses can be minimized.[29] The geometry of the metaphyses allows the transfer of high loads applied at articular surfaces to compact bone of the diaphyses.[57] Attachment sites of ligaments and tendons on bone provide a means to transfer joint loads to the cortical shaft.[98]

The purpose of bone modeling is to modify the shape and adjust the mass of a bone so that the stresses of everyday activities can be withstood. Bone strength can be altered by changes in material and geometrical properties of bone. Material properties include the percentage of organic to nonorganic portions of bone, the number of cross-links among the collagen fibrils, and the orientation of collagen fibrils in relation to orientation of applied loads.[40] Geometrical properties represent the structural strength of bone, such as the amount of cortical and subperiosteal

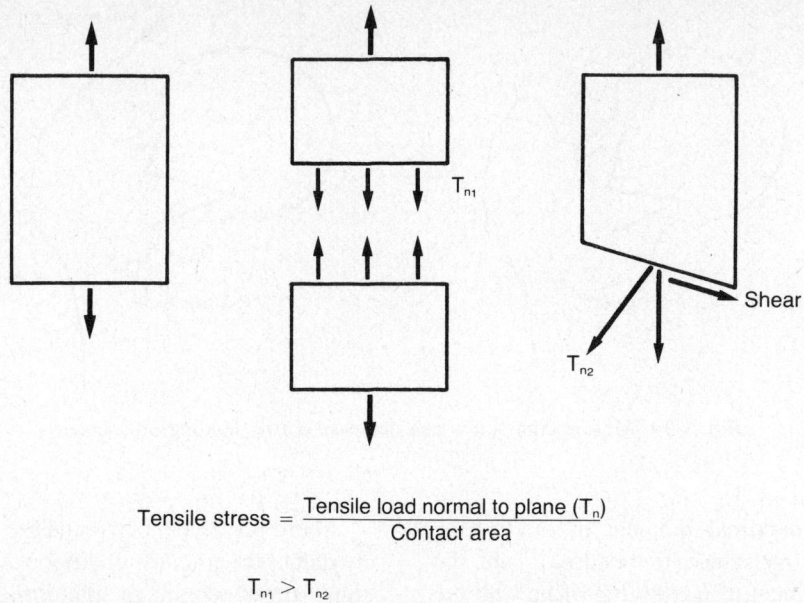

$$\text{Tensile stress} = \frac{\text{Tensile load normal to plane } (T_n)}{\text{Contact area}}$$

$$T_{n1} > T_{n2}$$

Fig. 1-33. Maximal tensile stress is located on a plane perpendicular to the tensile load.

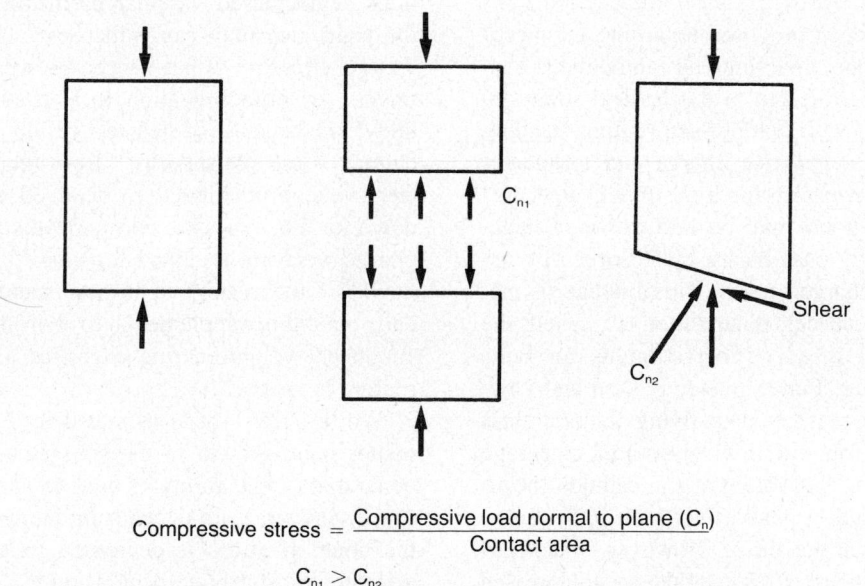

$$\text{Compressive stress} = \frac{\text{Compressive load normal to plane } (C_n)}{\text{Contact area}}$$

$$C_{n1} > C_{n2}$$

Fig. 1-34. Maximal compressive stress is located on a plane perpendicular to the compressive load.

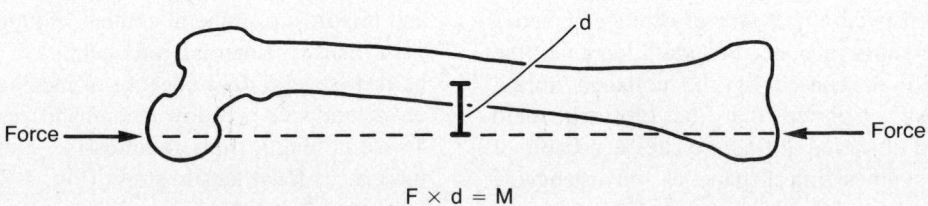

$$F \times d = M$$

Fig. 1-35. Calculation of the moment of force in an axially loaded bowed structure.

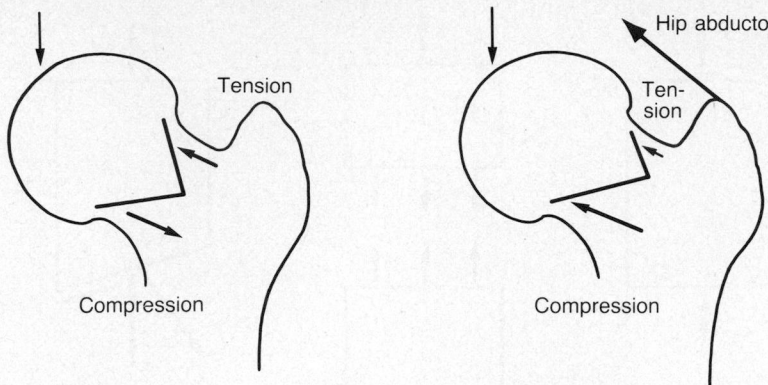

Fig. 1-36. Muscle contraction can decrease tensile loading on a bone.

area, the plane of the maximal moment of inertia (the plane with the greatest resistance to bending), and the plane of the minimal moment of inertia (the plane with the least resistance to bending). In some instances changes in material properties that would weaken the bone may be compensated for by changes in geometrical properties. This will be discussed in the section on age-related changes of bone.

Many theories have been proposed regarding the mechanism that stimulates bone modeling and remodeling. Bassett[6,7] states that bones subjected to mechanical strain develop electrical charges, with compressed regions (tending to be concave) having a negative charge and tensile regions (tending to be convex) having a positive charge. Because of this polarity, bone may be laid down in negatively charged regions by osteoblasts and resorbed by osteoclasts in positively charged areas. This linkage of mechanical strain and electrical polarization is called the *piezoelectric effect* and is a possible stimulus for bone modeling and remodeling. For example, Bassett and Pawlick[7] implanted a metal plate next to living femoral shaft bone in adult dogs and found that when optimal amperage was used, new bone was laid down at the cathode (negatively charged plate), with a peak effect seen in 2 weeks. No osteoclasis occurred at the anode. However, when Hert and Zalud[61] measured negative potentials on compressed bone surfaces and positive potentials on surfaces subjected to tensile strain in rabbit tibiae undergoing intermittent bending loads, they found that appositional bone growth occurred on both surfaces. They proposed an alternate hypothesis that negative and positive electrical potentials may constitute a nonspecific activator of osteogenic activity by inducing ion shifts in bone. Fukada[46] identified the piezoelectric activity as caused by the collagen fibrils. Becker and Murray[8] reported that the electrical field caused by stress and observed at fracture sites is capable of activating protein-synthesizing organelles in osteogenic cells in frogs. In addition, they claimed that the presence of the electrical field near polymerizing tropocollagen caused fibers to orient perpendicularly to lines of force.

Many researchers hypothesize that mechanical stresses modulate the growth, addition, or resorption of bone. Optimal stress within an appropriate range is essential for bone strength, since understressed or overstressed bone can become weaker.[47,57,84] Improper placement or tightening of plates, screws, nuts, or bolts in bone surgery may cause bone resorption, either from local stress concentrations or decreased vascular perfusion.[26,47] Plates that are too rigid also may cause increased bone atrophy.[112] Decreased stress on bones caused by weightlessness in space travel[74] or immobilization from casting a portion of the body[36] or because of bed rest results in a net loss of calcium[36,74] and phosphorus[36] from the body. When volunteers were immobilized in bivalved casts from the waist down for 6 to 7 weeks, normal levels of calcium and phosphorus were not regained for more than 6 weeks after removal of the casts.[36] It is now standard practice to give daily calcium supplements to astronauts and to require simulated weight-bearing exercises as part of their daily routine in space.[74]

Wolff's law (1884) as stated by Frankel and Nordin[41] relates bone growth to the stresses and strains placed on bone; that is, the ability of bone to adapt by changing size, shape, and structure depends on the mechanical stresses on the bone. If stress is decreased, resorption of periosteal and subperiostal bone occurs, with a subsequent decrease in strength and stiffness. If bone is subjected to high and consistent mechanical stress within a normal physiological range, hypertrophy of periosteal and subperiosteal bone can occur, with an increase in bone density. Bone will change in external shape (external or surface remodeling) and in porosity, mineral content, radiographic opacity, and mass density (internal remodeling).[47] These changes can be fast (several days because of increased output or uptake of mineral salts) or slow (months to years). Long bones increase in length from compressive stress and develop protuberances from tensile stress (Fig. 1-37).

Currey[29] believed that surface osteocytes received information via transient electrical fields or from the nerves entering the periosteum and initiated the adaptation or re-

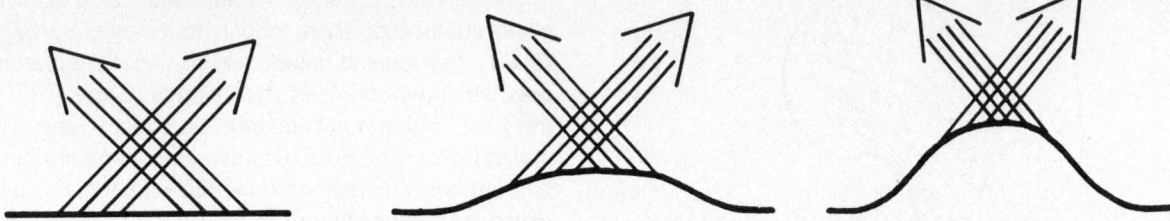

Fig. 1-37. Development of bony protuberances occurs as a result of tensile stress.

modeling process. However, direct innervation of bone may not be required for bone to react to stress, since Hert, Liskova, and Landrgot[59] found that compact bone reacted to intermittent stress by apposition of new bone whether the periosteum was innervated or not. Roux, as quoted by Fung[47] and reviewed by Roesler[47,90] and Pauwels,[85] formulated in 1895 two principles of bone remodeling: (1) functional adaptation (adaptation to function by practicing the function) and (2) maximum-minimum design (maximum strength is achieved with a minimum of material). Roux stated that pressure compression and tension are the functional stimuli that control modeling and that bony apposition and resorption are connected with the absolute value of local stress. Both Wolff and Roux proposed a trajectorial design for the trabeculae of the femoral neck; that is, that trabeculae subjected to compressive strain would be strengthened by the addition of bone (Fig. 1-38).

The work of Hayes and Snyder[58] supports this trajectorial theory of trabecular architecture; they found highly significant correlations between principal stress directions and trabecular orientation. They suggested that trabecular bone is most dense in regions of high shear stress (the principle of maximum difference in stresses causing shear), that trabeculae are aligned in the principal stress direction (45 degrees to the plane of maximum shear), and that trabecular orientation develops to minimize bending deformations in individual trabeculae. Lanyon[71] has shown that the direction of the trabeculae conforms closely to the direction of the greatest principal strains.

Frost[45] suggested that mechanical loads may control bone modeling in portions of bone between articulations and apophyses based on the amount of surface strain caused by the loads. Osteoclastic activity would arise on the convex surfaces and osteoblastic activity would arise on concave surfaces. Bone may drift toward the load-induced concavity and therefore minimize bending and maximize compressive stress (the flexural-drift law).[45] Frost also described internal remodeling, which involves adding or removing bone on osteons already in existence, as well as surface remodeling, which involves the deposition of new bone on periosteal and endosteal surfaces.[45,90] There has been an attempt to reduce flexural unit strains of lamellar bone tissue to or below a threshold level (minimum strain principle). Several recent studies have involved in vivo imposed loading of the bones of experimental animals.[27,71] Increased bone growth has been correlated with the type of loading; for example, compressive loading has a greater effect than loading in bending.[27] Bone growth has been correlated with the magnitude of loading,[27] with the strain rate during each loading cycle (the strain rate being more critical than the peak magnitude of strain),[71] and with the required number of consecutive loading cycles per day, which can be as few as 36.[71] The strain range is also important because it varies from expected strains connected with walking (0.001), running (0.001 to 0.002), and vigorous exercise (0.002 to 0.004) to strains that are large enough to create considerable fatigue, microdamage, and a strong remodeling stimulus.[16]

The biochemical activity of calcium may be involved in the modeling or remodeling process of bone. Justus and Luft[65] in 1970 found that when bone undergoes strain, there is an increased calcium concentration in the interstitial fluid. This increased concentration is due to a change in the solubility of hydroxyapatite crystals in response to stress.

The chain of possible events is shown in the flowchart below:

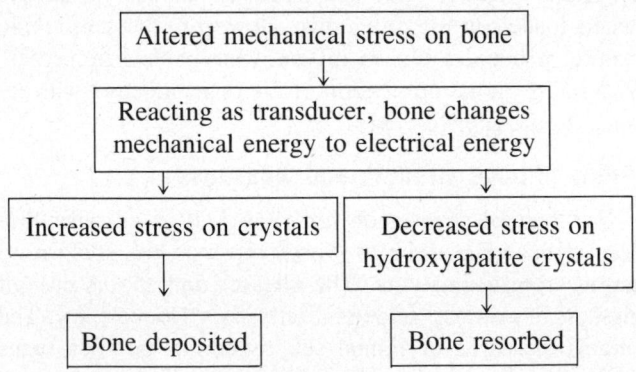

Alteration of the mechanical properties of bone can be explained by one of the remodeling theories presented, by a combination of theories, or perhaps by some process not yet fully understood. Because collagen fibers provide tensile strength, stiffness, and ductility, elastin fibers provide extensibility and brittleness, and GAGS provide compressive strength, an alteration in the percentage of these materials may considerably alter the mechanical properties of

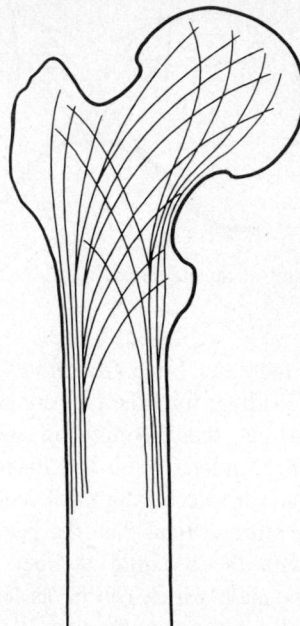

Fig. 1-38. Trajectorial design of trabeculae.

a tissue. The stress-strain curves of collagen and elastin demonstrate that collagen fibers can withstand 10% or less elongation, whereas elastin fibers can be elongated to 200% of their original length before they fail.[41]

Collagen and elastin fibers can vary a great deal in orientation within any connective tissue, including bone. Fibers can course parallel, perpendicular, oblique, or randomly to any applied load; they can course singly or in series; and they can be crimped (exist in a wavy state when relaxed and a straightened state when loaded). If all fibers were oriented equally in all directions, a tissue would be isotropic, that is, have the same mechanical properties when loaded in all directions. However, the anisotropic nature of bone results in different mechanical properties, depending on the orientation of the bone structure with respect to the applied load.[57]

Areas of bone strength and weakness

Mechanical stresses on bone (as well as on other biological materials, such as wood) more or less conform to engineering estimations. The stresses and strains on soft tissues, in contrast, seldom strictly obey Hooke's law. The strains measured in animal soft tissue can be 1000 times higher than the strains with which an engineer deals.

The strength of a composite material such as bone can be estimated by determining the stress-strain curves of the fiber and matrix materials.[56] If the fibers and matrix are well bonded and deform together, the load on the composite is shared between them in proportion to the cross-sectional area of each. Although many composite materials have a lower compressive strength than tensile strength, bone has a higher compressive strength.[47,56] The collagen

fibers provide flexibility within bone, and the whole organic component allows bone to be a good energy absorber. The mineral component provides rigidity and stiffness, about two thirds of the stiffness of steel.[56,66] Most of the load in a normal loading situation is carried by the mineral phase, because demineralized bone has only 5% to 10% of the strength of mineralized bone.[79] The microstructural organization of bone (i.e., the osteons and interstitial lamellae, having bonded at cement lines with ground substance) is partly responsible for some of the elastic and viscoelastic (time-dependent deformational) properties of macroscopic bone. In torsional loading, cement lines contribute significantly to the viscoelastic properties of bone.[66] Specific geometrical properties of bone reveal bone strength in specific loading patterns. Bone cross sections will be proportional to bone strength in axial loading, that is, loading in either tension or compression. With a bending or torsional load, the maximal and minimal moment of inertia will reveal bone strength or resistance to bending in two planes or to twisting in a third plane of motion, respectively.

Cement lines around the osteons and the planes between the lamellae in the haversian systems are generally weak areas in bone.[77] Bone stiffness is inversely proportional to osteonal size, the ratio of osteons to cement lines, and the size of haversian and Volkmann's canals.[31,66] Haversian bone has been reported to have 69% of the compliance of lamellar bone.[55,66] Compliance is the ratio of strain/stress, deformation/load, or length/force and is the inverse of stiffness, which is the stress/strain, load/deformation, or force/length ratio.

Bone strength is increased by a number of factors:

1. Increasing the bone density, with a correlation of $\rho = +.40 - .42$.[37,106]
2. Increasing the mineralization of bone to an optimal level.[106]
3. Increasing the percentage of small particles within bone.[106] This increases the surface area that is available for bonding. Small particles can account for as much as 30% of the total number of particles in bone. Their presence increases the tensile strength of bone.
4. Increasing the stiffness of bone.[106]
5. Increasing the length/diameter (slenderness) ratio of fibers within bone.[106] Apatite crystals join end to end to increase in length.
6. Increasing the cross-sectional area of bone.[41] This affects strength in tension, compression, bending, and torsion. Proportionality does not always exist, however; for example, a decrease in diameter by 20% may decrease the bone strength in torsion by 60%.[41]
7. Altering the distribution of bone tissue so as to increase the area moment of inertia.[41] This increases the strength in bending and torsion.
8. Increasing the strain rate.[32]

Bone stiffness can also be increased by a number of factors:

1. Increasing the density of bone.[37,66,106]
2. Decreasing the water content of bone, which increases the viscosity[106] and degree of mineralization.[66]
3. Increasing the speed at which bone is loaded.[41] During normal activity a small percentage of the total energy storage of a bone is used. This energy storage capacity varies with the speed at which bone is loaded.
4. Increasing the strain rate.[20,47]
5. Increasing the cross-sectional area of bone.[41]
6. Increasing the area moment of inertia.[41]

The shape of a bone as a whole and the orientation of fine trabeculae within it are determined both genetically and according to the stresses to which the bone is subjected.[41,99] For any of the weight-bearing bones, compression is caused by weight bearing, and bending is produced if the compression is eccentric to the neutral axis of the bone. Reduction of tensile stress and bending in cortical bone can result from the following factors:

1. Movement at joints eliminates the need for bone to bend as much within the shaft.[86] A decreased joint range of motion may lead to abnormal bending loads on the bone.
2. As mentioned before, some muscles, such as the gluteus medius, contract to reduce bending and therefore tensile stress. The protuberances help increase the mechanical advantage of the muscles.[79]
3. Since bone is weaker in tension than in compression,[56] the curve of a bone is in alignment with the predominant resultant force(s) acting on the bone. This increases the compressive stress on the bone but reduces the bending tendency and therefore the tensile stress. Bone will fatigue at lower bending stresses than axial stresses, so it is important to reduce bending stresses[29] (Fig. 1-39).
4. Bones are hollow, tubular structures.[84,86] The longer the bone, the greater the magnitude of the bending moment caused by the application of force. The stresses are proportional to the bending moment; that is, they are increased as the bending moment is increased. The tubular shape of bones and therefore the increase in the moment of inertia allow a lighter bone to have the same bending strength as a solidly filled structure.[41,84] Any bone will have a decreased tendency to fracture if the total amount of bone increases, but bone can be become unmanageably heavy as well.[29]

The polar moment of inertia is a quantity that includes information about a bone's cross-sectional area and distribution of bony material with regard to resisting torsion forces. Tubular bone allows even greater resistance to torsion forces than to bending forces. The resistance to the torsion force for circular sections such

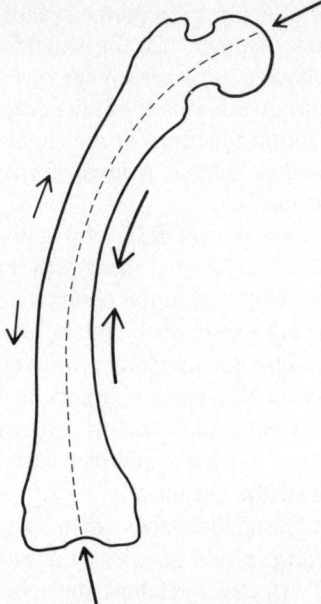

Fig. 1-39. Loading of a curved bone can result in decreased tensile stresses because of a decreased bending moment.

as long bones is proportional to the distance of the material from the neutral axis raised to the fourth power. Since the polar moment is most accurately used for circular cross sections, the circular shafts of bones are maximally effective for a given weight, and they decrease torsion and bending.[86]

Activities such as standing, walking, carrying, throwing, and pounding produce mainly tensile stress on the convex side of long bones as a result of bending stresses within the bone. Regions where net tension in a skeleton occurs during such functions include the following[83]:

1. Bony crests where opposing muscles have linear attachments on opposite edges, as on the cranial crests or the crest of the scapular spine. The temporal muscles, for example, pull laterally on the sagittal crest of the cranium. Usually humans and other species chew alternately on each side of the mouth, so that the sagittal crest area is not in marked net tension for a long period of time. Another example is the pull of the middle trapezius muscle, opposing that of the middle and posterior deltoid muscles, on the scapular spine and acromion process. The usual tensile stress produced by the middle trapezius muscle is much greater than that produced by the deltoid, and, in addition, these three muscles usually do not contract forcefully at the same time, thereby avoiding a large net tension at this site.
2. Thin bony plates where opposing muscles have surface attachments on either side. The infraspinatus and subscapularis muscles are good examples because they attach to opposite surfaces of the scapula. Both have

acute angles of application on the scapula, so that when they contract together, as for shoulder stabilization, they do not have a great percentage of their pull applied perpendicularly (or normally) to the scapula. They have opposing rotation functions at the shoulder as well. As a result, there is seldom a great tensile stress on the scapular surface.

When a bone is very thin, with muscles pulling on opposite sides, a fibrous sheet will exist instead of bone. This can be seen at the obturator foramen, where the internal and external obturators attach on opposite sides of the obturator membrane, as well as on the surrounding bone. Net tension occurs at the attachment site during external hip rotation—the main motion of both muscles—but the membrane instead of the bone resists some of the tension.

3. The patella. Sesamoid bones occur in tendons that are subject to compression stresses in a portion of the tendon. To be effective, tendons must be maintained in tension. In the patella, the quadriceps tendon and its continuation in the patellar ligament are maintained in tension.

The mechanical properties of cancellous bone and diploë depend on the orientation and distribution of trabeculae within the bone.[37] Trabeculae are arranged to provide maximal strength with a minimum of material. They are aligned according to the principal stress directions in a particular bone, taking into consideration the forces, quantities of forces over time, and direction of the forces. Park[84] has stated that the strength of bone is greatest in the direction of physiological loading, that is, according to principal stress directions. Most biological materials will have both compressive and tensile forces acting on them, but usually one will predominate. It is possible, however, that both combined tension and compression can be a principal stress on a bone.[83] The trabeculae in the proximal femur have been closely studied by many researchers, who have examined the thickness, spacing, and density of the trabeculae, which vary with the stress magnitudes to which the bone is subjected. Koch[70] states that the trabecular alignment is oriented predominantly according to principal compressive stresses. More recently, alignment of the trabeculae has been correlated with the direction of principal shear stresses.[58]

The strength of trabecular bone is less than that of cortical bone. Information about the mechanical stresses for cancellous bone appears in Table 1-4 and that for cortical bone appears in Table 1-5. The different specimens that are compared include longitudinal bone sections (sections cut parallel to the longitudinal axis of the bone), transverse sections (cut perpendicular to the longitudinal axis), radial sections (cut in the direction of the center of the arc formed by the longitudinal axis), and tangential sections

Table 1-4. Mechanical stresses in cancellous bone

	Compression	Tension	Shear
Strength	Trabeculae are aligned primarily according to compressive stresses[60]	Ultimate tensile strength is less than ultimate compressive strength[41]	Trabeculae may be aligned according to the direction of principal shear stresses.[49] Longitudinal sections loaded normally are stronger than transverse ones loaded in parallel
Strain	Sections cut and loaded in a lateromedial direction have the greatest amount of compressive strain	Ultimate tensile strain is less than ultimate compressive strain[41]	
Modulus of elasticity	Modulus is less with compressive loads than with tensile ones	Modulus is greater with tensile loads than with compressive ones. The E of trabecular bone is less than that of compact bone[41]	Sections cut and loaded in a lateromedial direction have the highest shear modulus
Energy absorbed to failure			Sections cut and loaded in a lateromedial direction have the greatest amount of energy absorbed to failure
Density			Sections cut and loaded in a lateromedial direction have the greatest amount of density

Based on data from Evans FG: Mechanical properties of bone, Springfield, Ill, 1973, Charles C Thomas, Publisher, except as noted.

(cut at a tangent to the longitudinal axis). These sections are diagramed in Fig. 1-40.

Longitudinal sections of cortical bone can absorb more energy to failure than transverse sections, which is logical considering the lower extremity bones, in particular, and their lines of weight bearing. In general, the stress and strain characteristics of cortical bone in adult human long bones are influenced by the duration and magnitude of the load applied, since the rate of plastic deflection of bone is proportional to the magnitude of the applied stress.[37] The measures of several mechanical strengths for different bones, as listed by Park,[84] are given in Table 1-6. Femoral strength has been reported as 160 MPa in bending and 54.1 MPa for ultimate shear as tested in torsion.[5,47]

Table 1-5. Mechanical stresses in cortical bone

	Compression	Tension	Shear	Bending	Torsion
Strength	Longitudinal sections are strongest, then transverse,[18,75] tangential, and radial, in order. Ultimate compressive strength is greater than ultimate tensile strength[41]	Longitudinal sections are eight times stronger than radial or tangential sections. Ultimate tensile strength is less than ultimate compressive strength[41]	Longitudinal sections loaded perpendicularly are twice as strong as transverse sections loaded in parallel		
Strain	Strain is greatest in transverse sections. Compressive strain is greater than ultimate tensile strain[41]	Ultimate tensile strain is less than ultimate compressive strain[41]			There is an initial short elastic region with torsional stress. Little torsional stress causes much nonelastic strain
Breaking load	There is greater ultimate compressive stress with increasing strain rates of loading	Longitudinal sections have greater ultimate strain than transverse sections		Longitudinal sections can withstand three times the bending load of transverse sections and six times that of radial sections in ox tibiae	
Deformation		Little or no plastic deformation occurs if the direction of a tensile load is perpendicular to the long axis of the bone[75]			
Modulus of elasticity	In the human femur longitudinal sections have twice the modulus of transverse sections and between one and two times the modulus of tangential and radial sections.[56] The modulus increases with increased strain rates of loading	In cattle bone, longitudinal sections have greater moduli than transverse sections. The modulus is greater with tensile loads than with compressive loads[41]	A single osteon has the greatest shear modulus. There is a decrease in the modulus with an increase in the number of osteons	Longitudinal sections have a higher modulus than transverse sections	

Based on data from Evans FG: Mechanical properties of bone, Springfield, Ill, 1973, Charles C Thomas, Publisher, except as noted.

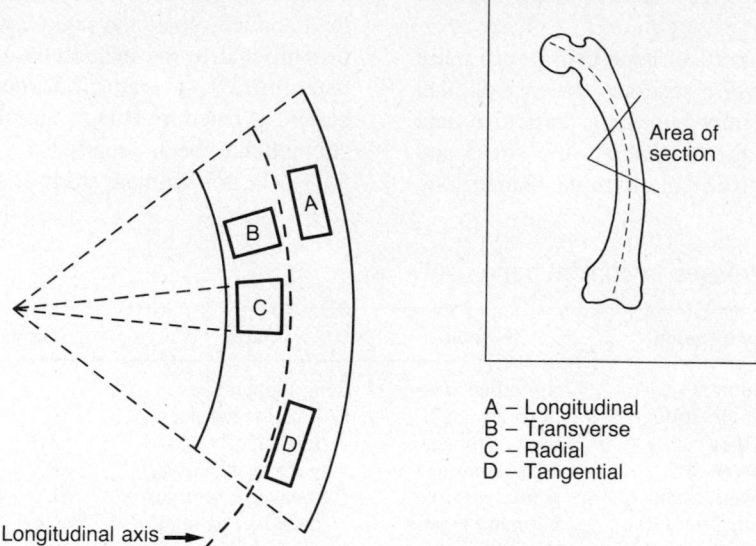

A – Longitudinal
B – Transverse
C – Radial
D – Tangential

Fig. 1-40. Different orientations of bone sections.

Table 1-6.

Bone	Test direction	Modulus of elasticity (GPa)	Tensile strength (MPa)	Compressive strength (MPa)
Femur	Longitudinal	17.2	121	167
Tibia	Longitudinal	18.1	140	159
Fibula	Longitudinal	18.6	146	123
Humerus	Longitudinal	17.2	130	132
Radius	Longitudinal	18.6	149	114
Ulna	Longitudinal	18.0	148	117
Vertebrae Cervical	Longitudinal	0.23	3.1	10
Lumbar	Longitudinal	0.16	3.7	5
Cancellous bone		0.09	1.2	1.9
Skull	Tangential	—	25	
	Radial	—		−97

The data in Tables 1-4 to 1-6 show that longitudinal sections have the greatest strength overall of the weight-bearing bones of the lower extremities. These bones have most of the external loading aligned more closely to the longitudinal axis than to any other axis. The vertebral segments have much loading along the longitudinal extent of the vertebral column as a whole but further from the axis. In the upper extremities, the main load taken by the major bones is in bending, characterized by such activities as throwing, pounding, lifting, and carrying. These loads cause primarily tensile stresses on the convex side of long upper extremity bones, which correspond to the posterior surfaces of the humerus, ulna, and radius. This loading pattern necessitates great strength in the upper extremity bones along the longitudinal axis to resist bending loads. A greater shear strength in the longitudinal sections of compact long bones is also required at the sites of muscle, tendon, and ligamentous attachment.

Decreased strain is withstood by compact bone as the number of osteons is increased. This is explained by the general weakness of cement lines, which increases as the number of osteons increases. This is particularly important to remember when a bone is loaded in shear because less strain will be tolerated before fatigue as the osteon number increases. Greater deformation is tolerated by compact bone loaded in torsion than by such bone loaded in tension, which is beneficial because the initial failure of compact bone loaded in torsion is in shear.

The compressive strength and modulus of elasticity for different types of osteons have been tested.[107] Three types of osteons were isolated. Type 1 osteons had lamellae with collagen fibers coursing predominantly in a transverse spiral direction. The collagen fibers in the lamellae of type 2 osteons coursed in a transverse direction in one lamella and a longitudinal direction in the next, whereas those in type 3 osteons had predominantly longitudinal fibers. Compressive strength was found to be greatest for the type 1 osteons and least for the type 3 osteons. Tensile strength is increased in bone with osteons that have collagen fibers that course longitudinally or are steeply spiraling as compared to bone having osteons with transverse fibers.[66]

The modulus of elasticity of cancellous bone is less than that of cortical bone.[47] The modulus (E) for tensile loading is intermediate between the values of E for collagen or apatite alone.[47] Therefore, bone strength is greater than that of either collagen or apatite individually, since collagen prevents apatite from brittle cracking and apatite prevents collagen from yielding. The modulus of elasticity and other mechanical properties, such as shear modulus, ultimate stress and strain, and viscoelastic properties, depend not only on the composition of bone—such as percentages of compact and cancellous bone, bonds between fibers, bonds between fibers and matrix, percentages of haversian and lamellar bone, and bone density—but also on bone structure or the geometric shape of different areas of bone.[2,3,47]

The mechanical properties of human bone can be affected by a number of other in vivo and in vitro factors, which include the following:[51,57]

1. Storage method—formalin, freezing, storage time, freezing rate
2. Specimen preparation procedures—machining methods, temperature during preparation, irrigation medium
3. Testing procedures—grip method, type of testing machine, deformation rate, uniformity of stress applied, environment
4. Individual characteristics—sex, age, height, weight, race, cause of death, activity before death, nutritional status before death, disease affecting the bone
5. Section of bone—right or left, variation in different portions of the bone

The mechanical properties of dried bone differ from those of embalmed bone, wet bone from a fresh cadaver, or bone in vivo. Drying affects all regions of the bone the same but affects each strength property differently.[3] Bone with the in vivo characteristic of being bathed in fluid can absorb more energy and elongate more before fracture than dry bone, because, unlike brittle materials, bone undergoes creep and stress relaxation.[39,41,84,103] The ultimate tensile and compressive stresses and modulus of elasticity for tension and compression are increased by drying.[41,77] Shear strength normal to the bone's long axis decreases with drying, and bone from an embalmed cadaver has an increased shear and decreased compressive strength.[41] The decrease in compressive strength with embalming has been reported at 13%.[3]

Stresses at epiphyseal plates

The stability of the epiphysis relative to the diaphysis depends upon the relationship of the epiphyseal plate to the internal stress pattern created by the most stressful activity over a majority of the time. Generally, the best position for an epiphyseal plate is transverse to the long axis of the parent bone. However, other advantages may outweigh this basic rule, depending on the individual bone.

Most epiphyseal plates are oriented parallel to the lines of principal stress, tension, or compression, so that shear stresses on the plate can be minimized. Proliferative columns of cartilage cells, however, bear no relationship to the stress patterns. They are oriented instead in the direction of the bone growth they produce. Cartilage cell columns may lie perpendicular or oblique to the plane of the epiphyseal plate. Only after primary diaphyseal bone trabeculae (those that form on the rods remaining after cartilage cell degeneration and erosion) have eroded and been replaced by secondary trabeculae can the structural alignment of the trabeculae according to stress patterns be seen. The epiphyseal plates will have their characteristic forms at birth,[99] so much of their general form is genetically determined. However, until the secondary trabeculae develop, the plates are exposed to shear stresses that tend to displace the plate on the diaphysis.

In areas of maximal compressive stress, plates are usually parallel to tensile stress lines and perpendicular to compressive stress lines. Exceptions are seen where the epiphyseal plate approaches the articular cartilage; there the plate often angles toward the diaphysis rather than remaining transverse to the long axis. When the epiphyseal plate deviates from its transverse course, muscles attaching near the joint attach to the epiphysis or apophysis instead of the diaphysis. If muscles were to attach to the diaphysis, the muscle attachment would have to move relative to the bone surface during growth, which is disadvantageous.[96]

Alteration of gravitational pull can markedly change the growth of the epiphyseal plates.[82] When 2-week-old chicks subjected to twice gravity's pull were compared with controls, they showed an increased width of cartilaginous layers in the proximal epiphysis and inhibition of both height and width of layers in the distal epiphysis.

Bone yielding and failure

Failure in bone can occur from trauma, degeneration, fatigue, or disease. Most fractures result from a combination of several loading modes occurring simultaneously.[41] The amount of energy absorbed before failure can be calculated by measuring the area under the stress-strain curve. If is important to be able to compute energy absorption, because most fractures arise from impact and are problems in energy absorption.[37]

Fractures can occur when the kinetic energy of a part undergoing impact is abruptly concentrated and converted to work that produces strain within the bone.[86] Since energy is released by the bone at the time of fracture, fractures can be considered low energy, such as the simple torsional ski accident; high energy, as often occurs in auto accidents; or very high energy, as can occur with a gunshot wound.[41]

Fractures occur in certain patterns because of the properties of bone. When bone is subjected to a steady load, plastic or viscous deformation caused by shear stress can occur, with a subsequent fracture if a crack appears and progresses. Conventional fracture mechanics assume that a crack or flaw in bone (or any solid) occurs and propagates, causing failure when the stress at the tip of the crack reaches a critical value that overcomes the forces of bone cohesion. Unlike other solids, bone is anisotropic and does not truly follow purely linear elastic characteristics in the initial portion of the stress-strain curve.[5]

Solid materials, including bone, have a great number of microscopic defects that usually do not progress into fractures unless available energy progresses the defects into larger and larger cracks. These defects explain why the stress-strain curve for bone differs slightly in linear elastic properties in the initial range of the curve.[5,41] To propagate a fracture, energy must rupture chemical bonds and create new surfaces. A propagating crack requires less energy to continue than a crack that has not begun to progress.[86] Fracture stress for crack growth in a brittle material is related to the initial crack depth by the following formula:

$$\text{Fracture stress}^2 = \frac{4 \times \text{Young's modulus} \times \text{Surface energy}}{\text{Depth of the crack}}$$

where

Surface energy = energy to progress a crack (determined in units of ergs, calories, or British thermal units)

However, since bone is a composite material, neither totally brittle nor totally ductile, the nonmineral components of bone can undergo a substantial plastic deformation before failure.[56] These components are also compliant and have good energy-absorbing characteristics (toughness) although bone crystals themselves are rigid, stiff, brittle, and fracture easily.[66] The composite characteristics of bone, plus the fact that the microfractures lead to various changes in bone based on the particular load, result in a large fracture energy (toughness) for bone.[56,86] The somewhat plastic behavior of bone has a strengthening or toughening effect. To determine the maximal stress on a simple beam before failure the following equation is used:

$$\text{Stress} = \frac{-My}{I}$$

where

M = Bending moment
y = Distance from the neutral axis to the extreme fibers
I = Moment of inertia

This formula is only valid for a linearly elastic material and holds true for a brittle material that has a ratio of elastic elongation to total elongation nearly equal to 1. However, if a material yields significantly (elastic elongation/ total elongation ratio is much less than 1), the equation cannot be used. Since bone is not totally brittle, a yielding effect must be considered.

Tensile stresses are particularly high at areas of stress concentration, such as where bone suddenly narrows—at grooves, notches, openings—or at any place where there is a change in the cross section.[86] The more abrupt the change, the greater the concentration of tensile stress. In a sharp, deep crack, tensile stresses can be concentrated by a factor of 10,000. However, only the component of the tensile stress that is perpendicular to the crack will progress the crack (Fig. 1-41).

When a crack in a bone has appeared, the weakest link within the bone will fail. The weakest links for stress concentration are haversian canals, canaliculi, lacunae, and cement lines. As shown in Fig. 1-41, tensile stresses perpendicular to the crack pull these areas apart, whereas compression stresses perpendicular to the crack discourage crack growth. The combined stress-strain curves for both tension and compression appear in Fig. 1-42.[14] As shown in Fig. 1-42, more compressive stress than tensile stress is required to produce an equal amount of strain. A bone fails sooner under a tensile load because tensile stress causes greater disruption of weak link areas, thus causing more strain and earlier fracture than will a compressive stress of equal magnitude.

If a fracture is produced by fatigue, the microscopic damage caused by repetitive loading stresses accumulates faster than bone healing can occur. Carter and Hayes[18-20] have suggested that bone yielding may be due to diffuse structural damage, such as debonding, microcracking, and fiber damage. It is possible that the microdamage may be the stimulus for bone remodeling.[17] During repeated loading, bone progressively loses stiffness and strength.[17-19,42] Fatigue life shortens as stress amplitude or temperature increases.[16,21,23] The load (force), number of repetitions, and frequency of loading are important factors to consider,[41] since an overuse syndrome can develop from a high repetition–low load situation or a low repetition– high load one.[89] An example of the former would be the runner who suddenly increases his or her mileage per day. An example of the latter is the high jumper who jumps a few times per day but with great effort at each jump.[35]

Remodeled (secondary or haversian) cortical bone is more compliant than primary bone and has about 83% of the Young's modulus of elasticity for primary bone.[16-19,66] The decreased fatigue resistance of secondary bone may be the result of the decreased density of haversian bone,[23] since a highly significant positive correlation exists between fatigue life and bone density.[16] Continuous strenuous activity not only fatigues muscle but it prevents neutralization of stress because the bone stores less energy when constantly stressed.[41] Fewer repetitions are required to cause a fracture as the stress per repetition approaches that which corresponds to the yield point on the stress-strain curve.

Within haversian bone, there is increased resistance to fatigue at the edge of an osteon. Even though openings in bone increase stress concentration around the opening, ce-

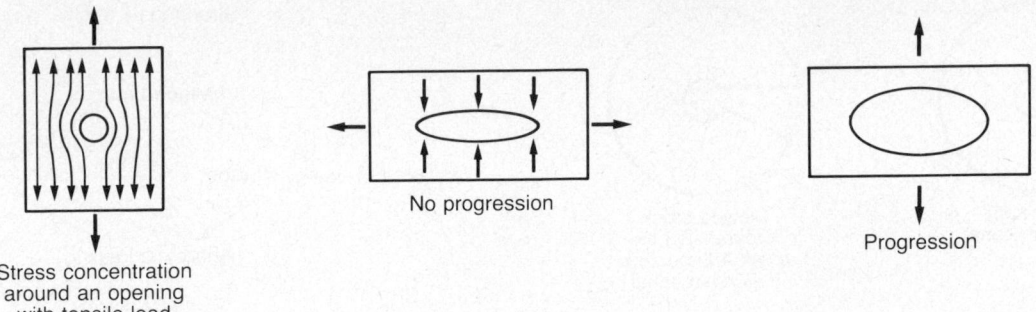

Stress concentration
around an opening
with tensile load

No progression

Progression

Fig. 1-41. Tensile stresses at the location of a crack will progress the crack, whereas compressive stresses will not.

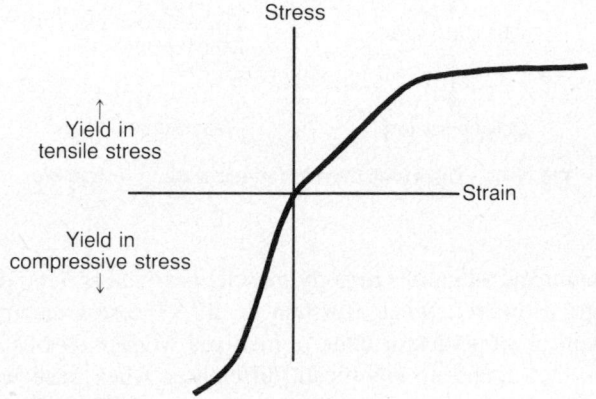

Stress

Yield in
tensile stress

Strain

Yield in
compressive stress

Fig. 1-42. Greater compressive stress than tensile stress is required to produce an equal amount of strain.

ment lines and haversian canals can act at times to slow the propagation of a crack. The cement lines can guide a crack longitudinally, which may cause less damage. Since the haversian canal has an increased radius of curvature, that is, an edge that is not as sharp as the crack edge, higher stresses are required to progress the crack at the canal[86] (Fig. 1-43).

Speed of loading is also important in determining fatigue. The higher the speed of loading, the more energy can be stored in the bone and the more load can be withstood before failure.[41] With increasing speeds, the load to failure can almost double, whereas the deformation changes little. The speed of loading not only influences the fracture pattern, but also affects the amount of soft tissue damage at the fracture. When bone fractures after being loaded at a slow speed, energy can often dissipate by the formation of a single crack, and there is little soft tissue damage or damage to the rest of the bone. If a fracture occurs when bone is loaded at a high speed, extensive soft tissue damage can occur, with the breaking of the bone in many places.[41] Cracks, or fractures, resulting from slow loading tend to propagate preferentially along osteon boundaries and not through osteons.[66]

Muscle fatigue tends to increase the possibility of fa-

tigue fractures.[41] As mentioned before, muscle contraction can decrease or even eliminate tensile stress from bending by producing a compressive stress that partially or totally neutralizes the tensile stress.[41] The theory of muscle fatigue leading to fracture as a sequential series of events[41] is outlined in Fig. 1-44.

Bone failure is controlled by strain magnitude and stress magnitude. Fatigue fractures can occur in servicemen and servicewomen during basic training; in ballet dancers, runners, or other athletes; or in people who abruptly begin a vigorous exercise program or too quickly progress through an exercise routine.[17,19,20] Military personnel may incur fatigue fractures at the metatarsal level when they are instructed to march long distances, hence the common term, "march fracture." Fatigue fractures of the upper third of the fibula may occur when basic training involves performing full deep knee bends and walking from that position.[101] During this maneuver, the soleus, posterior tibial, peroneus longus, and flexor hallucis longus muscles pull forcefully on the fibula. A forceful contraction of the ankle plantar flexor and toe flexor muscles pulls the tibia and fibula together, which could be the mechanism for fibular fracture here and in runners as well.[101]

Fatigue fractures occur more commonly at particular bony sites in the elderly, specifically at the femoral neck region in elderly women, the distal radius, vertebral bodies, and the surgical neck of the humerus. As bone density decreases with age and osteoporosis occurs, trabecular fractures increase.[42] The earliest and most striking decreases in bone density occur in trabecular bone, with the trabeculae becoming thin and sparse.[94] Microdamage accumulation occurring at a faster rate than healing seems to be the main failure mechanism, since an increased number of trabecular failures have been located in the same site as the gross fractures in the subcapital femoral neck area.[42]

Cortical bone is stiffer than cancellous bone and therefore can withstand more stress before failure but less strain. Cortical bone fractures when the strain is greater than 2% of the original length of the segment, whereas cancellous bone fractures only after a strain of greater than

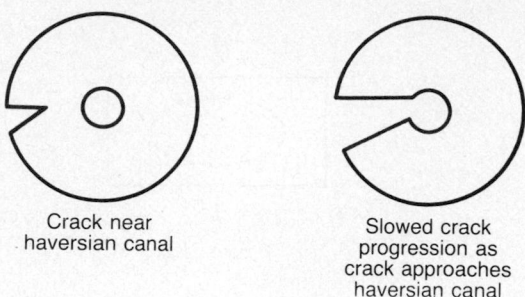

Fig. 1-43. Progression of a crack is slowed at the site of a haversian canal.

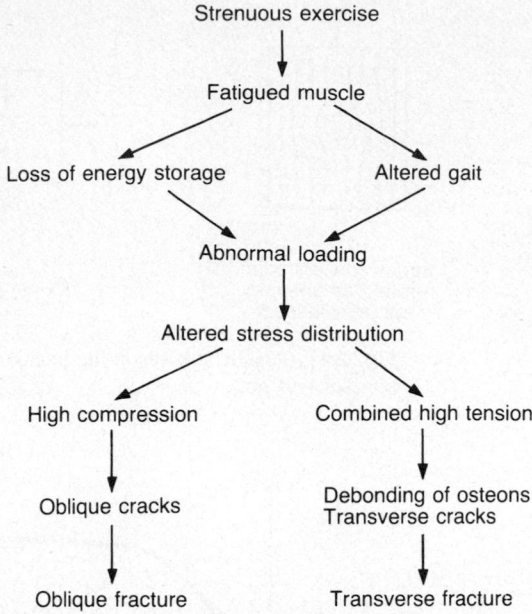

Fig. 1-44. Theory of muscle fatigue leading to fracture.

7%. As a result, cancellous bone is said to have a high-energy storage capacity. Table 1-7 lists the ultimate strength properties of bone for different types of stress or load.

Bone healing

Bone healing after fracture begins with clotting of the blood that surrounds the bone fragments and soft tissue. The clot is invaded by a loose meshwork of capillaries and fibroblasts.[15,109] Cells that will proliferate and differentiate into fibrous connective tissue, fibrocartilage, hyaline cartilage, and bone are supplied by the torn ends of the periosteum, endosteum, and bone marrow. The tearing of the periosteum strongly stimulates cell proliferation in the deeper periosteum and new bone formation can begin within 48 hours in young people. Callus, the substance formed by the proliferating cells at the fracture site, is composed of a combination of bone and cartilage.[62]

If the fracture site has adequate oxygen, bone will be formed preferentially from the undifferentiated cells. If the oxygen supply is inadequate, cartilage will be formed preferentially, since cartilage requires less oxygen for its viability. Mature cartilage callus later is replaced by bone in a similar manner to initial endochondral ossification.

The time required for bone healing is directly proportional to the total volume of injured bone and the extent of the damage. If the fractured segments are in contact, bones such as the humerus, radius, and ulna may unite in 3 months; union of femoral and tibial fractures may require twice that time. Spiral fractures tend to heal more quickly than transverse fractures. Healing time increases with age.

Differences in mechanical properties of bone for men versus women

Bone strength is greatest in the direction of physiological loading, that is, where maximal loads occur for the greatest percentage of time. Bone strength will increase to meet increasing demands. Some researchers believe that bone strength in men is greater in most mechanical properties than it is in women, perhaps because men are subject to higher stresses from a more active life[84] or because of

anatomical variations in body muscle mass and skeletal design. However, when Burstein et al.[13,14] tested the mechanical properties of bone in men and women ages 21 to 86, they found no significant differences when bone was tested with tensile, compressive, and torsional loads. A comparison of the mechanical properties of bone for men and women is found in Table 1-8.

Data have been gathered regarding differences in bone composition for mice raised under different gravitational forces.[114] Although comparison of animal studies to human studies should be done with caution, any information learned in this area has great significance for astronauts who are subjected to gravitational forces other than that of the earth. Following centrifugation (which increases gravitational force) for 1 to 8 weeks after the fifth week of life, the bone size of both male and female mice was greater than that of the control mice, who experienced normal gravitational force.

Age-related differences in mechanical properties of bone

Throughout life, significant changes occur in the dimensions of various portions of bone. Subperiosteal bone grows rapidly postnatally by appositional growth. It markedly decreases in growth rate at about 6 months, grows more rapidly during both juvenile and adolescent growth spurts, and continues to grow at a slow rate via appositional growth throughout life[48] and therefore becomes relatively stronger with advancing age.[22] After an initial endosteal resorption to form the medullary canal, changes in endosteal bone include an initial (juvenile) phase of resorption, a second steroid-mediated phase of apposition,

Table 1-7. Ultimate strength properties of bone

	Tension	Compression	Shear	Bending	Torsion
Ultimate strength	Failure of bone is closely associated with planes of maximal stress,[13] usually caused by bending or torsion[86] Tensile strength is greater in bending than axial loading[13] Load to failure in axial tension is proportional to cross-sectional area of bone[41] Cortical bone can withstand greater tensile than shear stress[41] Fatigue fracture from tensile stress results in transverse crack and may fracture rapidly and completely[41] Ultimate strength of wet bone is about 13,818 psi, whereas that of dry bone is about 19,939 psi (as compared to that of collagen— 80,000 psi)[77]	Load to failure in axial compression is proportional to cross-sectional area of bone[41] Cortical bone can withstand greater stress in compression than tension[41] Fatigue fracture due to compression stress proceeds more slowly than one due to tension and may not completely fracture[41]	Fracture from torsional stress begins with crack parallel to neutral axis due to shear[41]	Fracture in bending begins on tensile side at outside fibers or where groove, crack, etc., is present Crack proceeds transversely[86] Fractures are commonly due to three- and four-point bending[41] With three-point bending, fracture occurs at middle force; with four-point bending, fracture occurs at weakest part of bone[41]	During torsional loads, tensile deformation causes fracture[86] Fracture due to torsion occurs where bone has smallest polar moment of inertia[41]
Fracture healing				During healing, callus increases area moment of inertia so bone strength and stiffness increase; this resists deformation due to bending; callus is gradually resorbed[41]	During healing, callus increases polar moment of inertia, which increases bone strength and stiffness; this resists deformation due to torsion; callus is gradually resorbed[41]
Mechanism of failure	Widely distributed fractures accumulate; these lead to delamination of haversian systems and debonding at weak osteon/matrix interfaces (cement lines), with subsequent erosion of osteons[41,42,56]	Fracture occurs from oblique cracking of osteons[41,42]	Bone can deform by kinking mechanism, initiated by shear of matrix; since interfaces are weak areas within composite materials, any stress that causes shear at interfaces results in premature failure of composite[56]	Bone is more resistant to fatigue with bending loads than with uniaxial loads[22]; During bending, more microdamage is found on compressed side than side under tension[16]	Residual microscopic strain results from: 1. Nonelastic deformation of collagen initially and then deformation of crystals; crystals can support greater loads 2. Shearing along interfacial region between collagen and crystals[56]

Continued.

Table 1-7. Ultimate strength properties of bone—cont'd

Tension	Compression	Shear	Bending	Torsion
In uniaxial tensile loading, tensile strength decreases faster than does compressive strength with uniaxial compressive loading[22]				Torsional stresses cause spiral fractures, as longitudinal fibers are stretched by distortions due to shear; shearing initiates crack parallel to bone's neutral axis; tensile deformation then causes crack growth along plane of maximal tensile stress,[41,86] which is greatest at 30- to 45-degree angle to axis of torsion[86]

and an adult phase of resorption. An initial neonatal gain of cortical bone until the age of 6 months is followed by an infantile loss, a juvenile gain, an adolescent spurt, a slight adult gain to the fifth decade, and then a decline.[48] The reported decrease in cortical bone density (including subperiosteal bone) with advancing age is probably related to an increase in average bone porosity, since bone mineralization increases with advancing age.[22]

Differences in osteonal properties are seen with aging.[64] Children have increased bone formation and resorption and therefore an increased turnover rate of bone. (Density is comparatively low, since the number of forming osteons and resorption cavities is increased.) The turnover rate for bone in young adults is decreased, and most osteons are not fully mineralized. Bone material strength decreases after age 30 because of increased porosity from an increase in the number of vascular channels. The osteonal picture parallels the general increase in endosteal resorption in the later years. From age 60 on, the number of osteons that are less than three-fourths closed, especially in endosteal bone, sharply increases. The osteons simply do not completely close. From age 70 on, up to 25% of the bone surface may be occupied by resorption cavities.[64]

Changes in the collagen fibers and bone ash also occur with age.[33] Collagen fibers increase in stability with age as more bonding occurs. Bone ash increases markedly between ages 2 to 17, less rapidly from 26 to 48, and only slightly until age 80. The decreased ash content in the bones of children may explain both the increased plastic deformation and the increased energy absorption before failure, as well as the lower modulus of elasticity and bending strength in this age group.

The tensile strength, tensile strain, and failure in infant femoral bones compare with the values for adult femoral bones, although the modulus of elasticity is considerably lower. It would seem that weight bearing may not be critical for tensile strength and strain, because these properties would be increased by bending moments of bone and by muscular traction forces. Since an infant cannot walk until Young's modulus is high enough—that is, until the bones have adequate stiffness (which is determined by stress and strain measurements)—it is possible that the modulus may not develop until walking is attempted.[37]

A summary of the findings on various mechanical properties of bone as a variable of age is found in Table 1-9. In general, mechanical and material properties of bone tend to decrease with age, but changes in the geometrical properties of bone may compensate for changes in intrinsic bone properties. Traditionally, static tensile strength has been used as the criterion in judging the overall quality of bone, whether to determine age effects on bone, effects of sex on bone quality, or the effects of nutrition on bone.[51]

Ultimate tensile strength declines with advanced age and at times the decline is quite rapid. A rapid decline does not appear to be caused by properties of collagen fibers, which do not change quickly, or the degree of preferred orientation of the apatite crystals, which also changes little during life. The decline is more likely caused by differences in mineral particle size distribution within a bone. Any radius change in particles affects bone strength, since the effect of a particle on strength dimensions is a function of its distance cubed from the neutral axis of the bone.[106] The percentage of small particles in the mineral (apatite) phase of bone—the high modulus portion—increases to the fourth decade and then decreases.

Table 1-8. Comparison of mechanical properties of bone in men and women

Mechanical property	Comparison
Cortical human bone	
Tension	
Tensile strength	Greater in men or equal
Ultimate strength	Equal
Percentage of elongation	Equal or greater in women
Mean deformation at failure	Equal
Modulus of elasticity	Greater in men or equal
Compression	
Compressive strength	Greater in men
Modulus of elasticity	Equal
Bending properties	Equal
Torsion strength	Greater in men
Density	Increases with age in men; decreases with age in women
Cancellous human bone (vertebral bodies)	
Tension	
Tensile strength[14,37]	Equal
Tensile strain	Equal
Compression	
Mean ultimate compressive stress	Greater in men
Compressive strength	Controversial
Compressive strain	Equal or greater in women
Compressive modulus of elasticity	Greater in men
Torsion	
Torsional strength[14,37]	Equal
Breaking torsional moment	Greater in men
Energy absorbed to failure	Greater in men
Density	Greater in men

Based on data from Evans FG: Mechanical properties of bone, Springfield, Ill, 1973, Charles C Thomas, Publisher, except as noted.

The subperiosteal and endosteal changes in bone affect men and women differently. Both sexes have endosteal resorption of bone with advanced age as the walls of cancellous bone become progressively thinner.[49] This endosteal resorption is greater in women, particularly after menopause. Men and women also have subperiosteal bone growth (men more than women), which could increase the moment of inertia[48,49] and bending stiffness.[91] However, the increase in subperiosteal diameter is later and longer in men.[48] Men also experience a larger subperiosteal change in their late teens.[48] This subperiosteal expansion may be a compensatory mechanism for bone loss caused by endosteal resorption and cortical thinning.[90] This expansion of the subperiosteum in men offsets endosteal resorption of cortical bone, whereas cortical bone in women undergoes a net decrease with advancing age (i.e., the subperiosteal expansion does not offset the endosteal resorption)[48,91] and therefore a net decrease over time in the ability of the bones of women to resist failure.[48,75,91] In terms of femoral changes, the most profound differences between men and women are seen at the ends of the femur. Although femoral material strength decreases with age for both men and women, the increased moment of inertia in men compensates for the decreased material strength.[75] In women the subperiosteal expansion is not significant enough, in view of the endosteal resorption, to increase the moment of inertia. There is, in effect, an actual decrease in the moment of inertia, which, with the decreased material strength of the bone with age, weakens the femur.[75]

The strain characteristics of the older adult bone differ from those of younger bone. Bones of the elderly can withstand about half the strain of those of younger adults. The bones of the elderly are less ductile and less able to store energy to failure.[41] From a structural viewpoint, the decrease in plastic strain and therefore in ultimate strain is the most important age change in bone.[13,14] The decrease in ultimate strain refers to the inability of the bone as a whole to bend. The weakening of the femur in females because of decreases in the moment of inertia, material strength, and subperiosteal expansion in the femoral neck compared with the remaining femur,[100] coupled with the knowledge that women live longer than men and have marked hormonal change,[44] explains why elderly women have so many fractured femurs. Although many people with fractured femurs believe they must have tripped or stumbled, but cannot remember the incident distinctly, many have spontaneous fractures while standing or walking and fall as a result.[42,100,104]

All of these changes related to aging should be viewed in the context of the more sedentary life-style of most older people and the possibility that many of the changes are in fact due to inactivity.

Adaptation of bone to exercise stress

Original bone modeling and remodeling involve the reaction of bone to stresses from gravity, joint position, dynamic motion, and genetic influences. Bone adaptation may be stimulated by microdamage, piezoelectricity, surface strain, some combination of stimuli, or an as yet unknown mechanism.[76] Ruff and Hayes[92] suggest that bone stress and strain caused by exercise seem important as stimuli for subperiosteal appositional growth and skeletal modeling in adults. For example, metaphyseal regions of long bones are not as subject to high bending and torsional stresses in vivo as are diaphyseal regions. Hence, there is not as much stimulus for subperiosteal expansion. In general, the regions near the ends of bones are mechanically weaker; that is, they are more prone to fail under high bending or torsional loading. The extent to which exercise can maintain bone integrity in these areas can be evaluated by comparing the percentage of hip fractures in women from nonindustrialized societies with the percentage in industrialized societies. Women in the former group have fewer hip fractures,[24] partially because of their more active

Table 1-9. Mechanical properties of bone as a function of age

Mechanical property	Bone	Characteristics
Cortical bone		
Tensile strength	Femur Tibia Fibula	Those over 60 have less tensile strength than those under 60; there is no significant difference in the amount of calcium, organic tissue, or ash content (mineral content)
	Femur, unembalmed	Mean tensile strength decreases up to 10% with age except in women 15 to 19 years old, in whom it increases; maximal tensile strain occurs at 10 to 19 years old and then decreases to a minimum between ages 60 to 79; no changes occur in Young's modulus
	Fibula	Microhardness of fibular cortical bone increases to age 30, then plateaus
	Tibia, embalmed	Mean tensile stress and strain are maximal between ages 20 to 39, then decrease; Young's modulus is maximal at ages 40 to 59, then decreases gradually; same is true for shear modulus
	Femur	Shear modulus is maximal at ages 20 to 39, then decreases between ages 40 to 59 and plateaus
	Femur	Progressive loss of tensile strength occurs with age (21 to 86 years)[14]
	Tibia	No decrease in loss of tensile strength with age[14]
	Femur	The mean tensile stress and strain to failure for infant femoral bone are within same range values as for adult femoral bone but with much lower modulus of elasticity; mean tensile strength and strain for 14-year-old are greater than those values for adults; tensile properties of cortical bone are greatest from ages 20 to 29, with leveling or slight decrease to age 39, then more rapid decrease; ultimate tensile strength is greater in small bones (in order of greater to lesser strength—radius, ulna, fibula, tibia, humerus, femur)[115]
Compressive strength	Femur (posterior shaft)	Mean ultimate strength is maximal at ages 20 to 39 and decreases 15% with age to minimum at ages 60 to 79; no changes occur in Young's modulus; compressive properties of cortical bone are greatest from ages 20 to 29, with leveling or slight decrease to age 39, then decrease[115]
Bending strength	Femur	Bending strength is maximal at ages 24 to 32, then decreases to minimum at ages 70 to 80; mean ultimate fiber strength steadily decreases; energy absorbed to failure and modulus of elasticity decrease in elderly
	Cortical bone	Bending properties of cortical bone are greatest from ages 20 to 29, with leveling or slight decrease to age 39, then specific decrease[115]
	Femur	Bending strength of whole bone decreases in elderly, although tissue specimens have increased bending strength[104]
Torsion	Embalmed bone	Maximal torsional stress occurs at ages 20 to 39, then decreases to minimum at ages 60 to 79; torsional shear, shear modulus, and energy absorbed to failure show no specific trend with age
	Cortical bone	Torsional properties of cortical bone are greatest from ages 20 to 29, with leveling or slight decrease to age 39, then more rapid decrease[115]
		Torsional strength is maximal at ages 25 to 35, then decreases; modulus of elasticity in torsion decreases with age[38]
Plastic deformation	Femur Tibia	From ages 20 to 80, plastic part of stress-strain curve increases with age, in femur more than tibia
Elastic deformation		There is increased stiffness of femur compared with that of tibia
Cancellous bone		
Compression	Femur	Maximal compressive stress, modulus of elasticity, and energy absorbed to failure decrease after age 70; compressive strain at failure increases with age to 70
	Inferior calcaneal tuberosity	Compressive stress at failure decreases with age

Based on data from Evans FG: Mechanical properties of bone, Springfield, Ill, 1973, Charles C Thomas, Publisher, except as noted.

life-styles. Women in industrialized societies have a more sedentary life-style and more hip fractures because the inactivity fails to stimulate the geometrical changes in bone, which could help compensate for the decreasing bone material strength with advanced age.[75] The subperiosteal ap-

position and therefore the increased moment of inertia that would be caused by the exercise stimulus do not occur in sedentary individuals.

Mechanical considerations—such as the moments produced around a joint, joint forces, the duration of exercise, and bony alignment (particularly of weight-bearing joints)—are important in understanding the adaptation of bone to exercise. Mechanical characteristics are often discussed broadly in terms of multiples of body weight loads occurring at a joint. During normal walking, for example, forces two to four times body weight usually occur at the hip, with forces six to nine times body weight occurring during a fast walk. Landing from a jump of 1 m would cause a compressive load of about 24 times body weight at the knee joint.

General training variables include the type of training undertaken (continuous or intermittent), the intensity of training (mild, moderate, or intensive), and the duration of training (times per day and number of weeks, months, and years), taking into account such factors as the person's age, health, and previous immobilization.[52,60,72,110] Exercise can have a specific effect, as seen by increased cortical thickness in the forearm bones of the dominant side in tennis players,[113] or a generalized effect as seen with an overall increase in bone mineral content in cross-country runners.[34] (The increase was measured in the forearm bones of the runners.) Because most of the experiments with different training intensities have involved animals, it is difficult to extrapolate the exercise intensities to humans. However, Woo et al.[113] have suggested that 40 km per week be considered moderate training for running, with additional distance constituting intense exercise.

Bone will respond differently to low or moderate exercise compared with intense exercise. Goodship, Lanyon, and McFie[53] performed ulnar ostectomies on young male pigs and found that within a 3-month period of free movement, the cross-sectional area of the radius of the operated side equalled that of the radius and ulna of the nonoperated side. Chamay and Tschantz[25] reported similar effects. Woo et al.[113] exercised year-old pigs in a running routine that was gradually increased over a year to a moderate level. Results of the exercise included an increase in cortical thickness (17%), increased energy absorbed to failure, increased bone mass, decreased endosteal bone, and increased calcium content in the bone—all of which added to bone strength. Bony adaptations in mice exercised by running at low or moderate levels have included increased bone mass in the limb bones,[68] longer bones,[67,68] and heavier bones.[67,68,96] Rats made bipedal at birth developed femurs with increased breaking strengths and densities.[95] Anderson, Milin, and Crackel[4] noted that pigs exercised by running at a moderate level had a decreased hydroxyproline content in their urine, indicating an increased hydroxyproline retention in the bone and probably an increased collagen synthesis.

Intense exercise in experimental animals has been shown to inhibit bone growth in length and girth. Al-though the operational definitions of mild, moderate, and intense exercise varied among investigators, the exercise intensities generally consisted of about 50 to 80 minutes of running a day as moderate exercise and more than 120 minutes per day as intense exercise, with speed varied according to the size of the animal. Kiiskinen and Heikkinen[67,68] exercised mice via a running program to an intense level and reported shorter and lighter limb bones, decreased bone volume, and a decreased hydroxyproline content in bone as compared to controls. The decreased hydroxyproline content probably indicated a reduced rate of collagen synthesis in the bone. These inhibitory effects on bone growth could reflect a slower rate of the bone's repair of microdamage than the actual microdamage rate. The effects seen in varying exercise intensity may be altered by factors such as the age and size of the experimental animal.[11,102]

The differing effects of continuous and intermittent exercise were reported by Hert, Liskova, and Landrgot[59] who loaded rabbit tibias by inserting two wires through the metaphyses of the bone. Long-term continuous bending of the adult bone resulted in an absence of reaction, even after 12 months of loading, although some effects were seen in growing animals.[59] Intermittent loading within physiological limits along with freedom of movement by the rabbits resulted in an increase of bone growth in areas of great stress.[54,73] Maintenance of lower extremity bone structure has been attempted for people who are unable to stand or walk by using a tilt table. A person can be secured to the table, which is tilted vertically at a varying rate and to a varying extent. The stimulus to bone from simulated weight bearing is a continuous one. Although the tilt table may have other functions, such as stimulation of mechanisms needed for blood pressure regulation, its value for maintaining bone integrity may well be questioned.

BONE GROWTH AND LOADING OF THE LOWER EXTREMITY BONES

Long bones of the lower extremities are the structural supports for the body.[66] The main function of the femur and tibia is weight bearing, whereas that of the fibula is to serve as an attachment for muscle.[37] These bones are subjected to asymmetrical loading modes. A comparison of material strengths of the three bones is listed in Table 1-10. In general, the fibula is strongest in tensile loading, which is logical considering the many muscular traction forces it has to withstand. The femur has a higher modulus of elasticity than the tibia because of the greater bending loads it must withstand.

These findings are based on relatively few studies, however, some of which are controversial. Further data are needed to verify findings and clarify contradictions.

Table 1-10. Comparison of material strengths of the femur, tibia, and fibula (human, unembalmed bone)

Load	Mechanical property	Material strength
Cortical bone		
Tension	Average tensile strength	Adult men: Fibula and tibia are stronger than femur; femur is stronger than humerus
	Tensile strain	Adults 20 to 39 years old: Fibula can withstand more strain than tibia, which can withstand more than femur[14,37]
	Young's modulus	Fibula has higher or equal modulus to tibia; both have higher modulus than femur; overall, tibia is stiffest and femur is most flexible[37,99]
Compression	Average compressive strength	Tested along long axis, tibia is stronger than femur[14] (two specimens)[37]; in another study of 26 specimens, femur was stronger than tibia and tibia stronger than fibula
	Compressive strain	Tested along long axis in 20- to 39-year-old adults, fibula can withstand more or equal strain than tibia, whereas tibia can withstand more than femur[14,37]
Shear	Shear strength	Relative shear strength is controversial
	Ultimate displacement	Fibula can withstand greater ultimate displacement than tibia, which can withstand more than femur
Bending	Strength	Femur is stronger than tibia in men, whereas tibia is stronger than femur in women (no age ranges given)
	Young's modulus	Femur has higher modulus than tibia
Fatigue life (cycles to failure)	Strength	Femur is stronger than tibia, which is stronger than fibula (results are not considered statistically significant)
Cancellous bone		
Young's modulus		In both tension and compression, fibula equals tibia and both have higher modulus than femur

Based on data from Evans FG: Mechanical properties of bone, Springfield Ill, 1973, Charles C Thomas, Publisher, except as noted.

Femur

In the standing position, the femur is subjected to tensile stresses. These occur especially at the sites of muscular attachment for the hip extensor, knee extensor, and plantar flexor muscles. On the lateral[86] and anterior diaphyseal regions, tensile stresses (as a result of weight bearing) exist.[75]

The shape of the femur is such that bending loads from weight bearing produce the forces A and D; their respective components are shown in Fig. 1-45. Forces E and B tend to bend the femur in one direction, whereas forces C and F tend to bend the femur in the opposite direction. The bending from weight bearing tends to bow the bone so that the convexity is on the lateral femur. Since the resultant forces D and A are aligned to the neutral axis of the femur, forces E and B can counter the bending moment caused by C and F. Comparison of material strengths of various portions of the femur is given in Table 1-11. As can be seen, even with relatively incomplete data collected regarding femoral strength throughout different portions of the bone, the greatest strength occurs in the areas subjected to the most stress, where bone has been modeled and remodeled to conform to those stresses. Examples are the high tensile strength in the middle third of the shaft—the lateral quadrant—which is subject to high tensile stresses because of weight bearing, and the great compressive strength in the femoral neck area adjacent to the lesser trochanter, which is subject to great compressive stresses (Fig. 1-46).[93]

Increased bone density can lead to strength in some mechanical properties and weakness in other properties. In compact femoral bone, for example, the presence of secondary osteons tends to increase the maximal shear stress, shear modulus, and energy absorbed to failure, whereas increased porosity decreases these properties. However, osteons also can decrease the amount of bone tissue available to support a load and therefore can weaken bone. The presence of haversian canals is more significant in weakening bone in torsion than are the canaliculi or lacunae. All three will increase the porosity of bone and can contribute to a decreased tensile strength as well. An increase in the number of secondary osteons, and therefore an increased number of cement lines and a decreased amount of interstitial lamellae, is associated with an increased ultimate tensile strength. This occurs because the cement lines form areas of weakness by developing microfractures as a result of tensile and bending stresses.

Fracture of the femur can occur from lack of material strength, but fracture of the whole bone is often associated with planes of maximal tensile stress, which are usually the result of torsion or bending.[14,86] Femoral neck fractures may occur as a result of osteoporosis and muscle fa-

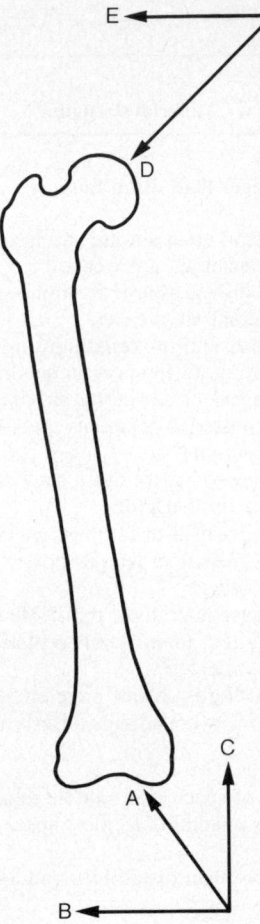

Fig. 1-45. Forces caused by bending loads in weight bearing.

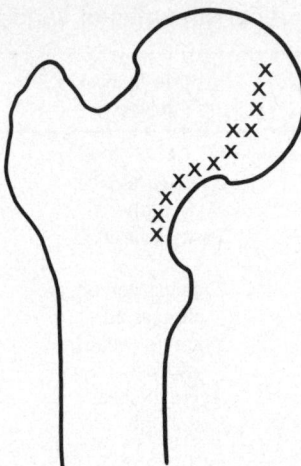

Fig. 1-46. In the femoral head and neck, the *xs* mark the areas of increased average compressive strength.

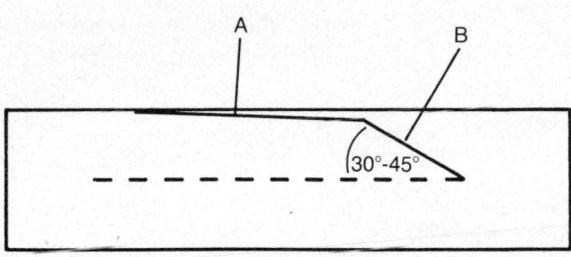

Fig. 1-47. Fractures from torsional stress exhibit initial bone failure in shear *(A)* and then follow the plane of maximal tensile stress *(B)*.

tigue (especially that of the gluteus medius), which combined cannot prevent high tensile stresses from forming on the superior femoral neck.[41,100] Compressive fractures, on the other hand, can occur near the hip joint when abnormally high compressive stresses are caused by strong co-contraction of the hip muscles. These stresses can be produced during electroconvulsive shock therapy and can result in a subcapital fracture of the femoral neck.[41] Shear fractures can occur at the femoral condyles.[41] As seen in Fig. 1-47, fractures from torsional stress exhibit initial bone failure in shear *(A)*, parallel to the neutral axis. The fracture line then tends to follow about a 30- to 45-degree angle to the neutral axis *(B)*, which corresponds to the plane of maximal tensile stress.[41,86]

It is interesting to note the location of the epiphyseal plates in relation to the lines of compression and tension lines within the femur. In Figs. 1-48 and 1-49, the thin solid lines represent the compressive stress lines and the dotted lines depict tensile stress lines during weight bearing. The thicker solid lines are the epiphyseal plates.[99] When the femur bears weight, the shaft bends anteriorly

and laterally, subjecting the anterior and lateral portions of the femur to tensile stress and the posterior and medial portions to compressive stress. Muscle groups help reduce the tensile stress; for example, the quadriceps act on the anterior femur. The aligning of the epiphyseal plates to these tensile and compressive trajectories results in decreased shear stress on the epiphyseal plates. Trabeculae will orient to these trajectories as well.

Tibia and fibula

The tibia is a weight-bearing bone, as is the femur. It has similar mechanical properties but generally has better mechanical stability than the femur.[13,14] Tibial bone has a faster turnover rate than that of the femur, and, as a result, a better chance for faster bone repair when microfractures occur. The plastic portion of the tibial stress-strain curve is more consistent, which indicates more rapidly forming new collagen in the tibia.[14]

Tibial fractures can occur as a result of many different mechanisms. The energy required to fracture the average tibia is about 1/10,000 of the kinetic energy of an 80 kg

Table 1-11. Material strengths of various portions of the femur

Load	Mechanical property	State of human bone (if known)	Material strength
Cortical bone			
Tension	Average tensile strength	Unembalmed	Middle third is stronger than distal third
	Tensile strain	Embalmed, wet	Middle third and lateral quadrant are strongest, and proximal third and anterior quadrant are weakest
	Greatest percentage elongation	Embalmed, wet	Middle third and medial quadrant are strongest and distal third and posterior quadrant are weakest
	Young's modulus (stiffness)	Embalmed, wet	Middle third is stiffest, and proximal third most flexible (lowest modulus); there are no differences in quadrants
Shear	Average shear strength	Embalmed, adult, wet	Middle third is strongest, followed by proximal third, then distal third; medial and posterior quadrants are stronger than anterior and lateral quadrants
Bending	Bending strength	Unembalmed, adult, wet	Lateral quadrant is strongest, followed by medial, anterior, and posterior quadrants, in that order
Torsion	Torsional shear stress	Embalmed, adult, wet	Middle third is stronger than distal third; medial quadrant can withstand greater stress than lateral, posterior, and anterior quadrants, in that order[37,38]
	Shear modulus	Embalmed, adult, wet	Middle third is stronger than distal third. Medial quadrant can withstand greater stress than lateral, posterior, and anterior quadrants, in that order[37,38]
	Energy absorbed to failure	Embalmed, adult, wet	Middle and proximal thirds absorb more energy than distal third; medial and lateral quadrants absorb more than anterior quadrant[37,38]
Percentage of spaces in bone			Greatest percentage of space is in middle third and least in distal third; posterior quadrant has most space, with lateral quadrant the least[38]
Complete osteons			Middle third has more than distal third and anterior quadrant[38]
Complete secondary osteons			Lateral quadrant has most[38]
Interstitial lamellae			Anterior quadrant has most and lateral quadrant least; distal third has most and proximal third least[38]
Cancellous bone			
Compression	Average compressive strength	Unembalmed, adult	In area outlined by *xs* in Fig. 1-46, average strength is greater than in rest of head and neck
	Young's modulus (stiffness)	Unembalmed, adult	In order of possessing high to low modulus are femoral head, lateral condyle, medial condyle, and greater trochanter, with inconclusive data regarding femoral neck
	Compressive strain	Unembalmed, adult	In order of high to low strain withstood are femoral head, lateral condyle, greater trochanter, medial condyle, and femoral neck
	Energy absorbed to failure	Unembalmed, adult	In order of most to least energy absorbed are femoral head, femoral neck, lateral condyle, medial condyle, and greater trochanter
			Elderly frequently have femoral osteoporosis and fracture as result of loss of bone mass; there is increased diameter of middle third of femur, with decreased cortical and trabecular thickness and decreased femoral density[100]
Bone in general	Plastic deformation		Ultimate deformation decreases 5% per decade after adulthood[13]

Based on data from Evans FG: Mechanical properties of bone, Springfield, Ill, 1973, Charles C Thomas, Publisher, except as noted.

skier traveling at 10 ms (24 mph).[86] Fractures resulting from shear stress occur in the tibial plateaus. They can occur from three-point bending, such as when a skier falls forward so that the body weight causes a moment at the proximal tibia and the ground causes an equal moment dis-

tally. The fracture is initiated posteriorly at the top of the boot where maximal tensile stress occurs.[41] With torsional loads on the tibia, the distal part of the bone often fractures first because the distal bone is closer to the neutral axis. There is a decreased polar moment of inertia and less

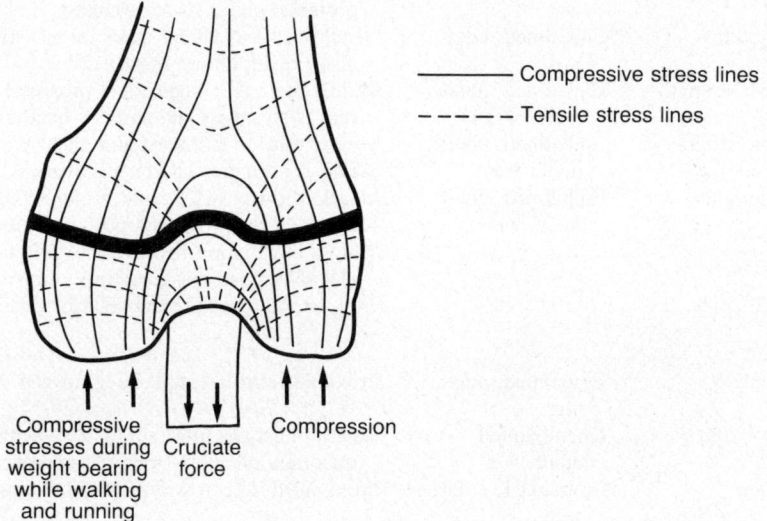

Fig. 1-48. Compressive and tensile stresses on the distal femur in relation to the epiphyseal plates during weight bearing, anterior view. (Modified from Smith JW: J Anat 96:58, 1962.)

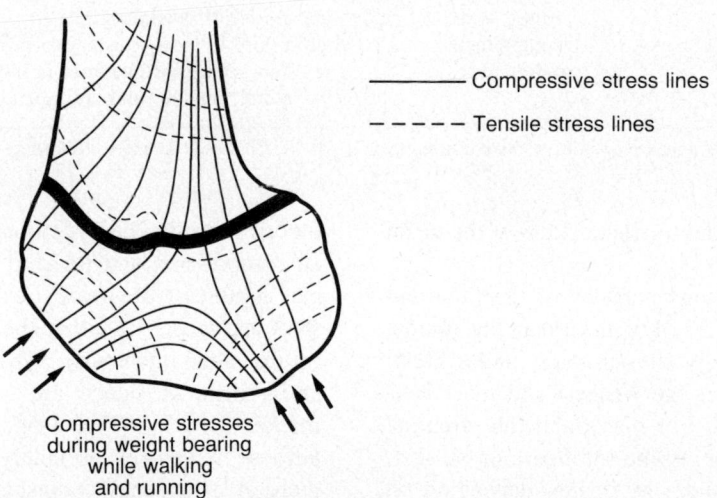

Fig. 1-49. Compressive and tensile stresses on the distal femur in relation to the epiphyseal plates during weight bearing, lateral view. (Modified from Smith JW: J Anat 96:58, 1962.)

Table 1-12. Material strengths of various portions of the tibia and fibula

Load	Mechanical property	State of human bone (if known)	Material strength
Tibia			
Tension	Tensile strength	Embalmed, adult, wet	Middle third and anterior quadrant are strongest; proximal third and medial quadrant are weakest
	Tensile strain	Embalmed, adult, wet	Middle third and anterior quadrant are strongest; proximal third and posterior quadrant are weakest
	Young's modulus	Embalmed, adult, wet	Distal third and lateral quadrant are stiffest; proximal third and anterior quadrant are most flexible
Compression	Compressive strength	Embalmed, adult male, wet	Middle third is strongest and proximal third weakest; medial quadrant is strongest and anterior quadrant weakest
	Compressive strain	Embalmed, adult male, wet	Middle third is strongest and distal third weakest; posterior quadrant is strongest and lateral quadrant is weakest
	Young's modulus	Embalmed, adult male, wet	Middle third is stiffest and proximal third is most flexible; anterior quadrant is stiffest and posterior quadrant is least stiff
Fatigue life[14]	Strength		Middle third is most resistant to fatigue and proximal third is least resistant; posterior quadrant is most resistant, followed in order by lateral, medial, and anterior quadrants
Fibula			
Tension	Tensile strength	Embalmed, adult, wet	Proximal third has most strength and distal third least
		Unembalmed, adult, wet	Middle third has most strength and proximal third least; posterior quadrant has most strength and anterior quadrant least
	Tensile strain	Embalmed, adult, wet	Proximal third can withstand most strain and distal third least
		Unembalmed, adult, wet	Anterior quadrant can withstand most strain and posterior quadrant least
	Young's modulus	Embalmed, adult	Middle third is stiffest and distal third most flexible
Shear	Shear strength	Embalmed, adult, wet	Middle third is strongest and distal third weakest
Bending	Bending strength	Unembalmed, adult, wet	Medial quadrant is strongest, followed in order by lateral, anterior, and posterior quadrants
Fatigue life	Strength	Unembalmed, adult, wet	Middle third is most resistant to fatigue and proximal third least resistant; posterior quadrant is most resistant, followed in order by lateral, medial, and anterior quadrants

Based on data from Evans FG: Mechanical properties of bone, Springfield, Ill, 1973, Charles C Thomas, Publisher, except as noted.

ability of the bone to resist the torsional stress at the distal tibia.

Material strengths of various portions of the tibia and fibula are given in Table 1-12. For the tibia, the middle third of the bone is generally the strongest and stiffest, whereas the proximal third is the weakest and most flexible for the properties listed. For the fibula, the proximal or middle third of the bone is the strongest or stiffest. There are significant differences in results, depending on whether the tested specimens are embalmed or unembalmed. In either case it would appear logical for the fibula to have great tensile strength in the middle or proximal third because of the number of muscles (as well as the interosseous membrane) that produce tensile stresses in those areas. Likewise, great tensile strength is required in the posterior quadrant, since so many muscle fibers attach to that area.

The proximal epiphyseal plate of the tibia corresponds to the lines of greatest tensile and compressive stress over time. In the standing position, the tibia is subjected to axial compression and forward bending, resulting in principal compressive stresses extending along the posterior shaft and mostly to either the lateral condyle or the region of the tibial tuberosity. These and the principal tensile stress lines in stance are seen in Fig. 1-50. The area marked 2 to 3 in Fig. 1-50, *B*, is subject to shear stress because it courses obliquely to both axes. As a result, there is a tendency to displace the epiphysis proximally and posteriorly on the diaphysis. Areas between 1 and 2 are aligned with principal tensile stress lines and are subject only to compression. The distal dip of the anterior part of the epiphyseal plate allows adaptation of the plate to large tensile stresses.

The epiphyseal plates actually conform most closely to the lines of stress incurred during walking and running (Fig. 1-51).[99] As seen in Fig. 1-51, *A*, the plate is subject to shear stress from points 1 and 2. However, since there is increased tension in the posterior cruciate ligament, the

STANCE

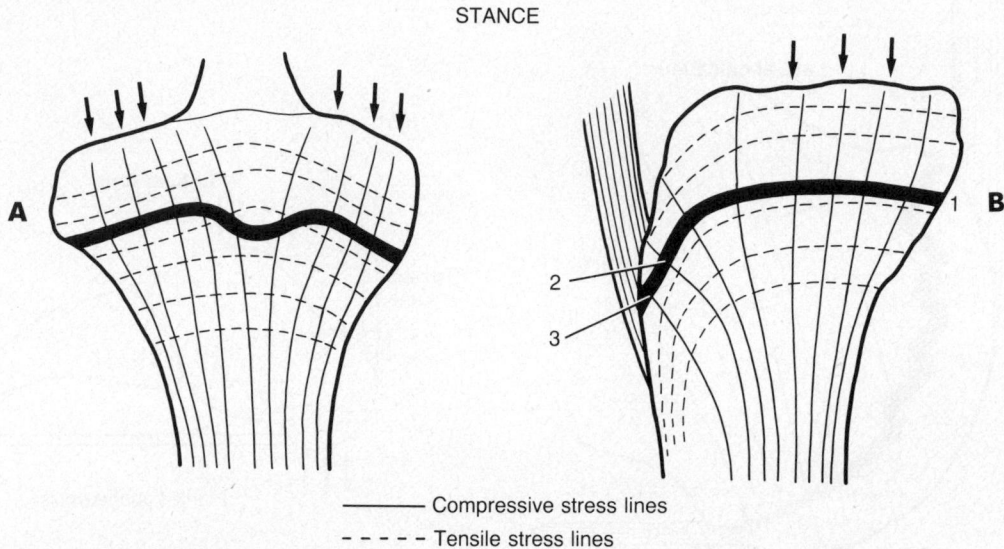

—————— Compressive stress lines

- - - - - Tensile stress lines

Fig. 1-50. Compressive and tensile stresses on the proximal tibia in relation to the epiphyseal plates during stance. **A,** Anterior view; **B,** lateral view. (Modified from Smith JW: J Anat 96:58, 1962.)

STANCE PHASE OF WALKING AND RUNNING

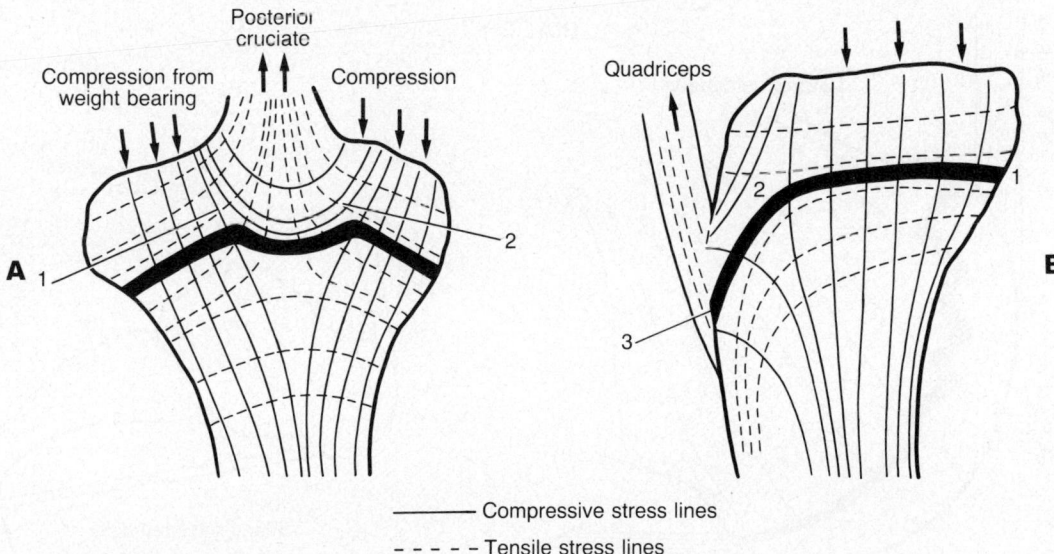

—————— Compressive stress lines

- - - - - Tensile stress lines

Fig. 1-51. The epiphyseal plate conforms more closely to the lines of compressive and tensile stress during stance phase of walking and running. **A,** Anterior view; **B,** lateral view. (Modified from Smith JW: J Anat 96:58, 1962.)

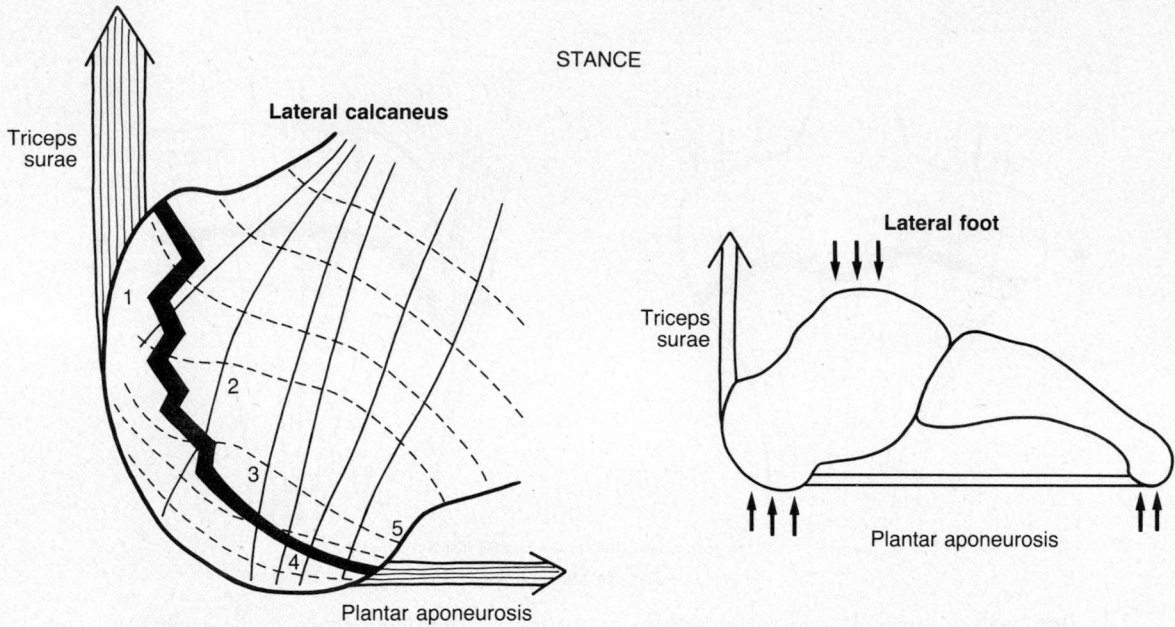

Fig. 1-52. Relationship of the epiphyseal plate of the calcaneus to the principal lines of tensile and compressive stress in stance. (Modified from Smith JW: J Anat 96:58, 1962.)

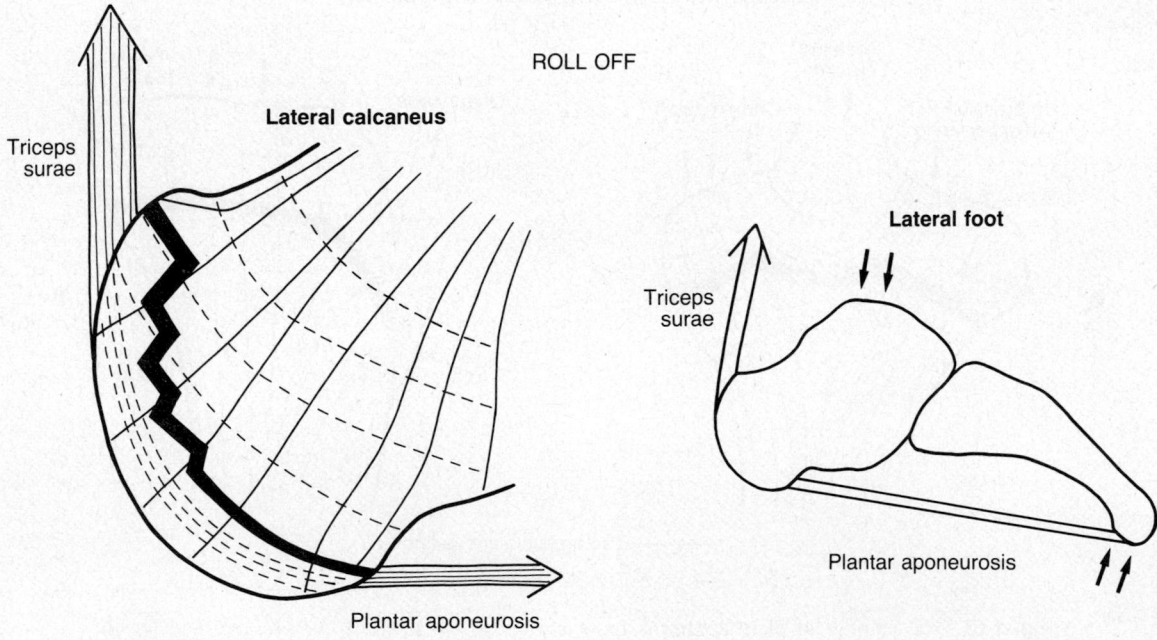

Fig. 1-53. The epiphyseal plate conforms more closely to the principal lines of tensile and compressive stress in the roll-off part of the gait cycle. (Modified from Smith JW: J Anat 96:58, 1962.)

central deflection of the plate adds to the stability of the epiphysis on the diaphysis. The fact that the central deflection exists suggests that the posterior cruciate ligament is significant in shaping the epiphyseal plate. The area of the plate from *B* to *C* in Fig. 1-53, *B,* still does not conform to the principal stress lines. However, the epiphyseal plate in that area is composed entirely of collagen fibers that are aligned with the principal tensile stresses and can transmit these tensile loads between the epiphysis and the diaphysis.

Foot

Orientation of the calcaneal epiphyseal plate occurs to accommodate maximal stress on the calcaneus (Fig. 1-51, 2 to 3). The plate of the calcaneus courses anteriorly on the inferior calcaneus and allows both the triceps surae tendon and the larger plantar muscles to gain attachment to the epiphysis.[99] The relationship of the plate to principal tensile and compressive stress lines in stance can be seen in Fig. 1-52. The general forces on the foot in stance or the early support phase of gait appear also in Fig. 1-52. The epiphyseal plate lies parallel alternately to the principal lines of compression, then tension, so that there is shear only at each bend point and not through most of the length (3 through 5) of the plate. This allows the plate to adapt to the growth requirements of the epiphysis. When compared during stance and roll off in gait (heel off to toe off) (Figs. 1-52 and 1-53), the plate corresponds to the principal stress lines in roll off. Roll off occurs when the forward motion of the body weight causes the longitudinal arch to flatten and plantar tissues to produce tension to stabilize the calcaneus.[99] In stance, the more vertically directed body weight vector produces an equal and opposite ground reaction force through the calcaneal tuberosities, and the plantar aponeurosis tightens to resist depression of the longitudinal arch. These stresses are not as great as in roll off. In stance, the compression lines are more vertical because of the vertically directed ground reaction vectors, whereas those in roll off in walking or push off in running are obliquely directed to align parallel to the ground reaction vectors accompanying these actions.

SUMMARY

Although the general shape of bone is genetically determined, bone itself is highly adaptable, depending on the types of stresses imposed upon it. Genetic considerations affect bone strength throughout life, in men differently than in women. It is hoped that future research will reveal an increased depth of knowledge as to those stimuli that will best strengthen normal bone tissue and those that will most efficiently and effectively help deformed or fractured bone approach or return to normal.

REFERENCES

1. Alexander RM and Bennet-Clark HC: Storage of elastic strain energy in muscles and other tissues, Nature 265:114, 1977.
2. Amtmann E: The distribution of breaking strength in the human femur shaft, J Biomech 1:271, 1968.
3. Amtmann E and Schmitt HP: The distribution of density in compact human femoral shaft bone and its significance for the determination of the breaking strength of bone, Z Anat Entwicklungsgesch 127:25, 1968 (English abstract).
4. Anderson JJB, Milin L, and Crackel WC: Effect of exercise on mineral and organic bone turnover in swine, J Appl Physiol 30:810, 1971.
5. Andrew EH: Fracture. In Vincent JFV and Currey JD, editors: Mechanical properties of biological materials, Symposia of the Society for Experimental Biology, Number XXXIV, Cambridge, England, 1980, Cambridge University Press.
6. Bassett CAL: Electrical effects in bone, Sci Am 213(4):18, 1965.
7. Bassett CAL and Pawlick RJ: Effects of electric currents on bone in vivo, Nature 204:652, 1964.
8. Becker RO and Murray DG: The electrical control system regulating fracture healing in amphibians, Clin Orthop 73:169, 1970.
9. Bjurholm A, et al: Innervation of bone tissue by sensory nerve fibers, Proceedings from the Orthopaedic Research Society, Trans Orthop Res Soc p 179, 1987.
10. Bloom W and Fawcett DW: A textbook of histology, Philadelphia, 1975, WB Saunders Co.
11. Booth FW and Gould EW: Effects of training and disuse on connective tissue, Exerc Sport Sci Rev p. 83, 1975.
12. Burr D, et al.: Bone remodeling to in vivo fatigue microdamage, J Biomech 18(3):189, 1985.
13. Burstein AH, Reilly DT, and Martens M: Aging of bone tissue, mechanical properties, J Bone Joint Surg 58A:82, 1976.
14. Burstein AH, et al: The ultimate properties of bone tissue: The effects of yielding, J Biomech 5:35, 1972.
15. Carter DR, Blenman PR, and Beaupre GS: Mechanical stress and vascular influences on fracture healing, Proceedings from the Orthopaedic Research Society, Trans Orthop Res Soc p 99, 1987.
16. Carter DR and Hayes WC: Fatigue life of compact bone. I. Effects of stress amplitude, temperature and density, J Biomech 9:27, 1976.
17. Carter DR and Hayes WC: Compact bone fatigue damage. II. A microscopic examination, Clin Orthop 127:265, 1977.
18. Carter DR and Hayes WC: Compact bone fatigue damage. I. Residual strength and stiffness, J Biomech 10:325, 1977.
19. Carter DR and Hayes WC: The compressive behavior of bone as a two-phase porous material, J Bone Joint Surg 59A:954, 1977.
20. Carter DR, Hayes WC, and Schurman DJ: Fatigue life of compact bone. II. Effects of microstructure and density, J Biomech 9:211, 1976.
21. Carter DR, Schwab GH, and Spengler DM: Tensile fracture of cancellous bone, Acta Orthop Scand 51:733, 1980.
22. Carter DR and Spengler DM: Mechanical properties and composition of cortical bone, Clin Orthop 135:192, 1978.
23. Carter DR, et al: The mechanical and biological response of cortical bone to in vivo strain histories. In Cowin SC, editor: Mechanical properties of bone, Joint ASME-ASCE Applied Mechanics, Fluids Engineering, and Bioengineering Conference, Boulder, Colo, June 1981.
24. Chalmers J and Ho KC: Geographical variations in senile osteoporosis, J Bone Joint Surg 52B:667, 1970.
25. Chamay A and Tschantz P: Mechanical influences in bone remodeling: Experimental research on Wolff's law, J Biomech 5:173, 1972.
26. Cheal EJ, et al: Stress analysis of compression plate fixation and its effects on long bone remodeling, J Biomech, 18(2):141, 1985.
27. Churches AE and Howlett CR: The response of mature cortical

bone to controlled time varying loading. In Cowin SC, editor: Mechanical properties of bone, Joint ASME-ASCE Applied Mechanics, Fluids Engineering, and Bioengineering Conference, Boulder, Colo, June 1981.

28. Crelin ES: Development of the musculoskeletal system, Clin Symp 33(1):1, 1981.
29. Currey JD: The adaptation of bones to stress, J Theor Biol 20:91, 1968.
30. Currey JD: The mechanical properties of bones, Clin Orthop 73:210, 1970.
31. Currey JD: The mechanical adaptation of bones, Princeton, NJ, 1976, Princeton University Press.
32. Currey JD: Properties of bone, cartilage, and synovial fluid. In Dowson D and Wright V, editors: Introduction to the biomechanics of joints and joint replacements, London, 1981, Mechanical Engineering Publications, Ltd.
33. Currey JD and Butler G: The mechanical properties of bone tissue in children, J Bone Joint Surg 57A:810, 1975.
34. Dalen N and Olsson KE: Bone mineral content and physical activity, Acta Orthop Scand 45:170, 1974.
35. Davies GJ, Wallace LA, and Malone T: Mechanisms of selected knee injuries, Phys Ther 60:1590, 1980.
36. Dietrick JE, Whedon G, and Shoor E: Effects of immobilization upon various metabolic and physiologic functions of normal men, Am J Med 4:3, 1948.
37. Evans FG: Mechanical properties of bone, Springfield, Ill, 1973, Charles C Thomas, Publisher.
38. Evans FG: Relations between torsion properties and histology of adult human compact bone, J Biomech 11(4):151, 1978.
39. Evans FG and LeBow M: Strength of human compact bone under repetitive loading, J Appl Physiol 10:127, 1957.
40. Evans FG and Vincentelli R: Relation of collagen fiber orientation to some mechanical properties of human cortical bone, J Biomech 2:63, 1969.
41. Frankel V and Nordin M: Basic biomechanics of the skeletal system, Philadelphia, 1980, Lea & Febiger.
42. Freeman MAR, Todd RD, and Pirie CJ: The role of fatigue in the pathogenesis of senile femoral neck fractures, J Bone Joint Surg 56B:698, 1974.
43. Frost HM: Bone remodeling and its relationship to metabolic bone diseases, Springfield, Ill, 1973, Charles C Thomas, Publisher.
44. Frost HM: The laws of bone structure, Springfield, Ill, 1973, Charles C Thomas, Publisher.
45. Frost HM: Orthopaedic biomechanics, vol 5, Springfield, Ill, 1973, Charles C Thomas, Publisher.
46. Fukada E: Mechanical deformation and electrical polarization in biological substances, Biorheology 5:199, 1968.
47. Fung YC: Mechanical properties of living tissues, New York, 1981, Springer-Verlag, Inc.
48. Garn SM: The earlier gain and later loss of cortical bone. In Nutritional perspective, Springfield, Ill, 1970, Charles C Thomas, Publisher.
49. Garn SM, et al: Continuing bone growth throughout life: A general phenomenon, Am J Physiol Anthropol 26:313, 1967.
50. Garnett ES, et al: A photon scattering technique for the measurement of absolute bone density in man, Radiology 106:209, 1973.
51. Ghista DN: Osteoarthromechanics, Washington, DC, 1982, Hemisphere Publishing Corp.
52. Goldstein SA, et al: Experimentally controlled trabecular bone remodeling: Effects of applied stress, Proceedings from the Orthopaedic Research Society, Trans Orthop Res Soc p 461, 1987.
53. Goodship AE, Lanyon LE, and McFie H: Functional adaptation of bone to increased stress, J Bone Joint Surg 61A:539, 1979.
54. Goodship AE, et al: The effect of different regimens of axial micromovement on the healing of experimental tibial fractures, Proceed-

ings from the Orthopaedic Research Society, Trans Orthop Res Soc p 98, 1987.
55. Gottesman T and Hashin Z: Analysis of viscoelastic behavior of bones on the basis of microstructure, J Biomech 13:89, 1980.
56. Harris B: The mechanical behaviour of composite materials. In Vincent JFV and Currey JD, editors: Mechanical properties of biological materials, Symposia of the Society for Experimental Biology, Number XXXIV, Cambridge, England, 1980, Cambridge University Press.
57. Hayes WC and Carter DR: Biomechanics of bone. In Simmons DJ and Klunin AS, editors: Skeletal research: An experimental approach, New York, 1979, Academic Press, Inc.
58. Hayes WC and Snyder B: Toward a quantitative formulation of Wolff's law in trabecular bone. In Corwin SC, editor: Mechanical properties of bone, Joint ASME-ASCE Applied Mechanics, Fluids Engineering, and Bioengineering Conference, Boulder, Colo, June 1981.
59. Hert J, Liskova M, and Landrgot B: Influence of the long-term, continuous bending on the bone, Folia Morphol 17:389, 1969.
60. Hert J, Sklenska A, and Liskova M: Reaction of bone to mechanical stimuli. V. Effect of intermittent stress on the rabbit tibia after resection of the peripheral nerves, Folia Morphol 19:378, 1971.
61. Hert J and Zalud J: Reaction of bone to mechanical stimuli. VI. Bioelectrical theory of functional adaptation of bone (in Czech), Acta Chir Orthop Traumatol Cech 38:280, 1971.
62. Hettinga DL: Normal joint structures and their reaction to injury, J Orth Sports Phys Ther 1(1):16, 1979.
63. Johnson KE: Histology: Microscopic anatomy and embryology, New York, 1982, John Wiley & Sons, Inc.
64. Jowsey J: Age changes in human bone, Clin Orthop 17:210, 1960.
65. Justus R and Luft JH: A mechanochemical hypothesis for bone remodeling induced by mechanical stress, Calcif Tissue Res 5:222, 1970.
66. Katz JL: The structure and biomechanics of bone. In Vinsant JFV and Currey JD, editors: Mechanical properties of biological materials, Symposia of the Society for Experimental Biology, Number XXXIV, Cambridge, England, 1980, Cambridge University Press.
67. Kiiskinen A: Physical training and connective tissue in young mice: Physical properties of Achilles tendons and long bones, Growth 41:123, 1979.
68. Kiiskinen A and Heikkinen E: Effects of physical training on the development and strength of tendons and bones in growing mice, Scand J Clin Lab Invest 29(suppl 123):20, 1972.
69. Kobayashi TK and Pedrini V: Proteoglycans: Collagen interactions in human costal cartilage, Biochim Biophys Acta 303:148, 1973.
70. Koch JC: The laws of bone architecture, Am J Anat 21:177, 1917.
71. Lanyon LE: The measurement and biological significance of bone strain in vivo. In Corwin SC, editor: Mechanical properties of bone, Joint ASME-ASCE Applied Mechanics, Fluids Engineering, and Bioengineering Conference, Boulder, Colo, June 1981.
72. Lester GE, et al.: Relationship between physical activity and bone density in Caucasian women: A 1- to 2-year follow-up, Proceedings from the Orthopaedic Research Society, Trans Orthop Res Soc p 464, 1987.
73. Liskova M and Hert J: Reaction of bone to mechanical stimuli. II. Periosteal and endosteal reaction of tibial diaphysis in rabbit to intermittent loading, Folia Morphol 19:301, 1971.
74. Mack PB, et al.: Bone demineralization of foot and hand of Gemini-Titan IV, V, and VII astronauts during orbital flight, AJR 100:503, 1967.
75. Martin RB and Atkinson PJ: Age and sex-related changes in the structure and strength of the human femoral shaft, J Biomech 10:223, 1977.
76. Martin RB and Burr DB: a hypothetical mechanism for the stimula-

tion of osteonal remodeling by fatigue damage, J Biomech 15(3):137, 1982.

77. Melick RA and Miller DR: Variations of tensile strength of human cortical bone with age, Clin Sci 30:243, 1966.
78. Moore K: The developing human, Philadelphia, 1977, WB Saunders Co.
79. Moore K: Clinically oriented anatomy, Baltimore, 1980, Williams & Wilkins.
80. Murray MP, Seireg A, and Scholz RC: Center of gravity, center of pressure, and supportive forces during human activities, J Appl Physiol 23:831, 1967.
81. Murray PDF: Bones, Cambridge, England, 1936, Cambridge University Press.
82. Negulesco J and Kossler T: Responses of articular and epiphyseal cartilage zones of developing avian radii to estrone treatment and a 2-G environment, Aviat Space Environ Med 49:489, 1978.
83. Oxnard CE: Tensile forces in skeletal structures, J Morphol 134:425, 1971.
84. Park JB: Biomaterials: An introduction, New York, 1979, Plenum Publishing Corp.
85. Pauwels F: Biomechanics of the locomotor apparatus, New York, 1980, Springer-Verlag, Inc.
86. Radin E, et al: Practical biomechanics for the orthopedic surgeon, New York, 1979, John Wiley & Sons, Inc.
87. Reilly DT and Burstein AH: The mechanical properties of cortical bone, J Bone Joint Surg 56A:1001, 1974.
88. Robinson RA: Bone tissue: Composition and function, Johns Hopkins Med J 145(1):10, 1979.
89. Rodahl K, Nicholson JT, and Brown EM, editors: Bone as a tissue, New York, 1960, McGraw-Hill Book Co.
90. Roesler H: Some historical remarks on the theory of cancellous bone structure (Wolff's law). In Cowin SC, editor: Mechanical properties of bone, Joint ASME-ASCE Applied Mechanics, Fluids Engineering, and Bioengineering Conference, Boulder, Colo, June 1981.
91. Ruff CB and Hayes WC: Changes with age in cortical bone geometry and mineral mass in the human lower limb, Trans Orthop Res Soc 7:320, 1982.
92. Ruff CB and Hayes WC: Subperiosteal expansion and cortical remodeling of human femur and tibia with aging, Science 217:945, 1982.
93. Rybicki EF, Simonen FA, and Weis EB, Jr: On the mathematical analysis of stress in the human femur, J Biomech 5:203, 1972.
94. Salter RB: Textbook of disorders and injuries of the musculoskeletal system: An introduction to orthopaedics, rheumatology, metabolic bone disease, rehabilitation, and fractures, Baltimore, 1970, Williams & Wilkins.
95. Saville PD and Smith R: Bone density, breaking force, and leg muscle mass as functions of weight in bipedal rats, Am J Phys Anthropol 25:35, 1966.
96. Saville PD and Whyte MP: Muscle and bone hypertrophy, Clin Orthop 65:81, 1969.
97. Silver P: Personal communication (course in biomechanics and biomaterials), Boston, Spring 1981, Boston University.
98. Singh I: The architecture of cancellous bone, J Anat 127:305, 1978.
99. Smith JW: The relationship of epiphyseal plates to stress in some bones of the lower limb, J Anat 96:58, 1962.
100. Smith RW and Walker RR: Femoral expansion in aging in women: Implications for osteoporosis and fractures, Science 145:156, 1964.
101. Symeonides PP: High stress fractures of the fibula, J Bone Joint Surg 62B:192, 1980.
102. Tipton CM, Matthes R, and Maynard J: Influence of chronic exercise on rat bones, Med Sci Sports Exerc 4:55, 1972.
103. Torzilli PA, et al.: The material and structural properties of maturing bone. In Cowin SC, editor: Mechanical properties of bone, Joint ASME-ASCE Applied Mechanics, Fluids Engineering, and Bioengineering Conference, Boulder, Colo, June 1981.
104. Vose GP, Stover BJ, and Mack PB: Quantitative bone strength measurements in senile osteoporosis, J Gerontol 16:120, 1961.
105. Wainwright SA, et al.: Mechanical design in organisms, Princeton, NJ, 1976, Princeton University Press.
106. Wall JC, Chatterji SK, and Jeffrey JW: The influence that bone density and orientation and particle size of the mineral phase have on the mechanical properties of bone, J Bioenerg Biomembr 2:517, 1978.
107. Warwick R and Williams P, editors: Gray's anatomy, ed 35, Philadelphia, 1973, WB Saunders Co.
108. Weiss PA: Cellular dynamics, Rev Mod Phys 31:11, 1959.
109. Werntz JR, et al.: The osteogenic potential of bone marrow to heal segmental long bone defects, Proceedings from the Orthopaedic Research Society, Trans Orthop Res Soc p 441, 1987.
110. Whalen RT, Carter DR, and Steele CR: The relationship between physical activity and bone density, Proceedings from the Orthopaedic Research Society, Trans Orthop Res Soc p 463, 1987.
111. Winter DA: Biomechanics of human movement, New York, 1979, John Wiley & Sons, Inc.
112. Woo SL-Y: The relationships of changes in stress levels on long bone remodeling. In Cowin SC, editor: Mechanical properties of bone, Joint ASME-ASCE Applied Mechanics, Fluids Engineering, and Bioengineering Conference, Boulder, Colo, June 1981.
113. Woo SL-Y, et al.: Effect of prolonged physical training on properties of long bone: A study of Wolff's law, J Bone Joint Surg 63A:780, 1981.
114. Wunder C: Femur-bending properties as influenced by gravity: Sex-related weakness after 4-G mouse growth, Aviat Space Environ Med 48:1023, 1977.
115. Yamada H: In Evans FG, editor: Strength of biological materials, Baltimore, 1970, Williams & Wilkins.

Chapter 2

AFFERENT NEUROBIOLOGY OF THE JOINT

Mark J. Rowinski

Man, in contradistinction to lower forms of life, relies for his existence upon an integration of systems from within and without. Man reacts to his environment to bring about alteration of body movements and function by using a receptor system to stimulate response. The excitation of the receptors of the proprio-ceptive field, in contradistinction from those of the extero-ceptive field, is related only secondarily to the agencies of the environment. Proprioceptive receptors receive their stimulation from some action, e.g., a muscular contraction, which was itself a primary reaction to excitation of a surface receptor by the environment. The primary reaction is excited in the majority of cases by a receptor of the extero field, that field so rich in the number and variety of its receptors. Reflexes arising from proprioceptive-organs come therefore to be habitually attached and appended to certain reflexes excited by extero organs. The reaction of the animal to stimulation of one of its extero-ceptors excites certain tissues, and the activity thus produced in these latter tissues excites in them their receptors, which are the proprioceptive-receptors. Thus, in a muscular movement induced by a stimulus to the skin of the spinal dog, the change in form and tension of muscles, and the movements of the joints, etc., excite the receptors in these structures, and these in turn initiate a reflex in their own arcs, and their reaction often has an "allied" relation to the reflex reaction excited from the skin.

C.S. Sherrington, 1906[72]

Having tentatively differentiated ourselves from other organisms on the basis of intellectual adroitness, manipulative capabilities, and technological flexibility, we humans view our own skeletomuscular system in fair likeness to our bipedal and even quadripedal mammalian relatives. We claim equality to our wild vertebrate relatives in the realm of perfection of locomotive skills but find ourselves continually seeking to extend the "limits" of human locomotive performance. In actuality, the real limitations on motor skill performance are set by the anatomical and physiological constraints of the systems involved—the skeletal, muscular, and nervous systems. The biomechanical structures of the skeleton, joints, and muscles seem universally fashioned to optimally meet the organisms' needs for maintaining stability and producing motility. The structural specialization of the joint provides for the interdependent requirements of rigid stability, shock absorption, and adaptable mobility, which are specific for survival of the species. It has been stated that "the joints are adapted to the range of motion that is required of them in the characteristic activities of any particular animal form."[81]

In seeking to understand the limitations of biomechanical function, scientific analyses have included invasive anatomical and physiological studies of tissue components and functional relations underlying freedom of action in some of our mammalian relatives. These highly controlled experimental efforts have yielded great insight into many features of normal and abnormal joint structure and function, and attempts have been made to relate these studies to the human arthroarchitecture. In addition, psychophysical studies of human position sense under normal and pathological conditions have contributed much information regarding cognitive functions related to joint activity in the human. Findings from gross morphological and detailed histological examinations of cadaver or amputated human articular structures have been done and detailed neuronal interrelations ascertained.

Articular tissues are endowed by the nervous system with a direct afferent innervation; that is, information about the degree of mechanical distortion of the articular structures is sent toward the central nervous system (CNS) through this innervation primarily to alert central neuron populations of current mechanical conditions. Such joint neural information contributes to *proprioception,* a term introduced by Sherrington[72] to describe all neural inputs originating from the joints, muscles, tendons, and associated deep tissues. Sherrington's explanation does not imply that this neural information relates to conscious perception, but only that the CNS conveys information from these tissues. The afferent information from the joint is therefore projected to central processing centers in the brain for some nonperceptual reflex and motor control mechanisms, as well as for some limited perceptual sensory activities. The status of articular tissues is conveyed in neural impulse code to many levels of the CNS so that information regarding static or dynamic conditions, equilibrium or disequilibrium, or biomechanical stress/strain relations may be ascertained. This information can influence muscle tone, motor execution programs, and cognitive somatic perceptions.

Precise knowledge of the relationships between afferent neural signaling capacity, central neuronal response functions, articular morphology and action, and skeletomuscular mechanical function is required for an understanding of the structural adaptation of the joint in all its functional and pathological implications. In recent years, an explosion of investigative efforts in the neural sciences has led to revisions in many of our long-held, empirically derived beliefs regarding innervation of the joint and its role in biomechanical pathology. Furthermore, within the last 10 years, since an excellent review of the subject by Skoglund,[74] there has been a major revision in the commonly held view of the importance of joint versus muscular innervation with regard to kinesthesia and static position sense. This chapter explains recent advances in scientific investigation regarding the neurobiology of the joints, building on other previous reviews of the subject.[7,10,58,74,75]

This chapter includes a description of the filtering and segregating mechanism related to joint tissue distortion that occurs at the primary afferent receptor level and an explanation of how this information is conveyed to the CNS. Reference is also made to the extent to which the human consciousness uses this information and the clinical relevance of this analysis regarding normal and abnormal joint action. Knowledge of articular neurology is of prime importance in physical therapy in order to guide voluntary and preprogrammed motor activity associated with motor skills, the reflexive modulation of muscle tone, the sequential activation and coordination of synergistic and antagonistic muscle groups, and some limited features of somatic sensation and perception.

GENERAL ORGANIZATION AND PHYSIOLOGY

The joint, or arthron, contains bone, cartilaginous inserts, and all the soft tissue structures between the rigid skeletal components and the adjacent pertinent muscular elements. Much of the early study of joint function has been reviewed in depth by Gardner,[26] who included a review of the initial studies on joint innervation.

The highly innervated soft tissues of the synovial joints include the fibrous and subsynovial capsule, the extrinsic and intrinsic ligaments, and the articular fat pads. Cartilaginous components of the joint—such as the disks, menisci, and articular hyaline cartilage that covers the articular facets of the bone—are commonly believed not to be innervated.[45] Earlier studies in the literature suggested that the outer edge of the meniscal tissue received direct innervation.[59,82] However, it now appears that only the immediately adjacent perimeniscal capsular tissue received direct innervation.[45] There is also some disagreement in the literature regarding the afferent innervation of the synovial membrane. One group of investigators denies its existence,[18,25,83] whereas other studies[31,45] and practical clinical considerations attest to its importance in contributing to neural information emanating from the joint. It is known that subchondral bone is well innervated,[55,64] but whether articular activity excites nerve endings at this site is unclear.

The nerve supply to most appendicular joints occurs by way of specific articular nerves that proceed to the joint capsule region as independent branches of larger peripheral nerves and also by way of nonspecific articular branches of related muscle nerves that reach the joint by traversing the muscles and interfascicular connective tissue.[83] Some joints may also receive articular "twigs" from cutaneous and periosteal nerve branches.[63] The vertebral joints likewise appear to receive a dual innervation, with the primary innervation occurring via the posterior rami of the segmental nerves and an accessory innervation supplied by branches of nerves to the deep paravertebral muscles.[76,86]

An example of the degree of spatial organization inherent in multiinnervated joints has recently been provided by Kennedy, Alexander, and Hayes[45] for the human knee joint. Their study consistently found that the knee was innervated by a posterior group of nerves (the posterior articular and obturator nerves) and by an anterior group (the articular branches of the femoral, common peroneal, and saphenous nerves). Each of the constituent nerves appears to have a particular spatial territory and, in some instances, the territory includes diverse periarticular tissues, such as the capsule and ligaments. Each nerve should therefore be considered multimodal and territorially specific. Nerve damage would necessarily result in spatially specific deficits across several information channels emanating from a particular joint. This model serves as a guide to the multiple sources of innervation of a specific joint and is an excellent source of information for the orthopaedic surgeon and therapist whenever procedures affecting periarticular innervation are considered.

Generalized duality of innervation suggests that primary and accessory nerves to the joint may have different compositions and functional roles. It is therefore difficult to draw general conclusions about joint innervation based on a limited sampling of information transmitted via primary joint nerves or muscle nerves alone, without attending to the distinction between muscular versus joint-originated signals. Such a caution, however, has not been heeded in many of the research endeavors in the past.

Embedded in the connective tissue of the joint are mechanoreceptors or specialized neuroepithelial cell aggregates that transduce the mechanical distortion of the tissues into electrical activity belonging to the neural element of the receptor complex. Since these receptors are specifically sensitive to changes originating in tissue rather than changes in external energies, they are appropriately categorized as proprioceptors. As mentioned previously, input from the receptors in itself does not imply that receptors participate in conscious appreciation of body sense. The typical mechanoreceptor ending is surrounded by specialized epithelial cells that are responsible for many of the response properties of the receptor complex.[4] However, some free nerve endings are not intimately "encapsulated" by epithelial cells, and these are believed to be either mechanically or chemically sensitive.

The intensity of mechanical distortion of the receptor ending or the concentration of the specific excitatory chemical agent—coupled with such factors as the (1) previous history of such stimulation, (2) adaptability of surrounding tissues to distortion,[12] and (3) specific sensitivity of the receptor ending itself—determines the amount of electrical change across the membrane of the receptor ending.

Thus distortion of the periarticular tissue triggers a change on the membrane of the specialized receptor ending whose amplitude has been modulated by the above listed factors. The potential change is referred to as the *receptor,* or *generator;* potential of the ending. As of this date, no recordings of isolated joint receptor potentials have been reported, but it must be assumed that the mechanism of receptor potential generation does not differ significantly from the basic mechanisms occurring in similarly configured somatosensory receptors in other body tissues.[71] The gradual receptor potential change then excites the axonal portion of the peripheral afferent neuron, eliciting a barrage of impulses in the parent axon (i.e., the primary afferent fiber). The rate of impulse production, termed the *discharge rate,* or *response frequency,* is mathematically related to the absolute amplitude of the generator potential, which in turn is directly proportional to the intensity of stimulation. The manner in which the afferent fiber's discharge rate is related to the overt activity of the joint is what determines the fiber's response type and serves as a convenient classification method of the receptor/primary afferent fiber complex.

Specific primary afferent units have been distinguished through recent correlations of receptor structure and parent axon response type (Fig. 2-1 and Table 2-1). Anatomical classification according to general receptor morphology therefore should be used provisionally along with fiber response type to specify the innervation of discrete joint regions or specific tissue components. It is important to realize that classification of receptor/fiber morphology and physiology involves a simplification and reductionistic approach, which all too often ignores fine gradations in unit typology that have been elucidated by previous detailed study.[63]

The articular soft tissues not only biomechanically stabilize the bony structures of the joint, but also the tissues. The extensive afferent nerve supply of articular soft tissues serves as a valuable and highly specific information source upon which tissue property modification can be based.

JOINT RECEPTORS

Summaries of the types of neural receptors invested in periarticular tissues are available in the literature.[7,74,83] Most of the early studies that contributed to these reviews were based on indirect correlations between structure and function. More recent neurophysiological recording techniques, involving single, peripheral afferent axon isolation, have greatly clarified the concept of joint innervation and its purpose. Such microphysiological and histological scrutiny of the stimulated tissue has yielded important information on the specificity of the neural code, which arises from the periphery.

The periarticular receptors are subject to distortion by mechanical forces associated with soft tissue elongation, relaxation, compression, and fluid tension changes. Each type of nerve ending serves as a selective filter for a specific kind of stimulus energy and grades its activity within that energy spectrum according to the intensity of soft tissue distortion. The micromechanical status of the joint must be rapidly and accurately conveyed to the CNS so that such information (1) can influence the activity of those

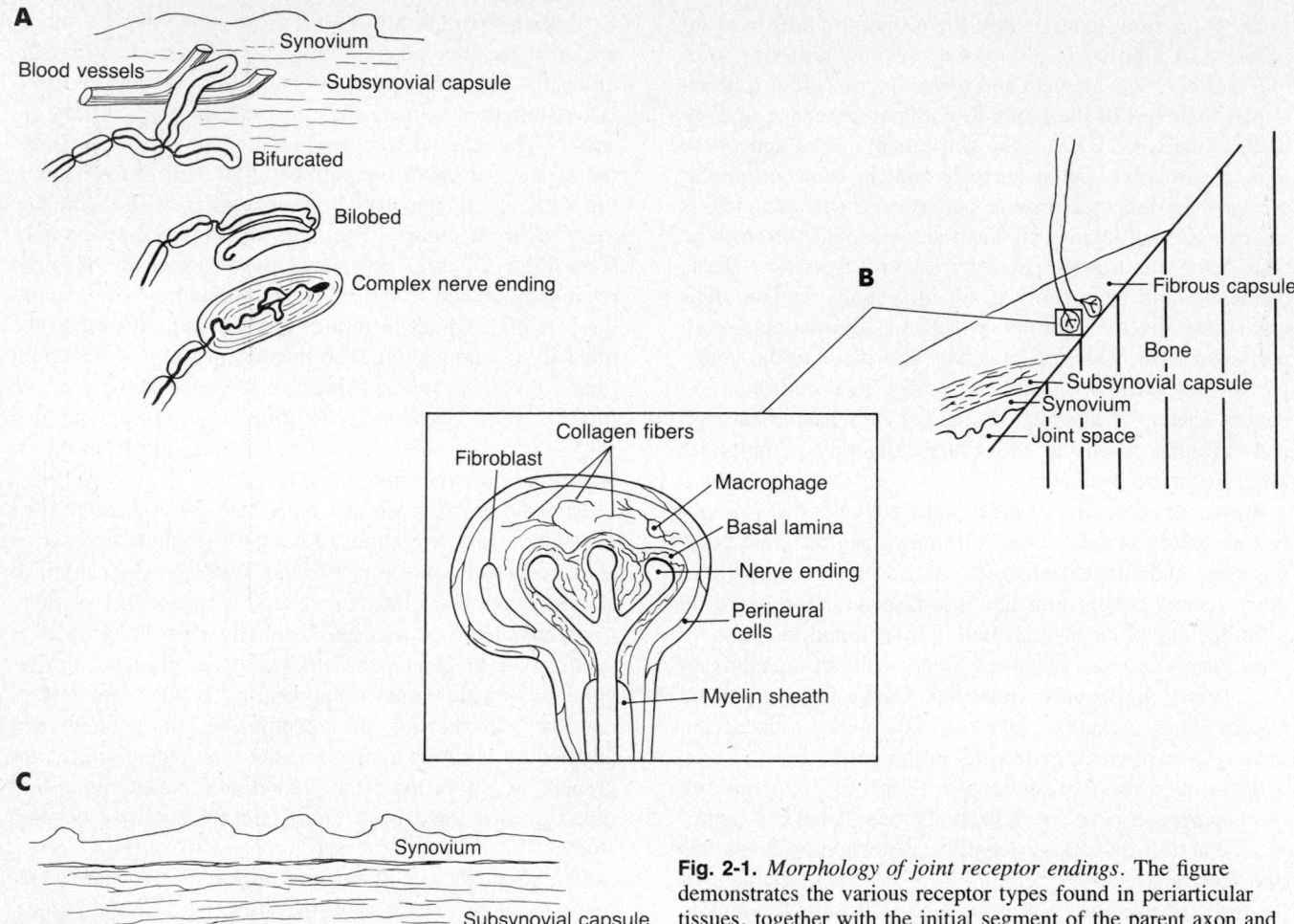

Fig. 2-1. *Morphology of joint receptor endings.* The figure demonstrates the various receptor types found in periarticular tissues, together with the initial segment of the parent axon and the typical ending cluster pattern: **A,** pacinian corpuscle; **B,** Golgi-Mazzoni corpuscle; **C,** Ruffini endings; **D,** Golgi ligament ending; **E,** free nerve endings (noxious and nonnoxious); **F,** composite diagram of total joint innervation pattern, showing interrelations of afferent receptors. The sources of information on which the figure is based are presented in Table 2-1.

motor units that regulate the joint aperture, position, and angulation; (2) can influence upper motor neurons that govern the patterns and coordination of muscle activity at the joint; and (3) can influence the activity of those neural pathways that mediate perceptions associated with awareness of joint condition.

Functionally, this neural information protects the joint from damage by movement beyond its normal physiological range, (2) determines the appropriate balance of synergistic and antagonistic forces (i.e., muscular action necessary for voluntary smooth joint movement), and (3) participates with other proprioceptive afferent receptors from the tendons and muscles to generate a somatosensory image within the CNS. Most joint afferent receptors are active only near the end range of motion and thus probably only contribute to reflexive and motor control mechanisms of body movement and position, that is, a type of self "end feel."[10]

Table 2-1 incorporates the most recent findings available in the literature on receptor and primary afferent fiber functional relations and attempts to consolidate these data with previously presented classification schemes. Most of the properties of a receptor type are determined by assuming that the receptor is linked to a given primary afferent fiber and that response characteristics are learned from experimental invasive studies of the fiber's response to controlled mechanical stimulation of its assumed receptor ending. For this reason, most of the discussion of functional

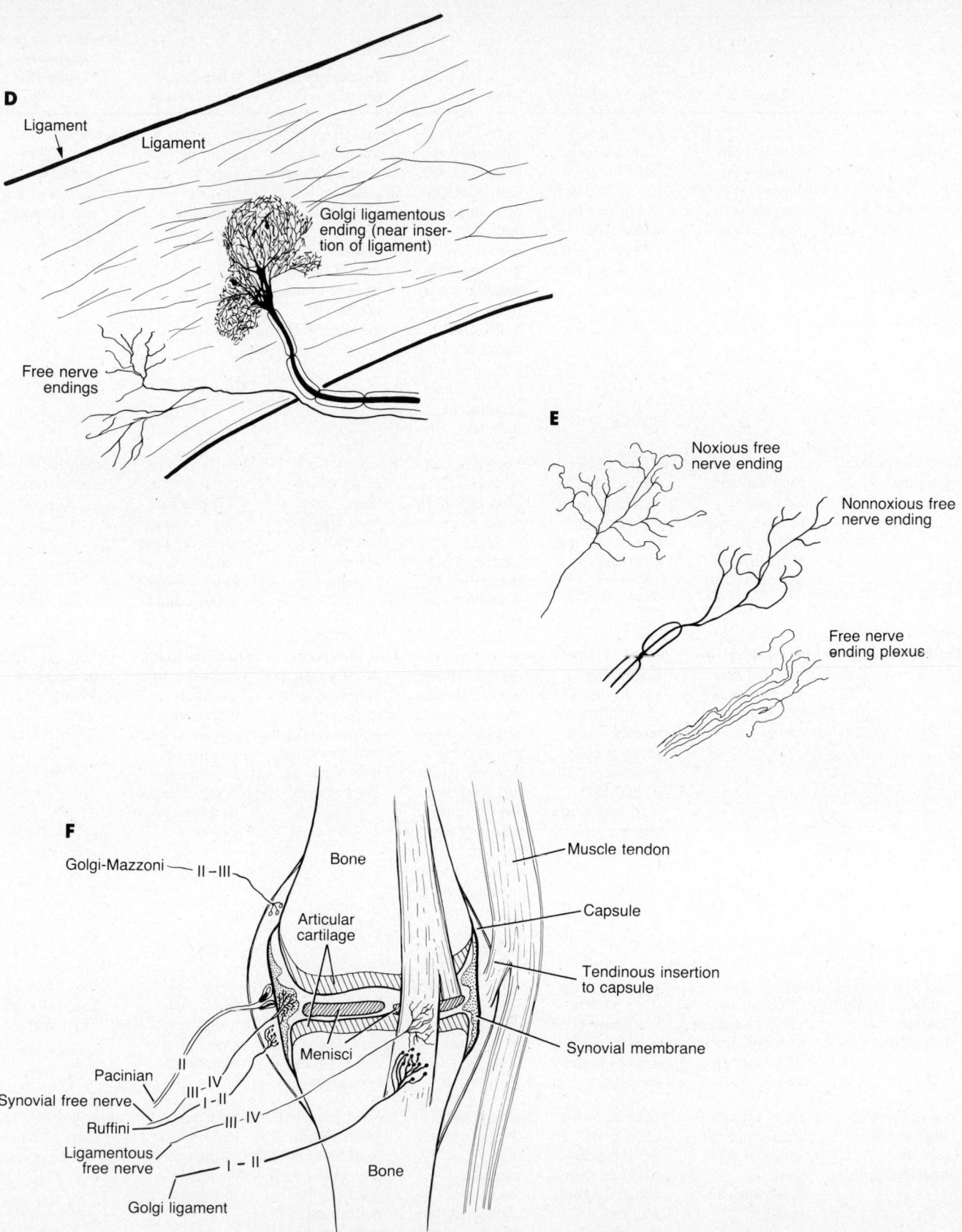

Fig. 2-1, cont'd. For legend see opposite page.

Table 2-1. Joint receptors

Receptor	Location	Description	Sensitivity	Distribution (of receptor type)	Functional classification	Parent axon (fiber diameter, conduction velocity)
Pacinian corpuscles	Fibrous layer of capsule, on capsule-synovium border, close to small blood vessels	Single terminal within lamellated encapsulation; appears in clusters of five or less (20-40 × 150-250 μm cylindrical)	Sensitive to high-frequency vibration (> 60 Hz), acceleration, and high-velocity changes in joint position; possible sensitivity to hemohydraulic, transient events and rapid contractile events of adjacent muscles	Found in all joints examined; sole corpuscular receptor in laryngeal and middle ear joints; greater density in distal than in proximal joints	Very rapidly adapting (RA); very low mechanical threshold	Group II (8-12 μM, 49 ms); terminal branch at 3-5 μm diameter
Golgi-Mazzoni corpuscles	Inner surface of joint capsule between fibrous layer and subcapsular fibroadipose tissue	Multiple terminating endings within thin encapsulation (30 × 200 μm cylindrical)	Sensitive to compression of joint capsule in plane perpendicular to its inner surface; insensitive to stretching capsule	Knee joint and many others likely; may have specific distribution within joint capsule	Slowly adapting (SA); response is linear function of compressive stress on capsule; low mechanical threshold	Group II-III (5-8 μm; estimate ≈ 30 ms)
Ruffini endings	Fibrous layer of capsule; few present in extrinsic ligaments	Spray-type terminal endings within thin encapsulation, having investment of collagen fibers (300 × 300-800 μm, two to six endings per axon)	Sensitive to capsule stretching along either of its long axes within capsular plane, direction and speed of capsular stretch, intracapsular fluid pressure change, amplitude and velocity of joint-position change	Few present in distal joints; greater density in proximal joints; concentrated in capsular regions of most stress	Slowly adapting (SA); low mechanical threshold; response is linear function of axial components of capsular plane stress	Group I-II (13-17 or 8-12 μm, 51 ms)
Golgi ligament endings (Golgi tendon organlike)	Extrinsic and intrinsic ligaments; adjacent to bony attachments of ligaments	Thick encapsulation, profuse branching (100 × 600 μm total terminal spread)	Sensitive to tension or stretch on ligaments	Present in most joints except cervical vertebral, laryngeal, and ossicular ligaments	Slowly adapting (SA); low-to-high mechanical threshold	Group I (13-17 μm; estimate ≈ 51 ms)
Free nerve endings (nociceptive and nonnociceptive)	Fibrous capsule, ligaments, subsynovial capsule, synovium, fat pads	Thin, bare nerve endings of small myelinated or unmyelinated axons; profuse branching	One type sensitive to nonnoxious mechanical stress; other type sensitive to noxious mechanical or biochemical stimuli	Present in all joints examined but density varies with joint component; most joints have relatively higher density in ligaments	Slowly adapting (SA); low-to-high mechanical threshold	Group III-IV (2-5 μm, < 2 μm; 2.5-20 ms)

Based on data from references 2, 5, 6, 13, 25, 30, 37-40, 56, 63, 69, 70, and 88.

response properties is included in the following section on primary afferent fibers. Further clarification of the morphological appearance of joint receptors is provided in Fig. 2-1.

Several points regarding the localization of specific receptor types should be emphasized. First, Kennedy, Alexander, and Hayes[45] have recently traced free nerve endings into the synovial membrane of the human knee joint. These nerve endings are different from those innervating adjacent fat pads, capsular tissue, or intrinsic ligaments of the joint. The same study also emphasizes that meniscal tissue is not innervated as previously believed,[82] but is surrounded by highly innervated perimeniscal tissue. A previous study of the cat has also confirmed the presence of fine nerve endings in the inner layer of the capsule, adjacent synovial tissue, adventitia of the large blood vessels, and arteriolar tissue.[68]

Other studies provide adequate evidence for the existence of highly sensitive vibratory receptors—pacinian corpuscles—in close association with the blood vessels supplying the synovial membrane.[40] The receptors reside at the synovial-capsular border in the stratum synovium of the capsule. The exquisite mechanosensitivity of the pacinian receptors makes it very likely that they would discharge in response to rapid perturbations of the synovium and possibly to its perfusion pressure pulse under appropriate hydraulic conditions. This latter hypothesis, however, should not be taken as support of Grieve's suggestion[34] that the pacinian afferent receptors may subserve the function of throbbing joint pain, since a previous study[62] implicates pacinian afferent receptors in quite the opposite role of pain suppression. Detailed histological examination of the synovium reveals that it is highly vascularized, penetrated by lymphatic vessels, populated with adipocytes, and intimately bound to the subsynovial connective tissue and capsule.[4] It is therefore most probable that synovial mechanical distortion activates subsynovial mechanoreceptors as well. Thus the synovial membrane may be considered an important contributor to the arthroneural-dependent behavior of the organism, and its dysfunction or removal may affect neural function of the joint.

A second point to be highlighted is that identification of the receptor type present in a joint region is not sufficient of itself to determine the neural information content contributed by that tissue. In other words, conclusions about structural and functional relations of joint innervation may be ambiguous if based only on information derived from histological examination of receptor density and typology. Physiological study must accompany histological identification. Two major findings support this contention. Grigg, Hoffman, and Fogarty[38] have determined that the Golgi-Mazzoni corpuscle, which resembles the rapidly adapting (RA) pacinian corpuscle in morphology, gives rise to a slowly adapting (SA) response (Fig. 2-2) when transcapsular compression forces are applied. This receptor type is virtually the only receptor type found on the anteromedial aspect of the cat knee capsule just anterior to the medial collateral ligament.[28] Many previous histological analyses of receptors in this region, which had not examined the exact physiological properties of the fibers innervating these receptors, may have actually attributed pacinian-like RA characteristics to these slowly adapting structures.[25,58] As a result, the responsiveness of this tissue to sustained compressive forces was largely ignored.

A further recent advance in our understanding of the relationship of structure and function in joint innervation comes from the work of Schaible and Schmidt,[69,70] who have studied small-diameter axons of articular nerves. These experiments have demonstrated that at least some of the previously assumed noxious stimulus detectors associated with small-diameter fibers[58,84,85] are actually fairly sensitive nonnoxious mechanoreceptors. In other words, not all free nerve endings in joint tissue are nociceptive, and some may actually be among the most sensitive mechanoreceptors of the joint. This situation is similar to the fact that the quality of light touch is mediated by some of the free nerve endings of cutaneous tissue. Thus recent high-resolution experimental studies reveal that many of the classical assumptions about joint receptor function may have been overly generalized. Furthermore, the complexity and diversity of articular receptors match those reported for cutaneous mechanoreceptors.[2,13,39]

PRIMARY AFFERENT FIBERS: STIMULUS-RESPONSE RELATIONSHIPS

The mechanoelectrical transduction events taking place at the receptor level can be translated into the discharge rate of the primary afferent fibers. The activity of one fiber in isolation provides information about the mechanical events occurring in a very limited and discrete region of the joint, whereas the activity pattern of many afferent fibers describes the action of the joint as a whole. In other words, a single afferent fiber can signal to the CNS only what specific joint is moving and a very small bit of information about the distortion of a small portion of periarticular tissue of that joint. Some examples of the diverse response types characteristic of various articular afferent fibers as they relate to standard joint excursions are presented in Fig. 2-2. The figure demonstrates how different ranges of joint excursion can shift the neuron population response pattern by shifting into the sensitivity ranges of different types of receptors.

Rossi and Grigg[65] have recently described a model for activation of capsular afferent receptors. In the hip joint, certain afferent receptors discharge only when the joint is rotated in a specific plan. The type of excursion that activates joint afferent receptors and their corresponding afferent fibers is determined by three factors: (1) the location of the receptors in the capsule, (2) the geometry of the joint, and (3) the geometry of the capsule.

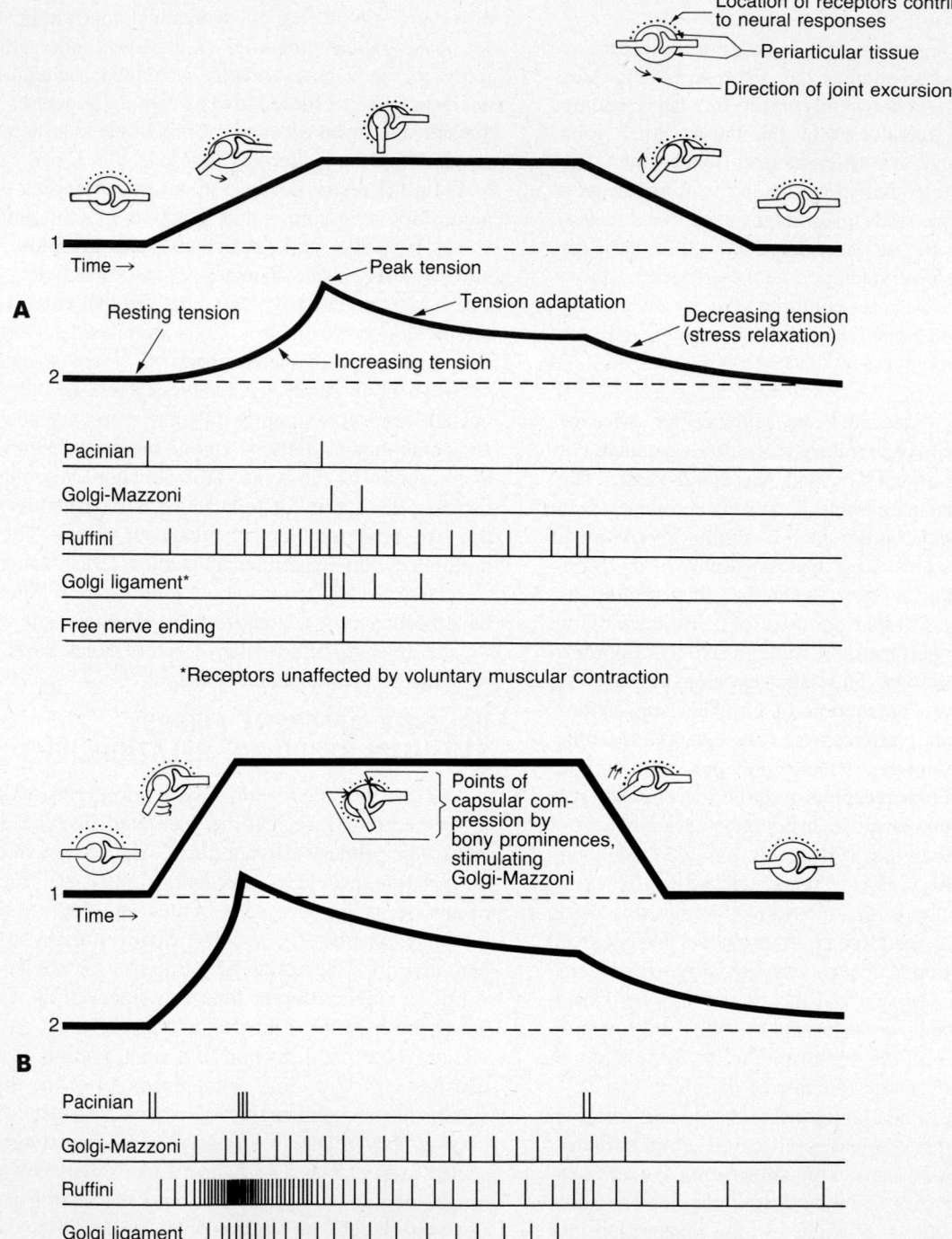

Fig. 2-2. *Physiological response types of various joint afferent fibers.* **A,** Typical responses of afferent fibers to moderate stimulation of the periarticular tissue. Excursion of joint is indicated by trace *1,* presumed tension generation in periarticular tissues by trace *2,* and neural responses by traces marked with appropriate afferent type. **B,** Same as **A** with the exception that more intense and rapid stimulus is applied to the joint.

For the hip, the most important movements appear to be internal/external rotation, which activates receptors of the posterior and anterior capsule, and abduction/adduction, which activates receptors of the inferior and superior portions of the capsule. Very few (2%) capsular receptors were found to be excited by flexion/extension of the hip. The study concluded that a joint's axis of rotation is signaled by the subpopulation of afferent fibers excited, whereas the extent of joint movement or excursion is signaled by the frequency of afferent fiber discharge. Capsular afferent fibers were generally not found to be active in neutral or intermediate limb positions.

Fiber spectrum

It has been reported that afferent fibers alone, among all of the traditionally defined afferent categories, innervate the periarticular tissues; that is, the fiber spectrum of joint innervation includes all fibers from the large group I myelinated range, the intermediate-diameter fibers, and the smallest unmyelinated group IV fibers. In Table 2-1 the fiber diameters and corresponding fiber classes are provided in relation to the receptors and tissues receiving the fibers.

Receptive fields

The area of the joint capsule, ligament, or other periarticular tissue whose mechanical distortion leads to excitation of a given joint afferent fiber is known as the *receptive field* (RF) of that afferent fiber. Recently, estimates of the size of articular afferent receptive fields have appeared in the literature. It has been determined that RFs of small-diameter fibers in groups III and IV are on the order of 25 mm^2, whereas larger diameter afferent fibers in group II may have smaller RFs or quite large RFs, ranging up to 100 mm.^{2}

The existence of joint afferent fibers with multiple RFs has recently been demonstrated by Schaible and Schmidt.[69] It is therefore possible that several receptor endings lying in spatially separate portions of a subregion of the joint capsule may be connected to one and the same parent afferent fiber. Alternatively, there may be regions of capsular heterogeneity that would contribute to differential sensitivity foci in a spatially compact receptor ending. The latter possibility may relate to posttraumatic periarticular receptor mechanisms, since scar tissue formation may be expected to cause significant distortion in the normal RF distribution of many joint primary afferent fibers.

Traditionally, it has been the custom to refer to the RF of a given joint afferent fiber in terms of the range of motion or joint excursion through which the afferent fiber is excited. For example, a given knee joint afferent fiber may begin to discharge only at 70 degrees of flexion and may increase its discharge rate up to a maximum of 135 degrees at the end of the range of joint flexion. The excursion RF of the neuron would therefore be considered to be 70 to 135 degrees, and the unit would be referred to as a *flexion-related unit* and would be assumed to have its receptor ending located on the anterior aspect of the knee joint capsule. This type of categorization of joint innervation fields is perhaps more clinically useful than focal definition of the afferent RF (in terms of the area of joint capsule, ligament, or other periarticular tissue), but the spatial RF should not be totally ignored, especially in cases of spatially specific joint trauma. The clinician must be well aware that individual or small populations of joint afferent neurons are activated by mechanical events in only a specific locus of the joint tissue, that this locus determines the range of motion or static posture through which the afferent fiber will be active, and that a peak sensitivity of the unit or neuron population occurs somewhere within that range of motion.

Force sensitivity

The sensitivity of joint mechanoreceptors to tissue tension is within the same range as has been demonstrated for other force-transducing receptors of the somatosensory system. Controlled mechanical stretching of capsular tissue in various planes has been used recently to ascertain the sensitivity of joint afferent fibers.

Force-pressure or tissue-tension mechanical thresholds of activation have been determined for afferent fibers of medium conduction velocity originating from the Golgi-Mazzoni receptors of the medial knee capsule in the cat.[38] Thresholds range from 1.5 to 25 gm/mm^2 (6.4 gm/mm^2, mean) for these afferent fibers when radially oriented (compressive) stress is applied to mimic normal capsular activation conditions. Ruffini receptor endings have been investigated in other studies[37] and have been found to be much more sensitive. Thresholds can be detected with axially or longitudinally oriented loads applied to the capsule and range from 0.13 to 6.3 gm/mm^2 (0.2 to 0.3 gm/mm^2, mode).

Mechanical thresholds have also been determined for less sensitive afferent fibers by less controlled techniques of force application to capsular tissue. For example, focal application of force directly to the center of the RFs of afferent fibers has been used to investigate the mechanical sensitivity of small-diameter fibers.[44] This method, which involves the use of fine-tipped probes (esthesiometers or von Frey hairs) to distort a punctate region of the total capsular RF of a unit under study, results in excitation of mechanoreceptors at lower than normal levels of force. Mechanical force thresholds determined in this manner for some group II and group IV joint afferent fibers have been found in the range of 0.3 to 22.5 gm, with the group IV fibers having the highest thresholds, that is, the lowest mechanical sensitivity.[69,70] It is expected that capsular loading under normal activity of the joint would have to be at least an order of magnitude higher than the above intensities to excite these fibers. The smaller diameter afferent fibers also tend to have a less steep slope (relating response to intensity or magnitude of force) than do the larger diameter fibers (Table 2-2). Since groups III and IV fibers represent the great majority of afferent fibers of a given articular nerve,[46] it is of great importance to understand their contribution to articular afferent mechanisms. Other major differences between groups III and IV joint afferent fibers relating to force sensitivity are given in Table 2-2.

Desensitization of receptors is possible under certain conditions of repetitive activation.[69] An example of such desensitizing stimulation would be the application of a suprathreshold stimulus such as 20 gm for 30 seconds at 1-minute intervals for four repetitions. This type of stimulation has been shown to reduce responsiveness of some group III and IV fibers.

Neuron population response and across-fiber pattern coding

Functionally, the activity of an individual joint afferent fiber by itself may not be meaningful to CNS mechanisms, since its relation to the function of the joint as a whole may vary. It is the temporal and spatial response patterns of many joint afferent fibers discharging in concert that informs the CNS about what the joint is doing. The importance of this concept is emphasized by the fact that any single afferent fiber, discharging throughout a particular range of motion, may discharge differently when that motion is accomplished actively versus passively. Furthermore, the increased soft tissue tension that may be associated with a slight degree of torsion superimposed on a uniplanar joint excursion may significantly alter the stimulus-response relation of a single unit. The former effect has been attributed to musculotendinous insertions into the capsule, which produce changes in capsule tension when muscle contraction occurs.[54] The latter effect is probably due to the increments or decrements in tissue tension arising from rotational tightening, deletion of slack, or the "windup" effect. Grigg and Hoffman[37] have demonstrated that many capsular afferent fibers respond to two or more directions of longitudinal capsular stress.

Therefore, evidence supports the argument that a somewhat tenuous relation exists between single-unit discharge and the absolute excursion of the joint, whereas the neuron population response pattern must be considered the neural encoder of periarticular stresses and strains. The neuron population response therefore must clearly reflect the following aspects of joint function: (1) the static joint angle, (2) the velocity of joint excursion, (3) the planes in which the joint excursion occurs, (4) the activity or passivity of joint excursion (i.e., whether joint movement is elicited by muscular contraction), and (5) the nature of internal or external compressive forces on the articular soft tissue.

Recent sensorineural theory advocates the across-fiber pattern as the important factor in nonambiguous transfer of information to the CNS. However, more detailed study is required before a final verdict can be reached regarding the informational impact of a single afferent fiber input, since it has recently been determined in humans that activity in a single cutaneous peripheral afferent fiber is adequate to elicit a conscious perception.[78,79] When coupled with the knowledge of how many afferent fibers usually participate in a functional joint response, the sensitivity of individual afferent fibers becomes an important factor in determining the minimal afferentation necessary to evoke adequate function of the joint neuronal information system.

Temporal response pattern

Two general patterns of joint afferent receptor sensitivity exist in relation to the time domain. The RA response of the pacinian afferent receptors consists of the occurrence of discharge of the receptor only during dynamic conditions involving rapid movement of the joint, that is, during high-velocity or accelerative phases of joint motion. It would be expected that very low amplitude vibrations (60 Hz or above) of the capsular or pericapsular tissue would be adequate to excite these afferent receptors.

Specific low-frequency vibration detectors, such as the Meissner corpuscle of cutaneous origin,[57] have not been found in periarticular tissues. However, SA articular afferent receptors such as the Ruffini, Golgi-Mazzoni, Golgi ligamentous, and free nerve ending type respond during both dynamic and static phases of stimulation. Therefore, low-frequency vibration and low-stimulus velocities are likely to be signaled in the initial discharge rate of SA af-

Table 2-2. Comparison of groups III and IV joint afferent fibers

Parameter	III	IV
Conduction velocity	2.5 to 20 ms	0.3 to 1.1 ms
Rotation > flexion/ extension needed to excite	30.5%	13%
Nonnoxious stimulation weakly excites; noxious stimulation strongly excites	19.5%	7.5%
Only noxious stimulation excites	28%	26%
Insensitivity to joint movement	22%	43.5%
Discharge frequency/ stimulation intensity slope relation	Steep	Less steep
Mechanical threshold	Low (<3 gm)	Some low, most high (some > 7.5 gm)

Based on data from Schaible HG and Schmidt RF: Activation of groups III and IV sensory units in medial articular nerve by local mechanical stimulation of knee joint, J Neurophysiol 49:35, 1983, and Responses of fine medial articular nerve afferents to passive movements of the knee joint, J Neurophysiol 49:118, 1983.

ferent fibers.[74] The traditional view has been that RA afferent receptors signal joint movement, and the SA afferent receptors specify static joint position. However, the neural code for static position and for low-velocity dynamic aspects of joint movement must rely heavily on the Ruffini, Golgi-Mazzoni, free nerve, and ligamentous afferent receptors and on different portions of their discharge pattern for unambiguity.

Grigg, Hoffman, and Fogarty[38] have recently determined that some SA afferent receptors of the knee joint capsule may present an RA-type response when stimulated off the focal point of their RF. This is analogous to what can be achieved by minimal stimulation of cutaneous afferent receptors at close to threshold strengths.[66] Large-amplitude movements to a given position therefore result in an entirely different sequence of neural information than does a sequence of small movements to the same position. Response variation as a function of the interplay of both intensity and stimulus sequence again requires that resolution of the mechanical events at the joint is encoded by the across-fiber pattern or spatial-temporal neural activity profile.[22] It is much too simplistic to relate joint movement detection to the RA afferent receptor channel and joint position to SA afference, especially since joint status is accompanied by status reports from the involved muscles and tendons. Whenever a joint assumes a particular position or is in the course of an excursion, it would be most fruitful to envision the myriad of impulses as arising from muscular, fascial, tendon, and bony receptors, as well as from articular receptors.

Quantitative stimulus-response functions

Two major types of stimulus-response functions have been determined for joint afferent fibers. Skoglund[73] initially observed afferent fibers whose maximal discharge rates were elicited at some intermediate or "best angle" of joint position. This type of stimulus-response relation, or "tuning" curve, is referred to as a *nonmonotonic response function*, since the response is maximal at some intermediate position of the range of motion curve and is submaximal on both sides of the best angle. This tuning curve is also referred to as "bell shaped" and has been studied in great detail by McCall et al.[50] If this were the case for all joint afferent fibers, then each angle would be specified in a unique neuron subpopulation of the total spectrum of joint afferent fibers.[75]

On the other hand, Burgess and Clark[8,9] found that practically all the afferent fibers in their studies exhibited a maximal discharge rate at one or the other of the extremes of the range of motion. These same investigators found the tuning curves of many afferent fibers to be very flat throughout the intermediate angles of the range of motion, meaning that little or no information about changing joint conditions could be signaled at these angles by the joint receptors.[14] This type of stimulus-response relation is viewed as monotonic, since maximal response coincides with maximal stimulus intensity; that is, there is no diminution of response as either extreme of the range of motion is approached. Ferrell[23] has recently concluded that the most common form of response function is in fact the monotonic form. Other authors have attempted to delineate the specificity of response function in terms of receptor types. The Golgi ligament ending, well studied by Andrew,[3] has been determined to have a monotonic type of relation, whereas Eklund and Skoglund[21] have attributed monotonic character to some Ruffini afferent receptors and nonmonotonic relations to other Ruffini receptors. Cohen[16] initially proposed that the monotonic type of relation for different joint afferent receptors helps to categorize each receptor as a flexion or an extension receptor.

EFFERENT MODULATION OF JOINT FIBER AFFERENCE: INFLUENCE OF MUSCULAR ACTIVITY

The relation between joint angle and excursion and joint afferent fiber discharge is in many instances subject to modification by the muscular tension exerted on the capsular tissue. Active muscular contraction resulting in joint angle change or isometric tension development is capable of inducing a response in the respective joint afferent neuron population. Millar[54] has suggested that one of the functions of muscle in proprioception may be to modulate joint afferent fiber discharge. Surely, certain muscles, such as the articular muscles of the knee and elbow (articularis genu and articularis cubiti, respectively),[81] seem to be specifically designed to generate periarticular tissue changes. Other more diversified muscles, such as the biceps, triceps, brachialis, pectoralis major, teres major, many of the forearm flexors, gluteus minimus, vastus lateralis, and vastus medialis,[54,81] also include tendinous insertions into joint capsules. These findings suggest that joint afferent fiber modulation by muscular tension development is a widespread and probably critically important physiological mechanism.

Grigg and Greenspan[36] demonstrated that few (<2%) of the primate knee joint afferent fibers tested in the posterior capsule (extension afferent fibers) were active at angles of more than 20 degrees of flexion from full extension. Many of the tested afferent fibers were sensitive to muscular contraction and exhibited a specific relation to the muscle group active around the joint. Force generation in the gastrocnemius muscle was primarily effective in activating 68% of the knee joint extension neurons, whereas force generation in the quadriceps muscle only elicited activity in 29% of these neurons. It was determined that torques on the order of 700 to 5,000 gm-cm (2,450 gm-cm, mean) were necessary to activate these capsular receptors. Muscular elicitation of knee joint activity was most likely at extreme joint extension, that is, in conditions of pronounced capsular leading, for afferent fibers that were generally sentient at intermediate joint angles. Evidence suggested a strong relation of joint afferent fiber discharge pattern to muscular force, since the decay rate of the SA discharge closely followed the rate of passive torque decay.

This modification of joint receptor activity may play a role in explaining the fact that accuracy of joint positioning is high for positioning a joint through active movement versus passive positioning of the joint as determined by subjective judgment testing.[60,61] Differences in joint afferent fiber activity with active and passive excursions may play a role in the postulated "sense of effort" or "feeling of innervation" that accompanies volitional muscular action.[52,53,67] Paillard and Brouchon[60,61] indicate that an acceleration afference would be critical in the superior estimation of active displacement to that position. It has already been mentioned that articular pacinian afferent receptors correspond to joint movement acceleration detectors. It would seem that this peripheral method for discriminating between active and passive body movements should complement any internal feedback mechanisms of motor command signal monitoring that provide the individual with knowledge regarding muscular contractions.[49,51,66]

One other mechanism to explain the increased receptor discharge that occurs between active and passive articular excursion lies in the additional receptor discharge from the component movements of rotation, roll, and glide, which occur with muscular control of the joint excursion, versus the lack of these component movement discharges when the joint is moved passively.

FUNCTIONAL IMPLICATIONS

The most important contributions of primary joint afference to CNS mechanisms include three distinct actions. At the lowest level, joint afferent fibers converge on spinal interneurons and are responsible for the eventual reflex activation, facilitation, or inhibition of motor neurons. This regulation of motor activity constitutes a control over the coordination of antagonistic and synergistic patterns of muscular contraction, establishing functional joint stability or mobilization. At the next level, afference from the neck, trunk, and limb joints is required by brain stem neuronal circuits for interaction with vestibular afference to facilitate postural and equilibrium maintenance. Finally, at the highest level, joint afference can mediate some aspects of cognitive awareness of body position and movement or at least modulate the perceptual impact of other somatosensory afference.

Spinal reflex action: intrinsic stability and mobility

Although the exact spinal termination pattern of primary joint afferent fibers has not been elucidated, the functional roles of the fibers has been determined by study of reflex motor effects and actions on spinally mediated

patterns of neural activity that subserve purposeful action. Periarticular tissue afference affects the following reflexes[74,77]: (1) a facilitatory effect on the ipsilateral flexion reflex,[27] (2) a facilitatory effect on the contralateral (crossed) extension reflex,[27] (3) effects opposite to the first two reflexes,[27] (4) facilitation of the ipsilateral group Ib or Golgi tendon organ reflex,[48] (5) modification of directional signs of cutaneous ambulatory reflexes, and (6) elicitation of reflex muscular splinting during conditions of abnormal stress about the joint.[11,45,80]

Kennedy, Alexander, and Hayes[45] have recently provided a scheme for understanding the manner in which posttraumatic abnormal joint afference can contribute to a loss of reflexive muscular splinting. They suggest that tonic or dynamic co-contraction of antagonistic muscles involved in dynamic stabilization of the joint may be inhibited by abnormal patterns of joint afference, resulting in an increased propensity for reinjury via destabilization.

Implied in the postulated loss of automatic motor control of a limb because of aberrant feedback from the articular receptors is the fact that therapeutic progression must incorporate a relearning paradigm, as well as a promotion of physical recovery factors. That is, joint injury represents a peripheral neurological dysfunction that triggers a new state of motor control factors in the nervous system. A portion of therapeutic recovery therefore must be devoted to reestablishment of an appropriate afference and development of motor skill on the basis of this new afference. This type of recovery program would seem to be most critical to avoid reinjury of the joint, primarily in the early stages of recovery. During the recovery/rehabilitation period, new sensory cues for motor guidance and retraining of appropriate muscle activation sequences may be required. It has been suggested that this relearning of normal function in an injured joint may involve several months.[29]

Less obvious but perhaps more important effects have been determined also regarding modification of motor neural activity patterns in the spinal cord and perhaps at higher CNS centers as well. Recent investigations have concluded that rhythmic limb movements, which occur in activities such as walking, depend upon a phase relationship between central neural activity patterns and feedback from the periphery.[1] According to this view, a centrally generated, locomotor neural activity pattern, primarily at local spinal levels, must be maintained by activity from periarticular receptors, which are stimulated by the locomotive actions. The relevant investigations have not, however, decisively determined whether joint afferent fibers from small muscles surrounding the joint (like the relationships of the pectineal muscle to the hip joint) are the major contributors to this input. It seems logical to conclude from these studies that joint afferent fiber response is necessary, if not sufficient, to "entrain" the central locomotive activity pattern and generate a dynamic equilibrium for the maintenance of a regular ambulatory activation pattern.

Aberrations in joint afferent fiber feedback may therefore serve to disrupt the phase relation between feedback and the central pattern and lead to secondary problems in gait. These problems may include increased sense of effort in the control of gait, deficiencies in developing high-velocity or accelerative components in the gait cycle, and an increased amount of total conscious involvement in ambulation. Since the CNS has been shown to be highly adaptable, it is reasonable to assume that abnormalities in the feedback and CNS pattern relations may require intelligently designed retraining exercises to foster more appropriate relations, especially in planning therapeutic programs.

Postural and equilibrium mechanisms

Joint afference is relayed to medullary and brain stem centers by way of the dorsal columns and the ascending somatosensory tracts of the dorsolateral fascicular, spinocerebellar,[47] and spinovestibular pathways.[24] Numerous studies have stressed the importance of this information for cerebral processing involved in motor control,[77] but its involvement in brain stem motor integration mechanisms is also critical. For example, the proprioceptors of the neck region include the cervical joint afferent receptors, which are involved in providing neck afference to the vestibular system of the head. The functional role of this afference includes (1) coordination of eye, head, and neck movements to stabilize retinal imagery for vision,[41,43] (2) maintenance of posture,[17,42] and (3) maintenance of coordinated movement patterns.[17,19]

Joint afferent fiber activity also assists the muscle spindle afferent fibers in inhibiting antagonist muscle activity under conditions of rapid lengthening and associated periarticular tissue distortion, both of which accompany unexpected postural perturbations. When simultaneous input arises from cutaneous, joint, muscle, and vestibular receptors, a unique pattern of afference is generated and elicits long-latency, nonvoluntary postural adjustments, acting to stabilize and bring the body center of gravity into a state of equilibrium.

It has not yet been determined to what extent joint afference responding to noxious stimulation impinges on brain stem neurons involved in the transmission and control of pain, but it is likely that the pathways and nuclei demonstrated for other afferent fibers are involved.[87] Patients frequently report that chronic pain localized to deep tissues of the spine or pelvis is alleviated or mitigated by movement, suggesting that the analgesic effect of joint mechanoreceptor stimulation may be quite powerful. The analgesia derived from selective activation of pacinian afferent receptors has been adequately demonstrated.

Proprioceptive and kinesthetic awareness

During the 1960s joint afferent receptors were viewed by many to be the unique determinants of position and movement sensation. The outright rejection of Sherrington's "muscular sensation" was fixed in vogue by numerous erroneous conclusions.[49] Recently, however, Burgess et al.,[10] having reviewed the literature and their own experimental and clinical findings, concluded that there is no valid evidence that the articular receptors of any joint are important for the conscious awareness of joint position. Two main types of studies contributed to this position: (1) local anesthetization of joint tissues did not reduce joint position awareness,[33,49] and (2) joint replacement surgery in humans in which most of the joint receptors were surgically removed resulted in little subsequent kinesthetic impairment.[35,49]

The suggested role in perception for the articular receptors involves their contribution to the feeling of deep pressure experienced by an individual near the limits of the range of motion of a joint.[10] This concept is supported by the fact that most joints, with the exception of the hip, have very few receptors that are activated either statically or dynamically in the middle of the range of motion; yet conscious appreciation of this part of the range is no more inferior than that near the end of the range.

The receptors that seem to be the most suited for a crucial involvement in joint position sense are the muscle spindle receptors.[20,32,33,49] These receptors are supported in this function by the activity of cutaneous and some joint receptors,[15] and all the afferent receptors together must be integrated with a corollary discharge from motor tracts in the brain at such centers as the cerebellum and the dorsal column nuclei.[49] Preliminary comparative investigations indicate that the joint afferent receptor channel may be subject to descending corticofugal modulatory influences to a greater extent than are other somatic afferent channels.[66]

SUMMARY

Knowledge of the relationship of structure and function in joint innervation is most critical for adequate prevention and treatment of maladaptation in the articular apparatus. Concentrating on the intricate balance of activity patterns arising from the joint afferent receptors, we can begin to appreciate the degree of focal specificity with which the nervous system operates. Physiological dissection of afferent channels of information emanating from each joint makes possible a new evaluative selectivity and provides the opportunity for the next quantum leap in therapeutic design. The future of physical medicine must be drawn by the magnetism of selective stimulation of specific afferent channels to facilitate appropriate biomechanical stabilization or mobilization processes. The interaction of muscular and soft tissue components of the articular system must be thoroughly understood before rational designs for therapeutic prevention of maladaptation, or optimal rate restitution of adequate function, may be achieved.

REFERENCES

1. Andersson O and Grillner S: On the feedback control of the cat's hindlimb during locomotion. In Taylor A and Prochazka A, editors: Muscle receptors and movement, New York, 1981, Oxford University Press.

2. Andres KH and von During M: Morphology of cutaneous receptors. In Iggo A, editor: Handbook of sensory physiology, vol 2, Somatosensory system, New York, 1973, Springer-Verlag New York, Inc.

3. Andrew BL: The sensory innervation of the medial ligament of the knee joint, J Physiol (Lond) 123:241, 1954.

4. Bloom W and Fawcett DW: A textbook of histology, ed 10, Philadelphia, 1975, WB Saunders Co.

5. Boyd IA: The histological structure of the receptors on the knee joint of the cat correlated with their physiological response, J Physiol 124:476, 1954.

6. Boyd IA and Roberts TDM: Proprioceptive discharges from stretch-receptors in the knee joint of the cat, J Physiol (Lond) 122:38, 1953.

7. Brodal A: Neurological anatomy, New York, 1981, Oxford University Press.

8. Burgess PR and Clark FJ: Characteristics of knee joint receptors in the cat, J Physiol (Lond) 203:317, 1969.

9. Burgess PR and Clark FJ: Dorsal column projection of fibres from the cat knee joint, J Physiol (Lond) 203:301, 1969.

10. Burgess PR et al.: Signaling of kinesthetic information by peripheral sensory receptors, Annu Rev Neurosci 5:171, 1982.

11. Cailliet R: Low back pain syndrome, ed 3, Philadelphia, 1981, FA Davis Co.

12. Catton WT and Petoe N: A viscoelastic theory of mechanoreceptor adaptation, J Physiol (Lond) 187:35, 1966.

13. Chouchkov C: Cutaneous receptors, Adv Anat Embryol Cell Biol 54:1, 1978.

14. Clark FJ and Burgess PR: Slowly adapting receptors in cat knee joint: Can they signal joint angle? J Neurophysiol 38:1448, 1975.

15. Clark FJ et al.: Contributions of cutaneous and joint receptors to static knee-position sense in man, J Neurophysiol 42:877, 1979.

16. Cohen LA: Activity of knee joint proprioceptors recorded from the posterior articular nerve, Yale J Biol Med 28:225, 1955/1956.

17. Cohen LA: Role of the eye and neck proprioception mechanism in body orientation and motor coordination, J Neurophysiol 24:1, 1961.

18. Dee R: Structure and function of hip joint innervation, Ann R Coll Surg Engl 45:357, 1969.

19. deJong P et al.: Ataxia and nystagmus induced by injection of local anaesthetics in the neck, Ann Neurol 1:240, 1977.

20. Eklund G: Position sense and state of contraction: The effects of vibration, J Neurol Neurosurg Psychiatry 35:606, 1972.

21. Eklund G and Skoglund S: On the specificity of the Ruffini-like receptors, Acta Physiol Scand 49:184, 1960.

22. Erickson RP: Parallel "population" neural coding in feature extraction. In Schmitt FO and Worden FG, editors: The neurosciences: Third study program, Cambridge, Mass, 1974, The MIT Press.

23. Ferrell WR: The adequacy of stretch receptors in the cat knee joint for signalling joint angle throughout a full range of movement, J Physiol (Lond) 299:85, 1980.

24. Fredrickson JM, Schwarz D, and Kornhuber HH: Convergence and interaction of vestibular and deep somatic afferents upon neurons in the vestibular nuclei of the cat, Acta Otolaryngol 61:168, 1965.

25. Freeman MAR and Wyke B: The innervation of the ankle joint: An anatomical and histological study in the cat, Acta Anat 68:321, 1967.

26. Gardner E: Physiology of moveable joints, Physiol Rev 30:127, 1950.

27. Gardner E: Reflex muscular responses to stimulation of articular nerves in the cat, Am J Physiol 161:133, 1950.

28. Gardner E and Noer R: Projection of afferent fibers from muscles and joints to the cerebral cortex of the cat, Am J Physiol 168:437, 1952.

29. Glencross D and Thornton E: Position sense following joint injury, J Sports Med Phys Fitness 21:23, 1981.

30. Godwin-Austen RB: The mechanoreceptors of the costovertebral joints, J Physiol (Lond) 202:737, 1969.

31. Goldie I and Wellisch M: The presence of nerves in patients synovectomised for rheumatoid arthritis, Acta Orthop Scand 40:143, 1969.

32. Goodwin GM, McCloskey DI, and Matthews PBC: The contribution of muscle afferents to kinesthesia shown by vibration-induced illusions of movement and by the effects of paralysing joint afferents, Brain 95:705, 1972.

33. Goodwin GM, McCloskey DL, and Matthews PBC: The persistence of appreciable kinesthesia after paralysing joint afferents but preserving muscle afferents, Brain Res 37:326, 1972.

34. Grieve GP: Common vertebral joint problems, New York, 1981, Churchill Livingstone, Inc.

35. Grigg P, Finerman GA, and Riley LH: Joint position sense after total hip replacement, J Bone Joint Surg 55B:1016, 1973.

36. Grigg P and Greenspan BJ: Response of primate joint afferent neurons to mechanical stimulation of knee joint, J Neurophysiol 40:1, 1977.

37. Grigg P and Hoffman AH: Properties of Ruffini afferents as revealed by stress analysis of isolated sections of cat knee capsule, J Neurophysiol 47:41, 1982.

38. Grigg P, Hoffman AH, and Fogarty KE: Properties of Golgi-Mazzoni afferents in cat knee joint capsule, as revealed by mechanical studies of isolated joint capsule, J Neurophysiol 47:31, 1982.

39. Halata Z: The mechanoreceptors of the mammalian skin: Ultrastructure and morphological classification, Adv Anat Embryol Cell Biol 50:1, 1975.

40. Halata Z: The ultrastructure of the sensory nerve endings in the articular capsule of the knee joint of the domestic cat (Ruffini corpuscles and pacinian corpuscles), J Anat 124:717, 1977.

41. Hikosaka O and Maeda M: Cervical effects on abducens motoneurones and their interaction with the vestibulo-ocular reflex, Exp Brain Res 18:512, 1973.

42. Igarashi M et al.: Role of the neck proprioceptors for the maintenance of dynamic bodily equilibrium in the squirrel monkey, Laryngoscope 79:1713, 1969.

43. Igarashi M et al.: Nystagmus after experimental cervical lesions, Laryngoscope 82:1609, 1972.

44. Kanaka R, Schaible HG, and Schmidt RF: Von Frey thresholds of mechanosensitive joint afferent units are related to conduction velocity, Pfluegers Arch 291:R44, 1981.

45. Kennedy JC, Alexander IJ, and Hayes KC: Nerve supply of the human knee and its functional importance, Am J Sports Med 10:329, 1982.

46. Langford LA and Schmidt RF: The medial articular nerve: An electron microscopic examination, Pfluegers Arch 394:R57, 1982.

47. Lindstrom S and Takata M: Monosynaptic excitation of dorsal spinocerebellar tract neurons from low threshold joint afferents, Acta Physiol Scand 84:430, 1972.

48. Lundberg A, Malmgren K, and Schomburg ED: Role of joint afferents in motor control exemplified by effects on reflex pathways from Ib afferents, J Physiol (Lond) 284:327, 1978.

49. Matthews PBC: Where does Sherrington's "muscular sense" originate? Muscles, joints, corollary discharges? Annu Rev Neurosci 5:189, 1982.

50. McCall WD Jr et al.: Static and dynamic responses of slowly adapting joint receptors, Brain Res 70:221, 1974.

51. McCloskey DI: Knowledge about muscular contractions, Trends Neurosci 3:311, 1980.

52. Merton PA: Human position sense and sense of effort, Symp Soc Exp Biol 18:387, 1964.
53. Merton PA: The sense of effort. In Porter R, editor: Breathing, Hering-Breuer Centenary Symposium, London, 1970, Churchill Livingstone, Inc.
54. Millar J: Joint afferent fibres responding to muscle stretch, vibration, and contraction, Brain Res 63:380, 1973.
55. Miller MR and Kasahara M: Observations on the innervation of human long bones, Anat Rec 145:13, 1963.
56. Molina F, Ramcharan J, and Wyke BD: Structure and function of articular receptor systems in the cervical spine, J Bone Joint Surg 58B:255, 1976.
57. Mountcastle VB et al.: Neural base for the sense of fluttervibration, Science 155:597, 1967.
58. Newton RA: Joint receptor contributions to reflexive and kinesthetic responses, Phys Ther 62:22, 1982.
59. O'Connor BL and McConnaughey JS: The structure and innervation of cat knee menisci and their relation to a "sensory hypothesis" of meniscal function, Am J Anat 153:431, 1978.
60. Paillard J and Brouchon M: Active and passive movements in the calibration of position sense. In Freedman SJ, editor: The neuropsychology of spatially oriented behavior, Homewood, Ill, 1968, The Dorsey Press.
61. Paillard J and Brouchon M: A proprioceptive contribution to the spatial encoding of position cues for ballistic movements, Brain Res 71:273, 1974.
62. Pertovaara A: Modification of human pain threshold by specific tactile receptors, Acta Physiol Scand 107:339, 1979.
63. Polacek P: Receptors of the joints: Their structure, variability and classification, Acta Fac Med Univ Brun 23:1, 1966.
64. Reimann I and Christensen SB: A histological demonstration of nerves in subchondral bone, Acta Orthop Scand 48:345, 1977.
65. Rossi A and Grigg P: Characteristics of hip joint mechanoreceptors in the cat, J Neurophysiol 47:1029, 1982.
66. Rowinski MJ and Stoney SD Jr: Specificity of cortical efferent modulation of somatosensory neuronal activity in the raccoon cuneate nucleus, Exp Neurol (in press).
67. Rymer WZ and D'Almeida A: Joint position sense: The effects of muscle contraction, Brain 103:1, 1980.
68. Samuel EP: The autonomic and somatic innervation of the articular capsule, Anat Rec 113:53, 1952.
69. Schaible HG and Schmidt RF: Activation of groups III and IV sensory units in medial articular nerve by local mechanical stimulation of knee joint, J Neurophysiol 49:35, 1983.
70. Schaible HG and Schmidt RF: Responses of fine medial articular nerve afferents to passive movements of the knee joint, J Neurophysiol 49:118, 1983.
71. Shepherd GM: Neurobiology, New York, 1983, Oxford University Press.
72. Sherrington CS: The integrative action of the nervous system, London, 1948, Cambridge University Press.
73. Skoglund S: Anatomical and physiological studies of the knee joint innervation in the cat, Acta Physiol Scand Suppl 36:124, 1956.
74. Skoglund S: Joint receptors and kinaesthesias. In Iggo A, editor: Handbook of sensory physiology, vol 2, Somatosensory system, New York, 1973, Springer-Verlag New York, Inc.
75. Somjen G: Sensory coding in the mammalian nervous system, New York, 1972, Plenum Publishing Corp.
76. Stilwell DL: The nerve supply of the vertebral column and its associated structures in the monkey, Anat Rec 125:139, 1956.
77. Tracey DJ: Joint receptors and the control of movement, Trends Neurosci 3:253, 1980.
78. Vallbo AB and Hagbarth KE: Activity from skin mechanoreceptors recorded percutaneously in awake human subjects, Exp Neurol 21:270, 1968.
79. Vallbo AB et al.: Somatosensory, proprioceptive, and sympathetic activity in human peripheral nerves, Physiol Rev 59:919, 1979.
80. Vrettos XC and Wyke BD: Articular reflexogenic systems in the costovertebral joints, J Bone Joint Surg 56B:382, 1974.
81. Williams PL and Warwick R, editors: Gray's anatomy, ed 36, Philadelphia, 1980, WB Saunders Co.
82. Wilson AD, Legg PG, and McNeur JC: Studies on the innervation of the medial meniscus in the human knee joint, Anat Rec 165:485, 1969.
83. Wyke BD: The neurology of the joints, Ann R Coll Surg Engl 41:25, 1967.
84. Wyke BD: Articular neurology: A review, Physiotherapy 58:94, 1972.
85. Wyke BD: Morphological and functional features of the innervation of the costovertebral joints, Folia Morphol 23:296, 1975.
86. Wyke BD: Neurology of the cervical spinal joints, Physiotherapy 65:72, 1979.
87. Wyke B: Neurological implications of low back pain. In Jayson M, editor: The lumbar spine and back pain, New York, 1976, Grune & Stratton, Inc.
88. Wyke BD and Polacek P: Articular neurology: The present position, J Bone Joint Surg 57B:401, 1975.

Chapter 3

Basic Biomechanics in Sports and Orthopaedic Therapy

Barney F. LeVeau

MECHANICS AND INJURY

Mechanics deals with the analysis of forces acting on an object. The study of biomechanics applies the principles of mechanics to human and animal bodies. All body postures are the result of muscular forces balancing the forces imposed upon the body, and all body movements are caused by forces acting within and upon the body.

Forces are also involved to some extent in all sports. Individuals working with musculoskeletal injuries must understand how forces affect the body structure and how forces control movement. Radin[33] states that of all the basic sciences, mechanics has the clearest direct application to injury therapy and functional recovery from musculoskeletal problems. Knowledge of mechanical principles therefore is essential for understanding the prevention, diagnosis, and treatment of orthopaedic and sports injuries.

Muscle mechanics

Biomechanics is the basis of musculoskeletal function. Muscles produce force that acts through the bony lever system. The bony system either moves or statically acts upon a resistance. If a load is applied to the lever system, the muscles react to control the load. Muscles have a variety of ways to control the body. The fiber arrangement of each muscle determines the amount of force the muscle can produce and the distance over which the muscles can contract. Muscles often act together to obtain a resulting force with the desired magnitude and in the desired direction. An individual muscle's attachment to the lever system affects lever arm length and angle of pull, which ultimately affects its force production. The distance the muscle attaches from the joint axis determines the muscle moment of force, whereas the angle of muscular pull controls the rotatory and nonrotatory components of the force. Within the body, muscles are the major structures controlling posture and movement. However, ligaments, cartilage, and other soft tissues also aid in joint control or are affected by body position or movement.

Mechanism of injury

Forces may directly or indirectly cause injuries. An injury may result from a single force of large magnitude or from repetitive forces of low magnitude. If the forces that cause an injury are known, personnel working with sports and orthopaedic cases can act to prevent or reduce the seriousness of the injury. The therapist or practitioner who knows the mechanism of injury is better able to evaluate the kind of injury involved and its extent. Several authors* have emphasized the value of accurate evaluation of the injury-producing force to aid early detection and prompt diagnosis. Garrick,[15] for example, indicates that the diagnosis of injuries can be a problem if the circumstances under which they occur are unfamiliar.

Evaluation of injury

Every time an injury is evaluated, the practitioner uses procedures based on the principles of biomechanics. For example, Noyes et al.[30] strongly believe that practical biomechanical concepts govern the successful interpretation of clinical laxity tests. Their study of knee ligaments demonstrates that an understanding of biomechanics allows for more accurate interpretation of knee injuries. In fact, several tests for knee joint problems use mechanics directly. For example, the three-point principle is used in valgus and varus testing, tension and compression are used in the Apley tests for ligament and meniscal problems, compression helps determine the presence of chondromalacia patellae, and tension is used in clinical drawer tests to determine joint laxity. Tests for other joints also make use of mechanical principles.

Treatment of injury

Most procedures used to treat or rehabilitate musculoskeletal injuries are based to a great extent on biomechanical principles. Surgical procedures, casting, bracing,

*See references 10, 17, 20, 31, 38, 40, and 48.

splinting, and exercise programs all depend upon correct application of forces to obtain satisfactory results. Several example of these procedures should be mentioned. Successful surgical realignment of the patella either proximally or distally depends upon the surgeon's knowledge of force application. Surgical treatment of a dislocated or subluxated (separated) acromioclavicular joint involves knowledge of forces and the strength of biological materials. Casting limits motion of debilitated joints in children with sports-related problems such as Osgood-Schlatter disease and chondromalacia patellae. Casts have been applied after knee surgery, bracing may be used for postoperative treatments, and splinting of fingers and hands is often used to limit motion and to protect them from further injury.

Exercise analysis

In addition to treating musculoskeletal injuries, sports medicine and orthopaedic practitioners must provide exercise programs for prevention and rehabilitation of injuries. Many types of exercise devices exist, each with its advantages and disadvantages. Knowledge of the application of resisting force and its effect on the muscle and joint is essential for the professional therapist to develop the best program for each individual.

Protective equipment

The design and proper use of protective equipment also requires the knowledge and application of biomechanical principles. Most sports use some sort of protective equipment, whether it is worn by the participant or located within the playing area. Sports such as cycling, hockey, kayaking, baseball, and wrestling require head gear. Often children with cerebral palsy wear headgear for protection. Protective padding is also worn by participants in such sports as riflery, football, lacrosse, soccer, and softball. Most sports, of course, require specially designed shoes to protect the foot and provide traction. Other examples of mechanically designed protective equipment include jumping pits, gymnastic mats, and treatment mats that must be fabricated to provide comfort and protection and yet provide sufficient firmness for reaction forces. Playing surfaces, such as gymnasium floors and football fields, should also be constructed based on mechanical principles. In the past, most equipment was developed by trial and error or practical experience. Now, however, mechanical theory forms the basis of equipment construction.

Mechanical analysis of movement

Knowledge of mechanical principles has proved to be essential for those practitioners working with joint replacement. The manner and materials of joint construction, surgical procedures such as positioning, and deciding which treatment method should be chosen all depend upon the elements of biomechanics.

BASIC TERMS AND CONCEPTS

Several terms and concepts must be learned before one can intelligently apply mechanics to sports and orthopaedic therapy. Many terms are misused daily. For example, the terms "strength," "pressure," and "power" are used frequently instead of the term "force." The term "load" is used to describe force as it is externally applied to an object, whereas internal reactions to load are referred to by such terms as "stress," "strain," "tension," "compression," and "shear." The strength of various materials is described by these internal reactions as forces or loads are imposed upon the materials. The practitioner must know which terms are synonymous and which are not. Terms and concepts within mechanics and medicine should be precise and accurate.

Force

The science of mechanics is concerned with forces. A *force* may simply be defined as a push or pull. An equation often used to define force is $F = ma$, where F is the force, m is the mass of the object, and a is the acceleration of the object. By this definition, force is an entity that tends to produce motion. Sometimes motion does not occur or the object is in equilibrium. The branch of mechanics dealing with this phenomenon is called *statics*. If motion does occur, the related branch of mechanics is called *dynamics*.

Force is composed of four specific characteristics (Fig. 3-1). The magnitude of force, often denoted by a capital letter, is the amount of push or pull. This amount of force acts along a line of application that in turn acts as a specific point of application. Force also must be defined by its direction, which is indicated by an arrowhead on the line of application.

The most common forces involved in sports medicine and orthopaedic therapy are muscular, gravitational, inertial, bouyant, and contact forces. The force produced by a muscle depends upon several factors. Two of these factors

include the speed of muscle contraction and the length of the muscle. (Other factors that relate to measuring muscular force will be discussed later.) The weight of an object is the result of gravitational force. The formula for defining gravitational force is $W = mg$, where W is the weight of the object, m is the mass of the object, and g is the constant acceleration caused by gravitational pull. The concept of inertia maintains that a body remains at rest or in uniform motion until acted upon by an outside force. Although not a true force, inertia acts like a force because it resists the change in motion (or lack of it) of an object. Bouyant force tends to resist the force of gravity. In water the magnitude of this force equals the weight of the water that the object displaces. Contact force exists any time two objects are in contact with each other. This type of force may be a reaction force or an impact force. In either case, the force can be further subdivided into a normal force perpendicular to the contacting surfaces and a shearing or frictional force that is parallel (or tangential) to the contacting surfaces. The magnitude of the frictional force, either static or dynamic, depends upon how tightly the two surfaces are pressed together (the normal force) and the kind of materials in contact, which establishes the coefficient of friction between the two contacting surfaces. The equation is $F_f = \mu N$, where F_f is the maximal frictional force, μ is the coefficient of friction between the surfaces, and N is the normal force.

Strength

The term *strength* is often used to mean the ability of muscle to produce or resist a force. When one states that an individual is strong, one means that the individual can lift or resist a great amount of weight. The greater the force produced by a muscle, the greater the strength of the muscle. This concept may be related to the ability of a muscle to overcome a load, such as occurs in a shortening contraction; to maintain a load, as in a static contraction; or to offer support to a load by muscle elongation, as in a lengthening contraction. In normal situations muscle strength, or the amount of force it can produce, cannot be measured directly. To determine muscle strength, the amount of resistance the muscle lever system can either overcome or maintain is measured.

Several biomechanical problems exist with this indirect method of determining a muscle's strength, however. These problems include the muscle angle of pull, the angle of application of resisting force, the muscle length, the speed of muscle contraction, and the speed of movement.

During shortening muscle contractions, the amount of weight moved can be no greater than the weakest point in the range of movement. Conventional isotonic exercises, such as "free weights," only provide sufficient resistance for an exercise effect or a testing value for this weakest area. Thus the strength of the muscle is not thoroughly

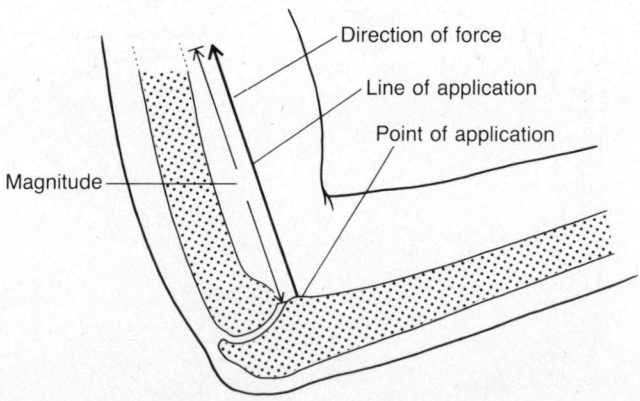

Fig. 3-1. The four characteristics of force.

Direction of force

Line of application

Point of application

Magnitude

evaluated. Several exercise devices attempt to account for the change in the mechanical factors of muscle contraction. These devices accommodate the resistance by matching the force applied and recording the resistance on a dial or graph for the full range of motion. Other devices provide cam systems or lever systems that vary the resistance through the range of motion so that less muscle force is needed in the weaker area. All of these devices attempt to provide an exercise effect or an indirect measure of strength throughout the entire movement.

Isometric muscle contractions indicate muscle strength at the tested joint position. The strength throughout the range of motion can be tested at several specific angles to obtain an idea of the strength throughout the range.[6] A tensiometer or dynamometer is the most common method used to indirectly test isometric muscle strength. Occasionally a free weight may be held to obtain a maximal determination of the static muscle strength. The actual strength of the muscle contraction can be estimated by using mathematical calculations.[23]

No valid or reliable method has been developed to measure eccentric, or lengthening, muscle strength, such as the quadriceps muscle contraction that occurs as one descends stairs or hamstring muscle contraction as the leg is decelerated during gait. Nevertheless, many muscle contractions are of the lengthening type.

The aspect of strength just discussed involves only a limited concept of strength. More information on strength is presented later in this chapter.

Pressure

Pressure defines how a force is distributed over an area. Although a force may often be represented by one line of application, it is distributed over the entire area of contact. This distribution of force over an entire area is called *pressure* and is measured in terms of force/unit area (e.g., pounds per square inch or N/cm^2). A large magnitude of force over a small area would have a relatively large amount of pressure, whereas a small force over a large area would have a small amount of pressure. On the other hand, a small force on a small area may have a greater amount of pressure than a large force distributed over a very large area. Pressure, then, is related to force but is not the same as force.

A striking example of the effect of a force on a small area occurs when a small piece of gravel becomes lodged in a runner's shoe. The force on the foot may be the same as when no foreign material is present in the shoe, but the area of the foot touching the gravel feels pain because of the reduced area taking the force. Damage to the foot may eventually occur. Often the pressure that develops is highly irritating even when the force is reduced as the runner slows to a walk. Similar pressure on the foot may result from wrinkled socks, a wrap, or tape. The athletic trainer must be careful not to allow wrinkles from a wrap

or tape on the area of the foot that will be taking a large force.

Also of concern is what may happen when a large force is applied to a small area over a period of time. Decubitus ulcers (pressure sores) result from soft tissue damage over the sacrum, heels, and ischial tuberosities when a person lies or sits in one position for an extended period.

Pads on braces and parts of casts and splints can cause the skin to break down if the area of contact is too small or the force on the contact area is too great. The following are examples of actions that may cause injury because they create forces over a very small area: being struck by a karate punch, being hit by a baseball or golf ball, or being stepped on by football cleats or track spikes. Extreme examples of high-pressure forces occur when a bullet or the tip of an arrow strikes an object.

Pressure also changes in the joints as they go through a range of motion and the joint configuration at contact changes. An important example of this is the change that occurs when a person goes from standing to a deep knee bend (Fig. 3-2). A decrease in the contact area between the femoral condyles and the tibia occurs, and the force produced by the quadriceps muscles increases greatly. The pressure in this situation also increases greatly and may even damage the knee if the action is done often enough with the individual holding a large weight. Pads help reduce pressure by distributing force over a larger area and thus reduce the chance of injury. Hip pads protect football players against a hip pointer injury, pads on the shoulders

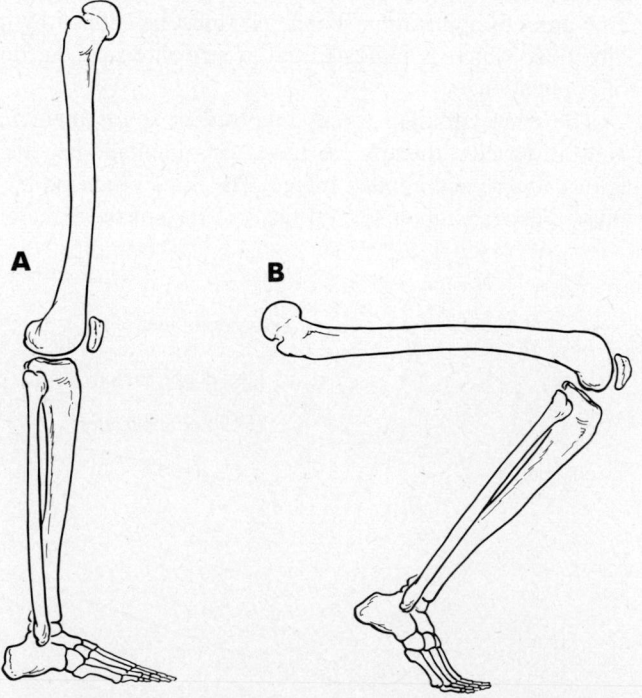

Fig. 3-2. Change in size of tibiofemoral joint contact area with **A,** knee extended, and **B,** knee flexed.

of lacrosse players and on the shins of soccer players protect against contusions, and helmets for children with cerebral palsy protect against concussions.

Power

The term power should not be confused with force. *Power* is the rate of doing work or dissipating energy. Two formulas for this entity expressed in terms of translatory (linear) motion are $P = Fd/t$ and $P = Fv$, where P stands for power, F for force, d for linear displacement, t for time, and v for linear velocity. Analogous formulas for rotatory motion are $P = T\Theta/t$ and $P = T \times \omega$, where T stands for torque, Θ for angular displacement, T for time, and ω for angular velocity. The combined terms—Fd and $T\Theta$—are part of the respective formulas for work in linear and rotatory movements. Some units of power are foot-pounds per second and newton-meters per second.

Force is contained within the concept of power but time is also an important aspect. An individual may be able to produce a great amount of force, but unless the force is produced rapidly, the amount of power may be low. Some sporting skills require force without regard to time; others emphasize the rate at which force is applied. Training for power activities can be quite different from training for events requiring strength. The type of injury that may occur can also be related to the rate of energy dissipation.

Any musculoskeletal activity that requires moving an object during a short period of time involves the concept of power. Common tests for determining power are the vertical jump, the standing long jump, and the softball throw. Each of these activities requires the movement of an object against resistance. Many exercise specialists believe that a rapid contraction of muscles, generating a large amount of force, provides a large magnitude of power as the body or ball is displaced.[23,44] The magnitude of displacement is considered to be an indirect measure of the individual's power.

Individuals who sprint, jump, or throw an object for speed or distance during a sport must have the strength to provide a large amount of force and the neuromuscular coordination to contract the muscles rapidly. Training for power is specific and the individual must train the muscle to contract rapidly against a heavy load. Thistle et al.[42] and Moffroid and Whipple[25] have discussed this concept in greater detail in several articles.

Load, stress, and strain

An outside force or group of forces acting on an object is called a *load*. A heavy box placed on a table provides an external force or load on the table. The same box carried by an individual places a load on that individual in several areas. The muscles resisting the load of the box place a load on the bone. The combined weight of the box and muscle forces place a load on the various joints. (The load and the reaction to the load must be evaluated separately

for each individual joint.) A blow to the thigh is a load to the soft tissue of the thigh. The compression caused by an elastic bandage in an attempt to reduce swelling is a load on the area covered. Adhesive tape applied to the ankle in an attempt to prevent injury is a load across the ankle joint. The exercise resistance provided by sandbags on the distal end of the leg is a load offered to the muscles in an attempt to strengthen them as they apply force across the knee. A load can act directly on a point or at some distance away from the point of application.

Forces within the loaded object react to the external load. These internal forces are distributed across an area within the object and are defined in terms of force/unit area, or $S = F/A$. The internal reaction or resistance to the external load is called *mechanical stress*. Often as an external load is applied to an object, deformation occurs. This deformation or change in dimensions is called *mechanical strain*.

Three principal stresses exist: tension, compression, and shear (Fig. 3-3). Tension occurs when the external forces (load) applied are colinear and act in opposite directions (away from each other). Compression is present when the external forces applied are colinear and act toward each other. Shear results when two parallel forces, opposite in direction and not colinear, cause one point on a surface of an object to slide past a point on an adjacent surface. A few examples of stress and resulting strain will be discussed.

Tension. Tension stress occurs within the lateral ligaments as the foot is excessively inverted, within the patellar tendon as the quadriceps muscles contract, within the anterior longitudinal ligament of the lumbar area during increased lumbar lordosis, and within the conoid and trapezoid ligaments as the arm is elevated. Sprains, strains, and avulsion fractures may result if the load exceeds the ability of the materials to resist.

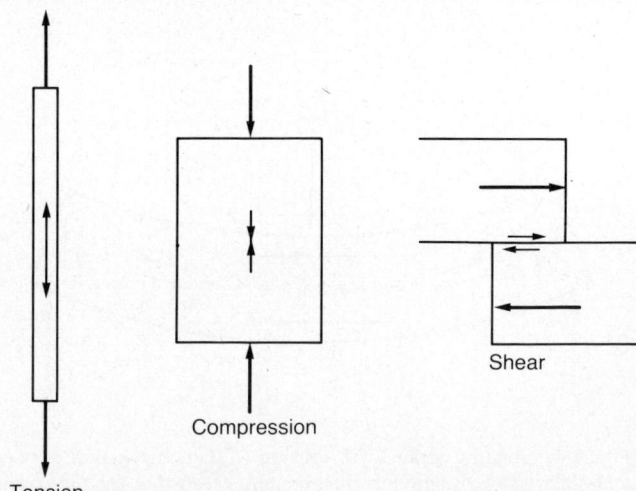

Fig. 3-3. The three principal stresses or strains.

Often individuals apply a load to obtain stretching of muscles or certain connective tissues. Tension strain occurs as the soft tissue elongates.

Compression. Compression stress occurs within the patella femoral joint as the quadriceps muscles contract, within the glenohumeral joint when the shoulder muscles contract, within a muscle or bone when struck directly, and within cartilage or bone when directly loaded. Some common results of this type of stress may be arthritic changes, contusions, fractures, or herniations.

Shear. Shear stress may exist in epiphyseal plates as the separate parts of the bones are loaded; between the sacrum, disks, and vertebrae as the psoas muscle contracts; and between the skin and underlying tissue as the skin is abraded. Epiphyseal breaking; apophyseal-type injuries, including Osgood-Schlatter disease and Sever's disease; spondylolisthesis resulting when a vertebra slides forward past an adjacent vertebra or the sacrum; and blisters, abrasions, and rips of the hand occurring as the skin is rubbed are all examples of shearing injuries. Shearing loads are often established in joint implants, which may fail as a result of too much shearing load.[47]

The three-point principle

In common three-point bending, loads placed upon a horizontal beam set up stresses within the beam (Fig. 3-4), causing it to bend or strain in flexure.[12] Compression stress develops parallel to the length of the beam on the concave portion, whereas tension stress develops parallel to the length of the beam in its convex portion. A neutral axis is located along the center of the beam where no compression or tension occurs. Shear stress is also produced maximally in two directions within the bending beam. One maximal shearing stress is parallel to the load and perpendicular to the compression and tension stress. The sum of this shearing stress results in the bending of the beam. The second shearing stress is parallel to the beam as the horizontal layers of the beam attempt to slide past each other.

A common karate demonstration can be set up according to these principles, with the supports as two points and the striking force as the third point. Gymnasts supported by the parallel bars, high bar, or uneven bars demonstrate the three-point loading principle in equipment. Several types of braces for the finger, wrist, and knee also employ this principle.

In cantilever bending one end of a beam is fixed, and the free end is loaded (Fig. 3-5). In this situation tension is created in the upper convex portion of the beam, whereas compression occurs in the lower concave part. Shearing stresses are established parallel to the load and parallel to the beam. In the supporting column, compression stress is added on the beam side to the compression caused by the load, and tension is created on the opposite side, which subtracts from the load's compression. Situations such as these occur often in athletics, as well as daily activities. Common examples are the loading of the proximal end of the femur and the lower limb when an individual is standing, and the hyperextended finger as an object strikes the end of the finger. A basketball player grabbing the rim of the basket may set up cantilever bending. Several other examples include the stress in a pole during vaulting, in a baseball bat during hitting, in a diving board in diving, in

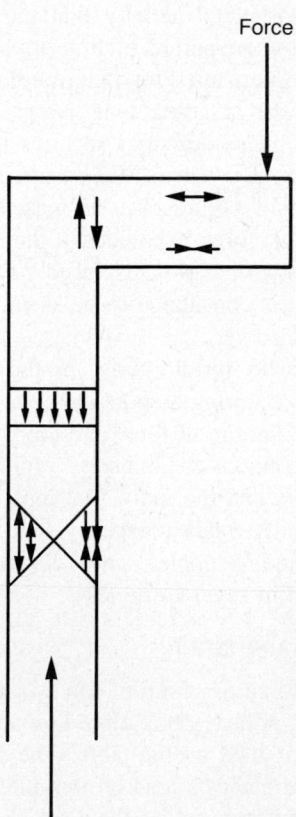

Force

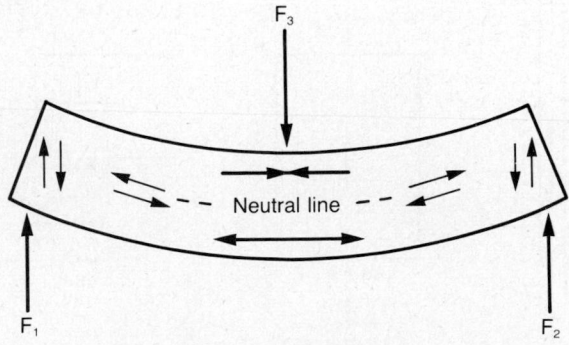

Fig. 3-4. Bending strain with tension (◯), compression (→←), and shear (⇆). Examples are bracing, greenstick fractures, and knee injury. This is the basic three-point principle (three forces: F_1, F_2, and F_3).

Fig. 3-5. Forces acting in cantilever bending, which result in strains of tension (◯), compression (→←), and shear (⇆). An example is the femur and lower limb as a whole.

several splints designed by therapists, and on the handle of a common cane in walking. Some protective equipment such as shoulder pads and face guards are examples of the cantilever design.

Torsion

In torsion loading of an object, stresses also develop (Fig. 3-6). Compression and tension occur in a spiral pattern at a 45-degree angle and perpendicular to the long axis of the object. Shearing stresses lie in two planes: one parallel to the long axis of the object and the other parallel to the applied load. Two common examples of torsion injuries are spiral fractures, which occur in the tibia during skiing and in the humerus during throwing.[43,50]

Stress at a point anywhere within an object is related to the bending moment established by the load, the distance the point is from the neutral axis, and the shape of the beam. Since the outer surface of the object is the greatest distance from the neutral axis, maximal compression or tension will occur at that location.[7-9,12,39]

Strength of materials

An important aspect of strength referred to earlier is related to stress, or the ability of an object to resist a load. A strong material can withstand a great load before it breaks. This type of material has a high level of stress. This aspect of strength has different measures, however. The ultimate strength of an object is the greatest load that the object can sustain. The breaking strength of an object is the load at the time the object fails. The yield strength occurs at the load level that produces a permanent deformation within the material.[27] Frankel and Nordin[11] present three different characteristics for determining the strength of an object: (1) the load the object can sustain before it breaks, (2) the deformation that the object can withstand before it breaks, and (3) the energy the object can store before it breaks.

The stress-strain curve (Fig. 3-7) shows the relationship between the internal resistance of a material to a load and to its own elongation and provides an illustrative graph of the strength properties of an object.[12,28] Each type of material has a unique curve. Certain characteristics of the curve, however, are similar for various types of materials. The first portion of the curve is a straight line that represents Hooke's law; that is, the strain is directly proportional to the ability of the material to resist the load. This portion of the curve, B, refers to the *elastic range*. If the load is released while the stress-strain curve is in the elastic area, the material will return to its original size and shape (elasticity). The ordinate point at which Hooke's law no longer holds is called the *proportional limit, A*, while the ordinate point beyond which the material will not return to its original size and shape is termed the *elastic limit*. These two points may be the same on the stress-strain curve. The region beyond the elastic limit to the point of rupture is called the *plastic range, C*. A material strained within this region of the curve remains permanently deformed. Some materials have either a small plastic range or none at all. Other materials have a plastic range that includes a yield point (Y) or an ordinate point at which an increase of strain occurs without an increase of stress, an ordinate point of ultimate strength (U), and a point of rupture of breaking strength (R).

Knowledge of the strength characteristics of certain materials is important in orthopaedic and sports medicine. Biological materials such as muscle, bone, ligaments, tendons, and cartilage may need improved strength to avoid breaking.[8] Knowledge of strength values and how much load will bring about these levels of stress within a material could be of great importance.

Increased strength in ligaments can help protect joints and prevent injuries. Some ligaments that contain more elastin are more extensible to allow increased range of movement, whereas other ligaments with more collagen elongate less to provide more stability. The strength of bone decreases with disuse such as prolonged bed rest. Care must be taken not to overload these bones until sufficient strength has been regained. Often treatment is performed to stretch joint tissues, break adhesions, or correct

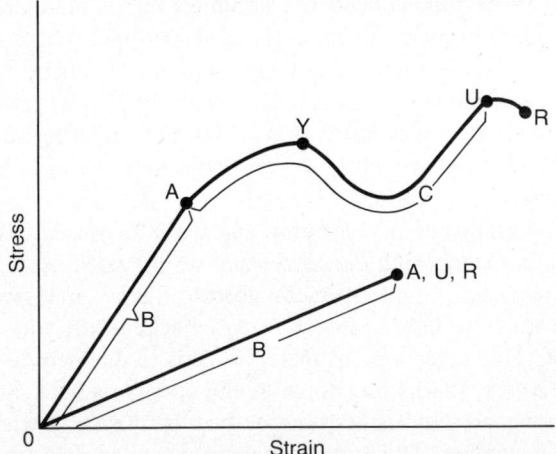

Fig. 3-7. Stress-strain curve showing elastic or proportional limit (A), yield point (Y), elastic range (B), ultimate strength (U), plastic range (C), and rupture or breaking strength (R).

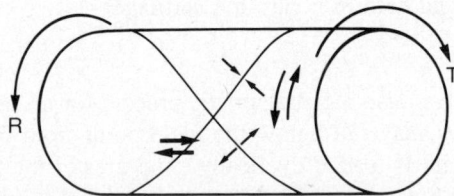

Fig. 3-6. Applied torque (T) and resisting torque (R) setting up resulting strains of tension (↻), compression, (→←), and shear (⇆). Examples are spiral fracture or twisting fractures.

deformities. Important questions are: How much force should be applied? Where? For how long? Without some knowledge of material strength, these questions cannot be accurately answered.

The stress-strain characteristics of building equipment and appliance materials also need to be known so that proper materials will be used for their intended purposes. Low strength in a cast, prosthesis, diving board, vaulting pole, or high bar could be disastrous. A certain amount of elasticity within these materials is essential. Knowledge of the elastic characteristics of materials for taping and wrapping allows the practitioner to intelligently select the necessary grade of tape or type of wrap to use. The differences between an elastic wrap and a cotton webbing wrap are important. In some cases as a body part swells the material must elongate (strain) but still resists the swelling with compression; in other instances a wrap to protect an injured ligament should have less ability to elongate or the ligament will not be protected sufficiently.

Resilience

Most materials have a certain resilience and toughness. These characteristics are related to the absorption and release of energy as a material is loaded rapidly on impact. The amount of work done on a unit volume of a material as a load is applied rapidly from zero to the proportional limit of the material defines the modulus of resilience for that material. The resilience of a material is its ability to absorb energy within the elastic range.[18]

As a resilient material is loaded, work is done on it and it will absorb energy. When the load is released, the energy is released and the material will return to its original shape. An excellent example of this concept is the resilience of a tennis ball. If it is highly resilient, it will bounce back from a hard surface to approximately the same height from which it was dropped (live ball). If it has poor resilience, it will not bounce as high (dead ball). Resilience seems to be time dependent. An object that is highly resilient tends to return to its original shape quickly and give off the absorbed energy quickly. A poorly resilient material tends to return to its original shape slowly and give off low-level energy as heat. Thus a common characteristic of resilience is the ability of an object to bounce back quickly.

The resilience of a playing surface is of major importance in determining the nature and severity of certain athletic injuries. Some surfaces absorb energy and give it back quickly. Others absorb energy but return it with less vigor. This latter type of material tends to dampen the applied force, dissipating some of the energy as heat. Some materials are not resilient but deform permanently when a load is applied. This type of material is called *analastic;* it is neither elastic nor resilient.[12] (An example would be a ball of bread dough dropped on the kitchen counter. The dough is deformed and does not bounce.) Playing surfaces

with this characteristic become permanently deformed and could easily be injurious to the athlete. A very muddy playing field covered with deep footprints is an example of an analastic surface. Knee and ankle injuries could result from playing on this type of field. A playing surface such as pavement, concrete, or tile that returns energy too quickly may also cause injury such as shin splints and stress fractures to the lower limb. Some surfaces such as wrestling mats, landing mats for gymnastics, and jumping pits should have limited resilience. They should absorb the energy and give it off slowly, but they should not become permanently deformed.

Toughness

The amount of work done on a unit volume of material as a load is applied rapidly from zero to the point of rupture defines the *modulus of toughness.* The ability of a material to absorb energy within the plastic range is called *toughness.* An important aspect of the toughness of a material is its ability to absorb energy without breaking.[28] Quite often practitioners in orthopaedics and sports medicine are concerned with the toughness of a material. The ability of ligaments, cartilage, bone, muscles, and tendons to absorb energy without rupturing is important for the prevention of injury. If too much energy is absorbed, however, the material may rupture violently, as occurs in some sprains, strains, and fractures.[29]

Creep

Creep occurs when a low-magnitude load, below the yield point and usually within the elastic range, is applied over a long period of time. This process is most obvious in metals and viscoelastic materials such as biological tissues. Creep occurs in all types of materials and with any level of load. The greater the load, however, the more rapidly the rate of creep progresses. Increasing the temperature also tends to increase the rate of creep. A load placed on an object for an extended period of time will cause the material to elongate. Eventually, permanent plastic deformation will result or the material may break.[8] This concept is applied during stretching exercises, which should have a prolonged duration with sufficient load to accomplish the desired effects. A warmed muscle should be more easily stretched. Posture and exercise positions held for a long period of time, such as yoga, may stretch ligaments and muscles and deform bones and cartilage.

Fatigue

Fatigue is also a characteristic process for all materials. A material may fail below the yield point from fatigue if the material is loaded cyclically. The greater the load applied, the fewer number of cycles are needed for the material to break. A minimal load, however, is necessary below which an infinite number of cycles will not cause failure of the material. This is called the *endurance limit* of that material.[8] A common example of fatigue failure is the breaking of a wire by bending it back and forth rapidly several times. Fatigue fractures in runners, dancers, and marching soldiers provide examples of mechanical fatigue.* Fatigue fractures (stress fractures) often develop in runners because of excessive mileage or poor mechanics of running style. A jogger with a 2-m stride will have 5,000 cycles on one lower limb while traveling 10,000 m. If the athlete is heavy, there will be an increased load and subsequent stress upon the lower limb. Daily jogging at this distance may cause a fatigue fracture in one of the bones of the lower limb. Common areas of fracture are the fibula, the metatarsal, the tibia, and the calcaneal bone.[46] A "march fracture" is another common example of fatigue fracture.

Several authors[21,34,35,49] have identified a fatigue fracture of the pars interarticular bone (spondylolysis) as a common cause of low back pain in athletes. Athletes participating in events requiring repeated hyperlordotic lumbar curves show the highest percentage of this condition.[35,36] The events include gymnastics, diving, weightlifting, wrestling, and jumping activities in track and field.

Equipment may also fail from mechanical fatigue. Usually safety factors are provided for in the construction of equipment, although safety factors for biological tissues are not known. Tissues can repair themselves, however, if the load is not too great.

COMPOSITION AND RESOLUTION OF FORCES
Resolution

A force is directed along one line of action. This force, however, may be divided into its effective components. Dividing a force into its components or replacing a single force by two or more equivalent forces is called the *resolution of force* (Fig. 3-8, *A*). Forces acting on a bone, such as the pull of a muscle or the weight of a load, most often occur as one component perpendicular to the bone and one parallel to the bone (Fig. 3-8, *B* and *C*). The perpendicular component is the rotatory component, whereas the parallel component is nonrotatory. The nonrotatory component compresses a joint or distracts the bone of the joint. Either effect may be useful or hazardous to the joint, depending upon the situation. Placing a large load of sandbags or a weighted boot on the foot to exercise the quadriceps muscles after a knee ligament injury may damage the injured ligament because of the distracting force. A distracting component of force, however, may be beneficial in reducing joint friction and the potential change of arthritis. Compression components may help stabilize the joint, but increased compression force may cause increased wear and tear on the joint surfaces. Forces directed through joints may occur as a normal (perpendicular to the surface) component and a shearing, or tangential (parallel to the sur-

*See references 2, 5, 32, 35, 46, and 48.

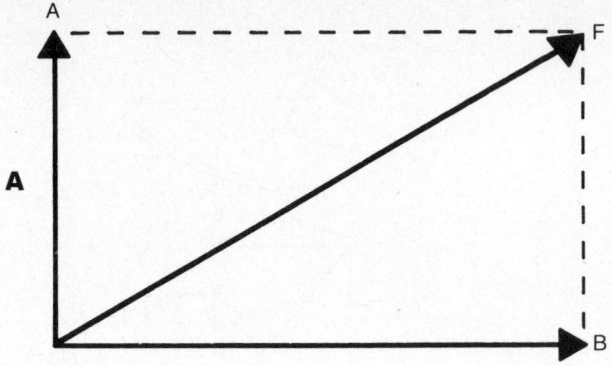

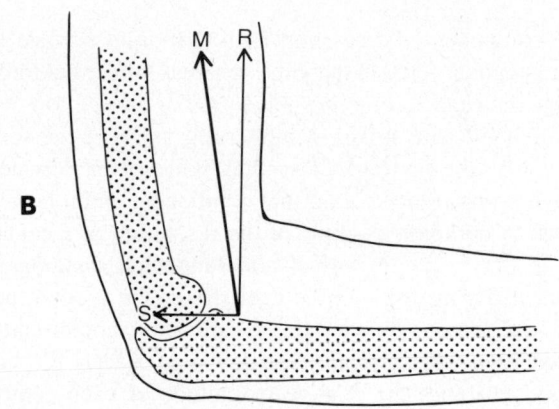

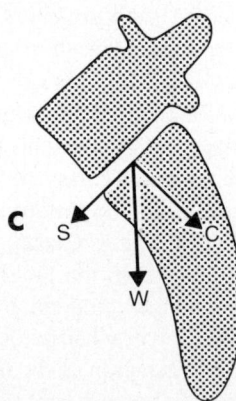

Fig. 3-8. A, *A* and *B* are rectangular components of force *(F)*. **B,** Rotary *(R)* and stabilizing *(S)* components of muscle force *(M)*. **C,** Compression *(C)* and shearing *(S)* force components of the superincumbent weight *(W)* at the lumbosacral junction.

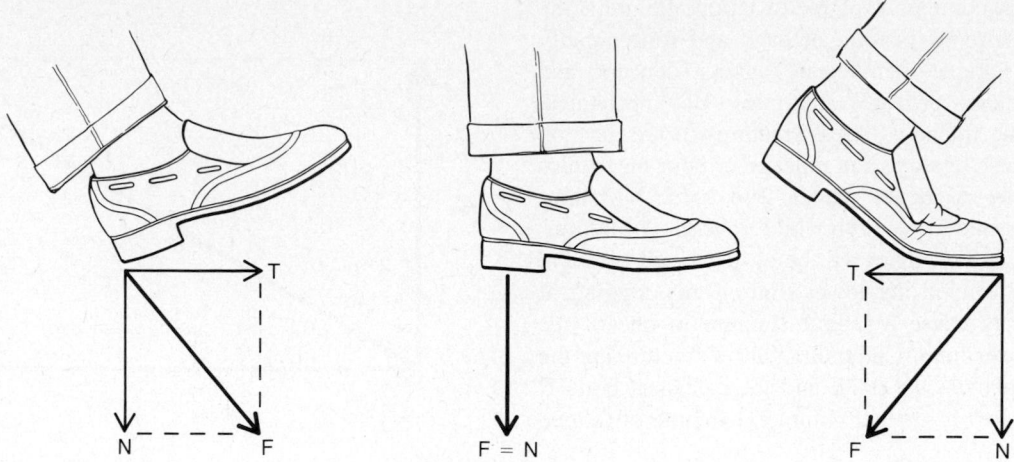

Fig. 3-9. Normal *(N)* and tangential *(T)* components of contact force *(F)* during gait.

face), component. Forces normal to the joint surface increase frictional force in the joint, whereas tangential forces increase the chance for joint subluxation or dislocation.

As a body part strikes a supporting surface, the force imparted by the body part also may be resolved (divided) into two components—a normal component and a tangential one. A common example of the resolution of a contact force is the resulting normal and tangential components that occur during gait. As the heel strikes the ground, part of the heel force is directed downward, and another part is directed along the ground. The angle at which the heel strikes determines the relative magnitude of each component (Fig. 3-9). A heel strike that is nearly perpendicular to the ground has little tangential force component. If the angle is more horizontal, however, the normal component is reduced and the tangential component is increased. A high coefficient of friction between the heel and ground is necessary if the angle is much less than 90 degrees. With a low coefficient of friction, such as occurs when a person is walking on ice, the steps should be short and almost perpendicular to the ground, or the heel may slip and the individual will fall. Similar situations exist if one walks on a wet locker room floor or plays on a wet gymnasium floor, a wet artificial grass surface, or a muddy grassy field. Understanding these force components is also important in changing directions while running and jumping. Cleats, spikes, and starting blocks allow an increase in the tangential component. Some athletes, such as high jumpers, need more normal force and less tangential force, whereas other types, such as long jumpers, need a combination of the normal component for height and the tangential component for distance.

Frictional force

The practitioner of sports and orthopaedic injury management must be aware of the contact force components and the interaction between the surfaces. Frictional force,

established when two objects are in contact, is the force component parallel to the surfaces at the point of contact. In curved objects the frictional component would be tangential to the surfaces.

Determination of the frictional force component is simple. The formula $F_f = \mu N$ states that the maximal friction force F_f equals the product of the coefficient of friction between the two surfaces (μ) times the normal force component (N). Different types of surfaces have different coefficients of friction. Moisture often reduces the value of the coefficient of friction. In specific situations, increasing or decreasing the coefficient of friction of the surfaces involved may reduce the chance of injury to the athlete.

Calculation of force components

The method to determine the magnitude of force components is based upon simple trigonometry and algebra, which can be reviewed in most kinesiology and physics textbooks.[1,23,34] Calculating these components may provide valuable information, such as the exercise effect of a load, the hazardous effects of certain exercises, or the advantageous position to place a body part in to gain a maximal result (e.g., the lower limb in a sprint start).

Composition

Often several forces acting on an object have a singular resulting effect (Fig. 3-10, *A*). This effect is called the *resultant force* and the process of determining this effect is called the *composition of forces*. Many examples of the composition of forces exist in the human body. Two or more muscles may act in different directions and along different lines of force to produce a desired motion. The combined pull of the muscles of the quadriceps provides a single resultant force that acts upon the patella (Fig. 3-10, *B*). The pull of the soleus muscle and the heads of the gastrocnemius muscle combine as one force upon the calca-

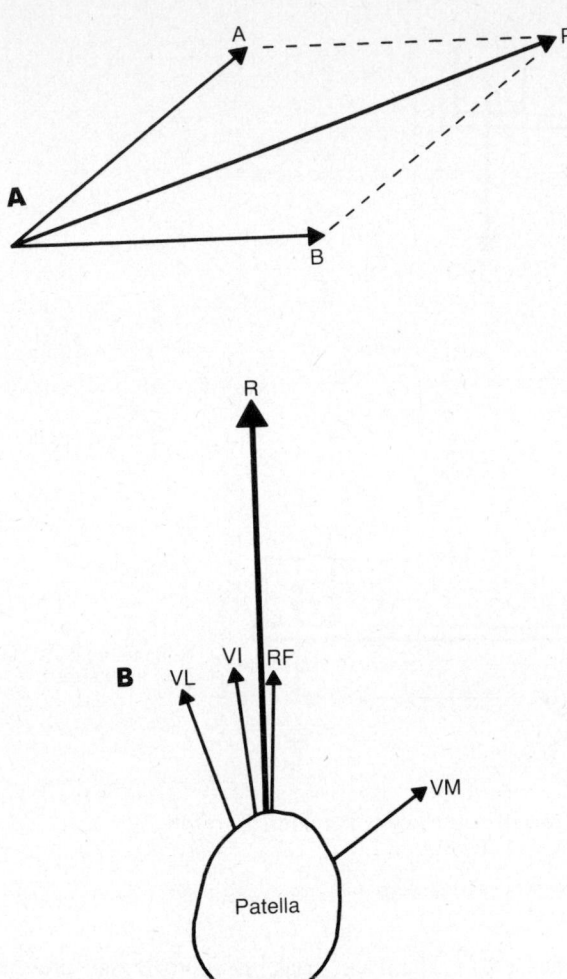

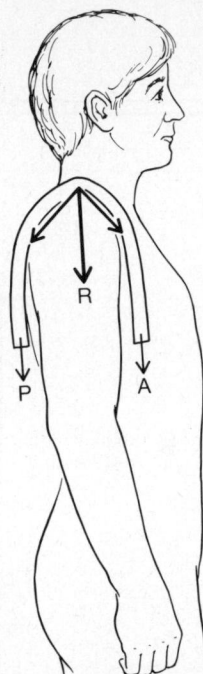

Fig. 3-11. Forces applied anteriorly *(A)* and posteriorly *(P)* to obtain a resultant force *(R)* on acromioclavicular joint.

Fig. 3-10. A, Forces *A* and *B* acting together to provide a resultant force *(R).* **B,** Resultant force *(R)* of the quadriceps muscle on the patella terminating in the combined forces of the vastus lateralis *(VL),* vastus intermedias *(VI),* rectus femoris *(RF),* and vastus medialis *(VM).*

neal bone. Other muscle combinations provide similar actions. Often the direction for making use of a single force is not practical for some reason. Therefore two or more forces are combined to give the desired single force. The acromioclavicular joint cannot easily be repaired to correct its subluxation. Forces may be applied anteriorly and posteriorly, however, so that a resulting force is applied in the desired direction on the joint (Fig. 3-11).

Injuries may also occur because of the combination of forces. Increased compression of the patellofemoral joint occurs as the forces from the quadriceps muscle group and the patellar tendon act on the patella.

MOMENTS OF FORCE
Torque

When a load acts on an object, it often acts at a distance (the lever arm) from a point of pivot or fulcrum. The prod-

uct of this distance times the force component perpendicular to the lever arm is the moment of force (Moment [M] = Force [F] × distance [d]). Thus the moment of force, or torque, developed depends upon the magnitude of force and the length of the lever arm (Fig. 3-12). The units of measure include foot-pounds and newton-meters.

Lever systems

A greater amount of force or a longer lever arm increases the moment of force. Leverage may be set up so that a small force applied to a relatively long arm can produce the same torque as a large force at the end of a short lever arm (Fig. 3-12, *A*). The reverse is also true. The same large force as on a short lever arm will only hold a small load at the end of a long lever arm (Fig. 3-12, *B*). The mechanical advantage (MA) of a lever system is the ratio of the length of the effort arm (dE) to the length of the resistance arm (dR), or MA = dE/dR. The effort arm is the distance of the applied force to the fulcrum, and the resistance arm is the distance from the fulcrum to the resisting load. If the effort arm is greater than the resistance arm, the mechanical advantage is greater than 1. If the resistance arm is greater than the effort arm, the mechanical advantage is less than 1.

Although a gain in force is often a reason for using a lever system, other effects may also be important. If the effort arm is shorter than the resistance arm (MA < 1), the resisting load will travel farther and faster than the point of application of the effort force. This result may be more

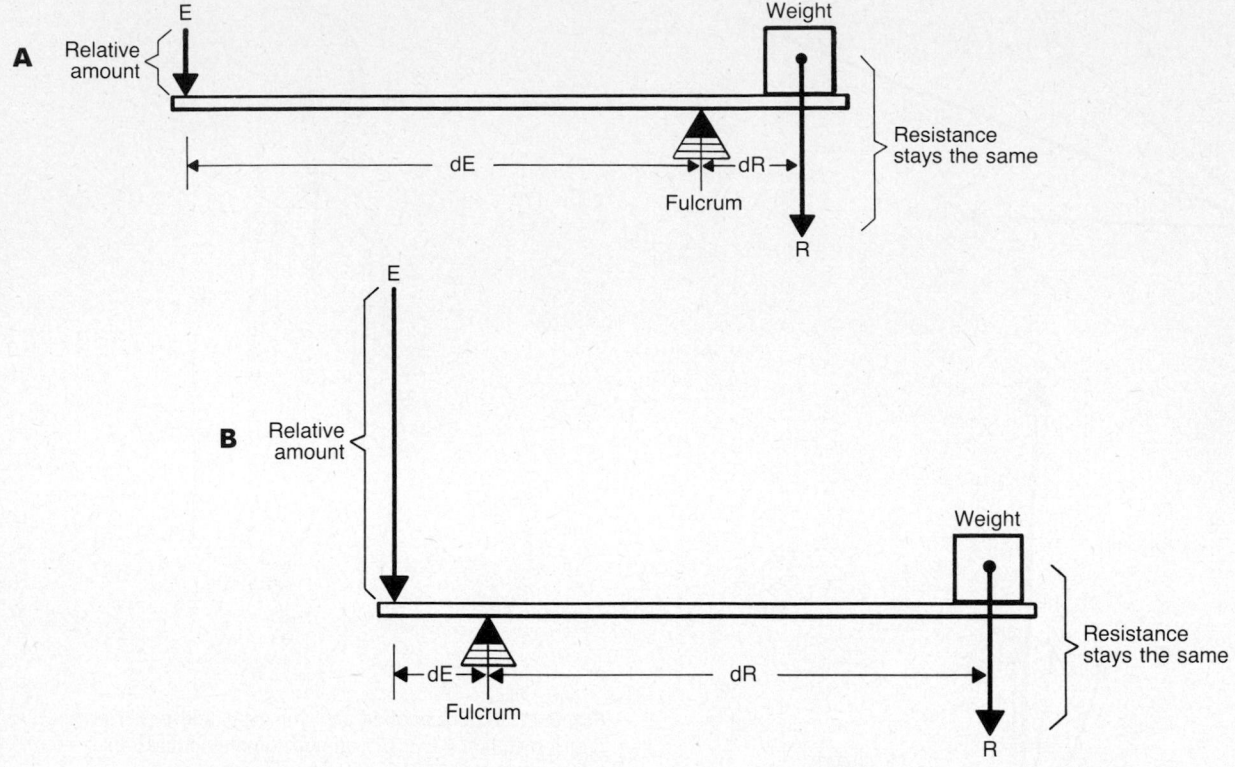

Fig. 3-12. Moment of force and mechanical advantage (MA) demonstrated with effort *(E)*, effort arm *(dE)*, resistance *(R)*, and resistance arm *(dR)*. **A,** MA > 1. **B,** MA < 1.

important than a gain in force. The lever systems of the human body generally have the effort arm much shorter than the resistance arm.

More than one effort force and more than one resistance force may be involved within a lever system (Fig. 3-13). These forces do not always act perpendicular to the lever arm. Therefore the force components perpendicular to the lever arm, or the calculated lever arm perpendicular to the line of action of each force, must be used to determine the moments of force. The effort forces and resistance forces are not the only forces involved in the lever system. An important force is that acting at the fulcrum. A reaction force in a joint occurs as a muscle contracts.

An example of a lever system that has several forces acting simultaneously is the forearm with a weight in the hand. The effort forces are the elbow flexors, mainly the brachialis, biceps, and brachioradialis muscles. The resisting forces are the weight of the limb and the weight held in the hand. The elbow joint reaction force can be determined by summing the components of forces acting on the forearm.

The length of an object and the force applied to that object are of great importance in musculoskeletal rehabilitation and injury prevention. Research relating to skiing injuries has shown that longer skis can produce more severe injuries.[7,26,50] The face mask in football has prevented several types of facial injuries, but the length of the bars protruding from the helmet provide an increased lever arm from which severe cervical injuries may result.[17] Exercise programs also make use of the principle of moments for gradation of the exercise effect. Bent-leg curls to strengthen the abdominal muscles may be made more difficult by having the individual move the arm position more distally from the hip. This maneuver will provide a longer resistance arm for the same force. Because the weight of the legs provides a long resistance arm, double leg-raising places a great load on the iliopsoas muscles, resulting in hazardous stress on the lower back. Placement of the practitioner's hands and the length of the client's limbs may affect the results obtained during manual muscle testing. Taller athletes, athletes with longer limbs, and athletes using longer rackets all make use of the principle of moment by having longer effort or longer resistance arms. Sometimes the situation may be advantageous; other times it may be a disadvantage.

Laws of equilibrium

Since there are abundant examples of moments in sports medicine, the practitioner should make a habit of evaluating moment situations and the mechanical advantage

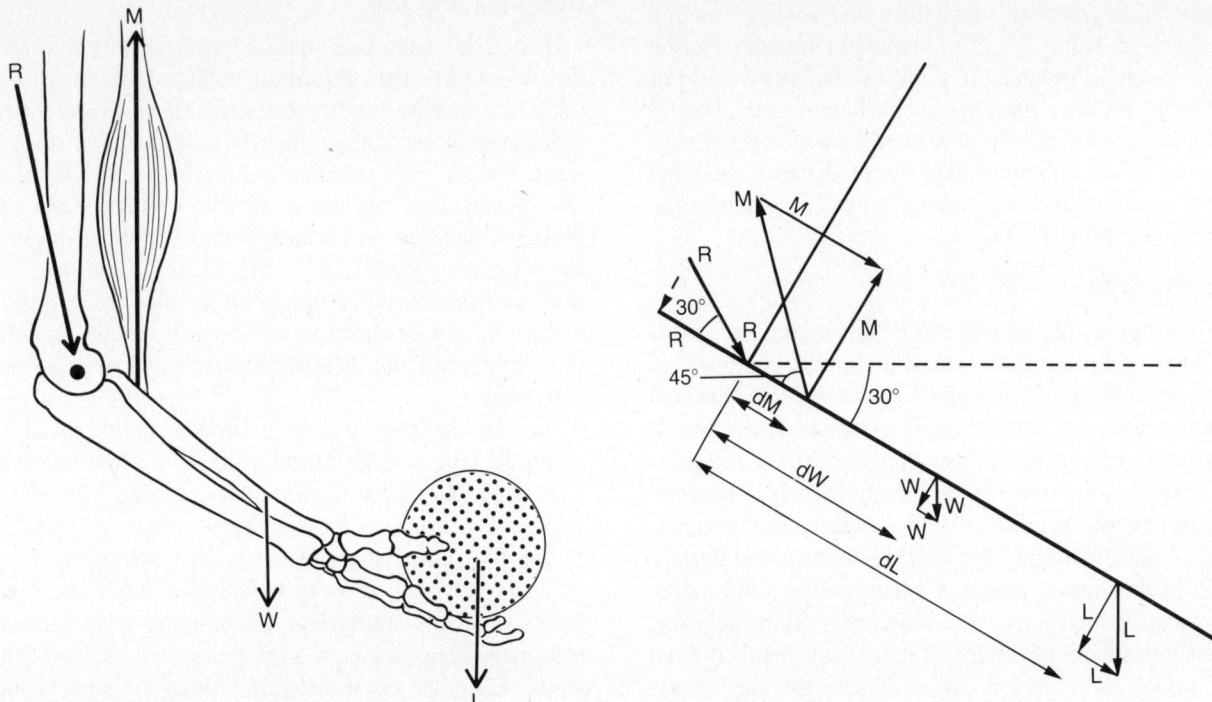

Fig. 3-13. Several forces involved on a lever system, including muscle force *(M)*, limb weight *(W)*, load *(L)*, and joint reaction force *(R)*. (Adapted from LeVeau B: Williams and Lissner biomechanics of human motion, Philadelphia, 1977, WB Saunders Co.)

present. To determine the forces acting on an object, the first and second conditions of equilibrium must be used. The first states that when the sum of all the forces acting on an object is zero, the object is in translational equilibrium $(\Sigma F = 0)$. This condition holds for all three cardinal planes so that $\Sigma F_x = 0$, $\Sigma F_y = 0$, and $\Sigma F_z = 0$.

The second condition of equilibrium states that when the sum of all the moments acting on an object is zero, the object is in rotatory equilibrium; that is, the clockwise moments will equal the counterclockwise moments and no angular motion will occur $(\Sigma M = 0)$. Calculations based upon accurate free body diagrams provide reasonable estimates of the forces involved in a situation. Once these estimates are determined, the situation may be more accurately assessed.

KINEMATICS
Motion

Forces tend to cause objects to move. Often, however, when an author describes the biomechanics of motion of a body part, only the ranges of motion are given, although biomechanics frequently includes several other characteristics. These characteristics are within the study of *kinetics,* which is concerned with the forces that effect motion. *Kinematics* is concerned with describing motion. Movement

in both translation (linear motion) and rotation (angular motion) must be considered.

Time, displacement, velocity, and acceleration

Motion is described by four terms: time, displacement, velocity, and acceleration. The concept of *time* is often used in gait analysis, as well as in the analysis of movement in various sporting activities. Time is also a vital part of velocity and acceleration.

Displacement is change in an object's position. It refers both to the distance between the original position and the final position and to the direction of the movement. Velocity is the time rate of change of displacement. It is how rapidly the object is moved. Displacement may be calculated by dividing the displacement by the amount of time elapsed. *Velocity* has both magnitude and direction. The term *speed,* however, has only magnitude. Often the terms velocity and speed are used interchangeably if direction is of no concern or is obvious.

Acceleration is the rate of change of velocity. It has magnitude and direction. Deceleration is the common term used for negative acceleration. As the magnitude or direction of velocity changes, the object will have an acceleration and will speed up, slow down, or change direction.

The symbols and equations for displacement, velocity,

and acceleration for both translatory and rotatory motion are presented in Table 3-1. The values for rotatory motion are often given in radians. If this is done, conversion of translatory to rotatory motion can be determined. The lever or tangential movement characteristics of a point on a rotating object can be determined by the distance the point is from the axis of rotation, or its radius, as given in the rotatory equations in Table 3-1.

Motion and injury

The description of motion can be invaluable to practitioners when determining the cause of injury, the extent of injury, and the effects of treatment. Knowledge of the normal characteristics of movement is essential. If the practitioner knows normal movement characteristics, the presence of abnormal motion can be determined. An abnormal running or walking pattern can cause injuries in several areas of the body, including the foot, knee, hip, and back.[41] Analysis of an injured person's gait provides information on the extent of the injury. The range of motion, velocity, and acceleration of the lower limb are all changed from normal values as a person limps. Treatment can be expected to bring these gait characteristics to within normal values.

Study of the acceleration and deceleration of the head during football activities provides information about injuries to the head and neck.[17-19] Similar studies have been done for hockey injuries.[38] Most descriptions of motion, however, concern the forces that affect the motion. Kinematics provides only a limited amount of information concerning motion. The study of kinetics, on the other hand, provides information about how forces affect the motion of an object.

KINETICS

The study of the forces that produce or affect motion is called kinetics. These are the same forces that have been discussed in the previous section. The laws of motion developed by Newton form the basis for the study of kinetics.

Table 3-1. Formulas for kinematic characteristics

Characteristic	Translatory motion	Rotatory motion*	Conversion of rotatory to translatory motion†
Displacement	d	Θ	$d = r\Theta$
Velocity	$v = \dfrac{d}{t}$	$\omega = \dfrac{\Theta}{t}$	$v = r\psi$
Acceleration	$a = \dfrac{v}{t}$	$\alpha = \dfrac{\psi}{t}$	$a_t = r\alpha$

*Θ, Angular displacement; t, time; ω, angular velocity; α, angular acceleration; r, radius.
†Units in radians (1 radian = 57.3 degrees).

Newton's first law

Force has often been defined as the entity that accelerates an object. This definition implies motion. The acceleration, either positive or negative, of an object is its rate of change of velocity, which is brought about by one or more forces. This concept is presented in Newton's first law of motion—the law of inertia—which states that an object remains in its existing state of motion unless acted upon by an outside force. Therefore a stationary object will not begin to move unless an unbalanced outside force acts on it, and an object in motion will remain in motion at the same speed and direction unless acted upon by an outside force.

Inertia can play a role in understanding head injury when damage is done to the brain by a blow to the skull. The skull may show little outward damage, but the brain may suffer severe injury. One theory explains that damage to the generally self-protected brain results from the skull being rapidly forced away by a blow, while the brain remains relatively stationary. The moving skull contacts the stationary brain, damaging the brain without fracturing the skull. A similar situation occurs when the head is moving rapidly, is suddenly stopped by a blow, and the brain continues moving until it contacts the skull. Mass movements of the brain in such instances can cause contusions on the blow side of the brain and tissue tearing on the opposite side.[18]

Once the muscles initiate the motion, inertia is a major cause of the continued motion of the swinging lower limb as an athlete is sprinting. An outside force is needed to decelerate and stop the leg (a strong contraction of the hamstring muscles). Hamstring strains could result if the force needed for deceleration is greater than hamstring muscle strength.

Lesions of the pitching arm are also related to the law of inertia. As the arm is drawn back in the cocked phase, a sudden strong forward motion is initiated by the internal rotator muscles to overcome the inertia of the arm and to accelerate the arm and ball. Immediate muscle or joint damage or humeral fracture may result.*

Newton's second law

Newton's second law of motion is the law of acceleration. It states that if an outside force acts upon an object, the object will change its velocity or accelerate in direct proportion to the force applied. The object will also accelerate in inverse proportion to its mass. Hence, mass tends to resist acceleration. The well-known formula $F = ma$ demonstrates this relationship, which, according to Newton's law, would be expressed as $a = F/m$.

The formula $a = F/m$ holds for objects moving in translation or linearly. The units for linear acceleration are ft/sec^2 or ms^2. An analogous formula exists for objects rotat-

*See references 3, 14, 16, 37, 40, 43, and 44.

ing around a point. This formula is $\alpha = T/I$, where α is angular acceleration, T is torque, and I is the moment of inertia of the object. The units for angular acceleration are radians/sec^2. As mass resists change in linear motion, the moment of inertia resists change in angular motion. In general, the equation for the moment of inertia is $I = \Sigma mr^2$, where Σ is the sum over all the particles of mass (m) of the object and r is the average radii of all the particles of mass. This formula indicates that the distribution of mass along the axis of motion is a major contributing factor for the resistance-to-change of angular motion.

A flywheel on a machine is an example of the moment of inertia. The term *radius of gyration* is related to "r" in the moment of inertia formula. It is similar to the term "center of mass." The radius of gyration is the magnitude of a radius such that the moment of inertia for the object would be unchanged if the entire mass of the object were located at that distance from the center of rotation. Most movements of the body, especially swinging limbs, are rotatory. Thus the angular formulas should often be applied when determining the characteristics of a moving body.

Newton's third law

Gravity is an outside force that is always acting on an object on the earth. To balance this increasing force, a second outside force must be introduced. An object resting on a table is acted upon by at least two forces: the force of gravity and the force exerted by the table. This example illustrates Newton's third law of motion of the law of reaction. An object will react with a force of equal magnitude and in the opposite direction to the first force. Thus as the object on the table is acted on by the pull of gravity, the table reacts to the force of gravity with an equal and opposite force.

Impulse and momentum

Manipulation of the acceleration formula reveals a relationship between force, resistance to change in movement, velocity, and time, which can be expressed by two formulas: $F = M\Delta v/t$ and $T = I\Delta\omega/t$. The terms $M\Delta v$ and $I\Delta\omega$ represent the momentum of the object either in translatory or rotatory motion. These basic equations determine the force or torque needed to cause the movement (M or I), change in velocity (Δv, $\Delta\omega$), and the time taken for the change of occur. Often these two equations are used when a collision of objects occurs. When two objects collide, their combined momentum after the impact is equal to their combined momentum before the collision.

Simply stated, the law of conservation of momentum states that the change of momentum of the first object is equal in magnitude and opposite in direction to the change of momentum of the second object, or $M\Delta v = -m_2\Delta v_2$ and $I\Delta\omega = -I_2\Delta\omega_2$. Further manipulation of the equations $F = M\Delta v/t$ and $T = I\Delta\omega/t$ yields two impulse-momentum equations, $Ft = M\Delta v$ and $Tt = I\Delta\omega$. The product of force or torque and time is known as *impulse*, which is equal to the change in momentum. A greater force applied or a force applied over a longer period of time increases the momentum of an object.

An athlete or leisure activity participant often attempts to impart a great amount of momentum to an object by applying large force over a long period of time. On the other hand, if the momentum of an object must be reduced, the shorter the time period needed for the reduction of the object's momentum, the greater the force required. This concept is of great importance in sports medicine and orthopaedic therapy. Less force is needed if a longer time is taken to absorb or reduce the momentum of a moving object. The give of the hands as a person catches a ball is a common example of taking time to absorb a force, whereas the sudden stop of a moving object requires a large amount of force. A large amount of force develops rapidly as an automobile strikes a wall. Restraints and padded dashboards are usually provided to reduce force on the occupants by allowing more time for the force on the occupants by allowing more time for the force to be absorbed. A person who lands on the ground abruptly with the joints in extension may be seriously injured because the body's momentum is stopped quickly. A step from a stair or a curb or walking or running without a small amount of knee flexion can cause an increased load on the weight-bearing joints. The usual landing surfaces in jumping and gymnastic events require more time to absorb the momentum of the body. Thus less force is taken by the body.[45]

Work

If the force on an object is related to the location of the object, the principles of work and energy become important. In mechanics work refers to the product of the force exerted on an object and the object's displacement parallel to the resisting force component of the object (Work [W] = Force [F] × distance [d]). This concept is different from that of moments, which is also a force times a distance. Work is accomplished as the force overcomes a resistance and moves the object in a direction parallel to the resisting force component. A moment or torque, as discussed earlier, is the force component perpendicular to the lever arm times the distance of the point of application of force from the point of rotation. A force that produces torque can do work in rotatory motion. In this situation, the displacement is angular and the equation would be $W = T\Theta$.

During weight training positive work is done as the weight is raised and negative work is done as the weight is lowered. A combination of the linear and angular work formula may be used if the exercise device has weights that move in a linear fashion. If the load is moved in an angular fashion, the angular work formula should be used.

Energy

Energy is the capacity to do work. Many forms of energy exist, but the ones that will be considered in this chapter are mechanical energy and heat. Heat is often considered the byproduct of other forms of energy or results when one form of energy changes to another. Increased heat occurs when molecules of the heated area increase their amount of motion.

Mechanical energy can be divided into two types: potential and kinetic energy. Potential energy is stored-up energy. It has the potential to be released and become kinetic energy, which is the energy of motion. The most common example of potential energy in mechanics is that energy related to the location of an object and the force of gravity exerted on that object. The formula to determine the potential energy of an object is $PE = mgh$, where m is the mass of the object, g is the value of gravitational acceleration, and h is the height of the object above a reference point.

As the object begins to fall, it loses potential energy. Since kinetic energy is determined by the formula $KE = \frac{1}{2} mv^2$, the falling object gains in kinetic energy as its velocity increases. When the object reaches a reference point, such as the floor, the height will equal zero so that the object will have no potential energy. However, the object's velocity will be maximal and it will have a maximal kinetic energy. If the object bounces, it will regain some potential energy and lose kinetic energy as it rises. As the object comes to rest, the mechanical energy will have been converted to heat.

Kinetic energy can also exist in rotatory motion. The formula for this type of motion is analogous to the formula for linear motion. The kinetic energy equals the product of one half the moment of inertia times the square of the angular velocity, or $KE = \frac{1}{2} I\omega^2$.

Using these formulas, Gainor et al.[14] determined that the amount of energy that develops in the arm of a pitcher is about 27,000 in-lb. This magnitude of energy is sufficient to cause severe damage to part of the throwing mechanism. Similar calculations to determine energy during an activity can be made to determine the safety of the activity. The energy developed at the hip and knee in kicking,[13] absorbed by the hip or upper limb in a fall,[9] created in the tibia as it is twisted by a ski, or produced on the hand by a karate blow all have potential to produce injury. Knowledge of how to prevent injury by absorbing the energy is of major importance. Using the energy formulas and relating them to the resilience of materials can help provide this information. For example, various helmets can be evaluated to determine their energy-absorbing abilities. Gurdjian, Roberts, and Thomas[18] found a linear relationship between kinetic energy and the degree of brain injury resulting from head collisions during football practice and games. They also found that helmet design and padding thickness affected the amount of energy absorbed by the head.

The energy involved in loading a tissue may determine the type and degree of injury that will result. A fast loading rate may produce a ligament rupture, whereas a slow loading rate may result in an avulsion fracture. If a bone is loaded rapidly, more load is needed to fracture it and more energy is absorbed before it breaks. It will fracture, however, with a high-energy explosion. Slow loading will produce a low-energy fracture.[29] Examples of high-energy injuries are bullet wounds and skiing fractures. Results of low-energy loads include stress fractures.

During locomotion the energy absorbed by the natural shock absorbers (bones, menisci, intervertebral disks, and joints) may lead to degenerative changes within these tissues. Methods to reduce the energy going to these body parts may delay, reduce, or prevent damage to these tissues.

BIOMECHANICAL EXAMPLES

Many different biomechanical principles are involved in movement and sports activities. Some examples of injuries, exercises, and treatment procedures will show how these principles are involved.

Injuries

A common injury in skiing is the spiral fracture. The long lever arm of the ski needs only a small force to produce a large torque within the tibia. Benedek and Villars[1] reported that a force component of only 25 to 35 pounds acting perpendicularly to the ski tip creates a twisting movement sufficient to fracture the tibia (Fig. 3-14, A). A spiral fracture results when failure occurs mainly in tension (Fig. 3-14, B). The ski is equipped with release bindings so that if the approximate strength of the tibia is known, the magnitude of torque that will cause the binding to release can be set to allow a safety margin and prevent injury. Zernicke,[50] however, has discussed several problems with bindings. They may be set too tightly, they may malfunction, or the axis of the binding and ski may not be in common. These problems will allow more torque than can be withstood by the leg and fracture may result.

An excellent review of the mechanism of knee injuries—their evaluation, rehabilitation, and protection—that incorporates these mechanical principles can be found in the December, 1980, issue of *Physical Therapy*.[4,24,30]

Exercise programs

Biomechanical analysis is essential for the proper development of exercise programs. With the variety of exercise equipment on the market, the practitioner must be able to evaluate the advantages and disadvantages of each type and determine the exercise effect and potential hazards of each exercise.

The practitioner must know the mechanical principles involved in the sports activity for which the individual is

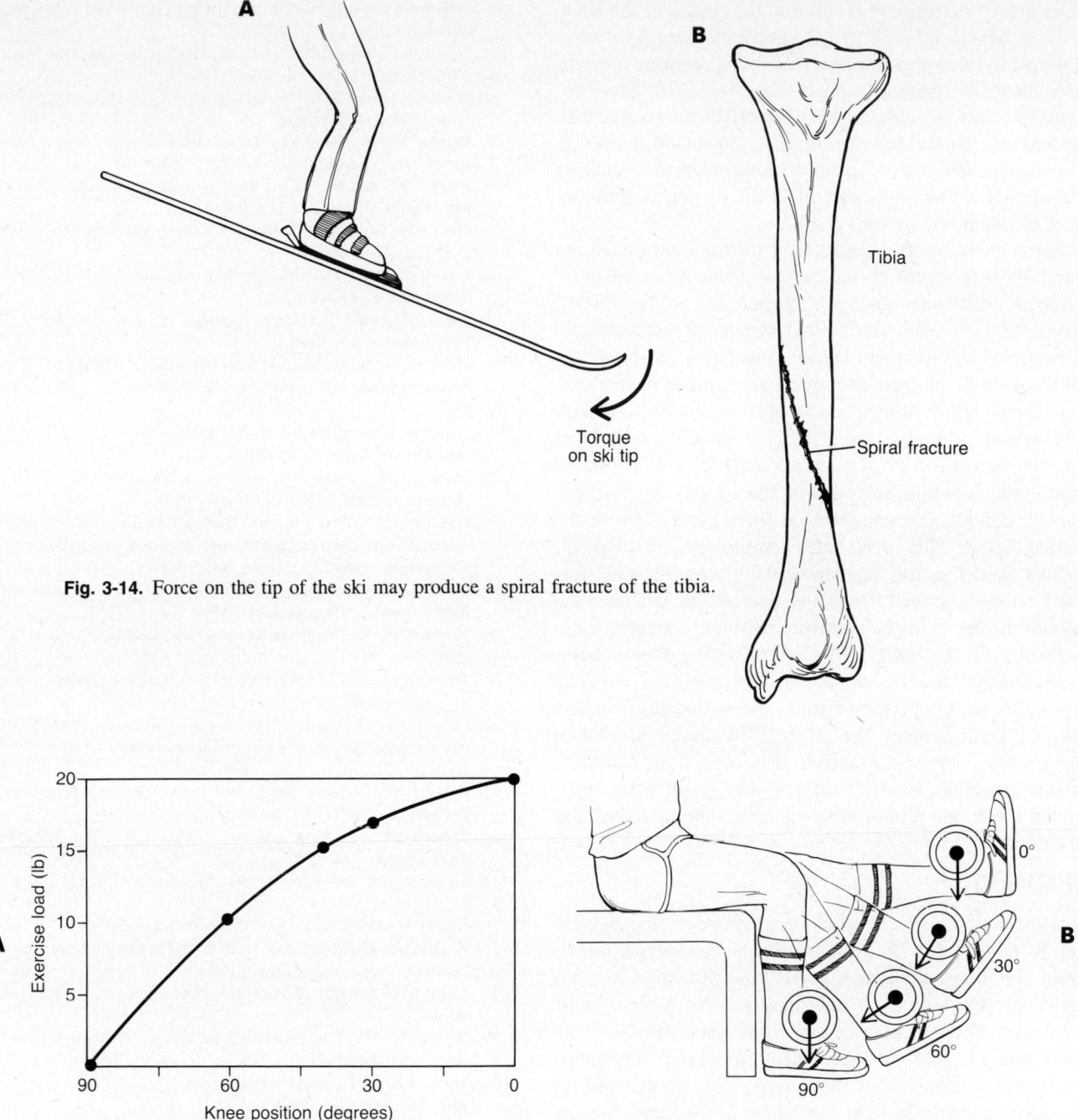

Fig. 3-14. Force on the tip of the ski may produce a spiral fracture of the tibia.

Fig. 3-15. A, Resisting force component of an isotonic boot exercise. **B,** Relationship between the resisting moment and the knee angle during a knee-extension exercise with a boot. (Adapted from LeVeau B: Williams and Lissner biomechanics of human motion, Philadelphia, 1977, WB Saunders Co.)

training. A sprinter should work on having the greatest-quadriceps muscle strength when the knee is flexed approximately 90 degrees to obtain the greatest force possible out of the starting blocks. A sprinter also needs a rapid muscle contraction for an explosive start. Therefore the sprinter should be trained in an exercise program that emphasizes a powerful contraction beginning at 90 degrees of

knee flexion and continuing into extension. The practitioner should be able to determine what exercises will provide this training effect most effectively.

Exercises for the quadriceps muscles using sandbags or a weighted boot provide the greatest effect when the knee is in extension. No exercise effect with these devices is present when the knee is in 90 degrees of flexion. The exercise effect increases in relation to the cosine of the angle of knee flexion (Fig. 3-15, *A*). Other devices have been designed to offer approximately the same resisting moment throughout the range of motion (Fig. 3-15, *B*). These devices can only provide an exercise effect no greater than the weakest part of the range of knee movement, however. Knowledge and use of certain biomechanical principles will allow the practitioner to select the proper exercise devices to obtain the desired result.

Some exercises frequently used may be harmful to the body. Most problems do not become evident immediately, however. Mechanical analysis of exercises provides information to the practitioner so that beneficial exercises may be designed and used and harmful ones avoided. Exercises for the abdominal muscles provide an example of this concept. Long-lying sit-ups and double-leg raises, although they provide a load to the abdominal muscles, may harm the lumbar spine.[22,27] The psoas muscles are tensed in most athletes while they are in the long-lying position. This tension places a compression and shearing load on the lumbar spine. The disks are compressed, lordosis increases, and the fifth lumbar vertebra tends to slide forward on the sacrum. When the exercise is initiated, the psoas muscles strongly contract, producing greater stress within the lumbar spine. If the exercises are done rapidly, even more stress is developed. If these exercises are done repeatedly over a period of time, the biological materials may fail from fatigue. The affect of forces can also cause deformities. Scoliosis, clubfoot, dislocated hips, and tibial torsion are examples of deformities that result when undesirable forces are produced by inappropriate body position or activity.

SUMMARY

Most mechanisms, evaluation, treatment, and prevention of injuries can be explained by biomechanical principles. This chapter has discussed basic principles and has given a few examples of how they are involved in sports medicine. The practitioner should become familiar with them and be able to apply them in various situations. Without a knowledge of these principles, no practitioner should be considered fully competent in the field of sports medicine or orthopaedic therapy.

REFERENCES

1. Benedek GB and Villars FMH: Physics: Mechanics, vol 1, Reading, Mass, 1973, Addison-Wesley Publishing Co, Inc.
2. Blazina ME, Watanabe RS, and Drake EC: Fatigue fractures in track athletes, Calif Med 97:61, 1962.
3. Cahill BR, Tullos HS, and Fain RH: Little League shoulder, J Sports Med Phys Fitness 2:150, 1974.
4. Davies GJ, Wallace LA, and Malone TR: Mechanisms of selected knee injuries, Phys Ther 60:1590, 1980.
5. Devas MB and Sweetnam R: Stress fractures of the fibula, J Bone Joint Surg 38B:818, 1956.
6. deVries HA: Physiology of exercise, Dubuque, Ia, 1966, Wm C Brown Group.
7. Dubravcik P and Burke DL: Ski fractures above and below the boot top, Can J Surg 22:343, 1979.
8. Dumbleton JH and Black J: An introduction to orthopedic materials, 1975, Springfield, Ill, Charles C Thomas, Publisher.
9. Frankel VH and Burstein AH: Orthopedic biomechanics, Philadelphia, 1970, Lea & Febiger.
10. Frankel VH and Hang YS: Recent advances in the biomechanics of sports injuries, Acta Orthop Scand 46:484, 1975.
11. Frankel VH and Nordin M: Basic biomechanics of the skeletal system, Philadelphia, 1980, Lea & Febiger.
12. Frost HM: Orthopedic biomechanics, Springfield, Ill, 1973, Charles C Thomas, Publisher.
13. Gainor BJ et al.: The kick: Biomechanics and collision injury, Am J Sports Med 6:185, 1978.
14. Gainor BJ et al.: The throw: Biomechanics and acute injury, Am J Sports Med 8:114, 1980.
15. Garrick JG: An introduction to orthopaedics. In Strauss RH, editor: Sports medicine and physiology, Philadelphia, 1979, WB Saunders Co.
16. Gregersen HN: Fractures of the humerus from muscular violence, Acta Orthop Scand 42:506, 1971.
17. Gurdjian ES, Lissner HR, and Patrick LM: Protection of the head and neck in sports, JAMA 182:509, 1962.
18. Gurdjian ES, Roberts VL, and Thomas LM: Tolerance curves of acceleration and intercranial pressure and protective index in experimental head injury, J Trauma 6:600, 1966.
19. Gurdjian ES et al.: Evaluation of the protective characteristics of helmets in sports, J Trauma 4:309, 1964.
20. Hirsch C: Biomechanics in motor skeletal trauma, J Trauma 10:997, 1970.
21. Jackson DW et al.: Stress reactions involving the pars interarticularis in young athletes, Am J Sports Med 9:304, 1981.
22. LeVeau BF: Movement of the lumbar spine during selected abdominal strengthening exercises doctoral dissertation, University Park, Pa, 1973, Pennsylvania State University.
23. LeVeau BF: Williams and Lissner biomechanics of human motion, Philadelphia, 1977, WB Saunders Co.
24. Malone TR, Blackburn TA, and Wallace LA: Knee rehabilitation, Phys Ther 60:1602, 1980.
25. Moffroid MT and Whipple RH: Specificity of speed of exercise, Phys Ther 50:1692, 1970.
26. Mortiz JR: Ski injuries, Am J Surg 98:493, 1959.
27. Nachemson A and Elfstrom G: Intravital dynamic pressure measurements in lumbar discs, Scand J Rehabil Med Suppl 1:5, 1970.
28. Nash WA: Strength of materials, New York, 1972, McGraw-Hill Book Co.
29. Noyes FR et al.: Biomechanics of ligament failure, J Bone Joint Surg 56A:1406, 1974.
30. Noyes FR et al.: Knee ligament tests: What do they really mean? Phys Ther 60:1578, 1980.
31. O'Donoghue DH: Injuries to the knee, Am J Surg 98:463, 1959.
32. Orava S and Puranen J: Exertion injuries in adolescent athletes, Br J Sports Med 12:4, 1978.
33. Radin E: Relevant biomechanics in the treatment of musculoskeletal injuries and disorders, Clin Orthop 146:2, 1980.
34. Rasch PJ and Burke RK: Kinesiology and applied anatomy, Philadelphia, 1974, Lea & Febiger.
35. Refior HJ and Zenker H: Wirbelsaule and Leistungsturnen, Munche Med Woch 112:463, 1970.
36. Rossi F: Spondylolysis, spondylolisthesis and sports, J Sports Med Phys Fitness 18:317, 1978.
37. Schwab GH et al.: Biomechanics of elbow instability: The role of the medial collateral ligament, Clin Orthop 146:42, 1980.
38. Sim FH and Chao EY: Injury potential in modern ice hockey, Am J Sports Med 6:378, 1978.

39. Slocum DB: The mechanism of football injuries, JAMA 170:1640, 1959.
40. Slocum DB: The mechanism of some common injuries to the shoulder in sports, Am J Surg 98:394, 1959.
41. Subotnick SI: Podiatric aspects of children in sports, J Am Podiatry Assoc 69:443, 1979.
42. Thistle HG et al.: Isokinetic contraction: A new concept of exercise, Arch Phys Med Rehabil 48:279, 1967.
43. Tullos HS and King JW: Lesion of the pitching arm in adolescents, JAMA 220:264, 1972.
44. Tullos HS and King JW: Throwing mechanisms in sports, Orthop Clin North Am 4:709, 1973.
45. Voloskin A and Wosk J: Influence of artificial shock absorbers on human gait, Clin Orthop 160:52, 1981.
46. Walter NE and Walf MD: Stress fractures in young athletes, Am J Sports Med 5:165, 1977.
47. Wilkins KE: The uniqueness of the young athlete: Musculoskeletal injuries, Am J Sports Med 8:377, 1980.
48. Williams JGP: Wear and tear injuries in athletes: An overview, Br J Sports Med 12:211, 1979.
49. Williams JGP: Biomechanical factors in spinal injuries, Br J Sports Med 14:14, 1980.
50. Zernicke RF: Biomechanical evaluation of bilateral tibial spiral fractures during skiing: A case study, Med Sci Sports Exerc 13:243, 1981.

Part Two

TRAUMA

Chapter 4

INFLAMMATORY RESPONSE OF SYNOVIAL JOINT STRUCTURES

Dixie L. Hettinga

The framework of the human body is essentially composed of a series of bones that articulate at joints and are moved by muscles. The joints form an integral part of this complex system since they allow motion to take place, hold parts of the bony skeleton together, or perform both functions.

Joints are frequently classified according to the type of motion they allow. Three groups are recognized: (1) synarthroses or immovable joints, (2) amphiarthroses or slightly movable joints, and (3) diarthroses or movable joints. Diarthroses—also known as synovial joints—comprise the majority of the body's articulations.[24]

SYNOVIAL JOINT STRUCTURE AND FUNCTIONS

The *synovial joint* is constructed to allow movement in one or more directions between two or more major segments of the human skeleton under either weight-bearing or non-weight-bearing conditions or both. The joint provides a low-friction articulation to enable movement of the body with minimal effort.[33,34,53] The articulating bony surfaces—termed *articular endplates*—are thin plates of dense cortical bone that overlay cancellous bone. Tightly adherent to the bony endplates is the *hyaline cartilage,* specialized connective tissue that acts as a bearing and gliding surface. The *joint cavity* is a tissue space, lined with the synovial membrane that contains only a few milliliters of synovial fluid.[24]

Joint mobility is provided by movement of the cartilaginous surfaces on one another. Joint stability, necessary to prevent movement in abnormal planes or excessive slippage under load, is provided by the bony configuration of the joint, the ligamentous and capsular support systems, the muscles controlling the joint, atmospheric pressure, and, for many joints, gravity. Each joint has unique load and positional requirements, which are reflected in its individual design. Uniaxial, biaxial, or polyaxial joint motion is possible, depending on the fit of the component at the various ranges.[17,24] To a certain extent, maximal strength and mobility are incompatible, and joints typically represent a compromise in which strength is somewhat sacrificed for mobility (e.g., at the shoulder) or mobility is somewhat sacrificed for strength (e.g., at the hip).[17]

The range of motion possible at joints is restrained by apposition of soft tissue, by limitations in the articular surface (impingement of bone against bone), and by muscles that are not long enough to allow an extreme movement in a direction opposite to which they normally act.[17] Accessory structures that maintain the integrity of the joint are the fibrous capsule and the ligaments. The *fibrous capsule* consists of dense connective tissue, which is invested in the entire joint and inserted into the bone, usually close to the articulating surfaces. Within the capsule are parallel bands of collagen fibers called *ligaments.* These, too, insert in the bony parts and vary in their tension from anatomical site to site, depending on the position of the joint.[24]

Within the joint capsule and defining the intraarticular space is the *synovial membrane* or *sac,* composed of *synoviocytes,* a specialized layer of connective tissue cells. Beneath this layer are varying amounts of highly vascular adipose, fibrous, or areolar tissue supporting the synoviocytes and allowing the sac to be appropriately loose in certain ranges of motion, without permitting the synovial folds to become entrapped between the joint surfaces. The synovial membrane replicates the inner surface of the capsule but is reflected at the capsular insertion into the bone, and then extends along the bone to the margin of the articular cartilage but does not cover the cartilaginous surfaces.[17]

The subsynovial tissue is endowed with nerve endings, which, along with those in the capsule and with spindles in the muscles and tendons, are responsible for proprioception and deep pain perception that protect the joint.[24] The nerve supply to a synovial joint is usually derived from several nerves, the general rule being that each nerve that innervates muscles acting across a joint gives at least one branch to that joint. Some of the nerves follow blood vessels and are apparently vasomotor.[17]

Some joints have a complete or incomplete fibrocartilaginous discoid partition known as a *meniscus*. The synovial membrane does not cover the avascular, aneural meniscus, which is firmly fixed to the joint margin by attachment to bone and to the ligaments or capsule, preventing abnormal movement or intraarticular displacement during joint function.[24]

Thus the essential components of a synovial joint are the synovial membrane, synovial fluid, articular cartilage, the joint capsule with associated ligaments, and, in some cases, intraarticular structures (Fig. 4-1). In the following discussion, the normal composition and function of each of these tissues will be delineated so that the structure's specific response to injury can be better appreciated.

THE INFLAMMATORY RESPONSE
Causes of inflammation

The body's response to injurious agents—inflammation—is almost always the same regardless of the location of the injury or the nature of the agent. Injurious agents can include physical injury; injury from heat, light, and laser beams; bacterial and viral effects; endotoxin shock; effects of antigen-antibody reactions; and chemical injury.[18] Joints are most often affected by physical trauma (direct or indirect), infections, metabolic disease (gout), neuropathies (tabes dorsalis, syringomyelia), systemic diseases (hemophilia, serum sickness), and local joint disturbances (aseptic necrosis).[50] For the purpose of this chapter, discussion will be limited to joint inflammatory responses initiated by physical injury.

Definition of trauma

The types of trauma that can cause insults to joints are as varied as the resulting injuries. Trauma can result from a direct blow to the joint area by an object or by a fall. This type of trauma may produce a sprain, subluxation, dislocation, fracture, or any combination of these injuries,

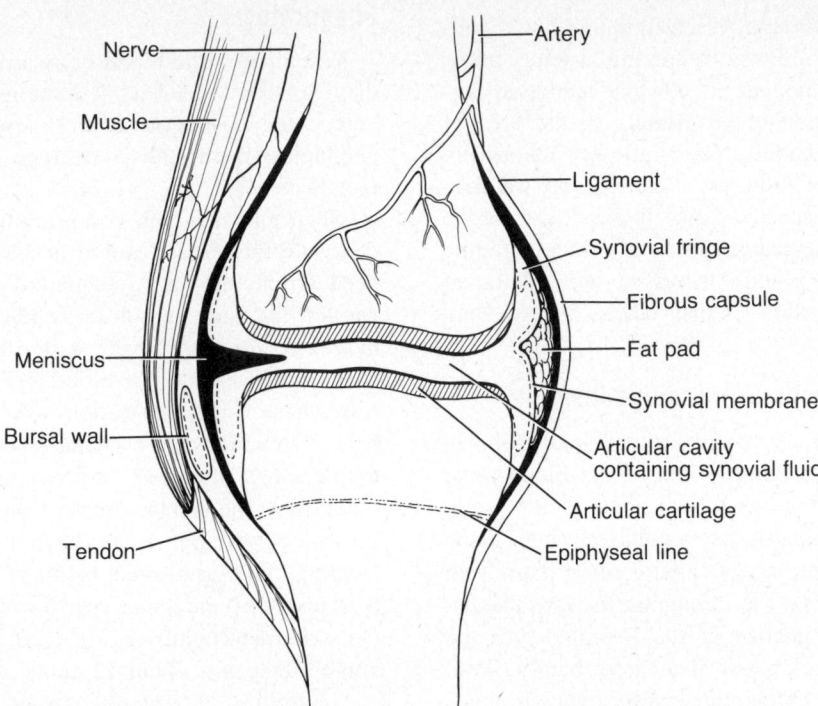

Fig. 4-1. A typical synovial joint. (From Wright V, Dowson D, and Kerr J: Int Rev Connect Tissue Res 6:105, 1973.)

depending on the force of the blow. Indirect trauma—from forcing a joint beyond its normal range of motion or causing an abnormal motion of the joint—may result in some degree of sprain, or it may result in a more severe injury, depending on the type, duration, and direction of the force.[8]

Types of trauma to the joints

The mildest form of joint injury is either a simple sprain of the ligaments or the joint capsule or both with no displacement of articular surfaces. A *sprain* is defined as the partial or complete rupture of the fibers of a ligament. In a first-degree sprain, the mildest form of ligamentous injury, a few fibers are torn but integrity of the ligament is maintained and the joint remains stable. In a second-degree sprain the fibers are torn in sufficient quantity to diminish the ligamentous function, but joint stability is still maintained. Some excessive joint motion is evident when compared to the contralateral joint, and some discomfort is elicited. Complete tearing of fibers with loss of integrity and evidence of joint instability constitutes a third-degree sprain.[8,33]

In more severe injuries there is not only excessive joint motion, but the articular surfaces are also displaced from their normal positions. If there is no contact between the surfaces, the joint is said to be *luxated* or completely dislocated. If there is some contact between articular surfaces, the joint is said to be *subluxated* or partially dislocated. Severe injury can also result in intraarticular fractures or a combination of a fracture and a dislocation.[33]

The inflammatory process

Acute inflammation in the joint demonstrates the same characteristic cellular responses of inflammation seen in other body cavities or tissues. Chemical, metabolic, and vascular changes occur along with alterations in permeability, followed by some form of repair.[20,39]

Effects of trauma

Trauma causes both direct and secondary injury. Trauma, whether produced by a direct blow or by stretching and tearing of joint tissues, results in direct damage to the cells of both structural tissues (muscles, tendons, and ligaments) and associated tissues (nerves, capillaries, and blood vessels). The torn vessels allow direct hemorrhaging into the interstitial spaces of the injured area. The cellular debris and red blood cells then organize to form a hematoma. Enzymes from the damaged cells can cause an inflammatory response in the tissues on the margin of the central injured area.[20]

In the case of trauma, cells sustain structural changes that may lead to cell death. When cells degenerate, they release substances capable of producing vascular changes. One of these substances, *histamine,* increases the permeability of capillaries. The endothelial cells in the vessel wall seem to contract, thereby pulling away from each other and leaving gaps through which fluid and blood cells can escape. Vessels that are torn by the initial injury allow hemorrhage into the immediate area while increased permeability occurs in nondisrupted vessels in the area of injury. Increased permeability also allows abnormally large amounts of plasma proteins, colloids, and water to pass into the interstitial spaces. Since the colloids are the major force for causing reabsorption of fluids into the capillaries, their effect is now reversed and additional fluid is pulled out of the vessels; edema or swelling results.[20]

"Walling off," margination, and diapedesis

The purpose of postinjury vascular events is to mobilize and transport the defense components of the blood—the white blood cells or leukocytes—to the injury site and to secure their passage through the vessel wall into tissue spaces. One of the first effects of inflammation is to "wall off" the area of injury from the remaining tissues. The tissue spaces and the lymphatics in the inflamed area are blocked by fibrinogen clots so that fluid barely flows through the spaces. The extracellular and lymphatic fluids clot because of the coagulating effect of tissue exudates on the leaking fibrinogen, one of the plasma proteins. Thus edema develops in the spaces surrounding the injured cells.[16]

As a result, blood flow decreases. This allows white blood cells to move to the margin of the vessel. They tumble along the margin for awhile and then adhere to the wall of the damaged capillary in a process called *margination*. The motile white blood cells then escape through the vessel walls, which are enlarged because of their increased permeability, into the tissue spaces. Some cells squeeze through the pores of the blood vessels by a process called *diapedesis;* only a small portion of the cell slides through the pore at a time, being momentarily constricted to the size of the pore. Once outside the vessel, the cells migrate to the injury site.[16]

Chemotaxis

A number of different chemical substances in the tissues cause the white blood cells to move either toward or away from the source of the chemical. This phenomenon is known as *chemotaxis*. Degenerative products of inflamed tissues, especially tissue polysaccharides, can cause white blood cells to move toward the area of inflammation. Chemotaxis depends on the existence of a concentration gradient of the chemotaxic substance. The concentration is greatest near the source, and, as the substance spreads by diffusion away from the source, its concentration decreases approximately in proportion to the square of the distance. Therefore the concentration of the chemotaxic substance is greater on one side of the white blood cell than the other, and this causes pseudopodia to project toward the source of the substance.[16]

Phagocytosis

When the white blood cells arrive at the site of injury, they remove the irritating material by *phagocytosis*. The leukocytes most involved in this process are the polymorphonuclear neutrophils (one type of granulocyte) and the monocytes.[16,20]

Neutrophils, which comprise 62% of the white blood cells, are formed and stored in the bone marrow; when the need arises, they are transported in the blood to various parts of the body. A substance known as *leukocytosis-promoting factor* is believed to be liberated by inflamed tissues. It diffuses into the blood and travels to the bone marrow where it has two actions. First, it causes large numbers of granulocytes, especially neutrophils, to be released within a few minutes to a few hours of its arrival into the blood from the storage areas of the bone marrow. Second, the rate of granulocyte production by the bone marrow increases, either as a direct result of the factor or as an indirect result of the bone marrow release of granulocytes. Once the neutrophils are released into the blood, their average life span is about 12 hours.[16]

Neutrophils entering the tissues are already mature cells that can immediately begin phagocytosis. On approaching a particle to be phagocytized, the neutrophil projects pseudopodia in all directions around the particle, and the pseudopodia meet each other on the opposite side and fuse. This creates an enclosed chamber containing the phagocytized particle. The chamber then invaginates to the inside of the cell's cytoplasmic cavity, and the portion of the cell membrane that surrounds the phagocytized particle breaks away from the outer cell membrane to form a free-floating phagocytic vesicle inside the cytoplasm.[16]

Monocytes comprise about 5.3% of white blood cells and may live for weeks or even months. They are discharged from the bone marrow into the blood as still immature cells. After the monocytes enter traumatized tissues, they begin to swell, often increasing fivefold in diameter. Extremely large numbers of lysosomes and mitochondria develop in the monocytes' cytoplasm. The monocytes are now called *macrophages*, representing a mature form of the cell. These macrophages are much more powerful phagocytes than the neutrophils, often capable of phagocytizing as many as 100 bacteria each before undergoing necrosis themselves. They have the ability to engulf much larger particles and often five or more times as many particles as neutrophils. They can even phagocytize whole red blood cells and necrotic tissue, the latter function being very important in chronic inflammation.[16]

Obviously, the neutrophils and macrophages must be selective in the material they phagocytize; otherwise, some of the structures of the body itself would be ingested. The process of phagocytosis is enhanced by at least two factors. If the surface of a particle is rough, the likelihood of phagocytosis is increased. Also, since most natural substances of the body have electronegative surface charges, they repel the phagocytes, which also carry electronegative surface charges. Dead tissues and foreign particles, on the other hand, are usually electropositive, making them more susceptible to phagocytosis.[16]

Once a particle has been phagocytized, lysosomes in the cell immediately come in contact with the phagocytic vesicle and their membranes fuse. Acid hydrolase enzymes of the lysosomes are dumped into the vesicle, which then becomes a digestive organ and immediately begins digestion of the phagocytized particle. Neutrophils and macrophages both have an abundance of lysosomes filled with proteolytic enzymes especially designed for digesting bacteria and other protein matter recognized as foreign matter.[16]

Sequence of events in inflammation

When an injury occurs and results in damage to cells, the first cells to respond are the *tissue histiocytes,* which are monocytes that have become fixed in the tissues. The tissue histiocytes, along with the lymphocytes, comprise the *reticuloendothelial system,* a nonmotile group of cells functioning to protect the body against foreign invaders. The histiocytes have the appearance of large macrophages, but, instead of moving freely through the tissues, they are entrapped by or adherent to the meshwork of the tissue. When an injury occurs, they develop ameboid motion and migrate chemotaxically to the area of injury. The numbers of histiocytes are few, but they provide the primary line of defense within the first hour of injury. The first motile white blood cells to arrive are the neutrophils, which have a predilection for destroying bacteria. Since there are usually no bacteria with most traumatic injuries, many of the neutrophils actually act as a deterrent to healing and die without assisting the process. They reach their maximum effectiveness in 6 to 12 hours, but by that time large numbers of monocytes have begun to enter the tissues. The monocytes evolve into macrophages and phagocytize neutrophil carcasses, cellular debris, fibrin, red blood cells, and any other particles, clearing the joint space for repair.[16,20] However, when neutrophils are destroyed, active proteolytic enzymes from their lysosomes are released into the surrounding inflammatory fluid. These enzymes can attack joint tissues as well. Thus, while the inflammatory response to trauma in a joint cavity may be nature's way of removing toxic or foreign materials, prolonged continuation of this response may also cause damage to surrounding joint structures.[39]

Repair

Once the inflammatory debris has been destroyed or removed, repair can begin. Cleanup by the macrophages and repair occur simultaneously, although enough of the debris must first be removed to permit ingrowth of new tissue. The amount of exudate present is directly related to the to-

tal healing time. If the size and amount of exudate are minimized, as in the use of cryotherapy, healing begins earlier and the total healing time is decreased.[20]

THE SYNOVIAL MEMBRANE

The synovial membrane, also referred to as the synovium, represents a condensation of connective tissue that covers the inner surface of the fibrous capsule and forms a sac enclosing the synovial cavity. The synovial membrane invests tendons that pass through the joint as well as the free margins of intraarticular structures, such as ligaments and menisci. The synovium is thrown into folds that surround the margin of the articular cartilage, but it does not cover the bearing surface of the cartilage.[5,33] In joints where the fibrous membrane of the capsule attaches some distance from the edges of the articular cartilage, the synovial membrane leaves the fibrous layer to be reflected back along the periosteum to the edge of the cartilage (Fig. 4-2).[17]

Morphology

Recent research on the synovial membrane has concentrated on its cellular structure, with emphasis on the cells found lining the inner synovial surface. The lining cells, called *synoviocytes,* are not in close proximity to each other, and there is no basement membrane separating the cells from subjacent cells and capillaries.[40,43] Cell processes that may interdigitate project from the cells toward the surface. Thin branching filaments, probably of reticular origin, rather than collagen fibers (which are usually absent), appear to serve as a supportive membrane for the cells.[24] This makes the synovium different in character from the mesothelium found lining the major serous cavities (pleural, pericardial, and peritoneal). The cellular lining of the joint cavity is therefore discontinuous; the interior of a synovial joint should be looked upon as a large tissue space rather than as a membrane-lined cavity.[5]

The absence of a basement membrane in the synovium ensures a continuation of morphology as well as function. The change from the highly cellular outer synovial lining to the subsynovial layer, which is relatively acellular and formed to thick intertwining bands of collagen fibers, is not abrupt. The cells below the synovial layer resemble lining cells, but there is more connective tissue. Underlying these, the cells appear more fibroblastic. Next fat cells increase in number, and larger blood vessels are seen. Then dense bands of collagen appear. The ligaments that span joints and confer stability on them are continuous with the outer layers of the capsule in many joints.[19]

Synovial lining or intima

The synovium can be divided into two layers: (1) the *intima* or synovial lining and (2) the *subsynovial tissue.*[5,19,24] The intimal portion of the synovial membrane consists of a layer of specialized fibroblasts known as synoviocytes, averaging one to three cells in depth (Fig. 4-3). These cells

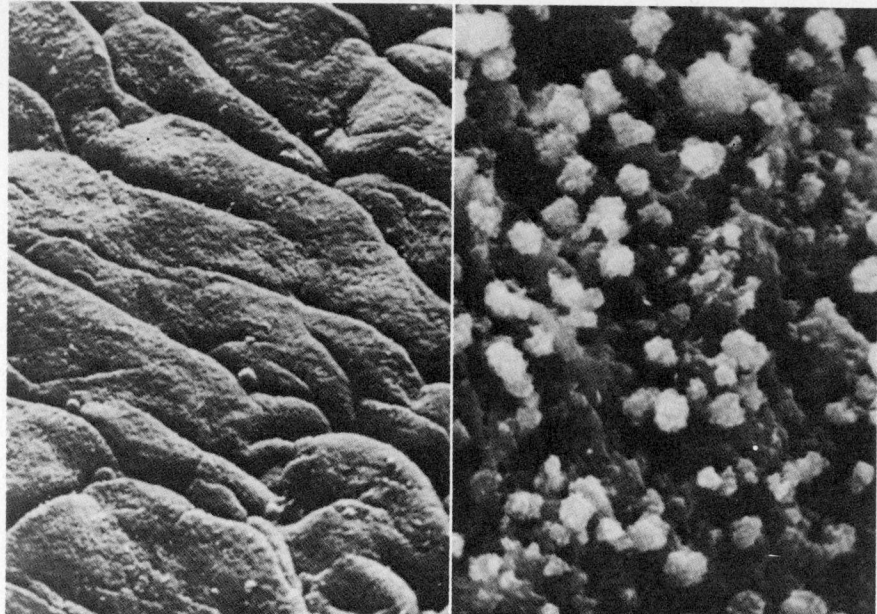

Fig. 4-2. Near normal human synovium (scanning electron microscopy). At low magnification *(left)*, the surface topography is arranged in a series of shallow folds that are capable of expanding during joint movement. At higher magnification *(right)*, individual synoviocytes are seen randomly distributed over the synovial surface. They are separated by wide areas, appear to be partially embedded within the intercellular matrix, and their surface exhibits folds and projections—the morphological expression of pinocytotic activity. (Courtesy Dr. C.R. Wynne-Roberts. Reprinted from The Primer of the Rheumatic Diseases, ed 8, copyright 1983, The Arthritis Foundation.)

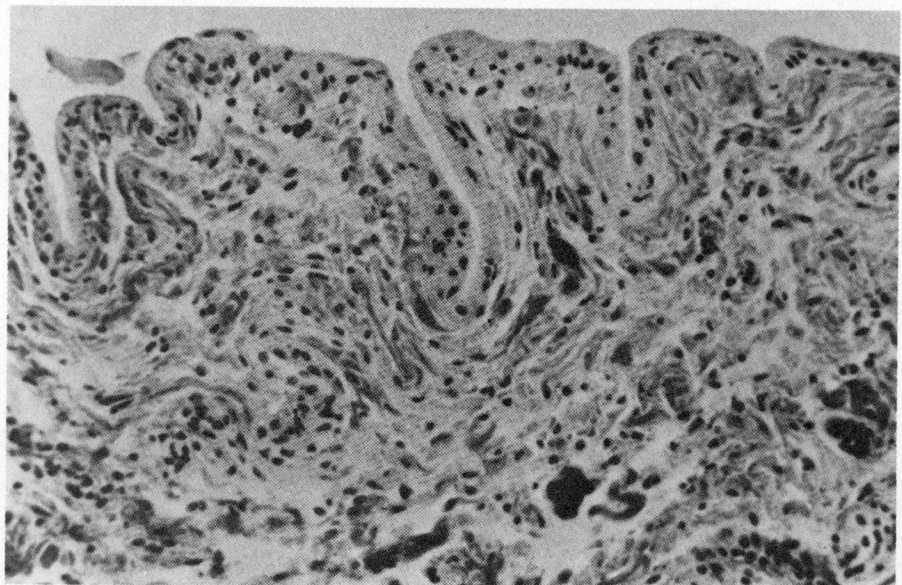

Fig. 4-3. Normal human synovium obtained from knee joint. Note small villi covered by layer of specialized synovial lining cells (synoviocytes), one to three cells in depth. The more superficial portion of the lining (stratum synoviale) consists of loosely textured, fibrous connective tissue containing numerous capillaries, while the deeper portion approaching the capsule (stratum fibrosum or subsynovialis) is made up of more compact fibrous tissue. (Courtesy Dr. C.R. Wynne-Roberts. Reprinted from The Primer of the Rheumatic Diseases, ed 8, copyright 1983, The Arthritis Foundation.)

must be able to synthesize hyaluronic acid, which becomes a major component of synovial fluid. They must also be able to phagocytize particulate debris and pinocytize soluble products of cellular and macromolecular catabolism. The debris diffuses through the synovial fluid to the borders of the joint space. (*Pinocytosis,* a process similar to phagocytosis, refers to the uptake of extracellular fluid and solutes into membrane-bound vesicles.)

The normal synovial lining is a thin, fine cellular aggregate overlying more dense subsynovial and capsular connective tissue. Grossly, the synovial membrane presents a relatively smooth surface with a variable number of villi and folds that project into the joint cavity and that are especially numerous in the region near the attachment of the capsule.[5,19,41] The normal membrane rarely contains blood vessels visible to the naked eye; these appear only when inflammation is present.[19]

Type A and B cells

Electron microscopy of the synovial lining cells reveals two functional types of cells based on ultrastructural and cytochemical characteristics.[5,33,43] *Type A cells,* which are more numerous, contain many mitochondria and are characterized by the presence of a richly variegated collection of cytoplasmic organelles, including lysosomes, smooth-walled vacuoles, and micropinocytic vesicles. They have a prominent Golgi complex situated near the apical aspect of the nucleus. Frequently, the cell processes stretching into the adjacent matrix are seen. Type A cells have little endoplasmic reticulum and are active in phagocytosis and secretion (Figs. 4-4 and 4-5). *Type B cells* possess an abundant endoplasmic reticulum and Golgi apparatus but relatively few mitochondria, vacuoles, vesicles, and cell processes. These cells are believed to be involved in synthesis of the hyaluronoprotein of synovial fluid (Figs. 4-5 and 4-6).[5,19,43]

However, attributing distinct functions to the A and B cells may be an oversimplification. It ignores the fact that one cell may have more than one function and that, in response to different stimuli, cells can modulate their internal structure as their function changes. A number of observations support this view:

1. *Type C cells,* representing an intermediate type of cell, have been described. They have both an endoplasmic reticulum and Golgi complexes and vacuoles (Fig. 4-7).
2. The use of stains for RNA on ribosomes (an acceptable index of synthetic function in cells) indicates that only a few cells stain positively in the normal synovium. Staining increases in intensity and appears in an increased number of cells only if a joint has been traumatized, and in severe inflammatory states no cells without a developed endoplasmic reticulum are observed.

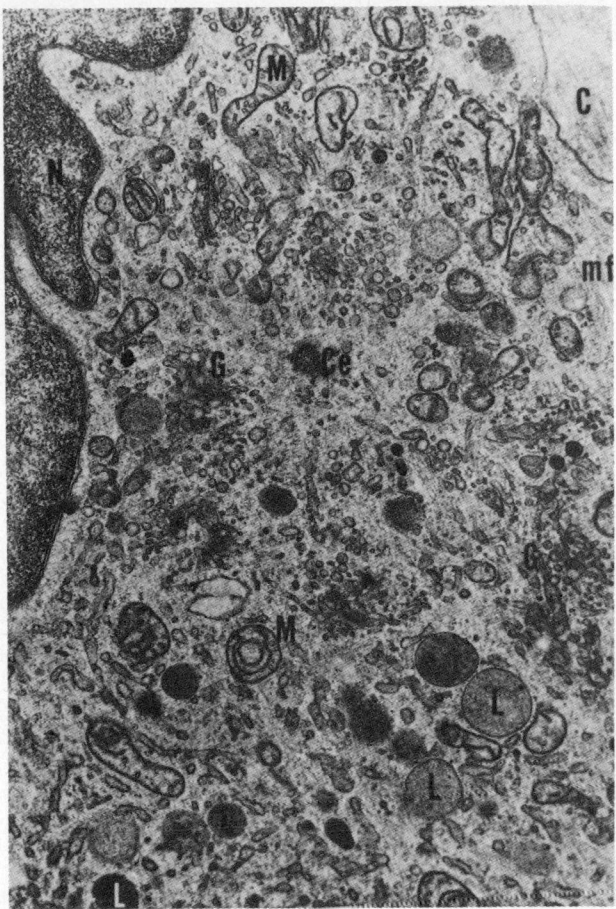

Fig. 4-4. Human synovium, type A cell. Cytoplasm of a type A synoviocyte demonstrating nucleus *(N)*, mitochondria *(M)*, a small centriole cut in cross section *(Ce)*, and several lysosomes *(L)*. The Golgi apparatus *(G)* is extensive and consists of lamellae and vesicles occurring in groups. Interspersed between the cytoplasmic organelles are fine microfilaments *(mf)*, and outside this cell lie a few collagen fibrils *(C)*. (Courtesy Dr. C.R. Wynne-Roberts. Reprinted from The Primer of the Rheumatic Diseases, ed 8, copyright 1983, The Arthritis Foundation.)

3. Synovial cells, which appear morphologically to be fibroblasts, will nevertheless demonstrate macrophage-like function in response to certain stimuli.
4. Evidence suggesting that type A cells may synthesize and secrete hyaluronic acid is mounting. The most convincing data are demonstratins by ultrastructural studies that hyaluronic acid is found both in the Golgi complex and in large secretory vacuoles of these cells.[19]

It may be reasonable to consider the synovial lining cell as one with multiple phenotypical possibilities and to resist categorizing it by its morphological resemblance at certain stages to other, better characterized cells. The A and B cells probably represent different functional phases of the same basic cell structure.[5,19,38]

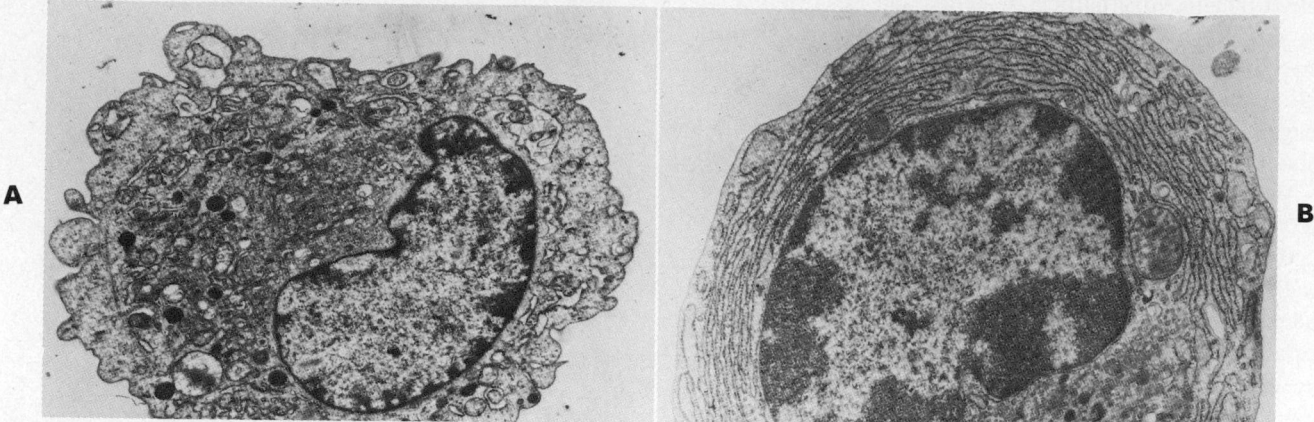

Fig. 4-5. A, Type A human synovial cell with many undulations in the cell membrane, vacuoles, and inclusions. This cell presumably has phagocytic capabilities and is thought of as a macrophage (×11,200.) **B,** Type B human synovial cell with a very well-developed endoplasmic reticulum. This cell presumably has capabilities for synthesis of protein (×17,500.) It must be emphasized that there are many synovial cells with organelles developed for both synthetic and phagocytic function. In addition, it is possible that individual cells may be modulated from cells with synthetic function to ones with phagocytic function. (From Kelley W et al: Textbook of rheumatology, Philadelphia, 1981, WB Saunders Co.)

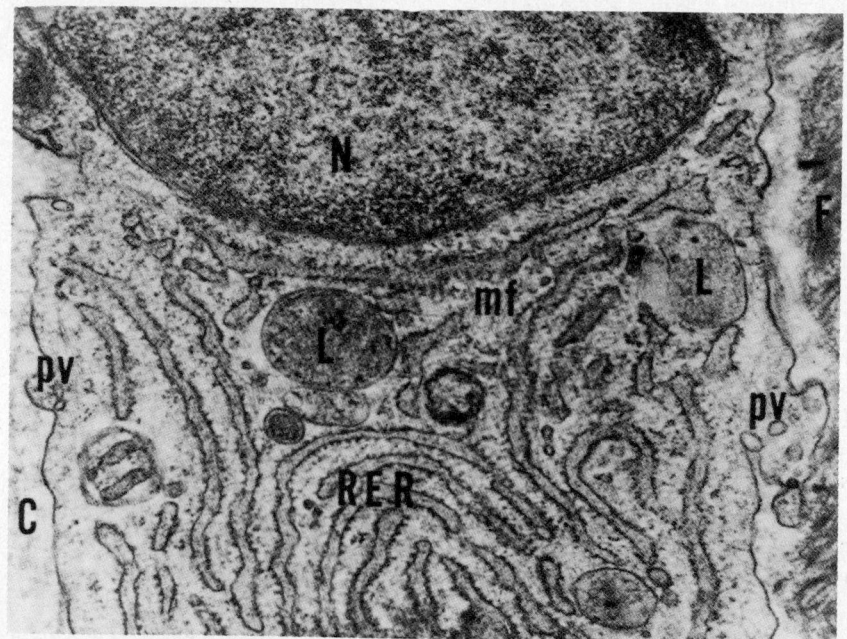

Fig. 4-6. Human synovium, type B cell. Part of a type B (synthetic) synoviocyte showing nucleus *(N),* well-developed lamellae of rough endoplasmic reticulum *(RER),* lysosomes *(L),* a few pinocytotic vesicles at the edge of the cell *(pv),* and a small group of microfilaments *(mf).* Some fibrin *(F)* and a small amount of collagen *(C)* lie outside the cell. (Courtesy Dr. C.R. Wynne-Roberts. Reprinted from The Primer of the Rheumatic Diseases, ed 8, copyright 1983, The Arthritis Foundation.)

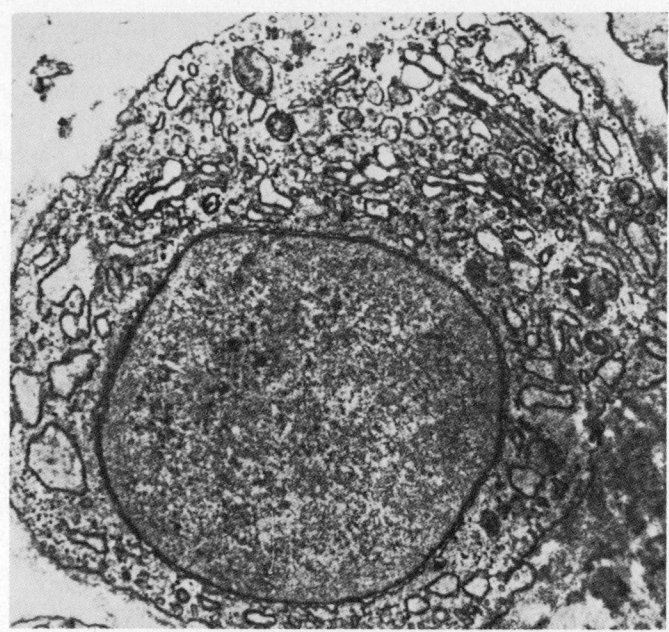

Fig. 4-7. Normal synovial cell, showing both prominent Golgi systems and abundant rough endoplasmic reticulum (intermediate type). (From Roy S, Ghadially FN, and Crane WAJ: Ann Rheum Dis 25:259, 1966.)

Subsynovial tissue

Beneath the synovial lining is a loose meshwork of richly vascularized fibrous connective tissue, known as *subsynovial tissue*. The cells of this tissue are more spindle-shaped than the lining cells and are spaced farther apart amid collagen fibrils, some fatty tissue, and a fine capillary network. These cells produce matrix collagen in moderate quantities. This subintimal portion of the synovial membrane differs in thickness and appearance from place to place within joints, being variously more or less fibrous, fatty, or areolar with elements of the reticuloendothelial system interspersed. This layer merges with the periosteum covering the bony components of the joint that lie within the confines of the capsule. At the margin of the articular cartilage, the conjoined tissue becomes continuous with the cartilage by means of a transitional zone of fibrocartilage.[5,19,24]

The synovium is richly endowed with a network of capillary vessels in the subsynovial layer. The vessels include some with thin walls and fenestrations that are adapted for rapid exchange of fluid and solutes (Fig. 4-8). Other vessels have thick walls with endothelial cells that can separate, producing gaps for the escape of cells and large particles.[5] Since there is no basement membrane separating the lining cells from the capillaries, the exchange of waste products and nutrients is facilitated (Fig. 4-9).[53]

The subsynovial layer is also supplied with lymphatics and nerve fibers. The nerve endings are few and are mostly in the capsule surrounding the outside of the synovial membrane.[40]

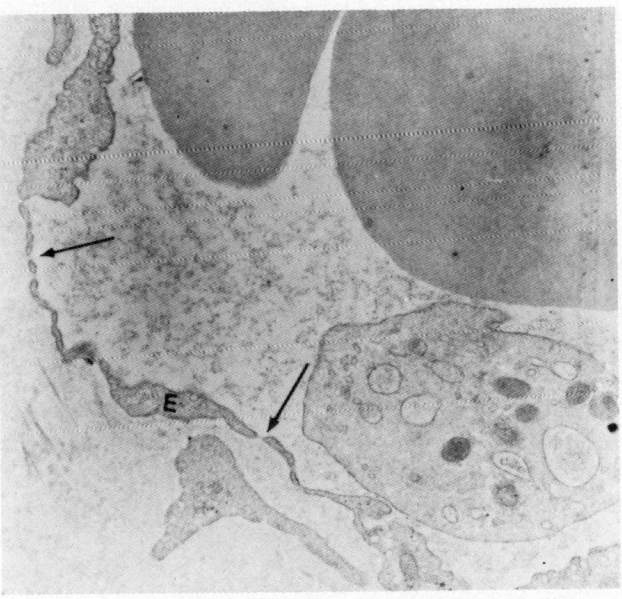

Fig. 4-8. Normal superficial synovial blood vessel. The endothelium *(E)* is thin and in some regions contains fenestrations *(arrows)* bridged only by a very thin diaphragm. (Electron micrograph.) (From Schumacker HR: J Sports Med 3:108, 1975.)

Functions

The synovium supports the normal joint in at least three physiological ways:

1. It provides a low-friction lining in itself and produces hyaluronic acid, which is the mucin component of synovial fluid.

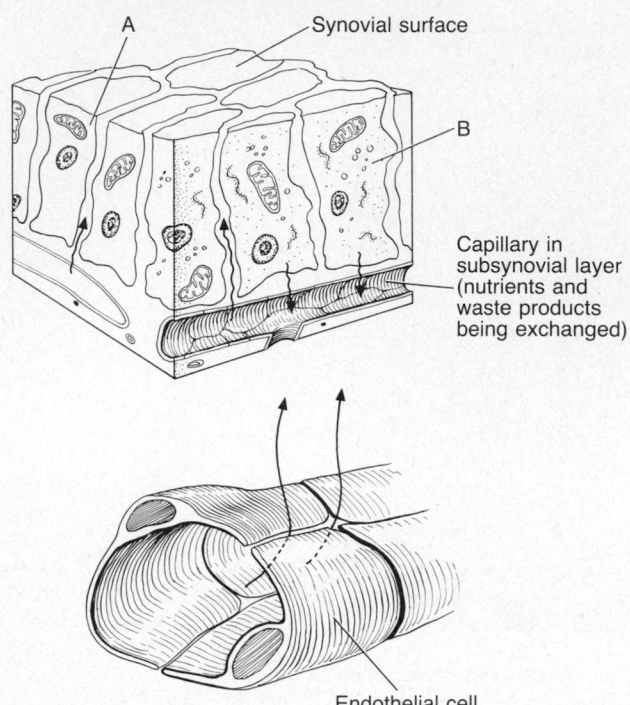

A — Synovial surface

B

Capillary in subsynovial layer (nutrients and waste products being exchanged)

Endothelial cell

Fig. 4-9. Schematic representation of synovium. *A,* macrophage type of cell. *B,* hyaluronate-synthesizing type of cell. (From Sledge CB: Orthop Clin North Am 6[3]:619, 1975.)

2. It transports needed nutrients into the joint space while it removes metabolic wastes through its capillary and lymphatic systems.

3. It plays an important role in maintaining joint stability.

In addition, the membrane, as a whole, regulates the entry of nutrients into the synovial fluid and inhibits the entry of serum proteins. The plasma in the capillaries is the source from which the dialysate fraction of the synovial fluid (synovial fluid except for hyaluronate) is derived, and the type A cells help keep the joint clear of debris by their phagocytic action.[42,48,53]

Joint lubrication

Since motion is the main function of synovial joints, the synovium must be able to adapt to the full range of positions permitted by the surrounding tendons, ligaments, and joint capsule. When a joint flexes and extends, for example, the synovium must correspondingly expand and contract. This process appears to be more consistent with a folding and unfolding than with an elastic stretching of the tissue.[42]

This expansion and contraction of the synovium takes place over unopposed surfaces of articular cartilage. For any joint to function as more than a simple pivot, there must be a disparity in the configuration of the surface areas of opposing cartilages. When the joint moves, the smaller area glides across or around the larger one. Cartilage not in contact with opposing cartilage will be temporarily covered by the synovium. As the cartilaginous surfaces return to their original positions, an effective lubrication system must prevent pinching of the highly vascular synovial tissue. Were this system to fail, repeated hemarthroses would rapidly incapacitate the affected individual. The hyaluronate molecules that render synovial fluid viscous may find their major role in lubricating the synovium, thus permitting the tremendous changes of internal geometry that occur within synovial joints during normal activity. This process is easiest when the volume of synovial tissue and fluid is at a minimum since the synovium must expand and contract within the confines of the joint capsule.[42]

Synovial transport. Synovial permeability or transfer of molecules across the synovium involves two processes—passage through an endothelial wall as well as diffusion through the intercellular spaces of the synovial membrane. After leaving the vessels, all molecules must traverse the synovial interstitium before they enter the synovial fluid. The tissue space appears to offer the most significant resistance, limiting the overall transsynovial exchange of most small molecules. For most compounds, synovial permeability is inversely related to the size of the permeant molecule. This proportionality suggests that most small molecules cross the synovium by a process of free diffusion. A specific transport system accelerates the entrance of glucose into normal joints, probably by facilitated diffusion. In the case of proteins, the microvascular endothelium is probably the major barrier blocking equilibration of plasma and synovial fluid protein (plasma contains large molecules, which are excluded from synovial fluid). In normal joints there is continual turnover of synovial fluid proteins. In contrast to the selectivity shown for entering proteins, all large molecules appear to leave the joints at equal rates. This clearance is thought to occur by lymphatic drainage.[42]

Role in joint stability. Only a film of synovial fluid separates the moving surfaces in normal joints. The intraarticular cavity is primarily a potential space with a subatmospheric intracavity pressure. Several investigators have actually measured intraarticular pressures in normal knee joints, with the average pressure being −4 mm Hg.[42]

This pressure differential may play a significant role in stabilizing joints. In concert with the action of tendons and ligaments, the suction will draw articulating surfaces into the best possible fit and will help to guide the surface contacts as the joint moves through its range of motion. Simple atmospheric pressure, aided by the surface tension of synovial fluid, is able to contribute tremendously to the stabilization and congruent articulation of large joints, especially in the shoulder and hip where ligaments play only a minor role in maintaining joint stability.[42]

THE SYNOVIAL MEMBRANE AND ITS REACTION TO INJURY

The basic inflammatory response in the synovial membrane is a proliferation of the surface cells, an increase in vascularity, and a gradual fibrosis of the subsynovial tissue. This can be seen as a gross thickening and development of a granular surface, while the effect of the changes is seen as an alteration of the synovial fluid.[23,33]

Posttraumatic synovitis

A clinical entity known as *posttraumatic synovitis* can be differentiated from other inflammatory and degenerative changes of the synovial membrane.[46] This represents the simplest response of the synovial membrane to minor trauma, such as might occur from a mild blow or a forced inappropriate movement. If such a simple mechanical disturbance occurs without too much bleeding, the synovial membrane is not microscopically disturbed, but it may have a severe vasomotor reaction. The capillaries of the synovial membrane dilate and filtration increases.[7] Protein leaks into the interstitium. As the extravascular concentration of protein rises toward the plasma level, there is a progressive diminution in the colloid osmotic pressure gradient between the two spaces. Since it is this pressure gradient that normally drives venular reabsorption of water, increased vascular permeability leads to edema in tissues and a traumatic exudate in the joint.[42]

Microscopically, there is only slight hyperemia of the synovial membrane and a slight cellular infiltration around the dilated capillaries. Later, the intima may multiply from three to five layers to eight or ten. This reaction of the synovial membrane disappears very quickly if the trauma occurs only once. The exudate disappears as the protein molecules are cleared by lymphatic drainage and the normal colloid osmotic pressure gradient is restored. The hyperemia lasts the longest but eventually decreases. The synovial lining then decreases to its original size.[7]

If the mechanical irritation is repeated, it can produce a characteristic posttraumatic synovitis. Studies by Bozdech[7] have revealed that, microscopically, the synovial lining becomes thicker and may contain up to 10 to 15 rows of cells. The synovial membrane is more infiltrated with lymphocytes, especially around the vessels, and the deeper cells of the synovial membrane show stronger activity. There is evidence of increased protein synthesis by the synovial cells, perhaps accounting for a portion of the excessive protein content in posttraumatic effusions.

Electron microscopy also reveals changes that occur in A and B cells. There are fewer A cells than are usually present in the normal synovial membrane because the A cells move into the synovial fluid as free macrophages. The synovial lining is also filled with fibroblasts that are usually deeper in the synovial membrane. These fibroblasts change into type B cells. A study by Roy, Ghadi-

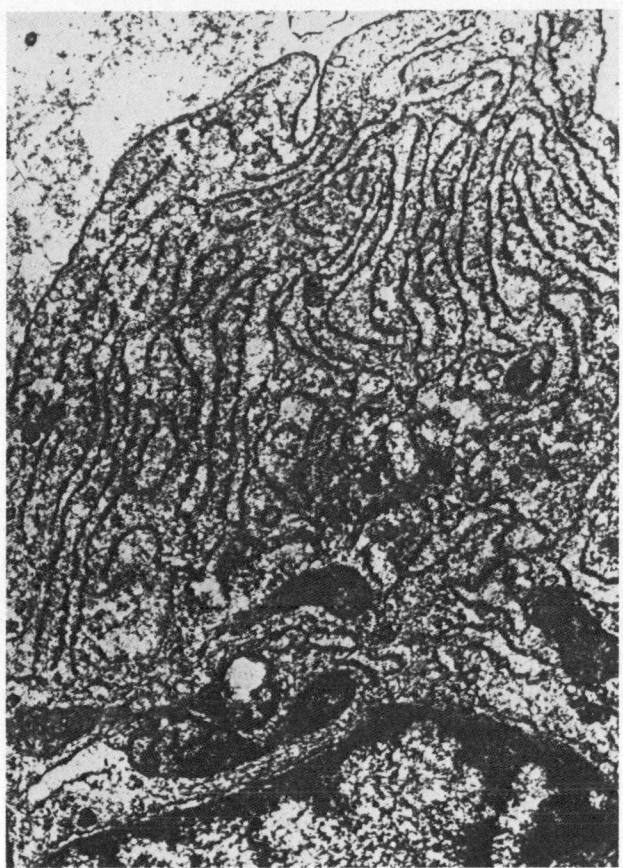

Fig. 4-10. Synovial cell from traumatic effusion, showing a marked hyperplasia of the rough endoplasmic reticulum. (From Roy S, Ghadially FN, and Crane WAJ: Ann Rheum Dis, 25:259, 1966.)

ally, and Crane[38] confirmed this reversal of the normal A:B cell ratio. Electron microscopy of the remaining cells in the synovial lining revealed that the distinction between type A and B cells was almost completely lost. The majority of cells instead contained rough endoplasmic reticulum in large amounts with dilated cisternae and complex Golgi systems. Of the remaining cells, the majority contained large amounts of rough endoplasmic reticulum (type B cells), while only an occasional cell had abundant Golgi systems and smooth endoplasmic reticulum (type A cells). The general impression was one of marked hyperplasia of the rough endoplasmic reticulum system (Fig. 4-10).

Changes in the synovial fluid, occurring as a result of these alterations in the synovial membrane, will be discussed in a following section. After the inflammatory reaction, synovitis can remain reactive for a long time. When the type A macrophages are destroyed by the neutrophils and monocytic macrophages, the latter cells ingest the lysosomes and proteolytic enzymes. The white blood cells, especially the neutrophils, die fast in the transudate and release proteolytic enzymes. These enzymes attack normal joint structures that are in close approximation. This results in a vicious inflammatory cycle. The process can keep a reactive synovitis alive for some time, even without further trauma.[7]

In studies by Soren et al[45,46] comparative light-scanning and transmission electron microscopic examinations were carried out in 35 cases in which trauma had occurred at least 4 months previously. In the first 6 months after trauma, a slight hyperplasia of the synovial lining was noted. During this early phase of posttraumatic synovitis, there was only a moderate polymorphy of the synovial cells and enlargement of the synovial surface by closely apposed tentacular cell processes (Fig. 4-11). A progressive sclerosis of the synovial membrane, starting about 4 to 6 months after trauma, was exhaustively demonstrated. A rather particular feature of posttraumatic synovitis became evident in a few instances when *hemosiderin* (the product of phagocytic digestion of iron derived from the blood) was observed and *siderosomes* (cells containing hemosiderin) were detected. The siderosomes were presumably partly dissolved and partly eliminated by the physiological desquamation of synovial cells. Without additional hemorrhages, the siderosomes vanished from the synovial

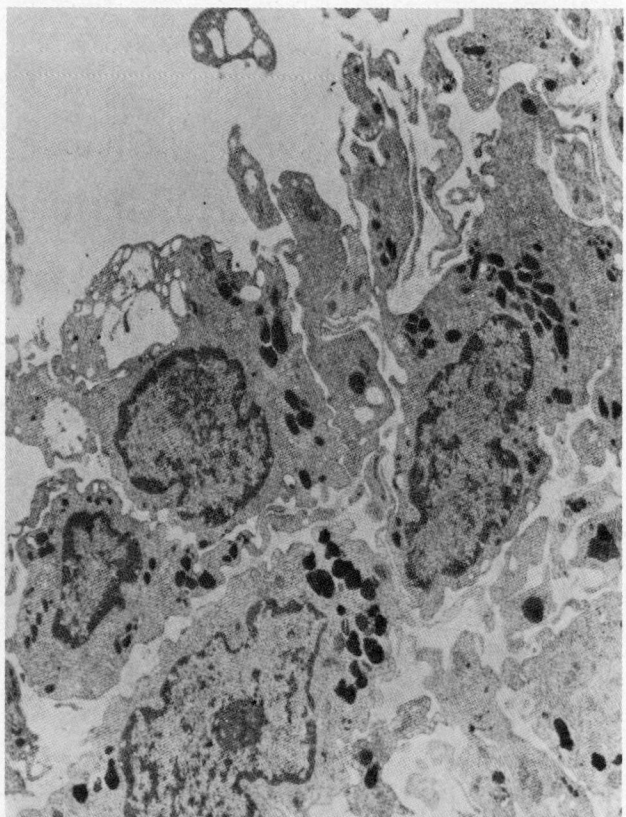

Fig. 4-11. Slightly polymorphic synoviocytes with siderosomes in posttraumatic synovitis. (From Soren A, Klein W, and Huth F: Clin Orthop 121:191, 1976.)

membrane after about 6 months, and proof of previous hemorrhage due to trauma disappeared. However, when posttraumatic joint symptoms continued beyond the first 6 months, a smooth rounding of synovial cells with loss of the tentacular processes was observed. A deviation of the previously outlined course of posttraumatic changes was noted in those cases in which the injury caused either a secondary laxity of ligaments with instability of the knee, hypermobility of the meniscus, or avulsions from the articular surfaces with formation of free joint bodies; these caused a chronic traumatization of the synovial membrane with resulting proliferative synovitis.[46]

Changes in blood vessels may be regarded as relatively characteristic for the posttraumatic reaction of the synovial membrane. In tissues removed in the first 6 to 12 months after trauma, changes usually consisted of swelling of the endothelium, proliferation of adventitial cells and extravasation of erythrocytes (observed by light microscopy), increased phagocytic activity, and formation of siderosomes in the endothelium and perithelium (observed by electron microscopy). With longer duration, sclerosing alterations of the vascular wall occurred, which were not observed as frequently in any other type of synovitis.[45,46] Also, fibrosis of the synovial membrane was noted with formation of mature, densely packed collagen fibrils up to the synovial surface. This sclerosis was associated with atrophy of the remaining synovial cells.[46]

For purposes of diagnosis it should be pointed out that inflammatory cell infiltrates rarely appear in the chronic posttraumatic synovial reaction. Therefore the concept of posttraumatic "synovitis" is justified only with some limitation. Also, aspirates of joint fluid rarely contain a significant increase in the number of inflammatory cells. The chronic posttraumatic joint effusions should be considered not as primarily inflammatory exudates but more probably as a sequel of the progressing sclerotic alterations of the synovial membrane.[46]

Clinically, onset of symptoms in uncomplicated posttraumatic synovitis occurs 12 to 24 hours after the trauma. The effusion is usually not associated with much warmth, erythema, or tenderness. Often the main complaint is a tight sensation. Effusions may linger 1 to 2 weeks.[40] The effusion should be aspirated to determine whether hemarthrosis is present and to aid in further examination of the joint. Hemarthrosis is usually present if fluid appears within 2 hours after injury; in about half the cases, swelling occurs within 15 minutes. With hemarthrosis there is usually more pain and at times a low-grade fever. Fractures, internal derangements, or major ligamentous tears must be ruled out by examination and radiographs, which should include stress, skyline, and intercondylar views. (In one series of clients with traumatic knee joint hemarthrosis, 66 had fractures or ligamentous rupture and 20 did not.)[32] There may be detachment or laceration of cartilage or capsular tears; however, they are not discovered in this manner. It has been suggested, on the basis of calcification that sometimes develops later in the median parapatellar area, that lateral subluxation of the patella and tearing of the medial retinaculum may be the source of joint hemorrhage in some cases.[32]

Minor joint trauma, causing initially slight symptoms that do not require medical care, may nevertheless be responsible for significant symptoms months afterward, even without additional traumatization.[45,46] This can be attributed to the phenomenon of reactive synovitis, which can keep the inflammatory process going for some time.

The subjective tight sensation felt after a joint has been subjected to mild trauma usually results from the presence of a joint effusion that causes the normally negative intraarticular pressure to become positive. Effusions deprive the joint of the stabilizing effects of subatmospheric pressure and substitute instead a distending force that increases stress on ligaments and the joint capsule. In contrast to normal joint, the pressures of effusions are greatest in joints in full flexion and extension, with minimal intraarticular pressures occurring at 30 degrees flexion.[42]

Conservative treatment with application of ice packs (or some other form of cryotherapy), rest and elevation of the affected joint when possible during the acute inflammatory stage, followed by contrast baths or heat treatment in the form of whirlpools or hot packs seems to be effective in most cases. Studies have shown that high-voltage galvanic stimulation is also effective in reducing edema, increasing circulation, and increasing tissue healing in acute injuries.[50] Compression dressings or posterior splints are also sometimes helpful. Graded quadriceps muscle exercises, in the case of the knee joint, can help reduce edema by muscle pumping action, which also prevents muscle atrophy. Repeated aspiration after the initial diagnostic aspiration may be necessary if significant volumes of fluid reaccumulate.[32] Analgesics and antiinflammatory medication (e.g., aspirin) can be used. The synovitis is usually self-limiting, but if it continues, intraarticular corticosteroid injections (one to three in number) can be given.[7,40] If the inflammatory process continues and the transudate becomes more inflammatory, a synovectomy will reduce the symptoms (Table 4-1).[7]

Pigmented villonodular synovitis

The synovium responds in a slightly different manner to recurrent hemarthroses. The most striking feature of synovial response to the injection of blood in experiments by Volz[51] was the production of a proliferative synovitis, known as *pigmented villonodular synovitis*. This synovial reaction was characterized by a villous and nodular hyperplasia of the synovial cells. Long villous projections of synovial tissue were seen extending into the joint. Associated with these changes was a prominent degree of subsynovial fibrosis. Also noted within the subsynovial layer were focal aggregations of round cells arranged in a pattern suggesting germinal follicles. Here and there giant cell formation was noted. Tissue stained with Prussian blue revealed moderate amounts of siderin pigment in the synovial layer (Figs. 4-12 and 4-13). The extent of these histological changes was observed to be roughly proportional to the number of injections of blood within the joint space. In no instance was there any suggestion of an inflammatory response.

Young and Hudacek (as cited by Volz[51] and Boyes[6]), in an experiment with dogs, demonstrated the correlation between blood injected into joints and the production of solitary nodular and pigmented villonodular synovitis characterized by an increased vascularity and hyperplasia of the synovium, diffuse depositions of siderin pigment, scattered giant cells, and subsynovial fibrosis. They observed blood clots floating free in the fluid, some of which were attached to the lining surface in varying degrees of organization. They theorized that the nodules were formed by the attachment of blood clots or by fusion of adjacent villi and

Table 4-1. Treatment of posttraumatic synovitis

Time elapsed after injury	Therapeutic techniques	Exercise	Medical intervention
First 24-48 hours	Ice, compression, elevation, high-voltage galvanic stimulation	Isometric contractions	Analgesics or antiinflammatory medications; diagnostic aspiration if large effusion
3-5 days	Contrast baths, whirlpools, hot packs, high-voltage galvanic stimulation	Gentle range of motion exercises, continued isometrics	Continued use of analgesics or antiinflammatory medications as needed
5 days-2 weeks	Whirlpools, hot packs, functional electrical stimulation	Range of motion exercises, strengthening exercises, progressive resistance exercises	
If symptoms persist >3-4 weeks >6-8 weeks	Continued use of modalities listed above (but less frequently)	Emphasis on range of motion exercises and isometrics	Repeated aspirations, corticosteroid injections Possible synovectomy

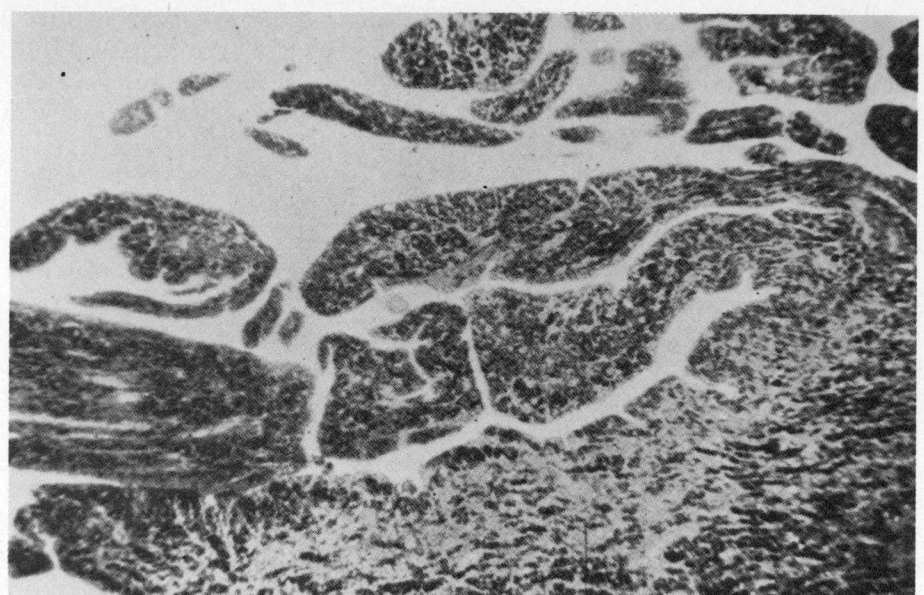

Fig. 4-12. Synovium displaying villonodular proliferative changes. Synovium was processed from a rabbit receiving 30 injections of iron. Note diffusely scattered multinucleated giant cells and siderin pigment. (From Volz R: Clin Orthop 45:127, 1966.)

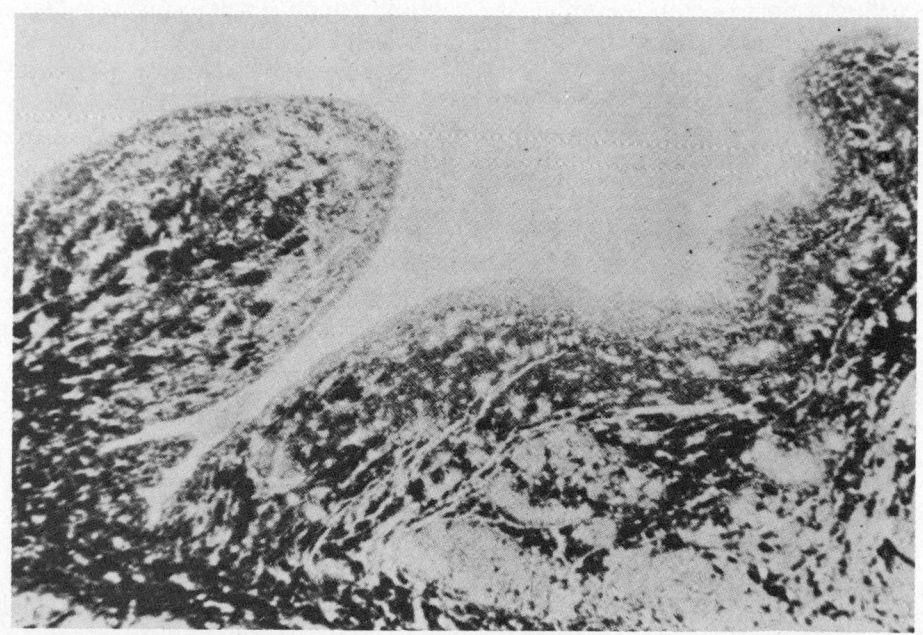

Fig. 4-13. Synovial tissue stained with Prussian blue. Darkly stained areas represent iron pigment deposits. (From Volz R: Clin Orthop 45:127, 1966.)

concluded that once villi are formed, the crushing of the nodule in joint motion may cause additional hemorrhage.

Volz,[51] in a study on the effects of repeated experimentally produced hemarthroses on the rate of absorption of blood from the rabbit's knee joint, discovered that the rate of absorption is related to the degree of reactive change in the synovium. The absorption rate after several closely spaced hemarthroses is delayed initially as the synovium finds itself unable to clear the joint of blood. As the synovium proliferates in response to repeated hemarthroses, the rate of absorption of blood markedly increases. With advanced reactive changes after repeated hemarthroses, the rate of absorption becomes greater than normal. The stimulus for the production of the proliferative synovitis would appear to be the iron released from the red blood cells. Iron has been shown to possess definite irritative properties, which attack the synovium and stimulate the production of a villous and a nodular synovitis. The histological features of this condition closely resemble those of pigmented villonodular synovitis.[48,51]

Solitary nodular synovitis

Cytological findings in *solitary nodular synovitis* are similar to those described for pigmented villonodular synovitis except in the degree of synovial cell proliferation and villous formation. Gross findings in an experiment by Boyes[6] revealed a solitary pedunculated nodule bathed in a serous effusion with associated lesions of the articular surfaces indicative of direct trauma. Within this vascular lesion were seen four basic cells: the giant cell, a polyhedral stroma cell, the lipophage, and the hemosiderin cell. Beneath the lining membrane of synovial cells in varying degrees of proliferation were masses of chronic inflammatory cells. Fibrin was seen in sheets, interspaced between the stroma cells, and undergoing necrosis.[6]

Regeneration of synovium

Synovial tissue has a remarkable capacity for regeneration, possibly stemming from its excellent blood supply and its origin from a single undifferentiated mesenchymal cell type. Within several months synovium completely regenerates into tissue that is indistinguishable from normal tissue. Synovial regeneration is actually the result of metaplasia of mesenchymal elements within the joint cavity rather than a hyperplasia of the residual synovial cells in the area. Further biochemical studies are needed to determine if new synovium is metabolically identical to the original tissue.[48]

SYNOVIAL FLUID

Synovial fluid, also called *synovia,* is essentially a dialysate of blood plasma with the addition of proteins and a mucopolysaccharide—hyaluronic acid *(hyaluronate).*[54] The entry of proteins is regulated by the synovial membrane, and the synoviocytes secrete hyaluronate.

Composition and characteristics of synovial fluid

Normal synovial fluid is clear and pale yellow in color. It does not clot since it lacks fibrinogen as well as prothrombin. Synovial fluid is quite sparse in normal joints; only about 0.5 to 4 ml can be aspirated from large joints, such as the knee. Menisci, intraarticular disks, fat pads, and synovial folds assist in joint lubrication by evenly spreading fluid throughout the joint and taking up dead space, thus economizing on the amount of joint fluid necessary.[48]

Synovial fluid is a viscous substance. Its viscosity is related to the presence of hyaluronoprotein, which is a complex macromolecule containing a large amount of hyaluronic acid.[5] The other constituents of synovial fluid appear to be derived from plasma. Certain larger proteins, including fibrinogen, are normally absent; if present are in markedly reduced concentration compared to plasma. Synovial fluid contains slightly less total protein than plasma but has an albumin:globulin ratio of about 4:1.[33] Molecular charge and shape, as well as molecular weight, appear to be important in determining the permeability of the synovium to different plasma proteins.[5]

Synovial fluid normally contains only a few white blood cells, numbering less than 200 per ml.[3] These consist chiefly of mononuclear cells believed to be derived from the lining tissue. Inflammation, trauma, and other pathological processes affecting the system can alter the composition, cellular content, and physical characteristics of synovia. Examination of this fluid plays an important role in the diagnosis of joint problems.[5]

Synovianalysis

Synovianalysis or laboratory examination of synovial fluid serves to divide the fluid into one of five categories: (1) normal, (2) noninflammatory (group I), (3) inflammatory (group II), (4) purulent (group III), or (5) hemorrhagic (group IV). Table 4-2 gives the range of values found for various tests performed on the first four categories.

Table 4-3 lists some of the possible etiologies of the various types of synovial fluid. Trauma produces a nonin-

Table 4-2. Gross analysis of joint fluid

Criteria	Normal	Noninflammatory (group I)	Inflammatory (group II)	Purulent (group III)
1. Volume (ml) (knee)	<4	Often >4	Often >4	Often >4
2. Color	Clear to pale yellow	Xanthochromic	Xanthochromic to white	White
3. Clarity	Transparent	Transparent	Translucent to opaque	Opaque
4. Viscosity	Very high	High	Low	Very low, may be high with coagulase-positive staphylococci
5. Mucin clot*	Good	Fair to good	Fair to poor	Poor
6. Spontaneous clot	None	Often	Often	Often

From McCarty DJ: Synovial fluid. In McCarty DJ, editor: Arthritis and allied conditions, Philadelphia, 1979, Lea & Febiger.
*Recent effusions do not give firm clot because of serum admixture.

Table 4-3. Examples of diseases producing fluids of different groups

Noninflammatory (group I)	Inflammatory* (group II)	Purulent* (group III)	Hemorrhagic (group IV)
Osteoarthritis	Rheumatoid arthritis	Bacterial infections	Trauma, especially fracture
Early rheumatoid arthritis	Reiter's syndrome	Tuberculosis	Neuroarthropathy (Charcot joint)
Trauma	Crystal synovitis, acute (gout		Blood dyscrasia (e.g., hemophilia)
Osteochondritis dissecans	and pseudogout)		Tumor, especially pigmented vil-
Aseptic necrosis	Psoriatic arthritis		lonodular synovitis or hemangi-
Osteochondromatosis	Arthritis of inflammatory bowel		oma
Crystal synovitis, chronic or sub-	disease		Chondrocalcinosis
siding acute (gout and	Viral arthritis		Anticoagulant therapy
pseudogout)	Rheumatic fever		Joint prostheses
Systemic lupus erythematosus†			Thrombocytosis
Polyarteritis nodosa†			Sickle cell trait or disease
Scleroderma			
Amyloidosis (articular)			

From McCarty DJ: Synovial fluid. In McCarty DJ, editor: Arthritis and allied conditions, Philadelphia, 1979, Lea & Febiger.
*As disease in these groups remits, the exudate (fluid) passes through a group I phase before returning to normal.
†May occasionally be inflammatory, usually when clinical picture is that of rheumatoid arthritis.

flammatory (group I) type of synovial fluid, which will be discussed in the next section.[26]

Viscosity of synovial fluid

Synovial fluid exhibits a property common to all mucinous solutions in that its viscosity varies in a non-Newtonian fashion: when the rate of shear is low, it is highly viscous, and as the shear rate increases, the viscosity decreases.[3,13,33] Synovial fluid acts as a viscous fluid in the low-frequency region (corresponding to the slowly moving joint) but assumes the properties of an elastic material in the high-frequency region (corresponding to a rapidly moving joint). Synovial fluid is essentially a liquid whose relaxation time falls in the range between normal motion and motion that is rapid enough to induce trauma.[28]

The viscosity of synovial fluid results from the presence of hyaluronic acid, also called hyaluronate or mucin. Hyaluronate polymerizes into long-chain polysaccharides of high molecular weight and high viscosity.[43,48] A solution of hyaluronic acid is particularly suitable for lubricating joints required to carry load at varying rates of movement. The viscosity is high at the lowest rates to shear so that the joint is able to support a high load even at a low rate of movement. At higher rates of movement, the viscosity falls so that the drag of the joint is lessened, but the load that it will bear is not reduced because the greater rate of movement more than offsets the fall of viscosity. Hyaluronic acid produces high viscosity at a low concentration without a large osmotic effect. These properties result from its high molecular weight and its random chain structure.[29]

Functions of synovial fluid

One of the functions of synovial fluid is to assist in lubrication of the joints. Weight bearing tends to squeeze lubricant out from between the contacting surfaces of opposing articular cartilages. This is resisted by the tenacious quality of the viscous synovial fluid and by the incongruent surfaces of diarthrodial joints. The latter effect allows contact of adjoining cartilage structures at a limited but changing number of regions as the joint moves through its range of motion. In the intervening area where the fit is not exact, synovial fluid forms films of greater thicknesses. The next result is the creation of a series of wedge-shaped fluid layers that act to force fluid over the entire cartilage surface. Thus a fluid film constantly separates the joint surfaces, thereby holding attrition of joint cartilage to a low level.[34,39] The film is probably composed mainly of hyaluronic acid. The voluminous, randomly coiled particles may be thought of as being trapped and squeezed, like sponges, between the two articular surfaces (Figs. 4-14 and 4-15).[3,29]

Hyaluronate, besides lubricating the surfaces of the articular cartilage, has been shown to lubricate the periarticular soft tissues. The rubbing surfaces of synovial joints are made up of cartilage, synovial membrane, and soft tissues. The soft tissues around a joint are actually responsible for over 99% of the joint's resistance to movement.[34]

Another function of the synovial fluid is to provide nourishment for about two thirds of the avascular articular cartilage bordering the joint space.[40] (The role of synovial fluid in stabilization of joints has already been indicated.)

SYNOVIAL FLUID AND ITS REACTION TO INJURY

In general, nonhemorrhagic synovial fluids show relatively little change from normal after trauma. Typical fluids, aspirated less than 3 months after injury, are clear and do not clot. The total nucleated cell count is usually below 1000 per mm^3, sugar concentration is essentially the same

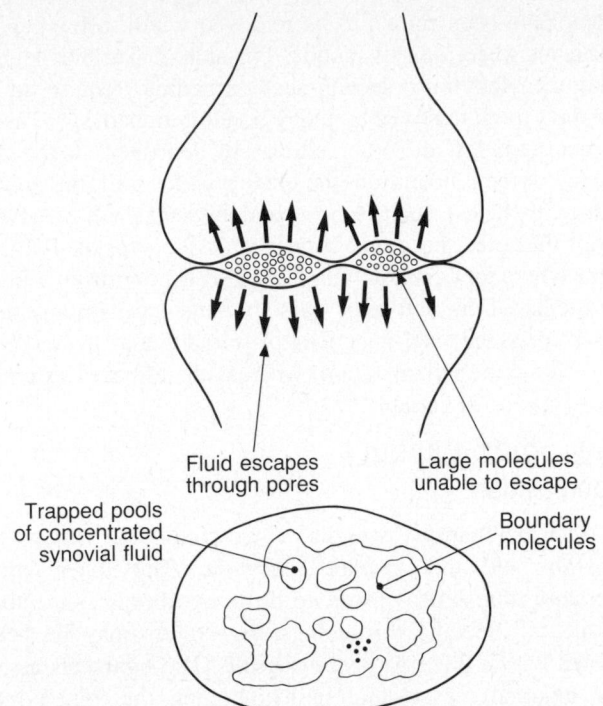

Fluid escapes
through pores

Large molecules
unable to escape

Trapped pools
of concentrated
synovial fluid

Boundary
molecules

Fig. 4-14. Pictorial representation of the lubrication of cartilage with synovial fluid. (From Dowson D, Wright V, and Longfield MD: Bio-medical Engineering 4:160, 1969.)

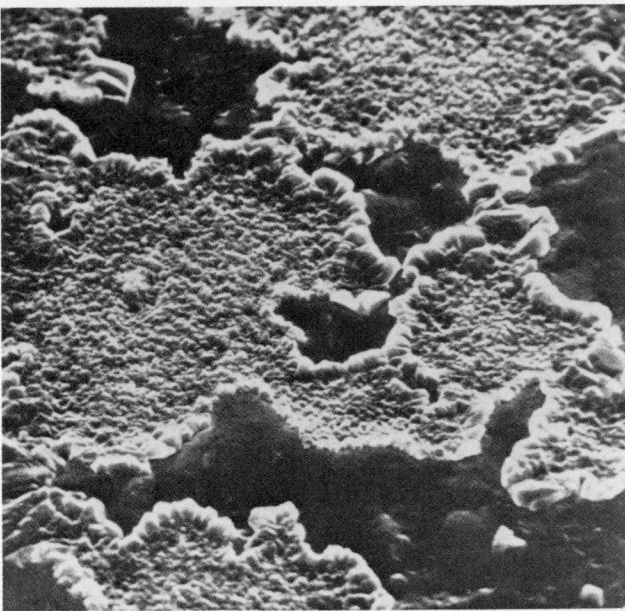

Fig. 4-15. Scanning electron microscope visualization of trapped pools of synovial fluid on the surface of articular cartilage. (From Dowson D, Wright V, and Longfield MD: Bio-medical Engineering 4:160, 1969.)

as that of serum, and there is good mucin precipitate.[12] In reactive synovitis, the percentage of protein is slightly elevated (from 2.7% to 3.4%), and the number of white blood cells is only slightly increased (from 100 or 150 to 300/mm³).[7]

Synovial fluid in posttraumatic synovitis

In synovitis of slightly longer duration or in posttraumatic synovitis, there is an increase in the white blood cell count to 600 to 2000/mm³ (some sources say 5000[10]).[7] The white blood cells, mostly mononuclear macrophages, comprise 80% to 90% of all cells. The amount of protein is about the same as mentioned for reactive synovitis.[7] This transudate is typical for posttraumatic synovitis and can be used for diagnosis.[40,47] If the posttraumatic synovitis lasts for a long time, more and more neutrophils are seen in the exudate, where they can reach up to 20% of all cells.

The synovial fluid reflects the inflammatory reactions going on in the synovial membrane. Thus the increased protein is probably derived from the synovial lining cells since one of the responses of the synovial membrane to trauma is an increase in type B cells that synthesize protein.[38] Also, as mentioned earlier, entry of small molecules into synovial fluid can be explained by diffusion between synovial lining cells, whereas factor-limiting protein entry is probably caused by the number and size of the fenestrations in the subsynovial capillaries. With inflam-

mation and increased synovial blood flow, protein entry may often increase out of proportion to the entry of small molecules. Therefore virtually all protein molecules found in plasma enter the joint; with increasing inflammation their concentration in synovia approaches the concentration of the plasma.[26] There is an increase in synovial fluid volume (often 10 to 20 times normal), resulting from increased production of exudate. The increase in white blood cells is a result of the inflammatory process, and the increase in total cell count also reflects the hypertrophy of the synovial membrane and the migration of type A cells into the synovial fluid.[33] There is also a decrease in viscosity due to a fall in the concentration of hyaluronate.[10]

After minor trauma, the joint shows only increased fluid volume with normal hyaluronic acid concentration and molecular weight. As the severity increases, the rate of fluid transfer to the joint surpasses the synthetic capacity of the synovial lining cells and hyaluronic acid concentration falls below normal. When the inflammatory process becomes sufficiently disruptive, joint lining cells not only fail to maintain hyaluronic acid concentration but also fail to maintain normal polymer weight.[10]

Synovial fluid in hemorrhagic effusions

Traumatic effusions that are hemorrhagic present a somewhat different picture. Sugar concentration is generally lower, the total nucleated cell count is higher, and the mucin precipitate is generally poorer. It is not uncommon to find small blood clots in a hemorrhagic effusion, but the majority of the blood remains fluid. Fibrinogen is not found in normal synovial fluid but occurs when there is bleeding into a joint. Because thromboplastic activity is absent or only slight in synovial and fibrous capsular tissue, it appears that local hemostasis after injury to a joint is effected chiefly by activation of the plasma thromboplastic system that enters the joint along with blood after injury.[12] With a grossly bloody fluid, there is the possibility of bleeding diathesis, pigmented villonodular synovitis, or tumor, as well as the suspected trauma. Bone marrow spicules or immature red blood cells in the fluid are often the first clue to a fracture. Blood is absorbed quickly by phagocytic cells in the synovial membrane so that blood may not be evident in the fluid if several days have passed after a hemarthrosis. However, an iron stain may show hemosiderin in synovial cells released into the synovial fluid.[40]

Synovial fluid containing fat globules

A recent traumatic effusion may also contain globules of free fat. When fractures are intracapsular, fat is liberated from the bone marrow; when there is cartilage and ligament injury, fat reaches the joint from the intracapsular, extrasynovial adipose tissue through a tear in the synovium.[4,12] In fractures of the knee, the joint may serve as a reservoir for fat so that the fat is absorbed slowly rather than discharged into the circulation in harmful amounts.[4]

Cloudy synovial fluid

If the aspirated fluid is cloudy, a variety of diseases should be considered. Cloudy fluids are usually caused by leukocytes (although cartilage fragments, crystals, red blood cells, fibrils, and "rice bodies" can occasionally be the cause). Leukocyte counts of greater than 2000 per mm^3 require careful evaluation for evidence of inflammatory joint diseases, such as gouty arthritis and rheumatoid arthritis. In the young, one should especially consider Reiter's syndrome, ankylosing spondylitis or colitis, viral or bacterial arthritis, as well as the collagen vascular diseases. Commonly, persons in the early stage of rheumatic disease associate the first swollen joint with trauma. Trauma can be shown to accentuate the severity of experimentally induced arthritis in rats and dogs.[40]

Reabsorption of traumatic effusions

The rate of absorption of solutions from the joint space is inversely proportional to the size of the particles—the larger the molecules, the slower the clearance. Diffusion and absorption are increased if the synovial fluid pressure is increased by intraarticular injection or movement. Small molecules are rapidly removed by osmosis and diffusion via the blood capillaries. Lymphatics remove larger molecules, such as proteins and colloidal solutions, from the joint space with minimal aid from the blood vessels. Solutions have been shown to be removed within a few hours from the knee joint of rabbits, but colloid particles larger than the globulin molecule, such as carbon, require up to 10 days to be removed by the regional lymphatics.[48] These larger particles are often ultimately deposited in the regional lymph nodes on the flexor surface of the joint. Large particles, such as iron and bismuth, are removed from the joint space and deposited in the subsynovial tissues where they remain. Clinically, absorption from a joint is increased by active or passive range of motion exercises, massage, and injections of intraarticular hydrocortisone for acute inflammation, whereas the effect of external compression is variable.[48]

THE JOINT CAPSULE
Composition

The joint capsule consists of two parts—*the stratum fibrosum* and the *stratum synoviale*. The outer layer (stratum fibrosum) is made up of dense fibrous connective tissue.[5,17] Specific thickenings, *ligaments,* may be contained within this part of the capsule. The ligaments assist the external musculature in maintaining the joint's mechanical integrity. The ligaments along with the rest of the joint capsule securely join the bones forming the articulation and serve to maintain the bones in apposition and influence the range of joint movement.[33] The stratum fibrosum also serves to protect and enclose the finely structured synovial membrane that lies within it.

Although there is some variation, the periarticular ligaments and capsule are fairly uniform in histological appearance, chemical composition, and tissue organization. The structures consist principally of parallel bundles or fascicles of collagen, sparsely populated with fibrocytes. Blood vessels traverse a tortuous course between the fascicles, and an occasional nerve fiber is noted, most frequently perivascular but occasionally free in the ligament or capsule. Together the fibrous proteins (collagen and elastin) account for 90% of the dry weight of the tissue.[24,53] The tough outer layer blends into the perichondrium and periosteum but does not extend over the surface of the articular cartilage within the joint. The ligaments and fibrous tissue are firmly united to the bone by collagen fibers, demonstrating a zonal organization. Parallel bundles of collagen first become invested with a fibrocartilaginous stroma and, as they near the bone, become calcified. The collagen fibers, continuous with the ligament, then enter the cortical osseous tissue in a manner analogous to Sharpey's fibers. The gradual transition of ligaments to mineralized fibrocartilage and then to bone enhances the ability of the insertions to distribute forces evenly.[24,33] The inner layer (stratum synoviale) consists of loose, highly vascularized tissue—the synovium (discussed in the first section of this chapter).[5,17]

Some joints are partially or completely subdivided by fibrocartilaginous disks or menisci that are attached at their periphery to the fibrous capsule. Fascia and other periarticular connective tissues blend with the joint capsule, adjacent ligaments, and the musculotendinous structures that pass over the joint, as well as investing the nerves and blood vessels entering the joint.[5]

Nerve and blood supply

The blood supply of the joint arises from vessels that enter the subchondral bone at or near the line of capsular attachment and form an arterial circle around the joint. These vessels subdivide into a rich capillary network that is especially prominent in the portions of the synovium immediately adjacent to the joint cavity.[5] Both capsules and ligaments have a poor blood supply but a very rich nerve supply with proprioceptive and pain endings.[33] Articular nerves carry both fibers derived from several spinal segments and autonomic and sensory fibers. The larger sensory fibers form proprioceptive endings that are sensitive to position and movement. Most of the smaller sensory fibers terminate in pain endings in the capsule, ligaments, and adventitia of blood vessels. The free nerve endings are particularly sensitive to twisting and stretching of these structures.[5] The capsule is thus the most generally receptive component of the joint tissues and is particularly sensitive to being stretched.[34] However, pain arising from the capsule or the synovium tends to be diffuse and poorly localized.[5]

Functions

Several functions of the joint capsule have already been mentioned. The stratum fibrosum, especially the ligaments, aids in holding together the bones that comprise the joint. Besides maintaining the bones in alignment, the ligaments serve to check movement occurring at a joint. Ligaments and capsular structures vary considerably in thickness and position, depending on the joint studied and the site within that joint. Structures range from the thin, redundant capsule of the shoulder joint to the thick, collagenous collateral ligament of the knee. In some joints, ligaments are condensations within the capsule, while in others, they are discretely separated from the capsule by an areolar layer. Capsular redundancy is an important aspect of joint function, particularly in relation to range of motion. The inferior medial portion of the shoulder joint capsule is a loose, redundant sac that becomes tense only when the shoulder is fully abducted or flexed. The posterior capsule of the knee is loose in flexion but so tight in extension that it becomes an important stabilizer. Ligaments that check movements often do so as the joint reaches the most stable position, and, as a consequence of being taut at that point, they frequently play a very important role in stabilizing the joint. Ligaments also sometimes guide movement at the joints. The stratum fibrosum protects and encloses the synovial membrane. The function of the stratum synoviale or the synovium has already been discussed.

THE JOINT CAPSULE AND ITS REACTION TO INJURY

The fibrous joint capsule reacts to trauma in a manner similar to the synovial membrane, showing an increase in vascularity and eventually the development of more fibrous tissue, resulting in a very thick capsule. The thickening of the joint capsule can often be palpated.[33]

Effusion into the joint cavity may lead to stretching of the capsule and associated ligaments. The elastic properties of the joint capsule can be expressed in terms of compliance. This compliance is given by relating the magnitude of a change in intraarticular volume to the associated change in intraarticular pressure (dV/dP). In general, a low-pressure effusion has been found to be associated with a hyperplastic synovial lining and a high-pressure effusion with an attenuated synovial surface. The physical properties of a particular effusion seem to be reflected in the changes in the synovium of the individual joint. The higher the hydrostatic pressure and volume of an effusion, the faster fluid reaccumulates after aspiration. This indicates that higher rates of transudation occur from synovial capillaries of such joints.[30]

A significant rise in intraarticular hydrostatic pressure contributes to joint damage by stretching the capsule and associated ligaments. In some cases the pressure level can be sufficient to exceed the elastic limit of the joint capsule.[30]

Sprains

Excessive or abnormal joint motion may cause injury to the ligaments or a sprain. Sprains are classified as first, second, or third degree and may vary from minor tearing of a few fibers without loss of integrity of the ligament to a complete tear of the ligament. Tears may be longitudinal, transverse, or oblique, each causing elongation of the remaining ligamentous fibers. Strain may be considered to be the physical force imposed on the ligamentous tissues, which exceeds normal stress but does not cause deformation or damage to the tissues. Physiological recovery can be expected. Experimentally, it has been shown that ligaments in which some fibers remain and in which there is good circulation regenerate well. With poor circulation, there is scar tissue formation rather than ligamentous growth.[8]

Enthesitis

Muscular insertions may also serve as reinforcing fibrous bundles in the joint capsule (as well as from tendon to ligament or between tendons). A continually recurring concentration of muscle stress at these points may provoke an inflammatory reaction known as enthesitis. There is a strong tendency toward fibrosis and calcification with this condition. Enthesitis can be differentiated from traumatic arthritis and periarthritis because only movements that bring into play the affected muscle are painful. Also, there is usually radiographic evidence of calcification at the insertion.[21]

INTRAARTICULAR FIBROCARTILAGE AND FAT PADS
Menisci

Fibrocartilage disks or menisci consist of a very dense, interwoven fibrous tissue with a scattering of mature fibrocytic cells. They are composed of complete or incomplete flattened, triangular, or somewhat irregularly shaped disks firmly attached to the fibrous capsules and often to one of the adjacent bones. Menisci normally occur only in the knee, temporomandibular, sternoclavicular, distal radioulnar, and acromioclavicular joints. Examination of menisci of the knee under polarized or light microscopy has shown that the collagen fibers are arranged circumferentially, presumably to withstand the tension of load bearing.[24,33,53]

The blood and nerve supply is from the joint capsule peripherally, and near the center of the joint, the menisci are virtually avascular. They presumably derive their nutrition from synovial fluid but also by diffusion from vascular plexuses, which are present in the soft tissues adjacent to their attachment to bone or fibrous capsule.[25,33,53]

Fat pads

Fat pads have a copious blood supply and consist of closely packed fat cells surrounded by fibrous tissue septa. These fibrous septa contain a considerable amount of elastic tissue. Besides the capillary network of the circulatory system, fat pads are liberally supplied with nerve endings. The fat pad as a whole is covered by a flattened layer of synovial cells.[52]

Functions

The menisci perform numerous functions[24,53]:

1. They help to fill in "dead" space between badly conforming bones. Serving in this way as physiological "packing," they tend to reduce the amount of play in the joint. They also provide better geometry for the appropriate wedge-shaped film of synovial fluid, characteristic of hydrodynamic lubrication, to be formed.
2. They act as shock absorbers, possibly because of the elastic nature of the disk, and serve to protect the articular surface.
3. They increase the congruity between articular surfaces, thereby improving joint stability.
4. They permit motion of bones relative to a joint-dividing disk as well as relative to each other.
5. They act as a chock to prevent undue forward gliding.
6. They provide a ball-bearing action (i.e., rolling of the lateral femoral condyle at the end of knee extension).
7. They improve weight distribution by enlarging effective contact area between the bones.
8. They also protect the joint margin.

Fat pads may act as packing—filling dead spaces in joint cavities—or as cushions, receiving the bony processes during extremes of movement. They may also assist in the generation of the lubrication wedge required for fluid-film or hydrodynamic lubrication.[53]

INTRAARTICULAR STRUCTURES AND THEIR REACTION TO INJURY
Meniscus injury

Mechanisms causing meniscus injury in the knee are numerous, but meniscus injuries are predominantly caused by compression and/or traction. The usual injury mechanism is rotatory stress on the weight-bearing leg. The stress is imposed by violation of internal rotation during flexion or external rotation during extension. Another mechanism that frequently causes injury to menisci is a forced valgus of the knee during flexion and an external rotation that opens the joint space and consequently entraps the meniscus.[8,9]

Symptoms are not caused by the cartilage tear per se but by stretching or tearing of peripheral attachments, which results in an acute synovial reaction within the joint space. Synovial effusion invariably accompanies meniscus tears and results from injury to the synovium, the capsule, or the ligaments. Tears in the substance of the avascular portion of the cartilage do not heal. Tears in the peripheral zones heal by invasion of fibrous tissue. If part of the meniscus is removed, it is replaced by dense collagen fiber from the remaining portion of the meniscus.[8,9]

Injury to fat pads

Fat pads may be impinged on by internal hemorrhage or increased effusion after trauma to a joint. Pain results and, in the knee, tenderness is felt just medial (or lateral) to the patellar tendon. Examination may reveal a hypertrophied fat pad. Bilateral injury to the fat pads in the same knee occurs more often when there is a concomitant degenerative arthritis. Injection of the pad with corticosteroids may be both diagnostic and momentarily therapeutic, but usually surgical removal is necessary.[9]

Intraarticular damage and osteophytes in osteoarthritis

Tissues not injured in the original trauma can be damaged as the inflammatory process in the synovial membrane progresses. In osteoarthritis there may be splitting and shredding of the menisci, especially the medial meniscus.[33]

Osteophytic proliferation occurs as the result of increased vascularity of the bone adjacent to the joint, including bone beneath the articular cartilage and at the articular margins. It is at the latter site that the osteophytes are most significant because they can be palpated there at an early stage and give the earliest indications of osteoarthritis that can be seen on radiographs. They contribute significantly to the overall increase in girth of osteoarthritic joints in addition to the thickened joint capsule, the inflamed synovial membrane, and other periarticular fibrosis.[33]

The periarticular *osteophytes* arise at the fibrocartilaginous transition zone between the synovial membrane and the joint capsule on one side and the articular cartilage on the other. The development is nodular at first, but as the disease progresses, the nodules coalesce to form large strips of cancellous bone usually covered with fibrocartilage, although grossly this often has the appearance of hyaline cartilage.[32]

The precise reason for the gross periarticular proliferation of osteophytes is not known. It would appear to be a logical response to locally increased blood flow and oxygen tension, but many theories advanced for the location of this reaction are either unsatisfactory or very difficult to prove.[33]

If their origin is obscure, then the clinical significance of osteophytes in the pathogenesis of the diseased joint is even more uncertain, apart from being an aid in diagnosis. They may be simply an indication of degenerate articular cartilage or generally increased blood flow. Occasionally, fragments of an osteophyte can become free in the joint and exacerbate the clinical signs, but this is rare. It is customary to remove the osteophytes when debriding a badly diseased joint to reduce stretching of the joint capsule and therefore irritation and pain.[33]

Joint bodies

Injury to joint regions may also cause formation of "free joint bodies," whose long-term effect is to enhance articular damage (like foreign bodies in a closed gearbox). Such joint "mice" may represent detached bits of articular cartilage, small osteoarticular fracture fragments, or marginal osteophytes. There are other sources of joint bodies—osteochondromatosis of the synovium or a focus of osteochondritis dissecans of the knee that has loosened and become free. Whatever the origin of joint bodies, they are nourished by the synovial fluid and grow slowly by the accumulation of layers of cartilage on their surfaces. Eventually, they become several times their original size. The cartilage component can become calcified, but ossification does not occur because this would require a blood supply.[23]

ARTICULAR CARTILAGE

The actual load-carrying surface of the synovial joint is covered by a thin overlay of specialized connective tissue referred to as hyaline cartilage. This layer is only about 1 to 7 mm thick in healthy joints.[53] The chief components of articular cartilage are collagen, protein-polysaccharides, and water. The physical properties of cartilage are determined by the chemical nature of its constituents as well as by their interactions and physical arrangement.[43]

Composition

The articular cartilage contains small numbers of chondrocytes, housed in lacunae, surrounded by a resilient, three-dimensional lattice of collagen fibrils that provides a large degree of the mechanical strength of the tissue. Between the collagen fibers lies the ground substance, comprising all of the noncellular and nonfibrous material present. This ground substance is a gel-like interstitial medium composed of sulfated polysaccharides associated with protein and an aqueous solution of electrolytes.[33,49,53]

The matrix of articular cartilage is hyperhydrated, with a water content varying from 65% to 80% of the total weight. This water plays an important role in joint lubrication inasmuch as about two thirds is extracellular and provides the vehicle for diffusion of metabolic substrates and products of the chondrocytes.[42] The solid matter of the matrix consists chiefly of two macromolecules that are synthesized by the chondrocytes—collagen and proteoglycans (protein-polysaccharides). Collagen fibers form over half the dry weight of the matrix. These fibers play a major role in the elasticity of articular cartilage. The remainder of the solids are made up largely of protein-polysaccharides, a family of molecules consisting of a protein core to which are attached long chains of negatively charged, repeating units of sulfated disaccharide. The protein-polysaccharides are highly viscous and strongly hydrophilic, properties that are of key importance in the resiliency of articular cartilage and the lubrication of its bearing surfaces under compressive loads.[5]

Nutritional supply

Articular cartilage is distinguished by a relatively low concentration of cells and a corresponding preponderance of intercellular material. Normal articular cartilage is devoid of blood vessels, lymphatic channels, and nerves. The tissue derives its nourishment largely from the synovial fluid that bathes its surface and to a lesser extent from the diffusion of blood substrates coursing through vessels in the underlying bony endplate.[2,5,33,49] Isolation from the body's vascular system dictates that nutrients must pass through a double diffusion process to reach the chondrocytes. Normally, materials in the bloodstream destined to reach the chondrocytic cells must first diffuse across the synovial membrane into the synovial fluid and then across the matrix of the articular cartilage to traverse the cell membrane. Diffusion of nutrients across the synovial membrane is a relatively simple process, and the constituents of synovial fluid are an ultrafiltrate of plasma to which the B cells have added hyaluronate. Diffusion across the articular cartilage surface is considerably limited not only by the electrical charge of the nutrient but also by the theoretical "pore size."[1] Because of the high degree of entanglement of protein-polysaccharide molecules, the tight packing of collagen, and the large amount of bound or structured water, cartilage behaves as a molecular sieve, with an effective pore size of about 60 Å in diameter. This excludes large molecules, such as hyaluronate, plasma proteins, and immunoglobulins in the joint fluid, and retains the chondroitin sulfate and other matrix components.[43]

The movement of fluid into and out of articular cartilage appears to be produced by diffusion and osmosis. Joint mobility and agitation of the fluid increase the rate of diffusion. In a mature joint there is no transfer across the bone-cartilage interface, whereas in an immature joint there is some diffusion. Investigation into the effect of alternate compression and relaxation on diffusion shows that such alternation adds very little to the normal diffusion rate.[25,54] At low pressures intermittent loading (compression) contributes little to the material transfer into cartilage, while at high pressures intermittent loading does lead to the transport of solutes into cartilage, but it cannot significantly increase the rate of transfer above that attributable to normal diffusion. Loading cartilage surfaces for prolonged periods without allowing intermittent relaxation can be expected to lead to a decreased diffusion, without any absorption of fresh fluid attributable to the action of a pump, and this would result in an overall decrease in the rate or penetration of substances into cartilage. A consistently maintained compression of cartilage results in the loss of fluid, which is taken up again on removal of the load.[25] The sloshing back and forth of fluid in and out of cartilage is essential for cartilage nutrition. Chondrocytes die in the face of absolute immobilization, excessive pressure, or lack of pressure on the joint, all of which prevent fluid flow.[34]

Zones of articular cartilage

Histological and ultrastructural examination of cartilage has revealed four zones: a *tangential or gliding zone* (zone 1), a *transitional zone* (zone 2), a *radial zone* (zone 3), and a *calcified zone* (zone 4) (Fig. 4-16).[26,50]

Zone 1, immediately adjacent to the joint space, consists of a very thin layer of small collagen fibers, lying parallel to the surface and covered by a fine, acellular, afibrillar membrane. The collagen fiber bundles are densely packed with little intervening ground substance, and the cells are small and of an elongated, elliptical shape with their long axes parallel to the articular surfaces.[33,43,53,54] At the periphery, the fibrous components merge with the fibrous periosteum of the adjacent bone.[50]

Zone 2, the intermediate or transitional zone, has collagen fibers that form a coiled, interlacing, open network. Ground substance is more abundant. Cells are more numerous than in the tangential zone and are spheroidal and dispersed but equally spaced.[50]

In the deep or radial zone, zone 3, the collagen fibers are thicker, form a tighter meshwork, and tend to run radially to the subchondral bone. The fibers are coiled and S-shaped with large spaces between while the spheroidal cells are arranged in columnar fashion, often in groups of

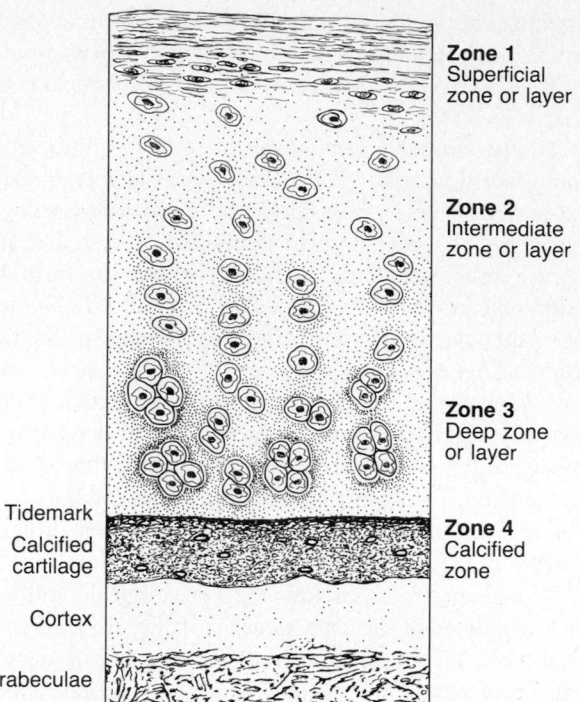

Fig. 4-16. The zones of adult articular cartilage. (From Turek SL: Orthopaedics: principles and their application, Philadelphia, 1977, JB Lippincott Co, Inc.)

two to eight cells. The radial zone is separated from the calcified zone by a wavy, basophilic, irregular line called the "tidemark."[50]

The deepest collagen fibers are embedded in the zone of calcified cartilage, zone 4, above the subchondral bone and help to secure the cartilage to the bone. The cells are sparser and smaller, and the matrix is heavily impregnated with calcium salts.* The fibers are of larger size and oriented perpendicularly with the meshwork more closely packed.[52]

The surface layer of circumferentially arranged fibers and featureless membrane remains very thin in all the joints studied, whereas the deeper zones vary in thickness from joint to joint and even at different points on one articular surface. This is reflected in a variation of thickness of the articular cartilage.[33]

Under static compressive loading, it appears that zone 1 provides a load diffusion effect in addition to a relatively smooth bearing surface.[52] Zone 2 and, to a lesser degree, zone 3 act as an area of deformability and energy storage—open meshwork becomes disrupted and the collagen fibers tend to orient perpendicularly to the direction of loading and to uncoil.[52,53] Zone 4 binds the tissue to the underlying bone and provides a degree of constraint.[52] The arrangement of collagen fibers and ground substance can account for the elasticity and compressibility of articular

*See references 33, 43, 50, 53, and 54.

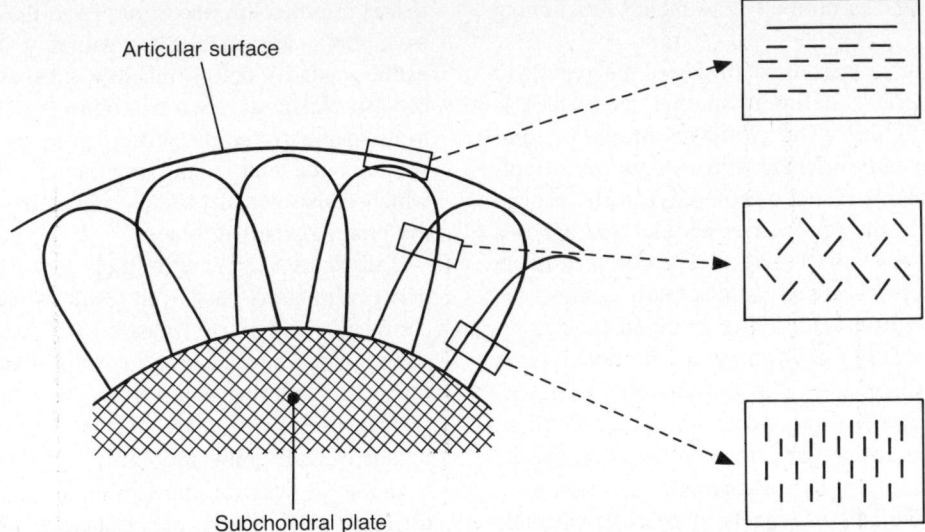

Articular surface

Subchondral plate

Fig. 4-17. Schematic representation of collagen-fiber orientation in articular cartilage. (From Sledge CB: Orthop Clin North Am 6[3]:619, 1975.)

cartilage, which is essential for the pumping of nutrients through the tissue to the chondrocytes and aids in proper joint lubrication.[33]

Taken as a whole, the collagen fibers are arranged at right angles to the surface of the subchondral bone to which they are attached, and they curve near the articular surface so as to run parallel to the surface (Fig. 4-17). This curve results in the formation of arches arranged to resist both shearing and direct compression forces. The collagen fibers add strength, whereas the ground substance provides firmness and smoothness to the surface. The gently curved shape of the bearing surface of the joints further provides for rapid, uniform dissipation of stress.[2]

Metabolic activity of articular cartilage

The articular cartilage in the adult is not simply a lining surface responsible for joint motion and tissue resiliency, but it is also an actively metabolizing tissue. Specifically, the chondrocytes synthesize the proteoglycans and collagen matrix. Turnover of at least a portion of the proteoglycans (estimated half-life, 8 to 17 days) is so rapid that it suggests the existence of an internal remodeling system. There is also ample evidence that the chondrocytes synthesize lysosomal enzymes presumably necessary for this internal remodeling system.[1,5,43] Normally, the cells cease their DNA synthesis at maturity but under a variety of circumstances may reinitiate this process, presumably to repair defects or respond to the chronic stress of osteoarthritis.[1]

Chondrocytes are metabolically very active cells, continuously utilizing both aerobic and anaerobic pathways. The chondrocytes from zones 2 and 3 of articular cartilage have extensive networks of rough-surfaced endoplasmic reticulum, dilated cisternae, vacuoles, and Golgi apparatus—suggesting that they actively synthesize protein, polysaccharides, collagen, and other components of the matrix. Metabolic studies using radioisotopes demonstrate that the chondrocyte cell synthesizes the components of macromolecules of proteoglycans and collagen, assembles them intracellularly, and then rapidly extrudes them into the surrounding matrix. The synthesis of proteoglycans is rapid, but the turnover rate of collagen is much slower.[50]

Functions of articular cartilage

Load carriage. *Load carriage* is the capacity of cartilage to sustain loads to which it is subjected without failing mechanically, to compensate for the gross incongruities and small asperities at the subchondral bone surface, and to reduce stress on the subchondral bone from dynamic loads. Cartilage compensates for bony incongruities by increasing the area of contact in the joint, thereby reducing the contact pressures on the bone.[50]

Articular cartilage seems to act primarily as a bearing surface and to distribute load rather than acting as a shock absorber.[1] The major contribution to peak force attenuation comes from the soft tissue structures and bone rather than from cartilage and synovial fluid.[34,35] Articular cartilage is about 10 times as effective in reducing peak loads as is an equivalent amount of subchondral bone. However, because the amount of articular cartilage present in joints relative to bone is so small, even with its greater efficiency, cartilage contributes a minor share to peak force attenuation.[36] The important role played by periarticular soft tissues, such as the joint capsule, in force attenuation is probably due to their elastic nature.[35] Active contraction of muscle against tension can also absorb tremendous amounts of energy and is normally the major functioning shock absorber.[1,34]

Articular cartilage is structured to resist the repetitive rubbing and considerable deformation that its surface is subjected to in a lifetime. The cartilage matrix is composed of a systematically oriented fibrous network of collagen and a set of highly charged proteoglycan molecules. The collagen fibers at the surface run parallel and act as a membrane holding the matrix together. The collagen fibers in the calcified zone run vertically and actually connect the articular cartilage with its underlying calcified bone, preventing shear failure during joint motion. The fibers in the midzone of the cartilage appear to be randomly oriented, but when the cartilage is subjected to axial compression, the fibers tend to line up perpendicular to the compressive force, the most advantageous arrangement in resisting a compressive load. The lack of vessels in articular cartilage appears to be of significant functional advantage. Under physiological conditions, articular cartilage can be compressed to as much as 40% of its original height. If blood vessels traversed it, they would be rendered useless.[24]

Stress applied to articular cartilage is dependent not only on the magnitude of the applied force but also on the rate of application of the force. When load is applied to articular cartilage, an instantaneous deformation occurs and is followed by a time-dependent creep phase, in which the indentation increases continuously with time although a constant load is maintained. The first stage of instantaneous deformation causes a change in contour but not in volume and results from a simultaneous bulk movement of the matrix and collagen fibers rather than from a flow of water through the matrix. During the second stage, cartilage deforms increasingly with the passage of time, even though the applied pressure is held constant. This is known as *creep* and is related to the flow of water through the matrix. This property determines the description of cartilage as a viscoelastic material. The ability of cartilage to deform elastically and then flow under load is followed by a reabsorption of fluid when the load is removed. These viscoelastic properties enable cartilage to perform one of its vital functions in the diarthrodial joints—that of limiting the stresses transmitted to the bone ends.[50,53,54]

When the load is removed, cartilage recovers its original thickness as a result of an initial instantaneous (elastic) recovery followed by a time-dependent recovery phase (reimbibition of water). Cartilage is considered to be capable of displaying an elastic or "springlike" deformation within 2 seconds after application of a load. Approximately 90% or more of the instantaneous deformation is instantaneously recoverable when the load is quickly removed. During the normal walking cycle the duration of the applied load is between 0.5 second and 1 second, and peak loads are applied for less then 0.5 second.[50]

Most weight-bearing joints are subjected to loads applied rapidly and high loads of short duration. Cartilage

assists in protecting the bones from these stresses by acting as a shock absorber (i.e., damping and attenuating dynamic loads by deforming to a substantial extent in a viscoelastic fashion). Two components of cartilage contribute to its load-carriage properties: proteoglycans, which retain water in the matrix and regulate its flow, and collagen, which resists tensile forces within the matrix and retains the proteoglycans in place.[50]

Lubrication. The extremely low coefficient of friction between joints is partly the result of the nature of articular cartilage—which is elastic and extremely smooth—although the surface roughness is about 10 times greater than conventional engineering bearing surfaces.[13,14] Its surface irregularities are elastic, becoming deformed and flattened with joint motions.[43] There is no one model available to describe lubrication at each point of the articulating cycle. There are basically two mechanisms involved in cartilage-on-cartilage lubrication.[24,50] *Boundary lubrication* means that each bearing surface is coated with a thin layer of molecules that slide on the opposing surface more readily than they are sheared off the underlying one. This is necessary for lowering frictional effects of cartilage on cartilage, but it ceases to function when loads are excessive.[50] Boundary lubrication functions primarily when joints move under a relatively light load. It involves the binding of a special glycoprotein found in synovial fluid, which is then affixed to the cartilage surfaces and keeps them from touching.[24] The second mechanism, *fluid lubrication,* produces synovial fluid film completely separating the opposing bearing surfaces, with resistance to motion arising from the viscosity of the fluid. A fluid film forms on the articular surfaces when cartilage is rubbed against cartilage under load in the presence of a lubricant. In the early phases of loading, fluid is trapped in the existing depressions in the surface of cartilage. The cartilage surface under load, because of its elasticity, undergoes deformation, creating a depression narrower at its periphery than at its center, trapping the fluid so that a phenomenon called *squeeze-film lubrication* results. *Squeeze-film lubrication* occurs when the approaching surfaces generate pressure in the lubricant as they squeeze it out of the area of impending contact between them. The resulting pressure keeps the surfaces apart. A fluid exudes from the cartilage and forms a film, termed the "squeeze film," in the transient area of impending contact.

Compressed articular cartilage also "weeps" fluid, mainly water and small ions. This fluid film produces *weeping lubrication,* a form of hydrostatic lubrication in which the interstitial fluid of hydrated articular cartilage flows onto its own surface when a load is applied to it.[50] Although the major part of water in cartilage is in the form of a proteoglycan-collagen gel, it is freely exchangeable with synovial fluid, and a significant portion can be liberated by pressure on the cartilage. Since in the adult there is little or no traversal of water through the subchondral plate nor a flow through the substance of the cartilage, the water displaced by cartilage compression will be expressed onto the surface of the cartilage, preferentially peripheral to the zone of impending contact. When the compression is released, the matrix within the cartilage contains enough of a fixed charge to osmotically attract the water and small solutes back into the matrix, and the cartilage regains its original height. The fluid film that exists between moving cartilage layers, therefore, consists of cartilaginous interstitial fluid, which is squeezed onto the surface as the cartilage compresses the already present synovial fluid trapped in the contact zone.[24] The cartilage acts as a self-pressurizing sponge; when the pressure is released, the fluid flows back into the cartilage. "Weeping" probably occurs beyond the area of contact, where counteracting pressure is lower. This mechanism has also been termed *self-pressurized hydrostatic lubrication.*[50]

The hydrostatic mechanism functions best under substantial loads, since under small loads there is little cartilage compression and little weeping of fluid onto the surface. Cartilage weeping may well be the most important mechanism for protecting the articular cartilage from damage in certain high-load situations.[37]

Cartilage lubrication is supplemented when hydrostatic pressure buildup in the interstitial fluid in cartilage during loading counteracts the pressure in the lubricant that has been trapped in the area of deformation at the surface. This prevents the lubricant from entering the pores in the cartilage, and the hyaluronate molecules left behind become concentrated and supposedly enhance lubrication *(boosted lubrication).*[14,50,53]

There is also a theory that in cartilage-on-cartilage bearings the surfaces are elastic enough so that the lubricant pressure that is generated by motion under a given load depresses the surfaces a distance greater than the height of their asperities. Consequently, fewer asperities come into contact, and the fluid film is more easily maintained. This is termed *elastohydrodynamic lubrication,* a form of fluid lubrication. This concept of cartilage lubrication, however, is not universally accepted.[50]

Thus synovial joints are lubricated by two complementary systems—a hydrostatic (fluid lubrication) system that functions primarily at high loads and a boundary system that is most effective at low loads.[24] Hyaluronate appears to have little place in cartilage-on-cartilage lubrication but does play an important role as the boundary lubricant for synovial tissue. Since the friction of cartilage rubbing on cartilage is very low (measured as little as .002 coefficient of friction), the preponderance of frictional resistance in joint movement is in the periarticular soft tissues, which also usually make up the bulk of the articulating area within the joint capsule. Resistance to motion is the result of stretching of soft tissues (ligaments, muscles, tendons) and of soft tissue fractional resistance (synovium-on-synovium, synovium-on-cartilage, cartilage-on-cartilage). Hyaluronate serves as a boundary lubricant in this system.[24]

ARTICULAR CARTILAGE AND ITS REACTION TO INJURY
Capacity for repair

Cartilage cells are quite active metabolically. The chondrocytes produce considerable amounts of collagen and mucopolysaccharides after injury. The numbers of chondrocytes and their metabolic rate may also increase. When an injury to cartilage is in an area close to some viable source of cells that are capable of metaplasia—such as synovium, subchondral bone, or perichondrium—cartilage heals by forming fibrocartilage, which is capable of maturing under appropriate circumstances.[34]

Substantial evidence exists to suggest that chondrocytes mitotically divide and that adult cartilage is capable, under certain circumstances, of repairing itself.[34] Experiments have shown that chondrocytes, isolated from mature individuals, grow readily and synthesize phenotypical glycosaminoglycans and collagen under proper conditions of culture in vitro. There is evidence for this in the release of the chondrocytes from their imprisoning matrix by enzymatic or other means. The matrix thus serves ordinarily to switch off the cell replicative mechanism. Although the rate of repair of articular cartilage is low, it may not be negligible over a period of time.[44] Whether the surface of articular cartilage continues to be slowly worn off in life and continuously replaced is still controversial.[34]

It has been suggested that the major shock absorber protecting cartilage is a reflexive neuromuscular response. Even in the presence of an intact neuromuscular system, the skeleton can be subjected to enough shock loading to microfracture the subchondral bone. Unexpected loads that present themselves in less then 65 msec (the natural response time) are not well dampened by the neuromuscular system. Substantial loads of a severe nature—such as might occur from auto accidents or skiing—can break bone. However, fracture is an excellent shock-absorbing mechanism, and, if the bone heals without malalignment and the break is distant from the joint, the cartilage is spared.[1]

Partial-thickness and full-thickness defects

Even when stress on a joint is insufficient to cause clinical fracture to the subchondral bone, damage may be found on microscopy. Articular cartilage—consisting of an elastic surface layer over a thin, calcified brittle one—is likely to slip at a plane between these layers, and the existence of such a plane of weakness at this level has been proven. Moreover, if there is a gap in the deeper tissue, the elastic cartilage may be expected to herniate into the opening. Such changes can be seen in sections without any other structural abnormality, sometimes near complete fractures but also independent of them; therefore it is reasonable to suggest that the changes are mechanical. Three stages, short of complete fracture, can be described: (1) splitting at the *tidemark* (a wavy line that marks the junction between calcified and uncalcified cartilage), (2) depression of cartilage into bone, and (3) fissuring of both calcified cartilage and bone along a vertical plane that permits blood vessels from the marrow to reach the cartilage.[22]

A trauma-induced defect in articular cartilage possesses a variable potential for repair. *Partial-thickness defects,* limited to the articular cartilage, adjacent to the synovial attachment or perichondrium, can undergo some degree of healing by proliferation and invasion from soft tissue. However, cartilage wounds at some distance from soft tissue do not heal well, although there is evidence of an intense biochemical response. Instead there is heightened synthesis of matrix components in such injuries and increased mitotic activity that is short-lived and ineffectual for healing. Nevertheless, there is complete repair in approximately 20% of the defects induced in experimental animals, involving a period of extraordinary cellular proliferation and cartilage growth. At first the surface is bridged by the layer of elongated compacted cells in a collagenous stroma. Then the defect is filled in rapidly by cellular fibroblastic tissue that changes, as it extends deeply, into chondroid tissues with cells irregularly arrayed in a homogeneous matrix. The reparative tissue consistently forms hyaline cartilage, which blends with preexisting cartilage.[50] However, in general, experimentally induced gaps in articular cartilage that do not penetrate into the subchondral vascular marrow show little tendency to be filled in with new cartilage.[44]

Repair of *full-thickness defects* (extending through the subchondral bone) takes place by proliferation of cellular tissue originating from the superficial layer that has bridged the defect at the surface and by rapidly invading osteogenic cells and granulation tissue from the narrow spaces at the base, resulting in a mixture of bony trabeculae, cartilage, and mostly fibrous tissue.[50]

The process begins when capillaries grow directly into the uncalcified cartilage without the mediation of any other cell to destroy the matrix ahead of them. There is physical splitting of the calcified cartilage behind them but no invasion or dissolution of it. The shape of the intruding mass into the cartilage is smoothly rounded. There is well-marked zonation around this mass—first, a chondrin-free ring next to the untouched cartilage; next, a ring where there is a gathering together of fine fibers to form a coarser set of strands; and finally, among the capillaries, the development of large and irregular fibers and the disappearance of cartilage cells (Fig. 4-18). When the process has gone on further, the degeneration of the hyaline cartilage is more complete. The hyaline cartilage loses its chondrin and reverts to fibrous tissue. The chondrocytes revert to fibrocytes and there is much more than normal collagen in the margin of the intrusion; this process represents not only the removal of one component of cartilage but includes excess production of another.[22] The final healed defect is represented by a slightly discolored and roughened pit or a superficial linear defect on an otherwise smooth surface of hyaline cartilage. This implies that full-

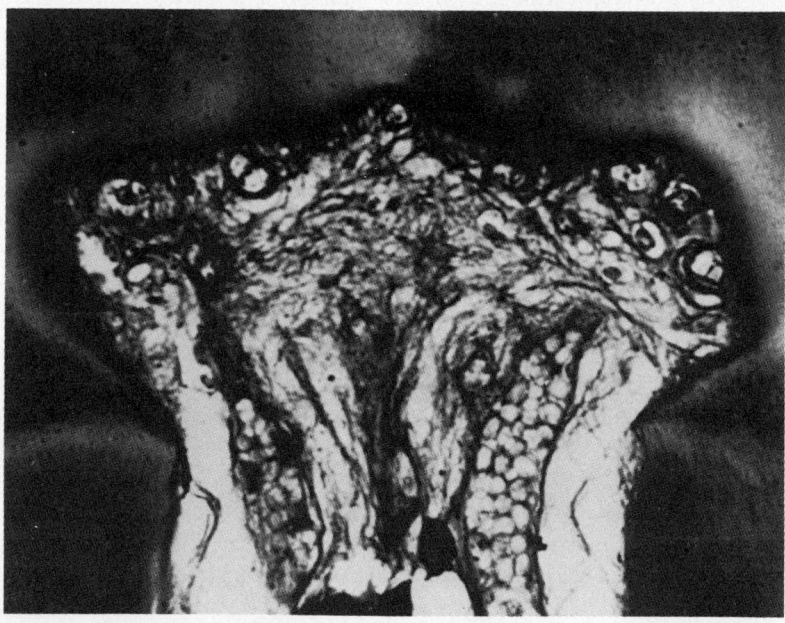

Fig. 4-18. Invasion of cartilage by capillaries from the bone below, with pale diffusion zone limited by a dark basophil ring. Cartilage cells and the aggregation of collagen fibers are well marked in the next zone; no adventitious cells. Process mechanically checked in the calcified zone but expands in the soft uncalcified zone; chemical changes stop abruptly at the tidemark. (From Landells JW: J Bone Joint Surg [Br] 38[2]:548, 1957.)

thickness defects will heal but only with fibrocartilage, a mechanically inferior tissue.[50]

However, the usual sequel of intrusion by capillaries in full-thickness defects includes early sealing off by ossification. This results in the formation of a nodule of bone in the deeper cartilage that, by fusion of adjacent foci, advances the bony articular lamella and thins the overlying cartilage in the middle of the joint; this impairs the cartilage's elasticity and favors further injury. At the edge of the cartilage, the process results in osteophyte formation.[22]

Cartilage formation is directly related to the nature of the stress that the tissue undergoes.[34] When a partial-thickness defect confined to the articular cartilage is subjected to constant joint motion, the differentiation toward hyaline cartilage is more pronounced. The main cartilaginous constituent forms nearer the surface. However, if the joint is immobilized, the defect fills with primitive connective tissue that includes little cartilage. When a full-thickness defect extends into the subchondral bone, granulation tissue rapidly invades from the vascular marrow spaces and healing is predominantly fibrous or fibrocartilaginous. Under conditions of continuous motion, the reparative tissue becomes more cartilaginous and restores a smooth articular surface, and the intercellular matrix fuses with the original cartilage.[50]

Complete fracture of articular cartilage

The changes in articular cartilage after complete fracture can be divided into three stages. Immediate changes may include a transverse fracture at the tidemark; vertical fractures elsewhere through the cartilage, calcified cartilage, and bone; and a narrow zone of dead cells around the injury site. Intermediate changes (3 to 14 days after injury) reveal no tendency of the cartilage to flake around the margin of the injury and little multiplication of cartilage cells exposed by the breach. The late stage of change and repair includes two events: (1) replacement of gaps left in the articular cartilage and (2) determination of the fate of the displaced fragments of such cartilage. Replacement is invariably by fibrous tissue, derived from granulation tissue emerging from the depths of the bone if the gap is central or from the synovial membrane if the gap is peripheral, or both. This fibrous tissue, if exposed to synovial fluid, is eventually impregnated with polysaccharides and may in several years come to resemble fibrocartilage and present a remarkably smooth surface, but the internal structure remains different from the original hyaline cartilage. Displaced fragments of cartilage change in several ways. When fibrous tissue grows over the surface of displaced cartilage and is itself nourished by synovial fluid, a new stratum of fibrocartilage may bury the old, which survives almost unchanged beneath it. More usually, however, cartilage perishes wherever it comes into contact with granulation tissue. The cells die and the chondrin is dissolved away before the actual invasion has gone far. Later, migrant fibrocytes penetrate the matrix and replace it with fibrous tissue, which may ossify.[22]

No specialized phagocyte appears to remove uncalcified cartilage. It is possible that the collagen is not removed but that the solution of the surrounding chondrin so changes the physical state of collagen that the fine fibrils dispersed in the gel come to form tight bundles. These take up little room, compared with their immediately adjacent pale diffusion ring, possibly because of the loss of much bound water as well as the acquisition of fresh interfibrillary bonds. In this vascular digestion, the adjacent calcified cartilage undergoes no internal change; its removal is always associated with the presence of multinucleate giant cells.[22]

The reaction that occurs in articular cartilage after trauma shows the importance of the normal balance between articular cartilage and its blood supply. The normal nutrition of cartilage is mainly synovial, although there is evidence of some vascular diffusion from bone. The presence of occasional blood vessels in the subarticular plane has been interpreted as important in the normal nutrition of cartilage, but such vessels are few in number and are insulated by a thin sheet of bone. If there are blood vessels present that do not have this sheet, abnormalities are visible in the cartilage. Examples of such contact may arise in several ways: (1) trauma may displace fragments into callus, (2) vascular tissue may grow over the cartilage surface, or (3) there may be intrusion of blood vessels through the articular lamella from trauma or erosion. In each case cartilage is being destroyed. A good blood supply is rapidly followed by complete disorganization of hyaline cartilage and its replacement by fibrous tissue, fibrocartilage, or bone.[22]

Osteoarthritis

Results of trauma to synovial joints can lead to subsequent development of some degree of a condition known variously as *osteoarthritis,* osteoarthrosis, hypertrophic arthritis, or degenerative joint disease. It is essentially a degenerative condition of articular cartilage with subsequent formation of marginal osteophytes, subchondral bone changes, bone marrow changes, inflammatory reaction of the synovium, capsular thickening, alteration of the synovial fluid, and damage to intraarticular structures.[8,33] Most authors distinguish between *primary* (idiopathic) *osteoarthritis* and *secondary osteoarthritis* (secondary to an infectious, traumatic, inflammatory, metabolic, or aging process). Often, however, the etiology of one type cannot be delineated from that of the other.[8,50]

Pathology and pathogenesis

The proteoglycan component of articular cartilage is readily susceptible to enzymatic degradation. This may occur after acute inflammation, synovectomy, immobilization, or even seemingly minor insults.[43] When subjected to increasing stress, the limiting effect of the pore size of articular cartilage is probably destroyed, and the ground substance (proteoglycan) leaks out. Lysosomal activity becomes marked.[34] The protease implicated is probably a cathepsin derived from the damaged cartilage cells. Enzymatic degradation of the ground substance and abrasive forces then release cartilage debris and mucopolysaccharide materials, which can lead to the secondary changes of osteoarthritis—spurs, cysts, and synovitis.[11] When the proteoglycan content is depleted, the physical properties of the cartilage change, rendering the collagen fibers susceptible to mechanical damage.[43] Along with degeneration of the mucopolysaccharide ground substance, there is loss of the fine superficial membrane and superficial cellular layer. When the disruption is confined to the tangential layer of the surface, the process is referred to as flaking; when the process extends to the deeper radial zone, it is described as fibrillation. The collagen fibers are thus exposed ("unmasked"), elasticity is impaired, and minor trauma is able to produce fissures and more fibrillation. This cracking of the surface is the earliest change visible to the naked eye and is followed by erosion of the tissue, often through to the subchondral bone, which may become smooth and shiny. There is no evidence of healing around areas of erosion and fibrillation.[33,44] Predilection for destruction of the joint surface is exhibited by those sites subject to the greatest load-bearing or shearing stress. Earliest fibrillation, however, is often present in regions that presumably carry low compressive stress.[44]

Where the cartilage is denuded and blood vessels reach the surface, there is a localized advance in the line of ossification.[23] New bone formation takes place in two separate locations in relation to the joint surface: in exostoses (osteophytes) at the margins of the articular cartilage and in the marrow immediately subjacent to the cartilage.[44]

The marginal osteophytes generally have one of two patterns of growth. One of these is a protuberance into the joint space; the other is a development within capsular and ligamentous attachments to the joint margins. In each circumstance the direction of osteophytic growth is governed by the lines of mechanical force exerted on the area of growth and generally corresponds to the contour of the joint surface from which the osteophytes protrude. Osteophytes consist in large part of bone that merges imperceptibly with cortical and cancellous tissue of subchondral bone. Osteophytic growth is frequently capped by a layer of hyaline cartilage and fibrocartilage that becomes continuous with the adjacent synovial lining.[44]

The proliferation of bone in the subchondral tissue is most marked in areas that have been denuded of their cartilaginous covering by osteoarthritic erosion. In these regions the articulating surface consists of bone that has been rubbed smooth. The glistening appearance of this polished sclerotic surface is the result of this process, termed *eburnation*. Most of the osteocytes in the eburnated surface undergo gradual degeneration, indicated by empty lacunae. This may result from frictional heat. In addition to this alteration, two other variants of new bone formation are seen in relation to the articular cartilage.[44]

"Cystic" areas of rarefaction of bone can be seen in radiographs immediately beneath the eburnated surfaces, most frequently in the hip joint. However, these lesions only infrequently contain pockets of mucoid fluid and thus are not truly cystic. The trabeculae in the affected areas disappear, and the marrow undergoes fibromyxoid degeneration. Fragments of dead bone, cartilage, and amorphous debris often are interspersed within them. In time, the entire area is encircled by a rim of reactive new bone and compact fibrous tissue. Minute gaps in the overlying articular cortex, resulting from microfractures, are commonly seen at the apices of the pseudocysts.[44]

The other type of new bone formation is a local ossific metaplasia of the base of the articular cartilage. This should be regarded as part of a general remodeling of the joint contour in which bone is added to a portion of the articular cortex, while other areas in the joint surface display focal resorption of the bone.[44] What exactly happens to the subchondral bone depends on whether there is motion in the affected joint or not—if there has been motion, the subchondral bone tends to become sclerotic; if there is no appreciable motion, the bone undergoes atrophy.[23]

Although degenerative joint disease by definition is not inherently inflammatory, focal areas of secondary chronic synovitis are usually present in advanced cases. This is generally characterized by small infiltrates of lymphocytes and mononuclear cells in the synovium. Occasionally the infiltration is sufficiently severe to raise a question of rheumatoid arthritis or the possibility of inflammation arising through autosensitization to joint detritus. A foreign-body reaction to detached fragments of cartilage also occurs and is probably responsible for pain and effusion in acute cases. Secondary synovial osteochondromatosis usually is minimal. However, villous hypertrophy and fibrosis of the synovium occur frequently in clinically obtrusive osteoarthritis. In the knee joint, cruciate ligaments and menisci become frayed and a degree of instability results. Fibrillation and fibrosis of the synovial surface and even mild cartilaginous metaplasia of the patellar tendon may occur in such cases. Minute tears in the capsular tissues appear as slender fibrous or vascular seams disrupting the principal axis of the collagen bundles.[44]

Under clinical conditions, there is little chance of protecting the defects from further wear and tear, and healing of the articular cartilage appears to be unlikely. Also, since degeneration of the ground substance leads to a loss of compressibility and elasticity, the normal pumping mechanism for the passage of nutrients through the articular cartilage is impaired and chondrocyte metabolism is decreased.[11,33] The ability of the tissue to manufacture enough permanent matrix to keep up with the increasing loss is reduced. Cartilage debris and excess ester sulfates released into the joint continue to produce synovitis.[11] Differentiation of the synovial changes in posttraumatic synovitis from those in osteoarthritis is possible to a very limited extent because similar changes with a similar rate of incidence can be observed in both conditions. This suggests that similar etiological agents, possibly macrotrauma and microtrauma, are the pathogenetic factors in common.[45]

Trauma can be implicated in several ways in the pathogenesis of osteoarthritis. Trauma may cause injury directly to the cartilage cells, setting off a cycle of cartilage degeneration. Trauma alone may also cause degenerative changes in healthy cartilage, and frequently repeated minor injuries in ordinary life can so affect the vascularity of cartilage that the degenerative changes of osteoarthritis will follow.[22] The events of cartilage degradation and repair can also be set off when there is loss of capacity to absorb impact energy. In this case overload is dissipated by fracturing of the trabeculae of the subchondral bone with consequent marginal joint remodeling and exposure of the articular cartilage to insult (Fig. 4-19).[1,31,45] Finally, in primary osteoarthritis minor traumatic effects will have a more serious impact if the cartilage has already degenerated.[22]

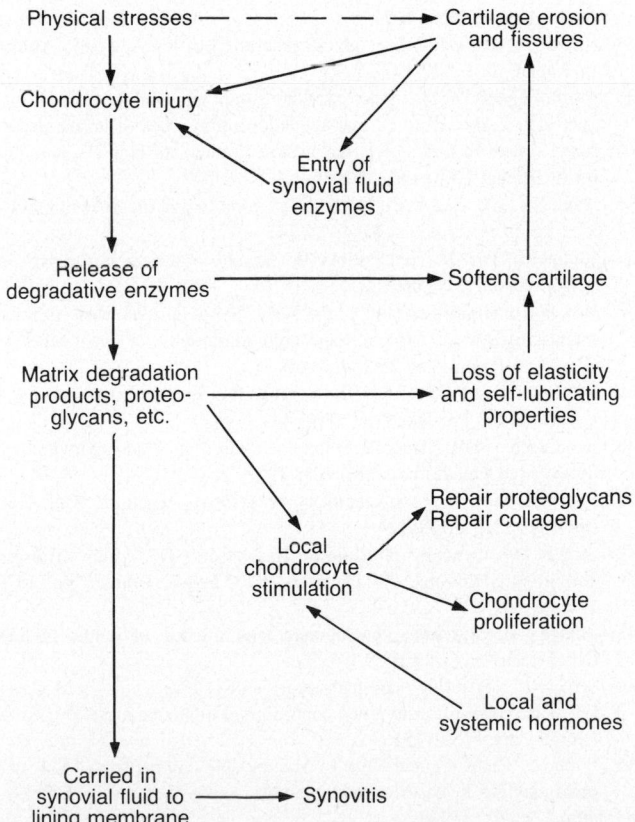

Fig. 4-19. A postulated final pathway of cartilage degeneration. (From American Academy of Orthopaedic Surgeons: Symposium on osteoarthritis, St Louis, 1976, The CV Mosby Co.)

Symptoms and treatment

Clinically, early degenerative changes may be asymptomatic until synovitis develops with effusion, stiffness, capsular thickening, and formation or marginal osteophytes. The osteophytes may cause excessive deformity of the articular bone ends, pain because of stretching of the periosteum, and limitation of movement. Other sources of pain include bony changes at sites of ligamentous attachment and protective muscle spasms that occur to immobilize the joint.[8]

Treatment includes heat application in the form of hot packs, diathermy, or ultrasound. During the initial acute exacerbation of synovitis, some form of cryotherapy may also prove effective. If the patient is overweight, weight reduction is mandatory. Evaluation of daily activities must be undertaken—low chairs should be avoided and sustained postures should not be maintained. Active flexion and extension exercises of the joint (e.g., the knee) should be done every morning before weight bearing is attempted. Walking is encouraged for daily activities but not forced for the sake of prolonged exercise as therapy. Deep knee bends should be avoided, and faulty posture that places a strain as a result of stance should be corrected if the involved joint is the knee or any other joint in the lower extremity or the back. In the case of knee involvement, exercises should include those to strengthen the quadriceps muscle group, hamstrings, and gastrocnemius-soleus muscles.[8] However, if 6 to 8 weeks of such therapy is not beneficial, analgesic and antiinflammatory drugs can be used, but the regimen of restricted exercise must be maintained. If conservative treatment is unsuccessful, surgical debridement of the joint is indicated. Osteophytes are removed along with any damaged intraarticular structures and/or villous projections of the synovial membrane.[33]

Traumatic arthritis

In some cases trauma may lead to a form of arthritis known as *traumatic arthritis*. Since trauma causes cracking or fibrillation of the intraarticular cartilage with subsequent atrophy, it may scar or weaken the intraarticular and extraarticular supporting structures, thereby decreasing the ability of the joint to withstand the physiological trauma that results from motion or weight bearing or both. Although it is relatively rare, arthritis may be precipitated by trauma.[15] More commonly, preexisting rheumatoid arthritis is aggravated by injury.[27]

SUMMARY

The synovial membrane, articular cartilage, joint capsule, and intraarticular structures each react to trauma in a characteristic way. Trauma to the synovial membrane, usually produced by a mild blow or overstretching of the joint capsule, may result in posttraumatic synovitis or pigmented villonodular synovitis, depending on whether the effusion is hemorrhagic or not. Repeated trauma to the articular cartilage may lead to osteoarthritis. All of these reactions can be observed by changes in the synovial fluid. The joint capsule can be injured directly (by overstretching) or indirectly (from effusion). Intraarticular structures can be damaged from a direct force or secondarily as a result of inflammatory processes occurring in nearby associated structures.

Beside gross, obvious damage in any injury to a joint (meniscus tear, sprain, subluxation, or dislocation), which may lead to decreased range of motion, increased temperature, edema, and decreased strength, one should be aware of changes that occur on a microscopic level and the clinical effects that can result. For example, the phenomenon of reactive synovitis can be responsible for damage to surrounding joint structures that were not involved in the initial injury.

Seemingly minor trauma can have its effect on the joint structures also and, if repeated or aggravated, can have serious consequences. There is an obvious implication to avoid mobilization techniques (which involve passive movements of the joint at the limit of its range) and vigorous exercising of an acutely injured or inflammatory joint.

REFERENCES

1. American Academy of Orthopaedic Surgeons: Symposium on osteoarthritis, St. Louis, 1976, The CV Mosby Co, pp. 1-7, 34-47.
2. Anderson CE: The structure and function of cartilage, J Bone Joint Surg (Am) 44:777, 1962.
3. Barnett CH: Wear and tear in joints: an experimental study, J Bone Joint Surg (Br) 38(2):567, 1956.
4. Berk RN: Liquid fat in the knee joint after trauma, N Engl J Med 277(26):1411, 1967.
5. Biology of connective tissue and the joints, JAMA 224(suppl 5):669, 1973.
6. Boyes JG: Solitary nodular synovitis: a traumatic lesion? South Med J 59:1212, 1966.
7. Bozdech Z: Posttraumatic synovitis, Acta Chir Orthop Traumatol Cech 43(3):244, 1976.
8. Cailliet R: Knee pain and disability, Philadelphia, 1972, FA Davis Co, pp. 40-44, 62-68, 97-99.
9. Cailliet R: Soft tissue pain and disability, Philadelphia, 1977, FA Davis Co, pp. 234-243.
10. Castor CW, Prince RK, and Hazelton MJ: Hyaluronic acid in human synovial effusions: a sensitive indicator of altered connective tissue cell function during inflammation, Arthritis Rheu 9(6):783, 1966.
11. Chrisman OD: Biochemical aspects of degenerative joint disease, Clin Orthop 64:77, 1969.
12. Curtiss PH: Changes produced in synovial membrane and synovial fluid, J Bone Joint Surg (Am) 46:873, 1964.
13. Dowson D: Lubrication and wear of joints, Physiotherapy 59(4):104, 1973.
14. Dowson D, Wright V, and Longfield MD: Human joint lubrication, Bio-Medical Engineering 4:160, 1969.
15. Gelfand L and Merliss R: Trauma and rheumatism, Ann Intern Med 50:999, 1959.
16. Guyton A: Textbook of medical physiology, Philadelphia, 1976, WB Saunders Co., pp. 72-74.
17. Hollinshead WH: Textbook of anatomy, New York, 1974, Harper & Row Publishers Inc., pp. 32-33.
18. Irwin JW and Way BA: Inflammation, Bibli Anat 17:72, 1979.
19. Kelley W and others: Philadelphia, 1981, WB Saunders Co, pp. 271-272.
20. Knight K.: The effects of hypothermia on inflammation and swelling, Athletic Training 11(1):7, 1976.
21. LaCava G.: Enthesitis—traumatic disease of insertions, JAMA 169:254, 1959.
22. Landells JW: The reactions of injured human articular cartilage, J Bone Joint Surg (Br) 38(2):548, 1957.
23. Lichtenstein L.: Disease of bone and joints, St. Louis, 1975, The CV Mosby Co., pp. 266-283.
24. Mankin HJ and Radin E: Structure and function of joints. In McCarty DJ, editor: Arthritis and allied conditions, Philadelphia, 1979, Lea & Febiger, pp. 151-164.
25. Maroudas A and others: The permeability of articular cartilage, J Bone Joint Surg (Br) 50(1):166, 1968.
26. McCarty DJ: Synovial fluid. In McCarty DJ, editor: Arthritis and allied conditions, Philadelphia, 1979, Lea & Febiger, pp. 51-67.
27. McCracken WJ: The role of trauma in arthritis, Industrial Med Surg 24:327, 1955.
28. Myers RR, Negami S, and White RK: Dynamic mechanical properties of synovial fluid, Biorheology 3:197, 1966.
29. Ogston AG and Stanier JE: The physiological function of hyaluronic acid in synovial fluid: viscous, elastic and lubricant properties, J Physiol 119:244, 1953.
30. Palmer DG: Dynamics of joint disruption, NZ Med J 78:166, 1973.
31. Pathophysiology of arthrosis: a review, Tidsskr Nor Laegef 96(32):1687, 1976.
32. Pinals RS: Traumatic arthritis and allied conditions. In McCarty DJ, editor: Arthritis and allied conditions, Philadelphia, 1979, Lea & Febiger, p. 986.
33. Pond MJ: Normal joint tissues and their reaction to injury, Vet Clin North Am 1(3):523, 1971.
34. Radin EL: The physiology and degeneration of joints, Semin Arthritis Rheum 2(3):245, 1972-1973.
35. Radin EL and Paul IL: Does cartilage compliance reduce skeletal impact loads? The relative force-attenuating properties of articular cartilage, synovial fluid, periarticular soft tissues and bone, Semin Arthritis Rheum 13(2):139, 1970.
36. Radin EL and Paul IL: Importance of bone in sparing articular cartilage from impact, Clin Orthop 78:342, 1971.
37. Radin EL, Paul IL, and Pollock D: Animal joint behavior under excessive loading, Nature 226:554, 1970.
38. Roy S, Ghadially FN, and Crane WAJ: Synovial membrane in traumatic effusion: ultrastructure and autoradiography with tritiated leucine, Ann Rheum Dis 25:259, 1966.
39. Schmid FR and Ogata RI: The composition and examination of synovial fluid, J Prosthet Dent 18(5):449, 1967.
40. Schumacher HR: Traumatic joint effusion and the synovium, J Sports Med Phys Fitness 3(3):108, 1975.
41. Sherman MS: The non-specificity of synovial reactions, Bull Hos Joint Dis 12:110, 1951.
42. Simkin PA: Synovial physiology. In McCarty DJ, editor: Arthritis and allied conditions, Philadelphia, 1979, Lea & Febiger, pp. 167-177.
43. Sledge CB: Structure, development and function of joints, Orthop Clin North Am 6(3):619, 1975.
44. Sokoloff L: Pathology and pathogenesis of osteoarthritis. In McCarty DJ, editor: Arthritis and allied conditions, Philadelphia, 1979, Lea & Febiger, pp. 1135-1151.
45. Soren A, Klein W, and Huth F: Microscopic comparison of the synovial changes in posttraumatic synovitis and osteoarthritis, Clin Orthop 121:191, 1976.
46. Soren A and others: Morphological examinations of so-called posttraumatic synovitis, Beitraege Pathol 150:11, 1973.
47. Sternbach GL and Baker FJ: The emergency joint: arthrocentesis and synovial fluid analysis, JACEP 5(10):787, 1976.

48. Stravino VD: The synovial system, Am J Phys Med 51(6):312, 1972.
49. Tallquist G: The reaction to mechanical trauma in growing articular cartilage, Acta Orthop Scand (suppl) 53:1, 1962.
50. Turek SL: Orthopaedics: principles and their application, Philadelphia, 1977, JB Lippincott Co, Inc., pp. 17-29, 147-169, 327-348.
51. Volz R: The response of synovial tissues to recurrent hemarthroses, Clin Orthop 45:127, 1966.
52. Wright V, editor: Lubrication and wear in joints, Proceedings of a symposium organized by the Biological Engineering Society and held at the General Infirmary, Leeds, on April 17, 1969, Philadelphia, 1972, JB Lippincott, Co, Inc., pp. 19, 41-48.
53. Wright V, Dowson D, and Kerr J: The structure of joints, Int Rev Connect Tissue Res 6:105, 1973.
54. Wright V, Dowson D, and Seller PC: Bio-engineering aspects of synovial fluid and cartilage, Mod Trends Rheumatol 2:21, 1971.

Chapter 5

FRACTURE STABILIZATION AND HEALING

Ivan A. Gradisar, Jr.

A *fracture* has been defined as *a severe soft tissue injury with an underlying bony defect.*[1] This definition is unusual in its emphasis on the soft tissue rather than on the bone, but it is particularly useful to those whose job it is to get the patient back to full function within a reasonable period of time.

In the past 10 years sophisticated advances have been made in some areas of fracture management. Despite these advances, it should be noted that the clinician can do little to increase the rate of fracture healing. Instead efforts must be made to remove significant deterrents to the healing process, and, in this endeavor, it is extremely important that the clinician better understand the ramifications of soft tissue damage.

SIGNIFICANCE OF SOFT TISSUE DAMAGE

Whereas damage to bone is often immediately obvious in the shortening or deformity of the fractured limb, the presence of severe, permanent damage to the soft parts, such as skin, muscle, tendon, ligament, vessels, and cartilage, is much more subtle and can easily escape attention in the early phases of fracture management. Damaged soft tissue can impede fracture healing in two important ways: First, it produces an increased metabolic burden, a poor source for vascular ingrowth, and thus a serious impediment to the process of repair because the tissues immediately surrounding the fracture act as a conduit for the new blood supply necessary to support the entire fracture-healing process. Second, it can prevent full recovery of function regardless of how well the fracture itself heals because the soft tissue elements, particularly muscle and tendon, are important musculoskeletal elements in their own right. In the long run, it is damage to the soft tissue that determines the speed of recovery and the ultimate functional level of the recovered patient.

Some soft tissue injuries are immediately apparent, as in cases of compound fracture in which bleeding or skin defects clearly signal damage to tissue. In other cases, however, soft tissue damage may not become apparent until the rehabilitation process has begun. In the early stages of rehabilitation following a long period of immobilization in traction or cast, it is not uncommon for a therapist to discover that a patient's fractured femur has been accompanied by a previously unnoticed disruption of the medial collateral ligament or tear of the meniscus. In 1980 Kennedy and Walker[3] reported on 26 cases of knee ligament damage associated with femoral shaft fractures and recorded a latency of 12.8 months before the ligament damage was noted. They found that 30% of 54 patients with femoral shaft fractures had "severe" ligament damage in the ipsilateral knee.

Belated discovery of soft tissue damage, which is sometimes unavoidable, often forces downward revisions of the rehabilitation timetable and ultimate recovery potential. Thorough appreciation of soft tissue damage surrounding a fracture at the time of the first evaluation can help prevent the need for such downward revisions and forestall the disappointment arising from them.

Soft tissue injury has serious implications for health and function long after a fracture has healed. A look at the pathomechanics of a fracture can be helpful in developing greater appreciation of the distribution of damage between bone and soft tissue when fracture occurs.

PATHOMECHANICS OF FRACTURE

The energy imposed on the human body by the forces of impact must be dissipated—preferably by non–injury-producing methods of absorption. Fig. 5-1 shows an idealized load-deflection curve generated in the laboratory by applying a load to bone and recording the deflection or bending that occurs as the load is increased.

The test begins at point A, where load and deflection are zero. As the load increases, the bone deflects along a portion of the curve designated as the "elastic zone." In this region deflection can absorb energy elastically and the bone will spring back to shape promptly when the load is removed. This is the loading range in which bones normally operate. However, when load is increased beyond point B, which marks the "proportional limit," tiny failures in bone substance begin to occur, creating permanent deformity as a consequence. Throughout the portion of the curve designated as the "plastic zone," progressive destruction occurs. If the load were removed at any point in the plastic zone, the bone would not return to its normal,

healthy state but would continue to contain small infarctions requiring repair. These defects, even when too small to be seen radiographically, may produce pain. During the repair process, the elaboration of callus can be seen radiographically even when frank fracture has not been observed at the time of first analysis and treatment of injury. This phenomenon often occurs in cases of stress fractures or march fractures—common among athletes.[5] In laboratory tests or actual occurrences, if the load applied to bone is increased to point C on the curve, the ultimate strength of bone is reached and the bone fails. This failure results in a classic bone fracture accompanied by all the clinical manifestations, including pain, deformity, false motion, and swelling.

Bone has a tremendous capacity for bearing load, often reaching 10 to 20 times body weight or up to 2000 to 4000 lbs.[7] In most instances of sudden impact, a portion of the load to be borne by the bone is external—applied by something outside the body, such as the ground or an athletic opponent—while another portion is internal—generated by the contractile forces of one's own muscles acting across the bone to control body position, as in jumping or falling. The total energy load imposed is usually applied only briefly, sometimes for no more than a fraction of a second. Nevertheless, the accumulated load of both external and internal forces must be absorbed so as to keep the load in the elastic zone if possible but below the ultimate strength load that causes fracture.

Forms of protective gear designed for athletic use, such as helmets, pads, and bindings that release, are meant to help absorb impact and reduce the load on bone, and sports like hockey, fencing, and tackle football cannot be played safely without them. Protective gear alone, however, is not adequate to absorb all the forces of impact imposed on the body. Load is transmitted through protective materials and absorbed in part by the body's own padding in the form of muscle bulk or fat but also by harder body components, such as cartilage and bone.

The principal energy-absorbing mechanism in the human body, however, is a lengthening contraction of muscle. This phenomenon can be visualized by considering, for example, the difference between jumping from a table and landing with hip, knee, and ankle locked in a fully extended position and landing in a flexed position so that an extending contraction of the gluteus muscle, quadriceps muscle, and gastrocnemius muscle can absorb the energy. In the former instance the impulse is delivered almost directly to the large bones and axial skeleton. When the energy is too great for the bone, articular cartilage, or intervertebral disks to absorb, overload occurs resulting in cellular damage. In its milder forms such damage may affect the articular cartilage, resulting in chondromalacia and other minor destructive changes clinically manifested by joint achiness or swelling and minimal pain. However, if overload is extreme, damage can

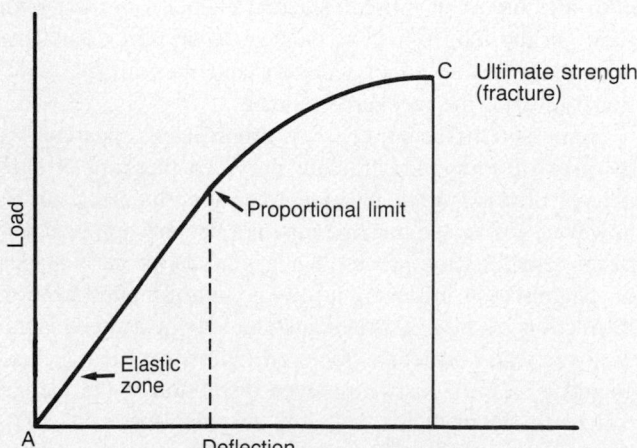

Fig. 5-1. Load-deflection curve representing idealized mechanical behavior of bone under slow loading. Point C represents fracture.

be severe, producing such injuries as vertebral compression fractures.

However, if one lands from a jump with hips, knees, and ankles flexed, energy is absorbed by muscle, creating a much broader margin of safety and a far smaller incidence of injury. Here, the leap from table to floor amounts to jumping to the squat position and "catching the force" with a lengthening contraction of the quadriceps and gastrocnemius muscles. This mechanism of protection is often recognized and encouraged by such phrases as "roll with the punch," "let your body 'give' with the fall," and "bend your knees when you ski."

Understanding the role of muscle in energy absorption forms the basis for today's strong emphasis on preparticipation conditioning in athletics. Clearly, many of the serious injuries that occur "out of bounds," during a "late hit," or to a "fatigued athlete" can be directly attributed to the player's inability to use muscle to absorb energy. This principle holds true for the general population as well. Strong muscles provide good protection from fracture.

Internally applied forces produced by voluntary or involuntary muscle contractions can be massive. Since bone is strongest when loaded in compression, the safest loading configuration is one in which the bone is symmetrically loaded by its accompanying musculature. If agonist and antagonist muscles are equally stressed, bending or torsional loads can be avoided. Unfortunately, a person cannot always accomplish symmetrical muscle loading, particularly in movements requiring rapid acceleration or deceleration or turning. If bending or twisting maneuvers exceed the strength of the bone, a fracture can result even in the absence of a collision or fall. The most common injuries of this kind are a "pull-off" fracture of the base of the fifth metatarsal, an "avulsion" fracture of the medial epicondyle of the elbow, or a spiral humeral fracture. In fact some element of asymmetrical loading is usually a factor in the pathomechanics of all fractures, especially those of the long bones. Muscles, on the other hand, can play opposing roles when people are injured. They can be protective agents in lengthening muscle contractures but causative agents in avulsion and other fractures. In either case the part of soft tissues in the prevention and rehabilitation of fractures cannot be overemphasized.

If the energy at the time of impact is more than can be absorbed by protective gear or lengthening contractures, injury occurs—first to the soft tissue in the form of a bruise or strain and then to bone and ligaments in the form of fracture or rupture. If the impact is severe enough and deformity occurs, vital soft tissues, such as arteries or nerves, can be damaged or destroyed. Always the energy of impact must be totally dissipated, whether that outcome is achieved by some or all of these mechanisms.

The reason why soft tissue injury so often accompanies fracture can be better appreciated if one thinks of the resemblance between the edges of a fractured tibia or humerus and the sharp, jagged edges of a broken piece of hardwood. Since the fractured bone may angulate 90 degrees or more at a very high rate of speed during the injury process and then return to a more normal position either spontaneously or as a result of deliberate repositioning, it is easy to imagine how soft tissue can be damaged. The rapid slicing of fracture ends through adjacent muscle damages the soft tissue and can cause extensive bleeding and swelling in the area surrounding the fracture. The extreme destructiveness of these events makes it easy to understand why volumes have been written on the emergency care of the fracture patient.

EMERGENCY FRACTURE CARE

Fracture management begins at the moment of first contact with the patient. The emphasis should be on *gentle,* nonforceful manipulation of the limb with immediate splinting so as to restore circulation and minimize the motion of the sharp fracture ends. This avoids additional soft tissue damage due to movement.

Emergency splinting[2]

First-aid efforts involving emergency splinting should be carried out or at least supervised by a physician or experienced technician. A brief but thorough survey of all body parts through "hands-on palpation" and inquiry should be carried out first. Throughout this initial on-site evaluation, the guiding principle is "fractures hurt." If squeezing or gently moving a body part does not produce pain, it can be safely assumed that the part is not fractured.

To be thorough in the use of the squeeze technique, the examiner should begin at the injured person's head and gently squeeze or palpate the skull, neck, shoulders, upper extremities, and so on, including the chest, pelvis, legs, and feet. Examination concludes with running the fingers down the victim's spine. The squeeze technique is reliable and fast: a complete examination can be completed in less than 10 seconds. A positive response is recorded when the victim complains of pain in response to a squeeze or when one palpates deformity in the bone or observes crepitation or false motion caused by a fracture.

If a fracture is found, emergency splinting is necessary before the patient can be transported elsewhere for medical attention. If possible, the deformed part should be gently returned to its proper anatomical position. If significant resistance to this return is met, however, the part should be splinted in the position in which it was found.

Sometimes emergency splinting in athletics calls for considerable ingenuity, as, for example, when an injured athlete is still wearing protective equipment, such as pads, boots, or helmet. In many such instances it is best to transport the patient with the protective gear still in place so as not to risk the chance of inflicting further injury.

Many kinds of devices are available to facilitate emergency splinting (Figs. 5-2 and 5-3). These include inflatable splints, cardboard splints, backboards, litters, slings, and portable traction devices, such as the Thomas splint and traction splints. If none of these happens to be available, improvisation is in order, and items such as skis, ski poles, pillows, or even rolled-up magazines can be used to fashion crude but effective emergency splints. In extreme cases the fractured leg can be splinted by binding it to the patient's uninjured leg; a fractured upper arm can be temporarily strapped to the chest.

Injuries to the neck require exceptional care. The patient with significant neck pain must, for safety's sake, be presumed to have suffered a neck fracture. In such cases splinting the injured area is necessary, and the patient should be transported as quickly as possible to a medical facility where a definitive evaluation can be made. The safest transport device for the neck- or back-injured victim is a backboard and sandbags or straps. A complaint of even mild or localized numbness, flaccidity, or any other neurological deficit—even if only of short duration—must always be interpreted as a contraindication to resuming activity until a complete evaluation of the injury has been made. This should include radiographs and a careful neurological examination.

When transporting the injured person, it is extremely important that the primary care group or the family send relevant information with the patient, either in writing or by word of mouth. This includes:

1. A report of associated or secondary injuries.
2. A description of the mechanism of injury.
3. A list of relevant prior injuries or medical conditions.

Some of these observations can be made only by the acute care group, but all are crucial to achieving complete and safe management of the patient. Too often a significant contributing factor to the seriousness of an injury has been ignored or poorly evaluated.

TYPES OF FRACTURES

Fracture can take several forms, depending on the position of the limb when fractured, the velocity of the injury, the position of protective pads or equipment, and the duration of impact. For example, high-energy, twisting injury that occurs to an alpine skier can produce a severely *comminuted* fracture, while a low-speed, bending injury may result in a *simple* transverse fracture. *Compound* fractures occur when sharp ends of broken bone protrude through the victim's skin, or when some projectile penetrates the skin into the fracture site.

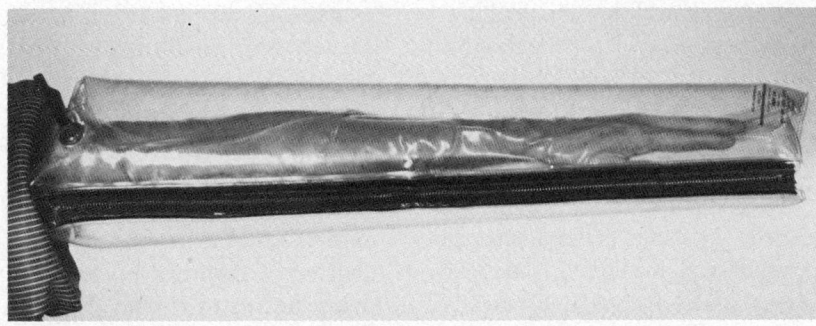

Fig. 5-2. Inflatable (air) splint for emergency immobilization of a fractured forearm.

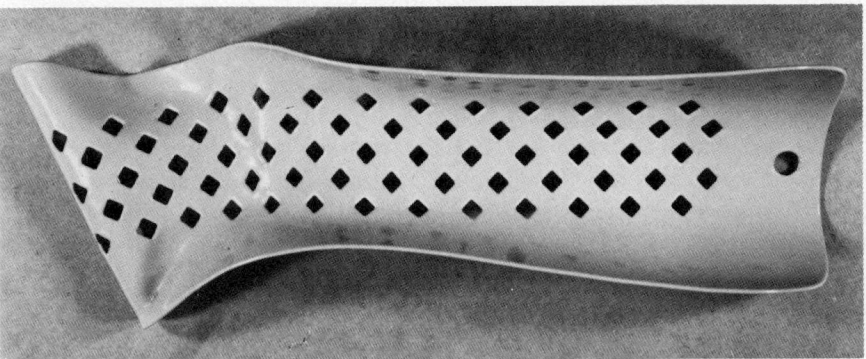

Fig. 5-3. Fixed forearm splint for emergency immobilization of fractured left forearm.

The presence of a compound fracture significantly alters fracture management and may negatively influence the likelihood of complete healing since it often signifies the presence of extensive soft tissue damage or contamination. A compound fracture that has become infected will not heal until the infection has been eliminated. Therefore, to prevent infection the limb with protruding bone ends should be covered with a sterile dressing and transported as is, without returning the bone end to its normal position inside the skin. This type of emergency treatment prevents the introduction of additional dirt and debris into the wound before the bone end can be cleansed and alerts the surgeon to the need for cleansing the injured area thoroughly. Fractures that involve joints and disrupt the "bearing surface" demand special attention. In the management of these fractures, it is essential to reduce the joint surface to its original smooth condition. Severely damaged articular cartilage or a residual step-off of bone at the joint may lead to premature degenerative arthritis.

NONUNION FRACTURES

Age and general health are two important factors influencing the rate of fracture healing. In an infant a fractured femur may heal in 4 weeks. The same fracture in a teenager may require 12 to 16 weeks to heal, and, in a 60-year-old person the healing may take 18 to 20 weeks. The presence of diabetes or some other medical problem, such as osteoporosis, will prolong the healing period or increase the incidence of fracture—or both. Taking certain medicines, such as steroids for allergy or other conditions, may have a similar slowing effect on the fracture-healing process.

When fractured bone has failed to reunite at the end of 5 months time, a nonunion is said to exist. In addition to the factors just described that are known to slow the healing process, two other factors often influence the development of a nonunion: contamination of the fracture site through a break in the skin and motion at the fracture site. Contamination is caused by foreign material, devitalized tissue, or bacteria, all of which inhibit the repair process and may prevent healing. Careful handling of tissue, thorough cleansing of the wound, surgical removal of devitalized tissue (debridement), and appropriate use of antibiotics can work to reduce the incidence of nonunion in compound fractures.

Motion at the fracture site is another leading cause, if not the leading cause, of nonunions. Motion can occur within a poorly applied cast or even with certain internally applied devices such as rods or plates. That is why a basic tenet of fracture management is to immobilize the fractured bone one joint above and one joint below the fracture site for a long enough time for the fracture to heal. Immobilization, however, can result in loss of muscle strength (atrophy) and bone strength (disuse osteopenia), and therefore the period of immobilization must last no longer than the time needed to produce a structurally safe union. This period is determined by radiographic evaluation and from experience.

Immobilization promotes healing by allowing the swelling to subside and permitting the formation of a healing "vascular swamp" around the broken bone that can bring in a rich blood supply to nourish callus first and then new bone.

A fracture management protocol must be individualized for each patient based on the type of fracture, the fracture location, and the method of stabilization.

The healing process is monitored radiographically and by clinical examination based on experience. Such planning and diligence minimizes the incidence of nonunion, but it continues to occur, even in the face of expert care and optimum circumstances.

Nonunions are prone to occur in bones where the blood supply is precarious. Two notorious examples are the femoral neck and the carpal navicular bone.

When a nonunion is identified, treatment consists of clearing an infection (if it exists), immobilizing the fracture (either by casting, plates and screws, rods, or other mechanical fixation techniques), and often bone grafting. Bone grafting consists of harvesting small quantities of bone from an area, such as the pelvis, in a manner that does not seriously weaken the site. This bone is then transferred to a location immediately around the nonunited fracture site. Bone taken from the patient himself is called *autograft,* and that taken from others or a cadaver is called *allograft.* The use of allographic bone requires very rigorous technique to avoid transferring infection or disease to either the donor or the recipient. Nonunion sites thus stimulated by bone graft usually go on to heal.

FRACTURES IN CHILDREN

Growth plates are disks composed of cartilage located close to the ends of long bones near all the major joints. Normally, this zone proliferates bone and causes the limbs to elongate, a process that accounts for normal bone growth throughout childhood and adolescence. After an individual reaches about 16 years of age, the growth plate closes solidly with bone and becomes less vulnerable. Until that time, however, damage to the cartilage cells in the growth plate—in the form of fracture, infection, or some other incident or process—may disturb growth and cause, for example, a crooked limb or even result in complete cessation of growth.

Although fractures in children's bones are common and growth disturbances rare, the outcome of a fracture through the growth plate is important. Unfortunately, a growth disturbance due to a fractured growth plate is diffi-

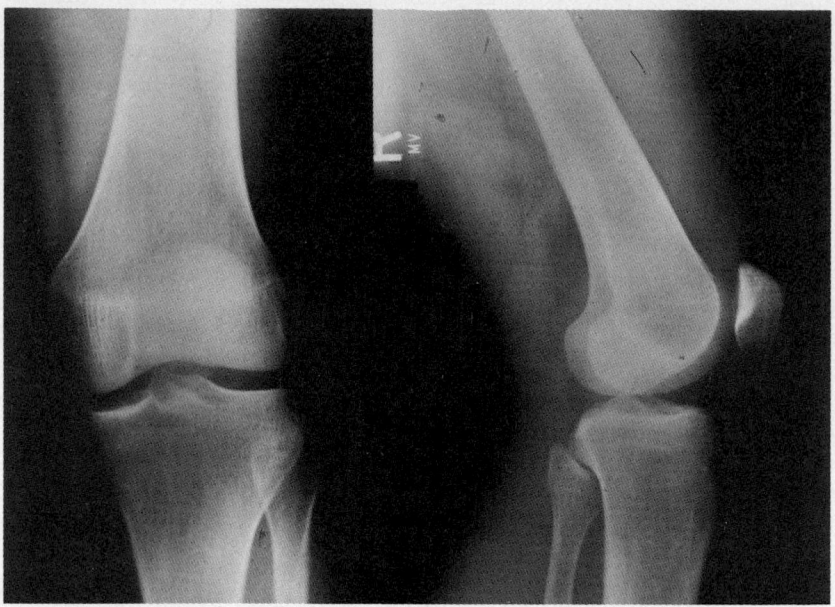

Fig. 5-4. Anteroposterior and lateral radiograph of an adult knee. Note articular cartilage interval between bones.

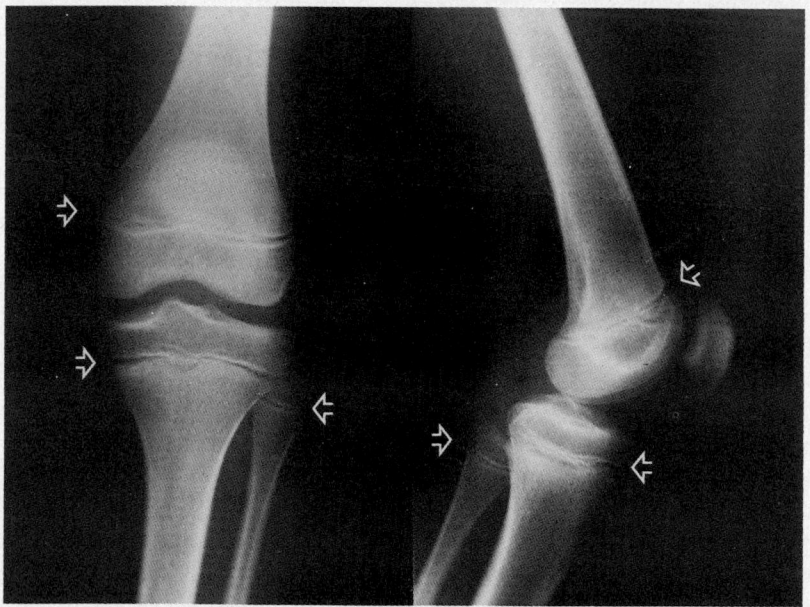

Fig. 5-5. Anteroposterior and lateral radiograph of a child's knee showing "open" epiphyseal growth plates *(arrows)*. These are disks of epiphyseal cartilage that produce longitudinal growth.

cult to diagnose. It reveals itself only gradually in the months following the injury as growth becomes increasingly and noticeably abnormal.

The growth plate appears on a radiograph as a lucent line near the joint, and a fracture through that line can easily be missed unless there is some disturbance in the alignment of the bone (Figs. 5-4 and 5-5).

A special case occurs at the knee where a fracture through the distal femoral or proximal tibial growth plates may be misdiagnosed as a ligament rupture. This kind of error can be avoided by a gentle stress radiograph when a growth plate fracture is suspected even though initial radiographs have been negative. If the knee opens at the growth plate rather than through the joint, a knee ligament injury should be ruled out and a growth plate fracture can be diagnosed.

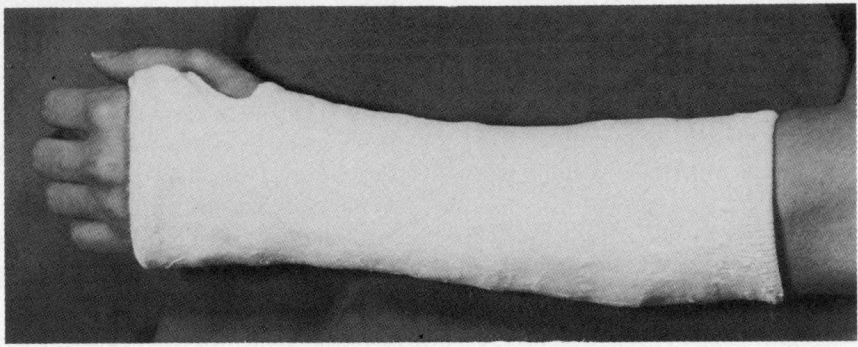

Fig. 5-6. Conventional plaster-of-Paris cast for wrist fracture.

When a fracture occurs in a growth plate, the patient's family should be alerted to the possibility of growth disturbance and the health professional should take special care to follow the healing process until the risk of growth disturbance has passed—at least 1 year. The younger the patient, the greater the growth potential remaining and, concomitantly, the greater the danger of significant growth disturbance. For these reasons special precautions are mandatory in the supervision of the very young fracture patient.

DEFINITIVE FRACTURE MANAGEMENT

The definitive management phase of fracture care usually begins in the hospital or clinic with a decision as to the most appropriate type of immobilization for the fracture in question. The selection process can be influenced by a number of variables, including the nature of the fracture (i.e., closed or open), its location, the physician's preference and skill in treatment, and the needs and preferences of the patient.

Today, such variables can usually be accommodated in several different ways, but occasionally an injury mandates a single treatment method. For example, a fracture that disrupts the joint surface requires that the bone fragments be held together so as to produce a smooth joint surface, which allows the fracture to heal and prevents the later development of degenerative arthritis. This means that the fracture must be either treated closed, as in a cast or traction, or open, with a surgical incision using plates, screws, or other internal fixation devices. The advantages of the former method, a closed reduction, are obvious: avoidance of surgery, reduction of the chance of wound infection, and, usually (except in the case of traction), a shorter hospital stay. Open reduction, on the other hand, may require subsequent removal of the metal devices, increases the possibility of infection, and lengthens hospitalization time.

Whatever technique is selected, however, premature return to the patient's prior activity level is never a good idea. The risk of permanent pain or deformity is simply too great.

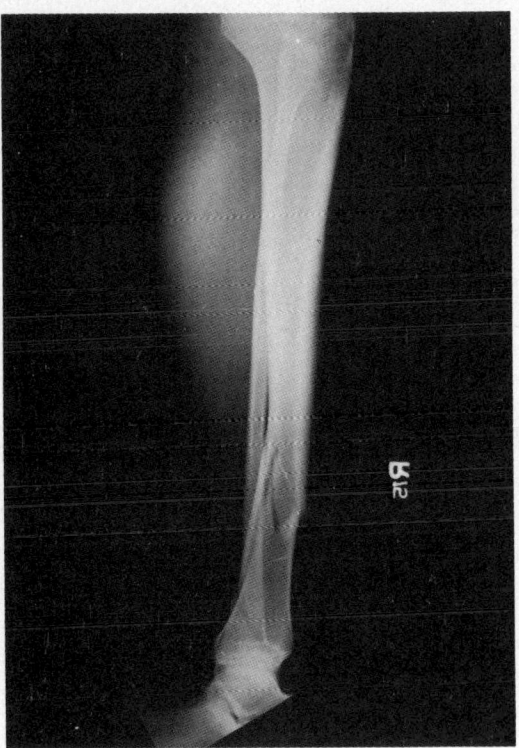

Fig. 5-7. Lateral radiograph of comminuted spiral distal tibial fracture.

Closed reduction

Closed reduction is the process of manually aligning the fracture, usually while the patient is under local or general anesthesia, and encasing the limb in a cast (Figs. 5-6 to 5-8).

The plaster cast is the most common fracture immobilization device and offers several advantages over other techniques: it is easily applied and removed, inexpensive, "breathable" (i.e., not airtight), nonallergenic, and noncombustible. The plaster cast consists of plaster-impregnated cloth rolls or sheets, which, when soaked in water, begin a heat-producing curing process lasting from

2 to 10 minutes. Usually the cast is applied over several layers of cotton sheeting laid directly on the skin. When dry, the cast can be cut and wedged or angled to align the fracture or split to expand and accommodate a swelling limb. It can be safely removed with an oscillating cast saw, and it can be fitted with hinges to allow the joint to move.

Today, however, despite numerous advantages, the plaster cast is only one of several forms of immobilizing devices available for the treatment of fracture. Casts made of resin or fiberglass tend to be more durable than plaster and are sometimes used to facilitate bathing and permit the

patient to continue exercising all body parts except the injured limb (Fig. 5-9).

It is usually safe for the patient to begin gentle range of motion exercises several weeks before the fractured limb is strong enough to return to normal weight-bearing function. For this purpose some casts are fitted with a metal or plastic hinged joint to permit early joint motion. Hinged casts are called cast braces and are extremely useful in shortening patient "downtime" as well as in facilitating early mobilization (Fig. 5-10).

In the later stages of fracture healing, prefabricated splints of plastic or fabric may be used. These can be worn to protect the fractured limb and can be taken off at intervals to permit joint mobilization or bathing (Figs. 5-11 and 5-12).

The range of immobilizing devices available to today's health professional permits the fracture-healing process to be staged. Rigid plaster immobilization for the first few weeks can be followed by a period during which removable splints facilitate joint mobilization. When the patient is ready to return to full activity, the chance of reinjury can be lessened by fitting him/her with a light protective splint or a brace. Even with a young person, 2 years or more may elapse before a seriously fractured bone is completely restored to its original, energy-absorbing functional level.

Open reduction (ORIF or open reduction-internal fixation)

Open reduction is the process of surgically opening the fracture site in order to align and secure the broken bone. This procedure has been known since medieval times, but only in the past 50 years has it been commonly employed (Figs. 5-13 and 5-14).

Bone-compression plating

One type of open reduction, bone-compression plating, was developed by a Swiss team of surgeons and engineers who founded a research group called the Association for the Scientific Investigation of Fractures (ASIF). In the 1960s and 1970s, the ASIF team designed plates, screws,

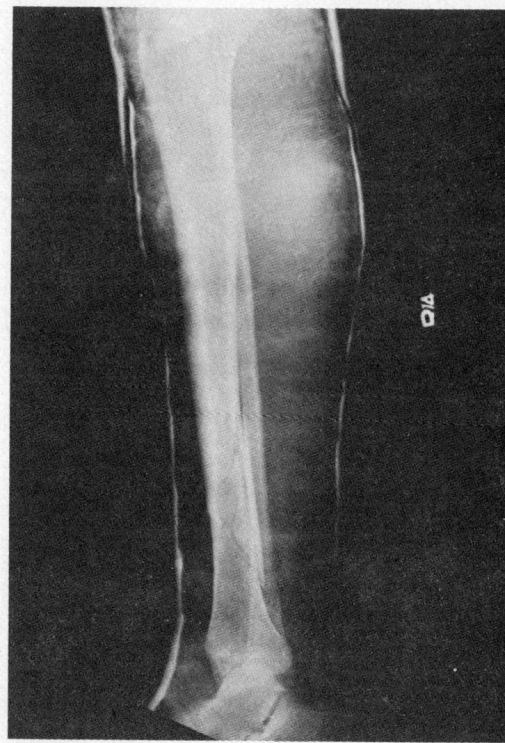

Fig. 5-8. Fracture, illustrated in Fig. 5-7, in excellent position in long-leg plaster cast.

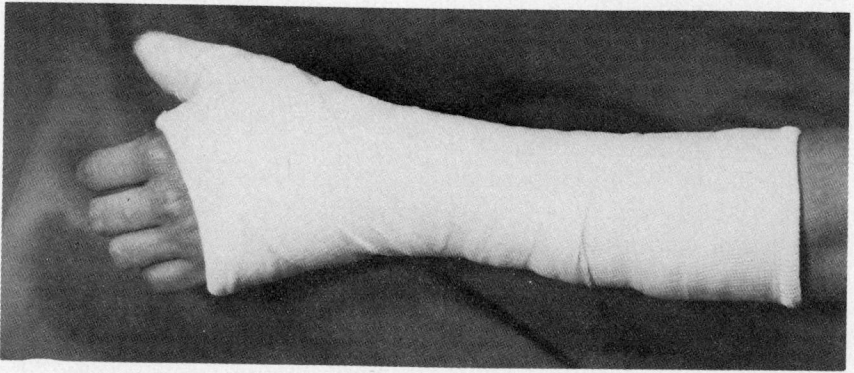

Fig. 5-9. Waterproof fiberglass cast.

and instruments to permit plating the fracture with metal and splinting the fracture so as to compress the bone ends together. Their approach was broadly inclusive, involving attention to important issues such as the proper care of soft tissue, reestablishment of the contour of joint surfaces, and aggressive rehabilitation of the patient (Fig. 5-15). The techniques they described are especially valuable in cases of joint fractures or very complicated shaft fractures, and their contributions have played a major role in advances made in fracture care around the world over the past 20

years. A principal goal of the ASIF group was to encourage the early return of function, a concept important to all patients, but especially to athletes and the elderly.

Compression plating involves the direct securing of the injured bone with metallic internal fixation devices, such as plates or screws. These are constructed of modern surgical-grade metals, such as stainless steel, cobalt chrome, and titanium alloys, which are well tolerated by the body and produce a very low incidence of tissue reaction. The fracture reduction procedure is undertaken by an ortho-

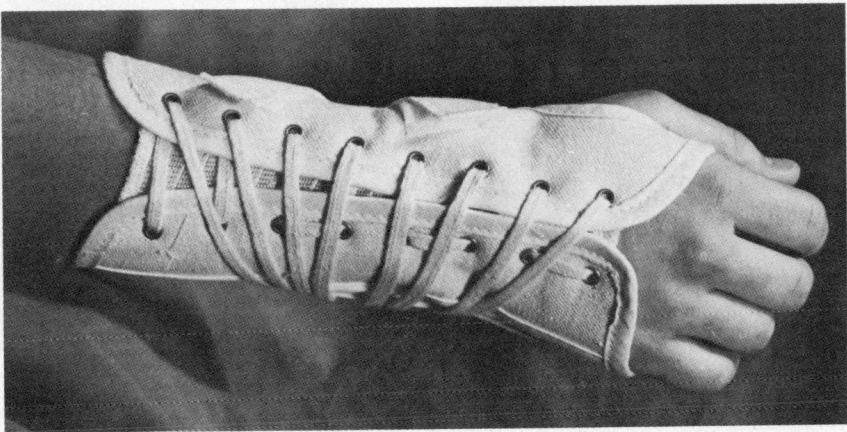

Fig. 5-10. Removable canvas wrist-splint used to treat wrist sprain or as protection during rehabilitation of wrist fracture.

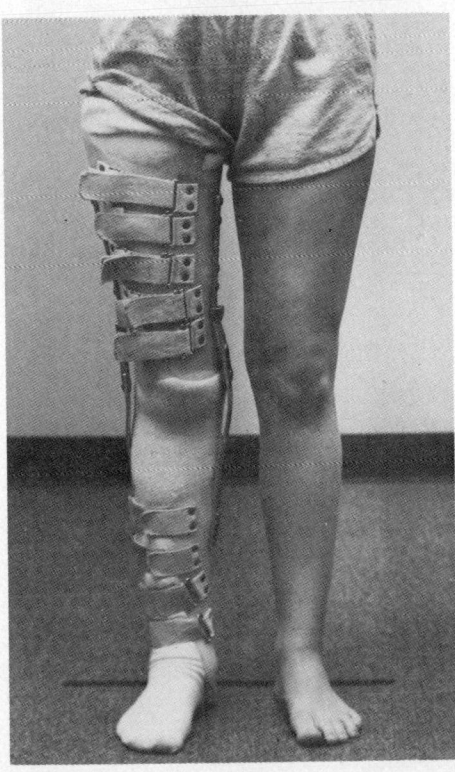

Fig. 5-11. Cast brace for fractured femur. Note adjustable thigh and calf bands and knee hinges. Note freedom of motion at knee and ankle.

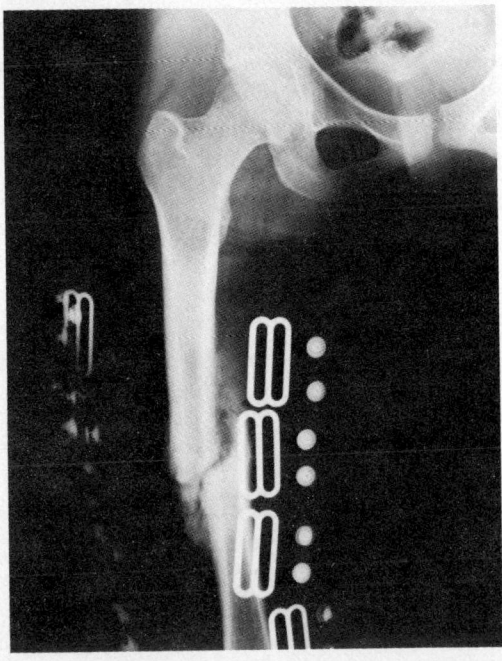

Fig. 5-12. Anteroposterior radiograph of right femoral fracture incurred by patient in Fig. 5-11. Note metal brace buckles and "cloud" of fracture callus.

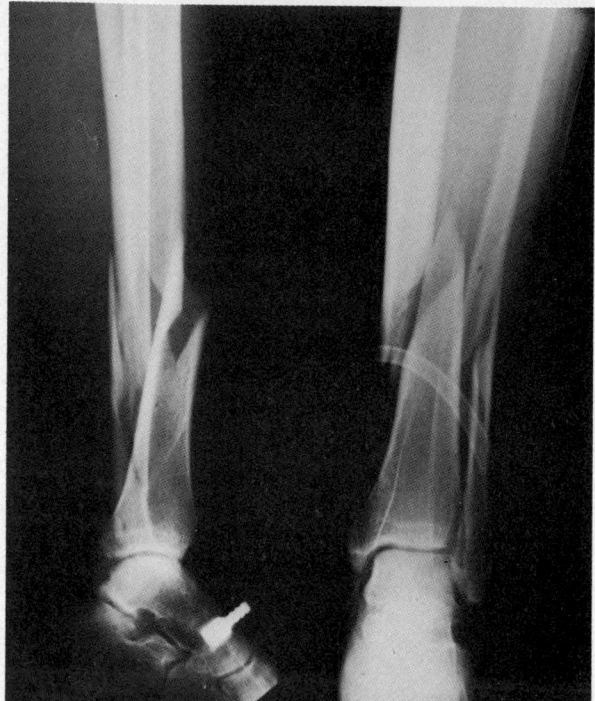

Fig. 5-13. Lateral and anteroposterior radiograph of distal tibial and fibular fracture. Note valve from air splint in lateral view.

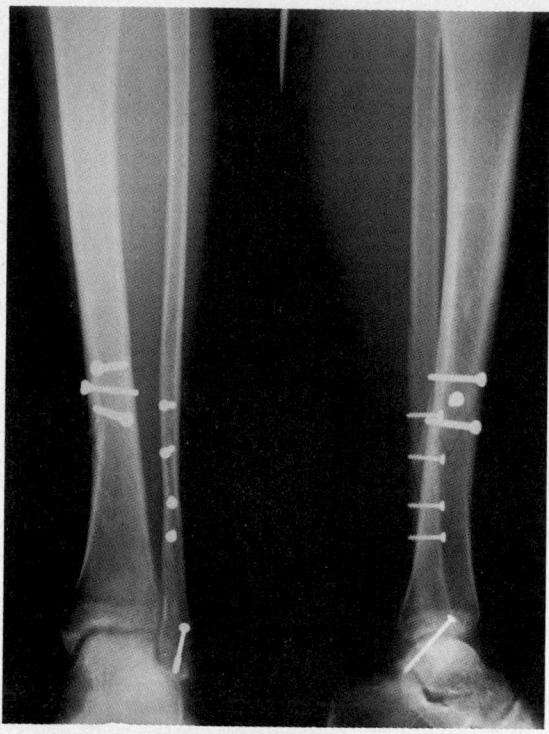

Fig. 5-14. Fractured lower leg illustrated in Fig. 5-13, repaired with interfragmentary screw fixation. Note: short-term plaster cast was also used.

paedic surgeon, usually on an elective basis after the fracture has been given a thorough preoperative assessment aided by radiographs. An appropriately shaped and sized device is selected, sterilized, and inserted through a surgical incision and secured to the bone with drilling and tapping techniques familiar to every experienced machinist. The main objectives are to restabilize the bone to its proper length and rotation, restore proper alignment, and, if a fracture has disrupted the joint, restore the joint surface to its normal smooth contour.

The normal joint is covered with a thin layer of articular cartilage, a highly specialized tissue that acts as a "biological bearing." Cartilage can withstand immense loads for many years, but once disrupted by a "step-off" irregularity, it roughens and can degenerate in a few months or years. This kind of joint destruction is called *degenerative arthritis,* and its prevention is one reason why smooth reestablishment of a fractured joint surface is so essential to the health of the joint.

Sometimes, particularly in the case of metal plates, the inserted metal must be removed after the fracture has healed (1 to 3 years). This is necessary because the end of the plate becomes a stress concentration or a focus for the forces of subsequent load on the bone at the end of the plate and increases the chances that a new fracture will occur. When plates and screws are removed, the bone experiences a temporary weakening while the screw holes fill in and the bone remodels. This effect may last from 6 to 12 weeks or longer, and, during this period, the patient

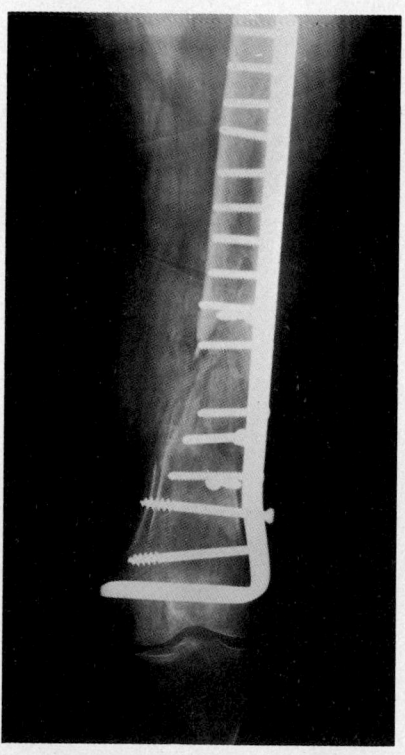

Fig. 5-15. Anterior radiograph of comminuted distal femoral fracture, secured with a condylar blade compression plate and multiple screws.

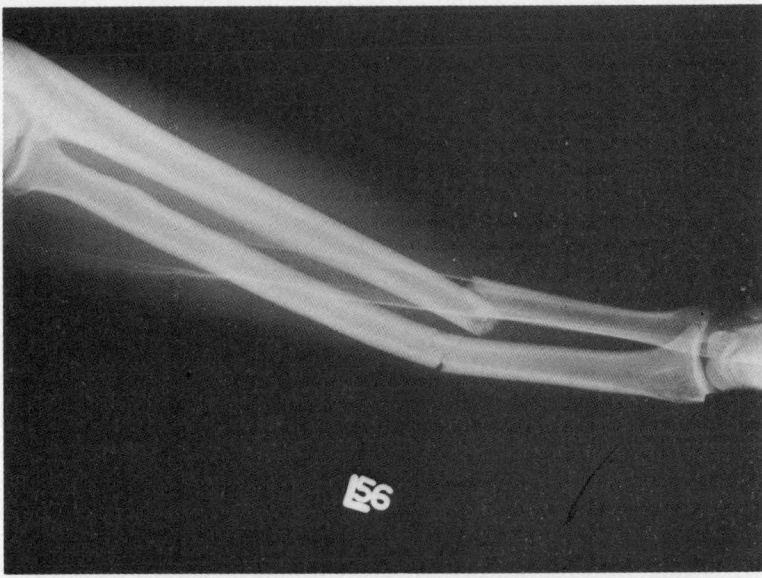

Fig. 5-16. Double bone fracture of distal forearm.

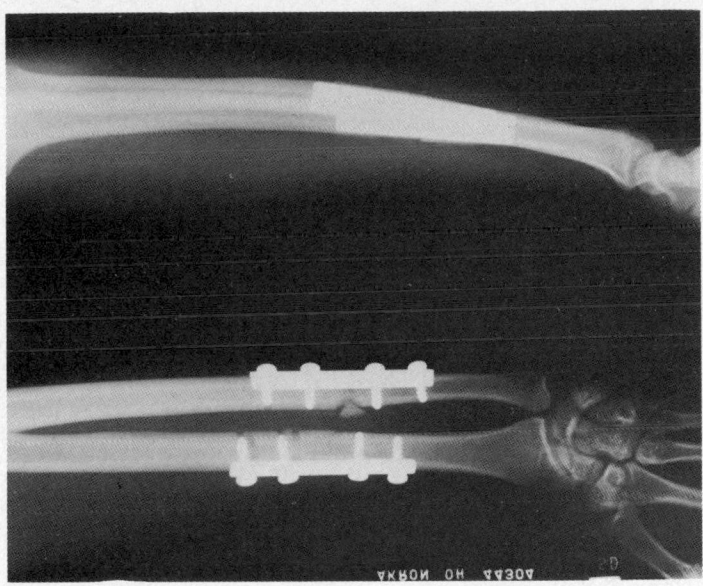

Fig. 5-17. Anteroposterior and lateral radiograph of fracture, illustrated in Fig. 5-16, with compression plates in place.

may need to use crutches or a splint and start a reconditioning process (Figs. 5-16 to 5-18).

Intramedullary rodding

Intramedullary rodding is another form of open reduction and is particularly useful in fractures of long hollow bones, such as the humerus, radius, tibia, or femur. In this technique the surgeon places a solid or tubular metal rod down the endosteal canal of the bone. In the case of the femur—the bone for which this technique is most often used—fixation can be secure enough to preclude the use of a cast, although crutches are often necessary until the frac-

ture unites. After the fracture heals, the rod can be safely removed through a small incision at the hip (Fig. 5-19).

Traction

Traction is a very old but effective method of fracture management. It involves keeping the patient in bed with the fractured limb immobilized and influenced by a system of weights and pulleys. Traction is usually established by percutaneously drilling a pin through the distal fracture fragment and employing a U-shaped clevis device that permits ropes and weights to pull the pin and bone in a direction that aligns the fracture. The patient's own weight sup-

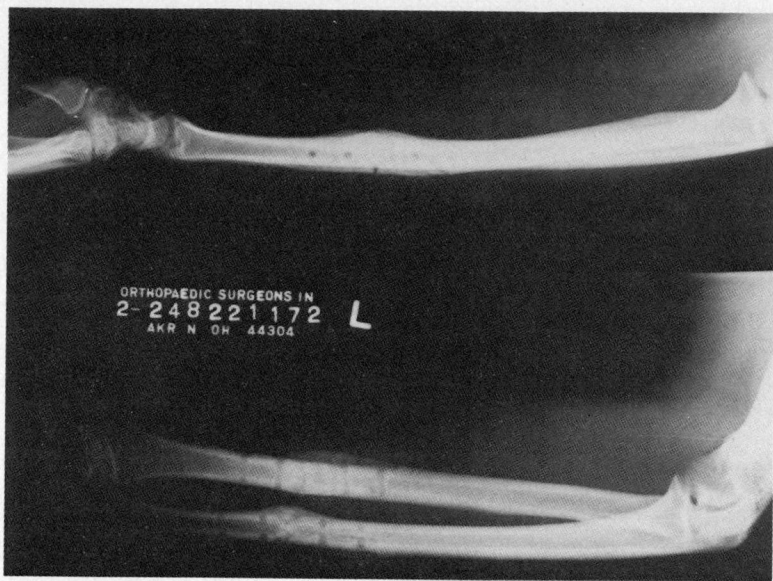

Fig. 5-18. Early remodeling phase of fracture seen in Figs. 5-16 and 5-17. Note: compression plates have been removed but drill holes are still evident 1 year after fracture.

plies the counterforce. The alignment process is assisted with a padded metal frame that gently supports the fractured limb.

The traction method takes advantage of the mass of soft tissues surrounding the injured limb. By pulling longitudinally on the limb, these surrounding muscles, ligaments, and tendons become taut (like the lines of a parachute shroud), thus correctly aligning the fractured bone they encircle.

Traction is maintained throughout the healing process, which usually takes several months. When the patient's injury is particularly complex (i.e., head trauma or abdominal injury), so that other forms of fracture management, such as surgery, are contraindicated, traction may be the only safe fracture management option available.

Rigid external fixation

Rigid external fixation involves the securing of each fracture segment with two or more metal pins percutaneously drilled through the limb and fracture fragment. Once in place, the pins, first, manipulate the fragments into correct alignment and then connect them to each other in a rigid external frame or a plaster casing. The injured limb looks as if it has been shot with arrows, but no incision need be made except for insertion of the pins. Thus the patient can be treated out of the hospital with the pins left in place until the fracture has healed. Rigid external fixation is especially useful in cases involving extensive damage to the skin because the orthopaedic surgeon and the plastic surgeon can work simultaneously on the patient (Figs. 5-20 and 5-21).

Bioelectrical stimulation

Bioelectrical stimulation is a relatively new fracture management technique that makes use of electrical stimu-

lation to help heal the fracture. To appreciate the particular value of this technique, it must be realized that sometimes a nonunion is really a fibrous connective tissue rather than bone. This fibrous tissue can be converted to bone by electrical stimulation.

One method of bioelectrical stimulation involves surrounding the entire limb at the fracture site with an electrical coil and inducing an electrical charge for 12 or more hours each day. This equipment is custom-designed and calibrated for each patient. A second method consists of surgically implanting tiny electrodes in the fibrous tissue at the nonunion site and connecting these to a power source, usually a lithium battery buried under the skin. A third method requires percutaneous insertion (under x-ray control) of Teflon-coated electrical wires into the nonunion site. The tips of the electrodes are bare and the wires are connected to a battery pack outside the skin. The fracture is then continuously electrically stimulated in the 20 Å range for 12 weeks (Figs. 5-22 to 5-24).

Most bioelectrical methods require the concomitant use of a cast and crutches throughout the process. The success rate of these methods applied to difficult cases of nonunion has been very good, approaching 80%.[4] To date, bioelectrical methods have been used to treat nonunions alone and are not currently indicated in the treatment of acute fractures.

Fracture rehabilitation

The rehabilitation phase is the last stage of fracture management. Adequate rehabilitation is usually determined by analysis of a combination of factors, including swelling, pain, joint mobility, and muscle strength. Much of the guesswork in determining completion of this phase

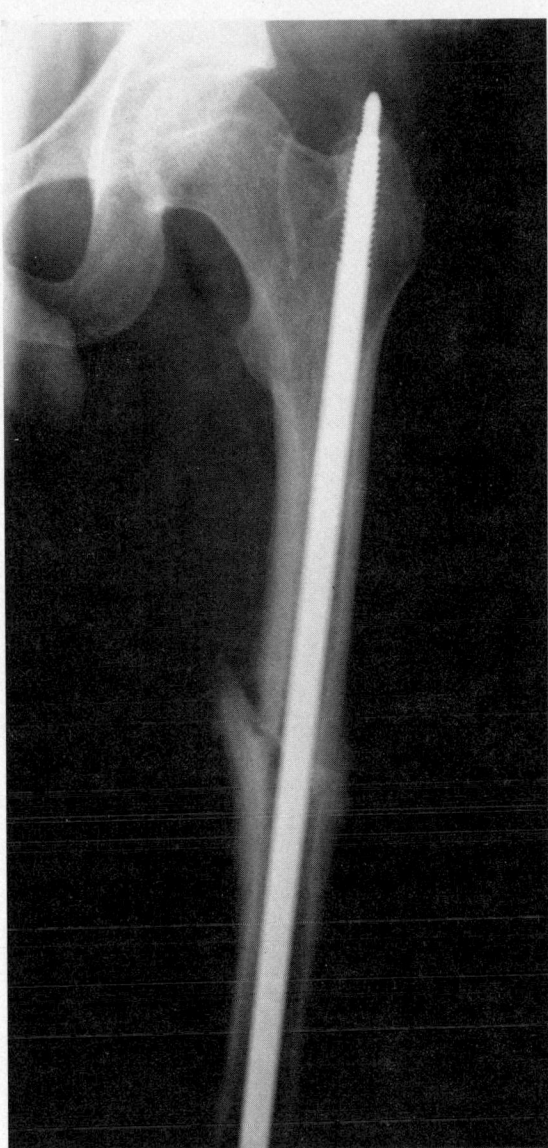

Fig. 5-19. Anteroposterior radiograph of a femur showing an intramedullary rod in the endosteal canal to secure a fracture.

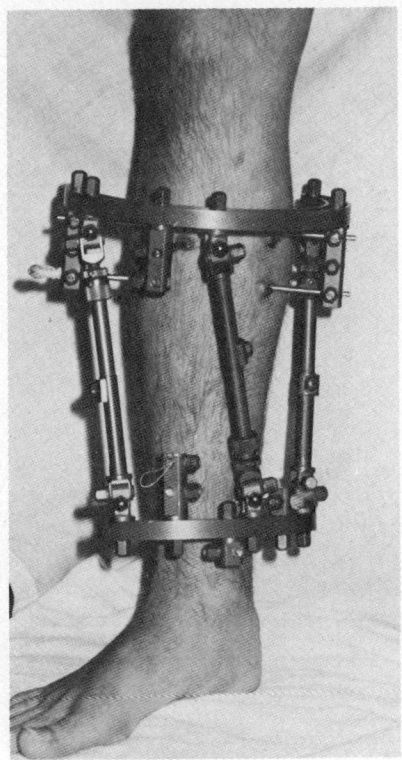

Fig. 5-20. External-fixation fracture device. Note percutaneous pins passing through bone.

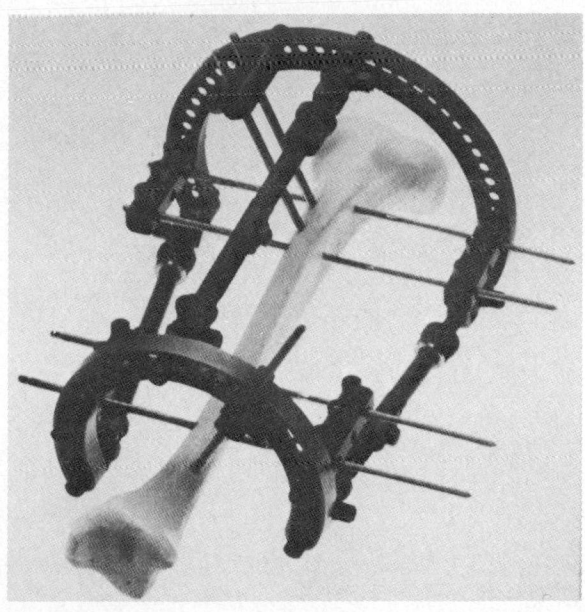

Fig. 5-21. Model illustrating relationship of external fixiter to pins that pass through bone to maintain bone alignment.

is eliminated by direct measurement and, in the case of fractured limbs, by comparison of the injured limb with its uninjured counterpart. Comparable limb diameter and joint swelling can be measured in inches, while joint motion is measured in degrees. Strength is measured by manual muscle testing or with an isokinetic machine* (when available) (Figs. 5-25 and 5-26) in radians per second or pounds per square inch at varying testing rates.

The patient's fractured limb is compared to its healthy counterpart (or, if necessary, to measurements of limb characteristics in a population of uninjured persons of similar age and build).

The decision to return a patient to his/her normal activity level is usually arrived at gradually with the return of strength and motion. It is a general rule of thumb that vig-

*Cybex, Ronkonkoma, N.Y.

orous activity can be resumed when the strength deficit is 15% or less, but today the decision is usually arrived at in a joint discussion between surgeon and therapist. It is modified immediately in the event of any regression during the early stages of the patient's return to full activity.

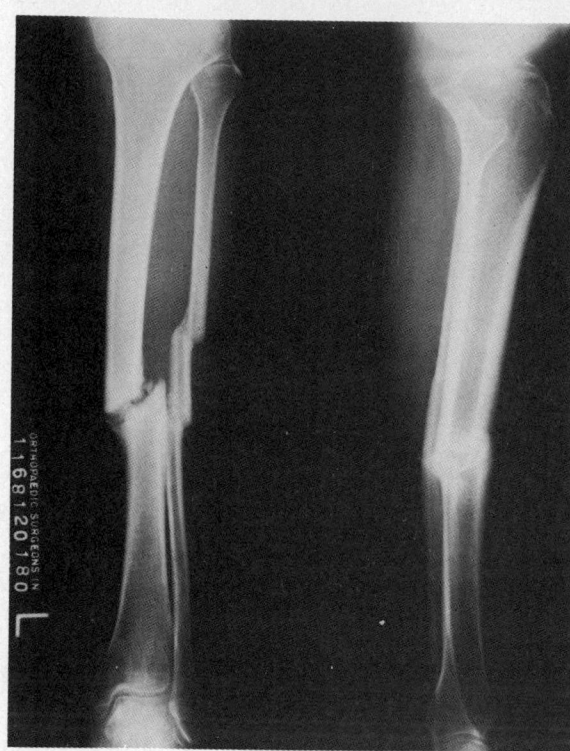

Fig. 5-22. Anteroposterior and lateral radiographs of a midshaft fractured tibia that has failed to heal because of tibial nonunion.

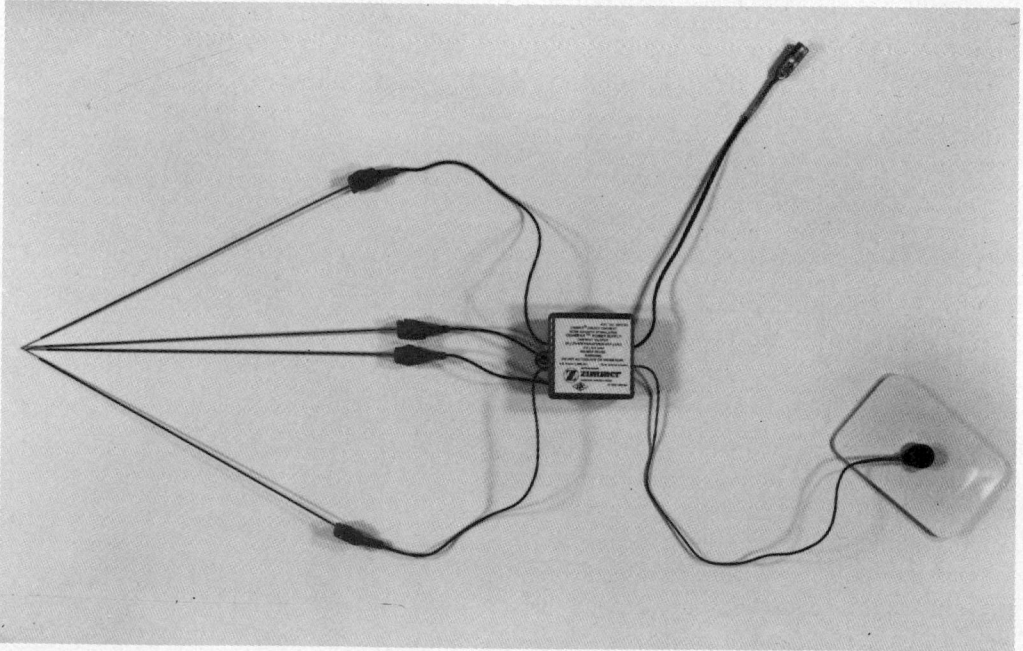

Fig. 5-23. Percutaneous bioelectrical bone stimulator used for treating delayed union or nonunion of bone. Note the four Teflon-coated electrodes and lithium battery pack with ground pad and reference electrode. (Courtesy Zimmer Corp., Warsaw, Ind.)

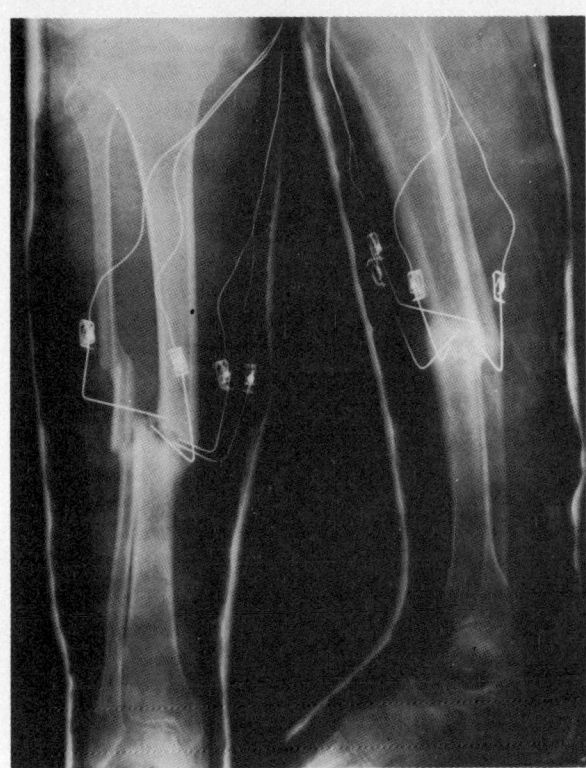

Fig. 5-24. Tibial fracture seen in Fig. 5-21 with percutaneous electrodes in place and electrode tips in fracture site.

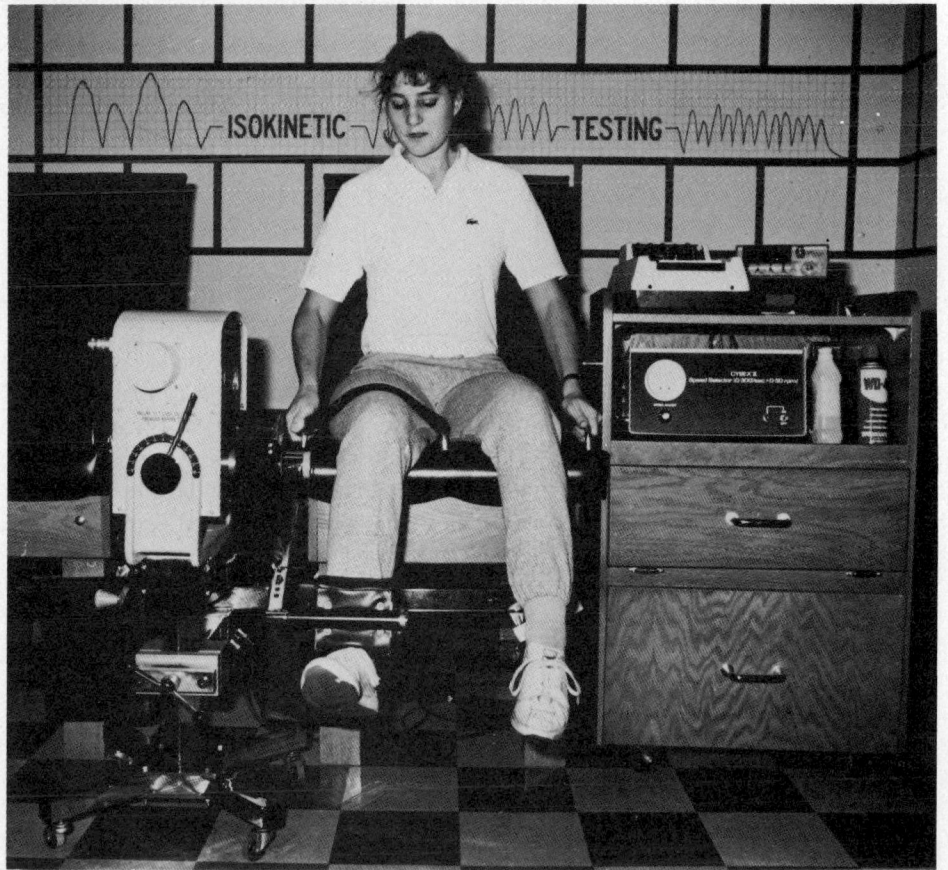

Fig. 5-25. Isokinetic (Cybex) machine testing muscle strength and endurance of the leg. (Courtesy Cybex, Ronkonkoma, NY.)

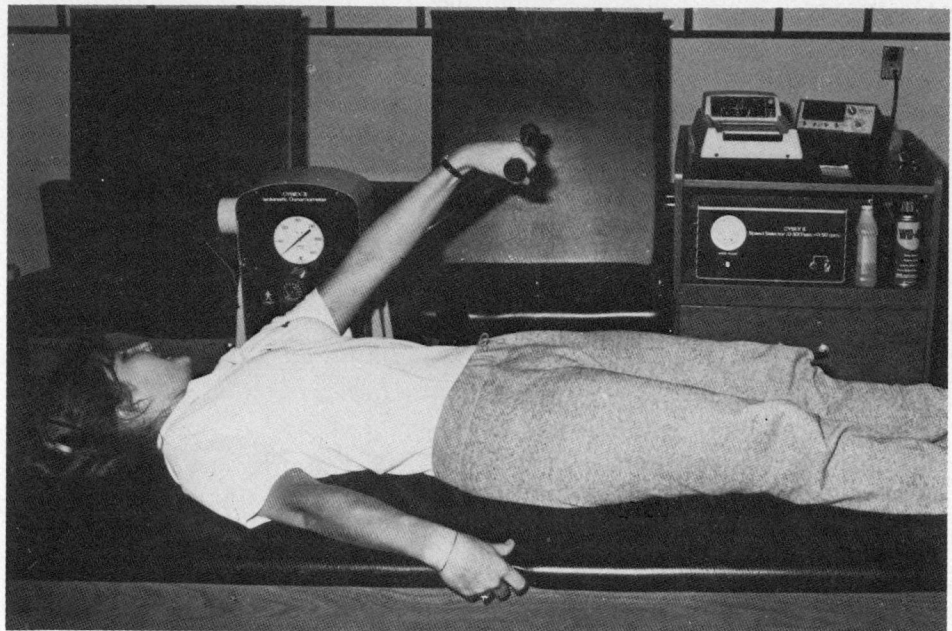

Fig. 5-26. Isokinetic (Cybex) machine testing muscle strength and endurance of the shoulder. (Courtesy Cybex, Ronkonkoma, NY.)

The patient's own assessment of readiness is usually evident in his/her level of confidence. Confidence is composed of a constellation of factors that are internally, unconsciously weighed on a daily basis and can be evaluated by comparison with the patient's preinjury confidence level. A therapist can and should help the injured person determine his/her own true level of confidence by helping the patient eliminate obscuring elements, such as peer or family pressure, inordinately intense ego drive, or inordinate fear. Even after careful measurement and management, determining the patient's confidence level is as difficult as determining whether someone's new shoe fits—only the person wearing it can be sure it is right. Failure to help the patient honestly develop confidence on the basis of good scientific rehabilitation principles can leave him/her in the perilous position of either never attaining full potential or plunging back into activity too quickly, thus performing inadequately and/or inviting reinjury.

Measurements of limb size or strength during the rehabilitation phase of fracture management tell much more about muscle strength and soft tissue repair than they do about bone strength. Even radiographic analysis provides only indirect information about the strength of the bone. The observation of a defect or failure in the bone is clear evidence of its weakness, of course, but the strength of bone under repair remains difficult to judge and extensive experience is necessary before one can feel confident of accurate analysis. Because of such considerations, motion, muscle strength, and atrophy are the principal determinates

of the progress of healing, coupled with the patient's own level of confidence.

Although the fracture site begins to demonstrate microscopic histological evidence of healing as early as 15 hours following injury, radiographic evidence of fracture healing in the form of callus is rarely seen before 4 weeks. In some bones, such as the small bones of the wrist or the neck, the appearance of callus is often skimpy, even in a fracture healing normally. The first radiographic evidence of callus appears about the fourth week following injury and continues for 10 weeks or more, to be followed by months of remodeling.

Remodeling is best defined by Wolf's law, which states: "Bone remodels along the lines of stress according to certain mathematical principles."[6] During the months of remodeling, the abundant callus is replaced by a progressively strong remodeled bone. It may be several years following the injury before the radiographic evidence of a fracture is gone.

The time factors related to fractures compose an interesting, if sometimes frustrating and disheartening, pattern. A fracture occurs in a matter of milliseconds, can force weeks of immobilization in a cast, requires months of rehabilitation time, and necessitates years before completion of the remodeling process. Throughout this time, a patient's return to activities and subsequent degree of participation are dependent on range of motion studies; evaluations of strength, pain, and swelling; and the health professional team's best guess as to the strength of the healing bone. Fortunately, accumulated clinical experience and modern methods of treatment and evaluation make this guessing a reasonably safe procedure.

SUMMARY

Great strides have been made in the diagnosis and management of fractures since Wilhelm Conrad Roentgen first showed the world a roentgen ray of the hand in 1896. However, such advances have brought with them myriads of new questions. Exactly how are bioelectrical and mechanical factors mediated? How does nutrition affect bone healing and remodeling? How can the detrimental effects of postmenopause hormonal changes on bone be reversed safely and conveniently? The answers to some of these questions appear to be just over the horizon. The quality of care for the fracture patient is improving daily.

REFERENCES

1. Curtiss PH Jr: Personal communication, 1966.
2. Hoyt WA Jr et al: Emergency care and transportation of the sick and injured, ed 3, Chicago, 1981, American Academy of Orthopaedic Surgeons.
3. Kennedy JD and Walker DM: Occult knee ligament injuries associated with femoral shaft fractures, J Sports Med Phys Fitness 8(3):172, 1980.
4. Khasigian HA: The results of treatment of nonunions with electrical stimulation, Orthopedics 31(1):32, 1980.
5. Radin E et al: Practical biomechanics for the orthopaedic surgeon, New York, 1979, John Wiley & Sons, Inc., p. 53.
6. Wolf J: Das Gesetz der Transformation den Knochen, Berlin, 1892, A. Hirschwald.
7. Yamada H: Strength of biological materials, Baltimore, 1970, Williams & Wilkins, p. 49.

Chapter 6

LIGAMENT AND MUSCLE-TENDON-UNIT INJURIES

James S. Keene

The functional stability of the many joints in the body is due, in part, to the intricate ligament systems and muscle-tendon units associated with each joint. This chapter details the basic principles of defining, classifying, and treating injuries to the ligaments and muscle-tendon units of the musculoskeletal system. The objectives of this discussion are to (1) define the terms that describe soft tissue injuries, (2) detail the process of detecting and diagnosing these injuries, and (3) discuss operative and nonoperative methods of treatment.

DEFINITION OF TERMS

Tendons are connective tissue structures that attach muscles to bones. *Ligaments* are similar connective tissue structures, but they arise from and insert into bone. However, despite their similarity, these two structures are quite distinct. Ligaments stabilize joints and serve to connect two bones but lack a motor component to move the joint. Tendons, on the other hand, are an integral part of the body's muscle-tendon units. A *muscle-tendon unit* refers to a complex unit formed by the muscle arising from bone, the muscle-tendon junction, and the tendon or tendons that insert into bone. Muscle-tendon units not only stabilize joints but provide the motor power to move them. Therefore injuries to muscles or tendons should not be considered isolated entities since they affect the muscle-tendon unit as a whole. Injuries to muscle-tendon units are referred to as strains, whereas injuries to ligaments are called sprains.

Strains

An injury described as a *strain* indicates that there has been some degree of disruption in the muscle fibers, the muscle-tendon junction, the tendon, or the bony insertion of a muscle-tendon unit. This disruption may be caused by (1) a direct blow (contusion), (2) excessive stretching (acute strain), (3) repetitive loading (chronic strain), or (4) a laceration.

The term *contusion* refers to an injury caused by a direct blow to the muscle belly of a muscle-tendon unit. This injury results in capillary rupture and bleeding into the muscle, followed by an inflammatory reaction. The severity of a contusion may be determined by the degree to which it limits motion of the joint(s) that the muscle-tendon unit crosses.

Acute and *chronic strains* occur when the muscular or tendinous portion of a muscle-tendon unit lacks the flexibility, strength, or endurance to accommodate the demands placed on it. Appreciating and evaluating these three qualities of the muscle-tendon unit are important to understanding the rationale for treatment and rehabilitation of these injuries. *Acute strains* are the result of a single violent force applied to the muscle-tendon unit. When the force is greater than the strength or exceeds the flexibility of the muscle-tendon unit, the muscle, muscle-tendon junction, or tendon will tear. In some instances the disruption occurs at the bony attachment of the muscle-tendon unit, resulting in an avulsion fracture (Fig. 6-1). *Chronic strains* occur when repetitive forces exceed the endurance of the muscle-tendon unit. If the muscle or tendon has not been conditioned for repetitive loading, a tear occurs. The tear propagates to adjacent portions of the muscle or the tendon if the precipitating activity is not curtailed. The term tendonitis is used to describe injuries to the tendinous portion of the muscle-tendon unit. *Tendonitis* is, in fact, a tear of the tendon that varies from microscopic to macroscopic levels. With acute tendonitis microscopic tears appear in the tendon, causing only localized swelling and tenderness. However, in chronic cases the tears may coalesce, causing a complete disruption of the tendinous tissue. The continuity of the tendon is maintained only by inflexible scar tissue.

Strains are graded as mild (first degree), moderate (second degree), or severe (third degree). With first-degree strains there is no gross disruption of the muscle-tendon unit. There is localized swelling and tenderness but no loss of strength in the injured unit or loss of motion in the adjacent joints. However, stretching and contractions of the injured muscle-tendon unit against resistance will elicit pain at the site of the injury. With second-degree strains there is some degree of gross disruption of the muscle-tendon unit, resulting in loss of strength in the muscle and limitation of active motion in the adjacent joints. However, clinical testing reveals that the muscle-tendon unit has not been completely disrupted. In third-degree strains one or more of the components of the muscle-tendon unit is completely disrupted and motion in the adjacent joints is severely restricted. Often, the site of this disruption is visibly evident. At other times, the defect may be palpated or documented by means of specific clinical tests. In ruptures of either the proximal or distal insertion of the brachial biceps muscle in the arm, the site of the disruption is usually evident (Fig. 6-2). Although a palpable defect is often present with third-degree strains of the Achilles tendon, these are best documented by the Thompson test, which is performed with the client in prone position with both feet extending past the end of the examination table. The examiner squeezes the calf muscles of the affected side (Fig. 6-3). If the tendon is intact, the foot will demonstrate plantar flexion. If the tendon is ruptured, the foot will not flex. Clients with this injury can still actively flex their ankles because the function of their posterior tibial, flexor digitorum, and flexor hallucis longus tendons is not impaired.

Sprains

The term *sprain* describes injuries to the ligaments. Sprains are caused by forces that stretch some or all of the ligament fibers beyond their elastic limit, producing some degree of rupture of the fibers and/or their bony attachment. As mentioned previously, ligaments are connective tissue structures that have no motor component to move joints but function to stabilize and prevent abnormal motion of a joint. The classification and grading of ligamentous injuries are based upon two factors: (1) the number of fibers disrupted and (2) the subsequent instability of the joint involved. The severity of the injury depends on the magnitude, direction, and duration of the forces applied.

Like musculotendinous injuries, ligament injuries are graded as mild (first degree), moderate (second degree), and severe (third degree). First-degree sprains produce localized tenderness and swelling over the injury site. Some ligament fibers are torn, but there is no demonstrable loss, clinically or functionally, of the integrity of the ligament. With second-degree sprains, many, but not all, of the ligament fibers are torn and there is clinical evidence of joint instability. However, stress-testing does not demonstrate complete functional loss of the integrity of the ligament. Third-degree sprains disrupt the ligament completely. This disruption occurs at the bony attachments or within the substance of the ligament.

Joint instability resulting from ligamentous injury is graded on a 0 to 3 scale. The degree of instability is deter-

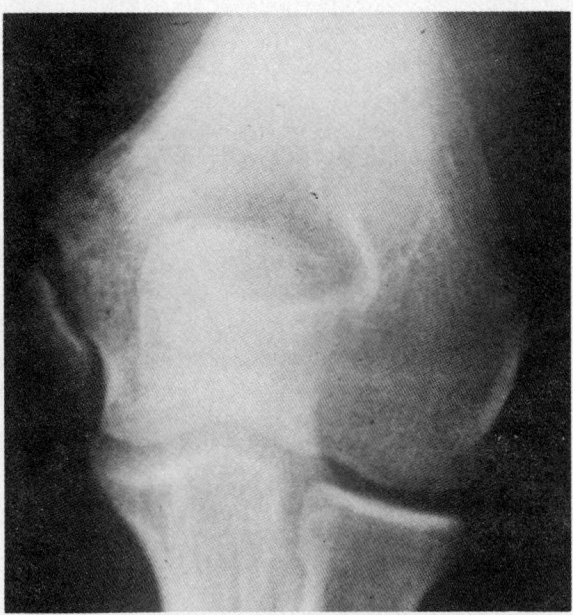

Fig. 6-1. Anteroposterior radiograph of elbow showing avulsion fracture at origin of extensor tendons.

mined by comparing the joint excursion permitted by an injured ligament with that permitted by its uninjured counterpart in the other extremity. The degree of instability is designated as 0, 1+, 2+, or 3+. Zero instability indicates that there is no difference between the amount of joint excursion permitted by the injured and uninjured ligaments. In a 1+, 2+, or 3+ instability, the difference between the laxity of the uninjured and injured ligaments is less than 0.5 cm, 0.5 to 1 cm, or greater than 1 cm, respectively.

CLASSIFYING INSTABILITY

In addition to grading scales, a standardized nomenclature and several classification systems have been developed to describe ligament injuries and instabilities.[51] In hinge-type (ginglymus) joints the instability is described as anterior, posterior, medial, or lateral. In joints that also have rotatory motion the nomenclature and classification system of ligament instability are more complex. The most elaborate classification system of ligament instability has been developed for the knee by Hughston et al.[22,23] Based on clinical tests and operative findings, it was concluded that knee instabilities are best classified as either straight (nonrotatory) or rotatory (simple or combined). The classification of straight instability is similar to that used for hinge-type joints and includes medial, lateral, anterior, and posterior instabilities. The classification of rotatory instability involves either anterior rotation of the medial tibial condyle or anterior and posterior rotation of the lateral tibial condyle. Three types of simple rotatory instability were found: anteromedial, anterolateral, and posterolat-

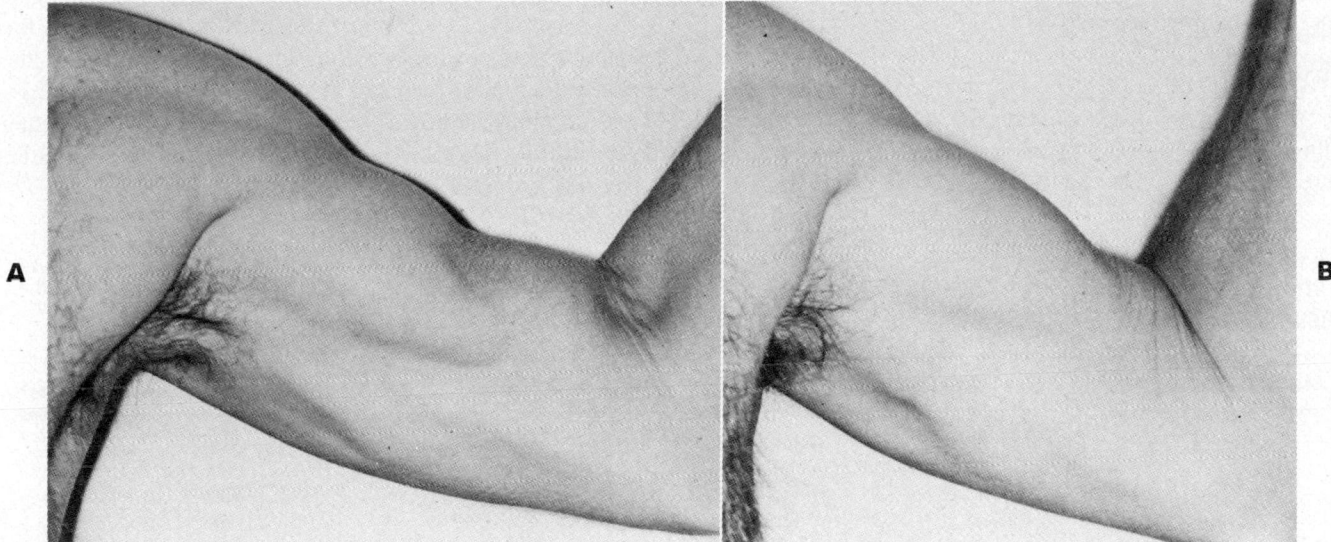

Fig. 6-2. Rupture of distal attachment of biceps muscle in right arm (**A**) is clearly evident when right and left arms (**B**) are compared.

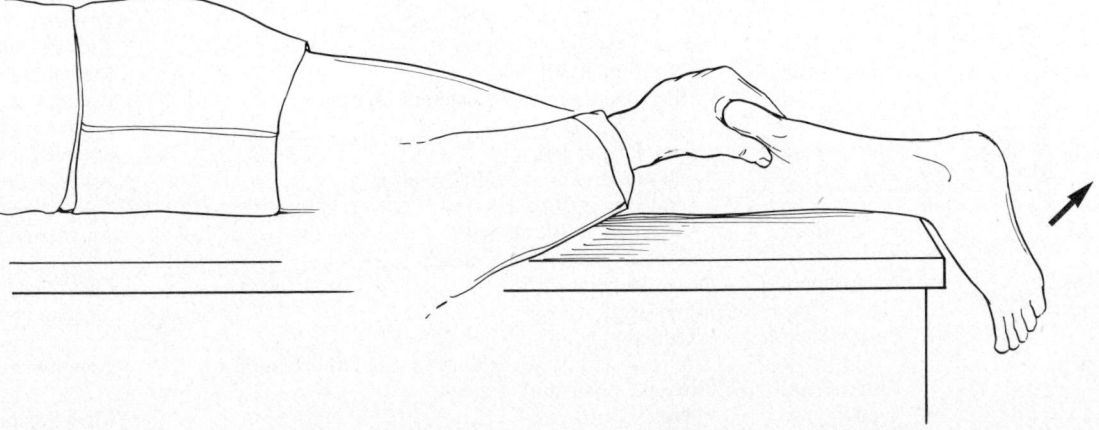

Fig. 6-3. Achilles tendon rupture diagnosed by Thompson test. If tendon is ruptured, foot will not plantar flex when calf muscles are compressed. If tendon is intact, foot will flex (arrow) with calf compression.

eral. It was also concluded that, although there were various combinations of the three types of rotatory instability, the two most common combinations were (1) anterolateral and posterolateral rotatory instability and (2) anteromedial and anterolateral rotatory instability. The clinical tests and the anatomical structures responsible for these types of instability are summarized in Table 6-1. Several of these tests are discussed in detail in subsequent sections of this chapter.

DIAGNOSIS

There are several important principles and aids for diagnosing ligament and muscle-tendon–unit injuries. These include (1) obtaining a detailed history, including the description of the mechanism of the injury, (2) performing a comprehensive physical examination, (3) using various radiographic techniques, and (4) evaluating the contents of the joint with an arthroscope.

History

A thorough history is often the key to understanding and appreciating which ligaments or muscles have been injured. Certain types of information should always be sought. Details of (1) the mechanism of the injury, (2) the timing and location of pain and swelling, and (3) the loss of function associated with the injury often provide important data necessary for developing a differential diagnosis.

Mechanism of injury

In the case of ligamentous injuries it is important to determine the direction and/or angle of the forces that caused the injury. Often, if the examiner is present when the injury occurs, the mechanism of injury can be observed directly. In a sport such as football the mechanism of injury can be determined from game films. However, if first-hand observation is not possible, one should question the individual regarding causes of the injury (e.g., contact with another person or an object) and angle of the impact. If the force was applied to the lateral aspect of the knee, for example, one should carefully evaluate the medial ligaments and meniscus. If the injury was caused by a blow to the anterior tibia, there should be careful examination of the posterior cruciate ligament and posterior capsule. If the injury occurred as the person fell or changed direction while running, one should be suspicious of an anterior or posterior cruciate ligament tear.

Table 6-1. Classification, positive stress tests, and injured ligamentous structures associated with various instabilities of the knee

Classification of instability	Type of instability	Positive stress tests	Injured ligamentous structures
Straight	Medial	Abduction at full extension	Medial compartment
			Posterior cruciate
		Abduction at 30° flexion	Medial compartment
	Lateral	Adduction at full extension	Lateral collateral
			Posterior cruciate
		Adduction at 30° flexion	Lateral collateral
	Anterior	Lachman's test	Anterior cruciate
		Anterior drawer	Anterior cruciate
			Medial compartment
	Posterior	Posterior drawer	Posterior cruciate
			Posterior oblique
			Arcuate complex
Rotatory	Anteromedial	Abduction at 30° flexion	Medial compartment
		Anterior drawer at 15° external rotation	Anterior cruciate
			Posterior oblique
	Anterolateral	Pivot-shift or jerk	Lateral capsular
		Anterior drawer at neutral rotation	Anterior cruciate
		Adduction at 30° flexion	
	Posterolateral	Adduction at 30° flexion	Arcuate complex
		External-rotation recurvatum	
Combined	Anterolateral and Posterolateral	Reverse pivot-shift	Lateral capsular
		Pivot-shift or jerk	Arcuate complex
		Adduction at 30° flexion	
		Anterior and posterior drawer at neutral rotation	Anterior cruciate
	Anterolateral and Anteromedial	Reverse pivot-shift	
		Pivot-shift or jerk	Medial capsular
		Anterior drawer at neutral and 15° external rotation	Lateral capsular
		Adduction at 30° flexion	Anterior cruciate
		Abduction at 30° flexion	

Symptoms, sounds, and swelling

The client's localization of pain is another key to determining the site of injury. Is the pain experienced acutely, or had there been some pain in the same area prior to the acute episode? The chronic intermittent pain of tendonitis that culminates in an acute episode may signify that a complete rupture of the tendon has occurred. Is the pain diffuse, or can the client point to the site of the pain with one finger? Diffuse pain suggests a muscle contusion or intraarticular ligament tear. Point tenderness is more commonly reported with disruption of the superficial ligaments and tendons. Did the client hear or feel a "snap" or "pop" when the injury occurred? These sounds and feelings often occur with cruciate ligament injuries of the knee and subluxating peroneal tendons at the ankle. Did the injured joint immediately "swell up," or was the onset of swelling slow? Immediate swelling of a joint, within the first hour of injury, is a hemarthrosis. An immediate, tense, bloody effusion in the knee (Fig. 6-4), for example, usually signifies that a rupture of the anterior cruciate ligament has occurred. Lesser effusions occuring over a period of many hours indicate a synovial effusion and are experienced with meniscal and collateral ligament injuries.

Loss of function

Often the severity of the injury can be determined by the effect it has on a client's or athlete's performance. After the injury occurred, could the athlete continue playing and bear full weight on the injured extremity, or did the extremity "give way"? First- and second-degree ligament injuries may allow the athlete to continue playing or walk off the field unaided, while third-degree injuries cause sufficient instability that the injured extremity buckles when weight is applied to it. Did the person experience "locking," and was he/she unable to move the injured joint through a full range of motion? Medial collateral, anterior cruciate ligament, and meniscal injuries of the knee often cause locking and the loss of 10 to 45 degrees of extension. Quadriceps muscle strains and contusions often limit flexion.

The importance of asking the appropriate questions and obtaining a thorough history cannot be overemphasized. History of the injury-producing event is the foundation on which physical examination of the various ligament and muscle injuries is based.

Physical examination

Ideally, ligament and muscle-tendon–unit injuries should be evaluated immediately after they occur; otherwise instability associated with the injury may quickly be masked by muscle spasm and joint tightness due to swelling. The examiner should first ascertain if the tenderness is localized or diffuse. Diffuse tenderness suggests more extensive soft tissue disruption. Next, one should perform clinical tests for the suspected specific joint instability involved (Table 6-1). If these tests are performed immediately after the injury, the degree of joint laxity can usually be accurately determined. If the examination is delayed, then stress-testing becomes increasingly unreliable because there is rapid onset of protective muscular resistance. If there is a suggestion of laxity but the examination is unsatisfactory because of muscular resistance, the injured joint should be examined with the client under a local or general anesthetic. The stability of the injured joint should always be compared to its uninjured counterpart. In this manner the client's normal physiological laxity will not be mistaken for laxity caused by the current injury. The results of the initial examination should be carefully recorded (Fig. 6-5) so that findings of subsequent examinations, and by other examiners, can be compared.

Radiographic evaluation

Although clinical tests for instability usually subjectively document (from the examiner's point of view) that

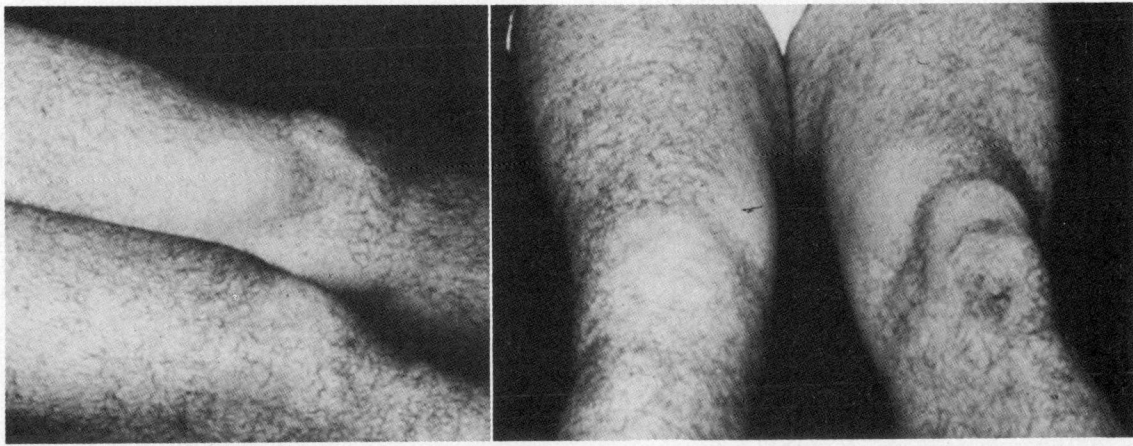

Fig. 6-4. Immediate, tense effusion is often associated with a third-degree anterior cruciate ligament disruption.

KNEE:　LIGAMENTOUS INJURIES

Client's name	History number	Preoperative		Anesthesia	
		R	L	R	L
Anterior drawer test					
External tibial rotation					
Neutral tibial rotation					
Internal tibial rotation					
Posterior drawer test					
External tibial rotation					
Neutral tibial rotation					
Internal tibial rotation					
Lachman's test					
Pivot-shift test					
Reverse pivot-shift test					
Abduction stress test					
Hyperextended					
0 degrees					
30 degrees					
Adduction stress test					
Hyperextended					
0 degrees					
30 degrees					

Diagnosis

Fig. 6-5. Evaluation form for recording clinical findings of examination of knees with ligamentous injuries.

laxity is present, standard radiographs should always be taken. They will indicate if the laxity is caused by an avulsion of the ligament with its bony attachment or by an epiphyseal separation. They will also demonstrate whether any other fractures are associated with the ligamentous injury. The standard radiographic evaluation should always include two exposures that are at right angles (90 degrees) to each other. If radiographs are taken in only one plane (e.g., only anteroposterior or lateral), the actual amount of displacement or malalignment of a fracture or joint cannot be ascertained. Ideally, all of the individual bony structures of the joint being examined should be radiographed in two planes, 90 degrees apart. There are several ancillary radiographic methods for evaluating ligament and cartilage injuries, including stress radiographs, arthrograms, and magnetic resonance imaging (MRI). MRI is an effective method for documenting injuries to tendons, ligaments, and cartilage, but because of its current cost the two ancil-

lary methods most often used to evaluate ligament injuries are stress radiographs and arthrograms.

Stress radiographs. Stress radiographs are obtained by applying the appropriate varus-valgus or anteroposterior stress to a joint as a standard radiograph is taken. Although stress radiographs are not routinely required for evaluating joint laxity, they have proved useful in documenting instabilities of the ankle and in evaluating epiphyseal injuries of the knee (Fig. 6-6). To obtain accurate information from stress studies, one must pay close attention to the positioning of the joint to be examined. Also, comparative views of the opposite uninjured joint should always be obtained.

Arthrography. Arthrography is another radiographic technique that is often helpful in evaluating soft tissue injuries. Arthrograms are used when the clinical history, physical examination, and standard radiographs do not clearly define the location and severity of the injury. Ar-

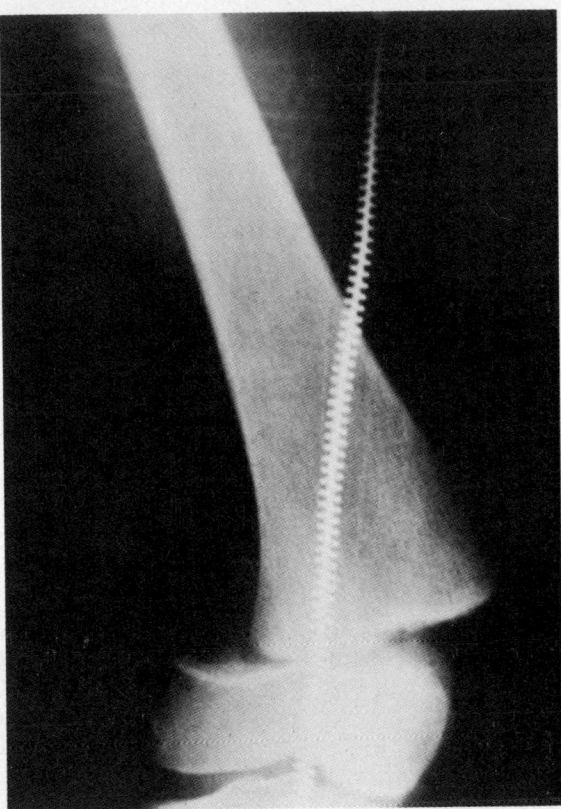

Fig. 6-6. Stress radiograph demonstrating separation of distal femoral epiphysis. Clinical stress-testing may suggest a medial collateral ligament injury rather than epiphyseal injury.

thrography is performed by injecting a joint with either a radiopaque liquid (Renografin) and/or room air. The procedure is called a *double-contrast arthrogram* when both air and liquid are injected and a *single-contrast arthrogram* when only liquid is injected. After liquid, air, or both have been injected into the joint, serial radiographs can be obtained at many different angles.

Although this technique has been applied to many joints in the body, it is most often used to evaluate meniscal and ligamentous injuries in the knee. A single-contrast arthrogram of the knee is performed by injecting the joint with 10 ml of Renografin and 5 to 10 ml of lidocaine (Xylocaine). The knee is then flexed and extended to distribute the Renografin. An elastic bandage is wrapped around the knee to force the dye out of the suprapatellar pouch and popliteal space, thus thoroughly coating the menisci and cruciate ligaments. Anteroposterior radiographs are then taken to evaluate the integrity of the medial and lateral capsular and ligamentous structures. Lateral radiographs with the knee flexed to 90 degrees are done with and without anterior stress on the tibia to evaluate the cruciate ligaments. Subsequently, serial tangential views of the medial and lateral meniscus are taken (Fig. 6-7).

Arthrography of the knee is employed for evaluation of knee injuries because of its accuracy in documenting meniscal lesions. Clinical accuracy in diagnosing meniscal injuries is usually reported to be approximately 70%.[30,47,49] Single- and double-contrast arthrograms in conjunction with a physical examination, and a client's history have improved the accuracy rate to 95%.[38,41,53,55] Single-contrast arthrography is usually the most effective technique for documenting cruciate and collateral ligament injuries (Fig. 6-8).

There are at least three significant limitations to the accuracy of knee arthrograms. The first limitation occurs in diagnosing collateral ligament injuries. If the arthrogram is not performed immediately after a third-degree or second-degree collateral ligament tear, the site of the disruption may be sealed by synovium or a clot and the dye will not leak out of the joint and will not localize the injury. The second limitation concerns the evaluation of lateral meniscal lesions. Evaluation of the posterior third of the lateral meniscus is extremely difficult because the popliteal tendon sheath, which crosses this area, fills with dye and obscures the outline of the meniscus. In addition, the posterior fifth of the lateral meniscus cannot be visualized on an arthrogram because it is obscured by the anterior cruciate ligament. The third limitation concerns evaluation of the anterior cruciate ligament. When this ligament is completely disrupted but its synovial sheath remains intact, the arthrogram will usually appear normal, even under stress. In general, whenever there are overlapping structures within a joint, the arthrogram is of limited value in assessing the integrity of either one or both of the structures.

Arthroscopy

Arthroscopy is another adjunctive diagnostic procedure that often is employed for the assessment of intraarticular soft-tissue injuries. With this technique an arthroscope, a cylindrical stainless-steel tube with a diameter ranging from 2 to 5 mm and optical lenses at both ends (Fig. 6-9), is inserted into a joint. With the aid of a continuous flow of sterile saline solution through the tube, a fiberoptic light source attached to the scope, and a small television camera, the structures within the joint can be examined directly. The "state of the art" of arthroscopy has progressed to the point where most joints in the musculoskeletal system can be examined in this manner. The scope often has to be inserted at multiple sites (the polypuncture technique) for complete examination of the larger joints.

Arthroscopy has proved to be a valuable adjunct in the evaluation of knee injuries. In a study of 100 clients with internal derangements of the knee, DeHaven and Collins[12] found that (1) the correct diagnosis could be made arthroscopically in 94 of the cases; (2) clinically and arthrographically, diagnoses were incorrect or conflicting in 39 of the cases; and (3) arthroscopy demonstrated unexpected disorders instead of the expected lesions in 25 of the cases. However, they concluded that clinical examination, ar-

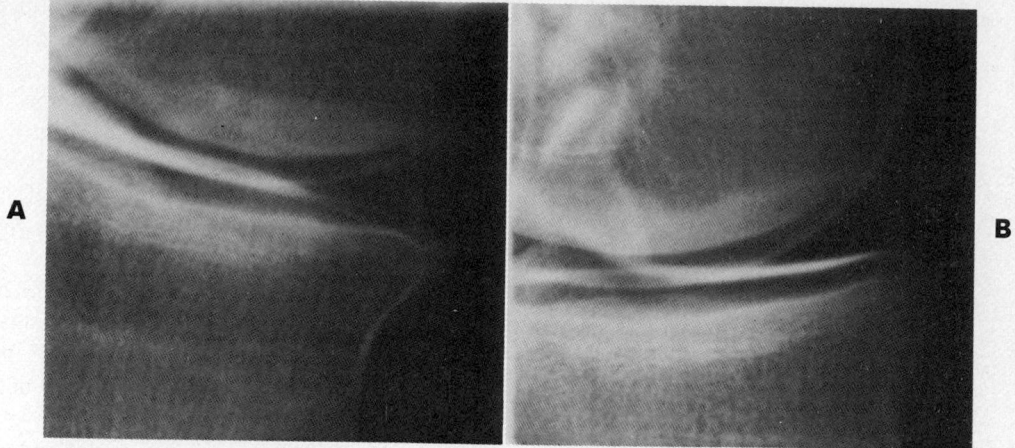

Fig. 6-7. Right knee arthrogram. **A,** Tangential views of medial meniscus demonstrate vertical tear. **B,** Normal meniscus.

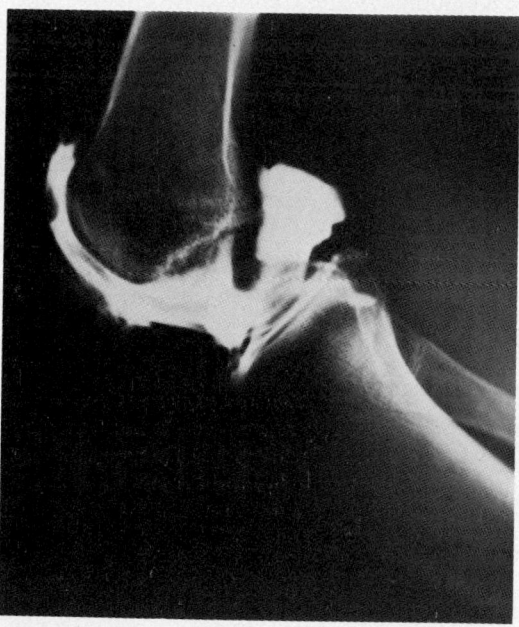

Fig. 6-8. Lateral view of single-contrast arthrogram of knee, demonstrating normal anterior and posterior cruciate ligaments.

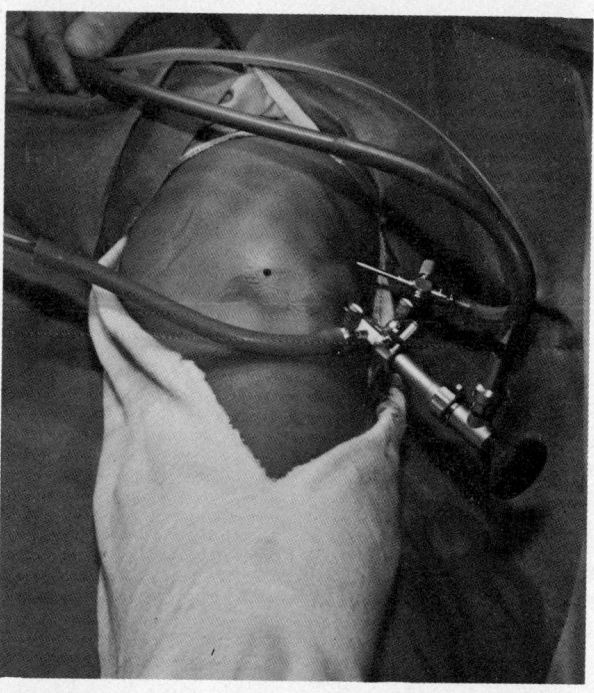

Fig. 6-9. A 170-degree, 5-mm arthroscope. The arthroscope is shown within the knee with fiberoptic light source and irrigation tubing in place.

thrography, *and* arthroscopy in combination provided a more accurate diagnosis than any modality did individually.

It has been my experience that arthroscopy has particular advantages over arthrography in the evaluation of patellar, anterior cruciate, and lateral meniscal injuries. The articular surface of the patella can be clearly visualized and manipulated arthroscopically, but it is difficult to evaluate arthrographically (Fig. 6-10). In addition, the patellar ar-

ticular surface can be debrided and abraided as necessary by inserting the appropriate instrument through another portal in the knee and then observing the surgery directly through the scope. Third-degree anterior cruciate ligament injuries are also better evaluated with the arthroscope. The ligament may appear to be continuous on an arthrogram because of an intact synovial sheath. With the scope, however, the ligament can be readily visualized and evaluated. The integrity of the ligament is determined by placing a

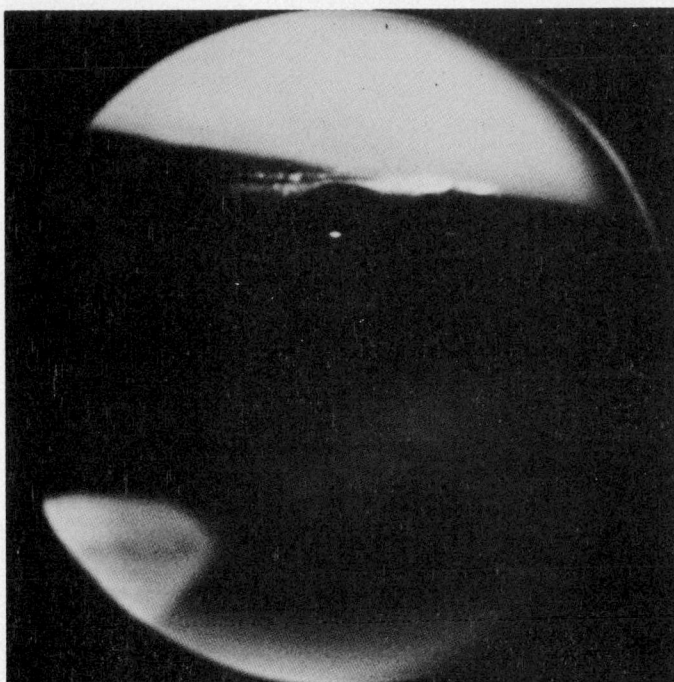

Fig. 6-10. Undersurface of normal patella as viewed through the arthroscope. Drainage cannula is evident beneath articular surface of patella.

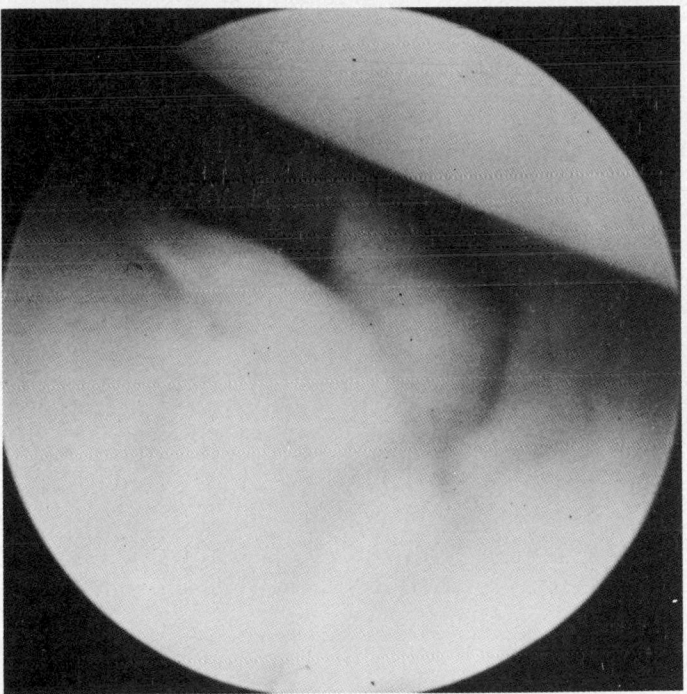

Fig. 6-11. Normal anterior cruciate ligament as viewed through the arthroscope. Ligament is the structure running obliquely along left side of photograph. Femoral articular surface is evident in upper right-hand corner.

probe (Fig. 6-11) into the joint through another portal and then manipulating the ligament under direct visual inspection. Similarly, lateral meniscal tears that are obscured on the arthrogram because of dye in the popliteal tendon sheath are easily evaluated with the arthroscope (Fig. 6-12). The lateral meniscus can be seen in its entirety, including the posterior attachment, which, as mentioned previously, is not visualizable on the arthrogram. In addition, most meniscal surgery is now performed with the arthro-

scope. As with the other procedures discussed, various cutting and grasping instruments can be inserted into the joint through separate portals or through the scope itself. All or part of the torn meniscus can then be freed from any remaining soft tissue attachment or, when indicated, repaired under direct visualization. Excised fragments are removed from the joint through one of the puncture wounds (Fig. 6-13).

Most arthroscopic procedures can be performed with lo-

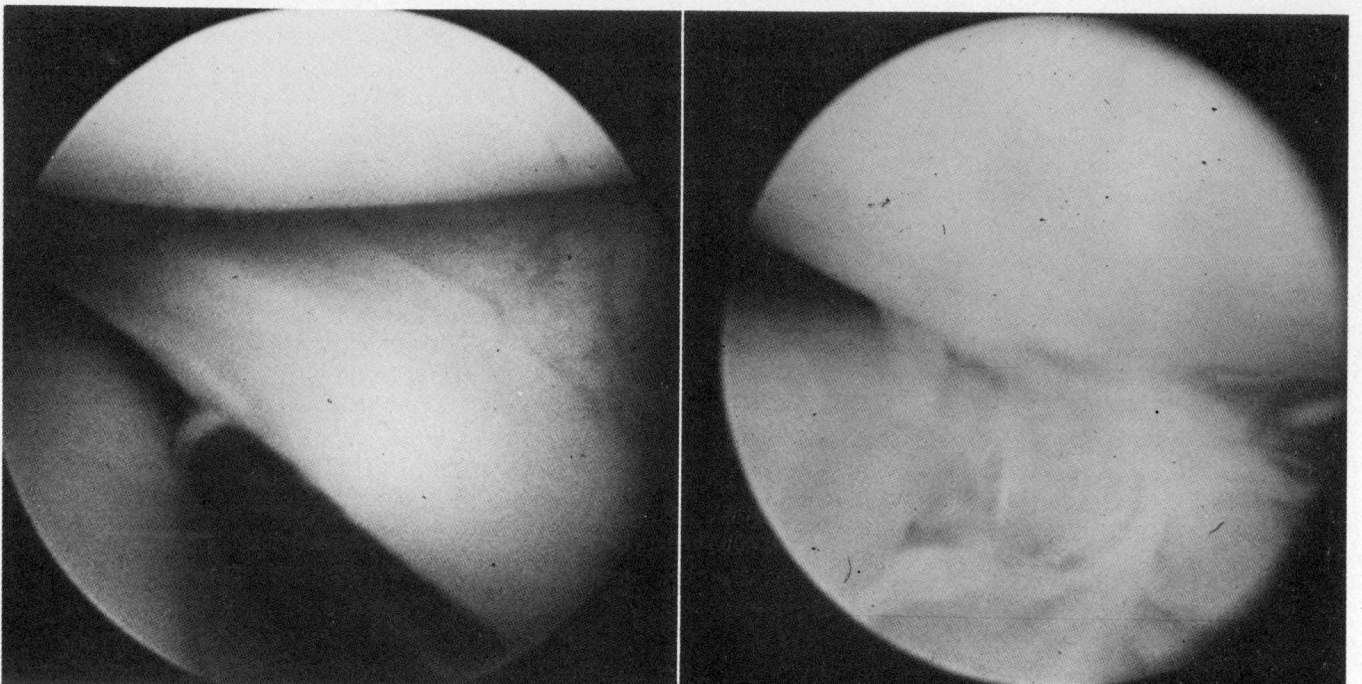

Fig. 6-12. Arthroscopic evaluation of lateral meniscus. **A,** Normal meniscus. **B,** Flap tear.

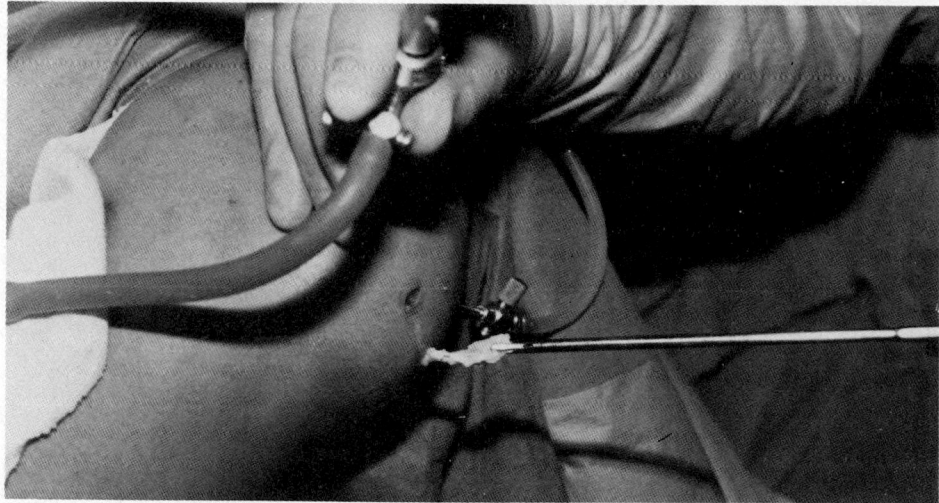

Fig. 6-13. Segment of torn lateral meniscus is removed through one of the puncture wounds. Excision of the meniscal tear was accomplished arthroscopically.

cal anesthesia. As can be imagined, the cost savings to both the client and the health care delivery system are remarkable. Also, the client does not need to be hospitalized, is not exposed to the risks of general or spinal anesthesia, and requires lower levels of narcotic analgesia in the postoperative period. The rehabilitation-recovery period—possibly including time on crutches and time to return to work and/or sports—has been markedly reduced with arthroscopic surgery as compared to an open arthrot-

omy of the joint. Most clients are no longer using crutches in 2 to 5 days, and many have completed a rehabilitation program within 3 weeks. This rapid recovery appears to be, in part, a result of less postoperative joint pain and swelling.

Summary

The key to establishing a diagnosis of ligament or muscle-tendon–unit injury includes: (1) obtaining a detailed history, (2) performing a thorough physical examination, and (3) utilizing, when appropriate, the adjunctive radiographic and/or arthroscopic techniques that are currently available. The importance of obtaining a detailed history must be stressed because certain points in the history—most often the mechanism of injury—will help the examiner form a provisional diagnosis and direct attention to specific aspects of the physical examination. The physical examination, if performed immediately after the injury has occurred or with anesthesia, will usually localize the site of the injury and document the resulting loss of function and/or the joint instability. When the location and severity of the injury cannot easily be determined from the history and physical examination, arthrography and/or arthroscopy should be performed. One should not, however, rely solely on either the history, the physical examination, or the radiographic and arthroscopic findings when evaluating ligament and soft tissue injuries. These methods of evaluation complement each other, and only by using them in combination can the most accurate diagnoses be achieved.

TREATMENT
General principles

The basic goals in the treatment of muscle strains and ligament sprains are to (1) regain full motion and stability of the joint involved, (2) facilitate normal neuromuscular patterns of movement, (3) restore the strength, flexibility, and endurance of the muscles involved, and (4) return the client to full function with minimal risk of reinjury. The method of achieving these goals is determined, in part, by the severity of the injury.

Muscle-tendon-unit injuries

In general, first- and second-degree strains are treated nonoperatively. Third-degree strains that occur in the tendinous portion of the muscle-tendon unit are treated operatively. (The term *nonoperative* is more descriptive than the term *conservative* because nonoperative treatment of some injuries, particularly third-degree strains, would be considered very radical and certainly not conservative.)

As mentioned previously, when a muscle strain occurs not only is the muscle and tendinous tissue torn but so are the adjacent blood vessels. Therefore the initial goals of treatment are to stop the interstitial bleeding and prevent further tearing of the muscle fibers. This is accomplished by applying a compression dressing, elevating and immobilizing the injured extremity, and placing ice on the injured area (five times per day for 20 minutes). This treatment is continued for 48 hours. During this period only minimal weight bearing should be permitted.

After 48 hours, gentle passive stretching of the injured muscle group is initiated. Subsequently, the individual is started on a more aggressive stretching program.[52]

Stretching program. The stretching program is performed on an individual basis or with a partner. (Exercises to stretch the knee will be used as an example.) If the affected muscle group is the quadriceps, adductors, or hamstrings, the stretching is performed in the following manner.

Step I—quadriceps stretch. The individual lies prone on a firm surface and flexes the knee on the injured side as far as possible. The partner kneels beside the individual's injured side and places one hand around the ankle and the other hand on the buttocks (Fig. 6-14, *A*). The individual then extends the knee against the resistance of the partner and holds the muscle contraction for a count of six. The partner then stretches the quadriceps muscle by gently pushing the individual's heel toward the buttocks (Fig. 6-14, *B*). This sequence is repeated three times.

Step II—adductor (groin) stretch. The individual sits on a firm surface, spreads his/her legs, and grasps the partner's wrists (Fig. 6-15, *A*).The partner sits facing the individual with knees bent, places his/her feet just above the individual's ankles, and grasps the wrists. The injured person then contracts the adductors by pressing his/her legs against the partner's resistance for a count of six (Fig. 6-15, *B*). The individual then relaxes as the partner pulls him/her forward while slowly and evenly spreading his/her legs. The sequence is repeated three times.

Step III—hamstring stretch. The individual lies supine on a firm surface with the knee of the injured extremity fully extended and the hip flexed to its limits. The opposite knee is also fully extended and the hip is extended so that it rests on the firm surface (Fig. 6-16, *A*). The partner then places the ankle of the individual's injured leg on his/her shoulder and grasps the anterior thigh, just above the knee, with both hands. The partner's opposite knee is placed on the individual's extended leg. The individual then extends the injured leg downward at the hip against the partner's resistance for a count of six (Fig. 6-16, *B*). The individual then relaxes as the partner stretches the hamstrings by pushing the leg upward toward the individual's head. This sequence is repeated three times.

Each stretch should be controlled and held steady for 30 to 60 seconds and the entire set of exercises should be performed three times per day until the individual can return to full activity. These exercises should evoke minimal pain when performed. Bouncing at the limits of the stretch (ballistic-stretching) should be avoided because this type of stretching may cause further tearing and will not increase flexibility of the muscle. The bouncing causes muscle contraction because it stimulates the muscle-tendon stretch reflex.

When the injured muscle group is able to move the adjacent joint(s) through a full range of motion without producing pain, running and weight programs can be started. Stretching is *always* performed immediately *before* and weight training immediately *after* the individual works on the running program.

Running program. The five step running program de-

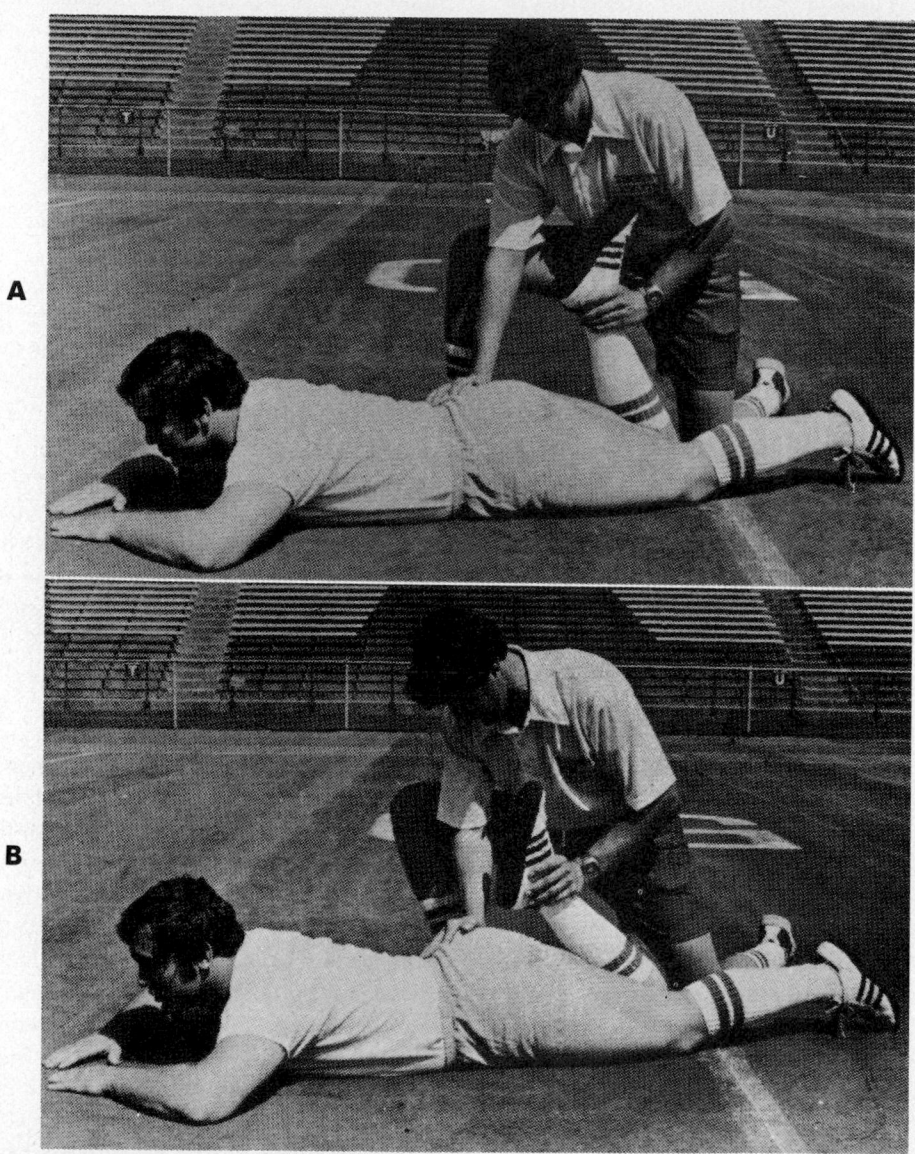

Fig. 6-14. Proprioceptive neuromuscular facilitation (PNF) stretching exercises of quadriceps muscles. **A,** Resistance-contraction phase; **B,** stretching phase. (Steps of exercise are explained in text.)

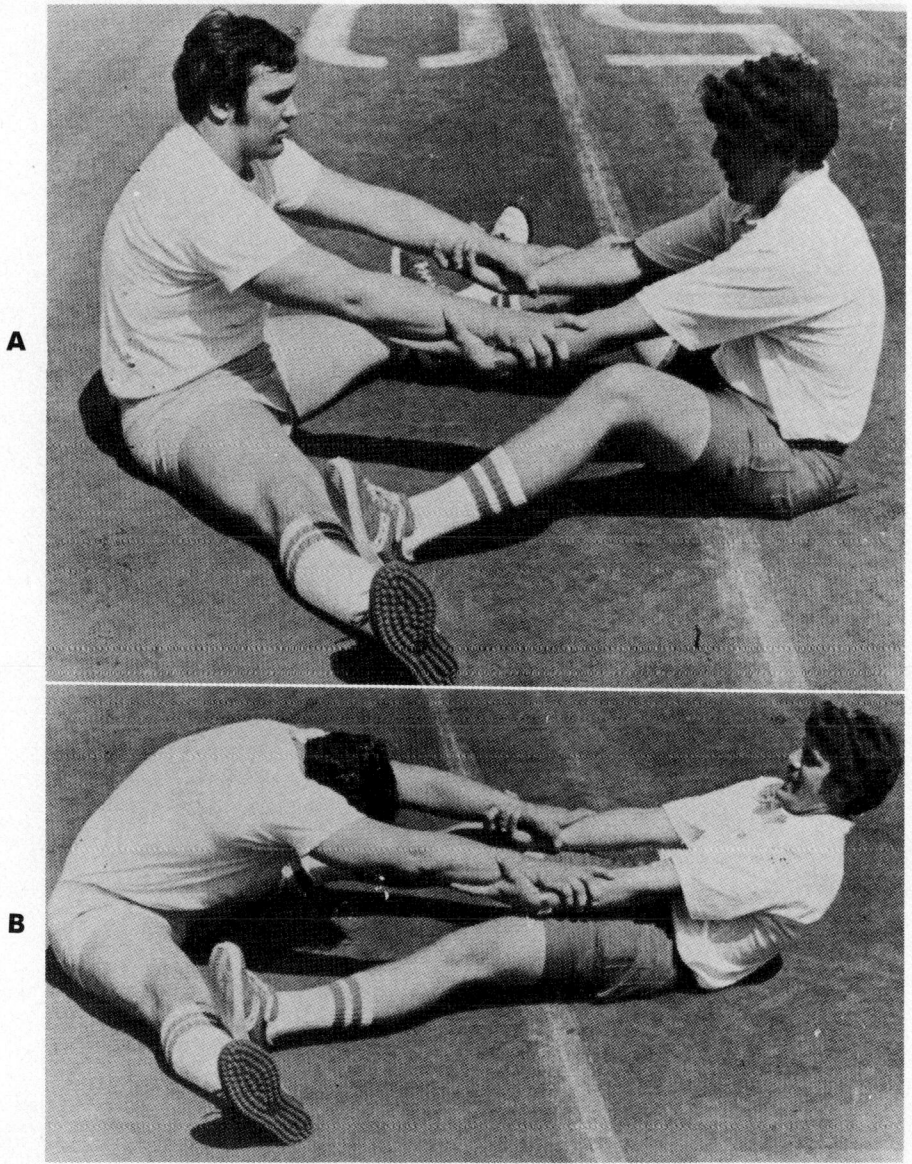

Fig. 6-15. PNF stretching exercises for adductors. **A,** Resistance-contraction phase; **B,** stretching phase. (Steps of exercise are explained in text.)

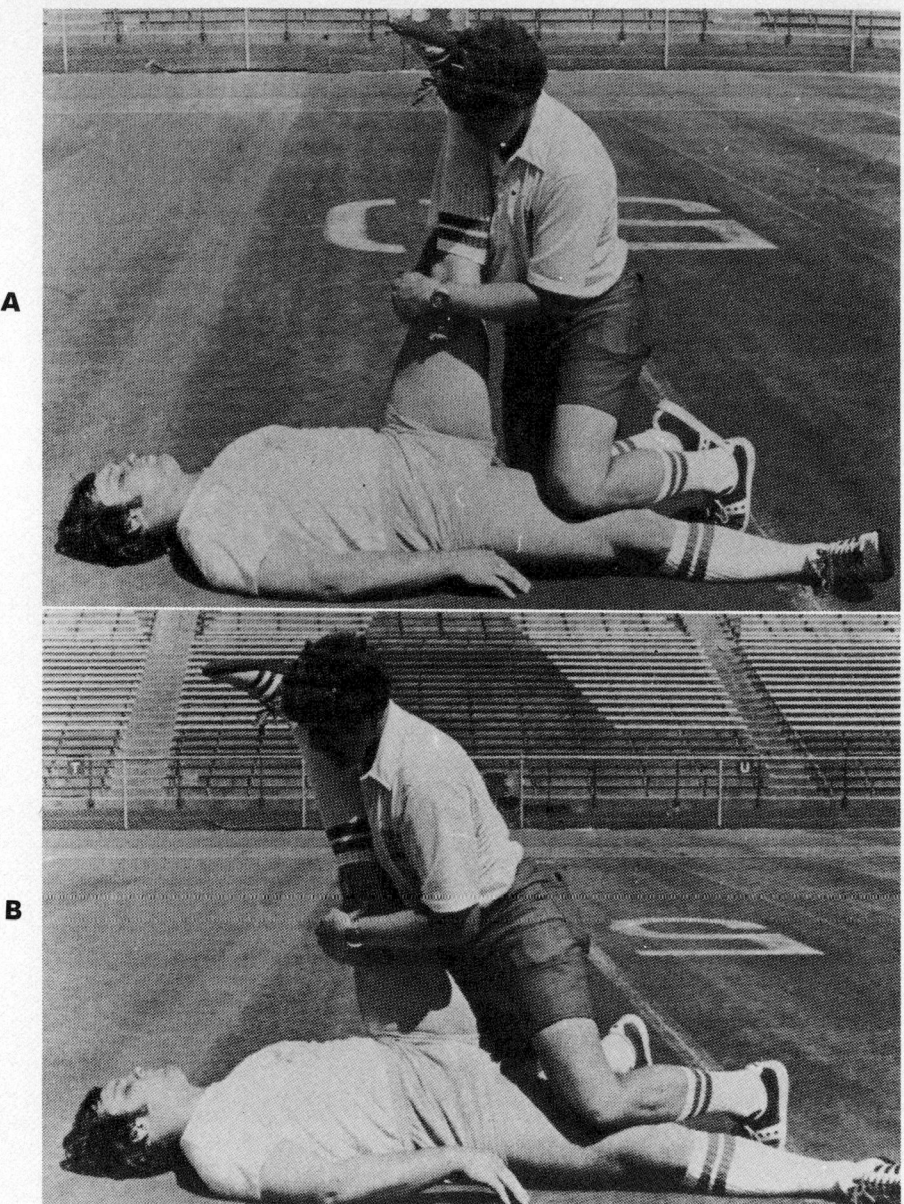

Fig. 6-16. PNF stretching exercises for hamstrings. **A,** Resistance-contraction phase; **B,** stretching phase. (Steps of exercise are explained in text.)

scribed hereafter and summarized in Table 6-2 is the one used at the University of Wisconsin.

The individual performs the running program daily, beginning at step I, until he/she can complete all five steps without developing pain or a limp. If an individual develops pain or a limp during any phase of the program, he/she must start the next day at step I. After completing the program, the individual, if an athlete, is put through various agility tests that are specific for his/her sport and position. These may include running figure eights, the carioca, back peddling, hopping, lateral crossover running, and cutting around cones.

Weight program. The weight-training program sum-

marized in Table 6-3 is also part of the University of Wisconsin regimen. It is started when an individual begins the running program and should be done every other day immediately after running. The weight-training program is best accomplished with the aid of isokinetic machines.* However, it can also be completed with free weights.

Immediately after completion of the weight program, ice packs should be applied to the injured area for 20 minutes or ice massage should be done until numbness occurs in the injured area (usually 5 to 8 minutes). When the single maximum lift (SML) of the injured and uninjured mus-

*Cybex, Ronkonkoma, NY.

Table 6-2. The running program

Step	Activity	Conditions
I	Jog ¼-½ mile/day. Add ¼ mile every 2-3 days, until jogging at least 1 mile	No pain or limp
II	Run six to eight 80-yard sprints at ½ speed	Able to jog 1 mile with no pain or limp
III	Run six to eight 80-yard sprints at ¾ speed	Completion of step II with no pain or limp
IV	Run six to eight 80-yard sprints at full speed and do six fast starts	Completion of step III with no pain or limp
V	Run six to eight 80-yard sprints, cutting right or left every 10 yards to ¾ speed and then back up to full speed	Completion of step IV with no pain or limp

Table 6-3. Muscle-strengthening program (accomplished with free weights)

Step	Activity	Goal
I	Determine single maximum lift (SML) of muscle(s) in *uninjured* extremity	Establishes strength to be obtained by *injured* muscles
II	Determine single maximum lift (SML) of muscle(s) in injured extremity	Establishes weight to be used in steps III and IV
III	Do three sets of 10 repetitions with the weight equal to SML, minus 10 pounds.	Builds muscle strength
IV	Do one set of 20 repetitions with the weight equal to SML, minus 20 pounds	Builds muscle endurance

Table 6-4. Rehabilitation program for first- and second-degree sprains

Step	Activity	Duration
I	Ice, elevation, and immobilization	48 hours
II	Cold whirlpool for range of motion exercises	Days 2-3
	Warm whirlpool until full range of motion attained	Days 4-5
III	Running and weight-training programs (Tables 6-2 and 6-3)	Days 7-21

cles comes within 10 percentage points of being equal, the individual has completed the weight-training program.

Summary. Muscle strains occur because the muscle-tendon unit lacks the strength, flexibility, and/or endurance to withstand the forces applied to it. The stretching, running, and weight-training programs outlined will correct these deficiencies. The individual who has completed all three programs may return to normal function or, if an athlete, to competition with a minimal risk of reinjury.

Ligament sprains

In contrast to muscle strains, ligament injuries or sprains may cause some degree of joint instability. For this reason the treatment of ligament disruptions requires a specific period of immobilization. The length of immobilization is determined by the severity of the injury. In first-and second-degree sprains the length of immobilization may be only a matter of days. With third-degree sprains the ligament is usually either surgically reconstructed or immobilized for several weeks. Although a period of immobilization is necessary for the injured or repaired ligament to heal, it is detrimental to the uninjured ligaments of the joint involved.

Noyes et al[43] have demonstrated that in monkeys an 8-week period of immobilization decreases the maximum failure load and the energy-absorption-to-failure ratio of uninjured anterior cruciate ligaments by 39% and 32%, respectively. They also found that after 20 weeks of reconditioning after immobilization the maximum failure load and energy-absorption-to-failure ratio had recovered, respectively, to only 86% and 84% of the normal range. Their results suggest that functional capacity of healing ligaments remains impaired for much longer than previously realized and evoke the question as to whether the length of time allowed for ligament healing, particularly in athletes, is long enough. In many cases athletes return to full competition before their injured ligaments have reached even 90% of normal strength.

Rehabilitation program. The basic rehabilitation program for first- and second-degree sprains is described in the following steps and is summarized in Table 6-4. Individuals with healed or repaired third-degree sprains should start the program at the warm whirlpool phase of Step II.

Step I. Immediately after the injury, and for the ensuing 48 hours, the injured joint should be elevated and immobilized. Cryotherapy is applied to the injured area five times a day for 20 minutes. As previously mentioned, radiographs should be obtained to rule out avulsion fractures and epiphyseal injuries.

Step II. After 48 hours, and for the next 2 to 3 days, the injured joint should be placed in a cold whirlpool for 20 minutes and range of motion exercises should be performed as tolerated. After 4 to 5 days, warm whirlpool treatment is initiated and continued until full range of motion is achieved.

Step III. When the client (1) has achieved a full range of motion, (2) has minimal swelling, and (3) can bear full weight and jump up and down on the injured extremity without pain, a running and weight-training program, as described previously, is instituted. If an individual, particularly an athlete, completes these programs, he/she is able to return to full competition.

The following sections of this chapter deal with the diagnosis and treatment of specific ligament and/or muscle-tendon–unit injuries.

Contusions

Contusions most commonly occur in the biceps muscle of the arm and the quadriceps muscle of the thigh. They are produced by a direct blow to the muscle, causing localized bleeding and edema but not resulting in complete disruption or total loss of function of the involved muscle. Quadriceps muscle contusions are most commonly caused by direct blows from either an athletic opponent's headgear or knee or from an individual striking his/her thigh against a fixed object. The individual may not appreciate the severity of the injury until the next day when knee motion is restricted and the quadriceps muscle is sore and swollen.

Quadriceps muscle contusions are graded as mild, moderate, and severe. Because it takes at least 24 hours for these injuries to stabilize, the severity of the injury is determined from clinical findings after 48 hours. Mild contusions are characterized by local tenderness, at least 90 degrees of knee motion, and no alterations in gait. The person can perform a deep kneebend test. Moderate contusions cause diffuse swelling and tenderness of the muscle mass, permit only 45 to 90 degrees of knee motion (Fig. 6-17), and alter one's gait. The person cannot perform a deep kneebend and experiences severe pain while climbing stairs or rising from a sitting position. Severe contusions produce such marked tenderness and swelling that the contour of the muscle is difficult to define. Also knee motion is restricted to less than 45 degrees, and a severe limp develops.

Treatment. Moderate and severe contusions are treated in three phases. During the first phase the goal is to minimize the interstitial bleeding. This is accomplished by applying ice and a compressive wrap to the affected area and by immobilizing and elevating the injured extremity.

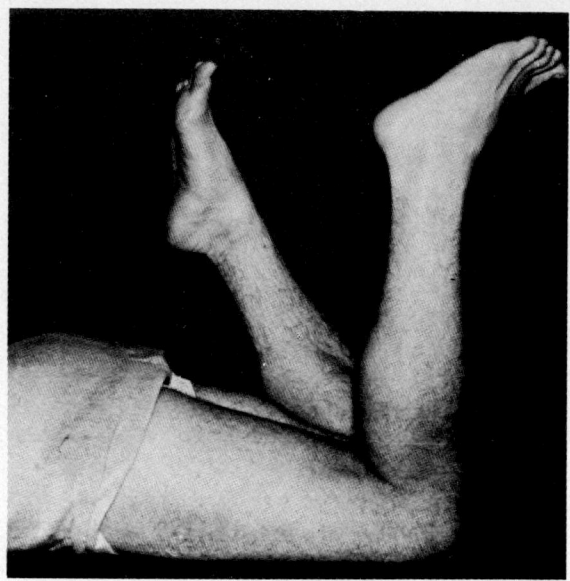

Fig. 6-17. Quadriceps contusions. Active knee motion is measured in the manner shown 48 hours after contusion occurred to determine severity of injury.

This phase of treatment usually lasts 24 hours for mild contusions and 48 hours or more for moderate to severe contusions. During this phase of treatment isometric quadriceps muscle exercises are permitted, but massage, heat, and range of motion exercises are not recommended.

After the swelling has stabilized and the person has regained quadriceps muscle control, range of motion exercises of phase two are initiated. The goals of this phase of treatment are first to gain full extension of the muscle and then slowly to restore flexion. Active flexion and extension exercises are started in the prone position (Fig. 6-17), and the rate of progress is determined by the pain experienced by the individual. During this phase of treatment crutch ambulation with touch-weight bearing is permitted. If swelling recurs, the person is immediately returned to phase one of the treatment program. Phase two is completed when there are at least 90 degrees of knee motion and the individual has a normal gait.

In the final phase of treatment progressive resistance exercises are performed until there is full motion and strength. During this phase the person is required to complete the running and weight training program outlined previously. When full motion, strength, and agility have been restored, the individual, if an athlete, can return to full competition.

The variable outcomes for clients with contusion injuries have been determined by Jackson and Feagin.[27] During a 9-month period they diagnosed and treated 65 quadriceps muscle contusions in 65 male military academy cadets. They found that the average time of disability for the 47 cadets with mild contusions was 6½ days, while the average time for the 7 with moderate and the 11 with severe

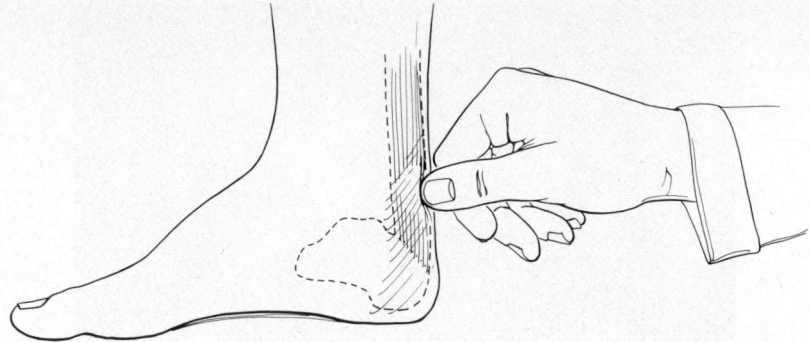

Fig. 6-18. With acute Achilles tendonitis, there is tenderness to palpation over a 1-inch area, 1 to 2 inches above proximal tip of calcaneal bone.

contusions was 56 and 72 days, respectively. They also found that 13 of the 18 cadets with moderate or severe injuries developed heterotopic bone formation (myositis ossificans) in the injured quadriceps muscles within 2 to 4 weeks of the injury. However, all 13 returned to athletic competition in an average of 73 days, none required surgery, and their return was not dependent on resorption of the heterotopic bone. Lipscomb, Thomas, and Johnson[34] reported similar results in treating this injury. However, they found it necessary to operatively excise the heterotopic bone in four individuals who were seen 5 to 7 months after the contusion. They had limited motion and persistent pain. All four returned to athletics after surgery.[34]

Summary. Improperly treated quadriceps contusions can severely disable a person. To properly treat these injuries, prevent reinjury, and shorten the period of disability, one must (1) recognize and accurately classify these injuries, (2) admit individuals with severe contusions to a hospital for phase I of treatment, and (3) educate the injured persons regarding the severity of the injury and temper their enthusiasm to return to normal function too rapidly.

Tendonitis

Although many persons participating in sports are prone to developing tendonitis, runners and other track athletes have a particularly high incidence of this injury. The most commonly affected tendon is the Achilles tendon. Brubaker and James[1] and Clancy[6] have reported that of 109 and 310 track injuries treated, respectively, 12% were tendonitis, and in 69% of these cases the Achilles tendon was involved.

The symptoms of Achilles tendonitis usually have an insidious onset. The person first notices a dull, aching pain in the Achilles tendon after running. If the individual continues running without treatment, he/she experiences pain in the Achilles tendon that is present on the initiation of running and is increased with sprinting. Eventually, the individual has pain when walking and is unable to run. These three phases of symptoms represent the acute, suba-

cute, and chronic stages of Achilles tendonitis. In the acute stage—symptoms of less than 2 weeks' duration—the pain resolves rapidly with rest. On examination, the tenderness is limited to a 1-inch area, 1 to 2 inches above the calcaneal attachment of the Achilles tendon (Fig. 6-18). The soft tissues around this area may be slightly edematous, suggesting an increased width of the injured tendon with respect to its uninjured counterpart. This stage of Achilles tendonitis is usually resolved with 2 weeks of rest, oral antiinflammatory agents, and a heel-lift. When the acute inflammation subsides, the individual is placed on an Achilles stretching program (Fig. 6-19) and is allowed to return to running when there is no localized tenderness and full flexibility has returned.

In the subacute stage—symptoms of 3 to 6 weeks' duration—the pain is more diffuse and occurs during running. The clinical symptoms are similar to those of the acute stage with the addition of crepitus noted during active dorsiflexion and plantar flexion of the ankle. Treatment is similar to that for acute tendonitis, but this stage of Achilles tendonitis requires at least 6 weeks of rest before the person can resume running.

In the chronic stage—symptoms over 6 weeks' duration—the pain is present over an even larger area and the person is unable to run effectively. On clinical examination, the tendon is found to be markedly thickened and often nodular. The treatment program outlined for the acute and subacute stages may not be effective. Clancy,[7] Fox et al[17] and Snook[50] have documented surgical findings in chronic Achilles tendonitis. The pathological changes range from thickening and microscopic disruption to partial- and full-thickness tears. Clancy concluded that surgical intervention should be considered when symptoms persist after 6 to 8 weeks of nonoperative treatment. He recommended releasing the tendon sheath, excising the scar tissue, and repairing the tears. He has performed this surgery in 22 cases of chronic Achilles tendonitis. In all but one case the clients have returned to running without symptoms.[5]

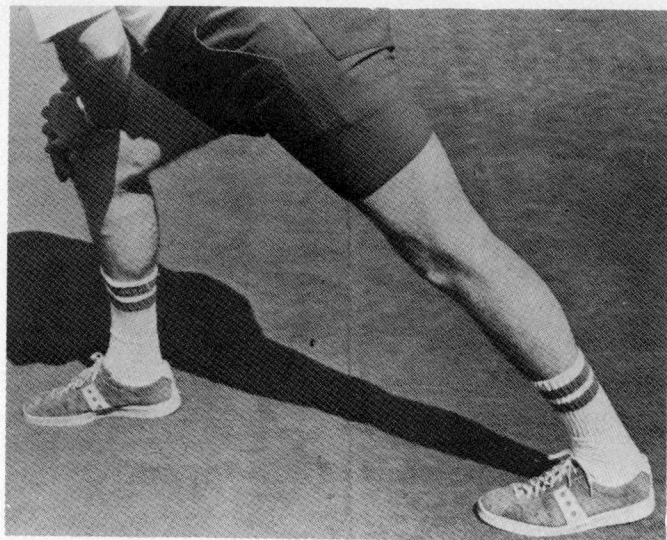

Fig. 6-19. Achilles tendon is stretched by keeping heel of side to be stretched on ground while the opposite knee is progressively flexed.

Collateral ligament injuries

The collateral ligaments of the knee and ankle are those most commonly injured by athletes. This section deals with current concepts regarding the diagnosis and treatment of medial and lateral collateral ligament injuries of the knee. However, the rationale for the clinical stress-testing used in diagnosing these injuries can be understood only if one has a basic understanding of the normal anatomical and biomechanical properties of these structures.

Medial ligamentous stabilizers of the knee. The ligaments that provide medial stability for the knee include (1) the superficial (medial) ligament, (2) the deep capsular ligaments (meniscofemoral and meniscotibial), and (3) the posterior oblique fibers. However, as Warren and Marshall[57] have demonstrated, these ligaments should be considered only as condensations within tissue planes and not as discrete structures (such as the cruciate ligaments).

The superficial tibial collateral ligament is a broad, triangular-shaped ligament that is attached proximally to the medial epicondyle of the femur and distally to the tibia as far anterior as the tibial tuberosity. The posterior fibers of the superficial ligament blend with the deep ligament and are firmly attached to the posterior horn of the medial meniscus. The deep medial ligament lies beneath the superficial tibial collateral ligament and is divided into meniscofemoral and meniscotibial components. The meniscofemoral component originates on the femur, just distal to the origin of the superficial ligament, and inserts in the midportion of the peripheral margin of the meniscus. The meniscotibial component, the coronary ligament, originates from the midportion of the peripheral margin of the meniscus and inserts on the tibia. The anterior and midmedial parts of the deep medial ligament are separated from the superficial ligament by one to three bursae. The posterior portion of the deep medial ligament, designated as the posterior oblique ligament by Hughston and Eilers,[21] blends with the superficial ligament as described previously.

The superficial medial ligament is the primary stabilizer of the medial side of the knee. Warren, Marshall, and Girgis[56] have demonstrated that the anterior portion (parallel fibers) of the superficial ligament is the primary medial stabilizer against valgus and rotatory stress from 0 to 90 degrees of flexion. Grood et al[20] found that the superficial ligament provided 57% of the total medial restraint at 5 degrees of knee flexion and 78% at 25 degrees of knee flexion. In contrast, they reported that the deep medial ligament (including the posteromedial portion) provided 25% of the total medial restraint at 5 degrees of flexion and only 8% at 25 degrees of knee flexion. In addition, they found that the combined restraint of the anterior and posterior cruciate ligaments was only 15% and 13% of the total at 5 degrees and 25 degrees of flexion, respectively.

Lateral ligamentous stabilizers of the knee. The ligaments that stabilize the lateral aspect of the knee include the (1) lateral (fibular) collateral ligament, (2) short collateral (fabellofibular) ligament, (3) lateral capsule, and (4) iliotibial tract.

The lateral (fibular) collateral ligament extends from the lateral femoral epicondyle to the fibular head. Unlike the posterior portion of the superficial medial ligament, the lateral collateral ligament has no attachments to the lateral meniscus. The short collateral ligament lies deep to the lateral collateral ligament and also extends from the femur to the fibular head. This ligament is of significant size only in individuals with a lateral fabella (8% to 16% of the population). It is then called the *fabellofibular ligament*.[29] The lateral capsule can be divided into three components. The anterior third originates from the lateral border of the patellar tendon and is reinforced by the lateral patellar retinaculum of the quadriceps tendon. The anterior portion of the capsule inserts into the articular margin of the proximal tibia and has no femoral attachment. The middle third of the capsule attaches proximally to the lateral epicondyle of the femur and distally at the articular margin of the proximal tibia. The middle third of the capsule, like the deep medial ligament, has meniscofemoral and meniscotibial components. The posterior third of the capsule has femoral, meniscal, and tibial attachments that are similar to the middle third, but it also has an area of condensed and thickened fibers, which is called the *arcuate ligament*. This ligament reinforces the posterolateral corner of the knee. The femoral-tibial portion of the iliotibial tract supplies static support and reinforces the middle third of the capsule. The tract inserts proximally into the lateral femoral epicondyle and distally into Gerdy's (lateral tibial) tubercle.

The lateral (fibular) collateral ligament is the primary lateral restraint to varus forces. Grood et al[20] have demonstrated that the lateral collateral ligament provided 55% of the total lateral restraint at 5 degrees of knee flexion and 69% at 25 degrees of flexion. The anterior and midlateral capsule provided only 4.1% and 3.7% of the restraint at 5 degrees and 25 degrees of flexion, respectively. The values for the posterior third of the capsule at the same degrees of flexion were 13% and 5%, respectively. The combined restraint of the anterior and posterior cruciate ligaments was 22% at 5 degrees of flexion and 12% at 25 degrees of flexion.

Medial and lateral ligament injuries. Medial collateral ligament injuries occur when there is an excessive *external* rotatory and/or abduction force applied to the flexed, weight-bearing knee. Lateral collateral ligament injuries are caused by excessive *internal* rotatory and/or abduction forces. In the case of a medial collateral ligament injury, the individual has pain to palpation over the medial epicondyle of the femur, the middle third of the medial joint line, and/or the tibial insertion of the ligament beneath the pes tendons. With lateral collateral injuries, the pain is localized to the fibular head or lateral femoral epicondyle. With first- or second-degree sprains, an athlete is usually able to walk off the field unaided. The amount of swelling and pain that ensues usually varies with the severity of the injury. In third-degree sprains the complete disruption of the capsule and ligaments allows the fluid and blood to run out of the joint and thus lessens the swelling and the pain. With medial collateral injuries the athlete may be unable to fully extend the knee. This represents "pseudo-locking" of the knee since the block is not caused by a displaced meniscus but occurs because the medial collateral ligament is put on greatest stretch in the last 10

to 15 degrees of extension. Thus fully extending the knee greatly increases the individual's pain. If the blocking is not a result of a meniscal lesion, full extension can often be obtained by injecting the femoral attachment of the medial collateral ligament with 1% solution of lidocaine (Xylocaine).

The severity of medial and lateral collateral ligament injuries is best determined by performing adduction and abduction stress tests, respectively. These tests should first be performed on the uninjured knee to establish the individual's normal physiological laxity. The abduction stress test is performed with the individual supine (Fig. 6-20). The extremity to be examined is abducted at the hip so that the thigh rests on the examining table and the quadriceps and hamstring muscles are relaxed. The knee is then flexed to 30 degrees over the side of the table as the leg is grasped with one hand about the lateral aspect of the knee and one hand on the foot or ankle. Abduction stress is then slowly and gently applied to the knee up to the point of pain. If the test is performed in this manner, the examiner will be able to accurately document the amount of instability. The adduction stress test is performed with the individual in the same position, but one hand is placed around the medial aspect of the knee and adduction stress is applied. These tests will not accurately evaluate the integrity of the medial or lateral collateral ligament if they are performed with the knee in full extension because the cruciate ligaments and the medial and lateral capsular structures provide 43% and 45% of the medial and lateral restraint, respectively, to straight varus and valgus testing.[20]

There is one interesting situation that occurs with lateral collateral ligament injuries. On occasion, the meniscotibial portion of the midlateral capsule will be avulsed from the tibia with part of the tibial bony attachment included. The fragment varies in size from a faint fleck to several millimeters in size and is evident on a routine anteroposterior radiograph (Fig. 6-21). This radiographic finding, which has been called the "lateral capsule sign,"[58] has great clinical significance because it not only indicates that there has been a severe lateral capsular injury, but it is usually associated with a third-degree anterior cruciate ligament injury and varying degrees of medial collateral ligament injury.

Treatment. When the abduction or adduction stress-testing reveals that the athlete has sustained a first- or second-degree collateral ligament disruption, the injury is treated nonoperatively. Third-degree sprains can also successfully be treated nonoperatively if there is no anterior cruciate injury.[24] It has been the experience of many therapists that operative treatment of second-degree and third-degree collateral ligament injuries will not improve stability. The laxity associated with second-degree and third-degree injuries is not altered by surgical attempts at tightening the ligament. Therefore recommended treatment of first-, second-, and third-degree medial and lateral collateral ligament injuries involves a three-phase therapy pro-

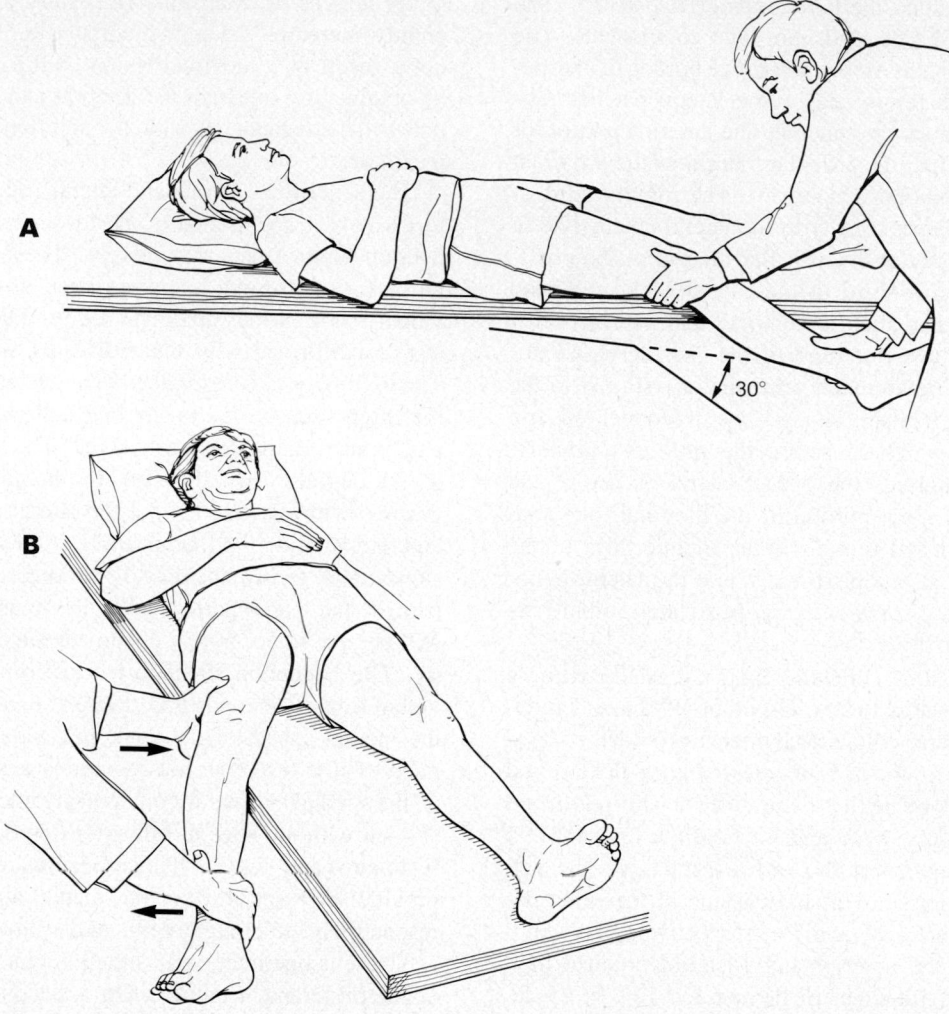

Fig. 6-20. A, Abduction stress-testing of knee. **B,** Abduction stress is slowly and gently applied. (Details of test are explained in text.)

gram. (Surgically treated third-degree injuries begin the program at the warm whirlpool stage of Phase II.)

PHASE I (days 1 to 3)

1. Crutch ambulation with touch-weight bearing
2. Compression dressing around the knee
3. Ice applied three or four times per day for 10-minute periods
4. Quadriceps sets—three sets of 20 repetitions, three times per day
5. Straight-leg lifts—three sets of 20 repetitions, three times per day
6. Knee immobilizer worn at night

PHASE II (days 4 to 7)

1. Continue quadriceps sets
2. Whirlpool for range of motion exercises (bike-riding motion); cold water for first 3 to 4 days, then warm water

3. Swimming (as an alternative to whirlpool, if available), 30 to 45 minutes, flutter kick only, trying to bend the knee
4. Weight-lifting program consisting of straight-leg raises done with maximum weight that can be raised 12 times. Three sets of 12 repetitions in hip extension, hip flexion, and hip abduction. Knee must be kept fully extended and no hip adduction strengthening should be attempted at this time
5. Crutch ambulation with knee immobilizer worn at night

PHASE III (days 8 to 14, 90 degrees of knee flexion obtained)

1. Continue quadriceps sets
2. Continue whirlpool and swimming for range of motion exercises
3. Exercise bike for 15 minutes at 60 rpm
4. Cybex or Orthotron machine—speed 5, three sets of

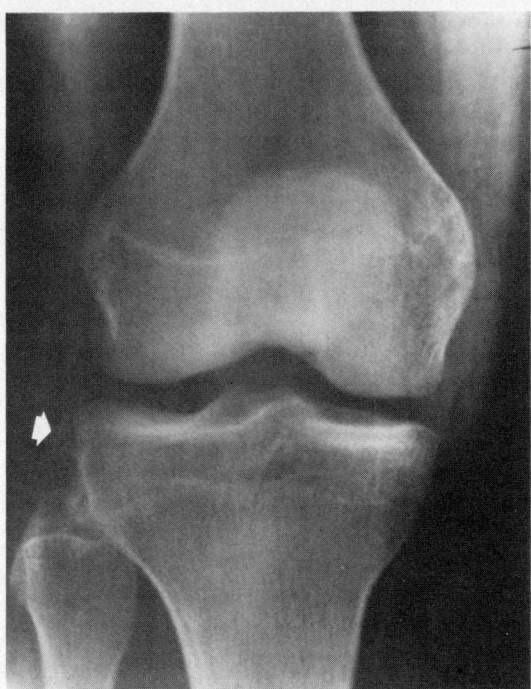

Fig. 6-21. "Lateral capsular sign." This anteroposterior radiograph demonstrates avulsion of bony attachment *(arrow)* of meniscotibial portion of lateral capsule. (Significance of this sign is explained in text.)

10 repetitions. Universal or Nautilus weights—three sets of 12 repetitions with maximum weight for both quadriceps and hamstrings

PHASE IV (day 14 to completion, if full flexion and extension present)

1. Whirlpool warm-up
2. Exercise bike for 15 minutes at 60 rpm
3. Orthotron machine—three sets of 10 repetitions at speed 3, three sets of 10 repetitions at speed 5, then (when equal to opposite side), three sets of 10 repetitions at speed 7. Universal or Nautilus weights—three sets of 12 repetitions with maximum weight for quadriceps and hamstrings
4. Start running program (see Table 6-2, page 151)

The athlete may return to competition when (1) no local tenderness is apparent (2) full range of motion has been restored, (3) quadriceps and hamstring muscle strength are within 90% of the normal leg, and (4) the running program has been completed.

Intraarticular ligament injuries

The most commonly injured intraarticular ligaments of the musculoskeletal system are the anterior and posterior cruciate ligaments of the knee.

Anatomy. The anterior and posterior cruciate ligaments are strong, rounded connective tissue cords located within the knee joint capsule between the femoral condyles but lie outside the synovial cavity of the joint. They are positioned between the medial and lateral synovial compartments and behind the posterior wall of the anterior synovial cavity.

The detailed anatomy of the cruciate ligaments has been documented by Girgis, Marshall, and Monajem.[19] The anterior cruciate ligament arises from a depression on a 30 mm long nonarticular area of the tibia, anterior to the intercondylar eminence. Its origin blends into the anterior attachment of the lateral meniscus. The ligament passes posteriorly and laterally to insert on the posterior nonarticular aspect of the medial surface of the lateral femoral condyle. The posterior cruciate ligament arises from a 13 mm wide depression behind the posterior articular surface of the tibia and is attached to the posterior horn of the lateral meniscus. The ligament passes anteriorly and medially to insert on the posterior aspect of the lateral surface of the medial femoral condyle. These ligaments cross each other between their femoral and tibial attachments and, thus, are called *cruciates*. They are also named for their tibial attachments. The average length of the anterior and posterior cruciate ligaments is 3.8 cm.

Girgis, Marshall, and Monajem[19] and Kennedy, Weinberg, and Wilson[33] have demonstrated that, except for the anterior medial portion, the majority of the fibers of the anterior cruciate are loose in flexion. In extension, however, all the fibers are under tension. The majority of the fibers of the posterior cruciate are taut in flexion except for the posterior portion. In extension, the posterior fibers are taut, but the majority of other fibers are lax. This variation in tension of the various parts of these ligaments may occur because they are multifascicular structures. The individual fasciculi are either directed in spiral fashion around the long axis of the ligament or pass directly from their femoral to tibial attachments. The major blood supply to the anterior and posterior cruciate ligaments comes from branches of the middle genicular artery.

The biomechanical functions of the cruciate ligaments have been best documented by Butler, Noyes, and Grood.[2] They found that the anterior cruciate ligament was the primary restraint to straight anterior stress placed upon the knee joint. The ligament provided 85% and 87% of the total restraint at 90 degrees and 30 degrees of flexion, respectively. The posterior cruciate ligament was the primary restraint to straight posterior forces placed on the knee joint. The posterior cruciate ligament provided 94% of the total restraint at 90 degrees and 30 degrees of flexion.

Anterior cruciate ligament injuries. Anterior cruciate ligament injuries are caused by a variety of mechanisms. These include (1) external rotation, abduction, and straight anterior forces applied to the tibia, (2) internal rotation of the femur on the tibia, and (3) hyperextension of the knee. Injuries most commonly occur in noncontact situations.[44]

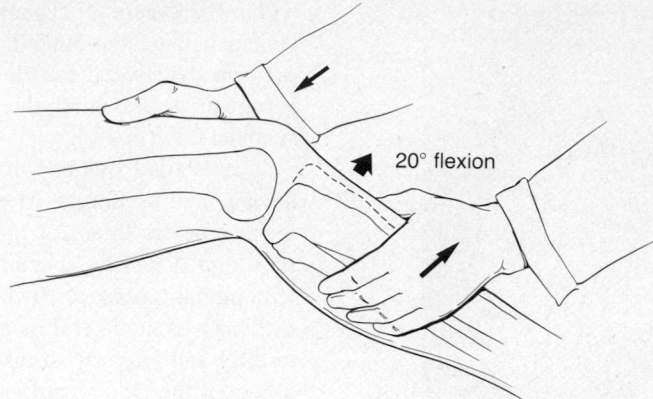

20° flexion

Fig. 6-22. Lachman's test shows position of examiner and examiner's hands with knee in 15 to 20 degrees of flexion. Anterior stress is applied to tibia. If test is positive, tibia will slide forward on femur and examiner will experience no, or a "mushy," end-feel. (Details of test are explained in text.)

Diagnosis. Regardless of the mechanism of injury, the athlete is usually (85% of the time) unable to continue competing and will experience immediate swelling of the knee, posterolateral knee pain, and varying degrees of knee instability. The effusion becomes tense within 24 hours and "pseudo-locking" (as described previously) occurs. Presence of a tense bloody effusion (hemarthrosis) (see Fig. 6-4) and a positive response to Lachman's test (Fig. 6-22) are the keys to diagnosing acute injuries. De-Haven[11] and Noyes et al.[44] have arthroscopically evaluated athletes with a hemarthrosis from an acute knee injury. They found partial or complete anterior cruciate tears in 72% of such cases, two thirds of which also had associated meniscal lesions. DeHaven also documented solitary meniscus tears in 15%, osteochondral fractures in 6%, posterior cruciate tears in 3%, and no demonstrable lesion in 4%. In arthroscopically evaluating over 100 athletes with hemarthrosis, I have observed similar findings and percentages.

On clinical examination, the knee with an anterior cruciate disruption has a tense effusion. Stress-testing of the knee, with adequate muscle relaxation, reveals a positive response to Lachman's test but only occasionally produces a positive anterior drawer test.

Lachman's test, as described by Torg, Conrad, and Kalen,[54] is performed in the following manner (Fig. 6-22). The client lies on the examining table or surface. The examiner stands to the outside of the knee to be examined. One of the examiner's hands firmly grasps the thigh just proximal to the patella. The other hand firmly grasps the leg at the level of the tibial tubercle. After the knee is gently flexed 20 degrees, the examiner pulls the tibia forward on the femur. The test is positive when the tibia can be subluxated forward with no, or a "mushy," end-feel. The examination of the injured knee must be compared to the uninjured knee, and the hamstrings must be relaxed. When

the uninjured knee is tested, the examiner should experience a solid end-feel as the tibia is pulled forward. If the hamstrings of the injured knee are adequately relaxed, the test will accurately (100%) document third-degree tears of the anterior cruciate ligament.[11,54]

However, the anterior drawer test is often negative with acute injuries because of a ball-valve action of the menisci, hamstring spasm, or a hemarthrosis.[54] The anterior drawer test is positive only when other ligamentous structures are acutely disrupted or when these secondary restraints become lengthened, as seen weeks to months after an anterior cruciate ligament injury.

Standard radiographs of the acutely injured knee usually only demonstrate hemarthrosis. This is because the great majority of the anterior cruciate ligament tears occur within the substance of the ligament not at their bony attachments. Kennedy and Fowler[32] reported that 72% of 50 clients with anterior cruciate disruptions documented by arthrotomies had midsubstance tears. Noyes, Delucas, and Torvik[42] concluded from primate studies that the high strain rates experienced with athletic trauma should cause midsubstance tears. They found that lower strain rates produced tibial and, to a much lesser extent, femoral bony avulsions.

These findings reflect my experience with this injury. Often clients are evaluated in an emergency room, and, when radiographs are negative, they are told that they have a "sprained knee." The diagnosis is partially accurate in that they often have a sprain of their anterior cruciate ligament. However, the initial instability caused by this injury deserves further investigation and, more importantly, proper treatment.

The individual with an acute third-degree anterior cruciate injury should be examined to determine if there is also anterolateral rotatory instability. This is important because McDevitt and Muur[39] and Marshall and Olsen[36] have demonstrated in dogs and Slocum et al[48] and Jacobsen[28] have shown in humans that anterior cruciate insufficiency and anterolateral rotatory instability of the knee is associated with the development of degenerative arthritis.

There are many diagnostic tests for detecting anterolateral rotatory instability.* These tests include (1) the pivot-shift, (2) the jerk, (3) flexion-rotation drawer, and (4) Losee. I prefer the pivot-shift test as described by Galway, Beaupre, and MacIntosh.[18] The pivot-shift test is performed in the following manner (Fig. 6-23). The client lies supine on the examining table with the knee in full extension. The tibia of the affected knee is grasped at the level of the tibial tubercle by the examiner's right or left hand. (The right hand should grasp the tibia in this location to examine the left knee, and the left hand should grasp the tibia in this position if the right knee is being examined.) The opposite hand grasps the ipsilateral ankle and applies maximal internal rotation (Fig. 6-23, *A*). The knee is then flexed as the proximal hand applies a valgus stress to the knee (Fig. 6-23, *B*). During this maneuver the examiner will feel and the client will experience a sudden shift (jerk) of the tibia on the femur if the test is positive. The validity of this test for anterior cruciate and anterolateral rotatory instability has been confirmed by Fetto and Marshall.[16] They found that sectioning of the anterior cruciate produced a positive pivot-shift sign in 33 of 37 cadaver knees. However, they also observed that excessive physiological soft tissue laxity may cause a false-positive result.

Treatment. When the diagnosis of a third-degree anterior cruciate ligament injury has been confirmed, there are several avenues of treatment. First, one should ascertain if there is an associated meniscal injury. A single-contrast arthrogram is usually obtained for this purpose. Second, one should determine what degree of anterolateral rotatory instability has occurred. This is accomplished by performing one or more of the tests listed above. If muscle spasm or a loss of knee motion occurs, the examination should be performed with the patient under general or spinal anesthesia. If the client is anesthetized for the examination, the joint should be arthroscopically evaluated to assess, particularly, the lateral meniscus because it is not well evaluated by an arthrogram. Also, the arthroscopic examination should determine whether the torn cruciate is blocking knee motion. It has been my experience and that of others[40] that the torn cruciate can become lodged under the medial or lateral femoral condyles and block knee extension. If this is the case, the offending portion of the ligament is resected via the arthroscope.

If it is determined that there is only minor or moderate (1+ or 2+) anterolateral rotatory instability, the knee is immobilized for several days and subsequently rehabilitated with the programs outlined previously. It has been my experience that individuals with minimal clinical and

*See references 2, 18, 35, 45, and 47.

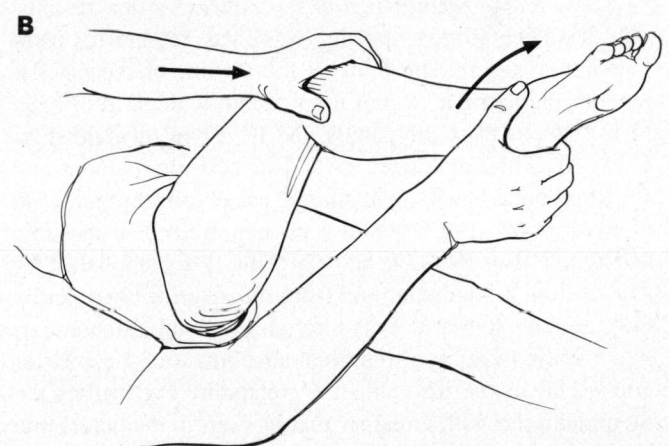

Fig. 6-23. Pivot-shift test performed on right knee. **A,** With knee in full extension, examiner's left hand grasps tibia at level of tibial tubercle and applies a valgus stress. Then examiner's right hand grasps and maximally internally rotates ankle or foot. This subluxates tibia anteriorly. **B,** Right hand then slowly flexes knee. If test is positive, examiner and client will note a sudden posterior "shift" of tibia on femur. (Details of test are explained in text.)

functional instability do very well if they complete the rehabilitation program and maintain quadriceps and hamstring strength equal to or greater than their uninjured extremity. Also these individuals are usually fitted for a derotation brace to be used for sporting activities.

If the stress-testing demonstrates gross (3+) anterolateral rotatory instability in the acute situation or if the individual develops gross instability subsequently, an anterior cruciate ligament reconstruction is recommended. In acute injuries midsubstance tears should also be reconstructed because the results of primary repair have been quite discouraging. Feagin and Curl[15] found that fewer than 10% of 32 clients had an asymptomatic stable knee 5 years after a primary repair. Many surgical procedures for correcting anterior cruciate ligament insufficiency have been proposed. However, these procedures can be classified as either extraarticular,[13,18,35] intraarticular,[4,14,26,46] or both.[9,37] A procedure that includes an intraarticular reconstruction of the ligament is preferred. The intraarticular reconstruction is performed in acute and chronic cases and is accomplished by substituting part of the patellar ligament with its bony attachments for the anterior cruciate ligament. It is my experience and that of others[3] that there are several advantages to using part of the patellar tendon as the substitute: (1) it is the strongest of the biological substitutes proposed to date, (2) it has been shown to revascularize and attain sufficient tensile strength,[8] and (3) its use does not require sacrificing other significant structures that are important to knee-joint function. Anterior cruciate reconstruction is described in the following section (Figs. 6-24 and 6-25).

Arthroscopic reconstruction procedures. After the knee joint has been arthroscopically examined, the graft is fashioned from the middle third (9 to 10 mm) of the patellar tendon, including a 25 mm long, 9 mm wide strip of bone (4 mm deep) from the patella and the tibial tubercle (Fig. 6-24, *A*). Three holes are drilled in both the patellar and the tibial bone blocks, and sutures are placed through each of these holes. Bony tunnels are then created in the tibia and femur (Fig. 6-24, *B* and *C*). This is accomplished by first drilling a Steinmann pin from the anterior tibial cortex into the joint so that it exits through the tibial articular cartilage at the location of the tibial attachment of the anterior cruciate ligament. The tunnel is created by overdrilling the Steinmann pin with a reamer that is 1 cm in diameter. In a similar manner a tunnel is created in the lateral femoral condyle (Fig. 6-24, *C*). The intraarticular portion of this tunnel is appropriately located at the femoral attachment of the anterior cruciate ligament. The tunnel exit is located extraarticularly on the lateral aspect of the lateral femoral condyle. The bone blocks of the graft are then passed into the tibial and the femoral tunnels, and the graft is put under maximal tension as the sutures are tied over unicortical cancellous screws (Fig. 6-25).

Postoperative care. After surgery the extremity is placed in a knee immobilizer, which is kept on for 3 weeks. During this time the client ambulates with crutches, bearing partial weight and is instructed to perform active range of motion exercises on a daily basis. Three weeks from the date of surgery, the client is instructed to progress to full weight bearing. At 6 weeks the knee immobilizer is removed, and the client may bear full weight on the extremity as tolerated and may discard the crutches if secure without them. Immediately after surgery the client is allowed and encouraged to remove the knee immobilizer each day and to begin range of motion exer-

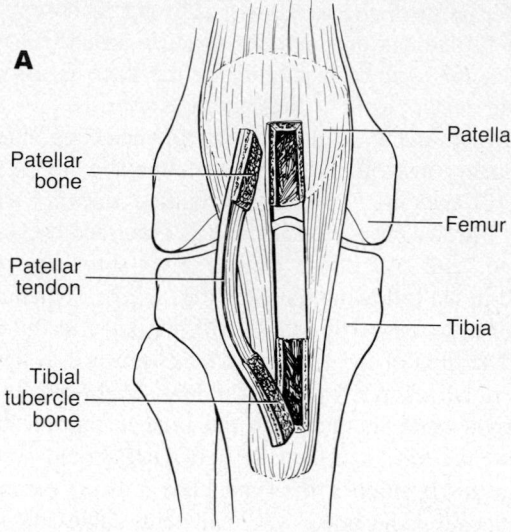

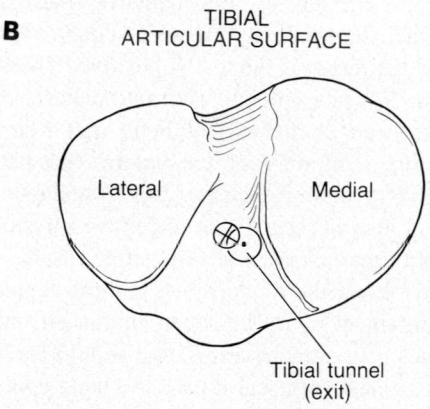

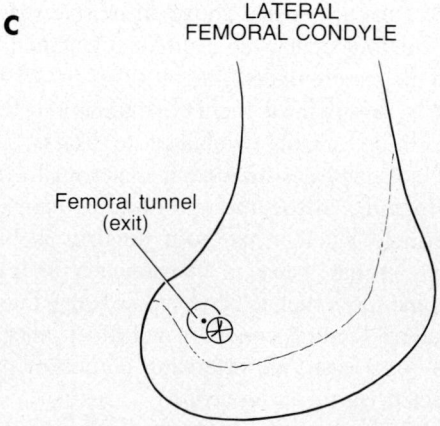

Fig. 6-24. Anterior cruciate ligament reconstruction. **A,** Harvesting of patellar bone, patellar tendon, tibial bone graft. Intraarticular location of the tibial, **B,** and femoral, **C,** tunnels. (Details of procedure are explained in text.)

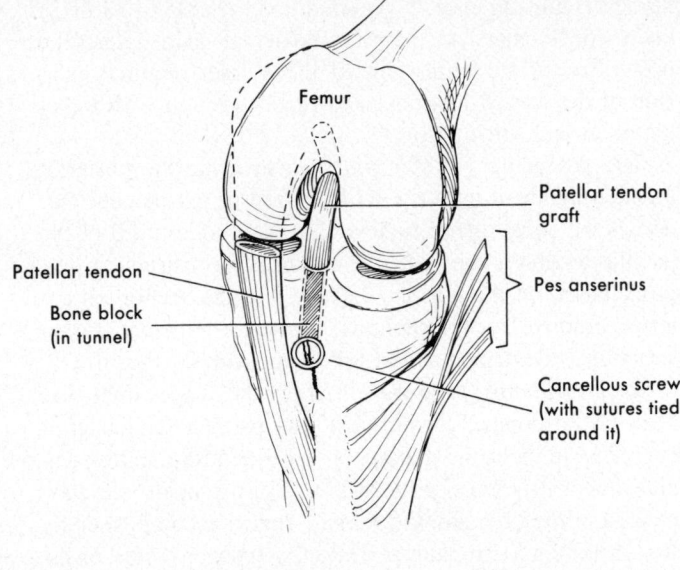

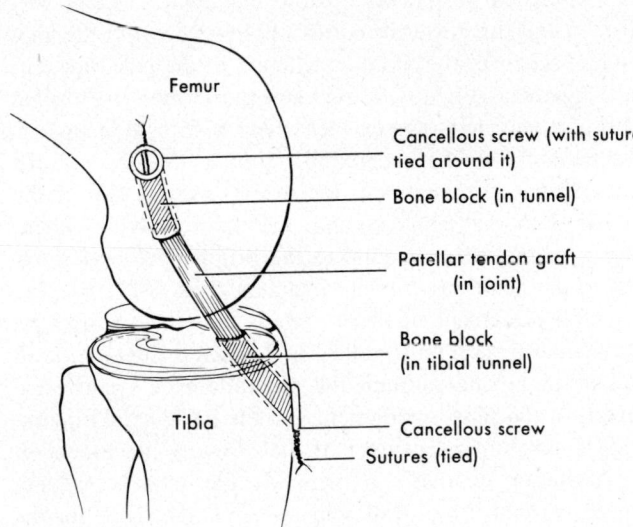

Fig. 6-25. Anterior cruciate ligament graft passed through bony tunnels and positioned within knee joint. Graft is put under tension and secured by tying sutures from bone blocks around cancellous screws.

cises. The swimming or whirlpool program as outlined previously is initiated 3 to 6 weeks after surgery and should be maintained for the next 2 to 3 months.

During the first 4 months after surgery the client is placed on quadriceps sets and straight-leg lifts for strengthening the hip extensors, flexors, and abductors. Nine weeks after surgery he/she is encouraged to do the straight-leg lifts (three sets of 10 repetitions, two to three times per day) with the maximum amount of weight tolerated.

Four months after surgery the client starts the progressive resistance exercise or weight programs outlined previously. This is continued until the individual regains full

strength. At 6 months the client is placed on a rope-jumping program and is instructed to jump rope 2 minutes per day the first week, 5 minutes per day the second, and 10 to 15 minutes per day the third and fourth weeks. At this point the client may start the running program, which requires jogging ½ to 1 mile every third day and jumping rope the 2 days in between. Four weeks into the running program the patient should be jogging every other day.

If at 6 months the client is not steadily increasing range of motion and does not have 90-degree flexion or lacks 10- to 15-degrees extension, a knee manipulation under anesthesia is recommended. At this time arthroscopic excision of intraarticular scar tissue may also be necessary. Athletes are not allowed to participate in contact sports until at least 9 months after such surgery.

I have performed 250 anterior cruciate reconstructions over the last 7 years. In 1982 Clancy et al[9] reported results from 50 clients that had been followed for at least 2 years. None of these clients had experienced episodes of instability with activities of daily living or with recreational activities. Six clients had returned to highly competitive intercollegiate or international sports. Six individuals considered the healed knee to be normal, 42 felt it was improved, and two thought the knee was worse. There were 30 (60%) excellent, 17 (34%) good, 1 (2%) fair, and 2 (4%) poor results. The procedure proved to be very effective in providing functional stability for the unstable anterior cruciate-deficient knee.

Posterior cruciate ligament injuries. The majority of posterior cruciate injuries are caused by one of two mechanisms: (1) the individual either falls on his/her knee with the ankle in forced plantar flexion, or (2) the individual is struck on the anterior aspect of the tibia and the tibia is forced posteriorly. Regardless of the mechanism of injury, an athlete with an acute injury usually is able to continue competition and may experience only minimal swelling, some posterior knee pain, and varying degrees of knee instability. The effusion does not become tense within the first 24 hours, and the individual does not experience the "pseudo-locking" that is associated with anterior cruciate ligament tears, but there is marked posterior pain. Individuals with chronic posterior cruciate insufficiency often complain of instability and disability with activities of daily living.

Diagnosis. In the acute and chronic posterior cruciate injuries, the clinical examination is diagnostic. Individuals with acute injuries have (1) a very mild bloody effusion but definite posterior pain, (2) a posterior subluxation of the involved tibia, seen best from the side with the knee flexed to 90 degrees (Fig. 6-26), (3) loss of the normal anteromedial and anterolateral prominence of the tibial plateau, beneath the femoral condyles, determined by palpation with the knee at 90 degrees of flexion, (4) a 2+ posterior drawer sign with the tibia in neutral and external rotation, and (5) a negative Lachman's test. Individuals with

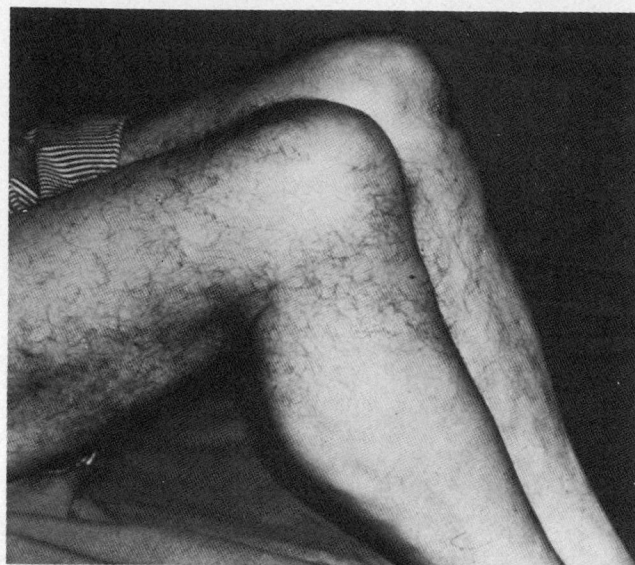

Fig. 6-26. Posterior cruciate ligament insufficiency. With third-degree posterior cruciate ligament injuries, there will be posterior sag of involved tibia on femur. This is best assessed by viewing client's knees from side with both knees in 90-degree flexion.

chronic injuries usually do not have an effusion but have greater posterior subluxation and laxity with stress-testing. The examiner must pay close attention to detail when performing the posterior drawer test. With the knee flexed to 90 degrees, the tibia of the knee with a posterior cruciate ligament injury will usually sag posteriorly. However, if the examiner does not recognize this subluxation, the anterior drawer test may be falsely interpreted as positive as the tibia is pulled forward and reduced. This mistake can be avoided if one observes the relationship of the tibia and femur from the side and documents the absence of the normal anterior tibial prominence before the stress-testing is performed.

Standard lateral radiographs of the acutely injured knee may demonstrate the posterior subluxation of the tibia on the femur if they are taken with the knee in 90 degrees of flexion. An arthrogram will also display this posterior sag, particularly if a posterior stress is applied to the tibia when the lateral views are obtained. The posterior cruciate, like the anterior cruciate, usually sustains an interstitial tear. Therefore standard radiographs rarely display an avulsion of one or the other of its bony attachments.

Treatment. When operative treatment of a third-degree posterior cruciate ligament injury is performed, a reconstruction, not a repair, is recommended. This recommendation is based on my experience and that of others.[9,31] In 1980 Kennedy[31] reported on 57 clients who had been treated nonoperatively for third-degree tears of their posterior cruciate ligament. Twenty-five of these 57 clients (44%) had developed degenerative changes in the knee joint within an average of 61 months from the injury. Al-

though Hughston et al.[23] reported good results in 13 of 20 knees (65%) that had primary repairs of acute interstitial posterior cruciate tears, nine of these cases required excision of the frayed ligament and reconstruction with a medial meniscal substitution.

The procedure I prefer for reconstructing the posterior cruciate ligament uses the middle third of the patellar tendon as the substitute. I believe that the middle third of the patellar tendon is the best substitute for reconstruction purposes based on the reasons discussed in the section on anterior cruciate reconstructions. Posterior cruciate reconstruction is described in the following section (Fig. 6-27).

Reconstruction procedure. After the knee joint has been arthroscopically examined, the patellar tendon graft is created in the same manner as described for anterior cruciate reconstructions (Fig. 6-24). Bony tunnels are then created in the tibia and the femur. This is accomplished by first drilling a Steinmann pin into the anterior cortex of the tibia just distal to the medial tibial tubercle. The pin is then advanced posteriorly, below the tibial articular surface, to exit the posterior cortex slightly lateral to the anatomical center of the tibial attachment of the posterior cruciate ligament (Fig. 6-27, *A*). The pin is then overdrilled with a cannulated reamer measuring 9 mm in diameter. The femoral tunnel is created in a similar manner, with the intraarticular portion being located at the junction of the medial femoral condyle and the intercondylar notch, slightly anterior and medial to the original femoral insertion of the posterior cruciate ligament (Fig. 6-27, *B*). The eccentric placement of these tunnels is necessary because the patellar tendon graft is flat, and, when under tension, it will lie along the supramedial circumference (anatomical center) of the tibial attachment and the infralateral circumference (anatomical center) of the femoral attachment of the posterior cruciate ligament. If the tunnels are not placed correctly, the graft will fail as a substitute for the posterior cruciate ligament.

The bone blocks, tendon graft, and sutures are then passed through the tibia and femur and put under tension as described for the anterior cruciate ligament (Fig. 6-28, *A* and *B*).

Postoperative care. After surgery the extremity is placed in a knee immobilizer with the knee in full extension. Full extension puts the graft under the least tension while it is being vascularized and consolidated. The remainder of the postoperative care and rehabilitation program is as described for the anterior cruciate ligament repair.

I have performed 25 posterior cruciate reconstructions over the last 4 years, and Clancy et al[10] reported on the results of 20 clients, 11 with acute and 9 with chronic instability, who were followed for at least 2 years. The 11 clients with acute instability had clinical findings similar to the posterior cruciate ligament injury described previously and all had at least a 2+ on the posterior drawer test. Post-

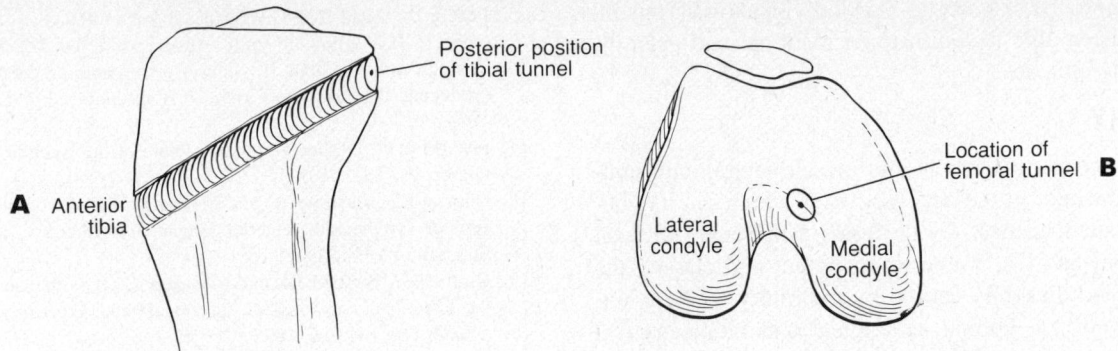

Fig. 6-27. A, Tibial tunnel created for posterior cruciate ligament reconstruction. **B,** Intraarticular location of femoral tunnel.

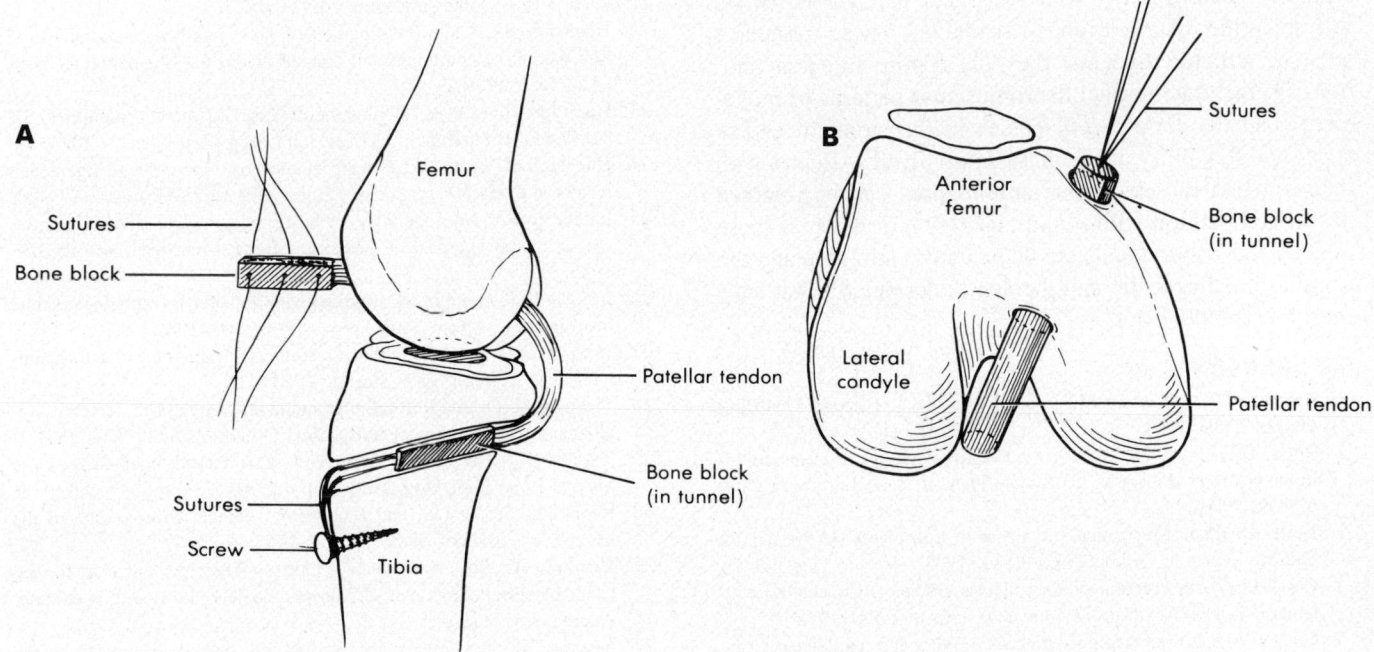

Fig. 6-28. Posterior cruciate ligament substitute has been passed through tibia (**A**) and femur (**B**). Tension is placed on graft by tying sutures over buttons. (Details of procedure are described in text.)

operatively, none exhibited posterior sag or loss of the tibial plateau step-off that they had preoperatively. Four clients had 0, four clients had a trace, and three clients had a 1+ result on the posterior drawer test. All returned to their previous level of athletic activity, including three who returned to intercollegiate football and one who returned to professional baseball. The results were similar for the nine clients with chronic instability.

Summary. The anterior and posterior cruciate ligaments of the knee are the most commonly injured intraarticular ligaments. The anterior cruciate ligament is the primary restraint against abnormal anterior displacement of the tibia on the femur. The clinical history (immediate, tense, bloody effusion) and positive results on clinical stress tests (Lachman's, pivot-shift) are usually diagnostic. If the results of a clinical examination are not conclusive, the client's knee should be examined under general anesthesia and should also be arthroscopically evaluated. Anterior cruciate ligament reconstructions with a patellar-tendon, bone-block graft have been very successful.

The posterior cruciate ligament is the primary restraint against abnormal posterior displacement of the tibia on the femur. Clinically, individuals with this injury will have a mild effusion, 2+ to 3+ result on a posterior drawer test, and posterior subluxation (loss of the normal tibial plateau prominence) of the tibia. The clinical examination is diagnostic. Posterior cruciate reconstructions with a patellar-tendon, bone-block graft have either eliminated the instability or improved stability so that individuals with this injury have been able to return to recreational and even intercollegiate athletics.

SUMMARY

The diagnosis of ligament and muscle-tendon-unit injuries is predicated on the accuracy with which one (1) obtains a detailed history, (2) performs a thorough physical examination, and (3) is able to document and classify the instability and disability caused by the injury. A basic understanding of the normal anatomical and biomechanical properties of an injured ligament or muscle-tendon unit is of paramount importance for understanding the various operative and nonoperative treatment regimens that have been discussed. Rehabilitation of these injuries can be successfully accomplished with programs that are based on the scientific data currently available. These programs must be structured so that they (1) restore full joint motion, (2) facilitate normal neuromuscular patterns of movement, and (3) correct deficiencies in the strength, endurance, and flexibility of the muscles involved. Athletes with ligament and muscle-tendon-unit injuries can be returned to full competition with a minimal risk of reinjury if those treating these individuals are dedicated to applying and expanding the diagnostic and therapeutic principles that have been presented.

REFERENCES

1. Brubaker CE and James SL: Injuries to runners, J Sports Med Phys Fitness 2:189, 1974.
2. Butler DL, Noyes FR, and Grood ES: Ligamentous restraints to anterior-posterior drawer in the human knee, J Bone Joint Surg (Am) 62:259, 1980.
3. Butler DL et al: Mechanical properties of transplants for the anterior cruciate ligament, Orthop Trans 3:180, 1979.
4. Cho KO: Reconstruction of the anterior cruciate ligament by semi-tendinosis tenodesis, J Bone Joint Surg (Am) 57:608, 1975.
5. Clancy WG: Lower extremity injuries in the jogger and distance runner, Phys Sports Med 2:46, 1974.
6. Clancy WG: Personal communication, 1984.
7. Clancy WG Jr, Neidhart D, and Brand RL: Achilles tendonitis in runners: a report of five cases, Am J Sports Med 4:46, 1976.
8. Clancy WG Jr et al: Anterior and posterior cruciate ligament reconstruction in Rhesus monkeys, J Bone Joint Surg (Am) 63:1270, 1981.
9. Clancy WG Jr et al: Anterior cruciate ligament reconstruction using one-third of the patellar ligament augmented with extraarticular tendon transfers, J Bone Joint Surg (Am) 64:352, 1982.
10. Clancy WG Jr et al: Posterior cruciate ligament reconstruction: preliminary report of a new technique, J Bone Joint Surg (Am) 65:310, 1983.
11. DeHaven KE: Diagnosis of acute knee injuries with hemarthrosis, Am J Sports Med 8:9, 1980.
12. DeHaven KE and Collins R: Diagnosis of internal derangements of the knee: the role of arthroscopy, J Bone Joint Surg (Am) 57:802, 1975.
13. Ellison AE: Distal iliotibial band transfer for anterolateral instability of the knee, J Bone Joint Surg (Am) 45:905, 1963.
14. Ericksson E: Sports injuries of knee ligaments: their diagnosis, treatment, rehabilitation, and prevention, Med Sci Sports Exerc 8:133, 1976.
15. Feagin JA Jr and Curl WW: Isolated tear of the anterior cruciate ligament: 5-year follow-up study, Am J Sports Med 4(3):95, 1976.
16. Fetto JF and Marshall JL: Injury to the anterior cruciate ligament producing the pivot-shift sign, J Bone Joint Surg (Am) 61:710, 1979.
17. Fox JM et al: Degeneration and rupture of the Achilles tendon, Clin Orthop 107:221, 1978.
18. Galway RD, Beaupre A, and MacIntosh DC: Pivot shift: a clinical sign of symptomatic anterior cruciate insufficiency, J Bone Joint Surg (Br) 54:763, 1972.
19. Girgis FG, Marshall JL, and Monajem A: The cruciate ligaments of the knee joint: anatomical, functional, and experimental analysis, Clin Orthop 106:216, 1975.
20. Grood ES et al: Ligamentous and capsular restraints preventing straight medial and lateral laxity in intact human cadaver knees, J Bone Joint Surg (Am) 63:1257, 1981.
21. Hughston JC and Eilers AF: The role of the posterior oblique ligament in repairs of acute medial (collateral) ligament tears of the knee, J Bone Joint Surg (Am) 55:923, 1973.
22. Hughston JC et al: Classification of knee ligament instabilities. I. The medial compartment and cruciate ligaments, J Bone Joint Surg (Am) 58:159, 1976.
23. Hughston JC et al: Classification of knee ligament instabilities. II. The lateral compartment, J Bone Joint Surg (Am) 58:173, 1976.
24. Hughston JC et al: Acute tears of the posterior cruciate ligaments: results of operative treatment, J Bone Joint Surg (Am) 62:438, 1980.
25. Indelicato PA: Non-operative treatment of complete tears of the medial collateral ligament of the knee, J Bone Joint Surg (Am) 65:323, 1983.
26. Insall J et al: Bone-block iliotibial band transfer for anterior cruciate insufficiency, J Bone Joint Surg (Am) 63:560, 1981.
27. Jackson DW and Feagin JA: Quadriceps contusions in young athletes, J Bone Joint Surg (Am) 55:95, 1973.
28. Jacobsen K: Osteoarthritis following insufficiency of the cruciate ligaments in man: a clinical study, Acta Orthop Scand 48:520, 1977.
29. Kaplan EB: The fabellofibular and short lateral ligaments of the knee, J Bone Joint Surg (Am) 43:169, 1961.
30. Keats TE, Scaatz DS, and Bailey RW: Pneumoarthrography of the knee, Surg Gynecol Obstet 94:361, 1952.
31. Kennedy JC: Posterior cruciate injuries. Paper presented at the interim meeting, American Orthopedic Society for Sports Medicine, Atlanta, Feb. 1980.
32. Kennedy JC and Fowler PJ: Medial and anterior instability of the knee: an anatomical and clinical study using stress machines, J Bone Joint Surg (Am) 53:1257, 1971.
33. Kennedy JC, Weinberg JW, and Wilson AS: The anatomy and function of the anterior cruciate ligament, J Bone Joint Surg (Am) 56:223, 1974.
34. Lipscomb AB, Thomas ED, and Johnson RK: Treatment of myositis ossificans traumatica in athletes, Am J Sports Med 4:111, 1970.
35. Losee RE, Johnson TR, and Southwick WO: Anterior subluxation of the lateral tibial plateau: a diagnostic test and operative repair, J Bone Joint Surg (Am) 60:1015, 1978.
36. Marshall JL and Olsen S: Instability of the knee: a long-term experimental study in dogs, J Bone Joint Surg (Am) 53:1561, 1971.
37. Marshall JL et al: The anterior cruciate ligament: a technique of repair and reconstruction, Clin Orthop 143:97, 1979.
38. McBeath AA and Wirka HW: Positive-contrast arthrography of the knee, Clin Orthop 88:70, 1972.
39. McDevitt CA and Muur H: Biochemical changes in the cartilage of the knee in experimental and natural osteoarthritis in the dog, J Bone Joint Surg (Br) 58:94, 1976.
40. Monaco BR, Noble HB, and Bachman DC: Incomplete tears of toe, anterior cruciate ligament and knee locking, JAMA 247:1582, 1982.
41. Nicholas JA, Freiberger RH, and Killoran PJ: Double-contrast arthrography of the knee, J Bone Joint Surg (Am) 52:203, 1970.

42. Noyes FR, Delucas JL, and Torvik PJ: Biomechanics of anterior cruciate ligament failure: an analysis of strain-rate sensitivity and mechanisms of failure in primates, J Bone Joint Surg (Am) 56:236, 1974.
43. Noyes FR et al: Biomechanics of ligament failure, J Bone Joint Surg (Am) 56:1406, 1974.
44. Noyes FR et al: Arthroscopy in acute traumatic hemarthrosis of the knee, J Bone Joint Surg (Am) 62:687, 1980.
45. Noyes FR et al: Flexion rotation drawer: a sensitive test for anterior cruciate laxity. In press.
46. O'Donoghue DH: A method of replacement of the anterior cruciate ligament of the knee: report of twenty cases, J Bone Joint Surg (Am) 45:905, 1963.
47. Sach MD, McGaw WH, and Rizzo RP: Studies in the scope of pneumography of the knee as a diagnosis aid, Radiology 54:10, 1950.
48. Slocum DB et al: Clinical test for anterolateral rotatory instability of the knee, Clin Orthop 118:63, 1976.
49. Smillie IS: Injuries of the knee joint, ed 4, Edinburgh, 1970, Churchill Livingstone, Inc, p. 93.
50. Snook GA: Achilles tendon tenosynovitis in long distance runners, Med Sci Sports Exerc 4:155, 1972.
51. Standard nomenclature of athletic injuries, Committee on the Medical Aspects of Sports of the American Medical Association, Madison, Wis., 1968.
52. Stoddard GA: The Stoddard warm-up: a preventive exercise program for increasing strength and flexibility, Madison, Wis., Guild Printing, 1978.
53. Tongue JR and Larson RL: Limited arthrography in acute knee injuries, Am J Sports Med 8:1923, 1980.
54. Torg JS, Conrad W, and Kalen V: Clinical diagnosis of anterior cruciate ligament instability in the athlete, Am J Sports Med 4:84, 1976.
55. Wang JB and Marshall JL: Acute ligamentous injuries of the knee single contrast arthrography—a diagnostic aid, J Trauma 15:431, 1975.
56. Warren LR and Marshall JL: The supporting structures and layers on the medial side of the knee: an anatomical analysis, J Bone Joint Surg (Am) 61:56, 1979.
57. Warren LR, Marshall JL, and Girgis F: The prime static stabilizer of the medial side of the knee, J Bone Joint Surg (Am) 56:665, 1974.
58. Woods GW, Stanley RF, and Tullos JS: The lateral capsule sign: x-ray clue to a significant knee instability, Am J Sports Med 7:27, 1979.

Part Three

EXAMINATION, REHABILITATION, AND PREVENTION

Chapter 7

Evaluation of a Musculoskeletal Disorder

H. Duane Saunders

The role of the physical therapist in the examination and treatment of musculoskeletal conditions has developed into a position of greater responsibility in the medical field. With direct access to physical therapy services, it is incumbant on the therapist to prepare a proper data base from which to plan and conduct the treatment of a musculoskeletal problem.

The important aspects of evaluating a musculoskeletal disorder are discussed in this chapter. Although most of the specific examples refer to the spine, the examination processes are applicable to all parts of the musculoskeletal system.

THE PHYSICAL THERAPY APPROACH

Physical therapy is not just the application of individual modalities but the adoption of a total system of care that includes client examination, client assessment, treatment planning, treatment application, assessment of the treatment effect, modification of the treatment program in accordance with changes in the client's signs and symptoms, and client education.

THE EVALUATION PROCESS

In physical therapy evaluation is an ongoing process. Thus even though it may be possible to complete a full and thorough evaluation during the client's first examination, signs and symptoms must be rechecked continuously during the course of treatment to determine the client's progress. This ongoing evaluation and assessment form the basis for treatment modification.

The need to continue the evaluation process is also a key factor in client management. The initial examination, no matter how thorough, cannot be expected to provide all the answers. A trial treatment should be administered and then assessed to determine whether a more definitive treatment program is necessary.

CLIENT EXAMINATION

The examination is the foundation on which effective treatment rests. The examination findings should guide the therapist in selecting appropriate treatment techniques. Because many different tests, measurements, and sequences for collecting the required data are available, the format chosen largely depends on individual preference. However, a methodical and complete examination is essential.

When performing the musculoskeletal examination, the therapist should adhere to one method. This will allow full development of the therapist's intuitive skills. Several recognized methods of evaluation are taught in orthopaedic and sports physical therapy settings. While there are some differences in the order of questioning and emphasis, the essentials do not differ. The emphasis, of course, should always be on thoroughness and accuracy.

The only exception to performing a complete examination and assessment of the client's status on the initial visit is in the case of acute, severe pain. In this case a physician must determine if the problem is of a musculoskeletal nature, ruling out such things as fracture or dislocation if trauma is involved. In clients with acute, severe pain a complete history should be taken and, if it does not contraindicate the objective information available, the therapist should proceed with trial treatment of the symptoms both to reduce the pain and to expose its underlying etiology. When the symptoms of acute pain have subsided sufficiently, the therapist must carry out a complete evaluation.

Collecting data

In performing an evaluation it is important for the physical therapist to collect relevant, accurate, and measurable data and to measure and record the data as objectively as possible. For example, it is essential to document a positive straight-leg raise in degrees and to take actual circumference measurements and state restrictions of movement in degrees or inches. These data need to be accurately determined since they will be used later to assess changes brought about by treatment.

Any subjective information must be collected and recorded in an objective manner also. This can be accomplished by recording some objectively measurable factor that correlates with the subjectively described symptoms—such as length of time the symptoms persist after a certain activity or the distance the client can walk before the onset of symptoms.

Subjective questioning protocol and objective tests must be individualized by the therapist to maximize the information obtained. The therapist should ask the client only purposeful questions directed at determining the client's problem. In addition, the objective tests used should be geared to the therapist's individual size, dexterity, physique, and experience. Similarly, certain questions and tests will have more or less meaning to individual clients. For example, the results of an individual test or question can lead to further questioning and testing to determine the relevance of the item to the present signs and symptoms.

It is important that the therapist refrain from jumping to conclusions during the data collection phase of the evaluation process. Only careful, accurate, and thorough data collection will ensure correct assessment and treatment.

Recording data

In performing an examination it is important to record data in a format that can be easily interpreted by other health professionals. An example is the SOAP format (Fig. 7-1), which can be used for all clients requiring physical therapy. It contains subjective and objective examination sections, an assessment section that lists prob-

lems with treatment goals, and a planning section that consists of an outline of the treatment plan and prognosis.

Progress notes and the discharge summary should follow the SOAP format. The notes and summary, in combination with the initial examination, assessment, and treatment plan, become the complete physical therapy record for most clients. Special tests that require an additional form—such as a complete muscle test or a nerve conduction study—can be attached to the initial evaluation, and in some instances a separate data base and/or problem list will be needed.

In record keeping the use of dictation equipment and typewriters and word processors aids efficiency and clarity. The examination can be an effective communication instrument if it is concise and clear. A handwritten examination is seldom as neat, easy to read, concise, and complete as one that is typewritten. Also, physicians and other health care personnel are less likely to read an evaluation over one page in length. However, thoroughness should not be sacrificed to keep the written evaluation brief. Material should always be arranged in the same order so others will know where to find certain information, and reference must be made to negative as well as positive findings.

To ensure that all important parts of the evaluation are performed and recorded, a worksheet should be used (Fig. 7-2). Even the most experienced practitioner may not recall all the pertinent questions and tests that are necessary for a complete and thorough examination. The worksheet is also used as a reference when the formal written examination is dictated.

Testing sequence

When conducting an examination, the therapist should follow a sequential list of tests and questions to avoid unnecessary movement of the client (see boxed material). This sequence lists all tests done in standing, sitting, supine, side-lying, and prone positions. It ensures that all the tests conducted in one position are completed before moving to the next position. This sequence also ensures that nothing is overlooked or forgotten, and it keeps the therapist moving along in an organized and efficient manner. This sequencing should be applied to examination of all major musculoskeletal areas, and data gathering sheets should be developed for use as a reference to ensure thoroughness in testing.

The SOAP format

The SOAP examination format consists of two parts: the subjective examination and the objective examination. During the subjective examination the therapist questions the client concerning his/her perception of the condition and its behavior or symptoms. The objective examination consists of actual observation during the various tests and diagnostic procedures used to evaluate the signs of the condition.

PHYSICAL THERAPY RECORD
(Client data)

Client's name: _____

Subjective:

Objective:

Assessment:

Plan:

Physical therapist _____

Physician _____

Fig. 7-1. Physical therapy record, containing initial evaluation subjective and objective sections, (which should include assessment of problem[s] and problem lists); treatment goals (assessment section); and treatment plan and prognosis (plan section).

Subjective examination (symptoms). Each musculoskeletal disorder presents a unique history. The physical therapist must possess a thorough understanding of musculoskeletal pathology and the clinical picture that each disorder presents. Even with this in mind it is a mistake to consider treating a pathological condition, such as degenerative disk disease, by a routine approach. The signs and symptoms of a specific condition in one client may differ significantly from those in another, or signs and symptoms may alter from treatment to treatment in the same client.

It is essential to good practice to sit down with the client in the examination room and obtain a detailed history of the condition and events that led to the onset of symptoms. With the history completed the therapist can leave the room to finish recording the history, review the notes from the subjective examination, and plan the objective examination.

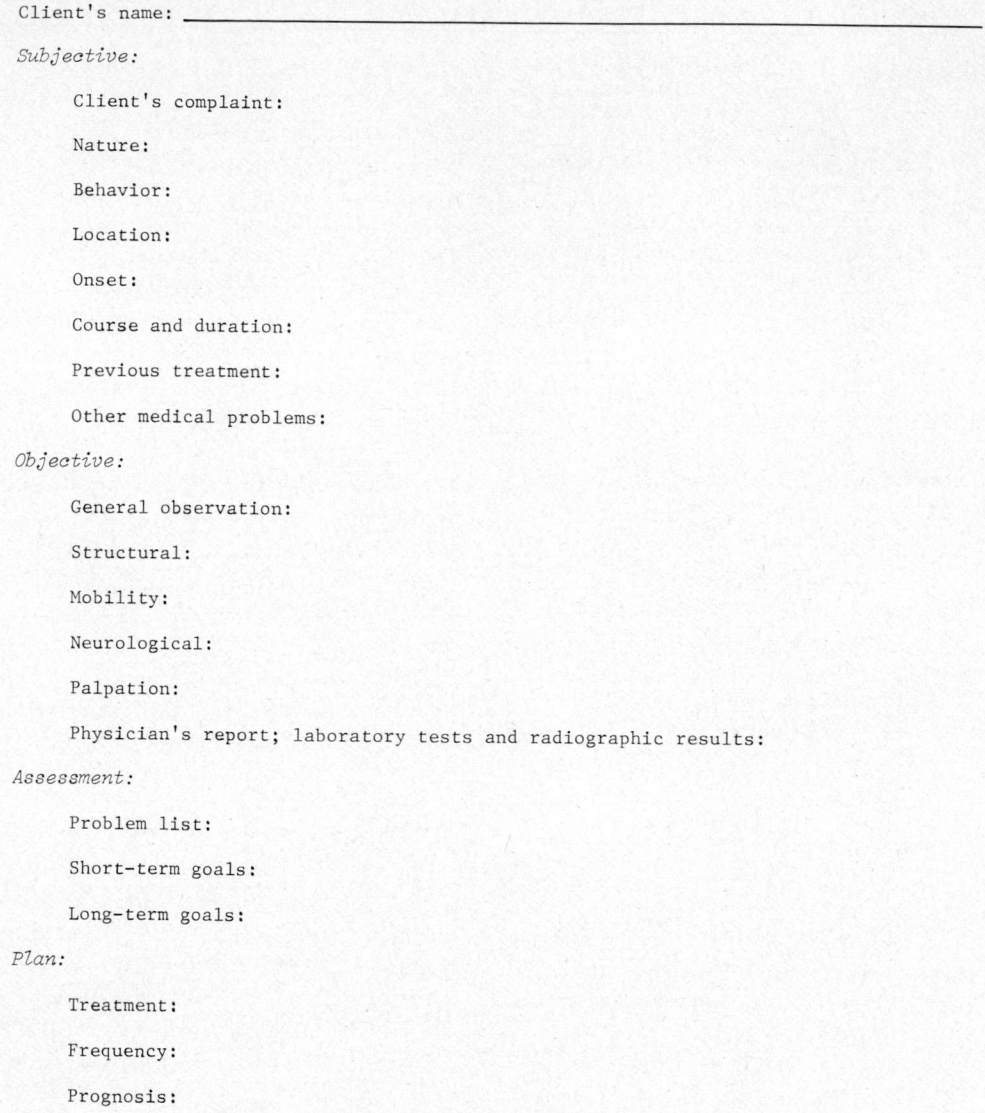

PHYSICAL THERAPY RECORD
(Worksheet)

Client's name: _____

Subjective:

    Client's complaint:

    Nature:

    Behavior:

    Location:

    Onset:

    Course and duration:

    Previous treatment:

    Other medical problems:

Objective:

    General observation:

    Structural:

    Mobility:

    Neurological:

    Palpation:

    Physician's report; laboratory tests and radiographic results:

Assessment:

    Problem list:

    Short-term goals:

    Long-term goals:

Plan:

    Treatment:

    Frequency:

    Prognosis:

Fig. 7-2. Worksheet used to record findings during evaluation. The physical therapist dictates the physical therapy record from this worksheet, which is then discarded.

Following is a step-by-step description of some common areas of questioning that should be asked by the therapist during the subjective examination to obtain an accurate client history.

Client's complaint. When taking the history, the first question to ask is simply: "What is your complaint?" This gives the client a chance to tell in his/her own words anything that is thought to be important. This first question facilitates conducting the rest of the interview by placing both the therapist and the client at ease.

Nature of symptoms. If the client has not mentioned the nature of his/her symptoms in answering the therapist's first question, it is important to find this out now. Pain, weakness, numbness, stiffness, and hypersensitivity are common symptoms. The therapist should ask for a specific description of the symptoms, such as "constant deep ache," "intermittent pain," or "sharp stab of pain."

It is important to carefully differentiate between "pins and needles", "tingling" or "numbness" descriptions. The client should be asked if there is an area of skin that can be pinched or pricked with a pin and not be felt. If so, nerve-root impingement or peripheral nerve entrapment is a probable cause. "Pins and needles" and "tingling" are often nonspecific descriptions that many clients use regardless of the disorder involved.

Weakness that is present without pain suggests a neurological deficit, unless it is generalized and associated with prolonged disuse. Painless weakness associated with a peripheral nerve entrapment or spinal nerve root compression often follows a specific nerve or myotome distribution. If weakness is present with pain, it is difficult to determine if the pain alone is causing the weakness or if there is also an underlying neurological deficit.

Behavior of symptoms. Closely related to the nature of the symptoms is the behavior of the symptoms. Are the symptoms brought on by certain activities or positions? Does the client wake up with the pain in the morning? Is the pain worse while sitting? Does the weakness appear only after walking? The client should be asked to explain how the symptoms are aggravated and how they are eased. The patterns of the symptoms over 24 hours also should be reviewed. Musculoskeletal symptoms are usually aggravated by certain movements and positions and relieved by others. If the symptoms are unrelated to movement or position, one should suspect a systemic disease or visceral disorder and should consult a physician.

The effect of position can be an important clue to the cause of pain. For example, spinal pain arising from the disk is aggravated by sitting and forward bending, whereas walking gives relief. Pain arising from the facet joints is often relieved by sitting and forward bending, but walking tends to be painful. Pain associated with acute injury and/or inflammation is often present if a joint is moved in any direction, whereas simple joint dysfunction and disk pain are often aggravated by movements in only one or two directions.

Pain occurring while resting suggests the presence of an inflammatory process. Night pain is suggestive of bone tumor. Peripheral nerve entrapments, such as carpal tunnel and thoracic outlet syndromes, are also often worse at night.[6] Combinations of symptoms that do not fit the normal musculoskeletal symptom pattern require further diagnostics.

Location of symptoms. The therapist should remember that the location of the pain is not necessarily a reliable indication of the area of true disorder.[1] However, the client should be asked the location of the symptoms because it can be useful in finding some patterns. For example, most disk or nerve root syndromes cause bilateral pain in the spine, while most spinal joint problems are unilateral. Pain limited to one spinal segment suggests joint or nerve root disorder, whereas pain over several spinal segments is more descriptive of muscle, inflammatory, or systemic disorder.

Pain and other symptoms are often referred distally but can, rarely, be referred proximally. For example, cervical pain is often felt in the upper trapezius muscle, shoulder pain in the upper arm, and low back pain in the buttocks and posterior thigh.

Pain that migrates from one joint to another suggests a systemic disease rather than a musculoskeletal disorder.

Pain that spreads from the original site to the surrounding muscles is usually caused by inflammation and/or muscle spasm, both of which are often secondary reactions to the primary musculoskeletal disorder.

Onset of symptoms. The original onset of symptoms as well as the most recent episode should be considered. Knowing the exact mechanism of injury can be helpful. For example, joint locking is caused by a sudden, unguarded movement, whereas sprains and strains involve aggravation or trauma. Inflammatory and systemic disorders present a more subtle onset. Disk conditions usually have an insidious onset caused by repeated activities related to slump sitting, forward bending, and lifting; however, the client may perceive the onset as sudden and related to the particular activity engaged in when the pain was first noticed.

It is important to realize that the client will always try to remember an incident that caused the problem. This may not be reliable, and it is often misleading to place too great an emphasis on the onset described by the client. The client may also attempt to relate present complaints to old injuries, which may be unrelated. This can be very misleading.

Course and duration of symptoms. It is important that the therapist consider the length of time since the onset of the symptoms because this can help determine whether the condition is acute, subacute, or chronic—a diagnosis that influences selection of treatment.

The natural progression of the condition should also be considered. Was the pain greatest when the injury first occurred, or did it get worse the second or third day? Has there been improvement? Has the client continued to work since the onset of the symptoms? Is a workman's compensation claim or litigation involved?

Effect of previous treatment. It is important to know the effect of any previous treatment. If the client has been to a chiropractor or other medical practitioner, did the treatment affect the condition? If the client has had a previous episode of this condition and a certain treatment helped, it should be considered as a possible means of treatment again. Medication and home treatment are also important to note at this time.

Other related medical problems. Special questions involving other medical problems, such as general health, bowel and bladder problems, any relevant recent weight loss, and any recent illnesses, must also be considered.

Objective examination (signs)

Screening examination. Sometimes the exact location of the disorder is unclear. The client complaining of arm symptoms may have a cervical disorder. Leg symptoms may be referred pain from the lumbar spine or hip joint. The screening examination should be a quick overview of several areas to provide the therapist with enough information to decide what specific areas must be examined in detail. If the screening examination proves negative, it must be repeated since there is the possibility that something was missed. If no abnormalities are found, the therapist should consult a physician and further medical diagnosis should be pursued.[2]

Upper quarter screening examination. The upper quarter screening examination consists of a series of mobility and neurological tests to identify problem areas in the cervical spine, shoulder, elbow, wrist, and hand (see boxed material). The testing is done with the client sitting in a straightback chair or on the edge of a treatment plinth.

First, a postural assessment is made, then the cervical spine is taken through active range of motion as the therapist watches for pain, muscle spasm, and/or limited movement. If no signs or symptoms are observed with active range of motion and passive overpressures, the joints of the cervical spine are considered "clear" and not the etiological structures.

Next, resisted pressures should be exerted in all planes of motion with the cervical spine held in a neutral midrange position. If the isometric resisted muscle tests produce no pain and no weakness is observed, the musculature of the cervical spine is considered "clear." Resisted rotation of the cervical spine is also a neurological test of spinal nerve C-1. Resisted shoulder elevation is a test for disorder in the upper trapezius, levator scapulae, and rhomboid muscles and for neurological involvement of the spinal nerves C-2 to C-4.

The client is then asked to hold his/her arms abducted to 90 degrees while downward resistance is applied to test the deltoid and supraspinatus musculature and spinal nerve C-5. This is followed by active shoulder flexion and external and internal rotation with overpressure to "clear" the shoulder. Resisted elbow flexion and extension tests the musculature of the upper arm and spinal nerves C-6 and C-7. Active range of motion completes "clearing" of the elbow. Resisted testing of wrist flexion and extension,

thumb extension, and finger abduction "clear" the wrist and hand and test spinal nerves C-7 to T-1. The upper quarter screening is completed by doing a Babinski reflex test for upper motor neuron involvement.

Lower quarter screening examination. The lower quarter screening examination consists of a series of mobility and neurological tests to identify problem areas in the lumbar spine, sacroiliac area, hip, knee, ankle, and foot (see boxed material). The examination begins with the client standing so that posture can be observed. The lumbar spine is taken through active forward, backward, and lateral bending as the therapist watches for signs of pain, muscle spasm, and/or limited movement. Heel and toe walking is then completed to neurologically test spinal nerves L-4 and L-5 (heel) and S-1 (toe). It also "clears" the ankle and foot when no pain or limitation of movement is observed.

Active lumbar rotation is checked with the client sitting. The client is asked to extend the arms forward with his/her hands held together and then to "twist" to the right and left as far as possible. If no signs or symptoms are observed with active range of motion, passive overpressures are applied. If rotation, along with forward, backward, and lateral bending, produces no signs or symptoms when done both actively and with passive overpressures, the joints and muscles of the lumbar spine are considered "clear" for those movements.

Next, the client performs straight-leg raises in supine position to neurologically test spinal nerves L-4 to S-1. Spring tests for sacroiliac involvement are also done at this time.

The hip is "clear" if passive flexion, medical and lateral rotation, and resisted hip flexion do not produce any signs or symptoms. Resisted hip flexion is also a neurological test of spinal nerves L-1 and L-2.

Resisted knee extension is a neurological test of spinal

Summary of upper quarter screening examination

Postural assessment
Active range of motion of the cervical spine
Passive overpressure if spine is symptom free
Resisted muscle tests of the cervical spine (rotation C-1)
Resisted shoulder elevation (C-2 to C-4)
Resisted shoulder abduction (C-5)
Active shoulder flexion and rotation
Resisted elbow flexion (C-6)
Resisted elbow extension (C-7)
Active range of motion of elbow
Resisted wrist flexion (C-7)
Resisted wrist extension (C-6)
Resisted thumb extension (C-8)
Resisted finger abduction (T-1)
Babinski reflex test for upper motor neuron involvement

Summary of lower quarter screening examination

Posture assessment
Active forward, backward, and lateral bending of lumbar spine
Toe walking (S-1)
Heel walking (L-4, L-5)
Active rotation of lumbar spine
Overpressure if spine is symptom free
Straight-leg raise (L-4 to S-1)
Sacroiliac spring tests
Resisted hip flexion (L-1, L-2)
Passive range of motion of hip
Resisted knee extension (L-3, L-4)
Knee flexion, extension, and medial and lateral tilt
Femoral nerve stretch
Babinski reflex test for upper motor neuron involvement

nerves L-3 and L-4. "Clearing" of the knee is completed by passively testing flexion, extension, and applying varus and valgus stresses.

A femoral nerve stretch in the prone position may be indicated if the client has described symptoms in the anterior hip, thigh, or groin area. The lower quarter screening is completed by doing a Babinski reflex test for upper motor neuron involvement.

Detailed objective examination of a specific area. Areas of specific complaint or areas that have shown some questionable signs during the screening examination should be examined in detail.

General observation. The detailed objective examination begins with general observation and inspection of the client. The way the client responds to the therapist's questions should be noted. For example, what kind of attitude does the client seem to have toward his/her condition—apprehensive, resentful, or depressed? Since the behavioral attitude of the client often has a bearing on the success of the treatment, the therapist should consider this important aspect of the client's condition.

How does the client walk? Does he/she seem to be in excruciating pain? Are there any obvious abnormalities in the way the client moves and carries himself/herself? It is important for the therapist to note such observations because they may later tell more about the client's progress than direct questioning.

Structural examination. The structural examination involves a closer, more specific inspection of the area of complaint. It is essential that the areas being examined are adequately free of clothing.

Inspection involves the observation of bony, joint, and muscular structures in the affected areas. When examining the extremities, the examiner usually has an advantage because there is a "normal" side to use for comparison.

Next the size of the specific muscles should be inspected. A muscle or muscle group that appears smaller than usual may be a clue to peripheral nerve injury or entrapment, spinal nerve impingement, or disuse atrophy. The musculature around the scapula, shoulder, hand, and thigh is most often subject to atrophy that is visible during inspection. Muscle spasm and guarding can also be seen during visual inspection. A muscle or tendon rupture can be seen as a knot or lump in the soft tissue.

Each joint should be inspected, and any deviations from normal surface anatomy should be noted. Clues to degenerative joint disease can be observed in the sternoclavicular joints and in the elbows, fingers, knees, and toes. If the acromioclavicular joint is separated, it can often be detected by visual inspection. A subluxation of the glenohumeral joint can also be seen in many cases. The classic deformities of rheumatoid arthritis, such as ulnar drift of the fingers and enlarged proximal interphalangeal joints, should be noted during the structural examination.

Obvious joint deformities of the lower extremities include genu valgus or genu varus, pronated feet, fallen arches, and hammer toes. The sole of the foot should be examined for callous formation—a clue to abnormal gait patterns—or other foot problems, such as a fallen metatarsal head.

The lumbar and cervical spine should show a mild lordotic curve and the thoracic spine a mild kyphotic curve. Absence of any of the curves may indicate restriction of mobility, whereas excessive lordotic or kyphotic curves may indicate the presence of any of a variety of structural and postural problems. Many pathological processes present certain predictable changes in lordosis and kyphosis and can be important aids in diagnosis.[4,8]

Lateral curves in the spine are abnormal and are classified as either functional or structural or as caused by a specific pathological process. A structural scoliosis is caused by a defect in the bony structure of the spine, such as wedging of the vertebral bodies, and is characterized by the fact that it does not "straighten" during forward bending of the spine. Because lateral bending is always accompanied by an equal amount of rotation, the client will have a "lumbar bulge" and/or "rib hump" when he/she bends forward if a structural scoliosis is present. A functional scoliosis may be caused by a nonspinal bony defect, such as unequal leg length, muscle imbalance, or poor postural habits, and generally will straighten during forward bending.

McKenzie[4] states that a lumbar scoliosis (lateral shift) may be caused by the posterolateral movement of the nucleus pulposus. Fennison[3] also describes a lumbar scoliosis (protective scoliosis) that results when the client shifts the spine to one side to take the spinal nerve root off the bulge of a disk protrusion.

Close attention should also be paid to the sacral base during the structural examination. With the client standing straight—feet slightly spread apart and weight equally distributed—the height of the iliac crests, posterior superior iliac spines, anterior superior iliac spines, trochanters, gluteal folds, and fibular heads are checked to determine if the sacral base is uneven and, if so, where the discrepancy lies. For example, if the posterior superior iliac spines are uneven and the trochanters are even, the discrepancy lies between these two structures. In this case the sacroiliac joint, hip joint, and angulation of the femoral neck are possible areas of discrepancy.

The sacral base should be checked closely, even in clients with complaints of the cervical spine, because compensatory scoliotic curves are often present in the cervical spine that may need to be treated by correcting the sacral base. The shoulders and the base of the cervical spine (C-7) should also be examined to determine if they are level.

Leg length is assessed with the client in the supine position by comparing the relative position of the medial malleoli. This position may then be compared with the client in the long-sitting position. If a difference is observed between the supine and long-sitting leg-length tests, it is an indication of a rotational defect in one of the sacroiliac joints.

Any special assistive devices or supports, such as a knee brace, lumbar corset, cervical collar, or cane, that the client uses should be noted at this time. The device should be carefully assessed to ensure that it has been properly fitted and is being used correctly.

Mobility examination. The mobility examination consists of passive, resisted, active, special mobility, and strength tests. It is done to determine which joints and/or muscles are affected and to what extent. During the mobility examination the therapist looks for either joint hypermobility or hypomobility, flexibility, and any change in symptoms caused by movement. The examination must include all tissues from which the client's symptoms might arise. Tension must be applied to all these tissues to note which movements provoke or change the client's symptoms or otherwise seem abnormal.

The tissues may be divided into two groups: noncontractile and contractile. The noncontractile tissue group includes capsules, ligaments, bursae, nerves and their sheaths, cartilages, intervertebral disks, and dura mater. These structures can have tension applied to them by passive stretching (passive movements). The contractile tissue group includes muscles and tendons with their attachments. These structures may also have tension applied to them by passive stretching, but it is more effective to make them contract maximally as a result of resisted movement.[1] Active movements test the client's willingness to move. They combine joint range of motion (passive) and muscle contraction (resisted).

Resisted movements are maximal static contractions, usually done in a comfortable neutral position within the available range of motion. If no movement is observed at the joint, the muscle group (contractile) has been tested, and the inert structures have not been disturbed. If contractile tissue is at fault, the appropriate resisted movement will be painful.

Passive movements test the specific range of motion available in a joint or spinal segment. These tests determine if the joint range is reduced (hypomobile), increased (hypermobile), or normal. If noncontractile tissue is at fault, passive movements may be painful.

Mobility examination of spine and sacroiliac joints. Examination of the spine and sacroiliac determines the extent of joint and muscle involvement.

ACTIVE MOVEMENTS. Active range of motion of the spine is performed to give the therapist a general assessment of available range of motion and should be done only within the limits of pain. The specific level of hypermobility or hypomobility cannot be determined, but a general impression of problem areas can be gained. Pain arising from active movements may occur in certain predictable patterns, which are helpful in determining the origin of such pain.

For example, a painful recovery from forward bending is usually of muscular origin, whereas pain only at the end of range is more indicative of joint restriction.

RESISTED (ISOMETRIC) TESTS. Resisted movement tests determine muscle involvement. The joints are placed in a neutral midrange position, and the client is asked to hold against resistance in each direction. The therapist attempts to elicit a strong muscle contraction with very little or no joint movement. If the test causes increased pain, the muscles are primarily implicated. While this method of testing is helpful in examining the extremity joints, it has little application in testing the lumbar and thoracic spine because of the difficulty in isolating muscle contraction without joint movement in these areas. Resisted muscle tests are generally more helpful in determining muscular involvement in the cervical spine.

PASSIVE MOVEMENTS. Passive movement testing is an extremely valuable procedure because it provides the therapist with specific information about each individual spinal segment. It requires considerable practice by and experience of the therapist before competence is achieved. Passive range of motion tests assess movement at the specific segmental level.

Mobility examination of extremities. In most cases clients with a musculoskeletal problem in an extremity will have an uninvolved side that can be used for comparison. Testing of the uninvolved side and comparison should always be done when doing the mobility examination. It not only gives the therapist an assessment of the client's normal mobility; it demonstrates the test or procedure to the client and puts him/her at ease before the involved extremity is examined. This is especially important when examining joint play movements, because the client may be unfamiliar with these procedures and may be apprehensive.

ACTIVE MOVEMENTS. Active movements combine joint range of motion (passive) and muscular contraction (resisted). If a client has pain or other symptoms with active movements, the examiner cannot determine if the joint, the muscle, or both are at fault.

Active movements do test the client's willingness to move. If a client is symptom free with both passive and resisted movement testing but has symptoms with active movements, there may be a question concerning the client's willingness to perform the movement. In such cases consideration should be given to psychogenic causes for the client's complaint.

RESISTED (ISOMETRIC) TESTS. Resisted movements are strong static contractions done in a comfortable neutral position within the available range of motion. No movement should be allowed at the joint when performing resisted tests. If pain is produced with resisted tests, there is probably a disorder within the muscle, tendon, or tendinous attachment (contractile group), resulting from injury (muscle strain, contusion, or strain of the tendon insertion) or inflammation (myositis or tendonitis). Prolonged muscle guarding and spasm may cause circulatory stasis and retention of metabolites, which will in turn cause the muscle to be tender to palpation and the resisted tests to be painful. This must be considered when determining whether muscular dysfunction is the primary problem.[2]

If a resisted muscle contraction is strong and painless, there is nothing wrong with the muscle, tendon, or the tendinous attachment. If the contraction is strong and painful, there is a disorder in the contractile group. If the contraction is weak and painless, there is a neurological deficit or the muscle is weak from disuse. If the contraction is weak and painful, there is a dysfunction in the contractile group, but it is impossible to determine by this test alone if the weakness is a result of the pain or if a neurological deficit is present.[2]

PASSIVE MOVEMENTS. Passive range of motion tests the noncontractile structures of the joint, including the capsule, ligaments, bursae, nerves and their sheaths, and cartilages. Passive movements are conducted in the supine position with the client as relaxed as possible. The passive movement is carried through full functional range, gently if necessary, to determine if there is a limitation of range, and if so, whether it is painful. If noncontractile tissue is at fault, passive movements are painful and there may be limitation of movement.

Although passive movement tests are primarily done to find noncontractile joint involvement, they also passively stretch the muscles that surround the joint. If pain is found with passive movements, it must not be assumed that it is arising from the joint. The location of the pain will often help the therapist determine which structure is involved. Also comparison of the passive range of motion findings to those of the resisted muscle tests should determine which structures are implicated.

Special mobility tests. Normal range of joint movement is that movement which is available to a normal joint as a result of normal muscle action. These voluntary movements cannot be achieved unless certain well-defined accessory movements are present. Accessory movements (joint play) are independent of the action of voluntary muscles. Painless, full, voluntary range of motion is dependent upon the presence of these very small, precise accessory movements.[5]

Accessory movement tests. Accessory movements are assessed by special mobility tests. The examiner first tests the accessory movement on the uninvolved side to determine the amount of joint play that is normal for that particular client. The involved extremity is then examined, and an assessment is made as to whether the accessory movement is excessive, resulting in a joint that is hypermobile, less than normal, indicating a joint that is hypomobile, or normal.

Muscle-strength testing. Specific muscle-strength testing may be done if weakness is suspected. It is important that muscle-strength testing be measured as objectively as possible using manual muscle-testing procedures. More elaborate procedures, such as isokinetic muscle testing, are also available to aid in diagnosis and to establish a more accurate data base.

Neurological examination. The neurological portion of a musculoskeletal evaluation consists of a series of tests to determine if there is impingement or encroachment on a spinal nerve root or entrapment of a peripheral nerve.

Resisted (isometric) muscle tests. Resisted (isometric) muscle tests determine whether there is either muscular or neurological involvement. If resisted muscular contraction produces pain, there is a disorder within the muscle, tendon, or the tendinous attachment. When weakness is also present with the painful contraction, the therapist cannot be certain if the muscle is weak because of a neurological deficit or because of the pain itself. If pain and/or immobilization has been present for an extended period of time, the muscle may also be weak because of disuse. Specific muscular weakness that is not associated with pain or disuse is considered a positive neurological finding.

Resisted muscle tests are done bilaterally at the same time, if possible, because this makes it easier to determine slight differences in strength. Resisted tests can be conducted on machines that give graph readings of muscle strength.

Muscle-stretch reflexes. Muscle-stretch reflexes are often helpful in locating neurological deficits. As a general rule hyperactive reflexes indicate upper motor nerve disorder, and hypoactive reflexes indicate impingement, entrapment, or injury of a lower motor nerve (spinal nerve root or peripheral nerve). Normal reflexes vary a great deal from person to person. Occasionally reflexes are difficult to elicit or appear hypoactive in some clients, while other clients appear to have hyperactive reflexes. If these findings appear bilaterally, they are probably "normal" for those clients. It is when a reflex appears hypoactive or hyperactive when compared to the opposite side that the results are significant.

The client should be questioned closely during the subjective examination concerning absence of skin sensation. If the client indicates a sensation deficit, the therapist should use a pinprick test to determine the extent and exact location of involvement. An area of numbness that follows a dermatome pattern or is distributed along a peripheral nerve indicates spinal nerve root impingement or peripheral nerve entrapment or injury. If the area of numbness involves the entire circumference of an extremity (glove or stocking effect), a sensory nerve deficit resulting from vascular insufficiency is probably involved rather than a disorder of a musculoskeletal nature.

Pain that follows a dermatome, scleratome, or myotome pattern does not necessarily indicate nerve root impingement or peripheral nerve entrapment. Pain may be referred from muscles, joints, and/or other structures that are innervated by the same spinal nerve level or peripheral nerve.[1,7]

As a general rule pain is referred distally from the affected structure and is rarely referred proximally. It is therefore from the proximal ends of longer segments that diffuse pains usually arise.

Referred pain can also cause increased muscular activity in the area where the pain is felt. This increased muscular activity can in turn have an inhibitory action on the antagonist muscle group. For example, pain arising from a disorder in any pain-producing structure* in the lower lumbar spine can be felt as pain down the posterior aspect of the thigh. This referred pain may cause increased muscular activity in the hamstring muscles, which in turn may inhibit the quadriceps muscle. This inhibitory action on the quadriceps muscle may cause a hypoactive muscle-stretch reflex. The implication is that certain muscle-stretch reflex changes can be caused by referred pain as well as by spinal nerve root impingement or peripheral nerve entrapment.[5]

STRAIGHT-LEG RAISE TEST. The client is positioned supine for the straight-leg raise test, which determines if there is impingement of the spinal nerve root. As the straight leg is raised, the sciatic nerve is progressively stretched, which in turn stretches the spinal nerve roots. If there is an impingement on the spinal nerve root, the symptoms will be increased or aggravated by this test. Straight-leg raising also stretches the hamstring muscle, so if the test increases pain in the posterior thigh, it must be determined whether this indicates tightness in the hamstring muscle or a true positive neurological deficit. If the only sign is increased pain in the posterior thigh, it is unlikely to be a true neurological sign. It is also helpful to do hold-relax muscle stretching of the hamstring if there is some doubt. If the hold-relax stretching seems to increase the range of motion, the pain and restriction are probably in the hamstring. If, on the other hand, the hold-relax stretching has no effect, spinal nerve root impingement is probably involved. Another useful variation of the straight-leg raise test is to have the client do it with and without raising his/her head. When the head is raised, the dura is pulled superiorly, putting an added stretch on the spinal nerve root, thus increasing any positive sign of the straight-leg raise. Dorsiflexion of the ankle also stretches the sciatic nerve and, if it is added to the straight-leg test, will often increase the positive sign if true nerve root impingement is involved.

Normally, a positive straight-leg raise test indicates a more severe disorder if it occurs at 20 to 40 degrees of hip flexion and a less severe disorder if it occurs at 50 to 70 degrees of flexion. It is difficult to interpret a straight-leg raise as positive at ranges over 70 degrees of flexion. The degree of flexion present when the symptoms occur should be recorded so comparison can be made later to determine if progress has been made.

*Pain-producing structures in the lower lumbar spine are (1) paraspinal musculature, (2) facet joint capsule, (3) dura mater, (4) outer ring of the annulus of the intervertebral disk, and (5) spinal ligaments.

Occasionally, a positive straight-leg raise test is seen when the opposite leg is raised, which may indicate a disk herniation medial to the nerve root. Another indication of this condition is if pain is relieved when the client leans toward the side of symptoms rather than away from the side of symptoms.

A sitting straight-leg raise test should be done to determine if the client's reaction to the supine straight-leg raise test is genuine. The malingering client may be familiar with the supine straight-leg test and may exaggerate the pain during the test. However, the client may not be aware that straight-leg raise testing is being done while sitting and will not know when to exaggerate the pain. The therapist should do the sitting straight-leg test while checking the resisted muscle tests at the knee so as not to call attention to the test. If the sitting straight-leg raise is pain free or causes very little reaction and the supine straight-leg raise causes considerable more reaction, the client is probably exaggerating the symptoms.

FEMORAL NERVE STRETCH. Femoral nerve stretch is done with the client prone. As the femoral nerve is stretched by flexing the knee and hyperextending the hip, the spinal nerve roots L-1 to L-3 are stretched across their respective intervertebral foramen. If there is impingement of one of these spinal nerve roots, the symptoms will be increased as this test is performed. One must be careful to distinguish between a painful quadriceps muscle and a true nerve root sign. If nerve root impingement is present, the symptoms will extend into the lateral aspect of the hip and into the upper lumbar spine as well as the anterior thigh.

TRACTION AND COMPRESSION TESTS. As traction and compression are applied to the spine, certain symptoms may be altered, indicating a possible spinal nerve root impingement. If traction relieves and compression aggravates the client's symptoms, it is an indication that a spinal nerve root is impinged. Acute facet joint pain can also present similar findings with this test, and therefore it is not a completely reliable indication of spinal nerve root impingement. The test is most valuable because it gives an indication of when traction might be an effective treatment or when it might aggravate the client's condition.

PERIPHERAL NERVE ENTRAPMENT TESTS. Tests to determine peripheral nerve entrapment syndromes should also be included in the neurological examination. The tests for the three thoracic outlet syndromes—the carpal tunnel syndrome, the piriformis syndrome, and common perineal nerve syndrome—are most often used.

BABINSKI REFLEX TEST. The neurological examination is completed by doing a Babinski reflex test, which is performed by stroking the sole of the client's foot from the heel, along the lateral aspect, and across the ball with a blunt instrument. A positive reaction consists of extension of the great toe, usually associated with fanning (abduction and slight flexion) of the other toes. This indicates upper motor neuron disorder.

ELECTRODIAGNOSTIC TESTS AND OTHER NEUROLOGICAL TESTS. Electrodiagnostic studies and sophisticated neurological testing are required when symptoms suggest a neurological basis that cannot be explained by a basic neurological examination, such as the Babinski reflex test.

Palpation examination. During the palpation examination an inexperienced examiner frequently uses a single palpation procedure to gain information concerning tenderness, muscle tone, and position of the bone. A better approach is to study each element of the palpation examination as a separate procedure. The elements considered should be the skin, subcutaneous tissue, peripheral circulation, muscles, ligaments, and bone.

The skin is palpated and examined for tenderness, color, temperature, moisture, and texture. Because pain is often referred, the site where the client reports pain may not be the site of the primary disorder. The position where there is tenderness to palpation is a more reliable indication of the site of a primary disorder, but prolonged muscle guarding and spasm in response to referred pain can fool the inexperienced examiner. Temperature changes are helpful in finding areas of dysfunction. For instance, a warm area may indicate acute inflammation or a cool area may mean chronic disorder, such as joint hypomobility. A dry, smooth, shiny skin is indicative of a chronic condition, whereas a slight rise in moisture may indicate an acute condition.

The subcutaneous tissue is palpated for abnormal amounts of fat, tissue fluid, tension, localized swelling, and nodules. Normally the skin can be rolled over the spine freely and painlessly. If there are pathological changes in the subcutaneous tissue, there will be tightness and pain when the skin-rolling test is done. Any moles on the skin are examined to determine if they are superficial or deep in nature.

The dorsalis pedis and posterior tibial pulses are felt in the foot to assess peripheral circulation. Muscle tenderness is examined, and careful interpretation is given to any positive findings. Muscle guarding and/or muscle spasm is noted. Next the condition of the palpable ligaments is noted. They may be tender if the joint is injured, inflammed, or thickened, and coarse if joint hypomobility is present.

The position of the bones is felt to rule out dislocation, subluxation, or joint locking. The examiner must not assume that all bony abnormalities are pathological, since some may be congenital and unrelated to the client's present complaint.[9]

Because of the depth of many of the structures of the spine, palpation of the skin may not reveal temperature or color changes even though inflammation may be present.

When palpating the spinal joints, the examiner can only feel the spinous processes and the supraspinous ligament. However, what can be felt through these structures is surprisingly valuable. The supraspinous ligament is normally "springy" and "supple," so if it is thickened and hardened the segment may be hypomobile. When palpation between the spinous processes elicits pain, it is an indication that the spinal segment (facet joints and/or intervertebral disk) is involved.

The positions of the spinous processes are felt to determine alignment of the spine. Changes in position of the bone suggest the presence of facet joint locking or facet joint hypomobility. Positional changes may also be congenital in nature and by themselves do not necessarily mean a joint is locked or hypomobile. Mobility testing must confirm that a segment is locked or hypomobile before the final assessment is made.

Palpation is an especially valuable evaluation tool for examining the extremities. Many of the joint structures, muscles, and tendons are more superficial and easier to identify in the extremities than in the spine.

Correlation with other reports. On completion of the examination, the therapist correlates the findings with other information that is available, such as medical diagnosis, radiology reports, and laboratory and other tests. In order that the evaluation is done without bias, the correlation should be done at the conclusion of the evaluation rather than at the beginning.

Assessment

The assessment can be made in two ways: It can be a list of problems (signs and symptoms) found in the subjective and objective examinations, or it can be a statement of the impression or conclusion that the therapist has drawn.

Realistic goals should be established based on the assessment and recorded in the assessment portion of the evaluation.

Plan

The treatment plan is based on the findings of the subjective and objective evaluation and the assessment. The treatment plan should specifically state what treatment is planned, including estimated frequency and duration. Client and family education should be noted in detail, and any plans for long-term follow-up should be recorded. The client's reaction to the first treatment is also recorded.

It should again be emphasized that the entire evaluation process is ongoing and is expanded each time the therapist sees the client. As new facts are presented, assessment is continued and treatment modifications are made as necessary. It is not until the client's problem is resolved that the assessment process is concluded.

SUMMARY

The examination is the foundation on which effective assessment and treatment rest. It is an ongoing process. The major components of evaluation are the subjective examination (symptoms) and objective examination (signs). Some of the many questions, tests, and measurements that are available for evaluation have been presented. Based on educational background and experience and practice setting, each therapist must determine which of these procedures can be best used to collect the data needed to successfully manage the client's disorder.

REFERENCES

1. Cloward R: The clinical significance of the sinuvertebral nerve of the cervical spine in relation to the cervical disk syndrome, J Neurol Neurosurg Psychiatry 23:321, 1960.
2. Cyriax J: Textbook of orthopaedic medicine, vol 1, Baltimore, 1969, Williams & Wilkins.
3. Fennison B: Low back pain, Philadelphia, 1973, JB Lippincott Co.
4. McKenzie R: The lumbar spine, Waikanae, New Zealand, 1981, Spinal Publications.
5. Mennell J: Joint pain, Boston, 1964, Little, Brown & Co.
6. Mennell J: Differential diagnosis of visceral from somatic back pain, J Occup Med 8:477, 1966.
7. Mooney V and Robertson J: The facet syndrome, Clin Orthop 115:149, 1976.
8. Saunders H: Orthopaedic physical therapy: evaluation and treatment of musculoskeletal disorders, Minneapolis, 1982, Meyers printing.
9. Zohn D and Mennell J: Musculoskeletal pain, Boston, 1976, Little, Brown & Co.

Chapter 8

PHYSICAL AGENTS AND MUSCULOSKELETAL PAIN

A. Joseph Santiesteban

The effective treatment of musculoskeletal pain and dysfunction requires a broad knowledge of physical agents. Physical agents, termed *modalities* by some, include a long list of techniques and devices that employ heat, cold, sound, and various categories of the electromagnetic spectrum, such as light and electricity.

The task of explaining the mechanisms and uses of all the physical agents employed in treating musculoskeletal pain and dysfunction would necessitate a discussion beyond the scope of this chapter. Instead, selected physical agents are described. Electrotherapy receives the greatest attention because, although not new, it has recently undergone a resurgence. Among the physical agents described under electrotherapy are transcutaneous electrical nerve stimulation (TENS), electroacupuncture, iontophoresis, and high-voltage and medium-frequency current stimulation. Superficial thermotherapy and deep heat are also dis-

cussed briefly, and some new techniques are suggested for shortwave diathermy. Phonophoresis, an extremely effective ultrasound technique, is also described. Many of these physical agents are new and apparently clinically effective.

However, a few misconceptions about the effectiveness of physical agents should be mentioned at the onset of this discussion. Many physical agents are used with success in reducing pain and improving the activities of daily living. Yet seldom are physical agents *cures*. Biomechanical dysfunction that causes pain may require other therapeutic approaches in addition to the application of physical agents. Overuse syndromes may require rest and prescriptive exercise as well.

Physical agent effectiveness can be improved by careful application of the selected technique over the target tissue. For instance, a general or haphazard application of ultrasound over the thoracic spine will not be as effective as concentration of the sound waves over the facet joint exhibiting the dysfunction. Of course, it must be stressed that a thorough physical evaluation, including a history and subjective and objective examinations, must be performed before the prescription and application of any physical agent.

TRANSCUTANEOUS ELECTRICAL NERVE STIMULATION

The development of transcutaneous electrical nerve stimulation (TENS) has revolutionized the nonmedicinal approach to the treatment of pain. TENS is the application, via surface skin electrodes, of low-intensity, pulsed, alternating or direct currents. These pulsed currents have been shown to reduce the pain of muscle sprains, ligamentous damage, nerve root irritations, and surgery.*

TENS is based on the early theoretical work of Melzack and Wall.[34] This theory suggests that peripheral stimulation of large-diameter cutaneous afferent nerve fibers can block pain sensation at the spinal cord. Thus blocked, pain sensation does not reach the conscious brain. Later research shows that other mechanisms may also be at work. The endogenous opiate system found in the midbrain, spinal cord, and pituitary also appears to block pain and alter certain systemic functions.[51] This system is activated, at least in part, by noxious or near-noxious ambient stimuli, such as peripheral electrical stimulation. The interested reader is encouraged to review Bishop's synopsis of pain mechanisms.[4]

The effectiveness of TENS in the management of musculoskeletal pain is well documented in literature on the subject. Ersek[14] found TENS to reduce both chronic and acute low-back pain. Of 35 clients treated, 23 had 50% to 89% pain relief, while the remainder reported almost complete relief. In another study of low-back pain, neck pain, and headache, Indeck and Printy[24] observed that TENS appeared useful in reducing a wide variety of chronic musculoskeletal pain syndromes. As might be expected, TENS has found wide acceptance in the world of sports medicine. Roeser et al[38] report that they have used TENS for a number of conditions including (1) hip pointer injury, (2) elbow epicondylitis, (3) mild sprains, (4) shoulder dysfunction, (5) cervical strains, (6) and other injuries.

Postoperative use of TENS

Postoperative use of TENS is also well documented. After studying 40 clients who have undergone total-hip replacement, Pike[37] reported that TENS was effective in reducing the dosage of pain medication they needed. A TENS plus p.r.n. medication group was compared to a medication-only control group. The TENS p.r.n. group required fewer doses of medication than the control group during the first 24-hour postoperative period.

Stabile and Mallory also have reported on knee and hip joint replacement clients assigned to a TENS plus p.r.n. medication group or to a medication-only group.[46] Forty-three clients were assigned to the experimental TENS p.r.n. group, and 42 clients were assigned to the control group. The majority of the experimental group clients (86%) reported significant relief with TENS.

TENS has been shown to be effective in controlling pain with various surgical procedures of the knee, including total knee replacements, meniscectomies, arthrotomies, and synovectomies.[21] The narcotic medication dosage prescribed and the length of hospital stay were reduced significantly for clients using TENS.[21]

Foot surgery clients have also been shown to benefit by

*See references 1, 14, 21, 24, 46, 50.

the use of TENS.[1] Clients were assigned to a TENS group, a TENS control group, or a no-TENS, medication-only control group. The TENS group reported significantly less pain than either the TENS sham or the control group. The TENS group also used fewer narcotic medications administered p.r.n.

TENS stimulation variables

A review of the literature has shown that TENS is not always effective. TENS effectiveness can be maximized by careful selection of stimulation variables, electrode placement, and type of equipment. In this section stimulation variables will be examined.

A controversy exists concerning the correlation between TENS effectiveness and a combination of pulse rates, waveform, pulse widths, and output intensities. Early in the history of TENS, client perception of a comfortable electrical stimulus was thought to be the best indicator of effectiveness in treatment. Devices were developed that allowed for low-voltage, higher frequency, low pulse-width variables, which were perceived by the client as being comfortable. The pain control record of these stimulators was good but not outstanding. In more recent years stimulators have been developed that produce a more noxious stimulation-variable combination. Extended pulse width, low pulse rate, and higher output intensities are currently being recommended for the treatment of both acute and chronic pain. This new approach, based on the concept of acupuncture, involves the cutaneous and subcutaneous insertion of the needle, which evokes some discomfort. It appears probable that recommendations to keep the pulse rate low will predominate in TENS application theory.

Frequency. Low-frequency electrical currents are those with frequencies of 1,000 Hz or less. Yet when TENS is discussed, low frequency is often defined as a frequency of less than 10 Hz. Some clinicians suggest that for both chronic and acute pain a low frequency of 2 Hz is effective in reducing nociception. In certain acute cases a slightly higher frequency of 8 Hz, because it may produce less discomfort, may be better tolerated by the client.

Pulse width. A low-frequency current should have a greater pulse width. A greater pulse width permits the current to be in the tissues for a longer time, thus allowing the depolarization of smaller-diameter afferent nerve fibers because of the strength-duration characteristics of these fibers. It has been suggested that the small-diameter afferent fibers facilitate increased production of endogenous opiates. Currently available portable TENS devices have pulse widths adjustable from 40 to 250 microseconds. Pulse widths of 200 microseconds or more are favored by some clinicians because these longer pulse widths are able to depolarize C and delta nociceptor neurons more readily at lower output intensities.[50]

Output intensity. Output intensity is the third important stimulation variable. Sufficient current must be available so that the proper afferent nerve fibers are depolarized. Depth of penetration of the stimulus is also dependent on the strength of output intensity. The TENS unit selected should have sufficient output intensity to drive four electrodes.[41] Each electrode must be able to facilitate a muscle contraction. Minimal muscle contractions may be used as a reference point for determining an adequate output intensity setting.

In summary, therefore, the TENS unit selected should have low-frequency compatibility, a wide pulse width, and sufficient output (at least 50 mA). Another consideration in selecting the unit is determining whether a modulated set of stimulation variables is available. Modulated variables, such as pulse width or frequency, should be alterable over time by the unit. Instead of a constant pulse width or a set frequency, the unit should be able to change either of these two variables. This modulation tends to prevent the client from accommodating to the stimulus. When accommodation occurs, the effectiveness of the TENS treatment is probably reduced.

Waveform. Waveform may also be important for maximizing TENS effectiveness. All TENS devices have the capability of producing muscle contractions and nonnoxious stimuli. So all TENS waveforms appear to be at least adequate for their task. Yet it may be that particular waveforms are superior to others. Research in this area, however, continues with no definite recommendations possible at this time.

Electrodes. Electrodes come in a myriad of sizes, shapes, and compositions. The most common type is either a square or round carbon-impregnated rubber electrode. These are supplied with most TENS devices, and their chief advantages are that they are inexpensive and reusable. Carbon-rubber electrodes, however, tend to separate from the site of stimulation and do not conform well to the contours of the body. Disposable electrodes, although more expensive, tend to adhere better and conform more effectively than carbon-rubber electrodes. Disposable, sterile, post-surgical electrodes are also available.

Various types of electrodes should be available in a well-equipped facility. Carbon-rubber electrodes are useful for brief clinical applications or long-term home use. Disposable electrodes are suggested for treatments extending over a period of hours or days. Disposable electrodes may also be used during athletic activities. However, if stimulation is to be ongoing during contact activities, the device must be well shielded.

Electrode placement is the key to effective TENS pain management. Most TENS devices can energize at least four electrodes. These electrodes may be placed over the area of pain (Fig. 8-1), along dermatomes corresponding to the pain, or on selected acupuncture points. Pain relief appears to be best achieved with acupuncture point placement (Tables 8-1 and 8-2).[40] Dermatome placement appears to be the next best choice, although it provides

CROSSED AND UNCROSSED PLACEMENT OVER AREAS OF PAIN

	Ch 1		Ch 2
Crossed placement	———	Area of pain	———
	Ch 2		Ch 1

	Ch 1		Ch 2
Uncrossed placement	———	Area of pain	———
	Ch 1		Ch 2

	Ch 1		Ch 1
Uncrossed placement	———	Area of pain	———
	Ch 2		Ch 2

Fig. 8-1. TENS electrode configuration.

weaker stimulation than acupuncture point placement. Electrode placement over the area of pain is often not very effective in chronic pain management but is acceptable for acute pain relief.

TENS application

TENS may be effective in chronic and acute pain cases using the points described. Whenever possible the points should be stimulated bilaterally even though the pain may be unilateral. At least four points should be stimulated. Once the electrodes are in place, the therapist should adjust the TENS pulse width to the maximum, set the pulse frequency at 2 Hz, and increase the output intensity until a visible yet comfortable muscular contraction is observed. The client must be able to sense the stimulation. If the device being used does not in itself modulate the stimulation variables, constant post-application checks must be made. The output intensity should be increased if the client is accommodating to the stimulus.

For acute conditions TENS may be applied alone or with ice for 30 minutes once daily. As the acute condition resolves into a postacute stage, TENS may be continued and coupled with heat, contrast baths, or ultrasound. Chronic pain is more difficult to treat because it often implies a long-standing biomechanical problem. Stronger TENS therapy for a longer period of time is usually more effective in chronic pain cases. The TENS application may have a duration of 60 minutes daily. Output intensity should be increased to produce a stronger muscular contraction. TENS may be preceded by electroacupuncture at selected acupuncture points, and it may be followed by shortwave diathermy, traction, mobilization, or exercise.

For chronic and acute pain TENS is seldom a cure. It is an effective way of reducing pain without medication so that other treatments can be administered. In reference to medications there is some evidence that narcotic medication intake reduces the maximum effectiveness of TENS. Whenever possible the client should be on p.r.n. medications.

TENS effectiveness can be documented by recording

Table 8-1. Acupuncture points for extremity pain

Point	Location
Foot/ankle	
ST-41	Midpoint of transverse malleolar crease, between extensor digitorum longus and extensor hallucis longus tendons
ST-42	1½ body-inches* distal to ST-41, over highest point of the dorsum of the foot
GB-40	Anterior and inferior to lateral malleolus, in depression above calcaneocuboid joint
B-60	Dorsal to the most lateral point of lateral malleolus
Knee	
B-60	—
ST-35	With knee bent, in lateral depression just below patella
ST-36	3 body-inches below ST-35 and one finger breadth from crest of tibia
ST-34	In depression 2 body-inches above superior-lateral patellar margin
SP-10	2 body-inches above superior border of patella, over motor point of vastus medialis
Elbow	
LI-4	At the midpoint of second metacarpal, over motor point of first dorsal interosseus
LI-11	In depression at lateral end of transverse cubital crease when elbow is flexed
LI-10	2 body-inches below LI-11
LI-9	3 body-inches below LI-11
LI-14	Over the deltoid tuberosity
Shoulder	
LI-4	—
LI-11	—
LI-14	—
LI-15	Anterior and inferior to border of acromioclavicular joint, inferior to acromion when arm is in adduction
SI-9	With arm at side, 1 body-inch superior to posterior axillary fold
SI-12	In center of suprascapular fossa, in depression when arm is abducted

*A body-inch equals the width of a client's thumb interphalangeal joint.

Table 8-2. Acupuncture points for neck and back pain

Point	Location
Neck	
LI-4	At the midpoint of second metacarpal, over motor point of first dorsal interosseus
LI-10	2 body-inches* below LI-11
LI-14	Over the deltoid tuberosity
SI-14	3 body-inches lateral to lower border of spinous process of first thoracic vertebra on the vertical line drawn up from the vertebral border of the scapula
GB-21	Highest point of shoulder, motor point of upper trapezius muscle
GB-20	In depression between sternocleidomastoid and trapezius muscles, directly inferior to occiput
Low back	
B-60	Dorsal to the most lateral point of lateral malleolus
B-54	Midpoint of popliteal crease
GB-34	Distal to fibular head in the fibular fossa
GB-31	With arm at side, at the point just distal to middle fingertip
B-27	1½ body-inches lateral to S2 spinous process, at level of posterior superior iliac spine (PSIS)
B-23	1½ body-inches lateral to lower margin of L2 spinous process

*A body-inch equals width of a client's thumb interphalangeal joint.

stimulation variables, dosage and types of medications used, ambulation, mobility, rate of return to competition or activities of daily living, and subjective pain response. Such documentation allows for the development of improved treatment protocols. Documentation of all treatments and outcomes should be standard procedure.

ELECTROACUPUNCTURE

A special technique frequently performed in conjunction with TENS is *electroacupuncture* (EAP). EAP is performed by applying an intense electrical stimulus to acupuncture points. The pulse-frequency and pulse widths are similar to those used with conventional TENS. However,

the output intensity is perceived by the client as greater since the treatment electrode is approximately 1 mm in diameter. The passage of current through this small-diameter electrode is concentrated, and a potentially noxious stimulus is produced.[35] Some clinicians favor the following treatment protocol. Stimulation of points is initiated at the most distal point location from the pain focus, as described in the treatment formulas (Tables 8-1 and 8-2). Stimulation is performed bilaterally for approximately 60 seconds at each point and proceeds proximally to the area of pain. The level of stimulation (output intensity) is regulated according to the client's response. A slightly uncomfortable, but not painful, sensation should be reported by the client.

EAP is usually administered as the initial treatment and followed by TENS, traction, mobilization, or other treatments.[40] One treatment daily should be sufficient to reduce or eliminate chronic and acute musculoskeletal pain. After a few EAP treatments the effectiveness decreases.

Clinicians experienced with EAP have found that the output intensity tolerated by the client is an indicator of the client's painful state and rehabilitation progress. Those clients experiencing severe pain will tolerate less output intensity than individuals having less discomfort. As the painful condition subsides, the client will be able to toler-

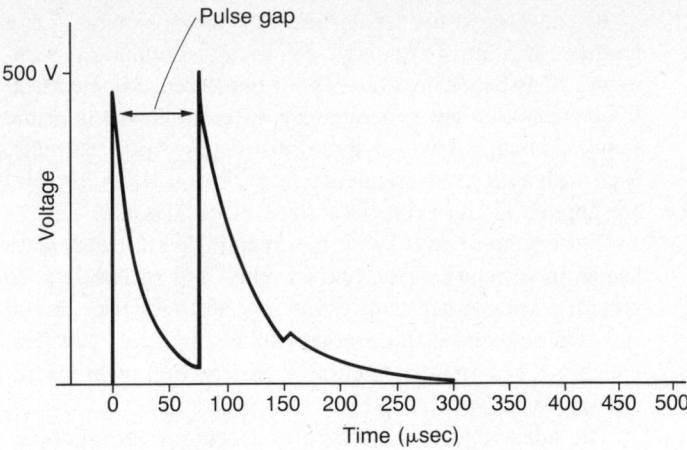

Fig. 8-2. High-voltage double waveform.

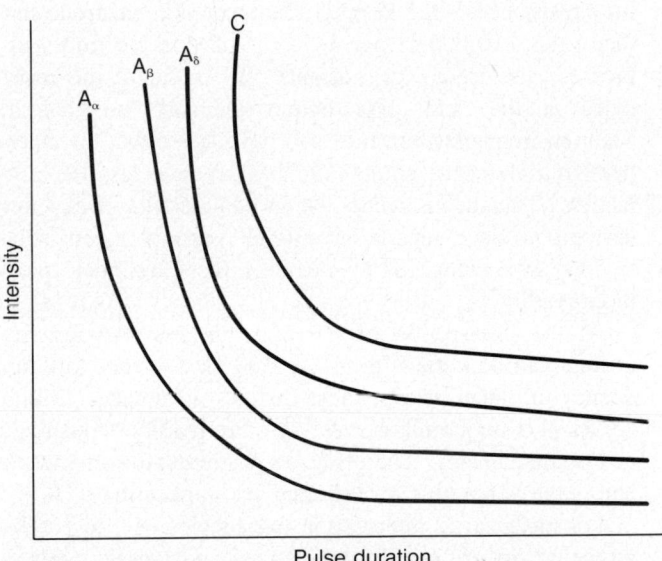

Fig. 8-3. Strength-duration curves for various neuron types.

ate an increased output intensity. A suggested method of documenting the client's progress is to record the output intensity as indicated on the device's meter at the 30-second mark. Each acupuncture point treated may have a different tolerance, so a record must be kept of each reading.

HIGH-VOLTAGE ELECTRICAL STIMULATION

A recent development in treating musculoskeletal problems involves use of a high-voltage electrical stimulator (HVS). The high-voltage electrical stimulator is defined as a device using a voltage greater than 150 V at medium frequencies. HVS has some reported advantages over low-voltage stimulators. Among these are the creation of a less noxious peripheral sensation because of the specific HVS waveform and deeper penetration.

According to basic electrophysiology, large- and small-diameter nerves respond differently to electrical currents. Large-diameter nerves, which innervate muscle fibers and certain afferent sensory structures, are depolarized at lower current intensities. Small-diameter nerves, such as pain

nerve fibers and autonomic nerves, require much higher electrical currents for depolarization.

Depolarization of nerves is also dependent on the rate of change in the electrical current and the length of time the current remains in the tissues. If a current has a slow rate of rise, a stronger intensity is required. The relationships between current intensity and pulse duration are demonstrated in Fig. 8-2. This figure describes standard strength-duration curves for different axon types.

Fig. 8-3 represents a typical HVS waveform. Twin pulses at a given voltage have a very rapid rate of rise. The high rate of rise and the brief peak duration of the HVS pulse may mimic the effects of medium-frequency currents. Depolarization of cutaneous afferent nerve fibers is minimized with this waveform so that increased output intensities are better tolerated by the client.

Little research is available on the effects of HVS. Yet clinicians are reporting good results when HVS is used for the treatment of myofascial pain, chondromalacia patellae, the edema of acute injury[26], and wound healing.[28]

A typical HVS treatment setup is pictured in Fig. 8-4.

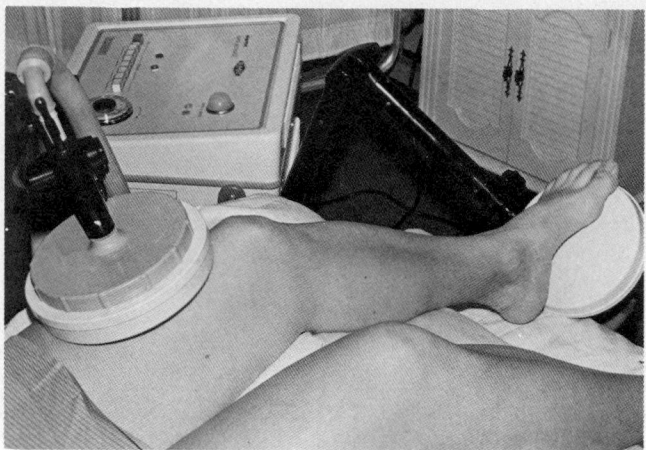

Fig. 8-4. Capacitive shortwave for lower extremity dysfunction.

The two active electrodes are placed on either side of the knee for the treatment of chondromalacia patellae or acute swelling. A dispersive pad is placed under the client's thigh or foot. The polarity of both active electrodes can be either positive or negative. The polarity of the dispersive pad alternates accordingly. The current can be made to flow between one active electrode and the dispersive pad and then the other active electrode and the dispersive pad. The rate at which this is accomplished is termed the *switching rate.*

Three other variables are adjustable. The output intensity, measured in volts, varies from 0 to 500 V. The pulse gap (Fig. 8-3) and the pulse frequency are also adjustable. As a general rule the pulse gap and frequency adjustments should be large for treating the initial acute injury or for those persons who are particularly sensitive to electricity. During the initial treatment the pulse gap and frequency can be reduced. This reduction will tend to make the stimulus stronger as more current per unit time is passed through the tissues. Chronic conditions often respond well to low pulse gap settings and low frequencies.

Most HVS units have great flexibility. With a hand-held applicator, electroacupuncture or galvanic massage can be performed. HVS can also be used for muscle reeducation in conditions such as medial meniscectomy and quadriceps muscle weakness. Low-back or neck muscle spasms can be effectively relaxed. A TENS treatment approach is also possible with HVS.

MEDIUM-FREQUENCY ELECTRICAL THERAPY

Medium-frequency electrical currents employ frequencies measuring between 1,000 and 100,000 Hz. Two such currents are the interference current (IC) therapy and the Russian technique for muscle stimulation best termed *neuromuscular stimulation* (NMS). Whereas the IC may be used for electroanalgesia first and muscle stimulation second, the NMS apparently has its greatest application in muscle strengthening.

IC, developed by the Austrian physicist Nemec,[47] is a unique, medium-frequency electrical stimulation technique. IC is based on a concept of interference in electrical frequencies that are generated by different channels of the same apparatus. Two (or three) distinct electrical currents, each with a different frequency (e.g., 4,000 Hz, 4,100 Hz) are applied to the skin via surface electrodes (see Fig. 8-1). For example, an IC with two such different frequencies has an intersection of the two currents, and an interference pattern is established that results in a net frequency of 100 Hz. Consequently, the target tissues receive 100 Hz, which is a low-frequency current, instead of a medium-frequency current of 4,100 Hz.

The advantages of this type of technique are multiple. Medium-frequency currents penetrate the skin with very little resistance— 125 Ω per 127 cm^2 of skin electrode surface versus 10,000 Ω per 127 cm^2 of skin electrode surface for low-frequency currents. By reducing the resistance at the skin, less output intensity is required. Medium-frequency currents also have less effect on superficial muscle-nerve complexes and produce less depolarization of cutaneous receptors. In contrast, low-frequency currents produce superficial muscle contractions and tend to depolarize cutaneous mechanoreceptors and nociceptors more readily.

At the intersection of the two currents, the net frequency can be varied from 0 to 100 Hz. A very low frequency stimulation has some distinct advantages. Motor nerves and autonomic nerves are more readily depolarized at low-frequencies. Therefore deep stimulation of muscle and nerve is possible by the selective application of IC.

For instance, at intersection frequencies of 0 to 10 Hz, motor nerves are readily depolarized and muscle contraction initiated. When stronger muscle contractions are desired, the IC can be adjusted so that the channels have current frequencies of 4,000 and 4,100 Hz. The initiation of muscle contractions is useful for muscle relaxation, muscle strengthening, and muscle reeducation. Smooth muscle surrounding blood vessels also responds well to stimulation at these lower frequencies. When excessive nerve irritability produces symptoms such as neuritis or root irritation, an intersection frequency of 90 to 100 Hz may be selected. The latter frequency also decreases autonomic system activity.

With IC, muscle spasms can be treated by repetitive, pulsed frequencies.[48] The effects are similar to those achieved with a low-frequency current but without the disagreeable peripheral sensation. Sympathetic tone can be altered at higher frequencies. This allows the therapist to treat edema effectively even in acute conditions. At frequencies of 1 to 100 Hz, TENS effects are possible and pain relief is readily achieved.

In 1977 Kots[29] described the strengthening effects of a medium-frequency current generator used on well-trained athletes. His method has become known as the Russian technique for muscle stimulation (NMS). NMS consists of employing sinusoidal current frequencies of 1,600 to 4,000 Hz, depending on the type of device used.

The frequency of pulses is modulated into 50 pulse-trains per second, which allows the muscle to achieve motor response and tetany when the output intensity is sufficiently high. Because of the nature of medium-frequency currents, cutaneous afferent nerve fibers are not readily depolarized. The client therefore may be able to tolerate increased current levels producing 60% of maximum muscle contraction in certain cases.

As a treatment for strengthening injured or normal muscle, Kots recommended a 10 seconds on, 50 seconds off stimulation cycle. He indicated that athletes treated in this fashion experienced significant muscle strength increases. Replication of his study has not been performed, and other researchers have not found such dramatic strength increases.[15,30] A review of electrical stimulation therapy used to improve muscle strength is offered by Kramer and Mendryk[30] and Currier.[10]

NMS may also be used to produce profound anesthesia under electrode surface area. Submotor response intensities for periods of 5 to 20 minutes produce numbness in these areas, and the client does not respond to pinpricks or other noxious stimuli. When strong nonvoluntary contractions are desirable, a preceding anesthetic treatment may allow the client to better tolerate high output intensities.

In an investigation of various electric currents on cutaneous sensation and joint proprioception, Santiesteban and Ostrow observed that a 2,500 Hz current at less than 20 mA produced decreased fine touch.[44] High-voltage current, low-voltage current (60 Hz), and 2,500 Hz currents did not appear to affect joint position sense.

Some nonpublished observations suggest that the greatest contractions of the quadriceps muscles are produced by placing a large electrode just distal to the inguinal region and another large electrode proximal to the patella and slightly medial to the rectus femoris. Constant current intensities up to 40 mA with this electrode configuration are tolerated by some clients.

NMS may be useful in exercising motor units that are innervated by the largest diameter efferents. These motor units may be classified as fast-twitch units; the larger the diameter of the axon, the easier depolarization occurs with electrical stimulation that is opposite of the size principle.[22] It has been postulated that heavier resistance to muscles is required to activate fast-twitch fibers. Many postoperative and posttrauma conditions prevent clients from exercising at heavier resistance. Therefore NMS may be a useful adjunct to exercise even though the patient may not be able to tolerate high current output intensities.

IONTOPHORESIS

Iontophoresis is the introduction of selected ions into the tissues. This technique has many applications, includ-

Table 8-3. Polar effects of direct current

Pole	Chemical effects	Physiological effects
Anode (positive)	Repels metal ions and other positive ions	Sclerotic; decreases nerve irritability
Cathode (negative)	Repels acid radicals and other negative ions	Sclerolytic; increases nerve irritability

ing the treatment of calcium deposits, inflammation, and pain.[26]

A working knowledge of iontophoresis requires a brief discussion of the effects of low-voltage direct current. Direct current has various polarity effects, which are listed in Table 8-3. The anode or positive pole repels positive ions, increases the irritability threshold of nerves, and has a sclerotic or tissue-hardening effect. Conversely, the cathode or negative pole repels negative ions, decreases the irritability threshold of nerves, and has a sclerolytic or tissue-softening effect.[45]

This brief description of the polarity effects of direct current indicates some very important applications and precautions. The cathode pole tends to be caustic, chemically and sensorially. Tissues may dissolve if the dosage is too great. The sensation perceived by the client will be slightly uncomfortable at recommended dosages and painful at higher dosages because of increased nerve irritability. The anode pole will not be caustic, and the sensation experienced by the client will be less uncomfortable.

Various substances that dissociate or form ions in solution have been identified as useful in treating soft tissue conditions. Most common and readily available among these substances are the salicylates, hydrocortisone, dexamethasone, and lidocaine. Table 8-4 describes various ions, sources of these ions, and their application in treating soft tissue problems. Calcium deposits,[25] myospasms,[26] plantar warts,[18] pain,[39] and inflammation are also treatable by iontophoresis and are discussed in the literature.

Because of the caustic and sclerolytic effects of direct current, iontophoresis offers a slight but ever-present degree of hazard to the client. Some simple procedural steps will ensure that the treatment is conducted satisfactorily. As a general rule the therapist should always maintain a 2:1 cathode-to-anode electrode surface area ratio since the effects of the negative pole (cathode) can be made less caustic if the cathode's relative surface area is larger than that of the anode. By increasing the surface area the negative charge is better dispersed over a greater area, thereby reducing current density. The ionic solution should be applied to a 4 × 4 inch gauze or towel, which is placed under the electrode or to an ointment rubbed onto the skin. The towel must be thoroughly soaked and all wrinkles removed. Wrinkling of the towel or gauze may concentrate

Table 8-4. Ions and their use

Ion	Substance	Pole	Use
Hydrocortisone	1% cream solution	Positive	Antiinflammatory
Lidocaine	5% cream solution	Positive	Anesthetic
Salicylate	Aspirin cream or ASA and water	Negative	Analgesic and antiinflammatory
Magnesium	Magnesium sulfate (epsom salts)	Positive	Antispasmodic
Calcium	Calcium chloride	Positive	Analgesic, and antispasmodic
Zinc	Zinc oxide	Positive	Tissue healing
Iodine	Iodex	Negative	Sclerolytic, for scar softening

See Kahn J: Low volt technique, Syosset, NY, 1976, for additional uses.

the current over these areas and increase the potential for a burn. It is suggested that specifically designed iontophoresis electrodes be used and that the current intensity be no greater than 4 mA. This intensity is sufficient in most cases. Additional current intensities may produce burns. During the treatment the current will tend to increase because of falling skin resistance, so the intensity should be checked frequently. The skin should have good sensation and should be free of cuts, scrapes, or significant amounts of hair.

How strong should the solution be? What is the dosage suggested for standard treatment? What is the acceptable depth of penetration for ions driven by iontophoresis? These are questions that the clinician must ask before the use of iontophoresis. An ionic solution or ointment should be in the 1% to 5% range. Such a weak solution allows for better dissociation of ions. The dosage for certain ions can be computed using the standard chemical equation

$$\text{current} \times \text{time} \times \text{ECE} = \text{dosage}$$

where ECE is the electrochemical equivalent. The ECE is defined as the mass liberated by the passage of a unit quantity of electricity.*

The dosage formula gives a very gross approximation of true dosage because the epidermis offers resistance to the passage of ions and deeper tissues have high ionic contents. Treatment duration for iontophoresis is usually 15 minutes. Griffin and Karselis[19] estimate that the ion depth of penetration by iontophoresis is less than 1 cm; whereas Glass, Stephen, and Jacobsen[16] indicate a 17 mm depth of penetration. These values may be too large, but effects on deeper tissues have been described. Possibly ions are carried to deeper tissues by circulatory currents or by slower diffusion pathways.

Recently new clinical iontophoresis devices have become available that are extremely convenient, although somewhat limited. The devices meter the ionic solution and drive it at 4 mA or less current intensities.

*Values for each ion listed in Table 8-4 can be found in older editions of Hodgman C, Weast R, and Salby S: Handbook of chemistry and physics, ed 37, Cleveland, 1955, Chemical Rubber Publishing.

SUPERFICIAL HEAT AND COLD

Topical applications of heat and cold have been popular treatment approaches for soft tissue dysfunction. Hot baths, moist warm towels, water bottles, infrared lamps, and hot packs have been traditionally used to treat chronic pain and muscle spasms. Ice bags, cold towels, ice massage, and ice compresses have been and still are often selected for the treatment of acute pain and swelling.

As might be expected, the treatment effects and the concomitant physiological changes are different for topical heat and cold. The local topical effects of heat are vasodilation and subsequent erythema, decreased fast nerve fiber sensation (touch), and, with prolonged exposure, decreased slow nerve fiber sensation (pain). The electrical resistance of the skin decreases as well. Local cooling produces an intense vasoconstriction followed by periods of vasodilation. Prolonged cooling decreases fast nerve fiber and slow nerve fiber sensation.[12]

The sensation of temperature is transmitted from unencapsulated nerve endings in the skin to the spinal cord via mostly unmyelinated nerve fibers for the warmth receptors and myelinated nerve fibers for the cold receptors.[31] Temperature sensation is then transmitted via the lateral spinothalamic tract to higher centers. Two parts of the hypothalamus are involved in thermoregulation.[7] The anterior hypothalamus initiates sweating and vasodilation of cutaneous vessels when temperature is increased. Decreased body temperature causes the posterior hypothalamus to initiate vasoconstriction of peripheral vessels, producing shivering and increased visceral activities.

Topical heat and cold have effects on muscle strength and endurance. With a muscle temperature of 27° C submaximal forearm contractions have been shown to be greatest when the forearm was immersed in a bath at 18° C.[9] Two-thirds maximal volitional contraction of the quadriceps muscle has been found to last longest at 26° C, and at lower temperatures endurance decreases.[13] Immersion of the forearm and hand in cold water significantly reduces the strength and proprioception of fine motor activities. It may be concluded from these studies that cool temperatures, not hot or cold, produce the best effects on muscle strength. However, as will be discussed later, deep heating of muscles may have an entirely different effect.

Moist hot packs are probably the most commonly used physical agent. The clay in the packs retains a large proportion of water that has been heated to 70° to 80° C. Hot packs are usually wrapped in Turkish toweling and applied to the client's skin for 15 to 20 minutes. This form of topical heat may be used prior to ultrasound or electrical stimulation or in preparation for exercise or traction. The rationale for using a moist pack is that it offers general superficial muscle relaxation and prepares the skin for a subsequent physical agent. While the skin heats up rapidly to about 43° C, tissues at a depth greater than 1 cm show little increase in temperature.[29] Certainly the muscles or joint capsules below 1 cm are not being heated significantly. Therefore the rationale for using hot packs to stimulate deep-seated muscles is probably invalid.

Topical cold can be applied to a local area by means of an ice massage or to a larger area by an ice bag. An ice massage may be performed by rubbing a cup filled with water that has been allowed to freeze over the target tissue for 3 to 7 minutes. An intense hyperemia and numbness result, decreasing pain and other sensations. Ice massage should not be performed over bony prominences since significant pain will be elicited. Ice bags usually consist of ice cubes or crushed ice placed in a plastic bag. A few milliliters of water and a pinch of salt can be added to improve the cooling effect. The ice bag is placed over the target tissue and is covered with toweling, which acts as an insulator. The ice bag is applied for 10 to 20 minutes or until gentle numbness is perceived by the client. Ice bags are effective in treating posttraumatic swollen joints and other tissues that exhibit the cardinal signs.

The application of cold in conjunction with compression is useful as an extension of the PRICE (protection, rest, ice, compression, and elevation) procedure treatment used in emergency care and sports medicine. An advantage of compression plus cooling is that it is more effective in reducing and preventing posttraumatic swelling than cold alone. The client's involved extremity is elevated, ice bags are applied to the traumatized area, and a compression device is attached. Intermittent compression at pressures below the diastolic blood pressure measurements is applied for 20 to 30 minutes. The theoretical basis for this type of treatment is that the cold will prevent further exudation from the injured capillary beds while the compression will help maintain a higher interstitial pressure. It may be argued, however, that prolonged or persistent use of cold will allow the proteins released into the interstitial spaces to coagulate. This coagulation will then produce distension of the interstitial spaces.

Local cooling is applied one to four times daily during the acute period. The acute period has been variously defined as the 24-hour period following injury, 72 hours after the insult, or the period that elapses until swelling and tissue temperature decrease to near normal.

It must be kept in mind that not all clients tolerate cold well. Some persons have neurovascular conditions, such as Raynaud's phenomenon, that make exposure to cold painful and dangerous. Others do not enjoy the sensation of cold. In these cases cold should not be applied; gentle moist heat may be substituted. No significant deleterious effects should occur as a result of the application of gentle heat in acute conditions unless there is a tendency toward hemorrhage.

DEEP HEAT

Ultrasound and shortwave diathermy are two types of effective deep heat therapy used in the treatment of musculoskeletal dysfunction. Microwave therapy will not be discussed since it has decreased in popularity among clinicians. Both ultrasound or shortwave diathermy serve as more than adequate substitutes.

Ultrasound

After hot packs ultrasound is probably the most frequently used physical agent in treating musculoskeletal pain. Ultrasound is a form of mechanotherapy, wherein a crystal embedded in a transducer (soundhead) is made to vibrate in response to the passage of an electrical current. As the crystal vibrates rapidly, sound waves are produced. Many ultrasound generators in the United States produce sound waves having a frequency of about 1 megacycle (1 million cycles) per second. This frequency is well out of range of human hearing. Sound waves can be transmitted through any of a number of media—the denser the medium, the better the transmission.[17] Ultrasound waves are transmitted more effectively through water, oil, or transmission gel than air. Therefore for clinical application a transmission medium is always required.

In normal biological applications 50% of ultrasound energy is transmitted to a depth of 5 cm.[17] This depth of penetration can be effectively employed in reaching deep tissues, such as joint capsules and deep muscles.

The more homogeneous the tissue, the less ultrasound energy is absorbed. So subcutaneous fat, which is very homogeneous, absorbs less energy than muscle, which is more heterogeneous. Metallic and synthetic implants are also homogeneous, and ultrasound waves produce very little increase in the temperature of these devices.[5] Therefore ultrasound can be safely used in the treatment of both obese individuals and clients who have implants.

Ultrasound waves tend to concentrate at the interface of dissimilar tissues. Therefore skin-fat and periosteum-bone interfaces experience a tissue temperature rise because of reflected energy. As a result, when one of the components of these interfacing tissues has a poor blood supply, the heat can become excessive and lead to pain. Prolonged sonation or sonation over very superficial interfaces can lead to tissue death.

Ultrasonic energy produces a number of physiological effects, which makes it a useful physical agent for the treatment of musculoskeletal problems. Sonation over peripheral nerves and nerve plexes has been found to increase the level of cortisol,[20,49] which functions to decrease the inflammation of trauma and overuse. As a result, ultrasound can be used to treat lumbosacral nerve root irritations, nerve-root impingements, and various types of neuritis. Sonation also has been reported to increase the extensibility of connective tissues, such as tendons, ligaments, and joint capsules, and it may be beneficial when limitations of range of motion are caused by contractures of ligamentous tissues.[32] Since ultrasonic waves penetrate deeply, structures such as spinal facet joints and hip capsules can be treated effectively. Bursae, which are specialized synovial membranes, are also reported to respond well to sonation.[3] Other synovia membranes, such as those lining the major joints, may also benefit from sonation. No published data have been found, however, to show that ultrasound is an efficacious agent for low-back pain.

Ultrasound, as a deep-heating agent, can influence the temperature of muscle. A 5-minute treatment over a muscle belly can elevate the tissue temperature by $1°$ to $2°$ C. This amount of tissue temperature rise is sufficient to cause muscle relaxation. Muscle spasms of a localized nature may therefore be effectively relaxed by sonation, either because of increased tissue temperature or because of micromassage effect.

Many standard ultrasound generators offer the versatility of either continuous or pulsed sonation. Continuous sonation means that the ultrasonic waves are constantly emitted from the transducer, while pulsed sonation means that the ultrasonic waves are emitted intermittently. This versatility may be used effectively in the treatment of both acute and chronic musculoskeletal disorders.

A continuous ultrasound treatment usually requires the application of a topical coupling agent. The coupling agent acts as a transmission medium for the ultrasonic waves. Water, mineral oil, and commercial transmission gels can be used effectively. Air bubbles should not be present in the coupling agent, because air interferes with ultrasonic energy. A sufficient amount of the transmission medium should be used so that the transducer and skin do not have any bare contact spots, which can reduce transmission effectiveness and produce excessive heat.

Continuous ultrasound also requires that the transducer be kept in constant motion while the crystal is vibrating. Slowing or stopping the transducer may produce excessive heat buildup. In employing continuous ultrasound it is recommended that a dosage of 1 W/cm^2 to 1.5 W/cm^2 for 5 minutes be used as a standard treatment. If the area to be treated is larger, the time of treatment can be increased; however, bony areas may require that the output intensity be reduced, while heavily muscled areas or deep target tissues may require greater output intensities.

Pulsed ultrasound is sometimes used in a stationary fashion. A coupling agent is used also, but the intensity is less and the duration of treatment more. It is not uncommon to treat an acute ligamentous or muscular problem at 0.5 W/cm^2 for 10 minutes. Since the ultrasonic energy is pulsed, there is less tissue temperature buildup. This limited heat increase makes pulsed ultrasound useful when heat is contraindicated.

Other conditions that are reported to respond well to pulsed ultrasound treatment are hematomas, hypertrophic scars, and muscle tears. In this last case the sonation, because of the mechanical disruption, may assist the healing tissues to align longitudinally along the long axis of the muscle. Ultrasound in this case can be compared to the deep-friction massage techniques advocated by Cyriax.[11]

Underwater ultrasound is a special technique used for treating irregular and bony body parts, such as feet and hands, which lack substantial flat surfaces. In this technique the body part is immersed in water and the transducer is slowly moved over the target tissue at a distance of about 2 cm. Intensity levels may need to be reduced or the skin-transducer distance increased. Care must be taken to reduce the potential for electrical shock when ultrasound is performed in an electrically grounded whirlpool. A ground fault interrupter, into which both the whirlpool and the ultrasound are plugged, reduces the hazard of electrical shock. As previously stated, air bubbles in the coupling medium disrupt ultrasound waves, so the whirlpool water should not be agitated before sonation.

There are a few contraindications and precautions in using ultrasound that must be mentioned. Using ultrasound in the lumbar or abdominal region at frequencies and intensities used for musculoskeletal treatment is contraindicated in pregnant clients. Ultrasound should not be used on malignancies unless the client is selected for hypothermic cancer therapy. Intense sonation over bony growth plates should probably be avoided. As a final precaution the physical therapist should be aware of the sensorial-perception characteristics of the client since the dosage is, in great measure, determined by the client's ability to perceive heat and pain.

Phonophoresis

Phonophoresis is the driving of selected medications into biological tissues by the use of ultrasound. These medications, usually in the form of topical creams, are liberally applied to the skin over the target tissue. A coupling agent may be used in addition to the medications. Continuous sonation for periods up to 10 minutes effectively drives physiologically useful amounts of medication to a depth of about 5 cm.[19]

Three common medications used in the phonophoretic treatment of musculoskeletal conditions are hydrocortisone, lidocaine, and aspirin. Hydrocortisone in 1% or 10% concentrations is used in both acute and chronic inflammatory conditions, such as bursitis, tendonitis, and neuritis. Lidocaine, available in 5% preparations, can be used in conjunction with hydrocortisone or alone for its local anesthetic effect. Aspirin in a cream base is used for pain control and as an antiinflammatory agent. Although apparently less effective than hydrocortisone in treating inflammation, aspirin has fewer side effects and is available as an over-the-counter medication.

Combining phonophoresis and cold packs can be an effective approach to the treatment of acute conditions. Inertial neck injuries and muscle strains respond well to this approach. As yet, however, no controlled studies have verified these clinically observed assertions.

Phonophoresis should be used with care. A complete client history should be taken so as to rule out any potential complications because of allergies to the various medications.

Shortwave diathermy

As a deep-heating method, shortwave diathermy (SWD) is exceedingly effective. Large body parts, such as the back or thigh, and deep areas, such as the hip, can be treated well by SWD.

SWD generators most commonly used in the United States produce high-frequency electromagnetic waves with a length of 11 meters and a frequency of 27 megacycles. Biological tissues offer variable resistance to the passage of these waves. Certain tissues, such as fat, offer greater resistance than the other tissues to the electrical component of the electromagnetic wave. Therefore these tissues get proportionately hotter when the composition of the electromagnetic energy has a high electrical component. Conversely, muscle has a high electrolytic content and conducts the electrical portion with less resistance and less heat production. However, the magnetic component produces vibration of molecules in tissues with a high electrolytic content and produces a higher rise in temperature. Fat, which has a low electrolyte content, experiences less heating at the passage of magnetic waves.

Condensor electrodes and induction electrodes, two types of SWD electrodes, favor electrical and magnetic components of the electromagnetic waves, respectively, and are useful for different types of client conditions.

The SWD generator uses a pair of condensor electrodes and the client as the dielectric to form the condensor or electrical field. High-frequency electrical energy oscillates between the electrodes, and the client as the dielectric offers resistance to the passage of the energy. Tissue heating over muscle is achieved with condensor electrodes. Where heat is needed in deep joints, such as the hip, condensor shortwave diathermy may be most effective.

Induction electrodes function independently and thus can be used singly or in multiples. The client is not part of the circuit in this SWD setup. Eddy currents generated in the coil induce energy absorption by the client's tissues. Induction electrodes allow for more superficial heating, and muscle tends to become warmer than fatty tissues. When heat to superficial muscles or joints is indicated, induction electrode shortwave therapy may be used.

A number of thermal and nonthermal physiological effects have been attributed to SWD. Among the thermal effects are the elevation of muscle temperature to 42° C after a 20-minute application.[19] Increased blood flow into heated muscle occurs, and a concomitant increase in metabolism and relaxation of contractile fibers is experienced. Continued treatment at thermal doses tends to produce muscle weakness.[8] Interestingly enough, however, a *brief* intense heat treatment, such as a 5-minute session, may produce increased muscular strength.[43] Also blood flow to the extremities can be increased by heating the abdomen.

Some nonthermal effects have been observed after SWD treatment. Experimental studies using animal models have shown that wound healing is accelerated after nonthermal SWD.[6] Other findings have corroborated that phagocytosis at the site of trauma is increased and that surgically induced hematomas resolve more rapidly. In a clinical study of foot surgery clients, it was observed that clients treated at nonthermal doses required fewer medications and experienced a shorter length of hospital stay.[44]

SWD is usually administered in chronic conditions for periods of 20 minutes at output intensities producing perceived gentle warmth. A more modern approach is to treat the chronic condition briefly at rather intense output intensities and then treat it for longer periods of time at nonthermal doses. A ratio of 1:3 or 5:15 minutes of a thermal to nonthermal setting is commonly used. The as yet untested rationale is that the intense thermal dose acts as a counterirritant and produces a great surge in circulation. The nonthermal dose slows the flow of blood and acts to reduce pain. The latter dose is termed the *cooldown*.

Electrode placement is exceedingly important in effective SWD use. Fig. 8-5 demonstrates an excellent way of arranging condensor electrodes for knee and leg dysfunction. The lines of electromagnetic energy will tend to follow the length of the leg. Another satisfactory arrangement would be to place electrodes on either side of the knee. Care must be taken not to place the electrodes too close together as the heating will become too superficial. Superficial low-back pain or neck pain may be effectively treated by placing an induction electrode over the area of pain.

SWD should not be used in clients suspected of being pregnant or for clients with pacemakers or superficial metal implants. Clients with deeper metal implants, however, have been treated at nonthermal doses.

All metal objects should be removed from the client and

the surrounding area. This includes chairs and beds. All electrical apparatus should also be removed from the immediate area, and no electrical device should be in contact with the client. These precautions reduce the hazard of burn or electrical shock.

New areas of the use of SWD include treating nonunion fractures,[2] accelerating poor wound healing, and providing hyperthermic treatments for cancer patients.[36] The future holds great promise for SWD.

SUMMARY

Various types of physical agents that are more commonly used in physical therapy clinics have been discussed in this chapter. Low-volt electrical stimulation, represented by TENS, medium-frequency currents, high-voltage currents, and superficial and deep thermotherapies have been described. The general thesis of this chapter has been that musculoskeletal pain can be controlled through the judicious use of physical agents. The improvement of functional activities, however, such as gait and posture, using neuromuscular stimulators has not been discussed.

It must again be emphasized that physical agents allow the physical therapist to control pain and improve other physiological functions. The clinician must then implement other treatment strategies to rectify the cause of the pain or dysfunction.

REFERENCES

1. Alm WA, Gold ML, and Weil LS: Evaluation of transcutaneous electrical nerve stimulation (TENS) in podiatric surgery, J Am Podiatry Assoc 69:537, 1979.
2. Bassett CA, Mitchell S, and Gaston S: Pulsing electromagnetic field treatment in ununited fractures and failed arthrodeses, JAMA 5:247, 1982.
3. Bearzy H: Clinical application of ultrasonic energy in treatment of acute and chronic subacromial bursitis, Arch Phys Med Rehabil 34:228, 1953.
4. Bishop B: Pain, Parts 1, 2, and 3, Phys Ther 60:21, 1980.
5. Brunner GD: Can ultrasound be used in the presence of surgical metal implants? Phys Ther 38:823, 1958.
6. Cameron BM: Experimental acceleration of wound healing, Am J Orthop 37:336, 1961.
7. Carpenter M: Core text of neuroanatomy, Baltimore, 1978, Williams & Wilkins.
8. Chastain P: The effects of deep heat on isometric strength, Phys Ther 48(5):543, 1978.
9. Clarke R, Hellon R, and Lind A: The duration of sustained contractions of the human forearm at different muscle temperatures, J Physiol 143:454, 1958.
10. Currier DP: Electrical stimulation for improving muscular strength and blood flow. In Nelson RM and Currier DP, editors: Clinical electrotherapy, Norwalk, Conn, 1987, Appleton & Lange.
11. Cyriax J: Textbook of orthopaedic medicine, vol 1, Baltimore, 1975, Williams & Wilkins.
12. deJesus P, Hausmanowa-Petrusewicz S, and Barchi R: The effect of cold on nerve conduction of human slow and fast nerve fibers, Neurology 23:1182, 1973.
13. Edwards R et al: Effect of temperature on muscle energy metabolism and endurance during successive isometric contractions, sustained to fatigue, of the quadriceps muscle in man, J Physiol 220:335, 1972.
14. Ersek RA: Low-back pain: prompt relief with transcutaneous neurostimulation, Orthop Rev 5:12, 1976, pp. 27-31.
15. Garret TR, Laughman RK, and Youdas JW: Strengthening brought about by a new Canadian muscle stimulator: a preliminary study, Phys Ther 5(60):616, 1980.
16. Glass JM, Stephen RL, and Jacobsen SC: The quantity and distribution of radiolabeled dexamethasone delivered to tissues by iontophoresis, Int J Dermatol 19:519-522, 1980.
17. Goldman DE and Heuter TF: Tabulator data on velocity and absorption of high frequency sound in mammalian tissues, J Acoust Soc Am 28:35, 1956.
18. Gordon-Weinstein A: Sodium salicylate iontophoresis in treatment of plantar warts, Phys Ther 49(8):869, 1969.
19. Griffin J and Karselis T: Physical agents for physical therapists, Springfield, Ill, 1978, Charles C Thomas, Publisher.
20. Griffin JE, Touchstone JC, and Liu AC: Ultrasonic movement of cortisol in peg tissues. II. Peripheral nerve, Am J Phys Med 41:20, 1965.
21. Harvie KW: A major advance in the control of postoperative knee pain, Orthopedics 2:129, 1979.
22. Henneman E, Somjen G, Carpenter D: Functional significance of cell size in spinal motoneurons, J Neurophysiology 28:560-580, 1965.
23. Hodgman C, Weast R, and Selby S: Handbook of chemistry and physics, ed 37, Cleveland, 1981, Chemical Rubber Publishing.
24. Indeck W and Printy A: Skin application of electrical impulses for relief of pain, Minn Med 17:305, 1975.
25. Kahn J: Acetic acid iontophoresis for calcific deposits, J Pi Theta Phi 26:357, 1956.
26. Kahn J: Calcium iontophoresis in suspected myopathy, Phys Ther 55(4):276, 1975.
27. Kahn J: Low volt technique, Syosset, NY, 1976, J Kahn.
28. Kloth LC and Feedar JA: Acceleration of wound healing with high voltage, monophasic, pulsed current, Phys Ther 68(4).503-508, 1988.
29. Kots YM: Electrostimulation. Paper presented at the Canadian-Soviet Exchange Symposium on electrostimulation of skeletal muscle, Concordia University, Montreal, December 6-10, 1977.
30. Kramer JF and Mendryk SW: Electrical stimulation as a strength improvement technique: a review, J Orthop Sports Phys Ther 4(2):91, 1982.
31. Kurilova LM: The skin temperature analyzer, Institute of Normal and Pathological Physiology, New York, 1972, Plenum Publishing Corp.
32. Lehmann JF: Effects of therapeutic temperature on tendon extensibility, Arch Phys Med Rehabil 51:481, 1970.
33. Lehmann JF et al: Temperature distributions in the human thigh produced by infrared, hot pack and microwave applications, Arch Phys Med Rehabil 47:291, 1966.
34. Melzack R and Wall PD: Pain mechanisms: a new theory, Science 150:971, 1965.
35. Outline of Chinese acupuncture, Peking, 1975, Peking Foreign Language Press.
36. Overgaard J: Biological effect of 27.12 MHz shortwave diathermic heating in experimental tumors, IEEE transactions of microwave theory and technique, vol MTT-26:93, 1978.
37. Pike PMH: Transcutaneous electrical nerve stimulation: its uses in the management of postoperative pain, Anaesthesia 33:165, 1978.
38. Roeser WM et al: The use of transcutaneous nerve stimulation for pain control in athletic medicine: a preliminary report, Am J Sports Med 4:5, 1976.
39. Russo J et al: Lidocaine anesthesia: comparison of iontophoresis, injection and swabbing, Am J Hosp Pharm 37:843, 1980.
40. Santiesteban AJ: Electroacupuncture and low back pain, Phys Ther 60(5):618, 1980.

41. Santiesteban AJ: Applications of transcutaneous electrical nerve stimulation for post-operative, cardiopulmonary, and obstetrics patients. In Wolf S, editor: Electrotherapy, New York, 1981, Churchill Livingstone, Inc.

42. Santiesteban AJ: Selected physiological properties of shortwave therapy, Phys Ther 61(5):738, 1981.

43. Santiesteban AJ and Grant C: Effects of pulsed diathermy following foot surgery, Phys Ther 59(5):560, 1979.

44. Santiesteban AJ and Ostrow D: Effects of electric currents on cutaneous sensation and joint position sense. Paper presented at APTA, June 1988.

45. Shriber WJ: A manual of electrotherapy, 1975, Philadelphia, Lea & Febiger.

46. Stabile ML and Mallory TH: The management of postoperative pain in total hip joint replacement, Orthop Rev 7:121, 1978.

47. Szeke E and David E: The stereodynamic interferential current: new electrotherapeutic technique, Electromedica 48(1):13, 1980.

48. Thom H: Stereodynamic interferential current therapy: fundamentals and initial results, Electromedica 48(1):18, 1980.

49. Touchstone JC, Griffin JE, and Kasparon M: Cortisol in human nerve, Science 142:1275, 1963.

50. Wolff MK, Lewis JA, and Simon RH: Experiences with electrical stimulation devices for the control of chronic pain, Med Instrum 9:5, 1975.

51. Zimmerman M: Peripheral and central nervous mechanism of nociception, pain, and pain therapy: facts and hypotheses. In Bonica J, editor: Advances in pain research and therapy, New York, 1979, Raven Press.

Chapter 9

BASIC CONCEPTS OF ORTHOPAEDIC MANUAL THERAPY

Tzvi Barak
Elaine R. Rosen
Roslyn Sofer

Orthopaedic manual therapy is one of the most rapidly growing specialty areas in the field of physical therapy today. The perspective from which therapists approach a client with a neuromusculoskeletal problem is rapidly chang-ing from following a set of prescribed exercises to performing a detailed evaluation from which a treatment plan can be formulated and directed toward restoring normal function.

Orthopaedic manual therapy can be defined as a systematic method of evaluating and treating dysfunctions of the neuromusculoskeletal system in order to relieve pain, increase or decrease mobility, and, in general, normalize function.

The purpose of this chapter is to help the reader develop a more comprehensive understanding of orthopaedic manual therapy.

HISTORY OF MANUAL THERAPY

Manipulation of the soft tissues is one of the oldest forms of physical therapy mentioned in ancient medical records. Hippocrates (460-380 BC) in his book, *Corpus Hippocrates,* listed methods of treatment that are comparable to mobilization techniques used today.[1] Speaking of articulation, he described how to reduce a fracture through the use of traction and mobilization by distending the part and then adjusting it with the palm of the hand.[4] In his chapter on surgery Hippocrates also indicated that exercise provided strengthening benefits and inactivity resulted in muscle wasting.[3,4] Teachings on fractures and dislocations by Galen (131-202 AD) surpassed even those of Hippocrates.[2] Galen recommended that an injured part be moved cautiously after the application of heat.[2] He also described how to treat outwardly dislocated vertebrae. His theories remained undisputed until the sixteenth century.[28]

However, it was Hippocrates who made the first mention of graded mobilization without producing pain. He suggested that a dislocated shoulder could be treated by "rubbing" it and moving it gently so as not to produce pain. He stated that this would heal a joint that was too "loose" and loosen a joint that was stiff.[3,4]

During the Renaissance Ambroise Paré, a well-known physician, described in detail how to treat dislocation by manipulation.[5] He advised a procedure in which an individual was tied prone on a board with ropes under the armpits and around the wrists and thighs. The person was then "pulled and stretched," and downward pressure was given to a kyphosis.[28]

In seventeenth-century England the practice of bone-setting became popular. Techniques of the bone-setters were kept secret within the family profession and were passed down from generation to generation. They believed in manipulation of the limbs and spine in order to relocate a bone that was out of place. The bone-setters were especially successful in treating six common types of disorders[28]:

1. Stiffness and pain in joints that were immobilized for a long period of time after fractures, dislocations, or sprains
2. Stiffness and pain resulting from disuse after soft tissue injuries
3. Internal derangements after rupture of the meniscus
4. Subluxations of small bones of the hands and feet
5. Ganglion development around the wrist
6. Treatment of neck and back disorders

In fact, medical literature from ancient times to the nineteenth century consistently advocated massage and manipulation but did not always clearly differentiate between the two. Graham (1884-1918) of Boston stated that massage denoted any procedure done by the hands and went on to mention friction and manipulation as examples.[28] William Merrell (1853-1912) of London defined massage as a scientific mode of treating certain forms of disease by scientific manipulation.[2] It is apparent that the term *massage* came to have multiple connotations, including passive range of motion, mobilization, and manipulation, during the course of medical history. In any case, whatever the meaning of the term, many in Europe advocated manipulation or passive movement, although orthodox medicine did not accept this view.[28]

Two categories of healers—osteopaths and chiropractors—developed in the United States. They were competitive and today are completely independent of each other. Initially both advocated treatment of all diseases by manipulation. This enraged the medical profession and caused it to disregard manipulation as a viable treatment technique.

Andrew Taylor Still (1828-1917) introduced osteopathy in 1871 in the United States.[26] His main tenets were that the body as a unit had the ability to fight off all diseases and that the cause of all disease was mechanical pressure on blood vessels and nerves produced by dislocated bones, abnormal ligaments, or contracted muscles in the back.[7,28] Still[7] called this mechanical pressure the osteopathic lesion, and it became the basis of his treatment system.

Daniel David Palmer (1845-1914) founded chiropractic in 1895. The original concept of chiropractic was to put bones back into place. Two groups developed—the "straights" and the "mixers." The "straights" hold to the original belief that disturbed nerve function is responsible for most illnesses and that structural adjustments are necessary to normalize nerve function, thereby restoring and maintaining health.[27] The "mixers" similarly believe in the science of treating human ailments by manipulation and adjustments of the spine and other structures of the human body, but they also advocate the use of other mechanical, physiotherapeutic, and nutritional measures, excluding drugs and major surgery.[27,28]

Within the last 100 years there have been major advances in the fields of medicine and surgery, but there has been resistance by the traditional medical community to the development and use of orthopaedic manual therapy. In spite of this, several schools of thought have developed within the past 50 years. Paris[26] has summarized the principal goals shared by these schools:

1. Relief of nerve-root pressure—relating only to the spine.
   a. Specific—chiropractors recommend the movement of one specific vertebra on another.
   b. Nonspecific—Cyriax[6,7] recommended general manipulation with traction.
2. Relief of pain—relating to the spine or extremities.
   a. Graded oscillations—Maitland[19,20] believes in mobilizations subthreshold to pain.
   b. Contrary movement—Maigne[18] recommends therapeutic movement in a direction exactly opposite to that which causes pain.
3. Normalization of joint mobility—relating to the spine or extremities.
   a. Osteopathy—osteopaths advocate specific techniques for mobilizing the spine and extremities.
   b. Treatment of stiffness—Kaltenborn[13] advocates the use of arthrokinematic principles to regain mobility without regard to pain.

There are many approaches to the treatment of musculoskeletal dysfunctions. The discrepancies usually relate to the cause of the dysfunction and treatment of pain. Chiropractors believe that all disturbances are caused by pressure on nerves and can be cured by adjustments. The medical profession, however, still reacts very negatively to this concept. Osteopaths, on the other hand, are concerned with maintaining and establishing normal structural integrity of the body through the use of diverse methods, including medication, nutrition, surgery, and possibly manipulation. In fact, they have changed their methods in accordance with medical advances and are now recognized as physicians by the allopathic medical profession in all states.

Cyriax,[6] a British orthopaedist, believed that almost all spinal pain arose from a disruption of disks, which could be reduced by manipulation and traction. He was an enthusiastic proponent of the use of manipulation by qualified physical therapists because of their training and expertise in understanding the musculoskeletal system. Maitland,[20] a physical therapist from Australia, has developed a system of dealing with a client's signs and symptoms through treatment with graded oscillations.[13] Kaltenborn and other members of a Scandinavian group of physical therapists categorize spinal dysfunctions into two main disorders: disk degeneration and facet dysfunction.[13] Treatment is determined by loss of mobility and the presence of pain. Pain is treated with standard physical therapy techniques, including thermal applications, electrical modalities, special massage methods, and contract-relax procedures. Loss of mobility is treated by localizing the level of the lesion, locking the joints above and below, and then delivering a thrust with minimum force in the direction of the limitation in order to normalize the movement of the joint. The divergence in focus of treatment between Maitland's and Kaltenborn's approaches may possibly be explained by the acuteness of the pain and dysfunction a client experiences when initially referred to physical therapy. McKenzie, a physical therapist from New Zealand, developed a method of classification of low back pain. It includes postural syndrome, dysfunction syndrome, and derangement syndrome. He proposed that the use of both passive extension and flexion be used for the treatment of cervical and lumbar pain. In addition, he is a great proponent of teaching patients self-reliance, so they can be responsible for their own care in the event of future exacerbations.[21]

Paris, a physical therapist from New Zealand, unlike Maitland and Kaltenborn, has advanced a concept of facet disorder as the primary cause of spinal dysfunction. In the early 1970s Paris initiated courses in mobilization and manipulation for physical therapists in the United States. His efforts brought about a drastic change in the thinking of physical therapists, from a traditional prescriptive mode to a more thorough examination and appropriate treatment mode.

CLASSIFICATION OF EXERCISES

Exercise can be divided into two basic categories: active and passive (Fig. 9-1).

Active exercise

Active exercises can be divided into three subcategories: isotonic, isometric, and isokinetic. *Isotonic exercise* involves movement through full or partial range of motion with the same weight used as resistance throughout the entire movement. *Isometric exercise* involves a buildup of

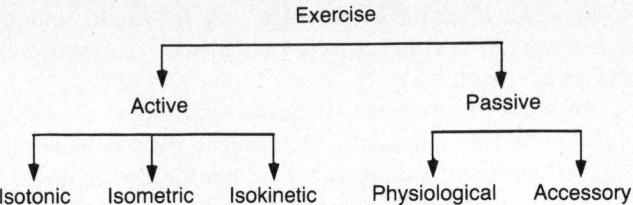

Fig. 9-1. Categories of exercise.

tone in a muscle group without movement of the body part through any portion of the range of motion. *Isokinetic exercise* is a method of exercising in which speed is held constant so that, as the force applied by the body part increases, the accommodating resistance encountered increases. Maximum resistance can therefore be achieved at finite points in the range of motion.

Passive exercise

Passive exercise can be divided into two subcategories: physiological movement and accessory movement. Passive *physiological movement* is the creation of motion within a joint by an outside force taking the body part through all or part of its range of motion. Passive *accessory movement*, on the other hand, is movement that occurs between the articulating surfaces of a joint that is involved in a physiological motion, either active or passive. Such movement is described by the words *glide*, *spin*, or *roll*, which will be discussed later in this chapter. Accessory movements cannot be produced actively—that is, the client cannot voluntarily perform the accessory movements of glide, spin, or roll. They occur automatically in conjunction with active physiological movement. Physiological movements, of course, can also be performed passively by the therapist. Accessory movements, when performed passively by the therapist, comprise a large portion of the manipulation done in manual therapy. However, there are, as yet, no standards of what is "normal" for accessory movement, as there are for physiological movement.

Physiological movement. Throughout the history of physical therapy the primary method used for improving range of motion has been passive physiological movement (i.e., passive range of motion). In this method the body part is moved through its range of motion by an outside force, such as the therapist or a pulley. In the past if a limitation of motion existed, there was usually no attempt to define the cause of the limitation. Attempts to improve range of motion were often done through sustained or oscillating stretch. However, this type of stretch can stimulate pain receptors and cause contraction of the muscles antagonistic to the desired motion. If the cause of the limitation was muscular, there was some chance of improving range of motion with "standard" techniques. However, if the cause of the limitation was tightness of the joint capsule or ligaments around the joint, full range of motion could never be achieved since the muscles would stop the movement before the capsule or ligaments reached their maximum length.

Accessory movement. Accessory movement can be divided into two categories: component motion and joint play. *Component motion* is the motion occurring in a related joint that allows the primary joint to function normally. For example, in order for full shoulder flexion to occur, there must also be specific movements occurring at the acromioclavicular, sternoclavicular, and scapulothoracic joints and the thoracic spine. If any of these movements are restricted, shoulder flexion will be limited and/ or painful. *Joint play* may be defined as the motion that occurs within the joint as a response to an outside force but not as a result of voluntary movement. For example, when a ball is gripped, the force of the ball against the fingers causes rotation of the metacarpophalangeal joints so that a spherical grip can be attained. This rotation is a joint play motion and does not occur in conjunction with flexion, extension, abduction, or adduction of the fingers.

Physiological movement comprises large ranges of motion that are measured in degrees. The position of the arm that is in humeral flexion is commonly understood and can be visualized. Accessory motion, on the other hand, although it has not been formally measured, can be thought of only in terms of millimeters.

Gradations of movement. In order to have a common ground for communication, the total accessory and/or physiological movement available in one direction can be determined, according to Maitland,[19] by five gradations of oscillations (Fig. 9-2, *A*):

1. *Grade I* is a small-amplitude movement conducted from the beginning of the available range of motion.
2. *Grade II* is a large-amplitude movement conducted within the range. It does not reach either end of the range of motion.
3. *Grade III* is a large-amplitude movement that does reach the end of the range of motion.
4. *Grade IV* is a small-amplitude movement conducted at the very end of the range of motion.
5. *Grade V* is a high-velocity thrust of small amplitude at the end of the available range of motion and within its anatomical range. It is usually accompanied by a popping sound and is called a *manipulation*. The accompanying pop or snap cannot be definitely explained, but there are a few theories. The popping sound could be caused by (1) the release of gases or fluids when joint surfaces are suddenly separated due to the internal negative pressure;[15,23] (2) Tearing of the adhesions;[26] or (3) Replacement of subluxation or replacement of disk matter.[26]

Although all five gradations of movement may be applied to either accessory or physiological movements, the grades most commonly used are II, III, and IV.

Therapists should remember that they are dealing with joints that have a limitation of movement (Fig. 9-2, *B*). As the limitation (point L) decreases, point L moves to the right. Therefore all the grades of movement also shift to the right toward the anatomical limit. However, the relationship between each grade always remains constant.

Since the introduction of the concept of accessory movement into the realm of physical therapy, treating restrictions of movement caused by tightness of joint structures has been revolutionized. Clinicians can now elongate joint structures by oscillating or stretching the joint in the direction of the accessory movement that is restricted. This type of stretching can provide the freedom of movement required to improve the physiological range of motion.

Joint mobilization, as the term is used today, can be defined as the attempt to improve joint mobility or decrease pain originating in joint structures by using selected grades of accessory movements. Table 9-1 is a comparison between accessory and physiological movement techniques.

When is it appropriate to use mobilization and/or manipulation techniques? Paris[26] has developed a system of classification of joint status that more clearly defines the indications and contraindications for mobilization and manipulation (Table 9-2).

CLASSIFICATION OF SYNOVIAL JOINTS

Since synovial joints are treated with the use of mobilization and manipulation techniques, it is important to know the characteristics of these joints and their different classifications.

An anatomical synovial joint is composed of two articular surfaces and their surrounding capsules, ligaments, and intraarticular structures. It can also be considered a physiological joint when the anatomical joint includes the

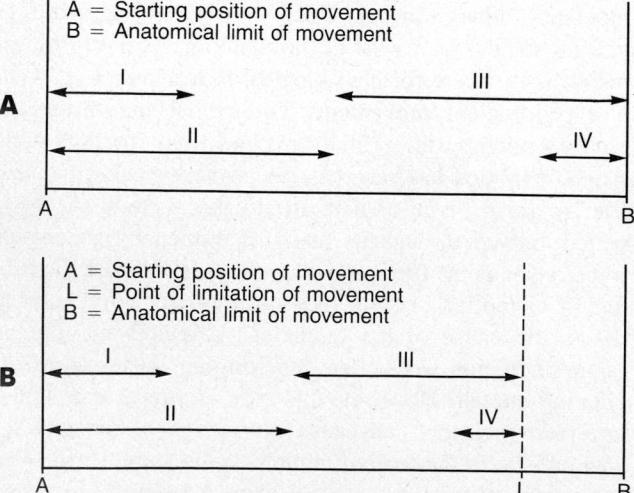

Fig. 9-2. A, Grades of oscillations used in manual therapy. **B,** Grades of oscillations used in manual therapy in relation to a joint with limited motion.

soft tissue around the joint—muscles, connective tissue, nerves, and blood vessels.[10] Anatomical synovial joints can be classified as simple, compound, and complex.[31] An anatomically simple joint is one that has only one joint space with two surfaces (one concave and one convex) and a single capsule—for example, the metacarpophalangeal joint. A compound joint has more than two articulating surfaces within a single capsule—for instance, the elbow. A complex joint, best exemplified by the knee, is an anatomically compound joint with a meniscus or intracapsular disk.[31]

In addition to being simple, compound, or complex, synovial joints have been classified according to their articular surface by MacConaill and Basmajian.[17] Four structural forms of joint-articulating surfaces have been delineated (Fig. 9-3):

1. *Unmodified ovoid*—ball-and-socket articulation in which the surface is spheroid, having three axes and allowing 3 degrees* of freedom of motion. The best examples of these articulations are the hip and the shoulder joints.
2. *Modified ovoid*—ellipsoid and sellar articulation where the surfaces are convex or concave in all directions. These joints have two axes and allow 2 degrees of freedom of motion. The best examples are the metacarpophalangeal joints.
3. *Unmodified sellar*—saddle articulation where the surfaces are convex and concave at right angles to one another. These joints have two axes and allow 2 degrees of freedom of motion. They are usually accompanied by a loose capsule, which allows an easy direction change. The best example of this type of joint is the first carpometacarpal joint.
4. *Modified sellar*—a hinge, ginglymus, or trochoid joint with one axis and 1 degree of freedom of motion. The best examples are the interphalangeal joints of the fingers, the ulnohumeral joint, and the knee.[12]

JOINT POSITIONS—CONGRUENCE

Analysis of joint positions is essential to understanding disorders of the joint and their treatment. Articulating surfaces are rarely, if ever, in total congruence. The area of weight bearing or use during any particular point in the joint's range of motion is relatively small compared to the total surface area. This allows for better lubrication and recovery time for the articular surfaces. As the articulating surfaces move through their range of motion, there will be times when very little of the surface area is in contact with the joint and the capsule is loose and other times when

*The term *degrees*, in this sense, refers to the number of available movements.

Table 9-1. Comparison of accessory and physiological movement

Accessory movement techniques	Physiological movement techniques
Used when primary resistance is encountered from the ligament and capsule of the joint and there is minimal muscular resistance	Used when primary resistance encountered is muscular
Can be done in any part of the physiological range of motion	Is effective only at the end of the physiological range of motion
Can be done in any direction (posteriorly, caudally, or anteriorly)	Is limited to one direction
Causes less pain per degree of range of motion gained	Causes more pain per degree of range of motion gained
Used for tight articular structures	Used for tight muscular structures
Is a safer method because it employs short lever-arm techniques	Is a less safe method because it employs long lever-arm techniques

Table 9-2. Classification of joint status

Grade	Definition	Possibilities for treatment
0	No movement, joint is ankylosed	No attempts should be made to mobilize
1	Extremely hypomobile	Use mobilization
2	Slightly hypomobile	May use mobilization or manipulation
3	Normal	No dysfunction; no treatment needed
4	Slightly hypermobile	Look for areas of hypomobility in surrounding joints (one above and one below). If found, treat the hypomobile joint. Exercise, taping, wrapping, or corset may be used to decrease hypermobile joint
5	Extremely hypermobile	Look for areas of hypomobility. Stabilize hypermobile joint using exercise techniques or splinting
6	Hypermobile to the point of instability	Bracing, splinting, casting, or surgery are possibilities for stabilization. Exercise is usually not effective in decreasing this amount of instability

Modified from Paris SV: The spine: course notebook, Atlanta, 1979, Institute Press.

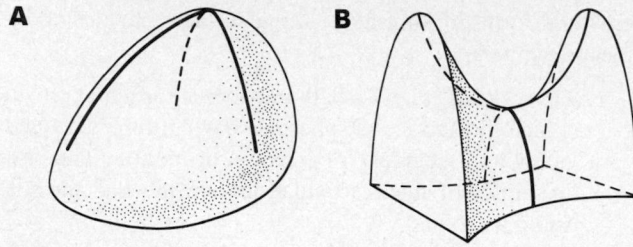

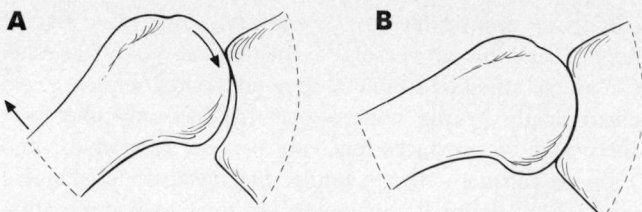

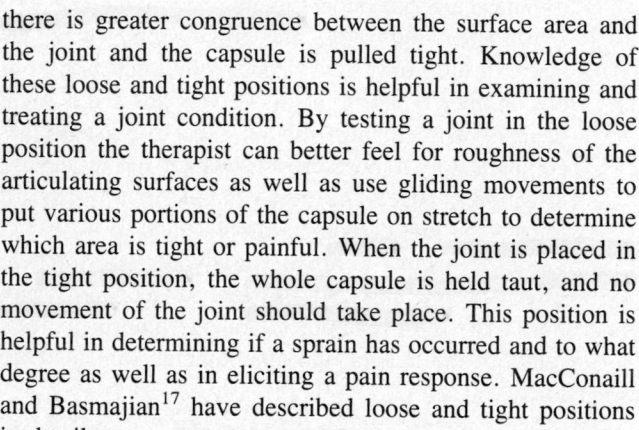

Fig. 9-3. Two basic types of articular surfaces: **A,** ovoid; **B,** sellar.

Fig. 9-4. The congruence of articular surfaces: **A,** loose-packed position; **B,** close-packed position.

there is greater congruence between the surface area and the joint and the capsule is pulled tight. Knowledge of these loose and tight positions is helpful in examining and treating a joint condition. By testing a joint in the loose position the therapist can better feel for roughness of the articulating surfaces as well as use gliding movements to put various portions of the capsule on stretch to determine which area is tight or painful. When the joint is placed in the tight position, the whole capsule is held taut, and no movement of the joint should take place. This position is helpful in determining if a sprain has occurred and to what degree as well as in eliciting a pain response. MacConaill and Basmajian[17] have described loose and tight positions in detail.

The *close-packed position* occurs when the joint surfaces are the most congruent—that is, a concave fits point for point in a convex (Fig. 9-4). In a close-packed position the major ligaments are maximally taut, the intracapsular space is minimal, and the surfaces cannot be pulled apart by traction forces. This position is used as a testing position but is never used for mobilization because there are no degrees of freedom of movement. Examples of the close-packed position are the knee in full extension, the interphalangeal joints in full extension, and the elbow in full extension with the forearm supinated.

The *loose-packed position* is any other position of the joint aside from the close-packed position. The maximal loose-packed position is known as the resting position. This occurs when the surrounding tissues are as lax as possible and the intracapsular space is at its greatest. The loose-packed position is the joint position that should be sought following joint trauma and subsequent effusion since this position allows room for maximal fluid accumulation. This maximally loose or resting position of the joint is the optimal position for joint mobilization. Examples of resting positions are the elbow flexed to 70 degrees and 10 degrees of supination or the knee in 30 degrees of flexion with a slight external rotation of the tibia. All joint-resting positions are described in Kaltenborn.[13]

OSTEOKINEMATICS AND ARTHROKINEMATICS

In order to have a more thorough understanding of mobilization techniques and assessment, it is necessary to be aware of the movements that occur in the joints and movements of the bones. Traditionally, kinesiology has dealt with gross movements of the limbs, controlled by muscles, around the cardinal axes. These anatomical movements have been referred to as flexion/extension, abduction/adduction, and internal/external rotation.

However, physiological bone movements are a combination of movements that are seen frequently in the activities of daily living—such as eating—and in therapeutic exercises that use diagonal patterns, such as proprioceptive neuromuscular facilitation (PNF). It was not until MacConaill and Basmajian[17] introduced a new classification of movement that clinicians became fully cognizant of bone movements as being independent of joint movements. Kinematics, the study of such movements, can therefore be broken down into two subdivisions: (1) osteokinematics, the study of movement of the bone, and (2) arthrokinematics, the study of movements at the joint.

Osteokinematics

MacConaill and Basmajian[17] have classified *bone movements*—osteokinematics—in two ways: spin and swing. *Spin* is described as a pure rotation around a mechanical axis. This rotation can be either clockwise or counterclockwise and is not accompanied by any other type of movement. A pure spin can occur only at the head of the femur, humerus, and radius.

Swing is any movement other than pure spin. It can be subdivided into (1) pure or cardinal swing and (2) impure or arcuate swing. In pure swing the movement is not simultaneous with a spin, and the movement, therefore, traverses the shortest route between two points. In impure swing rotation occurs simultaneously, and therefore the distance between two points is greater than in pure swing (Fig. 9-5).

A bone can move about one or more of the three mutually perpendicular axes: vertical, horizontal, and anteroposterior. (The number of available movements is known as the number of degrees of freedom available.) Even if the joint is multiaxial, it is still considered to have three degrees of freedom. For example, the shoulder joint is a ball-and-socket joint with 3 degrees of freedom: flexion/

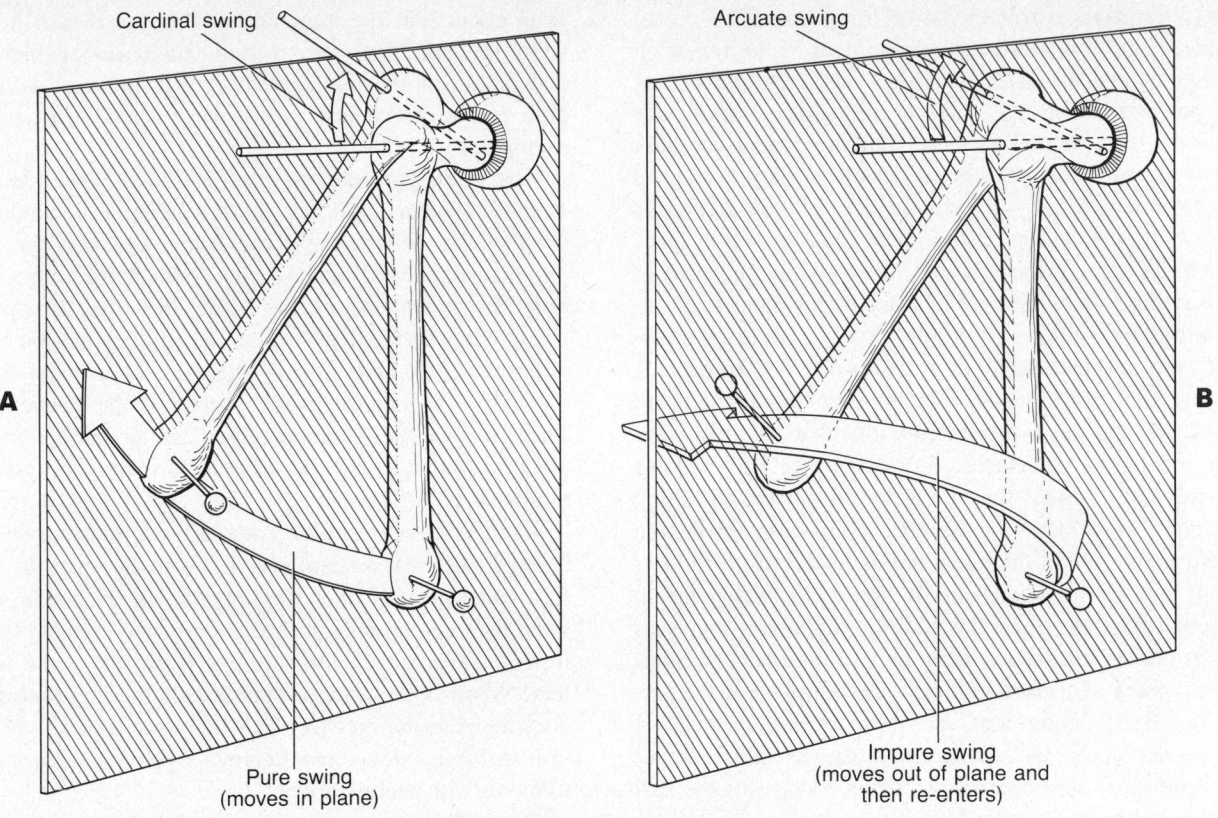

Fig. 9-5. MacConaill's classification of swing: **A,** pure swing; **B,** arcuate swing.

extension, abduction/adduction, and internal/external rotation. This freedom can only occur in the loose-packed position.

Arthrokinematics

According to *Gray's Anatomy* the conventional division of *joint movements* includes gliding, angular movements, circumduction, and rotation. Gliding or translation occurs when an arc surface simply slides over another surface without adding a component of angulation or rotation. Gliding is usually accompanied by some other motion but may take place purely in some carpal and tarsal articulations.[31]

Angular movement is the increase or decrease in the angle formed between adjacent bones, best illustrated in extension. Circumduction occurs when the bone follows a conical outline. *Rotation* is an imprecise term used to describe movement around a longitudinal axis.[31]

MacConaill and Basmajian[17] have described certain important *accessory movements* of the joint—arthrokinematics—as spin, glide, and roll (Fig. 9-6). *Spin* is rotation around a stationary mechanical axis and is similar to the spin in osteokinematics. *Gliding* or *sliding* occurs when one point on a moving surface comes into contact with new points on another surface. Pure gliding can occur only when the two surfaces are congruent and flat or congruent and curved. It only occurs as an involuntary motion and

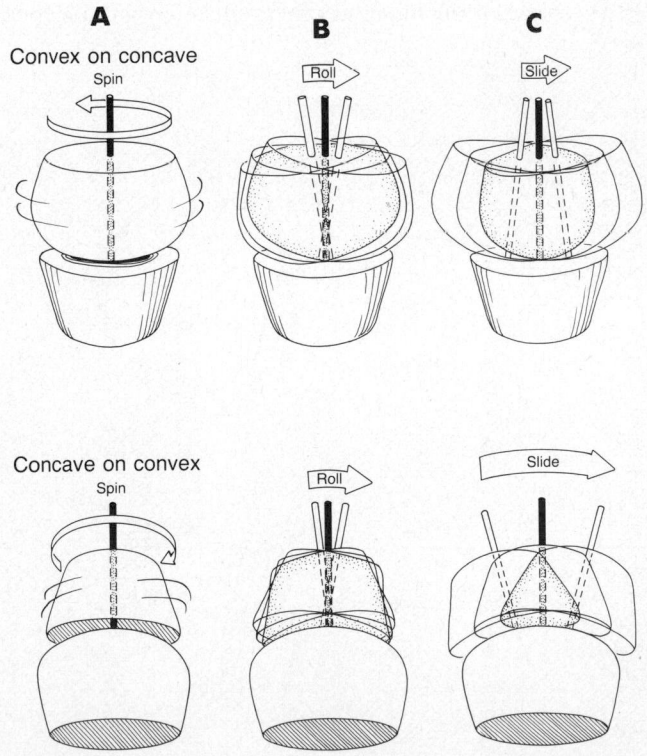

Fig. 9-6. MacConaill's classification of accessory movements: **A,** spin; **B,** roll; **C,** glide.

can be referred to as *translation* or *translatory glide*.[12] An example of glide would be the movement of the femur on the tibia during an anterior drawer test. *Rolling* occurs when new points on one surface come into contact with new points on a second surface. This movement can only occur if the surfaces are not congruent and is prevalent in joint movement when a convex surface rolls on a concave surface.[13] If pure rolling occurs, there is a decrease in space between the joint surfaces on the side to which the shaft of bone is going and an increase in space on the other side.

Rolling and gliding motions usually occur simultaneously but not necessarily in proportion to one another. A roll-glide joint movement combination occurs as the result of all active and passive bone rotations that take place between incongruent surfaces—for example, in the knee joint. Kapandji[14] notes that the proportion between rolling and gliding movements in the knee joint varies in flexion and extension. When the knee begins to flex from full extension, pure rolling occurs in the first 10 to 15 degrees on the medial condyle; then the sliding component increases until the end of the range, when pure sliding occurs. Kaltenborn[13] notes that more gliding will take place if the surfaces are nearly congruent and more rolling if they are more incongruent. The direction of the roll-glide movement depends on the convex or concave shape of the surface that is moving (Fig. 9-7).

The rolling portion of the combined roll-glide movement always follows the direction of the bone movement, regardless of whether the surface is convex or concave. For example, if the humerus moves in an upward direction

as in abduction, the humeral head will also roll in an upward direction. This pure rolling can cause compression or dislocation of the joint and is rarely found in a joint. A pure rolling movement is not used when mobilization is performed.[13]

The gliding portion of the combined roll-glide movement, however, follows a set pattern, depending on whether the moving surface is convex or concave. If the moving surface is concave, then both the gliding and the bone movement follow the same direction. However, if the moving surface is convex, the gliding motion will be opposite to the direction of the bone movement because the axis of rotation always occurs in the convex bone. Therefore in the shoulder joint, when abduction takes place, rolling occurs in an upward direction and gliding in a downward direction.

Convex-concave rule. All synovial joints are classified as either convex or concave. Even if the surfaces appear flat, cartilage will alter the contour. In a convex surface there is more cartilage at the center of the surface, whereas in a concave surface the cartilage is greater at the perimeters. When both surfaces appear flat, the larger surface is considered to be convex. The therapist should pay attention to these rules when treating a client who has a dysfunction with mobilization.

When the concave surface is stationary and the convex surface is moving, the gliding movement in the joint occurs in a direction opposite to the bone movement. This is because a particular axis of rotation is always being maintained in the convex bone. Therefore if the therapist wants

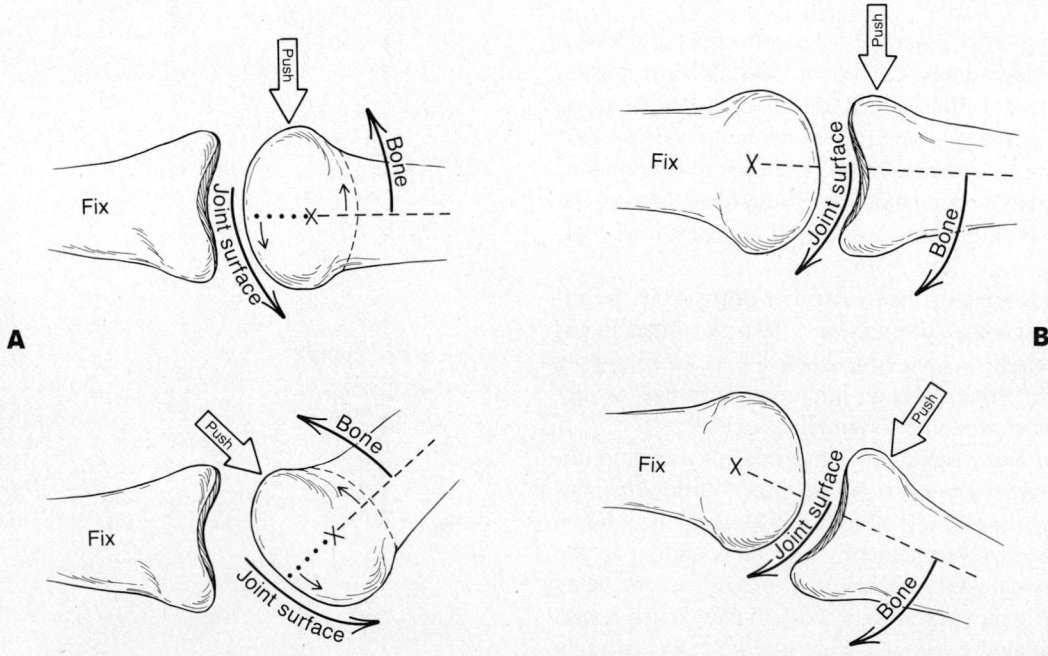

Fig. 9-7. A, Convex surface moving on concave surface. **B,** Concave surface moving on convex surface with a combination of roll, spin, and glide occurring in both simultaneously.

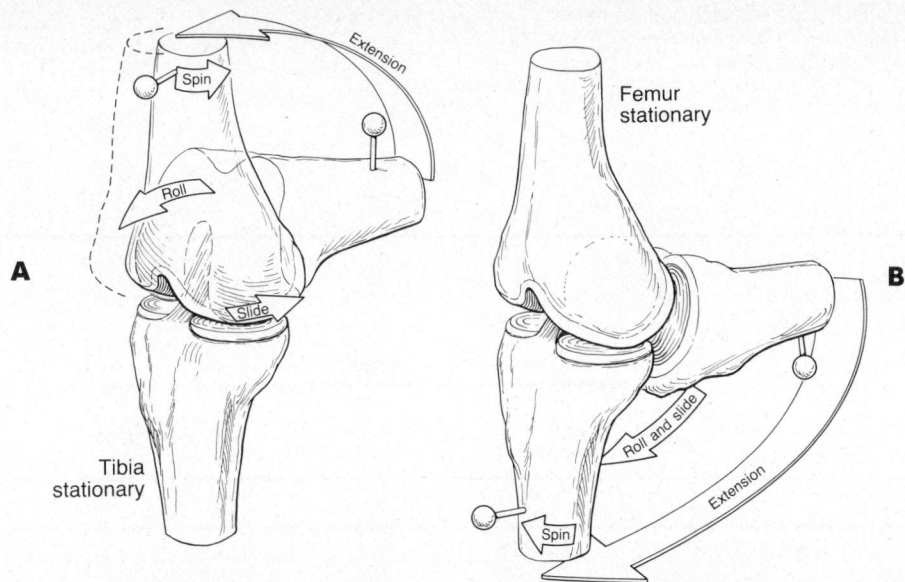

Fig. 9-8. Convex-concave rule: **A,** convex moving on concave; **B,** concave moving on convex.

to increase the range of motion of flexion in a hypomobile glenohumeral joint, the head of the humerus should be glided in a caudal or downward direction even though the humerus itself is moving upward (see Chapter 20 for specific techniques).

When the convex surface is stationary and the concave surface is moving, the gliding movement in the joint occurs in the same direction as the bone movement. This is also because of a particular axis of rotation that is always occurring in the convex bone so that the concave bone is moving along an established plane of movement. Therefore if the therapist wants to increase flexion in the knee joint, the proximal tibia should be mobilized in a posterior direction while at the same time the distal tibia is moving in a posterior direction (Fig. 9-8).

Traction. Traction can be divided into three stages or grades. Stage I[13] or grade I[19] is *piccolo traction,* which involves neutralizing pressure in the joint without actually separating the joint surfaces. This is used for pain relief and to prevent the trauma of grinding when performing mobilization techniques. Stage II[13] or grade IV[19] traction actually separates the joint surfaces and takes up the slack in the joint capsule. *Slack* is defined as the amount of looseness or play allowed by the capsule and ligaments in a normal joint. Stage II is also used to relieve pain. Stage III[13] or grade IV+,[19] traction involves an actual stretching of the soft tissues and is used to increase the mobility in a hypomobile joint. Traction and translatoric gliding can be applied separately or together in various mobilization techniques (Fig. 9-9).

Translatoric gliding can be used to increase mobility in a hypomobile joint by following the convex-concave rule after determining which specific movement is limited dur-

ing the examination. The translatoric glide is preceded by piccolo or grade I traction to eliminate the compressive forces (Fig. 9-10).

Traction as a treatment modality. Traction or long axis extension can be applied manually or mechanically.

Manual traction may be used as a treatment modality by following the principles mentioned in the previous section.

Mechanical units allow for the choice of intermittent, progressive intermittent, static, and progressive static traction.

Three-dimensional traction is a unique way of performing specific movement on a joint relative to all three cardinal planes. The therapist may specifically separate a facet joint by altering the client's position relative to flexion, lateral flexion, and rotation. This technique can be facilitated by using a multiaxial mobilization table.

Autotraction is a unique method of using three-dimensional positioning on a specially designed autotraction table that allows the patient to apply the traction force. The autotraction method was developed by Emil Natchev, M.D., a general surgeon from Stockholm.[25]

DIFFERENTIAL DIAGNOSIS OF SOFT TISSUE LESIONS

The proper use of mobilization hastens healing, reduces disability, relieves pain, and usually restores full range of motion.[33] A thorough, precise examination of the client's neuromuscular dysfunction must be performed by the physical therapist in order for an appropriate treatment program to be formulated. Dysfunction of the moving parts of the body occurs frequently and produces symptoms resembling any number of disorders. Each dysfunction requires a different treatment.

A = Beginning of range—joint surfaces approximated
L = Limitation of range due to dysfunction
B = End of normal anatomical range

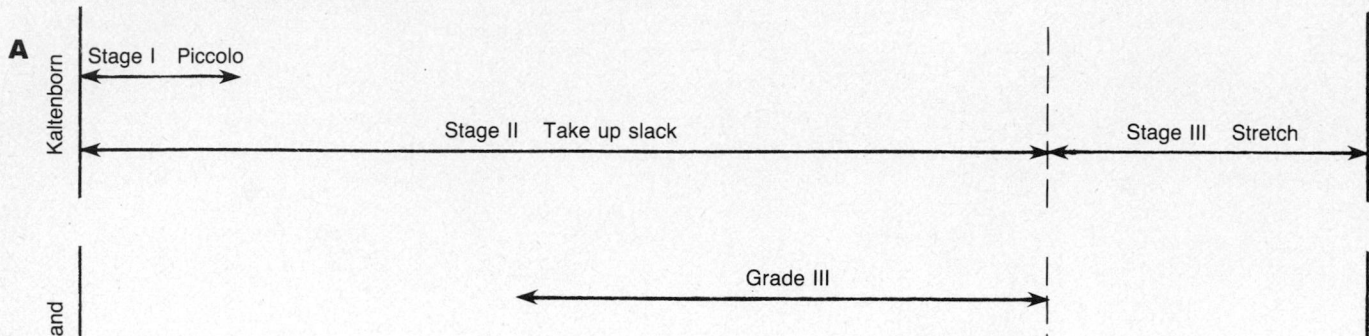

Fig. 9-9. Comparison of **A,** Kaltenborn's and **B,** Maitland's range of mobilization technique applications.

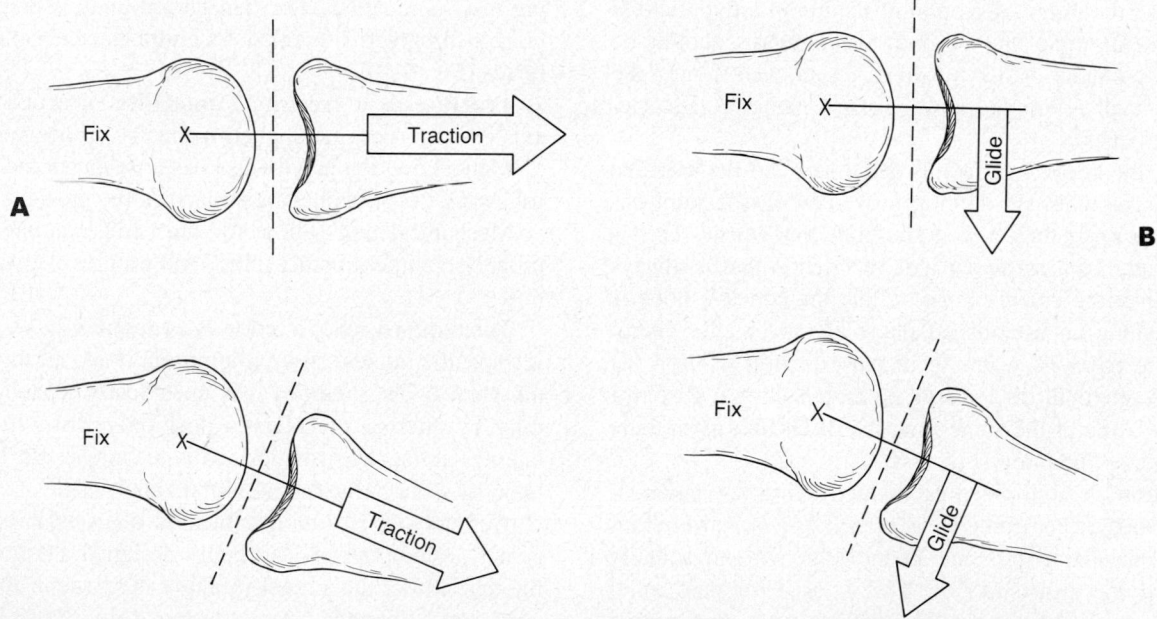

Fig. 9-10. A, Traction; **B,** glide.

Cyriax[6,7] described a system of examination that will usually reveal the origin of the dysfunction. In order to determine the origin of the dysfunction, the examiner must be able to reproduce pain that is consistent with the client's original complaint. If the examiner cannot reproduce the client's pain by physical testing, then the dysfunction is probably not of mechanical origin. Therefore the client should not be treated using mobilization techniques.

Soft tissue can be divided into contractile and noncontractile elements. Contractile elements are those structures that are a part of the muscle, its tendon, and/or its bony insertion.[6] Contractile elements are tested in midrange by isometric contraction against maximal resistance. Pain or weakness is considered a positive response; however, this is only a gross finding. Isometric contractions leave unclear whether the origin of the dysfunction is in the muscle belly, tendon, or the insertion of the tendon. Palpation and more specific testing are necessary to pinpoint the faulty structure.

Noncontractile elements are tissues that do not have the ability to contract or relax. Examples of tissues considered to be noncontractile are bursae, ligaments, fasciae, dura mater, and nerve roots. Both active and passive movements that create stretch may provoke pain in the noncontractile tissues. However, it must be remembered that active contraction also stresses contractile elements, and therefore only responses to passive stretch will implicate noncontractile elements. However, as with active tests, the examiner must do more specific testing—such as specific palpations, including spot tenderness, skin condition, skin temperature, sweating, swelling, skin rolling, and ligamentous stress tests—to determine which of the noncontractile elements is at fault. At the end of the evaluation a correlation of all symptoms and signs determines the treatment. Treatment cannot be based on one finding alone. Proper choice of treatment also depends on the phase of the client's disability at the time of the examination.

Mennell[22] divides dysfunction into two phases: healing and restorative. The goal of the healing phase is to prevent morbidity. This phase can be subdivided into (1) rest from function, in which the affected or pathologically involved structure is kept from having to conduct its normally stressful function and (2) maintenance or normal physiological status, in which the surrounding areas or structures are kept healthy through movement and exercise designed to avoid secondary effects.[33] Mennell[22] stresses the importance of rest from function but not rest from movement— "movement is life." The goal of the restorative phase is to restore function that has been lost during healing in the pathological state.[2]

EXAMINATION BY SELECTIVE TENSION[27]

The five parts of an objective selective tension examination for musculoskeletal dysfunction include testing for (1) active range of motion, (2) passive range of motion, (3) capsular patterns, (4) resisted movements, and (5) movements that are painful or have pain at one end of the range.

Active range of motion

Active range of motion gives the therapist a gross indication of the quantity and quality of movement that the client is willing to produce with regard to pain and limitation as a result of injury.

Passive range of motion

Passive range of motion gives an indication of the state of inert tissue. The physical therapist must pay particular attention to the sensations felt by the client at the end of the passive range. The sensations felt are called "end-feels" and can be classified as follows[6,14]:

1. Normal end-feels
   a. Soft tissue approximation—soft and spongy; occurs in elbow flexion.[6,26]
   b. Muscular—elastic reflex with some discomfort; occurs at the end of straight-leg raising or shoulder abduction.[2]
   c. Bone-on-bone or cartilaginous—abrupt halt without pain; occurs at the end of elbow extension.[6,26]
   d. Capsular—firm arrest of movement; occurs at the end of hip rotation.[6,26]
2. Abnormal end-feels
   a. Spasm—considerable pain that prevents completion of range.[6,26]
   b. Springy block or rebound—cartilaginous block; may occur with a torn meniscus in the knee.[6,26]
   c. Empty—considerable pain before end of range, and client actively resists movement; may occur with acute bursitis.[6,26]
   d. Loose—accompanies extreme hypermobility, may occur in cases of rheumatoid arthritis.[26]

In conducting passive movements the examiner should also take note of the sequence of pain and the limitation of range. If pain is felt before the end of the available range, it suggests an acute stage of injury. Stretching and manipulation are contraindicated. If pain is felt synchronous with the end of range, the client is in a subacute stage, and gentle stretching can be started cautiously.

Stretching

In order to obtain full ROM the therapist must ascertain if the tightness is in the skin, fascia, muscle, ligament, joint capsule, or any combination thereof. It is usually necessary to treat the soft tissue before addressing any joint involvement.[11]

It is generally accepted that soft tissue stretch be slow, steady, and prolonged in order to maximize its effectiveness.

If no pain is felt until after the available range is stretched, the client is in the chronic stage, and an aggressive treatment plan can be followed. This would include strong stretching, vigorous mobilization, and exercises.

Capsular pattern

When there is a lesion in the capsule or synovial membrane of a joint, limitation of active movement in characteristic proportions results. This sense of limitation at a joint is called a capsular pattern. A *capsular pattern* is found only in synovial joints that are controlled by muscles. There is no capsular pattern in joints such as the sacroiliac or others that rely primarily on ligamentous stability. Each synovial joint in the body has its own unique capsular pattern, but the overall capsular pattern is similar for individual joints. For example, the capsular pattern in all glenohumeral joints involves external rotation as the most limited movement, abduction as less limited, internal rotation still less limited, and flexion as the least limited movement.[6]

Noncapsular pattern

When limitation of movement does not follow the outline of the capsular pattern, it is labeled a noncapsular pattern. When a *noncapsular pattern* is found on examination, one must consider lesions that are outside the capsule. Cyriax[6] classified these as (1) ligamentous adhesions, (2) internal derangements, and (3) extraarticular lesions. These classifications are discussed in detail below:

1. *Ligamentous adhesions.* Adhesions following ligamentous injury may cause pain and/or a restriction of mobility. Usually one movement will be very limited, some will be painful near the end of range, and a few will be pain-free. The movements affected will depend on the location of extracapsular structures.
2. *Internal derangement.* Internal derangement is the displacement of a loose fragment within a joint. The onset is sudden, pain is localized, and movements that engage against the block are limited while all others are free.
3. *Extraarticular limitation.* Extraarticular limitation results from adhesions in structures outside the joint. Any movement causing a stretching of that adhesion will be limited; any movement not stressing that adhesion will be full and free of pain. For example, if the biceps adheres to the humeral shaft, elbow extension will be limited while elbow flexion will be full and free of pain.

Resisted movements

The fourth part of the selective tension examination involves resisted movement. This part of the examination gives the examiner information concerning the state of the contractile element of soft tissue, which includes muscle, musculotendinous junctions, the tendon, and the tendinous attachment to the bone. The client is asked to perform an isometric contraction against resistance provided by the examiner while the joint is maintained in midrange. The test must be performed so that primarily one muscle or group of muscles is tested. For example, to test the knee extensors, resistance should be applied proximal to the ankle joint but not to the foot.

Interpretation of response to resisted-movement testing is designated by Cyriax[6] as follows:

1. *Strong and painful*—indicative of a minor injury to some part of the muscle or tendon; this can be tendonitis or a first-degree strain.
2. *Weak and painless*—may indicate a full rupture of a muscle (third-degree strain) or a disruption of the nervous innervation to the muscle.
3. *Weak and painful*—may be a gross lesion, such as a fracture, or secondary deposits of cancer, or may be of psychological origin.
4. *All muscles (about a joint) painful*—may indicate an emotional or psychological problem or a very serious disorder.
5. *All muscles painless and strong*—indicates normal tissue.

Pain

Two other classifications of pain are important in diagnosing a musculoskeletal dysfunction: (1) painful arc and (2) pain at the extreme of range.

Painful arc. A painful arc is pain occurring at one point in the range of movement and disappearing on each side of that point.[29] Painful arcs are thought to occur because of pinching of tissues, usually bone approximating bone with a pain-producing tissue between. Pinching is not normal in a joint and is usually the result of a biomechanical fault but can also occur if there is metaplasia of the tissue between the bones that increases the tissue size. Painful arcs are found most commonly during active movements where muscle force approximates the joint surface, but they have also been noted on passive movements. Painful arcs can occur in all joints, both in the extremities and in the spine. The most common site of a painful arc is in the shoulder, where capsular restrictions cause biomechanical restrictions in gliding. This in turn creates impingement of the supraspinous muscle between the head of the humerus and the acromium on abduction and flexion movements that approximate 90 degrees.

Pain at the extreme of range. This type of response is also created by faulty biomechanics, but it is usually caused by shortening of the capsule or capsular ligaments, which creates increased tightness at end range. Shortening of the capsule creates an alteration of its movement pattern at the very end of the range, which in many cases is the close-packed position of the joint. Such altered mechanics also will create stretch and compression on structures that normally are not affected by movement to end range. Structures most commonly involved are ligaments and bursae. Restoration of normal mechanics by stretching the capsule in a neutral painless position usually resolves the symptoms.[27]

PRINCIPLES OF EXAMINATION

For purposes of examination the body is divided into four quarters, each consisting of an extremity and its adjacent spinal segments. The entire quarter should be addressed regardless of where the complaint lies.

The examination consists of two parts: subjective and objective. In the subjective part the therapist takes a history from the client and allows the client to describe the problem in his/her own words. In the objective part the therapist carries out evaluative tests, including range of motion, manual muscle testing, and a selective neurological examination.

Initial observation

The examination should start with an initial observation. The therapist should begin by watching the client's movements from the time he/she enters the examination area. The therapist should pay special attention to the client's gait pattern (including arm swing, cadence, and rhythm), posture (both sitting and standing), functional activities (such as removing articles of clothing), and the client's facial expressions (which can act as a key indicator of pain). The few minutes spent on this observation are invaluable to the clinician in assessing the client's total problem.

Subjective examination

The physical therapist should begin the subjective examination by interviewing the client. The therapist should listen to the client politely but at the same time extract relevant information so the history is concise and the client does not ramble.

The therapist should take a specific history of the client's present problem, including the date of onset, the mode of onset (insidious, spontaneous, or traumatic), the course of the dysfunction (improved, same, or worse), and any previous treatment. The past history of the same problem, including the initial bout (onset, duration, and treatment) and the number of bouts that have occurred since, must then be obtained.

Frequently the client has a great deal of difficulty describing the exact location of his/her symptoms. The examiner may also have a problem in trying to record the client's description accurately. It is very efficient to use a body chart to record information regarding the client's pain. The body chart may be used in two ways: either the client points to the area of pain on his/her own body and the examiner records it on the chart, or the client points to the area of pain on the body chart and the examiner records it (Fig. 9-11).

If there is more than one area that is symptomatic, the therapist should note the relative importance the client assigns to each area and whether a relationship exists between symptom areas. It is important to have a total picture of the pain—including the location, the quality of the pain (sharp, dull, etc.), the presence of areas of anesthesia or paresthesia, and whether the pain is constant or intermittent. This information is very useful because various tissues often emit symptoms that manifest themselves differently in terms of pain sensation. A burning pain may involve the nerve root, whereas a deep ache may involve a muscle.

The therapist must inquire about what brings on the pain and what relieves it. It is important to carefully determine if anything changes the quality of the pain. Often a client with some degree of continuous pain may not recognize that the intensity or the quality of the pain varies throughout the day. This information is valuable to the therapist in planning treatment and evaluating the client's progress.[5]

It is essential for the therapist to ask the client about the pain status of the areas above and below the major area of the pain and of the uninvolved side. The therapist should then place a checkmark over the corresponding areas on the body chart to indicate which are pain-free. This is im-

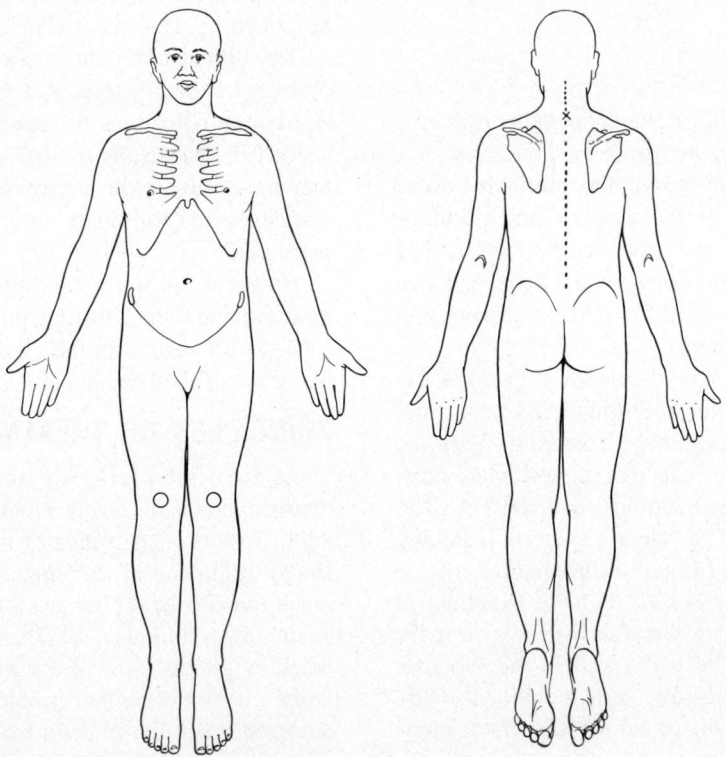

Fig. 9-11. Body chart.

portant since a client who originally complained of right shoulder pain may start to complain of left shoulder pain. Many times the therapist will not remember what the symptoms were at the time of the initial examination. If there is a checkmark on the body chart, the therapist can be assured that the left shoulder was pain-free initially and perhaps the client is now developing a new problem.

The examiner must also be concerned with the behavior of the client's symptoms. It is important to know (1) when the pain becomes worse or better, (2) if it is constant or intermittent, (3) if there is a limitation of function, and (4) how the pain behaves throughout a 24-hour cycle. The client should describe what the pain is like on rising, in the middle of the day, in the evening, and during the night. The examiner must also determine whether the client sleeps through the entire night and, if not, how many times he/she awakens. It is also essential to determine if the client is being awakened by the pain or by other factors, such as anxiety, noise, bad dreams, or urinary frequency.

Another function of the examination is to determine how easily pain is produced and how long it lasts. If the pain is brought on very easily and lasts a significant amount of time, the objective examination should not be done vigorously because it may create increased symptoms that will inhibit the completion of the examination.

Before terminating the subjective examination, the physical therapist must ask specific questions pertaining to the client's general health. These must include past medical history and information on any medications the client is presently taking.

Objective examination

When a client is examined for shoulder pain, it is necessary to determine if the symptoms are of shoulder or cervical origin. It is therefore imperative to examine the neck, shoulder, and arm as well as the anterior and posterior chest. For examination purposes the body therefore has been divided into four areas: two upper quarters and two lower quarters, each consisting of an entire extremity and its corresponding spinal segments.

The quarter examination should include a postural examination, "clearing" tests for the spinal segments that provide innervation to the extremity, "clearing" tests for the peripheral joints, and a selective neurological test, which tests the myotomes, dermatomes, and reflexes. The purpose of "clearing" tests is to "clear" or incriminate any of the joints or muscles being tested in the quarter. If, for instance, the cervical area is "clear" but the examiner is able to elicit a positive sign in the shoulder area, a more specific examination should be performed in the shoulder girdle (see Chapter 20). A positive sign is defined as the reproduction of the exact pain of which the client complains.

The first step in the objective quarter examination is a postural observation, in which the therapist observes the client from all sides. The examiner should look at tone, bulk, and symmetry of structure. This information may be recorded on the body chart for ease of visualization.

The examiner then proceeds to palpation. The examiner should be aware of the general condition of the skin, subcutaneous tissue, muscles, ligaments, and joint lines. Notation should be made of areas of sensitivity, warmth, moisture, and excessive histamine reaction when the area is scratched.

Active range of motion is then tested. The examiner should observe whether the client is using substitute patterns to complete the movement and how smoothly and rhythmically the motion is carried out.

The examiner then performs passive range of motion testing. As discussed before, this will provide information about the noncontractile elements in the joint. The examiner must pay attention to the pain-range relationship, involving the available range and the end-feel, once the end of the available range is reached.

Finally, the therapist should perform resisted testing. All testing is performed in the middle of the range to eliminate stress on the noncontractile elements and allow maximal isometric contraction of the contractile elements. The examiner must pay attention to the pain-strength relationship described earlier in this chapter.

When all physiological testing has been completed, mobility testing—including examination of the accessory movements of the specific joints—is performed as well as a neurological examination. (The specific techniques are described in subsequent chapters.)

The therapist should check recent radiographic reports or other laboratory tests to determine if there are any medical contraindications to treatment. If no further tests are needed or the results of the tests are negative, the examiner must review the information gathered during the examination and formulate an appropriate and specific treatment plan.

However, an understanding of the history of mobilization and individual testing procedures is not sufficient to successfully deal with the client's problem. One must also be aware of the principles of treatment application.

PRINCIPLES OF TREATMENT APPLICATION

As discussed previously, there are four grades of movements undertaken during mobilization. Grades I and II are applied short of the range of limitation, and grades III and IV go to the end of the range. Since grades I and II never reach the end of the range, they can never be effective as stretching techniques. Maitland[20] has developed a system whereby grades I and II are used as techniques when pain is the client's dominant problem, while grades III and IV are used when the client's main problem is stiffness.[20] A possible explanation for the effectiveness of grades I and II in dealing with pain is that there may be a neuromodulation effect on the sensory innervation within the joint, which involves mechanoreceptors and pain sensation receptors. This possibility has been extensively researched by Korr[16] and Wyke.[32]

Clients rarely have dysfunctions that are purely painful or stiff. There is usually a combination of these two factors. If pain is dominant, Maitland[19,20] believes it is necessary to deal with pain first. Once pain has diminished or disappeared, an underlying stiffness may be revealed and can be treated. Sometimes, in the course of treating stiffness, it is unavoidable that a certain amount of pain may result.

Maigne[18] believes in the rule of no pain and free movement. He states that the most useful maneuver is one that is carried out in the direction opposite to that which is painful or restricted. Therefore Maigne believes that pain should not be produced as a result of the treatment.

There are also conflicting theories regarding whether or not to treat a joint if it is stiff or asymptomatic. Kaltenborn[13] believes that restriction of movement should definitely be treated even if it is asymptomatic. His premise is that over a period of time a stiff, hypomobile joint will cause other structures to overtax their limits and become symptomatic. Therefore he feels that manipulation of hypomobile but asymptomatic segments helps prevent further problems. Maitland,[20] on the other hand, suggests treating a client's signs and symptoms when they occur. He feels that when stiffness is asymptomatic, it should not be treated unless recurrence of the symptoms results and can be correlated to the hypomobile area. Although these approaches, on the surface, seem to be at opposite ends of the spectrum, the key to both is the state of the symptoms when the client is first seen. Clients in acute stages of dysfunction will have pain as a major characteristic, but if the client is in a subacute state, stiffness will more likely be the dominant characteristic.

It is unwise to base selection of procedures on diagnosis alone because there are states of healing that must be taken into account. For example, a bursitis can be acute, subacute, chronic, or calcific and must be treated differently at each stage.

There is also universal agreement that the basic guidelines for treatment should be the client's signs and symptoms, and assessment of the treatment's effectiveness is based on changes in those signs and symptoms. After each technique or set of techniques is applied, the client should be reassessed regarding pain, range of motion, and function. In this way progress can be recorded and the therapist can decide on any changes to be made secondary to treatment.

Mobilization or manipulation is not a treatment to be carried out without careful planning. There are many situations in which precautions or even absolute contraindications exist to such treatments (Table 9-3). Physical treatment, however, can be modified from most gentle to very vigorous, which allows conditions that might contraindicate treatment to be divided into two groups: those that are absolute contraindications and those requiring extra care in selection and application of treatment.[11]

Absolute contraindications to manipulation include bone disease, neoplastic disease of skeletal or soft tissue in the area to be treated, old bony deformities or anomalies of the area to be treated, inflammatory arthritis, presence of central nervous system signs, vascular disease related to the area to be treated, and advanced degenerative changes.

Conditions precluding manipulation include hypermobility, joint irritability, and severe pain as well as the presence of protective muscle spasm or pregnancy.

Absolute contraindications to mobilization include malignancy of the area to be treated, signs and symptoms of central nervous system involvement, active inflammatory and infectious arthritis, and bone disease in the area to be treated.

Situations requiring extra care in the use of mobilization include the presence of neurological signs, rheumatoid arthritis, osteoporosis, spondylolisthesis, hypermobility, pregnancy, and previous malignant disease.

Table 9-3. Contraindications and precautions in mobilization and manipulation

Manipulation		Mobilization	
Absolute contraindications	**Relative precautions**	**Absolute contraindications**	**Relative precautions**
Bone disease	Hypermobility	Malignancy of area to be treated	Presence of neurological signs
Neoplastic disease of skeletal or soft tissue area to be treated	Joint irritability	Presence of central nervous system signs	Rheumatoid arthritis
	Severe pain		Osteoporosis
Old bony deformities or anomalies of area to be treated	Protective muscle spasm	Active inflammatory arthritis	Spondylolisthesis
	Pregnancy	Infectious arthritis	Hypermobility
Inflammatory arthritis		Bone disease of area to be treated	Pregnancy
Presence of central nervous system signs			Previous malignant disease
Vascular disease related to area to be treated			
Advanced degenerative changes			

New trends in physical therapy practice include a variety of osteopathic concepts:

Craniosacral therapy is one of the newest areas of interest in physical therapy. It was originally founded in the early 1900s by osteopath William G. Sutherland, and until recently had been exclusively practiced by osteopaths. Craniosacral therapy includes examination of the tissues and cerebral spinal fluid.[30] The gentle, noninvasive treatment tests movement and corrects appropriate restrictions. It has gained popularity in the treatment of chronic pain, temporomandibular joint dysfunction, and cervical and lumbosacral dysfunctions.

Muscle energy

Muscle energy, a term first suggested by Fred L. Mitchell Sr., D.O., describes an "osteopathic manipulative technique in which the patient uses his muscles on request, from a precisely controlled position, in a specific direction, against a distinctly executed operator counterforce."[8]

The techniques of muscle energy may be used to mobilize joints, strengthen weak muscles, stretch tight muscles and fascia, and increase local circulation.[5,9]

Myofascial release

The fascia is a connective tissue found throughout the entire body.

According to Dr. Ward of Michigan State University, myofascial release treatment addresses pain and mechanical problems simultaneously using the balance-barrier release concept. Barriers occur because of postural reflex and other changes. They create active effects and inhibit motion in single joints and joint complexes. There are two primary barriers: physiological and anatomical. Myofascial release treatment uses manually applied loads to assess and treat the barriers and asymmetries. The therapist should palpate and assess tissue and skeletal mechanics from the skin inward. Treatment is completed when areas of restriction have been released and appropriate balance achieved.[24]

It becomes apparent that the physical therapist, in order to approach and treat disorders holistically, must examine skin, fascia, adhesions, muscles, ligaments, joint capsules, nerve, dura, bone, and psyche. Each of these issues must be thoroughly addressed.

SUMMARY

This chapter has described the basic concepts of mobilization and manipulation used in treating musculoskeletal dysfunction. The importance of thorough and systematic evaluation and appropriate treatment have been emphasized.

The therapist should be constantly aware of the need for ongoing assessment in order to monitor the client's progress and make necessary changes in the treatment plan. It is advisable to use a minimal number of treatment techniques at each session in order to better focus on the effectiveness of each technique. The mobilization part of the treatment session may seem to be deceptively short because each technique is usually performed for only 20 to 60 seconds and repeated only four or five times. In actuality the oscillations are occurring at a rate of 2 per second or 120 per minute; therefore four 1-minute treatment sessions consist of 480 treatment repetitions—a large number in any rehabilitation program. Treatment should be continued with the same technique until no further improvement is noted. If after two or three treatment sessions the client does not demonstrate any noticeable improvement, the therapist must reevaluate the appropriateness of the technique chosen. If the therapist thinks that a manipulation should be performed, the results should be immediately noticeable.

It is recommended that treatment for a predominantly painful condition be carried out on a daily basis, whereas treatment for a stiffness problem should be carried out two to three times per week, allowing sufficient recovery time between sessions. The client with a stiffness dysfunction should be given a detailed home exercise program of self-mobilization techniques.

Although this chapter has emphasized mobilization, it is in reality only one part of the management of a client with a neuromusculoskeletal dysfunction. Physical therapists should develop expertise in the "laying on of hands" in a very broad spectrum. There is at the therapist's disposal a multitude of approaches that can be used to develop individualized treatment programs—massage (rolfing, connective tissue massage, Swedish massage, transverse friction massage), therapeutic exercise (proprioceptive neuromuscular facilitation, progressive resistive exercise, isometrics, isokinetics, and neurodevelopmental exercise), modalities (thermotherapy, electrotherapy, and hydrotherapy), as well as mobilization. The proper incorporation of all procedures is needed for effective treatment of musculoskeletal problems.

REFERENCES

1. Ackerknecht EH: A short history of medicine, New York, 1975, Ronald Press, pp. 65-72.
2. Beard G and Ward EC: Massage principles and techniques, Philadelphia, 1964, WB Saunders Co, pp. 3-5.
3. Bettman DL: A pictorial history of medicine, Springfield, Ill, 1962, Charles C Thomas, Publisher.
4. Bick EM: History of orthopedic surgery, New York, 1933, The Hospital of Joint Diseases, p. 212.
5. Bourdillon J: Spinal manipulation, Norwalk, Conn, 1987, Appleton & Lange.
6. Cyriax J: Textbook of orthopedic medicine, vol 1, Diagnosis of soft tissue lesions, London, 1969, Bailliere Tindall, pp. 5, 63-64, 70-73, 77-82, 85-86.
7. Cyriax J: Textbook of orthopedic medicine, vol 2, Treatment by manipulation, massage and injection, Baltimore, 1974, Williams & Wilkins, pp. 56-58, 61.
8. Glossary of Osteopathic Terminology, J Am Osteopath Assoc 80:552-667, 1981.

9. Goodridge J: Muscle energy technique: definition, explanation, methods of procedure, J Am Osteopath Assoc 81(4):13-18.

10. Grieve G: Mobilization of the spine, New York, 1965, Churchill Livingstone, Inc., p. 7.

11. Grieve G: Common vertebral joint problems, New York, 1981, Churchill Livingstone, Inc., p. 465.

12. Grimsby O: Fundamentals of manual therapy: a course workbook, Vagsbydgd, Norway, 1981, Sorlandets Fysikalske Institute.

13. Kaltenborn F: Mobilization of the extremity joints: examination and basic treatment techniques, Universitetsgaten, 1980, Olaf Norlis Bokhandel, pp. 9, 19, 21, 23.

14. Kapandji IA: Physiology of joints, vol 2, Lower limbs, Edinburgh, 1970, Churchill Livingstone, Inc. p. 88.

15. Kirkaldy-Willis WH: Managing low back pain, New York, 1983, Churchill Livingstone, Inc.

16. Korr IM: The neurobiologic mechanisms in manipulation therapy, New York, 1977, Plenum Publishing Corp.

17. MacConaill MA and Basmajian JV: Muscles and movements: a basis for human kinesiology, Baltimore, 1969, Williams & Wilkins.

18. Maigne R: Orthopedic medicine, Springfield, Ill, 1976, Charles C Thomas, Publisher, pp. 137-140.

19. Maitland GD: Extremity manipulation, London, 1977, Butterworth Publishers, pp. 5-10.

20. Maitland GD: Vertebral manipulation, London, 1978, Butterworth Publishers, pp. 84-85.

21. McKenzie RA: Mechanical diagnosis and therapy, Waikanae, New Zealand, 1981, Spinal Publications Ltd.

22. Mennell J: The spinal column: the science and art, Little, Brown & Co, 1952.

23. Mennell J: Joint pain: diagnosis and treatment using manipulative techniques, New York, 1964, Little, Brown & Co.

24. Michigan State University, School of Osteopathy: Tutorial on myofascial release technique, Level I, 1986.

25. Natchev E: A manual on auto-traction, Trycheribolaget, Sweden, 1984, Sundsvall.

26. Paris SV: The spine: course notebook, Atlanta, 1979, Institute Press, pp. 21, 30.

27. Paris SV: Extremity dysfunction and mobilization, Atlanta, 1980, Prepublication Manual, pp. 24-26.

28. Schiotz EH and Cyriax J: Manipulation: past and present, London, 1978, William Heinemann Medical Books Ltd, pp. 7, 13, 25, 38, 40, 53.

29. Stoddard A: Manual of osteopathic practice, London, 1969, Hutchinson Ross Publishing Co.

30. Upledger JE and Vredevogd JD: Craniosacral therapy, Chicago, 1983, Eastland Press.

31. Warwick R and Williams P: Gray's anatomy, ed 35, Philadelphia, 1973, WB Saunders Co, pp. 397, 399-400.

32. Wyke B: Articular neurology: a review, Physiotherapy 58:94, 1972.

33. Zohn DA and Mennell J: Musculoskeletal pain: diagnosis and physical treatment, Boston, 1976, Little, Brown & Co, pp. 3, 5-7.

ADDITIONAL READINGS

Cookson J: Orthopedic manual therapy: an overview. II. The spine, J Am Phys Ther Assoc 59:259, 1979.

Cookson J and Kent B: Orthopedic manual therapy: an overview. I: The extremities, J Am Phys Ther Assoc 59:136, 1979.

Kessler RM and Hertling D: Management of common musculoskeletal disorder: physical therapy principles and methods, New York, 1983, Harper & Row, Publishers, Inc.

Upledger JE: Craniosacral therapy II, beyond the dura, Seattle, 1987, Eastland Press.

Chapter 10

MOBILITY: ACTIVE-RESISTIVE TRAINING

Michael Sanders
Barbara Sanders

Active-resistive training (ART) can be classified as having either a conditioning or a rehabilitative effect. The procedures followed in both areas to enhance one's muscular strength, power, and endurance are essentially the same. The major difference between the two areas exists in the intensity of the exercise regimens used. ART for conditioning purposes should be as intense as safely possible while eliciting optimal gains. The goal of rehabilitation, on the other hand, is to restore the greatest possible function in the shortest possible time.

Mobility training, therefore, for whatever reason, must be restricted by individual limitations. An examination of specific physiological limitations will improve the therapist's and the individual's understanding of the complexity of ART.

LIMITING FACTORS IN ART

A major concern of this chapter is to describe the factors involved in mobility training. The effectiveness of ART depends on the current physical performance levels of each individual, but analyzing the factors that limit ART is a complex endeavor. To facilitate this task, an organizational paradigm (Fig. 10-1) was developed by Kearney.[14] The paradigm assumes that the core component of ART is physical performance, which involves three primary factors: skill, cardiovascular conditioning, and neuromuscular coordination. Five modifying factors—genetic predisposition, anthropometric characteristics, psychological-sociological variables, ambient environment, and pain tolerance—are also important considerations that affect physical performance. To illustrate the primary factors, an activity performance profile (Fig. 10-2) should be used; that is, one end of the neuromuscular continuum should be designed to show strength and power as dominant, while the opposite end stresses muscular endurance. An athletic performance profile is then established for certain activities by subjectively assigning a grade for each primary factor. From these primary factors certain physiological, neurological, and histological elements are ultimately determined as being responsible for limiting performance and, consequently, limiting ART.

In helping a client prepare to participate in a major sport, the main objectives the therapist should strive to achieve for depend on the preceding elements. The amount of preparation time for activities varies according to the demands of the sport. Marathon runners and swimmers are continually practicing their activity as they train, but their

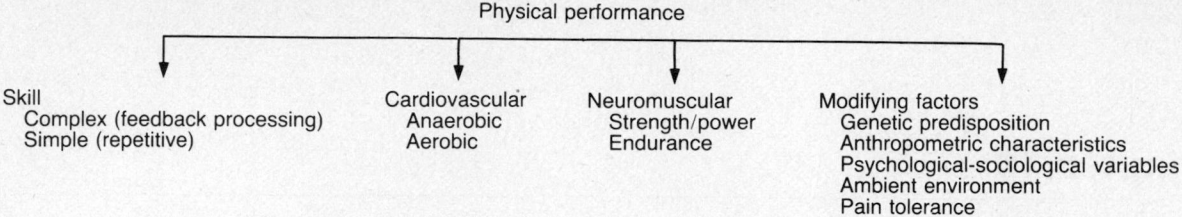

Fig. 10-1. Physical performance and its determining factors.

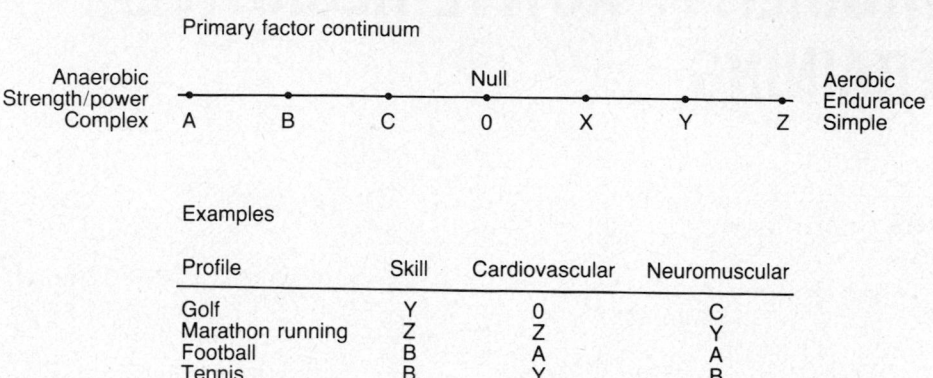

Fig. 10-2. Activity performance profile.

performance is primarily determined by their physical conditioning. Discus throwers and golfers do not require the high degree of physical conditioning needed by distance runners and swimmers, but they do need to devote a greater percentage of preparation time to skill development. This diversity in sports preparation can be represented on the neuromuscular continuum and illustrates the basic differences in the training required for each sport. For example, a golfer needs to strengthen arms, wrists, and shoulders by performing specific strength-training exercises rather than relying on the weight of the club alone to increase strength. However, much of a golfer's training consists of complex skill movements; which are mastered by continual practice of the sport.

Fig. 10-3 identifies factors that determine skill limitations. The logical progression of the skill continuum is from simple (repetitive) tasks to highly complex tasks requiring modification by proprioceptive feedback or response to opponent actions.

The items listed in Fig. 10-4 represent limiting factors in cardiovascular conditioning, which in the *anaerobic* spectrum include (1) fuel sources, (2) enzymatic activity, (3) muscle fiber types, and (4) oxygen debt capacity. The respective limiting factors in the *aerobic* spectrum are (1) maximum oxygen uptake, (2) distribution of blood supply, (3) muscle fiber type, (4) fuel sources, and (5) fluid and ionic balances.

Within this cardiovascular framework, energy (capacity or ability to do work) represents the bottom line. The human body must continuously be supplied with its own form of energy to do work. Adenosine triphosphate (ATP)

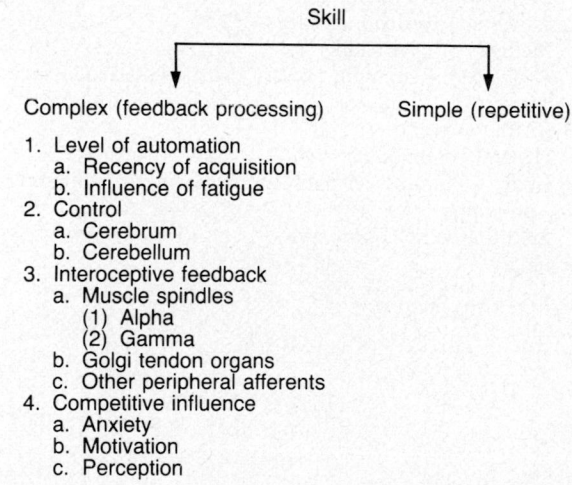

Fig. 10-3. Skill limiting factors.

is used for the immediate (anaerobic) activities and is continuously resynthesized for long-duration (aerobic) energy activities. The key to successful enhancement of the cardiovascular elements is to identify the predominant means of energy metabolism required for a desired area of performance and to train specifically to augment the capacity for that type of energy output.

Fig. 10-5 describes physiological factors limiting muscular strength and power. These include (1) total cross-sectional area of a muscle, (2) cortical control factors, (3) muscle fiber type, and (4) ambient conditions influencing the rate of muscle fiber shortening. Factors limiting mus-

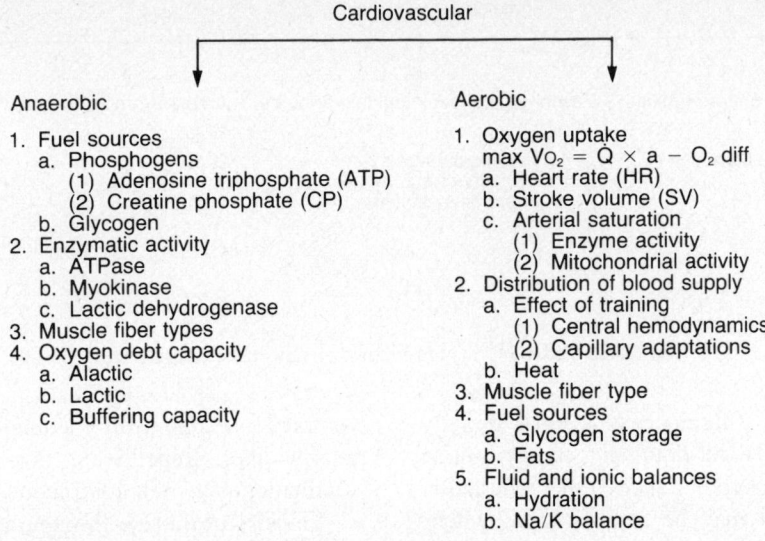

Fig. 10-4. Cardiovascular limiting factors.

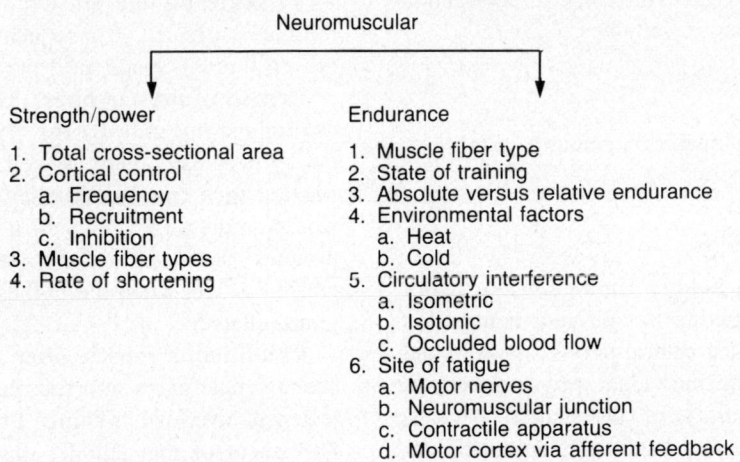

Fig. 10-5. Neuromuscular limiting factors.

cular endurance include (1) muscle fiber type, (2) state of training, (3) environmental factors, (4) circulatory conditions, and (5) type of activity involved.

Fig. 10-6 displays certain modifying factors that can enhance or restrict muscle performance. Of the factors cited genetic predisposition is potentially the most significant.

To make clear the relative importance of certain limiting factors in the paradigm, one specific activity should be closely evaluated. Marathon running is the ultimate challenge of aerobic power training, involving cardiovascular ability, muscular endurance, neuromuscular coordination, and simple skill movements. Modifying factors, such as genetic predisposition (high percentage of slow-twitch red fibers), anthropometric characteristics, and psychological and pain tolerance variables, also contribute to success in this activity.

With this information in mind potential limitations that may occur in ART can be demonstrated.

Physiological limitations

In addition to the preceding factors, there exist further specific physiological factors that ultimately limit the ability of an individual to function at the maximal possible muscular efficiency as well as the minimal balanced bilateral muscular efficiency. Much of the evidence accumulated on muscular efficiency suggests that limitations exist within the muscle fibers themselves.* Muscles are composed of varying numbers of motor units that contribute to such contractile properties as speed, power, and resistance to fatigue. Consequently, muscle fibers can be classified accordingly:

1. Slow-twitch red (slow oxidative glycogenolytic)
2. Fast-twitch red (fast oxidative glycogenolytic)
3. Fast-twitch white (fast glycolytic)

*See references 1, 4, 10, 13, 23, and 24.

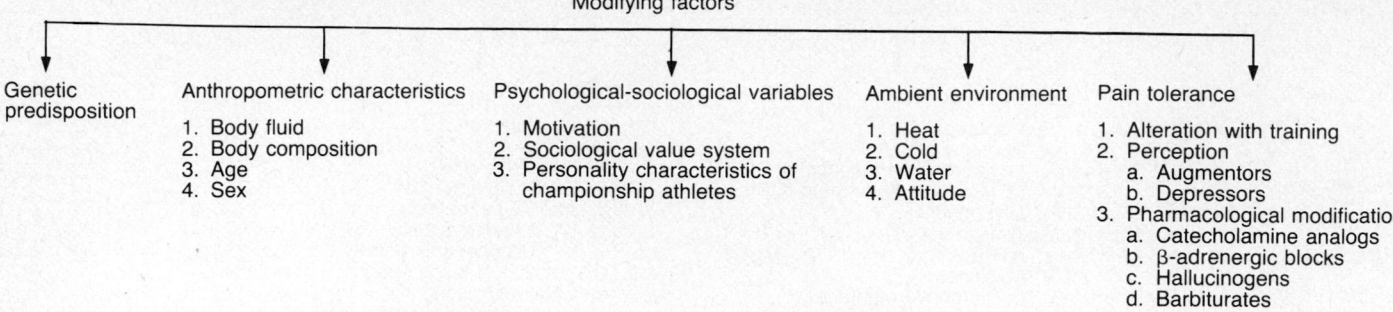

Fig. 10-6. Major modifying factors of physical performance.

There are two essential differences that exist initially between the fiber types: (1) the dominant energy source may be either aerobic or anaerobic, and (2) the contraction time of the particular fiber may be fast- or slow-twitch. However, the most important consideration in determining differences between fiber types is the tension that can be produced by a muscle fiber type. This force of contraction is ultimately dependent upon six variables:

1. Number of motor units firing
2. Size of motor units
3. Rate of firing of individual motor units
4. Velocity of muscle shortening
5. Length of muscle fiber
6. Condition of muscle fiber

Number of motor units firing. The number of motor units firing and thus contributing to muscular contraction depends on the integrity of the central nervous system and the motivational level of the individual. Coordination of movement is the responsibility of the central nervous system,* a fact that is important in understanding the development of strength. One theory is that with an intact central nervous system fewer inhibitory impulses are transmitted to different motor neurons, resulting in more motor units being activated at any one time.†

Size of motor units. Motor neurons may innervate less than 10 fibers or more than 1,000 fibers. The size of such motor units varies between muscles and within an individual muscle. The initiation of muscle contraction is precipitated by small-sized motor units. Recruitment of larger motor units is required as the demand for tension increases. The implications for ART are obvious: minimal contractions that elicit low muscle tension in effect activate tonic motor units. Consequently, a therapist knowing that a particular unit or fiber possesses a high resistance to fatigue could develop an exercise program requiring repeated submaximal contractions for long periods of time.

Rate of firing of individual motor units. A twitch

contraction is initiated by a single action potential within a muscle fiber. Repetitive action potentials can produce a summation of twitch contractions to produce tetanus.[2,12]

Velocity of muscle shortening. The velocity of muscle shortening decreases as the load increases until the velocity is zero and an isometric contraction is produced. As velocity decreases the tension that can be produced by a muscle is greater. Consequently, a heavier load can be moved through space until the load creates zero velocity.*

Length of muscle fiber. The length of muscle fiber is determined not only by the type of muscle fiber involved but by each sarcomere as well. During actual muscle contraction each crossbridge elicits a constant amount of tension regardless of the distance between the two contractile proteins, actin and myosin. It is theorized that maximal tension occurs when the highest number of crossbridges is interdigitated.†

Condition of muscle fiber. A number of physiological changes take place in a muscle when it is repeatedly subjected to overload training. Primary changes involve improvement of the neural pathways from brain to muscle and the tendinous attachment of the muscle to the bone, as well as the musculotendinous junction. Engaging in ART will result in improved efficiency of the neural pathways and a more effective application of force.‡

Although certain properties of muscle fiber function that determine contraction capability are shared by all fast-twitch red, fast-twitch white, and slow-twitch red fibers, a closer examination of histological, physiological, and biochemical properties can differentiate the fibers more clearly. Table 10-1 illustrates that slow-twitch red fibers have a high resistance to fatigue endurance and are adaptable to prolonged contractions since they rely on energy metabolism employing oxygen. The fast-twitch white fibers, on the other hand, are capable of strong, rapid contractions essential for dynamic movements, but they have a low resistance to fatigue. These fibers rely on an adenosine triphosphate and creatine phosphate pool for their energy.

*See references 1, 2, 4, 9, 11, 23, and 24.
†See references 1, 2, 12, 18, and 22.

*See references 2, 12, 17, 19, 22, and 23.
†See references 1, 2, 3, 17, 19, 23, and 24.
‡See references 1, 2, 12, 17, 22, 23, and 25.

Table 10-1. Properties of the various fiber types

	Slow-twitch red	Fast-twitch red	Fast-twitch white
Histological differences			
Size	Small	Intermediate	Large
Color	Red	Red	White
Myoglobin	High	High	Low
Sarcoplasmic reticulum and T tubules	Thin and sparse	Thin and sparse	Well developed
Nerve size (myelin)	Small	Medium	Large
Blood supply	High	High	Low
Mitochondrial density	High	Medium	Low
Sarcoplasm	Less	Moderate	More
Fibrils	Few	Moderate	Many
Fibers per motor unit	Low	Medium	High
Physiological differences			
Contraction time	Slow	Fast	Fast
Endurance	High	Medium	Low
Tension capacity	Low	Medium	High
Stretch sensitivity	Very sensitive	Moderately sensitive	Less sensitive
Biochemical differences			
K+ depletion	Slow	Moderate	Rapid
Metabolism	Oxidative	Both	Glycolytic
Myoglobin content	High	High	Low
Glycogen content	Similar	Similar	Similar
ATPase activity	Low	Moderate	High

RESISTIVE AND OVERLOAD TRAINING

Use of the overload principle in conditioning and rehabilitation facilitates an increase in muscular strength, power, and endurance. Simply stated, workloads for both conditioning and rehabilitation have to impose a demand on the organism, and, as adaptation to increased loading occurs, more load needs to be added. Exercise of this type is called progressive resistance exercise (PRE).

Methods of overloading

There are numerous ways to impose an overload on the muscular system. Most of the current therapeutic exercise equipment and many of the regimes employed use one or more of the following methods of overloading.

Increased weight/resistance. This is the most basic of all overloading techniques. The individual increases the resistance he/she is accustomed to, the muscular system is overloaded, and conditioning takes place. DeLorme[7,8] popularized this approach in the mid 1940s by using a weight boot and increasing the resistance as individual adaptation occurred.

Increased repetitions/sets. By increasing the number of times (repetitions) or group times (sets) an exercise is done, the individual can progressively overload the system. This regimen, also popularized by DeLorme,[7] is usually coupled with increased resistance to enhance overloading.

Increased frequency. This element of overloading is concerned with the number of times per week or per day that the individual trains. Studies of conditioning frequency indicate that significant levels of conditioning can be achieved if the frequency range is two to four times per week.*

Increased speed or rate of movement. The advent of speed training (isokinetic exercise) was popularized by use of Cybex† equipment manufactured by Lumex Corporation. Isokinetic movements are muscular contractions that occur at a constant speed through a full range of motion. The advantages of speed training are that the speed of contraction is fixed and a maximum of resistance is encountered through the full range of motion. No matter how much force is applied the velocity remains constant and the force accommodates[17,18] (Fig. 10-7).

Duration. Duration is the specific time element during which the individual is actually performing mobility exercises. The objective of the mobility training program determines the duration. Rehabilitation training may be conducted at lower intensities and for shorter time periods, while the opposite is true for conditioning training.

Rest interval. Overloading can be intensified or slackened by adjusting the length of the rest interval between

*See references 1, 3, 5, 8, 9, and 24.
†Cybex, Ronkonkoma, NY.

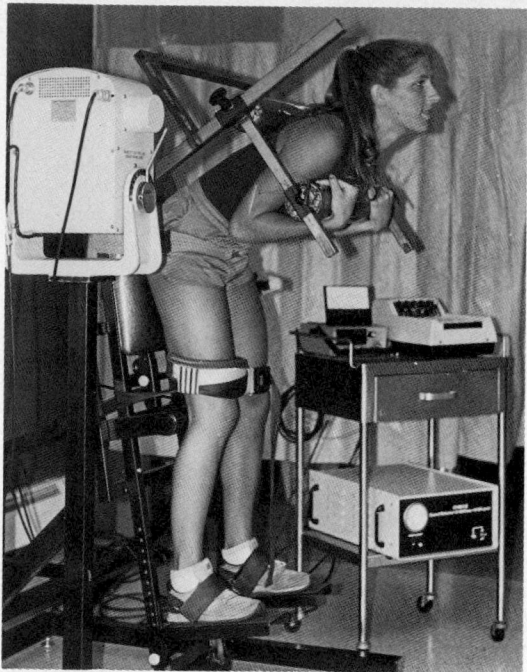

Fig. 10-7. Prototype Cybex back unit.

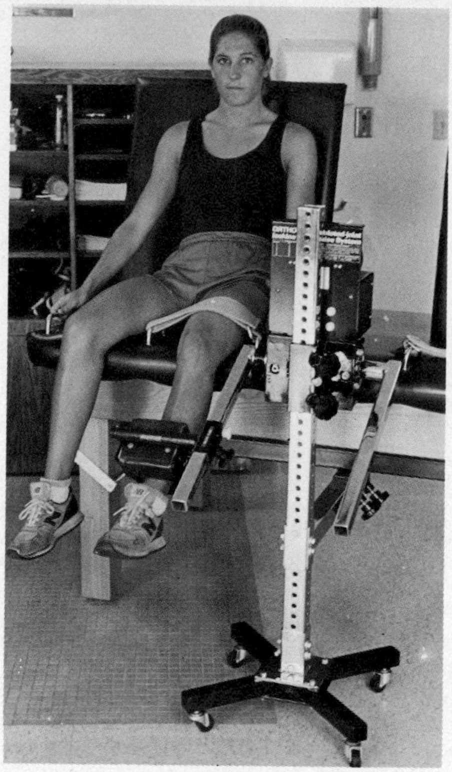

periods of intensity. An intense training session followed by a short rest interval before the next session causes a more extreme physical response:

1. Heart rate is higher
2. Oxygen debt is incurred earlier
3. Respiration rate increases
4. Exhaustion occurs sooner

This response is desirable for mobility training in some conditioning programs, but for early stages of rehabilitation intense training is not recommended.

Isolation of the muscle. Some proponents of mobility training advocate isolation of a specific muscle group to elicit optimal development. Nautilus,* Cybex, and numerous other types of training equipment incorporate this principle in their machinery. Basically, this approach tries to avoid the incidence of *synergistic response* (i.e., when an injured and/or weak muscle group performs a dynamic movement, the action of other muscles assist in the movement). Use of this type of equipment theoretically isolates the specific area to be strengthened (Figs. 10-8 to 10-10).

Range of motion. Range of motion is determined by the relative distance a body part traverses during an exercise. While performing mobility exercises for conditioning, it is desirable to perform the exercise through the full range of motion. For example, a barbell curl should begin from a position where the elbow flexors are in complete extension and finish with the elbow flexors in complete

*Nautilus, Deland, Fla.

Fig. 10-8. Lumex Orthotron unit.

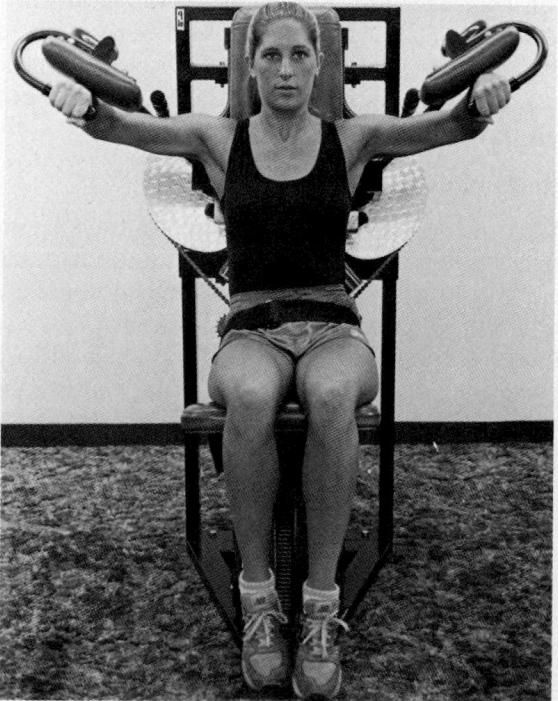

Fig. 10-9. Nautilus shoulder unit.

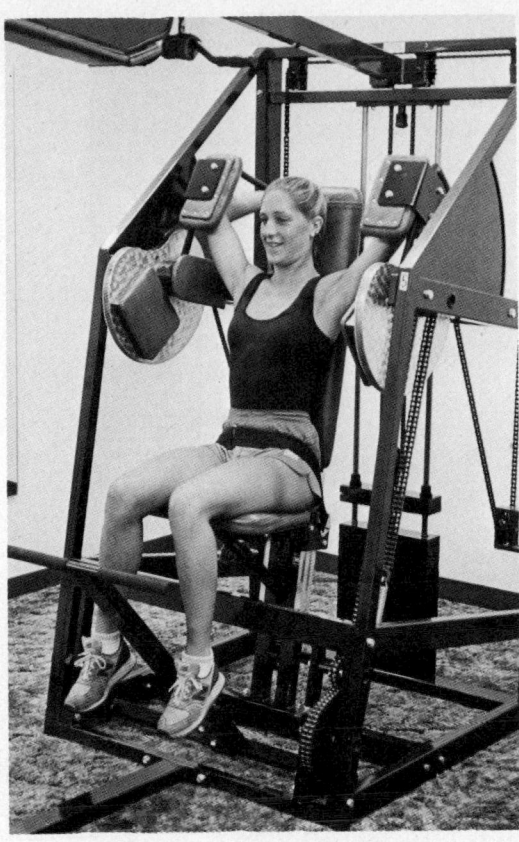

Fig. 10-10. Nautilus pullover machine.

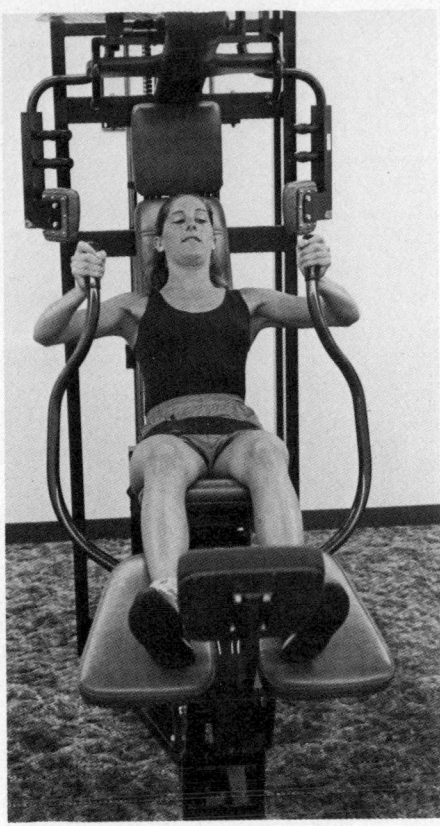

Fig. 10-11. Nautilus double chest machine.

flexion for proper overloading. Often, however, this is not possible immediately following an injury or surgery, but continued rehabilitation can gradually increase the range of motion so that there will be an increase in the overload of affected muscles and a consequent restoration of function (Figs. 10-11 to 10-13).

Principles of strength, power, and muscular endurance training

Providing a sufficiently descriptive semantic definition for strength, power, and muscular endurance has been an ongoing problem in recent years, especially with the advent of isokinetics. *Strength* appears to be a pure component, and, within the confines of the available training modalities, it can be defined in several ways:*

1. Strength is the maximum force that can be exerted against an immovable object (isometric strenght).
2. Strength is the heaviest weight that can be lifted against gravity (isotonic strength).
3. Strength is the maximal torque that can be developed against a preset, pre-limiting device at a slow contractile velocity (isokinetic strength).

*See references 1, 2, 9, 14, 15, and 18.

Although absolute strength is an important component of ART, *power* (force × distance) is dependent on the individual's level of strength. Time quantification of power has been achieved with the introduction of isokinetic equipment. Isokinetic devices, for instance, allow for an assessment of power from numerous muscle groups and joint motions by varying the speed at which the resistance moves. The implications for conditioning and rehabilitation are two-fold: (1) isokinetic devices provide a diagnostic tool for assessing muscular imbalances and/or deficiencies, and (2) they enhance an individual's ability to improve general power development. For definitive purposes muscular endurance can assume the same categories as strength.

Muscular endurance is the ability of a muscle to perform repeated contractions against an immovable object (isometric exercise), against gravity (isotonic exercise), and against a preset speed-limiting device (isokinetic exercise). Additionally, relative to dynamic or static movements, there can be both a concentric contraction and/or an eccentric contraction (Fig. 10-14).

A *concentric contraction* is the most common type of muscular contraction and occurs in rhythmical activities when the muscle shortens as it develops tension (Fig. 10-

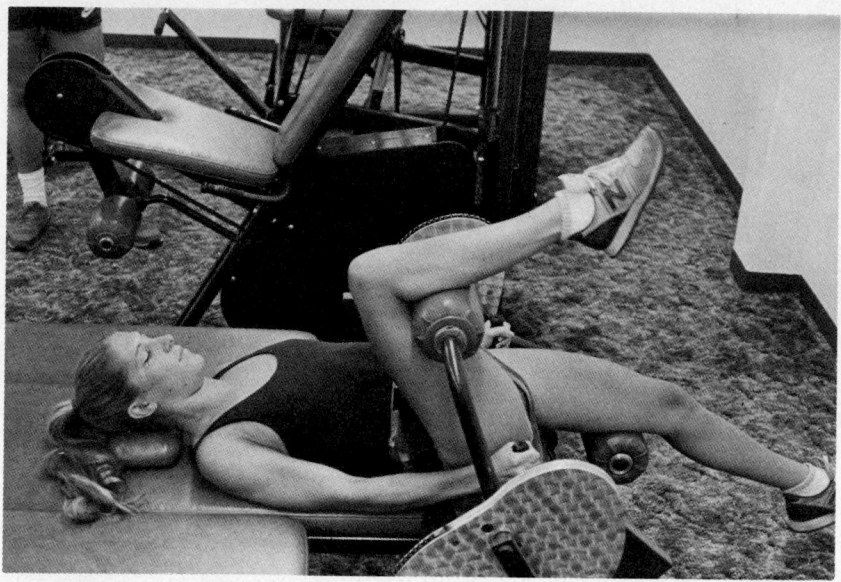

Fig. 10-12. Nautilus hip and leg machine.

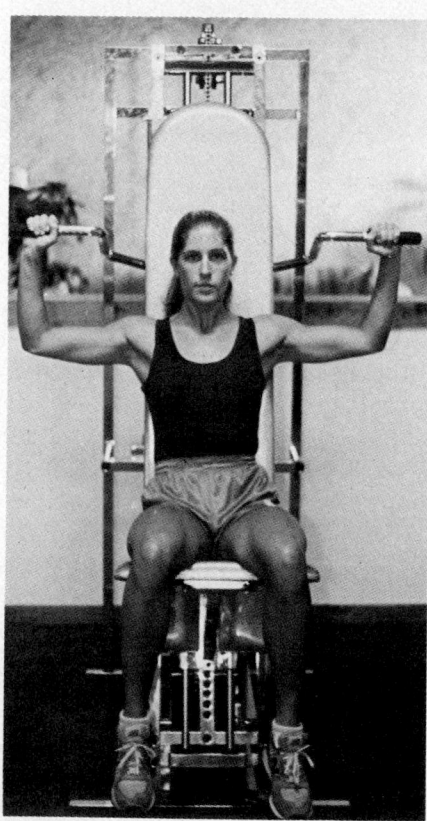

Fig. 10-13. Dynacam shoulder press machine.

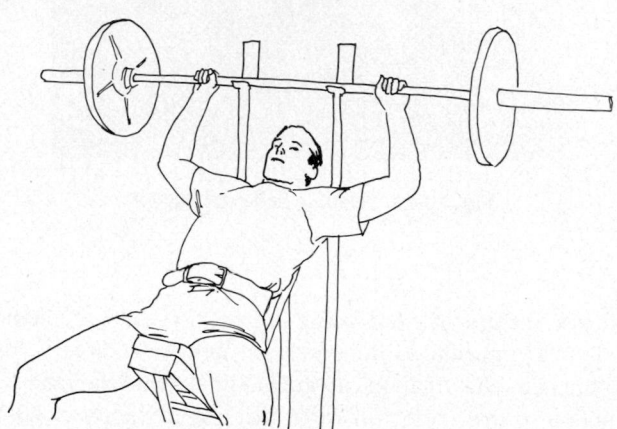

Fig. 10-14. Beginning phase.

The effect of ART on the muscular system primarily centers on hypertrophy, although strength, power, and endurance gains can be achieved without increases in the size of muscle fibers.[1,6,22,24] Table 10-2 compares the biological changes that result in an individual who engages in ART and one who engages in cardiovascular training. There are certain chemical and histochemical similarities that occur when various types of training are undertaken, and even cardiovascular training is a form of overloading.

THE ART PROGRAM

Selection of the proper exercise regimen for an ART program is essential for optimal benefits. The core element, whether the program is for conditioning or for rehabilitation, is the persistent reinforcement of effort to increase and improve muscle strength beyond prior limits. Resistive programs are varied and are designed for the

15). An *eccentric contraction*, on the other hand, entails lengthening of the muscle. This is achieved when a weight is lowered through a range of motion. The muscle yields to the resistance allowing itself to be stretched (Fig. 10-16).

Table 10-2. Physiological comparison between overload modalities in ART and cardiovascular training

Biological factors	Strength	Muscular endurance	Cardiovascular endurance
Collagen content	Increase	Increase	Increase
Connective tissue	Increase in density	Increase in density	Increase in density
Sarcolemma	Increase in density	Increase in density	Increase in density
Tendons and ligaments (volume)	Increase	Increase	Increase
Sarcoplasm	Increase	Increase	Increase
Contractile proteins (actin, myosin, troponin, tropomyosin)	Increase	Increase	Increase
Glycogen	Yes	Yes	Yes
Mitochondrion (size and number)	Yes	Yes	Very high
Fiber type response	Fast-twitch white (FTW)	Fast-twitch white (FTW) and fast-twitch red (FTR)	Slow-twitch red (STR)
Succinic dehydrogenase	Little	Little	Very high
Phosphorylase activity	Little	Little	Very high

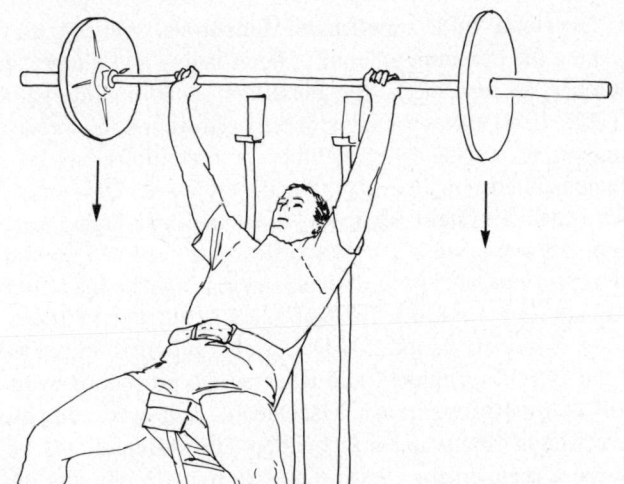

Fig. 10-15. Eccentric phase.

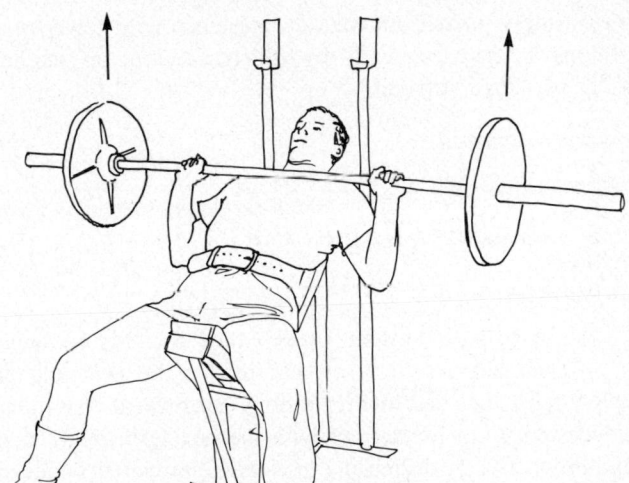

Fig. 10-16. Concentric phase.

cross section of individuals who engage in resistive training for whatever purpose. They include the following types of individuals:

1. Athletes—individuals who are interested in developing strength/power specific to their sport
2. Olympic and power lifters—individuals interested mainly in acquiring strength/power necessary to achieve success in respective lifts, such as Olympic (the snatch and the clean-and-jerk) and power lifting (squat, bench press, and the deadlift)
3. Body builders—individuals wanting to attain massive muscular development and definition
4. Those in need of rehabilitation—individuals who work with resistive exercise for restoration of function in injured areas
5. General physical fitness—individuals who desire general muscular toning.

General conditioning

Rasch and associates[3,18,19] describe the following programs that individuals can use to achieve optimal results in ART: set and repetition system, light-to-heavy system, heavy-to-light system, and circuit weight training.

Set and repetition system. This system was introduced by DeLorme[7] in the mid 1940s and is, by far, the most widely used method of training. Repetition refers to the number of complete and continuous executions of an exercise or the repetition maximum (RM) for a particular weight. A set constitutes the group number of repetitions of an exercise. If more than one set is performed, a short rest interval follows each set. This allows the person to quantify and objectively document the regimen.

EXAMPLE: EXERCISE:

Bench press, 100 lb × 10 RM (100%) × 1 set
Rest

Bench press, 100 lb × 10 RM (100%) × 1 set
Rest
Bench press, 100 lb × 10 RM (100%) × 1 set

The DeLorme method is characterized by doing an initial set at 50% of 10 RM, a second set at 75% of 10 RM, and progressing to a third set at 100% of 10 RM.

EXAMPLE: EXERCISE

Bench press, 50 lb × 10 RM (50%) × 1 set
Rest
Bench press, 75 lb × 10 RM (75%) × 1 set
Rest
Bench press, 100 lb × 10 RM (100%) × 1 set

Light-to-heavy system. In this system[24] the individual starts with a lighter weight, does a certain number of repetitions, rests, adds more resistance, does fewer repetitions, rests, adds even more resistance but does fewer repetitions, and continues this process until a certain weight and repetition goal is achieved. The regimen of imposing increasingly greater amounts of resistance with fewer repetitions is used frequently by athletes seeking to acquire great mass and strength.

EXAMPLE: EXERCISE

Bench press, 100 lb × 10 RM × 1 set
Rest
Bench press, 120 lb × 8 RM × 1 set
Rest
Bench press, 140 lb × 6 RM × 1 set

Heavy-to-light system. Also called the *Oxford technique,* the heavy-to-light system retains the principle of heavy resistance and low repetitions but reverses the light-to-heavy pattern by starting with the heaviest weight first and progressively decreasing the load. Zinovieff[26] believed that the DeLorme method was too fatiguing and that too great a strain was placed on the muscles.

EXAMPLE: EXERCISE

Bench press, 100 lb × 10 RM (100%) × 1 set
Rest
Bench press, 75 lb × 10 RM (75%) × 1 set
Rest
Bench press, 50 pound × 10 RM (50%) × 1 set

Circuit weight training. Circuit weight training involves a sequential arrangement of weight training exercises resulting in a system of continuous activity that brings about improvement of strength, muscular endurance, body composition, and aerobic capacity.[11] Circuit weight training requires the trainee to exercise in short, all-out bursts, followed by short rest intervals. A circuit of eight or more exercise stations is established with a specific time allotment and/or a required number of repetitions performed at each station. Exercises are arranged in the circuit so that there is an alternation of arm, leg, shoulder, and back movements to prevent fatigue of one muscle group before the circuit is completed.

EXAMPLE:

Exercise	Repetitions	Rest
Bench press	10 RM (100%)	30 sec
Squat	10 RM (100%)	30 sec
Upright row	10 RM (100%)	30 sec
Sit-up	10 RM (100%)	30 sec
Curl	10 RM (100%)	30 sec
Dead lift	10 RM (100%)	30 sec
Dip	10 RM (100%)	30 sec
Leg raise	10 RM (100%)	30 sec

Exercises are done one after another until the circuit is completed. After a rest period the circuit can be done two or three more times. To intensify the program the following can be done: (1) the rest interval can be decreased, (2) more repetitions can be added, and (3) more circuits can be completed. Regardless of the ART systems or methods of overloading used, progressively overcoming increased resistance is necessary for the development of muscular strength, power, and endurance.

Overload and repetitions. Numerous studies* concerning the optimum amount of overloading and the proper number of repetitions for maximum conditioning gains (Table 10-3) have been conducted. However, no precise amount of resistance or number of repetitions has been demonstrated conclusively as most effective. DeLorme[7,8] advocated a system of heavy resistance and high repetition, beginning with a light weight for a specified number of repetitions and progressively increasing the load from 50% to 75% to 100% for that specific number of repetitions. Zinovieff[26] modified DeLorme's progression, called it the Oxford technique, and reversed the procedure, while still doing 10 repetitions. MacQueen[16] surveyed competitive weight lifters and bodybuilders and differentiated between a regimen for eliciting muscle hypertrophy and one for developing muscle power. The study indicated that, generally, high repetitions and low resistance will result in increased endurance while low repetitions and high resistance will yield strength. The major practical implication that arose from this research was a definition of the effort required for muscular gains. RM, therefore, was defined as the maximum amount of weight a muscle can lift for that specific number of repetitions. Initially, determination of the RM was done on a trial-and-error basis.

Body weight percentages for beginning conditioning programs

Sanders[20] implemented a formula to determine starting weights in resistive programs based on percentage of body weight. These percentages represent median starting points for certain body parts and are used as a basic guidline in beginning programs. (Rehabilitative restoration of an injured area using ART, however, necessitates a somewhat modified approach to body weight percentage. Determination of the RM is not easy, and, because of pain or fear of

*See references 1, 3, 5, 8, 15, 19, 21, 22, and 23.

Table 10-3. ART programs

Programs	Rehabilitation	Conditioning
DeLorme[7]	B, I, A: 1st set × 10 repetitions × 50% of 10 RM 2nd set × 10 repetitions × 75% of 10 RM 3rd set × 10 repetitions × 100% of 10 RM	B, I, A: Same
Oxford technique (Zinovieff)[26]	B, I, A: 1st set × 10 repetitions × 100% of 10 RM 2nd set × 10 repetitions × 75% of 10 RM 3rd set × 10 repetitions × 50% of 10 RM	B, I, A: Same
MacQueen[16]	B, I, A: 3 sets × 10 repetitions × 100% of 10 RM A: 4-5 sets × 2-3 repetitions × 100% of 2-3 RM	B, I, A: Same A: Same
Sanders[20]	A: 4 sets × 5 repetitions × 100% of 5 RM (3 days/week) 1st day = 4 sets × 5 RM 2nd day = 4 sets × 3 RM 3rd day = 1 set × 5 RM 2 sets × 3 RM 2 sets × 2 RM	A: Same

B, Beginning (posttrauma); I, Intermediate; A, Advanced.

injury, the client may not understand the meaning of the maximum effort. It then becomes a problem of education and motivation on the part of the participant.)

The following percentages are recommended starting points for beginning lifters, doing three sets of 10 repetitions, and should serve only as a guideline for starting a weight-lifting program:

1. Barbell squat—45% body weight
2. Universal leg press—50% body weight
3. Barbell bench press—30% body weight
4. Universal bench press—30% body weight
5. Universal leg extension—20% body weight
6. Leg extension (weight boot)—20% body weight
7. Universal leg curl—10 to 15% body weight
8. Upright rowing—20% body weight

Table 10-3 presents various progressive loading systems that are currently in use. The programs are arranged under conditioning and rehabilitation heading to illustrate the adaptability of various systems to both areas. In addition, further information is given as to whether the programs should be implemented in the beginning, intermediate, or advanced phase of rehabilitation using the ART program.

The key to success in the various programs is always striving to increase resistance without sacrificing good mechanics. No matter what regimen is followed progressively increasing the resistance results in increased strength, power, and endurance for conditioning as well as for restoration of the injured area. Knight[15] introduced the concept of progressive resistance exercise (PRE) for post-surgical rehabilitation and also provided another means to determine whether a client is working at maximum levels. *Daily adjusted progressive resistance exercise* (DAPRE) is a technique that allows for individual differences in the rate at which a person regains strength in the injured area. Tables 10-4 and 10-5 depict the DAPRE technique of weight adjustment and progressive resistance exercise.

The number of repetitions performed during the third

Table 10-4. DAPRE technique

Set	Weight	Repetitions
1	50% RM	10
2	75% RM	6
3	100% RM	Maximum
4	Adjusted working weight	Maximum

Table 10-5. Guidelines for adjusted working weight

Number of repetitions performed during set	Adjusted working weight (fourth set)	Next exercise session
0-2	−5-10 lb	−5-10 lb
3-4	−0-5 lb	Same weight
5-6	Same weight	+5-10 lb
7-10	+5-10 lb	+5-15 lb
11	+10-15 lb	+10-20 lb

set and the weight guidelines described in Table 10-5 are used for determination of the adjusted working weight for the fourth set. Additionally, Table 10-5 gives the number of repetitions performed during the third set, determines the weight used in the fourth set, and indicates that the number of repetitions done in the fourth set is used to determine weight for the next exercise session.

Selecting various programs

The selection of various progressive systems and modalities is ultimately determined by availability and the current status and desire of the individual. Pathological conditions require a more moderate approach both in equipment and in progressive system approaches. Rehabilitation following injury is better accomplished when an exercise can be applied selectively and when resistance can be employed where it is most needed.

Logically, a progressive increase in load with decrease in the repetitions would be the most efficient approach for optimal strength, power, and endurance gains. Not only is the loading system important but so is the selection of exercises. A marathon runner doing a barbell squat of 550 lbs will find the exercise has little carry-over value for running 26.2 miles, while a shotputter performing the same exercise will experience a needed conditioning effect.

Physical conditioning for any sport should correspond with the physiological demands of the activity. The fact that many physiological factors play a role in athletic performance dictates that many combinations of loading systems must be employed.

A sample regimen that combines a circuit routine employing three sets of 10 RM (3 × 10 RM) would be suitable for both conditioning and rehabilitation, as long as the selection of exercises was correct. The use of a combination of overloading systems with repetition and set schemes is endless and presents a unique opportunity for the therapist and/or trainer to maximize an individual's muscular gains. Shown here is a combination program of circuit training and 3 × 10 RM.

CONDITIONING (BASIC PROGRAM)

1. Barbell squat
2. Bench press
3. Barbell upright rowing
4. Barbell curl
5. Hamstring curls (Universal)

REHABILITATION (KNEE EXERCISES)

1. Straight-leg raise
2. Side-leg raise
3. Standing front-leg raise
4. Standing knee flexion

To complete the regimen for the conditioning program the individual should perform the exercises in numerical sequence doing one set of 10 RM; then, after completing all five exercises, he/she should rest 2 minutes, repeat, rest, and repeat, consecutively, until three sets of 10 RM have been completed. The same procedure should be followed for the rehabilitation circuit. The severity of the workouts could be increased by (1) increasing the number of exercises, (2) repeating the circuit more times, (3) increasing the resistance, and/or (4) reducing the rest intervals between or at the end of each cycle. It is clear, therefore, that no matter what the desired outcome or situation, multiple ART programs can be designed and implemented.

SUMMARY

The basic underlying element in ART that is responsible for optimal muscular strength, power, and endurance gains is the progressive reinforcement of efforts to extend beyond limits already reached. Overloading presents numerous possibilities to the therapist/facilitator. There is, of course, no definitive exercise regimen that is applicable to all conditioning and rehabilitation situations. However, research has demonstrated that a number of specific procedures can be followed, and, for practical purposes, the 3 × 10 RM exercise regimen or some modification thereof is usually sufficient. What is also important is to understand that there are individual physiological limitations that might restrict advancement. The selection of programs and/or equipment becomes a problem of time, money, space, and the current status of the individual. Several methods can and should be used with each individual to maximize muscular strength, power, and endurance gains.

REFERENCES

1. Astrand PO and Rodahl K: Textbook of work physiology, New York, 1970, McGraw-Hill, Inc.
2. Basmajian JV: Therapeutic exercise: student edition, Baltimore, 1980, Williams & Wilkins.
3. Bjornaraa B: Weight training systematized, Stillwater, Minn, 1975, Croixside Press.
4. Burke EJ, editor: Toward an understanding of human performance: readings in exercise physiology for the coach and the athlete, Ithaca, NY, 1980, Movement Publications.
5. Capen EK: The effects of systematic weight training on power, strength, and endurance, Res Q Exerc Sport 21:83, 1950.
6. Clark DH: Adaptations in strength and muscular endurance resulting from exercise, Exerc Sport Sci Rev 1:73, 1973.
7. DeLorme TL: Restoration of muscle power by heavy resistance exercises, J Bone Joint Surg (Am) 27:645, 1945.
8. DeLorme TL and Watkins AL: Techniques of progressive resistance exercise, Arch Phys Med Rehabil 29:263, 1948.
9. de Vries HA: Physiology of exercise for physical education and athletics, ed 2, Dubuque, Iowa, 1974, William C. Brown Group.
10. Dons B and Bollerup K: The effect of weightlifting exercise related to muscle fiber composition and muscle cross-sectional area in humans, Eur J Applied Physiol 40:95, 1979.
11. Gettman LR and Pollock ML: Circuit weight training: a critical review of its physiological benefits, Physician Sports Med 9:44, 1981.
12. Jaeger L: Course syllabus for therapeutic exercise, Physical Therapy Program, University of Kentucky, 1976.
13. Katch FI and McArdle WD: Nutrition, weight control, and exercise, Boston, 1977, Houghton Mifflin Co.
14. Kearney JT: Limiting factors in physical performance, Paper presented at physical therapy seminar, University of Kentucky, April, 1976.
15. Knight KL: Knee rehabilitation by the daily adjustable progressive resistive exercise technique, Am J Sports Med 7:336, 1979.
16. MacQueen IJ: Recent advances in the technique of progressive resistance, Brit Med J 11:1193, 1954.
17. O'Donoghue DH: Treatment of injuries to athletes, ed 3, Philadelphia, 1976, WB Saunders Co.
18. O'Shea JP: Scientific principles and methods of strength fitness, Reading, Mass, 1969, Addison-Wesley Publishing Co, Inc.
19. Ryan AJ and Allman FL Jr: Sports medicine, New York, 1974, Academic Press, Inc.
20. Sanders MT: Unpublished study on resistive training, Collegeville, Minn, 1978, St. John's University.
21. Sanders MT: A comparison of two methods of training on the development of muscular strength and endurance, J Orthop Sports Phys Ther 1:210, 1980.
22. Schram DA: Resistance exercise. In Basmajian JV, editor: Therapeutic exercise, Baltimore, 1980, Williams & Wilkins.

23. Stone MH: Considerations in gaining a strength-power training effect (machines vs. free weights), Nat Strength Condition Assoc J 4:22, 1982.

24. Stone WJ and Kroll WA: Sports conditioning and weight training: programs for athletic competition, Boston, 1978, Allyn & Bacon, Inc.

25. Wilmore JH: Athletic training and physical fitness: physiological principles and practices of the conditioning process, Boston, 1976, Allyn & Bacon, Inc.

26. Zinovieff AN: Heavy resistance exercise, the Oxford technique, Brit J Physic Med 14:129, 1951.

Chapter 11

MOBILITY: CONDITIONING PROGRAMS

Donald T. Kirkendall

Work on this chapter was begun while the author was Director of the Research unit, La Crosse Exercise Program, University of Wisconsin–La Crosse.
I wish to acknowledge Cynthia Lee and Sandy Gilchrist for secretarial assistance and Glenn Street for proofing and editorial assistance.

This chapter discusses aspects of exercise physiology, a field that encompasses everything from heart-rate response in clients to subcellular adaptations in skeletal muscle of world-class athletes. It would be ideal if one conditioning program could encompass the spectrum from the general orthopaedic client to the elite athlete, but, unfortunately, it is not physiologically that easy. "Cookbook" programs are not effective in many cases, but the knowledge of basic principles is essential to establish individualized conditioning programs.

This chapter will not discuss what specific endurance or interval program should be used because this decision is made on the basis of individual goals, age, initial fitness level, level of competition (if any is desired), and activity to be performed. Training programs need to be tailored specifically for individuals and the activities they wish to perform. However, foundations for conditioning, metabolic pathways, muscle and fiber types, fatigue, and what responses are elicited by continual exercise (training) will be explained in this chapter to familiarize the therapist with effects of exercise physiology. The more familiar the overall picture of training, the greater the understanding of just what the body has endured to adapt to the training stimulus.

METABOLISM

Since all cellular activity depends on the metabolism of foodstuffs, it is appropriate to describe both the fuels for energy production and the metabolic pathways through which high-energy phosphate molecules, such as adenosine triphosphate (ATP), are produced. (The supply of energy-rich phosphate can be readily available for muscular exercise.) The subsequent effects of muscular training on

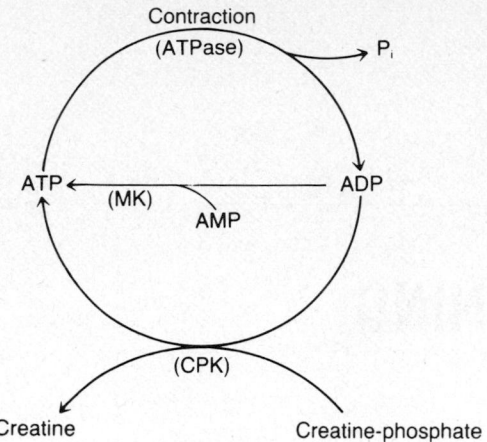

Fig. 11-1. Phosphagen replenishment of ATP.

availability and use of substrates along with the effects of training on the pathways themselves will also be discussed.

Anaerobic metabolism

Sarcomere, subsequent fiber, and whole muscle shortening is accomplished by use of the energy stored in the hydrolyzed bond that is created through hydrolysis of ATP to adenosine diphosphate (ADP) and inorganic phosphate (Pi). The cell must attempt to keep a supply of ATP available so that the process of contraction may continue. In the absence of oxygen ATP is supplied from the stored phosphagens and anaerobic glycolysis.

Phosphagens. The pathway for phosphagens is very simple because a stored high-energy molecule, creatine phosphate (CP), is hydrolyzed and the energy transferred to the new ATP molecule (Fig. 11-1). ADP and CP, in the presence of the enzyme creatine phosphokinase (CPK), will resynthesize the spent ATP molecule. In addition, two ADP molecules, in the presence of myokinase (MK), can produce an ATP molecule with an adenosine monophosphate (AMP) molecule remaining.

While these two methods serve as an immediate source of ATP during muscle contraction, this source of anaerobic energy is very limited and short term. The *power,* or rate of energy supply, of the phosphagens to supply ATP per minute is over 3.5 times that of aerobic metabolism, but the *capacity,* the amount of energy available independent of time, of the oxygen system is approximately 1,300 times as great as that of the phosphagens.[40]

One must realize that a great deal of anaerobic energy is available but not for a long period of time. Male and female athletes often have aerobic capacities of over 5 and 3 liters of oxygen per minute, respectively. While these are impressive amounts and the individuals can deliver ATP aerobically for contraction for extended periods, these amounts are still below the oxygen delivery needed for a 100-yard dash, were it an aerobic event, in which 45 to 60

liters of oxygen per minute (8 to 10 liters of oxygen per 10-second 100-yard dash) are needed. As a result, short-term, high-intensity, low-repetition events (e.g., 100-yard dash, shot put, and weight lifting) use phosphagens as the primary source of energy, while long-term, low-intensity, high-repetition activities, such as endurance running, rely on the aerobic pathway to supply energy for extended periods.

Data have been presented that demonstrate an increase in MK and CPK activity, in addition to increased levels of stored ATP and CP, with appropriate training. Training effectively increases the ability of the muscle to produce ATP more rapidly.[25,111] The results of this research should not, however, be construed to mean that fatigue can be delayed in performance of high-intensity exercises.

Anaerobic glycolysis. A second method by which the muscle can produce ATP in the absence of oxygen involves the process of carbohydrate oxidation through glycolysis in the cytoplasm (Fig. 11-2).

Entry of blood-borne glucose into the cell is facilitated by insulin. ATP is then needed for carbohydrate oxidation to proceed (step 1). The oxidation continues and another ATP is added (step 2). While many steps in metabolism are reversible, using the same enzyme, these two steps are not; a separate enzyme is needed to reverse the process. A 6-carbon molecule, fructose-1,6-diphosphate (F1,6-dip), is produced and then broken into two 3-carbon molecules. (Note that both 3-carbon molecules complete the path.) An inorganic phosphate is added, and an electron acceptor (NAD) is reduced to $NADH_2$ (step 6). In subsequent steps two ATP molecules are produced (steps 3 and 4). Thus four ATP molecules have been produced and two have been used during the oxidation of blood glucose to lactic acid, making a net yield of two ATP molecules. Finally, pyruvic acid is reduced to lactic acid (step 5), the end product of anaerobic glycolysis. The electrons for such a reduction come from the $NADH_2$ produced earlier (step 6). Therefore a ready, yet limited, supply of NAD is available for reduction further up the chain.

This lactic acid has three possible fates: (1) resynthesis to glycogen or glucose, (2) oxidation to carbon dioxide and water, or (3) conversion to various amino acids via pyruvate to alanine or various Krebs cycle intermediates. Lactate removal may occur in local fibers, nonworking muscles, or the liver. It was originally thought that up to 85% of the lactic acid was removed and resynthesized to glycogen.[6] Recent data by Hermansen[57,59] also support this thought. Brooks, Bravner, and Cassens[14,15] indicate that up to 75% of the lactate produced is oxidized through the Krebs cycle to carbon dioxide and water, 15% is converted to glucose by the liver, and the remaining 10% is untraceable by their technique. Stevensen et al[108] have demonstrated that glycogen deleted muscle perfused with an arterial solution high in lactate and absent in O_2 and glucose is capable of synthesizing glycogen from lactate.

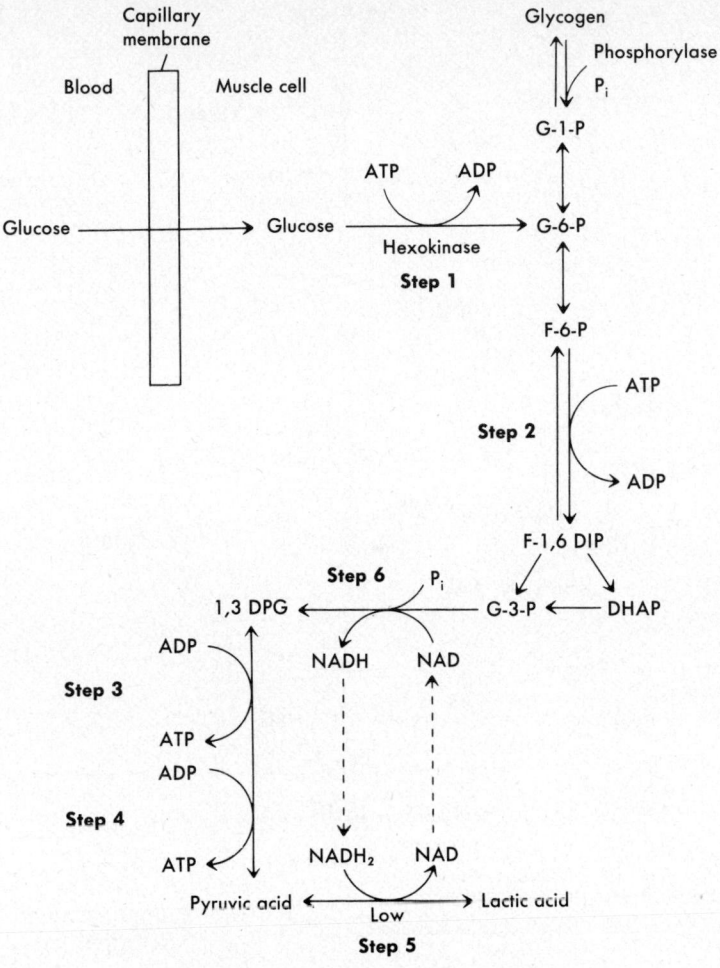

Fig. 11-2. Anaerobic glycolysis.

Endurance training appears to do little to increase the activity of the enzymes of glycolysis except for hexokinase (glucose→glucose-6-phosphate), which parallels oxidative enzymes.[62] Yet Costill's data showed increases in phosphorylase (glycogen→glucose-1-phosphate) and phosphofructokinase (fructose-6-phosphate→fructose-1,6-diphosphate), two enzymes generally thought of as rate limiters of glycolysis.[25]

Aerobic metabolism

Energy metabolism in the presence of oxygen, which occurs in the mitochondria, results in greater amounts of APT and waste products that are more easily eliminated, such as carbon dioxide and water. In addition, fats and proteins, along with carbohydrates, may be used as a fuel.

Carbohydrate metabolism. In the presence of oxygen, pyruvate reduction to lactate slows; via the pyruvate dehydrogenase enzyme complex, pyruvate is converted to acetyl coenzyme A (CoA), the common entry point to the Krebs cycle (Fig. 11-3). In the process carbon dioxide is produced and NAD is reduced to $NADH_2$. Also, the $NADH_2$ produced earlier in glycolysis has not been oxi-

dized, as lactate is thought not to be produced. Acetyl CoA then enters the Krebs cycle. In this process the 2-carbon acetyl CoA joins with the 4-carbon oxaloacetic acid. This 6-carbon molecule is then metabolized with two carbon dioxide, three $NADH_2$, one $FADH_2$ (another electron acceptor), and one ATP being produced. To develop the ATPs, the reduced electron acceptors ($NADH_2$ and $FADH_2$) are oxidized through the electron transport chain (ETC-cytochromes) with the final acceptor being oxygen. Thus the end products are water from the electron transport chain and carbon dioxide from the Krebs cycle. For each $NADH_2$ three ATPs are produced, and for each $FADH_2$ two ATPs are produced. This process occurs twice with two pyruvates being produced. Therefore a total of 38 ATPs are produced from one mode of glucose (Table 11-1).

Fat metabolism. Fat metabolism proceeds along a different path. Triglycerides in the blood or muscle must first be broken down to their component glycerol heads and the three free fatty acid (FFA) chains by a lipoprotein lipase. The FFA chain then proceeds through a process called beta-oxidation, so-called because the long FFA chain (14

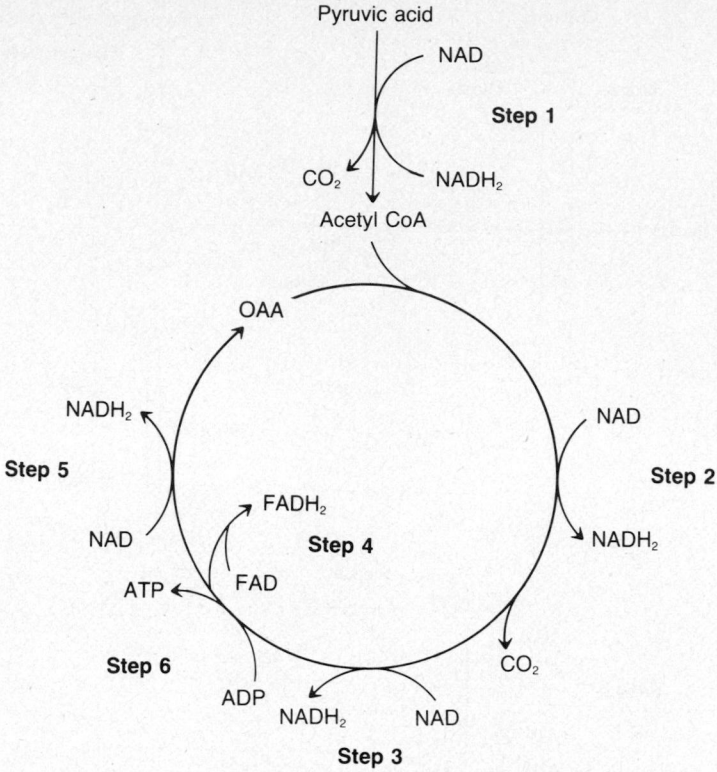

Fig. 11-3. Krebs cycle.

Table 11-1. Energetics of carbohydrate metabolism

Pathway	Method	Step	ATP produced
Glycolysis	$NADH_2$	6	6
(Fig. 11-2)	ATP	3,4	4
			10
	ATP utilization	1,2	−2
		NET	8
Krebs cycle	$NADH_2$	1	6
(Fig. 11-3)	NADH	2,3,5	18
	$FADH_2$	4	4
	ATP	6	2
			30
Total ATP—aerobic metabolism			38
Total ATP—anaerobic glycolysis			2

Modified from Harper HA: Physiological chemistry, Los Altos, Calif, 1973, Lange Medical Books.

to 18 carbons) is cleaved two carbons at a time and oxidized. In the process one $NADH_2$, one $FADH_2$, and one acetyl CoA are produced per beta-oxidation, with three and two ATPs, respectively, produced at the cytochromes for each electron carrier and 12 ATPs produced per turn of the Krebs cycle for each acetyl CoA. The energetics get tricky, but for a 16-carbon FFA chain, eight acetyl CoA are produced and seven β-oxidative processes occur. Eight

acetyl CoA multiplied by 12 ATPs per turn of the Krebs cycle equals 96 ATPs. Seven beta-oxidations with five ATPs from the two acceptors going through the cytochromes produce 35 ATPs. Therefore a total of 131 ATPs are produced with a net to the system of 129 (two ATPs are needed to initially activate the FFA chain). There are three FFA chains per triglyceride; therefore the number is multiplied by 3, since the 129 ATPs are from just one FFA chain, for a net of 387 ATPs. In addition to producing more ATP, the process is slightly more efficient than carbohydrate metabolism (41% versus 39%) in capturing the energy available from a molecule of substrate.

Protein metabolism. With respect to protein metabolism, it has generally been considered that carbohydrates and fats are the primary energy sources for exercise. Even the respiratory exchange ratio (RER, VCO_2/VO_2), routinely measured in metabolic studies to determine the fuel contribution in exercise (RER of 0.7 = fats as fuel; RER of 1.0 = carbohydrates as fuel), is a nonprotein factor: the value does not consider proteins as an energy source. There is research, however, that suggests that proteins may be more involved than previously assumed.[75]

The difference between protein, fat, and carbohydrate structure is that proteins contain a nitrogenous compound that must be removed before hydrolysis through metabolic pathways can occur. This hydrolysis can occur in skeletal muscle as well as in the liver. Excretion of nitrogen in

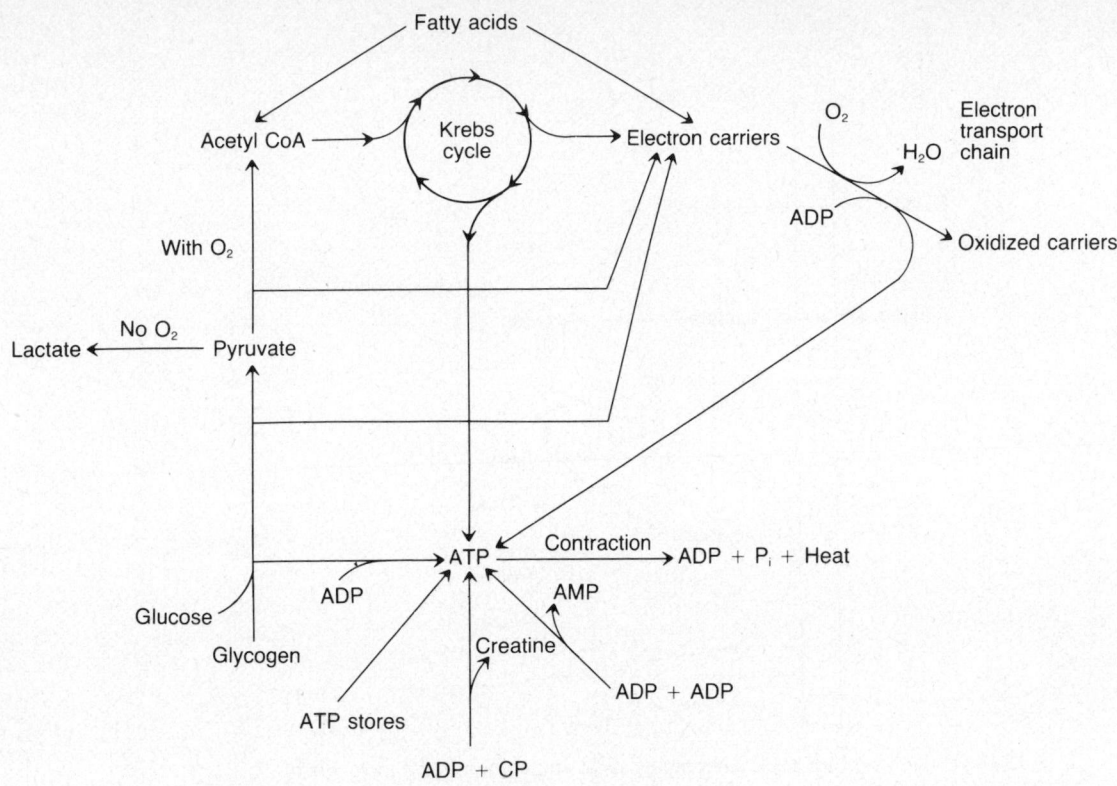

Fig. 11-4. Summary of ATP production.

sweat and urine as well as the presence of expired radioactive carbon dioxide from C-leucine illustrates the breakdown of proteins during exercise for use as an energy fuel.[16] Use of branched-chair amino acids (glucose-alanine cycle) is a major pathway for inclusion of proteins as an energy source.

While carbohydrates and fats are the primary fuels for activity, the contribution of proteins as a significant energy source and of dietary proteins during recovery from exercise cannot be ignored. For a thorough review of the topic, see Lemon and Nagle.[75]

Effects of training

It is well demonstrated that endurance training positively affects the enzymes of aerobic metabolism.[61-63] Succinate dehydrogenase (SDH) and malate dehydrogenase (MDH) are examples of marker enzymes of Krebs cycle activity that increase with training.[17,24,62,63] Cytochrome C, a marker of electron transport chain activity, also increases.[63] It has also been well documented that with training there is an increased reliance on fats as a preferred fuel for endurance exercise.[78,79] During submaximal work the endurance-trained person will use fats as the preferred fuel while an untrained person will use carbohydrates.[63,97] This appears to be caused by both an increased availability of FFA in the endurance-trained person and an increase in the activity of enzymes involved in lipid metabolism.[40]

Factors limiting metabolism

These metabolic processes are subject to control mechanisms that regulate metabolic rate. Obviously, substrate availability will affect metabolism and exercise. Costill[21] has demonstrated that in the absence of muscle glycogen, but adequate FFA, exercise is difficult, if not impossible, indicating a need for carbohydrates in some quantity. Another factor that limits metabolism is the rate-limiting enzyme of glycolysis, phosphofructokinase or PFK (step 2, Fig. 11-2). Products that indicate use of ATP, such as ADP, AMP, and P_i, and that have a low ATP/ADP ratio will encourage PFK activity, while high ATP and CP levels suggest adequate phosphagens and little need for increased levels and thus inhibit PFK. In addition, citrate, a Krebs cycle intermediate, and a low pH from increased lactate levels, for example, discourage PFK activity.[70] However, in an isometric model Sahlin, Harris, and Hultman[93] demonstrated that the glycolytic rate was maintained in spite of metabolic changes that might normally be considered negative influences on PFK. Various other enzymes are often discussed as controlling factors, such as hexokinase, lactate dehydrogenase, and pyruvate dehydrogenase.

Three methods of ATP production have been discussed: immediate sources (phosphagens), anaerobic glycolysis, and aerobic metabolism. Figs. 11-4 and 11-5 summarize ATP production and the integration of the pathways.

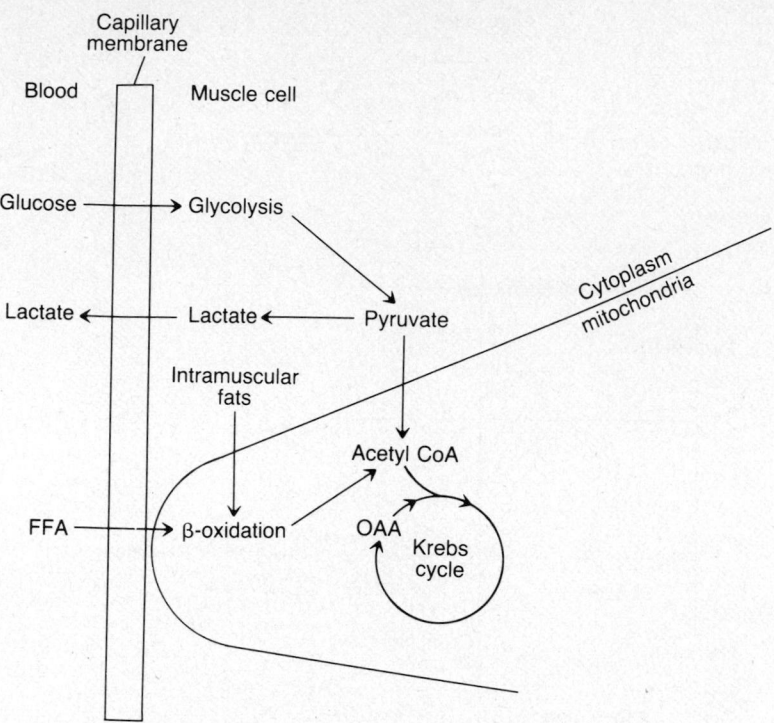

Fig. 11-5. Integration of fat and carbohydrate metabolism.

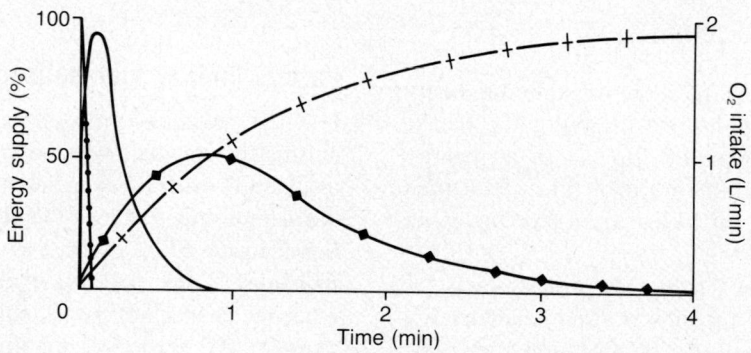

Fig. 11-6. Sources of energy at onset of exercise, showing initial short-lived breakdown of ATP and use of stored oxygen (●——●——●), breakdown of phosphoryl creatine (——), glycolysis (◆ – ◆), and aerobic metabolism (——+——).

Another question involves the integration of these energy sources for the performance of an activity. Since activities are a function of intensity, duration, and resistance to movement, an activity of short duration, high intensity, and low repetition (for example, resistance training) will require a rapid energy source for contraction; therefore these exercises use stored ATP and the ATP-CP network. Similar exercises of slightly longer duration (for example, a 400-meter run) require a large amount of ATP from stored phosphagens and glycolysis. Low-intensity, long-duration, and high-repetition exercise (for example, endurance running) requires a steady supply of ATP without buildup of a waste product, so the aerobic system plays the predominant role. The key is the time frame of the activ-

ity: the length of time one can perform the activity at the desired intensity. Fig. 11-6 illustrates the relationship between energy supply and time. This relationship is crucial for designing a training program. For example, knowing that endurance training increases the cell's ability to supply energy aerobically and that strength training improves the cell's anaerobic capacity, one can select a training method to correspond to the activity's nature (duration and intensity).

SKELETAL MUSCLE TISSUE
Structure

To better understand muscle function in exercise, a brief review of muscle structure and the contractile process

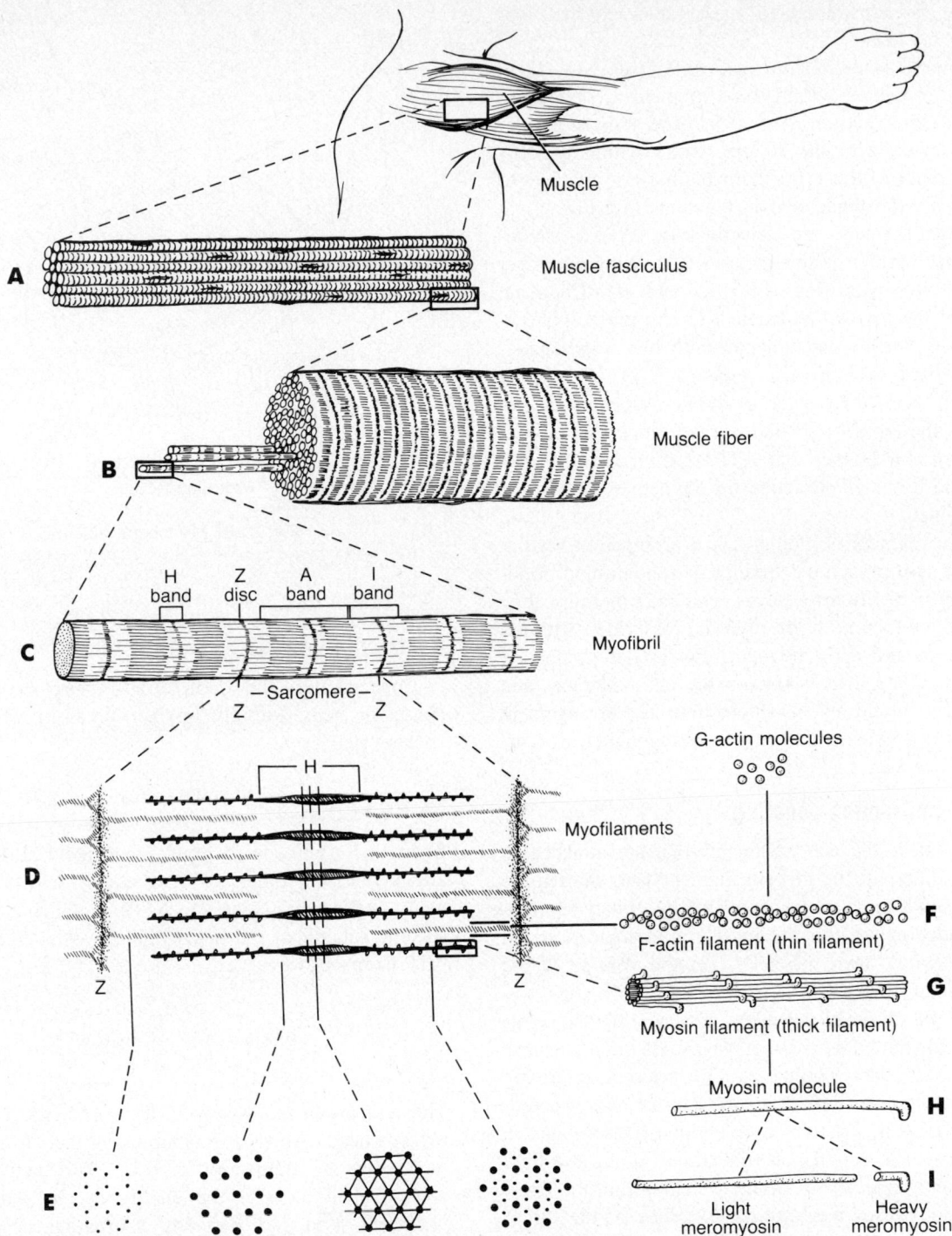

Fig. 11-7. Organization of a skeletal muscle from the whole muscle level to the level of the contractile proteins. **F** through **I** are cross sections of sarcomere taken from different levels. (From Bloom W and Fawcett DW: A textbook of histology, Philadelphia, 1975, WB Saunders Co.)

is appropriate. Muscle develops tension most favorably by shortening; that is, the muscle attempts to move one skeletal part toward another by pulling. Therefore an organized subcellular network must function to encourage tension development by shortening.

The muscle is arranged in fibers parallel to each other

and to the long axis of the muscle that facilitates shortening (Fig. 11-7, *A* to *E*). On observation the muscle appears striated, and examination of an individual myofibril will show an orderly arrangement of sarcomeres aligned end to end. Each sarcomere is capable of developing tension. When all sarcomeres shorten, this internal tension is transmitted to measurable external tension.

A sarcomere is deliniated by Z lines (see Fig. 11-7, *D* and *C*). Contained within the sarcomere are two contractile proteins—actin and myosin. The thin actin filaments are attached to the Z lines while within the sarcomere. Parallel to the actin filaments but not attached to the Z lines are the thick myosin filaments (see Fig. 11-7, *E*). These two filaments are collectively referred to as contractile units. Myosin filaments are made up of a number of myosin molecules (Fig. 11-7, *G* and *H*). Chemical treatment of the myosin molecule with the proteolytic enzyme trypsin cleaves the molecule into two fragments—heavy and light meromyosin (Fig. 11-7, *I*). The heavy meromyosin forms the portion of the myosin molecule referred to as the *crossbridge* and has two important biological properties: it houses that ATPase used for ATP hydrolysis, and it has an attraction for the active sites on the actin molecule.

The actin filament is globular, and arranged at regular intervals are two regulatory proteins—troponin and tropomyosin. These are referred to as regulatory because they regulate the interaction of the myosin crossbridge with the active sites on the actin filament. At rest, troponin and tropomyosin block active sites on the actin filament and thus inhibit actin and myosin interaction. The arrangement of the actin to myosin filaments is hexagonal: a 6:1 arrangement (see Fig. 11-7, *I*).

Excitation-contraction coupling

Simply stated, the actin filaments that are attached to the Z lines slide past the myosin filaments and shorten the sarcomere. With many sarcomeres simultaneously shortening and producing tension, the muscle in turn shortens and the cross-sectional area increases, yet the volume of the muscle remains constant.

For a muscle to develop tension, a nerve impulse is initiated and transmitted across the synapse of the motor unit (Fig. 11-8) via acetylcholine (ACh) vesicles migrating across the synapse to initiate a sarcolemmal action potential. The process is deactivated by cholinesterase bound in the end plate. The action potential travels along the fiber membrane and down the T tubule system within the fiber. This potential causes the terminal cisternae of the sarcoplasmic reticulum to become permeable to stored calcium ions, which can then pass into the sarcomere. Calcium cations combine, with particularly high affinity, with a subunit of troponin. This union causes the troponin-tropomyosin complex to "roll away" and open the actin active site, allowing actin and myosin interaction and the contractile process to continue. Therefore calcium ions have the ability to couple membrane excitation with muscular contraction. The term for this process is *excitation-contraction coupling*. For a detailed description of the process see Ebashi[34] or Katz.[70]

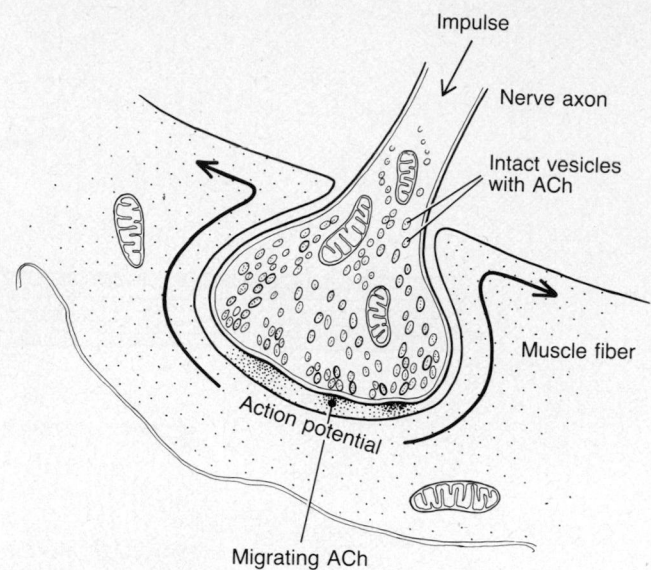

Fig. 11-8. Myoneural junction.

Contractile process

Conceptually, the contractile process occurs in five phases or steps. Initially, myosin binds to ATP to use its energy (step 1):

$$Myosin + ATP \rightarrow myosin—ATP$$

Since this affinity is so high, most likely all crossbridges are bound with either ATP or the hydrolytic end products—$ADP + P_i$. Next, the ATPase, which is housed in a specific subunit of the heavy meromyosin, hydrolyzes the ATP (step 2):

$$Myosin—ATP \rightarrow myosin \begin{array}{c} ADP \\ P_i \end{array}$$

The end products, however, do not dissociate from the myosin head. An active complex is then formed by the interaction of actin and myosin. This active complex is so named because the energy in the split ATP has not been used nor has any shortening occurred (step 3).

$$Actin + myosin \begin{array}{c} ADP \\ P_i \end{array} \longrightarrow$$

$$Actin-myosin \begin{array}{c} ADP \\ P_i \text{ (active complex)} \end{array}$$

The release of energy in this unstable complex causes a shift in the relationship of the crossbridge to the rest of the myosin molecule. This shift results in a new complex—a low-energy rigor complex (step 4).

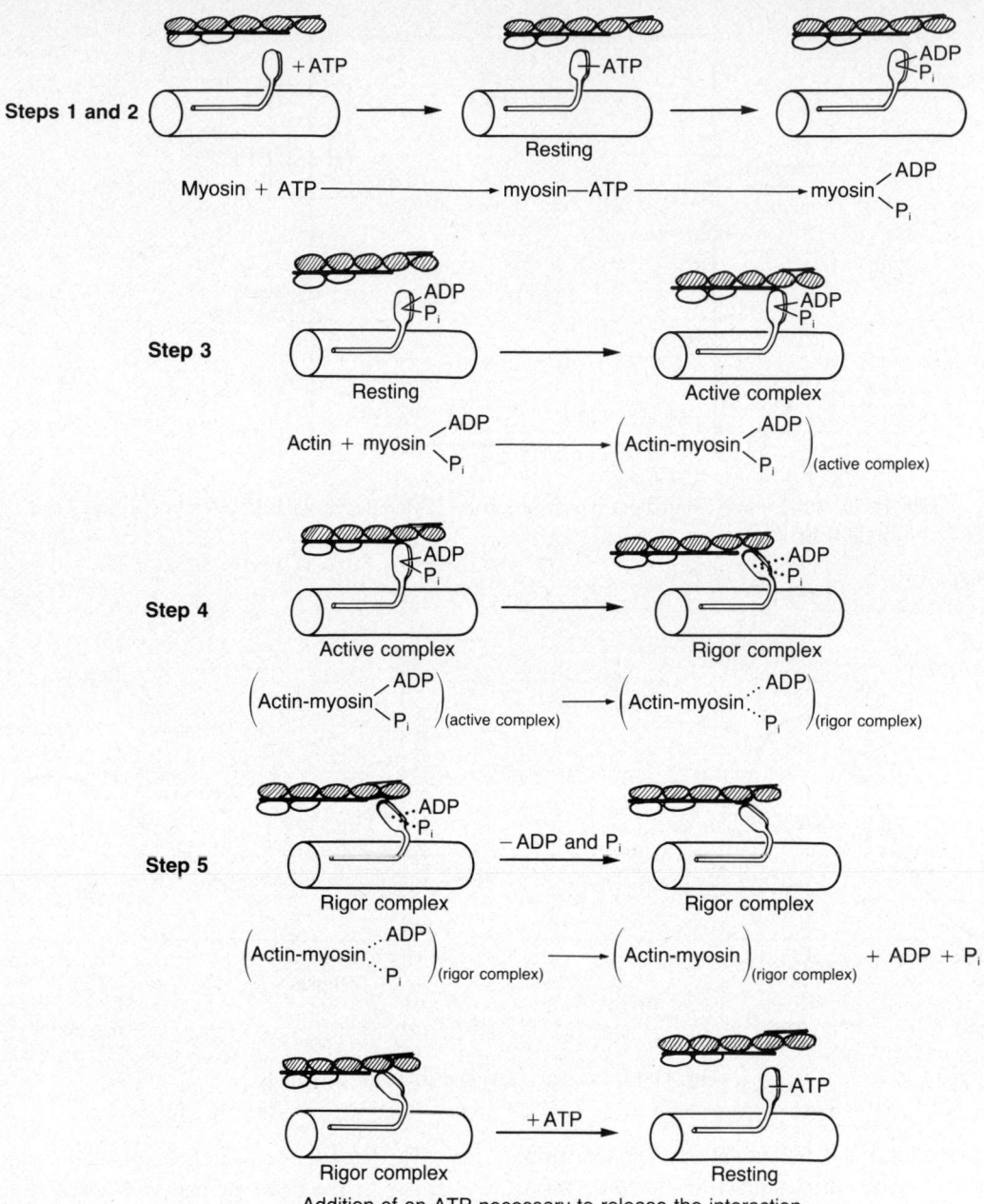

Fig. 11-9. Summary of steps involved in contractile process. (Adapted from Katz AM: Physiology of the heart, New York, 1977, Raven Press.)

Actin-myosin $\xrightarrow{\quad\quad}$
ADP
P_i (active complex)

ADP
Actin-myosin
P_i (rigor complex)

This shift changes the myosin head's relationship so that it draws the actin filament toward the center of the sarcomere. This last process entails the release of ADP and P_i from the myosin head (step 5). However, the actin-myosin interaction is highly stable and still is a rigor complex.

ADP
Actin-myosin
P_i (rigor complex)

Actin-myosin + ADP + P_i
(rigor complex)

These equations explain the contractile processes from binding of ATP and myosin to sarcomere shortening and release of ADP and P_i.

For the actin-myosin interaction to be released, an ATP must attach to the myosin head. Fig. 11-9 demonstrates the entire process.

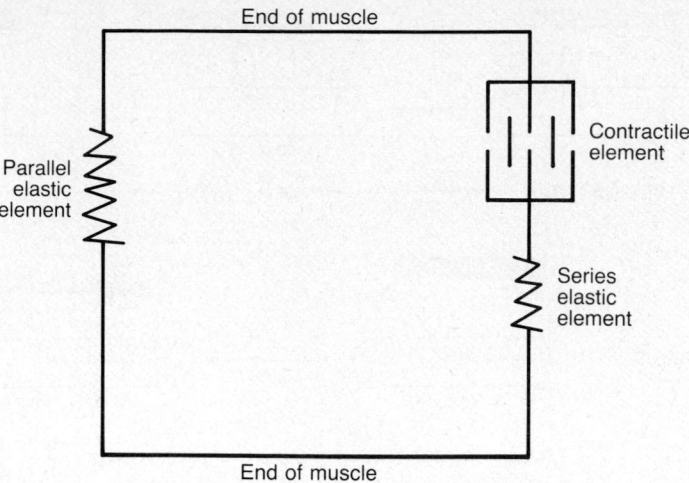

Fig. 11-10. Hill's three-component model of muscle. (Modified from Hill, AV Proc R Soc Lond [Biol] 126:136, 1938.)

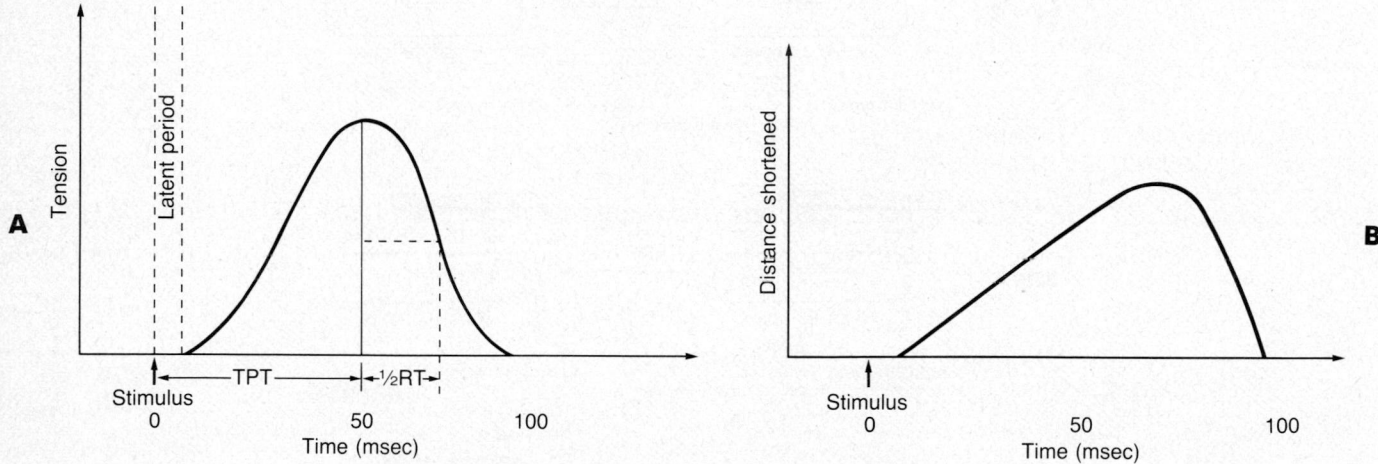

Fig. 11-11. Isometric (**A**) and isotonic (**B**) twitch.

Within this structural and functional arrangement three entities (elements) exist: the contractile element, series elastic element, and parallel elastic element[60] (Fig. 11-10). To illustrate the interaction of the elements, the basic response of a muscle—the twitch—will be discussed.

A twitch may be of two types: isometric (Fig. 11-11, *A*) or isotonic (Fig. 11-11, *B*). In an isometric twitch the muscle remains fixed at a constant length. In an isotonic twitch the muscle is allowed to shorten against a fixed load rather than a fixed length.

Fig. 11-11, *A* shows that after a stimulus, a brief latency period occurs. Then external tension is developed as the tension inside the sarcomere is transmitted to the ends of the muscle until a peak is reached. The sarcomeres then release their tension and the muscle relaxes. Characteristics measured include time to peak tension (TPT) and half relaxation time (½ relaxation time or ½ RT).

The latent period can be explained by looking at the interplay of the three elements. When a stimulus is applied to a muscle, the contractile element shortens but the tension developed in the sarcomere is not immediately realized at the end of the muscle (see Fig. 11-11, *A*), thus demonstrating the concept of an elastic element in series with the contractile element. When the series elastic element is stretched, tension will be visible at the end of the muscle. To use Vander's analogy,[114] imagine your arm as the contractile element, a brick as the load, and a spring from your arm to the brick as the series element. For you to lift the brick, a certain amount of tension must be generated and transmitted through the spring. Internal tension in your arm will continue to increase and the spring will stretch. When the tension developed exceeds the brick's weight, the brick will be moved. Obviously, the length of the latent period will vary with the weight of the load to be moved. With a cessation of contractile tension, the load

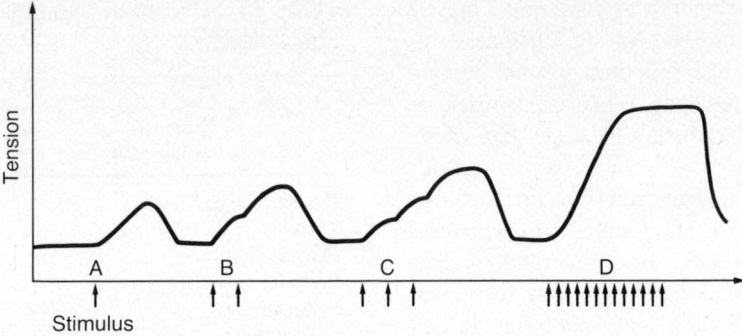

Fig. 11-12. Summation of twitches to tetany.

will be in excess of contractile tension and the muscle will reestablish its original length.

The location of the series elastic element is implied in Fig. 11-10 as being outside the contractile element. It appears that indeed some elasticity is present near and/or in the tendinous ends of the muscle. In addition, elasticity seems to be present in the myofilament crossbridges themselves.[70] The effect of the parallel elastic element will be discussed in the section or muscle mechanics.

The amount of tension produced by a muscle is partially determined by how the motor units are stimulated. Fig. 11-12 illustrates the tension produced in a single motor unit during four separate twitches *(A, B, C,* and *D),* with varying types of stimuli. Twitch *A* exhibits the resultant tension of a single stimulus (increased). Twitch *B* shows the tension produced when stimulus is added before relaxation; the total tension has been summated. Twitch *C* exhibits added summation with additional stimuli. Twitch *D* illustrates tetany, the maximal tension production in response to a barrage of impulses.

The central nervous system (CNS) can also regulate muscle tension by controlling the number of motor units recruited. For minimal tension requirements, relatively few motor units will be recruited, while for greater tension demands, more units will be recruited. The result is that muscle tension can be varied by two methods or a combination of both: by varying the rate of impulses to a muscle and/or by varying the number of units recruited.

Basic muscle mechanics

Two factors of muscle function will be explored by the relationship between muscle length and the tension developed and the relationship between force and velocity of contraction.

Length-tension relations. By varying the length of an isometrically stimulated muscle, different tensions can be produced. The mechanisms responsible can be described by detailing crossbridge interaction at the muscle's initial length.

At portion *A* of the curve (Fig. 11-13) crossbridge interaction is at its optimal level and has the greatest degree of

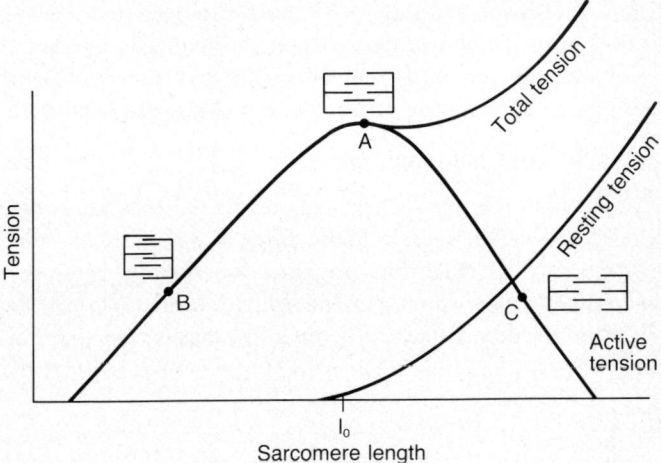

Fig. 11-13. Length-tension relationships.

actin-myosin communication possible. Setting a muscle at this length for an isometric contraction will produce its maximal tension. At area *B,* the muscle has been shortened to a level where two processes contribute to reduced tension: (1) the muscle's length has been reduced so that optimal crossbridge interaction is not possible, and (2) the muscle's cross-sectional area has increased distance between the myosin heads and actin filaments. Both of these factors reduce the tension achievable during optimal stretch *(A).* These two factors both affect the decreased tension development seen in area *A.*

As the length of the muscle is increased, the resting tension *(B)* increases. Since there has been no tension produced by the contractile element and the series elastic component functions in conjunction with shortening, as previously described, the origin of the tension lies within the third of Hill's three components—the parallel elastic component.[60] Increasing the length of the muscle increases the surrounding tension on the muscle.

The development of tension might be similar to the effects produced by the children's toy Chinese handcuffs. A finger is inserted in each end of a woven bamboo tube, and when one tries to pull the fingers out (increased muscle length), the web tightens (increased resting tension).

Crossbridge interaction is also less than optimal because the sarcomere has been stretched. When the muscle is stimulated (subtracting out the resting tension), less active tension is produced.

Force-velocity relations. The relationship between muscular force and velocity of shortening is a hyperbolic function (Fig. 11-14). Maximal force generation occurs during isometric conditions (velocity = 0), with force generation decreasing along the curve with increasing velocities. Maximal velocity of shortening would occur during a zero-load situation if that were experimentally possible. It should be noted that this curve was developed on excised muscle. Perrine and Edgerton[87] have demonstrated a deviation from the classic curve when shortening is measured isokinetically on intact human quadriceps muscle. Their results show a plateau of force at the slowest velocities.

Muscle fiber composition

To think that all skeletal muscle fibers are alike would indeed be naive. Muscle fibers differ in a number of characteristics that make muscle tissue functionally heterogeneous. The most common nomenclature used to classify fibers is based on contractile properties; that is, the speed at

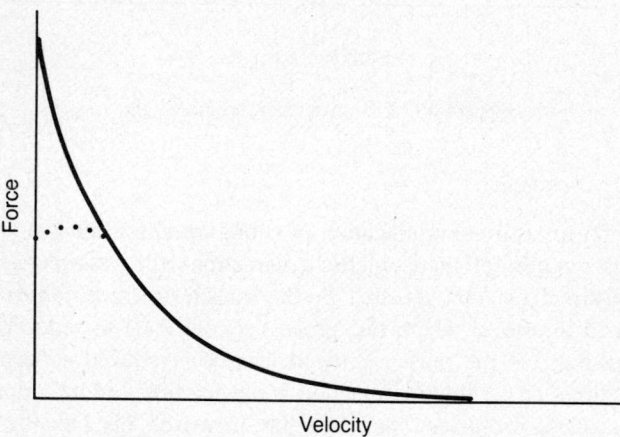

Fig. 11-14. Force-velocity relationships. (Modified from Perrine JJ and Edgerton VR: Med Sci Sports Exerc 10: 159, 1978.)

Table 11-2. Summary of muscle fiber nomenclature

	Type		
Tonic	Phasic		Reference
Slow twitch (red)	**Fast twitch (white)**		
Slow twitch	Fast twitch a	Fast twitch b	99
I	IIa	IIb	33
S	FR	FF	16
SO	FOG	FG	8

Table 11-3. Human skeletal muscle fiber characteristics

	Fiber type	
Characteristic	Slow twitch	Fast twitch
Cross-sectional area	Less	Larger
Time to peak tension	Slow	Fast
Fatigue resistance	High	Low
Enzyme activities		
Anaerobic	Low	High
Aerobic	High	Low
Capillary density	High	Low
Mitochondrial density	High	Low
Recruitment for:		
Short-term, high-intensity work	Less	Great
Long-term, low-intensity work	Great	Less
Innervation ratio (fiber/neuron)	Low	High

Modified from Lamb DR: Physiology of exercise: responses and adaptations, New York, 1978, Macmillan, Inc. and Armstrong, RB: Skeletal muscle physiology. In Strauss R, editor: Sports medicine and physiology, Philadelphia, 1979, WB Saunders Co.

which a fiber can produce its peak tension. Fast-twitch (FT) fibers are those that develop high tension rapidly, and slow-twitch (ST) fibers develop less tension more slowly. While this is the most recognized scheme for classifying fibers, other systems that recognize an intermediate fiber abound in the literature. Table 11-2 summarizes the commonly used nomenclatures. The simple ST, FT system will be used here.

Table 11-3 summarizes selected properties of fibers. FT fibers are those most suited to explosive activities—jumping, weight lifting, and sprints, to name a few. These activities call for rapid development of high tension. A single alpha motor neuron innervates many FT fibers, which are capable of developing short-term high tension with low fatigue resistance. These fibers predominantly use anaerobic metabolism for energy production since their aerobic capacity is poor; they have low levels of aerobic enzymes and low oxygen availability because of a low capillary density.

ST fibers, on the other hand, produce less tension, are highly resistant to fatigue, and have an adequate oxygen and enzyme activity. These fibers are used in activities of reduced intensity and extended duration, such as distance running.

Different muscles have varying percentages of each fiber type. Humans, being adaptable animals, have approximately equal percentages of each.[99] However, there are extreme cases. World-class endurance runners genetically inherit high percentages of ST fibers, while sprinters usually have high percentages of FT fibers. However, knowing a person's dominant fiber type is not reliable in predicting his/her athletic success or correct event or sport for participation. A coach could probably reach the same conclusion by having all the athletes perform a maximal 100-yard dash and a 2-mile run. Those athletes high in FT fibers will do better in the former and those high in ST fibers will succeed in the latter, saving the athlete and coach the expense and minor discomfort of a muscle biopsy. There are several good reviews on the topic of fiber composition. These should be consulted for further information.[6,16,24,99]

Effects of training on skeletal muscle

As previously mentioned, humans are superbly adaptable; stressing the body causes adaptations to occur that allow the organism to adjust to the new stress. Muscle will respond to repeated stress (training) by adapting to the specific stimulus. Two extremes of training will be considered: high-intensity, high-resistance, low-repetition training (strength training) and low-intensity, low-resistance, high-repetition training (endurance training). For a more detailed description of strength training, the reader is referred to Chapter 10.

Strength training. Research has confirmed that there is an association between large muscle and great strength—that is, strength is proportional to the cross-sectional area of that muscle.[51,66] Therefore, to increase the amount of tension produced by a muscle, the cross-sectional area of that muscle needs to increase. This may be accomplished by either increasing the size of the individual fibers (hypertrophy) or increasing the number of fibers (hyperplasia).

Hyperplasia, however, probably has little influence in increasing the cross-sectional area because the number of cells appears to be fixed.[4] Edgerton[35] published evidence to support the process of longitudinal fiber splitting in animals subjected to extreme conditions of overload, while the results of Gollnick's research[55] indicates the contrary. Evidence of a similar process occurring in humans has yet to be conclusively documented.

Hypertrophy results from an increase in the diameter of the myofibrils, along with increases in other muscle components[4,51] and enzyme activities.[25,111] In order for hypertrophy to occur, an overload must be imposed on the muscle. This overload needs to be exercise that will increase strength. The muscle must be stressed so that adaptations occur to accommodate a need for greater tension production. While both FT and ST fibers will hypertrophy, the FT fibers will exhibit a greater degree of change. Measurable strength, in normal adults, has been shown to improve via neural recruitment followed by fiber hypertrophy.[81,82] This model has not been tested on muscle recovering from immobilization. Endurance activities (low-resistance), like running, do not encourage muscular hypertrophy as significantly as strength training.

Most assuredly, while use will encourage hypertrophy, disuse will result in atrophy. This decrease in muscle size involves a mechanism opposite of hypertrophy—that is,

decreases in the diameter of the myofibrils, connective tissue, stored fuels, aerobic enzymes of muscle, number of sarcomeres, range of motion, and water content.[12] Immobilized limbs show visible atrophy with concomitant changes in contractile properties and metabolic profiles within 2 or 3 days.[11,16]

Endurance training. While the primary areas of adaptation in strength training deal with tension development, adaptation in endurance training results in resistance to fatigue. This resistance is accomplished through a number of mechanisms. An increase in the capillary-to-muscle fiber ratio occurs,[64] thus reducing the distance that oxygen molecules must diffuse to reach the working fibers. In addition, muscle myoglobin increases following endurance training.[86] Finally, major adaptations occur in the cells' ability to oxidize fuels. This includes an increase in both the size and the number of mitochondria[53,61-63,71] and the enzymes involved in oxidative metabolism of carbohydrates[8,61,79] and fats.[78,79] Changes in anaerobic metabolism also occur, including enhanced ATP and PC stores[68] and levels of selected enzymes.[54] Endurance training will also cause hypertrophy of ST but not FT fibers.[54]

These alterations, which occur only in the muscles used in endurance exercise, are obviously specific to an enhanced oxygen utilization system in the cells. Both FT and ST fiber types will increase their oxidative capacity. The metabolic profile of the FT fiber will appear to be more like the ST fiber than it was before training. However, it does not appear possible to convert FT to ST fibers or to change the FT fibers' contractile properties through long-term training.

It should be obvious that only the muscles and fibers stressed will exhibit tension or resistance development. Specific exercise and training, strength or endurance, will elicit a specific response resulting in FT or ST hypertrophy and anaerobic or aerobic adaptations in the specifically trained muscles. These responses will be lost through atrophy if the cell is not continually stressed.

For more detailed information on muscular adaptations to training (strength and endurance), the reader is referred to any one of several excellent reviews.*

AEROBIC TRAINING PRINCIPLES

Training for aerobic improvement involves the overload principle individually applied. Suggestions on the frequency, intensity, and duration of exercise are ideally based on a person's known capacity or maximal oxygen consumption (VO_2 MAX), age, and fitness level. Thus a nonindividualized program will be limited. Nevertheless, before embarking on a training program the client should complete a medical examination with an exercise test to screen for previously undetected heart disease.[2] This is especially important for inactive people over 35. In addition,

---

*See references 16, 19, 52, 63, 95, and 99.

the clinician should closely monitor the client for signs that might suggest the need for obtaining medical advice.

Overloading the aerobic system

Continuous inactivity conditions for just that: inactivity. Therefore the body must be stressed beyond its current level in order to adapt. Improvements in the body's ability to deliver and use oxygen may be achieved by walking, jogging, swimming, running, cycling, or other aerobic means, if performed regularly. Improvements in both submaximal capacity and efficiency as well as maximal capacity can be achieved. In order to do so, the heart rate, an easily monitored variable, must be elevated above the individual's threshold level. Less conditioned people will most likely work at a lower threshold, while athletes will want to work at higher levels of intensity, duration, and frequency.

Intensity, duration, and frequency are the variables manipulated in a conditioning program. *Frequency* (the number of workouts per week), *intensity* (the percentage of an individual's maximal capacity), and *duration* (the length of a workout) can all be manipulated when prescribing an aerobic program. Certain thresholds of each seem necessary to improve one's physical condition. Minimal guidelines have been established. A generally accepted threshold level is to exercise at least three times a week at a heart rate of 130 beats per minute for 10 minutes.[74]

However, to prescribe a singular training program to people of all ages might be too simplistic. This threshold level might be too intense for one person and not intense enough for another. For example, consider a 60-year-old person and a 20-year-old person. To estimate the maximal heart rate (MHR) for each, the following formula is used:

$$MHR = 220 - Age$$

The predicted MHR for the 60-year-old person would be 160 beats per minute, while the MHR for the 20-year old person would be 200 beats per minute. If each trained at the generally accepted threshold (130 beats per minute), the older person would be working at over 80% of predicted MHR while the younger person would be training at 65% of predicted MHR.

In addition, drugs may create further complications. Suppose the 60-year-old person is taking a beta-blocking agent that slows heart rate and depresses heart-rate response to exercise. Furthermore, suppose this person's MHR, measured during an exercise test, is 130 beats per minute not the 160 predicted by the age-adjusted method above. Our subject then would be exercising at 100% of the predicted MHR.

In order to set the appropriate training heart rate (THR), the Karvonen formula[69] can be used:

$$THR = RHR + 0.6 (MHR - RHR)$$

where

   THR = training heart rate
   RHR = resting heart rate
   0.6 = intensity of 60% (for intensity of 85% use 0.85)
   MHR = maximal heart rate

If we apply the formula to our examples, first using the age-adjusted MHR and setting RHR at 60 for each, the THR for each is determined as follows.

20-year-old person: THR = 60 + 0.6 (200-60)
THR = 144 beats per minute
60-year-old person: THR = 60 + 0.6 (160-60)
THR = 120 beats per minute

Therefore, for each person to exercise at 60% of his/her age-adjusted MHR, the 20- and 60-year-old would be working at 144 and 120 beats per minute respectively. Now, we can complete the formula using measured MHR and remembering that the 60-year-old person is taking a beta blocker.

20-year-old person: THR = 60 + 0.6 (190 − 60)
THR = 138
60-year-old person THR = 60 + 0.6 (130-60)
THR = 102

When we compare the results, the 20-year-old person's THR changes by 6 beats per minute (assuming a measured MHR of 190), a fairly small difference. Yet there is an obvious difference (120 versus 102 beats per minute) in the 60-year-old person's THR.

This points out two key factors to consider when figuring THR: (1) use measured MHR when possible (physician supervision of the test is essential when dealing with people with risk factors or those with suspected or known heart disease) and (2) assess people while they are taking the medications they will be taking during training. A change in medication status may necessitate reevaluation.

The intensity factor (0.6) used here is only an example. Intensity from 60% to 90% (0.6 to 0.9) of the reserve (MHR − RHR) is the range recommended by the American College of Sports Medicine (ACSM), with 70% to 85% as optimal.[2]

Frequency. For the greatest gains, exercise programs performed more often will result in the greatest degree of improvement. Fox et al[44] showed that less frequent exercise sessions—2 versus 4 days per week—produced less of an adaptation to the training program. ACSM suggests 3 to 5 days per week as the recommended frequency of training.[2] Many programs indicate exercising 4 days per week so that if 1 day is missed, the minimum ACSM guideline of 3 days per week is still met.

Duration. Continuous activity should be performed at the appropriate intensity for 15 to 60 minutes per exercise session.[40] Duration is also intensity dependent; that is, less intense activities should be performed for longer durations. While some might attempt to exercise at higher intensities for shorter periods, compliance problems, hazards, and injuries from excessive intensities are good arguments for less intense exercise for longer durations.[40]

Mode of exercise. The final consideration is exercise modality. The chosen mode of exercise should (1) involve a large muscle mass, such as the legs, (2) be maintained continuously, and (3) be aerobic and rhythmical. Some activities that satisfy these criteria are running, walking, swimming, skating (ice and roller), rowing, cross-country skiing, bicycling, rope skipping, dancing, and bench stepping. This list does not preclude the use of games, assuming they are played regularly and vigorously. In many cases mode of exercise is the most important consideration because enjoyment is paramount to adherence.

In summary any exercise program should be continuous in nature, use large muscle groups, and be done 3 to 5 days per week for 15 to 60 minutes at 60% to 90% of heart-rate reserve. For a more detailed discussion of the factors relating to exercise prescription, see the ACSM guidelines.[2]

Aerobic training may increase VO_2 MAX up to 30%.[90] There does, however, appear to be an individual ceiling for VO_2 MAX. Therefore someone with a low VO_2 MAX (20 to 30 ml/kg/min) may expect great gains, while a well-trained person with a high VO_2 MAX (60 to 70 ml/kg/min) may experience only minimal gains. Thus the person who knows he or she has a high VO_2 MAX should not expect the 30% or even the more classic 15% to 20% gains.[90]

Cardiorespiratory adaptations to training

Adaptations in the heart are evident at rest and during submaximal exercise. Endurance activities seem to cause hypertrophy of the heart by increasing the left ventricular cavity dimensions, while resistive training seems to cause hypertrophy by increasing ventricular wall thickness.[80] Yet the increase in left ventricular mass due to weight-lifting may simply be proportional to the increase in skeletal muscle mass while endurance training may result in a "true" hypertrophy[76]. Both endurance and resistive training result in decreased resting heart rate. This is the most visible effect of training and may be caused by an increased vagal tone, decreased sympathetic influence, or a combination of both. Evidence points toward increased vagal influence[45,112] because resting oxygen use and cardiac output do not change appreciably. It should be remembered that cardiac output (heart rate × stroke volume) and oxygen consumption are closely related. Therefore, with an unchanged cardiac output and a decreased resting heart rate, resting stroke volume must increase.

When identical submaximal exercise loads are compared before and after training, oxygen consumption may or may not decrease slightly after training and cardiac output changes little, if any. Submaximal heart rate decreases following training, a change most likely caused by a decreased sympathetic influence as a result of intracardiac or extracardiac mechanisms. Correspondingly, stroke volume must rise as heart rate is decreased and cardiac output is unchanged.

Training invokes an increased VO_2 MAX. In an initially untrained individual, increased cardiac output and other central factors account for about half the increase in VO_2 MAX.[100] The higher maximal cardiac output results from an increased stroke volume as the maximal heart rate may be slightly lower or equal to pretraining levels. Increased myocardial contractility and hypertrophy are suggested as a possible mechanism for increased stroke volume. This large stroke volume is a major discriminator between untrained and highly trained athletes.[98]

Biochemical adaptations of physical training

Aerobic adaptations. These changes are obviously related to the muscle's ability to use oxygen.

Myoglobin levels in trained muscles increase. Since myoglobin is responsible for binding oxygen in the muscle, it seems reasonable to expect that as myoglobin levels increase the stores of oxygen in the muscle would increase.[86]

The ability of the muscle to oxidize carbohydrates increases. This seems to be a function of both increased size and number of mitochondria and an increase in aerobic enzyme activity.[52,61] In addition, glycogen storage in the muscle is elevated.[52]

As fat is an aerobic substrate, it stands to reason that fat oxidation would also increase. This indeed occurs.[78,79] After training at any submaximal workload, there is an increased use of fats as a substrates. This appears to result from increased mobilization of fats and activity of the enzymes of fat metabolism. This results in muscle glycogen sparing.

Anaerobic adaptations. These adaptations occur in both ATP-CP and glycolytic systems. ATP-CP adaptations include increased stores of ATP and CP[62,67] and increased enzyme activity.[111] This represents an increased phosphagen availability and use.

Glycolytic changes include increased activity of selected glycolytic enzymes.[52] This would indicate an increased ability to produce ATP glycolytically.

The aerobic changes seem to occur in both FT and ST fibers, whereas the anaerobic changes seem to be more specific to the FT fibers.[52] Because the muscle has been overloaded, it will hypertrophy. However, the fibers that hypertrophy are specific to the training regimen (see box).

Physiology of intermittent work

If a person performs two identical bouts of work, one continuously and one intermittently, a reduced sensation of fatigue will be felt after the intermittent bout. The same applies if progressive work to maximum is performed in-

Summary of adaptation to physical training

REST

Cardiac hypertrophy
  ↑ ventricular cavity (endurance athletes)
  ↑ myocardial thickness (nonendurance athletes)
↓ heart rate
  ↑ parasympathetic activity
Stroke volume
  ↑ cardiac hypertrophy
  ↑ contractility

SUBMAXIMAL EXERCISE

No change or slight decrease in cardiac output and Vo_2
  ↑ stroke volume
    ↑ cardiac hypertrophy
    ↑ contractility
  ↓ heart rate
    ↓ sympathetic influence

MAXIMAL EXERCISE

↑ Vo_2 max
  ↑ cardiac output
    ↑ stroke volume
      ↑ hypertrophy
      ↑ contractility
    ↑ oxygen extraction
No change or slight decrease in heart rate
  ↓ sympathetic drive

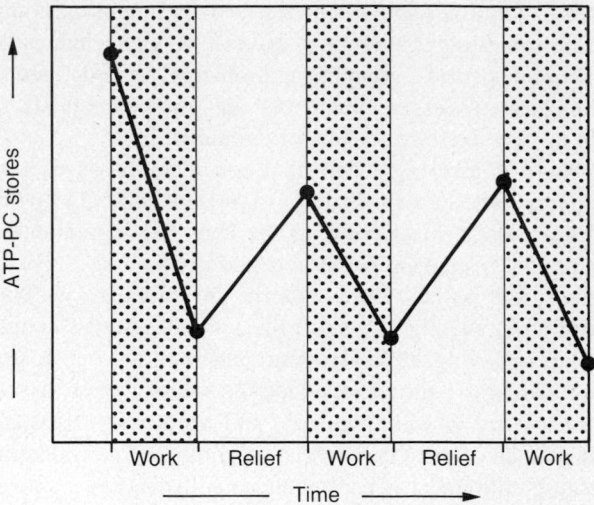

Fig. 11-15. In the relief intervals during intermittent work, muscular stores of ATP and CP depleted during preceding work intervals are partially replenished via aerobic system. (Modified from Fox EL and Mathews DK: Interval training: conditioning for sports and general fitness, Philadelphia, 1974, WB Saunders Co.)

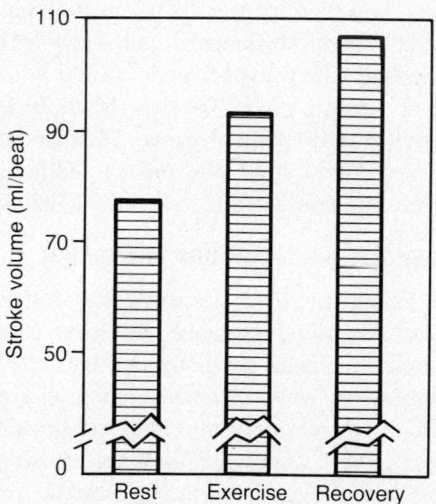

Fig. 11-16. Stroke volume is highest during recovery period from exercise. During interval training, stroke volume attains its highest level each work bout. (Data from Cumming GR: J Appl Physiol 32:575, 1982; modified from Fox EL and Mathews DK: Interval training: conditioning for sports and general fitness, Philadelphia, 1974, WB Saunders Co.)

termittently. The reason for the different sensations of fatigue can be explained metabolically through the difference in the use of the ATP-CP and glycolytic systems.

At the onset of work energy is supplied by the phosphagens, ATP-CP. After the work bout ATP-CP stores have been depleted. During the relief interval ATP-CP stores are being replenished as reflected by the elevated oxygen consumption. Had no relief interval occurred and work been continued ATP-CP stores would become depleted. Energy would then have to be supplied by glycolysis with its subsequent waste product of lactic acid and the limitations associated with lactate accumulation. With intermittent work the ATP-CP system is stressed, but use of glycolysis is limited, resulting in minimal lactate accumulation. With each relief interval ATP-CP is replenished and reused in preparation for the next work bout (Fig. 11-15).

This can affect control of the work interval in that increased work intensities can be tolerated without the fatigue associated with lactate buildup. Up to 2.5 times the intensity of work can be performed intermittently, as opposed to continuously. That is, blood lactate levels in continuous or intermittent work will be comparable at fatigue, but 2.5 times the intensity of work will have been performed intermittently.[40]

Just how much of the ATP-CP system is replenished depends on the duration of the relief interval. About 50% of the depleted phosphagens are restored within 30 seconds. All are restored after 3 minutes of recovery.[38,40,44] So the shorter the rest period, the less ATP-CP restoration will occur and the less the phosphagen stores available for the next work bout, resulting in a greater reliance on glycolysis in successive bouts. An added variable is whether activity occurs during the rest interval. If light work is per-

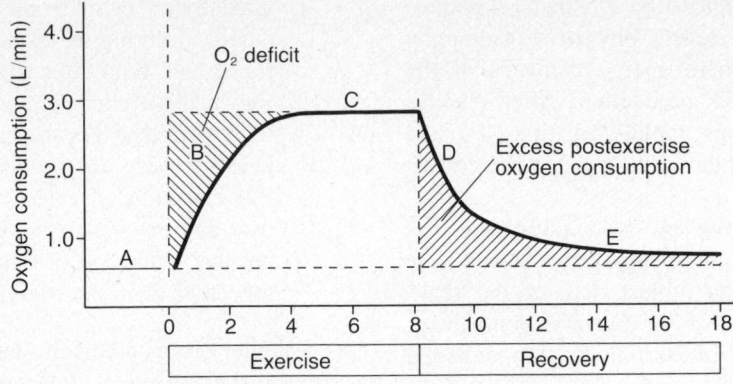

Fig. 11-17. Steady-state oxygen consumption.

Table 11-4. Guidelines for interval programs on basis of time

Area	Performance time	Energy system	Training time (hrs/min)	Repetitions per workout	Sets per workout	Repetitions per set	Work-relief ratio	Type of relief interval
1	30 sec	ATP-PC	0:10	50	5	10		Rest-relief (e.g., walking)
			0:15	45	5	9	1:3	
			0:20	40	4	10		
			0:25	32	4	8		
2	½-1½ min	ATP-PC glycolysis	0:30	25	5	5		Work-relief (light, mild exercise)
			0:40-:50	20	4	5	1:3	
			1:00-1:10	15	3	5		
			1:20	10	2	5	1:2	
3	1½-3 min	Glycolysis aerobic	1:30-2:00	8	2	4	1:2	Work-relief
			2:10-2:40	6	1	6		
			2:50-3:00	4	1	4	1:1	Rest-relief
4	3 min	Aerobic	3:00-4:00	4	1	4	1:1	Rest-relief
			4:00-5:00	3	1	3	1:½	

Modified from Fox EL and Mathews DK: Interval training: conditioning for sports and general fitness, Philadelphia, 1974, WB Saunders Co.

formed during the rest interval, there will be higher resting lactate levels[42] because the light work partially blocks phosphagen replenishment. Therefore increased reliance on glycolysis can be prescribed by either reducing the rest interval or working during the rest interval.

The physiology of intermittent work also encompasses a cardiac adaptation in addition to the discussed metabolic adaptations. The *stroke volume,* volume ejected per beat, is higher during the immediate recovery than during the activity.[27] Because intermittent programs contain numerous recovery periods, an increased stroke volume is an added adaptation (Fig. 11-16).

Stroke volume will also increase with continuous training but by a different mechanism. Continuous work has only one recovery period. However, a lower heart rate for any absolute continuous workload is seen after continuous training. With the exercise requiring the same energy expenditure and oxygen use, a lower heart rate will be compensated for by a higher stroke volume.

To construct an interval training program, one needs to know the energy system that is stressed in the sport or event and then design a training program around it. Then it is necessary to overload the trainee to observe improvements. Last, it is necessary to train specifically (i.e., swimmers need not run and shot putters need not run excessive distances).

The program is constructed around the work and rest interval, number of repetitions of the work bout, and the number of sets in the workout. Table 11-4 summarizes the manipulations of these variables. This table can aid in constructing the program using the time frame of the event and the energy system being stressed. If two thirds of the program comes from work effort areas 1 and 2 and one third from areas 3 and 4, the gains in all three energy systems will be realized for an untrained person.

CARDIORESPIRATORY RESPONSES TO STEADY-STATE EXERCISE

The cardiorespiratory responses to exercise are well documented.[6,40,74] As Fig. 11-17 demonstrates, from a resting level *(A)* of oxygen consumption, often referred to as 1 metabolic equivalent (MET) and subject to individual variability (1 MET is assumed to be 3.5 ml O_2/kg/min), toa submaximal exercising level, oxygen consumption rises *(B)* to a level *(C)* where energy demands of the body are met by aerobic ATP production. After exercise oxygen consumption declines rapidly at first *(D)* and then more slowly *(E)* until the resting value is reestablished.

Before discussing the curve one assumption is necessary. That is, the energy requirement for this steady-state exercise is the same when the subject steps on the treadmill as for all other portions of the exercise bout; therefore, the energy requirement of the first 10 seconds is the same as the middle and last 10 seconds.

If a bout is to be performed in which the energy requirements can be met aerobically, it would be advantageous if the body could adapt immediately from a resting steady state *(A)* to a new higher steady state *(C)*. However, this is not the case, and a lag *(B)* in the adjustment occurs. It takes time for the body to adjust to this new demand, yet energy must still be supplied to the exercising muscles. This supply comes from both stored phosphagens and anaerobic glycolysis, as previously described. Gradually, then, anaerobic metabolism decreases as the energy demands are met aerobically.

Oxygen consumption, heart rate, and pulmonary ventilation are all related to one another, so similar responses occur in the latter two variables; resting heart rate rises slowly to a steady state value, as does ventilation. Some people will occasionally refer to the attainment of this steady state as a *second wind*. The time it takes to reach a steady state varies with the individual and his/her training status. The more athletically fit person reaches steady state more rapidly than an untrained person.[40]

When a person concludes exercise, the body attempts to bring itself back to a resting condition. However, the body does not reestablish a resting state immediately. The excess oxygen consumed during recovery is used to alleviate the oxygen deficit incurred at the start of exercise. This excess postexercise oxygen consumption (EPOC) *(D and E)* is used to restore resting ATP and CP levels—50% of which is replenished in 30 seconds and all within 3 minutes—and to eliminate lactic acid. The first rapid decline is often referred to as the *alactacid portion* of recovery and the latter as the *lactacid portion,* both so named for their contribution to lactic acid removal.

Historically the term *oxygen debt* has been applied to the oxygen consumed in recovery. *Debt* is a poor word choice since recovery oxygen usually exceeds the estimated 0.6 liter of depletable oxygen (myoglobin and blood oxygen) by up to 30 times. Very little oxygen has been borrowed to necessitate a debt repayment. Therefore oxygen debt, while a recognized term, is mostly a misnomer because if a debt were to pay off a deficit, then the two would be equal. In addition, EPOC exceeds the calculated oxygen deficit incurred at the start of exercise for the following reasons:

1. Lactate may be taken up by inactive tissues and metabolized during the exercise, and lactate is released for up to 1 hour after some exercises.
2. Elevated body temperature increases metabolism.
3. Increased recovery heart rate and ventilation help keep recovery oxygen above rest.
4. Exercise-induced catecholamines stimulate metabolism and oxygen consumption. Thus oxygen debt is not just a removal of a deficit but also the oxidative processes from the exercise and recovery.

Another factor to be considered at the conclusion of exercise is fuel replacement. After exercise the depleted fuels need to be replaced. It appears that lactate produced from glycolysis[108] is not used to any great degree in glycogen replenishment but is oxidized through the Krebs cycle.[15] Glycogen replenishment is then a dietary function. While most people can replenish glycogen stores depleted by endurance exercise in up to 46 hours,[88] a person with a diet abundant in carbohydrates can replace depleted glycogen in less time.[21] In addition, if a person exercises and depletes the glycogen stores, continues to exercise for 2 or 3 days, and then increases carbohydrate intake, he/she can exhibit greater muscle glycogen storage than had the regimen not been followed.[9]

Several excellent reviews detailing various aspects of physical training on the cardiovascular system are available.[32,90,91,94,100]

PERIODIZATION OF TRAINING

It is common to see exercise programs based on the variables of frequency, intensity, duration, and mode. Rate of progression is typically a three-phase approach: initial, improvement, and maintenance. The conditioning athlete rarely follows such a simplistic approach. Typically, training is periodic, varying in volume and intensity in relation to the competitive year(s).

Periodicity of training is based on the concepts put forth by Dr. Hans Selye, who described the General Adaptation Syndrome (GAS). GAS recognizes that adaptation to stress followes a predictable pattern (Fig. 11-18, *A*). When stress is increased, there is an initial *alarm phase* when performance declines. This is followed by a period of rapid adaptation. If the stimulus is not modified further, a *plateau phase* occurs. However, if the stress is continually increased, there will be an *exhaustion phase,* evidenced by decreased performance.

When these principles are applied to a training program, the alarm phase may be the initial soreness that develops at the onset of a new training procedure. The adaptive stage then occurs with rapid improvement in performance as the body adapts to the imposed demands. A plateau of performance then occurs. Continuance of hard training can result in exhaustion or overtraining.

Stone, O'Bryant, and Garhammer[109] cite the model of Matveyev (Fig. 11-18, *B*). This generalized model divides

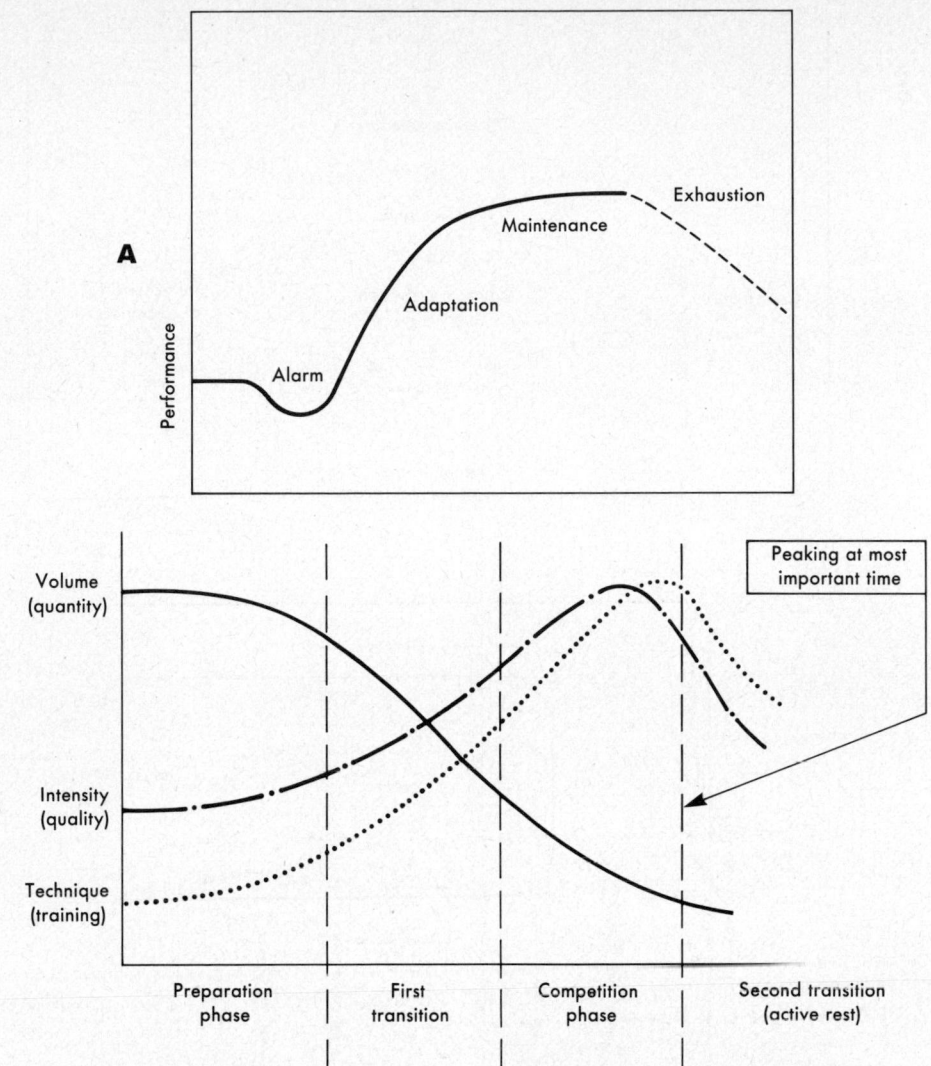

Fig. 11-18. A, General adaptation syndrome. **B,** Matveyev model.

training for competition into four stages. The preparation stage is typically high-volume and low-intensity exercise with little emphasis on technique. The relationship between these variables is gradually modified as the emphasis on intensity and technique is raised. As competition approaches, volume is drastically reduced while intensity remains high before being reduced in the immediate precompetition period. Following the focused competition is a period of active rest (i.e., doing activities other than the sport). The cycle begins again for the next competition.

Cycles are varied according to the competitive season and even to individual days of the week. This creates numerous microcycles within the larger macrocycle. This concept can also be applied to weight-lifting.[109]

DELAYED ONSET MUSCLE SORENESS

A common response to unaccustomed exercise is the feeling of muscular distress in the days following exertion. Typically, the discomfort peaks in the initial 24 to 72 hours postexercise and gradually decreases until the pain has disappeared, usually within 5 to 7 days postexercise.

Numerous mechanisms have been suggested to explain this phenonenon. These include structural damage resulting from increased tension, accumulation of toxic waste products, local effects of elevated temperature on muscle, muscle spasm, and a change in the neural control over muscles.

Structural damage

Pipes and Wilmore[89] reported that isokinetically trained subjects suffered less soreness than subjects training with free weights. Their conclusion was that lowering the load using free weights caused structural damage. In fact, they found that the easiest way to produce soreness was to perform eccentric exercise, such as running downhill. Eccentric contractions require fewer motor units to lower a weight; therefore the active cross-sectional area is re-

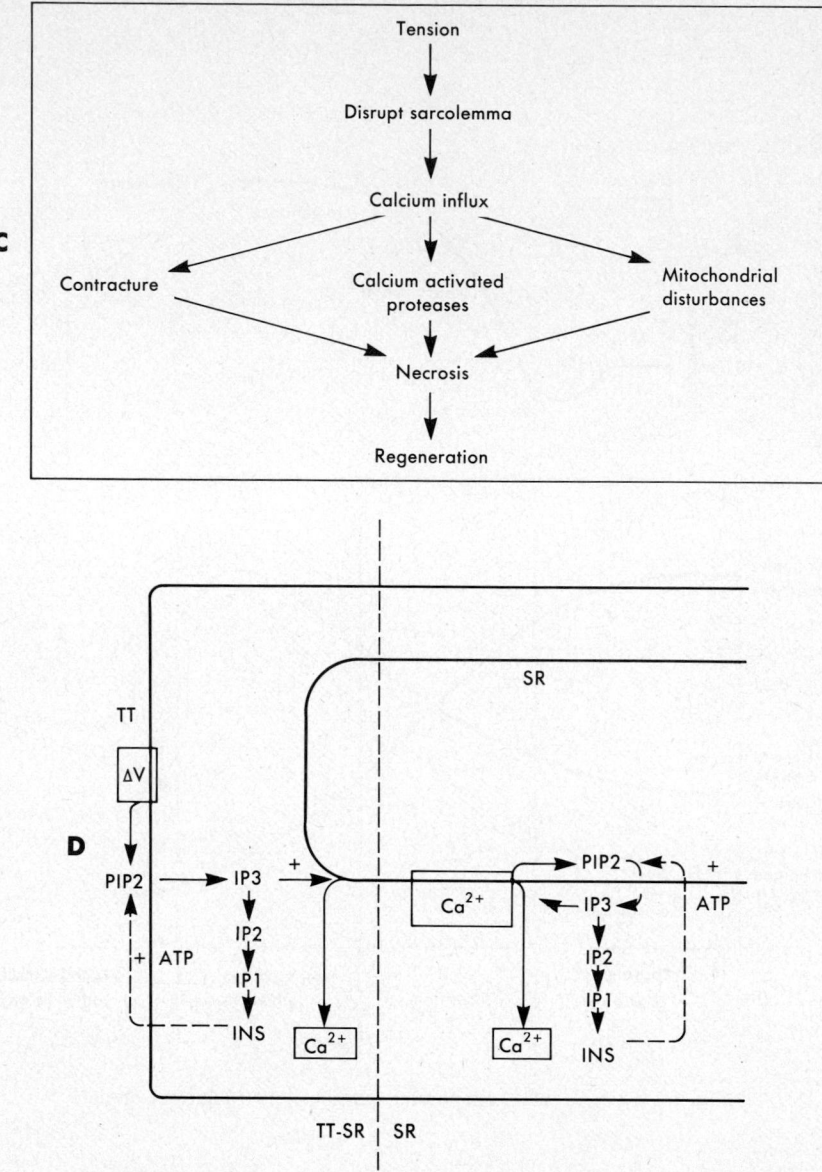

Fig. 11-18, cont'd. C, Proposed model of delayed onset of muscle soreness. **D,** Hypothesized mechanism of communication between sarcolemma and sarcoplasmic reticulum. (**B** from Stone MH et al: J Sports Med 21:342, 1981. **C** Modified from Armstrong RB: Med Sci Sport Exerc 16:529-538, 1984. **D** Modified from Donaldson SK: Acta Physiol Scand 128 (suppl 556):157-166, 1986.)

duced. The result is a greater tension per unit of active fibers. This appears to be the cause of structural damage.

Evidence for muscle damage can be verified by using serum enzymes, particularly CPK,[85] electron microscopy,[46,47] or other techniques. The damage appears to result in Z-line disruption, particularly at the muscle tendon junctions[46,47] or within connective tissue.[1]

Metabolic Waste Products

Probably the most popular theory involves lactic acid as a cause of soreness. There are, however, convincing argu-

ments against this theory. Eccentric exercise involves relatively lower energy expenditure and lactic acid production when compared with identical concentric power outputs.[28] Downhill running results in a lower oxygen requirement and less lactic acid production but evokes more soreness than level running.[101]

Temperature

Type II and III nerve endings are temperature sensitive, and heat production involved with the inflammatory process,[73] as well as the metabolic heat produced by eccentric exercise,[28,84] could be factors related to soreness.

Local spasm

DeVries[29] suggested that local muscle spasm resulted in a feedback loop that caused more pain. An inability to duplicate these findings[1] has led this theory to fall out of favor. Most of the discrepencies in the literature may be related to individual methods[81] and spasm may indeed be a real factor.

Neural factors

Pain is considered to be protective. Soreness occurs later, possibly at a time when the muscle needs rest.[5] However, exercise seems to relieve some of the soreness. This suggests that during peak soreness the muscle's ability to generate force has returned.[1] Type II and III nerves seem to be sensitive to mechanical, thermal, or chemical stimuli,[5] all of which occur following eccentric exercise. In addition, interstitial fluid pressure from exercise is elevated[46] and may offer an added mechanical stimulus to pain fibers.

Model of delayed onset muscle soreness Fig. 11-18, *C* summarizes the model of soreness as proposed by Armstrong,[5] Tension results in structural damage, which in turn may result in contractures, activation of proteases, or mitochondrial disruption (reduction of active calcium uptake by the sarcoplasmic reticulum), and necrosis and may lead to pain. Regeneration follows to protect the muscle from damage in the near future.

FATIGUE

Fatigue is characterized by an inability to maintain an expected power output. Fatigue should also be viewed as a protective mechanism that prevents the muscle from progressing to irreversible rigor. Many training programs are designed to delay the onset of fatigue. Yet the concept and causes of fatigue are usually not well understood by everyone prescribing training programs. For instance, is the fatigue experienced by a weight lifter a consequence of the same mechanism as the fatigue experienced by a distance runner, a wrestler, a sprinter, or a distance swimmer? The visible result is the same inability to perform, yet the cause may indeed be quite different. The causes to be examined will relate solely to muscular fatigue and will not encompass the very real area of psychological fatigue.

To understand fatigue, the sites, muscular and neural, where fatigue can occur should be detailed. Every site along the motor pathways, including the central nervous system (brain and spinal cord), the motor neuron and its synapses with both the descending cortical-spinal nerve and the skeletal muscle, and finally the muscle itself, have been under some scrutiny as possible areas of fatigue. Thus far, the only area that can be eliminated as a causative factor in fatigue is the motor neuron because it is quite difficult to voluntarily stimulate it to a level that the nerve fails to conduct an impulse. Some other link in the chain will most likely fail and precede neural fatigue.

Synaptic fatigue

Fatigue can occur outside the working muscle. It is methodologically difficult to trace the impulses from the brain to the appropriate spinal segment level in exercising humans. Yet in a study involving repeated contraction of the human fingers that led to fatigue, electrical stimulation of the motor nerve produced strong contractions, indicating that neither the myoneural junction nor the muscle was the site of fatigue.[103] Other studies, however, demonstrated that the myoneural junction may be a site of fatigue. Stephans and Taylor[107] showed similar decrements in electromyographic recordings from muscles under maximal voluntary contractions of electrical stimulation.[107]

Thus the inability to perform activities that call for high-tension outputs may result, in part, from the inability of the impulse to be transmitted across the synapse.

Fuel-related fatigue

Depending on the activity, availability of ATP can pose a threat to continued performance. This may be related to decrease in stored phosphagens (ATP and CP) or substrates (glucose or glycogen) used for the metabolic production of ATP. An underlying concept that might cause the fatigue is the time frame of the performance and the subsequent intensity of the activity. Therefore the possible fatigue mechanisms will be discussed as they relate to the time reference of the activity.

For activities of less than approximately 2 minutes' duration, aerobic metabolism is of limited importance for two reasons: (1) the ATP use is occurring too fast for the oxygen system to meet the required demands and/or (2) highly intense muscular contractions (60% to 70% of maximal strength) shut off muscle blood flow.[49] Therefore the ATP needed will be supplied by stored ATP and CP and anaerobic glycolysis.

Consider a contraction that can be maintained for less than 10 seconds. If glycogen, ATP, or CP depletion were the cause of the fatigue, then examination of their muscle levels should reveal serous depletion. However, little glycogen depletion is noticed, and only half the stored ATP and CP is depleted.[7] It appears then that somehow the rate at which ATP is made available from its storage areas in the mitochondria, sarcoplasmic reticulum, and other compartments to the crossbridges may not be able to keep up with the contractile demands.[30] As a result, the amount of work performed is not able to be maintained.

Now consider longer work bouts of up to 2 to 3 minutes, which will be less intense per unit of time. If one looked at the muscle levels of stored phosphagens and glycogen, one would find severely depleted CP stores of up to 90%, depleted ATP stores up to 50%, and relatively unchanged glycogen levels.[52,68] Because storage compartments of ATP do not allow total availability of ATP for contraction, the amount of CP available to resynthesize ATP may be a limiting factor.[74] Glycogen depletion is not excessive at pH values as low as 6.35,[58] but high lactate levels may inhibit rate-limiting steps of glycolysis.[6]

Last, consider a large category of exercises that exceed 3 minutes in duration. These activities, while fatiguing, are less intense per unit of time than the previous two examples. Oxygen delivery now becomes a more important factor. There are not sufficient amounts of phosphagens to sustain these exercises, and lactic acid accumulation could inhibit glycolysis, so aerobic metabolism plays a greater role. Muscle ATP, CP, and glycogen levels after approximately 25 minutes of exercise reveal 80% of the resting ATP level and 40% of the resting CP level, indicating adequate phosphagens.[68] Glycogen levels fall to 50% of resting levels.[97] Blood lipids or glucose contribute little as a fuel source. The fatigue factor for such activities is still under investigation and may lie in lactate levels, the membrane effect, or the muscular communication in the exercising muscles.

For extended activities of up to 3 hours, exercise-related glycogen depletion in muscles has been documented. Reduced or enhanced preexercise glycogen levels reduce or extend time to exhaustion, respectively, supporting a fatigue dependence on the muscle glycogen level. Thus for these activities, muscle glycogen depletion seems to play a major role in fatigue.[97] Strategies for increasing muscle glycogen,[102] conserving muscle glycogen,[22] or offering an alternative source[26] seem to assist delaying fatigue in this group of activities.

However, when 4 hours of activity is exceeded, muscle-glycogen depletion is less severe, but lower blood glucose and liver glycogen levels are found. As blood glucose is the major fuel for the CNS, fatigue may be of central origin since adequate fuels are available for the muscle.

pH and lactic acid

Lactic acid has been rightly or wrongly blamed as the primary culprit for fatigue. Consider that at physiological pH, lactic acid is nearly completely dissociated and almost all the H ions are buffered. The pH alterations are caused by only a few (<.001%) free hydrogen ions.[48,92]

Most people relate low pH as a negative feedback on the enzyme PFK (see Fig. 11-2). Yet AMP and fructose 6-phosphate can override the inhibition of PFK that occurs at low pH levels.[113] It has also been shown that, in the face of declining pH, the glycolytic rate was well maintained during voluntary isometric contraction.[93] What also increases is IMP and ammonia.[83] So while the glycolytic rate may be maintained in spite of a declining pH, a rise in ammonia may have effects centrally on the sarcolemna or the Krebs cycle intermediates.[83] To simply state that fatigue is a result of lactate accumulation and low pH is an oversimplification of a complex process.

Lactic acid cannot account for all types of fatigue. While the previous section has discussed this to some extent, added data suggest reduced importance of lactate as a cause of fatigue. It has already been mentioned that highly intense, short-duration activities do not show excessive lactate production. In addition, if one approaches an activity with decreased glycogen levels, exhaustion will occur sooner with less lactate.[65] Also, both older and younger people develop less lactate when exercising to exhaustion,[18] so to attribute all fatigue to lactic acid may be erroneous.

Changes in the electrical properties of muscle affect the ability of the fiber to conduct an action potential and contract. The membrane potential is dependent on a balance of intracellular and extracellular sodium and potassium and chloride concentration. Any shift of ions or water affects the concentration and the membrane potential.

Sjogaard[104,105] demonstrated that 2 hours of knee extensions at 50% of VO_2 MAX resulted in the expected rise in plasma potassium. Based on potassium and water shifts, the membrane potential changed from $-88mV$ at rest to $-80mV$. Exhaustive exercise (again knee extensions) further accentuated the potassium shifts out of the muscle and water into the fiber. This resulted in a change in the membrane potential from $-89mV$ to $-75mV$. A constant depolarizing stimulus has been shown to reduce propagation of an action potential.

Sjogaard, Adams, and Saltin[104-106] studied potassium that was absorbed by other tissues and rapidly delivered back to the exercising tissue during early recovery. This may relate to the rapid recovery of short-term power output while lactate levels remain high and pH is low.

Fatigue and excitation-contraction coupling

The communication of the surface of the muscle fiber to the sarcoplasmic reticulum has been of interest to researchers for quite some time. While calcium seems to be the coupling factor, additional methods of communication appear necessary. Donaldson[31] has proposed a mechanism of communication (Fig. 11-18, *D*) in which a transverse tubule polyphosphoinositol (PIP_2) is hydrolyzed to (IP_3) which diffuses to the SR and triggers calcium release.

It was also suggested by Donaldson[31] that PIP_2 hydrolysis could be more rapid than PIP_2 formation, thus reducing the calcium release to the fiber. It is also possible that the recycling of calcium may be slowed by a reduced availability of cytoplasmic ATP. Further work will define the function of this cycle and its interaction with exercise and fatigue.

Temperature

Exercise-elevated muscle and whole body temperature can have adverse effects on exercise performance. Temperature is related to the exercise intensity.[96] The more intense the exercise, the greater the heat that needs to be dissipated. Therefore blood must be shunted to the skin for heat loss. The result is a diminished blood flow to the working muscles and, hence, reduced oxygen availability.

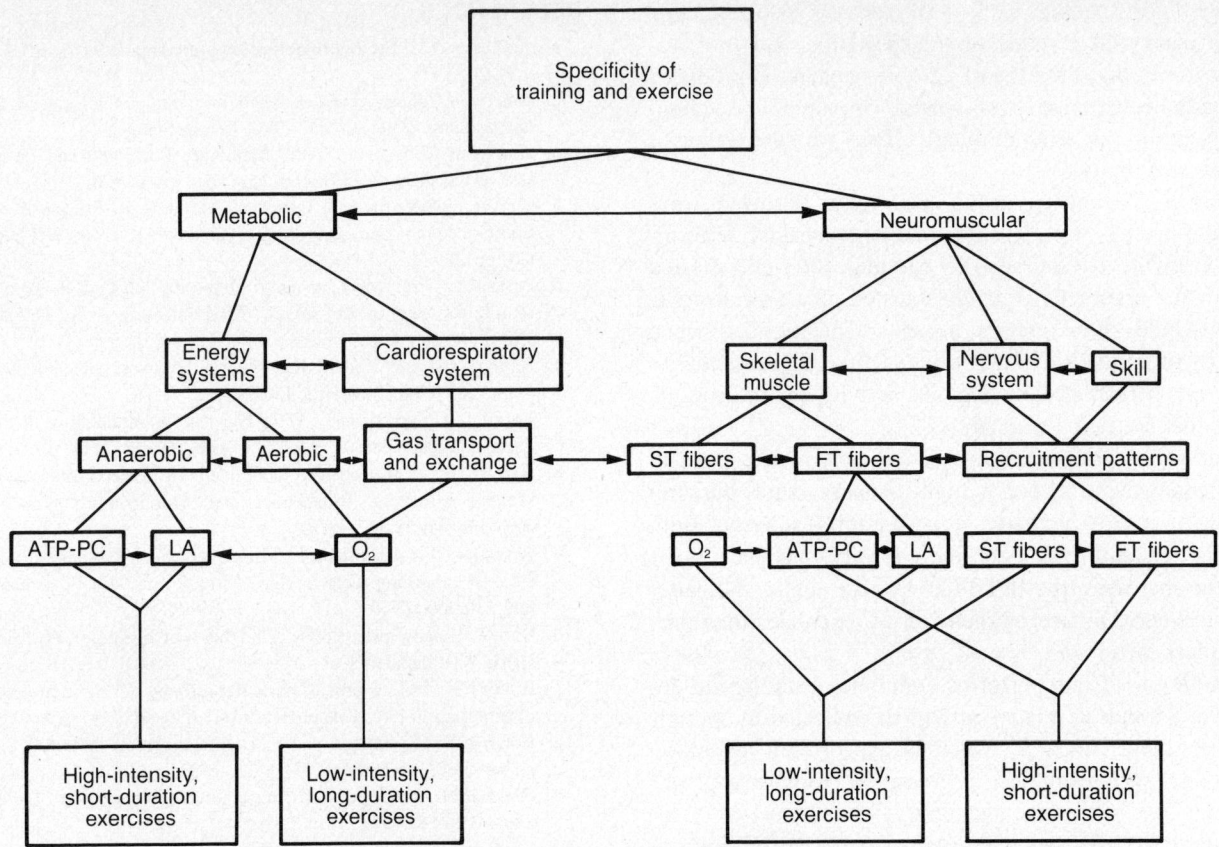

Fig. 11-19. Summary and interaction of physiological factors in specificity of exercise and training. (Modified from Fox EL and Matthews DK: Physiological bases of physical education and athletics, Philadelphia, 1981, WB Saunders Co.)

The effect is an increased reliance on glycolysis, thus causing production of lactate, which may in turn be an added factor in fatigue.[74] Also, environmental factors (ambient temperature and humidity, wind, clothing, etc.) will affect body temperature.[41]

Water and electrolyte disturbances

Loss of body water and electrolytes through sweating has also been examined as an influence in fatigue. With water loss, the body loses part of its ability to keep itself cool; that is, the core body temperature continues to rise.[20] In addition, electrolyte depletion from sweating may precipitate muscle cramps. The change in plasma volume caused by water loss may also place an added stress on the heart by forcing it to pump more viscous blood. Excellent reviews on both dehydration and rehydration are available.[20]

Blood flow and hypoxia

Diminished blood flow can deter performance in activities that require aerobic metabolism, while very short-term, high-intensity activities are not necessarily impeded. Blood flow, interrupted by contraction, is not essential to supply energy via the phosphagens. In addition, low in-spired oxygen tensions will reduce performance in all but anaerobic activities.[67]

• • •

What should be evident is that failure to perform an activity because of fatigue is not the result of a single factor. Fatigue is frequently defined in terms of failure but could also be viewed as a successful mechanism designed to prevent the muscle from irreversible damage. Water and electrolyte levels, ambient conditions, fuel availability, intensity-duration relationships, and selected processes in the contractile mechanism can all be construed as factors of fatigue. A specific exercise evokes not only a specific response and adaptation but also a specific culprit for fatigue.

SUMMARY: SPECIFICITY OF EXERCISE AND TRAINING

Throughout this section, responses to exercise and training have been discussed. Exercise responses have been described as being specific; that is, continuous exercise evokes one type of heart-rate response pattern and intermittent exercise produces another. The specificity concept can easily be described through some examples.

Since most people walk—an activity using a large muscle mass—as a mode of transportation, it is not surprising to see that the highest aerobic capacity is produced by treadmill exercise over seated or supine bicycling, bench stepping, or arm cranking.[13] Thus we have a type of exercise specificity.

There is also muscle-group specificity. If rowers, runners, and cyclists were tested for aerobic capacity performing their own event and also by running, the rowers tested on a rowing ergometer or cyclists tested on a bicycle ergometer, would show greater aerobic capacity than when tested by running.[41,110] Thus when testing, it is essential to assess the person performing the activity on the muscle groups that are being trained.

Training programs are also specific. It is important to train people using either a high-intensity, short-duration activity or a low-intensity, long-duration activity. Both programs increase one's aerobic capacity. Yet the former program increases the ATP-CP system while the latter trains the body to use oxygen during exercise, thus producing less lactic acid.[40]

In addition, if one performs endurance exercises, a decrease in ST muscle glycogen will be indicated by recruitment of those fibers,[50] whereas performing repetitive weight lifts will result in a decrease in FT muscle glycogen.[36,37]

As indicated before, exercise responses are specific to the type of exercise, the muscle groups trained, and the type of training program. These responses can be classified as metabolic and neuromuscular. The metabolic response encompasses two factors: cardiorespiratory (oxygen transport) and energy systems. It has already been noted that intensity and duration dictate the energy system used. It should be obvious by now that low-intensity, long-duration activities depend on the aerobic system. The cardiorespiratory system, which transports oxygen to the muscles and removes carbon dioxide from the muscles, is especially important in endurance activities but is of lesser importance in high-intensity, short-duration exercises.

Neuromuscular specificity is related to the CNS—the brain and spinal cord—and has to do with the recruitment of specific muscle fibers to perform an exercise that uses the special characteristics of the slow-twitch fiber. High-intensity, short-duration exercises use fast-twitch fiber and its unique characteristics.

The very obvious interrelationships between metabolic and neuromuscular factors are summarized in Fig. 11-19.[40]

Thus a specific type of exercise elicits a specific metabolic, neuromuscular, and related systemic response in specific muscle groups. Training using that exercise will result in specific adaptations of the various systems to that mode of training.

REFERENCES

1. Abraham WM: Factors in delayed muscle soreness, Med Sci Sports 9:11-20, 1977.
2. American College of Sports Medicine: Guidelines for graded exercise training, Philadelphia, 1980, Lea & Febiger.
3. American College of Sports Medicine: Position stand on weight loss in wrestlers, Med Sci Sports Exerc 8:xi, 1976.
4. Armstrong RB: Skeletal muscle physiology. In Strauss R, editor: Sports medicine and physiology, Philadelphia, 1979, WB Saunders Co, pp. 29-48.
5. Armstrong RB: Mechanisms of exercise induced delayed onset muscle soreness: a brief review. Med Sci Sport Exerc 16:529-538, 1984.
6. Astrand PO and Rodahl K: Textbook of work physiology, New York, 1977, McGraw-Hill, Inc.
7. Barklay JK and Stainsby WH: The role of blood flow in limiting maximal metabolic rate, Med Sci Sports Exerc 7:116, 1975.
8. Barnard RJ, Edgerton VR, and Peter JB: Effects of exercise on skeletal muscle. I. Biochemical and histochemical properties, J Appl Physiol 28:762, 1970.
9. Bergstrom J and Hultman E: Muscle glycogen synthesis after exercise: an enhancing factor localized to the muscle cells in man, Nature 210:309, 1966.
10. Bloom W and Fawcett DW: A textbook of histology, Philadelphia, 1975, WB Saunders Co.
11. Booth FW: Time course of muscular atrophy during immobilization of hindlimb in rats, J Appl Physiol 43:656-661, 1977.
12. Booth FW: Physiologic and biochemical effects of immobilization on muscle, Clin Orthop 219:15-20, 1987.
13. Bouchard C et al: Specificity of maximal aerobic power, Eur J Appl Physiol 40:85, 1979.
14. Brooks GA: Endpoints of lactate and glucose metabolism after exhausting exercise, J Appl Physiol 49:1057, 1980.
15. Brooks GA, Brauner KF, and Cassens RG: Glycogen synthesis and metabolism of lactic acid after exercise, Am J Physiol 224:1162, 1973.
16. Burke RE and Edgerton VR: Motor unit properties and selective involvement in movement. In Wilmore JH, editor: Exercise and sports science review, vol 3, New York, 1975, Academic Press, Inc.
17. Burke ER et al: Characteristics of skeletal muscle in competitive cyclists, Med Sci Sports Exerc 9:109, 1977.
18. Cerretelli P and Ambrosoli G: Limiting factors of anaerobic performance in man. In Keul J, editor: Limiting factors of physical performance, Stuttgart, 1973, Georg Thieme Verlag, pp. 157-165.
19. Close RI: Dynamic properties of mammalian skeletal muscles, Physiol Rev 52:129, 1972.
20. Costill DL: Water and electrolytes. In Morgan WP, editor: Ergogenic aids in muscular performance, New York, 1972, Academic Press, Inc., pp. 293-320.
21. Costill DL: Personal communication, 1980.
22. Costill DL, Dalsky GP, and Fink WJ: Effects of caffeine ingestion on metabolism and exercise performance, Med Sci Sports 10:155-158, 1977.
23. Costill DL et al: Water and electrolyte replacement during repeated days of work in the heat, Aviat Space Environ Med 46:795, 1975.
24. Costill DL et al: Skeletal muscle enzymes and fiber composition in male and female athletes, J Appl Physiol 90:149, 1976.
25. Costill DL et al: Adaptations in skeletal muscle following strength training, J Appl Physiol 46:96, 1979.
26. Coyle EF et al: Carbohydrate feeding during prolonged strenuous exercise can delay fatigue, J Appl Physiol 55:230-235, 1983.
27. Cummings GR: Stroke volume during recovery from supine bicycle exercise, J Appl Physiol 32:575, 1972.
28. Davies CTM and Barnes C: Negative (eccentric) work. II. Physio-

logical responses to walking uphill and downhill on a motor-driven treadmill, Ergonomics 15:121-131, 1972.

29. DeVries HA: Quantitative EMG investigations of the spasm theory of muscle pain, Am J Phys Med 45:119-134, 1966.

30. DiPrampero PE: The alactacid oxygen debt: its power, capacity and efficiency. In Pernow B and Saltin B, editors: Muscle metabolism during exercise, New York, 1971, Plenum Publishing Corp, pp. 371-382.

31. Donaldson SK: Mammalian muscle fiber types: comparison of excitation-contraction coupling mechanisms, Acta Physiol Scand 128(suppl 556):157-166, 1986.

32. Drinkwater BL: Physiological responses of women to exercise, Exerc Sport Sci Rev 1:125, 1973.

33. Dubowitz V and Brooke MH: Muscle biopsy: a modern approach, Philadelphia, 1973, WB Saunders Co.

34. Ebashi S: Excitation contraction coupling, Ann Rev Physiol 38:293, 1976.

35. Edgerton VR: Morphology and histochemistry of the soleus muscle from normal and exercised rats, Am J Anat 127:81, 1970.

36. Edgerton VR: Neuromuscular adaptations to power and endurance work, Can J Appl Sport Sci 1:49, 1976.

37. Edgerton VR et al: Overloaded skeletal muscles of a non-human primate (Galago senegalensis), Exp Neurol 37:322, 1972.

38. Fox EL: Measurement of the maximal alactic (phosphagen) capacity in man, Med Sci Sports Exerc 5:66, 1973.

39. Fox EL and Mathews DK: Interval training: conditioning for sports and general fitness, Philadelphia, 1974, WB Saunders Co.

40. Fox EL and Mathews DK: Physiological basis of physical education and athletics, Philadelphia, 1981, WB Saunders Co.

41. Fox EL, McKenzie D, and Cohen K: Specificity of training: metabolic and circulatory responses, Med Sci Sports Exerc 7:83, 1975.

42. Fox EL, Robinson S, and Weigman DL: Metabolic energy sources during continuous and interval running, J Appl Physiol 27:174, 1969.

43. Fox EL et al: Fitness standards for male college students, Int Z Angew Physiol 31:231, 1973.

44. Fox EL et al: Frequency and duration of interval training programs and changes in aerobic power, J Appl Physiol 38:481, 1975.

45. Frick M, Elovainio R, and Somer T: The mechanism of bradycardia evoked by physical training, Cardiologia 51:46, 1967.

46. Friden J, Sfakianos PN, and Hargens AR: Muscle soreness and intramuscular fluid pressure: comparison between eccentric and concentric load, J Appl Physiol 61:2175-2179, 1986.

47. Friden J, Sjostrom M, and Ekblom B: A morohological study of delayed muscle soreness, Experentia 37:506-507, 1981.

48. Fuchs F: Cooperative interactions between calcium binding sites on glycerinated muscle fibers: influence of crossbridge attachment, Acta Biochem Biophys Hung 462:314, 1977.

49. Funderburk GF et al: Development of and recovery from fatigue induced by static effort at various tensions, J Appl Physiol 37:392, 1974.

50. Gillespie CA, Simpson PR, and Edgerton VR: Motor unit recruitment as reflected by muscle fiber glycogen loss in a prosimian (bushbaby) after running and jumping, J Neurol Neurosurg Psychiat 37:817, 1974.

51. Goldberg A: Mechanism of work-induced hypertrophy of skeletal muscle, Med Sci Sports Exerc 7:185, 1975.

52. Gollnick PD and Hermansen L: Biochemical adaptations to exercise: anaerobic metabolism, Exerc Sport Sci Rev, p. 1, 1973.

53. Gollnick PD and King D: Effect of exercise and training on mitochondria of rat skeletal muscle, Am J Physiol 216:1502, 1969.

54. Gollnick PD et al: Effect of training of enzyme activity and fiber composition of human skeletal muscle, J Appl Physiol 34:107, 1973.

55. Gollnick PD et al: Muscular enlargement and number of fibers in skeletal muscles of rats, J Appl Physiol 50:936, 1981.

56. Harper HA: Physiological chemistry, Los Altos, Calif, 1973, Lange Medical Books.

57. Hermansen L, Hultman E, and Saltin B: Muscle glycogen during prolonged severe exercise, Acta Physiol Scand 71:129, 1967.

58. Hermansen L and Osnes JB: Blood and muscle pH after maximal exercise in man, J Appl Physiol 32:304, 1972.

59. Hermansen L and Vaage O: Lactate disappearance and glycogen synthesis in human muscle after maximal exercise, Am J Physio 233:E422, 1977.

60. Hill AV: The heat of shortening and the dynamic constants of muscle, Proc R Soc Lond (Biol) 126:136, 1938.

61. Holloszy JO: Effects of exercise on mitochondrial oxygen uptake and repsiratory enzyme activity in skeletal muscle, J Biol Chem 242:2278, 1967.

62. Holloszy JO: Biochemical adaptations to exercise: aerobic metabolism, Exerc Sport Sci Rev 1:46, 1973.

63. Holloszy JO and Booth FW: Biochemical adaptations to endurance exercise in muscle, Ann Rev Physiol 18:273, 1976.

64. Holloszy L and Wachtlova M: Capillary density of skeletal muscle in well trained and untrained men, J Appl Physiol 3:860, 1971.

65. Hultman E and Nilsson L: Liver glycogen as a glucose supplying source during exercise. In Keul J, editor: Limiting factors in physical performance, Stuttgart, 1973, Georg Thieme Verlag, pp. 179-189.

66. Ikai M and Fukuraga T: Calculation of muscle strength percent cross sectional area of human muscle by means of ultrasonic measurements, Int Z Angew Physiol 26:748, 1970.

67. Kaijser L: Oxygen supply as a limiting factor in physical performance. In Keul J, editor: Limiting factors in physical performance, Stuttgart, 1973, Georg Thieme Verlag, pp. 145-156.

68. Karlsson J et al: Muscle lactate ATP and CP levels during exercise and after physical training in man, J Appl Physiol 33:199, 1972.

69. Karvonen MJ, Kentala JE, and Mustala O: The effects of training on heart rate: a longitudinal study, Ann Med Exp Biol Fenniae 35:305, 1957.

70. Katz AM: Physiology of the heart, New York, 1977, Raven Press.

71. Kiessling K, Pichl K, and Lundquist C: Effect of physical training on ultrastructual features in human skeletal muscles. In Pernow B and Saltin B, editors: Muscle metabolism during exercise, New York, 1971, Plenum Publishing Corp.

72. Koslowski SE, Szczepanska E, and Zielinski A: The hypothalamo-hypophyseal antidiuretic system in physical exercises, Arch Int Physiol Biochem 75:218, 1967.

73. Kumazawa T and Mizumura K: Thin fiber receptors responding to mechanical, chemical and thermal stimulation in skeletal muscle of the dog, J Physiol (Lond) 273:179-194, 1977.

74. Lamb DR: Physiology of exercise: responses and adaptations, New York, 1978, Macmillan Publishing Co.

75. Lemon PWR and Nagle FJ: Effects of exercise on protein and amino acid metabolism, Med Sci Sports Exerc 13:141, 1981.

76. Longhurst JC et al: Echocardiographic left ventricular masses in distance runners and weight lifters, J Appl Physiol 48:154-162, 1980.

77. McDonogh CTM and Davies T: Adaptive response of mammalian skeletal muscle to exercise with high loads, Europ J Appl Physiol 52:139-155, 1984.

78. Mole P, Oscai L, and Holloszy JO: Adaptation of muscle to exercise: increase in levels of palmityl CoA synthetase, carnitine palmityltransferase and palmityl CoA dehydrogenase and in the capacity of oxidize fatty acids, J Clin Invest 50:2323, 1971.

79. Morgan T et al: Effects of long term exercise on human muscle mitochondria. In Pernow B and Saltin B, editors: Muscle metabolism

during exercise, New York, 1971, Plenum Publishing Corp, pp. 87-95.

80. Morganroth J et al: Comparative left ventricular dimensions in trained athletes, Ann Intern Med 82:521, 1975.

81. Moritani T and DeVries HA: Reexamination of the relationship between the surface integrated electromyogram (IEMG) and force of isometric contraction, Am J Phys Med 57:263-277, 1978.

82. Moritani T and DeVries HA: Neural factors versus hypertrophy in the time course of muscle strength gain, Am J Phys Med 58:115-123 , 1979.

83. Mutch BA and Banister EW: Ammonia metabolism in exercise and fatigue: a review, Med Sci Sport Exerc 15:41-50, 1983.

84. Nadel ER, Bergh J, and Saltin B: Body temperatures during negative work exercise, J Appl Physiol 33:553-558, 1972.

85. Newham DJ, Jones DA, and Edwards RHT: Large delayed plasma creatine kinase changes after stepping exercise, Muscle Nerve 6:380-385, 1983.

86. Pattengale P and Holloszy JO: Augmentation of skeletal muscle myoglobin by a program of treadmill running, Am J Physiol 213:783, 1967.

87. Perrine JJ and Edgerton VR: Muscle force-velocity and power velocity relationships under isokinetic loading, Med Sci Sports Exerc 10:159, 1978.

88. Piehl K: Time course for refilling of glycogen stores in human muscle following exercise induced glycogen depletion, Acta Physiol Scand 90:297, 1974.

89. Pipes TV and Wilmore JH: Isokinetic vs isotonic strength training in adult men, Med Sci Sports 7:262-274, 1975.

90. Pollack ML: The quantification of endurance training programs, Exerc Sport Sci Rev 1:155, 1973.

91. Rowell LB: Human cardiovascular adjustments to exercise and thermal stress, Physiol Rev 51:75, 1974.

92. Sahlin K: Muscle fatigue and lactic acid accumulation, Acta Physiol Scand 128 (suppl 556): 83-91, 1986.

93. Sahlin K, Harris RC, and Hultman E: Creatine kinase equiblibrium and lactate content compared with muscle pH in tissue samples obtained after isometric exercise, Biochem J 152:173-180, 1975.

94. Saltin B: Physiological effects of physical training, Med Sci Sports Exerc 1:50, 1969.

95. Saltin B and Gollnick PD: Skeletal muscle adaptability for metabolism and performance. In Peachey LD, Adrian RH, and Geiger SR, editors: Handbook of physiology, section 10, Skeletal muscle, Bethesda, MD, 1983, Am Physiol Soc, pp. 555-631.

96. Saltin B and Hermansen L: Esophageal, rectal and muscle temperature during exercise, J Appl Physiol 21:1757, 1966.

97. Saltin B and Karlsson J: Muscle glycogen utilization during work of different intensities. In Pernow B and Saltin B, editors: Muscle metabolism during exercise, New York, 1971, Plenum Publishing Corp, pp. 289-299.

98. Saltin B et al: Physical training in sedentary middle aged and older men. II. Oxygen uptake, heart rate, and blood lactate concentrations at submaximal and maximal exercise, Scand J Clin Lab Invest 24:323, 1969.

99. Saltin B et al: Fiber types and metabolic potentials of skeletal muscle in sedentary men and endurance runners, Ann NY Acad Sci 301:3: 1977.

100. Scheuer J and Tipton CM: Cardiovascular adaptations to training, Ann Rev Physiol 39:221, 1977.

101. Schwane JA et al: Is lactic acid relayed to delayed onset muscle soreness? Phys Sportsmed 11(3):124-131, 1983.

102. Sherman WM and Costill DL: The marathon: dietary manipulation to optimize performance, Am J Sports Med 12:44-51, 1984.

103. Simonson E, editor: Physiology of work capacity and fatigue, Springfield, Ill, 1971, Charles C Thomas, Publisher.

104. Sjogaard G: Electrolytes in slow and fast muscle fibers at rest and with dynamic exercise, Am J Physiol 245:R25-R31, 1983.

105. Sjogaard G: Water and electrolyte shifts during exercise and their relation to muscular fatigue, Acta Physiol Scand 128(suppl 556):129-136, 1986.

106. Sjogaard G, Adams RP, and Saltin B: Water and ion shifts in skeletal muscle of humans with intense dynamic knee extensions, Am J Physiol 245:R190-R196, 1985.

107. Stephans JA and Taylor AW: Fatigue of maintained voluntary contraction in man, J Physiol (Long) 220:1, 1973.

108. Stevensen RW et al: Lactate as substrate for glycogen resynthesis after exercise, J Appl Physiol 62:2237-2240, 1987.

109. Stone MH, O'Bryant H, and Garhammer J: A hypothetical model for strength training, J Sports Med 21:342-351, 1981.

110. Stromme SB, Ingjer F, and Meen ND: Assessment of maximal aerobic power in specifically trained athletes, J Appl Physiol 42:833, 1977.

111. Thorstensson A, Sjodin B, and Karlsson J: Enzyme activities and muscle strength after "sprint training" in man, Acta Physiol Scand 94:313, 1975.

112. Tipton CM: Training and bradycardia in rats, Am J Physiol 209:1089, 1965.

113. Trivedi B and Danforth WH: Effects of pH on the kinetics of frog muscle phosphofructokinase, J Biol Chem 241:4110-4114, 1966.

114. Vander AJ, Sherman JH, and Luciano DS: Human physiology: the mechanisms of body function, New York, 1980, McGraw-Hill, Inc.

Chapter 12

IMMOBILITY: LOWER EXTREMITY APPLIANCES AND PADS

Lynn A. Wallace
Gregory W. Kaumeyer

The application of appliances and pads has been an integral part of the care of musculoskeletal injuries for many years. The competent practitioner in orthopaedic and sports cases should maintain a knowledge of the current developments in appliances and protective pads. The clinician must be able to design and fabricate these devices or be able to procure them from other vendors.

An *appliance* is defined as a device that functions to support the musculoskeletal system (e.g., knee brace, ankle taping) or change the mechanical function of the system (e.g., foot orthotic) by balancing it. A *pad* is defined as a device used to provide a cushioning effect to absorb compressive forces. Examples of padding include a donut rubber pad over a blister and a thermoplastic bubble pad to provide protection from a hip pointer (iliac crest contusion).

The orthopaedic and sports physical therapy practice should provide services in the area of appliances and pads since this arrangement is advantageous to both the consumer and to the physician (if a physician is involved). The advantages to the client are convenience and familiarity; he/she is probably already seeing a therapist for a treatment program and therefore can conveniently see the same clinician for services in the area of appliances and pads. Therapists can render these services in a cost-effective manner. The advantage to the physician is that a licensed practitioner with knowledge of anatomy, biomechanics, and pathokinesiology will provide the most useful device for the client. In addition, the therapist is able to educate the client in the need for and use of the device.

APPLIANCES
Foot

Foot appliances are generally used to balance the foot, which means placing the rearfoot (subtalar joint) in a neutral position and bringing the ground up to the forefoot (posting). Thus the primary indication for use of a foot appliance is an intrinsically unbalanced foot. Forefoot and rearfoot varus and valgus are discussed in Chapter 14.

Treatment of the foot usually means orthosis. A foot orthosis is expensive, and the client has a right to expect a relative guarantee that the procedure will work. A good approach is to tape the foot in the appropriate position and have the client report on the effects of the taping. If the symptoms are relieved with taping, then progression is made to a foot orthotic device. A technique for taping the foot is described in the box on p. 255.

Techniques of fabrication. There are three techniques available for the fabrication of foot orthoses: free-form,

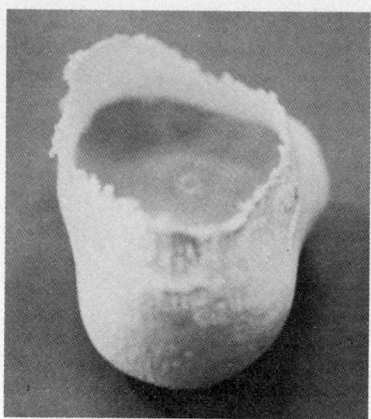

Fig. 12-1. Slipper cast.

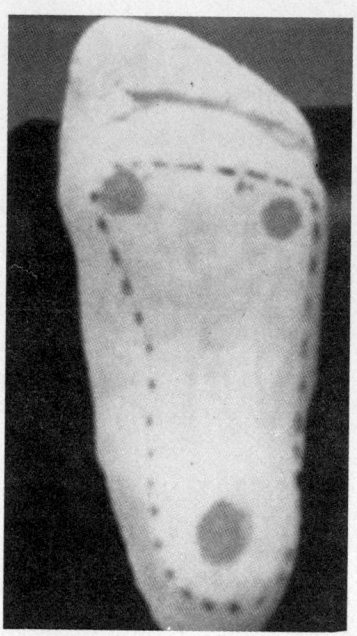

Fig. 12-2. Three-point suspension.

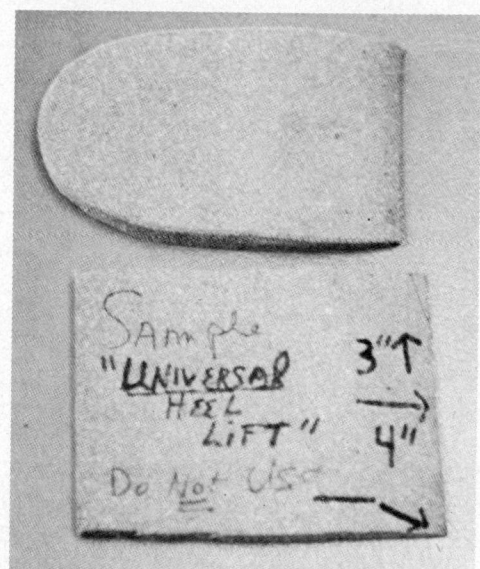

Fig. 12-3. Universal heel lift.

foam-box impression, and slipper-cast impression. In the *free-form technique* the orthosis is molded directly to the client's foot. The *foam-box impression* is made from a styrofoam-like material that the client steps into in either a semi– or a full–weight-bearing position. The impression created in the foam is then filled with plaster of Paris to form a positive model over which the orthosis is constructed. A *slipper-cast impression* is created by placing plaster gauze over the foot to create a slipperlike effect (Fig. 12-1). The cast can be applied in a non–, semi–, or full–weight-bearing position. The positive model is created by removing the slipper cast from the foot and filling it with plaster of Paris.

The advantage of the free-form technique is that it requires less material and time. The disadvantage is that no positive model is available to use for a more exact fabrication of a balanced orthosis. The foam- and slipper-cast techniques provide positive models that require more time and materials and are thus more expensive (see box on p. 256).

Materials. Many materials are used in the fabrication of foot orthosis, and each has advantages and disadvantages. It is incorrect to assume that the hardest material will provide the best foot control. The best control of the foot requires a three-point suspension system using the calcaneus and first and fifth metatarsal heads (Fig. 12-2). Hard materials (e.g., acrylics) must be discontinued proximal to the first and fifth metatarsal heads. Therefore softer materials that can extend up to the first and fifth metatarsal heads may provide more foot control (see accompanying boxes).

Heel lifts. Heel lifts are another form of foot orthosis. Frequently the cause of foot dysfunction is not intrinsic but extrinsic. Two common extrinsic causes are anatomical limb-length differences and decreased flexibility. An example of anatomical limb-length difference would be compensatory pronation on the long side in an attempt to functionally shorten that side. The most common flexibility deficiency affecting the foot is a tight gastrocnemius muscle,

which causes a compensatory foot pronation to secure additional dorsiflexion during the gait cycle. In either of these situations unilateral or bilateral heel lifts will change foot function.

The cork or corklike material used for heel-lifts is inexpensive, lightweight, and easy to apply. To save time in the clinic, use of a universal heel lift that is 3 × 4 inches with a beveled front edge (Fig. 12-3) is recommended.

This universal lift can be cut from large sheets of corklike material, and the front edge can be beveled on a grinder. The recommended heights are ¼ and ⅛ inch, but

---

Protocol for ankle taping

I. Materials
  A. Tincture of benzoin (tape adherent)
  B. Underwrap—polyurethane
  C. Tape—1 inch or 1½ inch
II. Rationale for use
  A. Excessive pronation—primary or secondary
    1. Demonstrates need for orthotic device
    2. Decreases pain
    3. Changes mechanics
  B. Sites causing client complaints
    1. Foot
    2. Shin
    3. Knee
    4. Groin
    5. Pelvis
    6. Back
III. Contraindications
  A. Allergy to tape or tape adherent
  B. Skin breakdown in area
IV. Procedure
  A. Preparation
    1. Long-sitting on table—feet in relaxed plantar flexion.
    2. Apply tape adherent to dorsal, plantar, and medial aspects of foot at level of first and fifth metatarsal heads.
    3. Roll two layers of underwrap around foot in this area. Secure with one small piece of tape.

B. Tape application
  1. Place tape on lateral aspect of head of fifth metatarsal and continue tape along fifth metatarsal around posterior calcaneus.
  2. *Before* placing tape on medial aspect of foot, measure amount of tape needed to extend to first metatarsal head. Tear tape from roll at this level.
  3. Longitudinally split tape (to be placed medially) back to calcaneus.
  4. Stabilize lateral four rays and plantar flex first ray.
  5. With first ray plantar flexed, secure upper half of tape strip on first ray up toward dorsum of foot as far as possible. (Do *not* place over the extensor tendon.) Be sure to pull tape taut before securing to foot.
  6. Repeat with lower half of tape strip, leaving ½-inch space between strips.
  7. Repeat steps 1 to 6, placing medial strips ½ inch lower on foot.
  8. Place half-circle strips from proximal calcaneus to level of first and fifth metatarsal heads.
    a. Start half-circle strips on lateral plantar aspect of foot, applying some gentle pressure and ending strips in middorsum of foot.
    b. Fill in open half-circle by applying strips beginning on lateral plantar aspect. *No* pressure should be applied to tape.
C. Reevaluation
  1. Foot and extremity posture in stance
  2. Foot and extremity posture in gait
  3. Does the procedure decrease symptoms?

---

other sizes can be created by gluing these heights together. When a lift is needed, the client should stand on the universal lift while the heel is traced. The outline can be quickly cut with scissors to fit into the shoe. Writing the words "bottom" and *right* or *left* on lifts when giving them to the client is recommended. Following are other suggestions for use of heel lifts.

1. If the limb-length difference is greater than ¼ inch, undercorrect with a heel lift and gradually increase the lift.
2. A difference of less than ⅛ inch is probably not significant.
3. A maximum of ⅜ inch of heel lift can be added inside the shoe. (If lift is placed outside the shoe, it must be added with a very lightweight material).
4. If a limb-length difference is over ¼ inch, the heel lift must be tapered up toward the metatarsal heads to prevent a midtarsal breakdown.
5. If a heel lift is used on a growing child, the child must be reevaluated in 3 to 4 months to determine if the lift is still needed.
6. If pressure on the calcaneus is a problem, a cutout can be added to the heel lift.

7. The client must be educated in the importance of using the heel lift in all shoes and in not wearing flat or low-heeled shoes.
8. Other treatments may be indicated, particularly stretching, if decreased flexibility is the primary cause of the foot dysfunction.

Plastic heel cups. Plastic heel cups (Fig. 12-4) can be helpful in the treatment of calcaneus pain. The heel cup pushes the fat pad under the calcaneus to increase the cushioning effect. This can provide partial or complete relief for clients with a contusion or spur. In clients with a spur or plantar fasciitis, control of abnormal pronatory forces with taping, orthosis, or heel lift may also be necessary.

Rocker bottom shoe. A rocker bottom is a modification placed outside of the shoe (Fig. 12-5) to decrease forces on the forefoot when a great toe sprain, amputation, or other abnormalities are present. A rocker bottom can be added to the outer sole of street shoes or can be added to the inner sole of a running shoe by heating the soles to loosen the glue between layers. After the layers are loosened they can be pried apart, the rocker added, and the soles reglued.

Protocol for slipper casting

I. Materials
   A. Slipper cast
      1. Dropcloth, newspapers
      2. Table
      3. 6-inch plaster gauze
      4. Basin, water
      5. Scissors (optional)
      6. Cast dryer (optional)
   B. Positive model
      1. Plaster of Paris
      2. Petrolatum
      3. Water, mixing bowl
II. Procedure—slipper cast
   A. Client position
      1. Long-sitting on table
      2. Foot in relaxed plantar-flexed position
   B. Plaster gauze application
      1. Unroll gauze and measure from base of first metacarpophalangeal joint to base of fifth metacarpophalangeal joint—double length.
      2. Dip gauze in water; remove excess water.
      3. Place gauze on posterior calcaneus. Fold lateral aspect across bottom of foot. Tuck excess under toes. Repeat with medial fold.
      4. Cut off plaster gauze to cover toe area—double length.
      5. Wet gauze and place over toe area.

   C. Drying—removal
      1. Allow foot to remain in relaxed plantar-flexed position.
      2. Rock slipper off foot.
III. Protocol—positive model
   A. Preparation of slipper cast
      1. Apply very thin coat of petrolatum to ensure easy removal of positive model.
      2. Step 1 can be ignored if positive model is removed 15 to 20 minutes after pouring.
   B. Mixing—pouring
      1. Measure plaster of Paris—use 30 ounces for one size 8 slipper cast.
      2. Ratio is 2 parts plaster to 1 part water; mix thoroughly and remove all lumps.
      3. Pour into slipper immediately after mixing.
      4. Move slipper back and forth to ensure that plaster is spread throughout slipper.
   C. Removal and cleanup
      1. Find a loose edge on slipper cast. Peel slipper away from positive model as you would peel a banana.
      2. Smooth off any rough edges on positive model with a towel.

Ankle

The ankle is without question the most common joint for application of protective external devices. Indications for application include protection of a recent injury (e.g., ankle sprain), prevention of injury in a high-risk sporting activity (e.g., basketball), or compensation for chronic joint instability. The use of an ankle support as a substitute for complete healing and/or rehabilitation is contraindicated.

Taping. Taping the ankle is an old but effective prevention technique, although the mechanism by which it functions is still questionable. It was originally postulated that ankle taping worked because it restricted range of motion. However, research[3,7,10] and observation have indicated that this cannot be a complete explanation for the effectiveness of ankle taping. Some more recent information seems to indicate that ankle taping may actually function more effectively if the tape is put on the ankle without excessive tension.[12] The explanation appears to be that tape applied with tension ruptures with lower forces. The effects of the tape on the proprioceptive system influence the results of this treatment.[13] Although it has been suggested that external support of the ankle joint will transmit forces to the knee joint, causing injury at that joint,[2] this claim has not been substantiated by research.[18] With the in-

creased cost of adhesive tape, alternative reusable materials, such as cloth ankle wraps, are being investigated. These appear to be effective for preventive purposes.[11,17]

When applying tape, the following should be considered:

1. There must be a need for the taping procedure.
2. The procedure must accomplish objectives with a minimal amount of tape.
3. The tape must look and feel good to the client.
4. The clinician must determine if the client is allergic to either the tape or the tape adherent before applying it.
5. The area to be taped should be shaved or covered with a pretaping material, such as polyurethane.
6. The client should be instructed to remove the tape within a reasonable period of time to avoid skin irritation.

Disadvantages of taping include cost, possible skin irritation, and the need for a skilled person for application. These disadvantages may necessitate the use of a brace.

Braces. Braces are practical because they can be used repeatedly and require no assistance for application. The effect of the brace depends on fit, type, and materials used. Elastic braces provide little support, although they

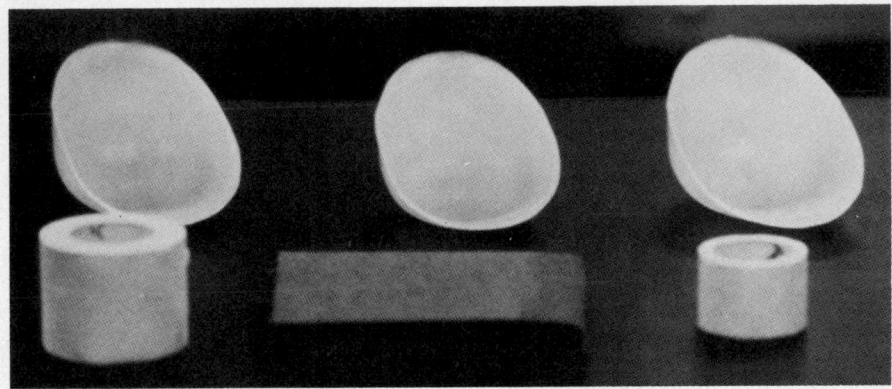

Fig. 12-4. Plastic heel cup.

may provide a stimulus to the proprioceptive system.[15] Cloth, leather, or a combination of materials provides considerably more support to the joint. The devices are commercially available from many sources. It is most desirable to find a company that can provide a variety of sizes, good quality control, prompt service, and guaranteed replacement if the product is defective.

The thermoplastic brace is made of heat-sensitive material, such as Orthoplast,* and fabricates a "horseshoe" to envelop the calcaneus and medial and lateral malleoli (Fig. 12-6). This device provides maximal stability and can be used on the injured ankle in place of a cast. Although the device appears ungainly and bulky, it can be used on an active client, even an athlete. The device can be used for a long time, applied by the client, and reheated and used on another client if desired. The protocol for fabrication of fiberglass protective pads is described in the accompanying box.

Recently a stock plastic splint, the Aircast,† has been introduced. In addition to the plastic "horseshoe," an air bladder on the inside can be inflated to conform to the client's ankle (Fig. 12-7). The advantages of the Aircast brace are ease of application for the clinician and adaptability to the client's ankle size provided by the air bladder.

Knee

The knee is one of the most frequently injured joints. The multitude of injuries to this area has resulted in the development of many appliances to protect and support the knee during activity. These appliances are not meant to replace the proper rehabilitation of an injured joint.

Knee appliances can be divided into three main categories: stock appliances for the knee, custom appliances for the knee, and stock appliances for patellar disorders. Both the stock and the custom appliances have advantages and disadvantages that must be considered when selecting a protective device for a client.

*Johnson & Johnson, New Brunswick, NJ.
†Aircast, Inc, 10 Friar Tuck Circle, Summit, NJ, 07901.

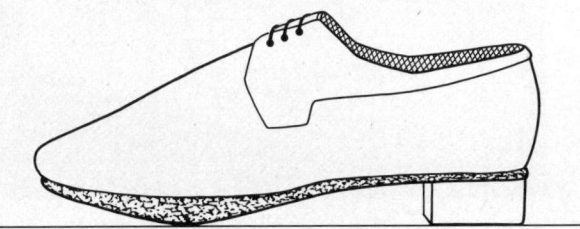

Fig. 12-5. Rocker bottom shoe.

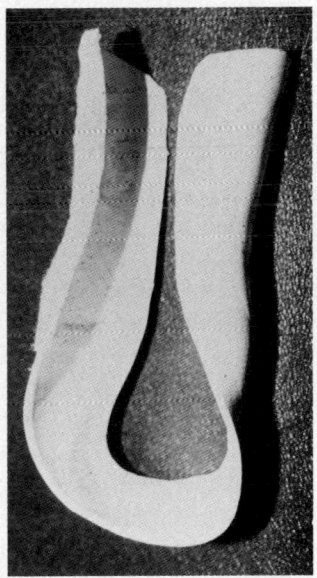

Fig. 12-6. Thermoplastic ankle splint.

Stock knee appliances. Stock knee appliances are available for immediate use by the individual and cost much less than a custom appliance. Although most stock appliances are available in different sizes, it is impossible to have a perfect fit for every individual. The support provided to the joint is therefore limited with this appliance.

The stock appliances are quite varied but can be classified into five types: knee sleeve (with modifications),

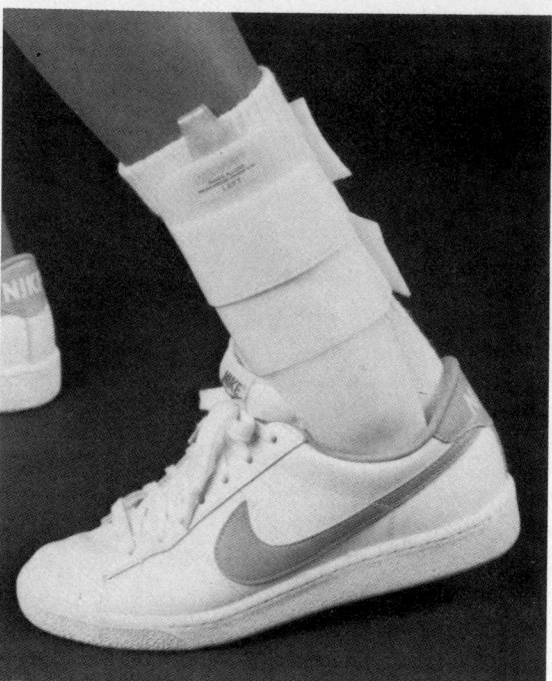

Fig. 12-7. Aircast ankle splint. (Courtesy Aircast, Inc, 10 Friar Tuck Circle, Summit, NJ 07901)

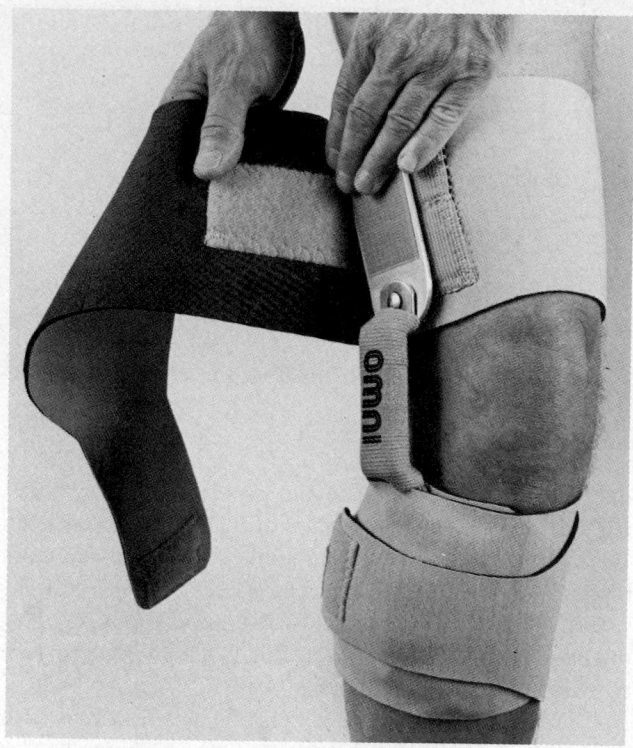

Fig. 12-8. Anderson Knee Stabler. (Courtesy Omni Scientific, Inc, PO Box 1307, Lafayette, Calif 94549.)

hinged-knee appliance, lateral stabilizer, derotation brace, and cartilage appliance.

Knee sleeve. The knee sleeve provides proprioceptive feedback to the individual[15] and mild compression around the knee joint.[4] This brace, available in elastic or rubber material, restricts knee movement the least but also provides very minimal support. The rubber sleeve is designed to provide a more uniform compression and retain body heat.[4] It does not slide easily on the skin and is therefore preferred by many athletes. The elastic knee sleeve, on the other hand, has been modified to provide more medial and lateral support. One modification of the elastic knee sleeve is the ribbed knee brace, which has flexible spiral stays on the medial and lateral sides and is designed to provide mild support while minimally restricting range of motion. The octopus brace, another type of knee sleeve, provides support with straps in a crossing pattern on the medial and lateral sides of the knee and is available in both elastic and rubber material. It has been our experience that the elastic or rubber sleeve remains in proper position much better than the nylon mesh appliances.

Hinged-knee appliance. The hinged-knee appliance is an elastic sleeve with medial and lateral steel or aluminum bars hinged at the axis of the knee joint. The hinged bars are stabilized proximally and distally with leather or Velcro straps. This appliance is also available with a lace-up front to facilitate control of circular compression and allow the brace to better conform to the "hard-to-fit" knee.

Lateral stabilizers. The lateral knee stabilizers are designed to provide rigid support to the collateral structures of the knee. The McDavid Knee Guard* consists of two padded, 2-inch wide concave plates that are hinged at a single pivot point. The plates are placed over the lateral side of the knee and the hinge positioned over the knee joint to allow full range of motion. This device is then taped to the individual's leg or can be secured with a rubber sleeve.

Derotation brace. The Anderson Knee Stabler† is a double-hinged lateral knee stabilizer (Fig. 12-8).[1] A rigid concave bar is connected to two foam rubber padded plates. The biaxial hinge is designed to accommodate the individual's knee and tracks the knee even with changes in alignment. This brace can be secured to the knee by tape, rubber bands, or a rubber sleeve.

The derotation braces were initially available only as a custom brace. The Lerman functional derotation brace‡ is the first brace in this category to be prefabricated. It consists of bilateral metal bars with polycentric knee hinges, bilateral condyle pads, and rubber bands with Velcro to secure the brace and control rotation.

Cartilage appliance. The cartilage knee brace is constructed of an elastic knee sleeve with horseshoe-shaped foam rubber pads, which are placed over the medial and lateral sides of the knee. This is designed to provide com-

*McDavid Knee Guard, Inc, P.O. Box 9, Clarendon Hills, ILL 60514.
†Omni Scientific, Inc, P.O. Box 1307, Lafayette, Calif. 94549.
‡All Orthopedic Appliances (AOA), 74 N.E. 75th Street, P.O. Box 380939, Miami, Fla. 33138.

pression to the joint line bilaterally. When combined with bilateral spiral ribs in certain braces, it provides more medial and lateral stability.

Custom knee appliances. There are now many custom knee braces available. Two frequently used custom knee braces are the Lenox Hill derotation brace* and the Can-Am brace†. They are custom made from a plaster cast of the knee and conform to the specific diagnosis of the knee injury. These braces are significantly more expensive than stock braces and require 2 to 4 weeks for construction. This type of brace is the only brace that will provide stability at the knee joint in an athletic event.

The Lenox Hill derotation brace (Fig. 12-9) consists of a single-joint hinged bar on one side and a rotating dial pad on the other. The bar from the rotating dial pad curves around the knee and attaches to the proximal and distal ends of the upright bar on the opposite side of the knee. The rotating dial pad is placed medially for a medial instability with an internal-rotation strap and laterally for a lateral instability with an external-rotation strap. In combined instabilities the rotating pad is placed on the side of the primary instability and both internal and external rotation straps are used. A hyperextension stop can be added to prevent the knee from going into recurvatum. This brace is used for presurgical and postsurgical control of instability of the knee and has been shown to reduce anterior laxity.[14]

The Lenox Hill derotation brace is fabricated from a negative cast of the knee. Stockinette is placed over the knee from midthigh to midcalf. The following areas are marked on the stockinette with an indelible pencil and are later transferred to the plaster cast (Fig. 12-10):

1. Anterior midline of thigh and leg
2. Outline of patella
3. Transverse line at midpatellar level
4. Outline of medial and lateral borders of tibia
5. Head of fibula (circled)
6. A transverse line placed 8 in proximal and distal to the midpatellar level

If there is atrophy of the thigh greater than 1 inch at the proximal transverse line, this should be noted on the order form.

A plaster cast is applied over the stockinette with the knee in complete extension. Once the plaster has dried, the cast is bivalved and the stockinette removed before the cast is shipped.

The Can-Am brace (Fig. 12-11) is constructed of bilateral aluminum bars with polycentric hinges that are stabilized on the thigh and leg with polypropylene plastic. This brace is designed to control ligament stability in all planes. It is custom made from a negative plaster cast of the individual's knee.

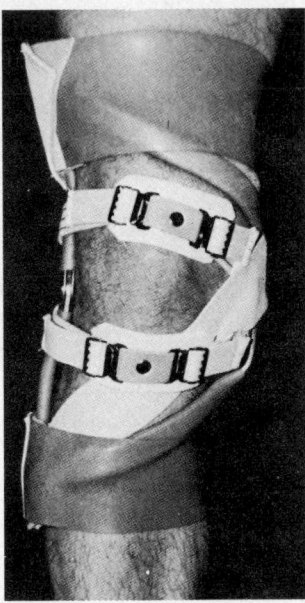

Fig. 12-9. Lenox Hill derotation brace. (Courtesy Lenox Hill Brace Shop, Inc, New York, NY 10028.)

The negative cast for the Can-Am knee brace is taken with the patient in full–weight-bearing position with the knee in the neutral position. A stockinette is placed over the leg. The following marks are made on the stockinette and later transferred to the negative cast:

1. Outline of patella
2. Circle on head of fibula
3. Vertical line through midpatella to extend 8 inches above and below
4. Horizontal line through midpatella

The plaster cast is made to extend at least 10 inches above and below the patella. Once the plaster dries, the cast is bivalved and shipped to the brace manufacturer.

Stock appliances for patellar disorders. There are many braces designed to stabilize or to allow normal tracking of the patella. This is not a new concept. A lateral pad to prevent lateral subluxation of the patella was described by Ober[8] over 40 years ago. There are two types of patellar appliances: those designed to control the movement of the patella by direct pressure and those designed to control patellar movement by pressure on the patellar tendon.

There are presently several designs of appliances to apply direct patellar pressure. A lateral V-shaped pad is incorporated in several rubber and elastic knee sleeves. This pad is further supported in some of these braces by a rubber circumferential strap to apply a dynamic, medially displacing force.[9] These appliances are available in several sizes for the right or left knee.

It is necessary to evaluate the comfort of these appliances during activity when fitting the client. Irritation of the popliteal space often occurs in certain individuals. The

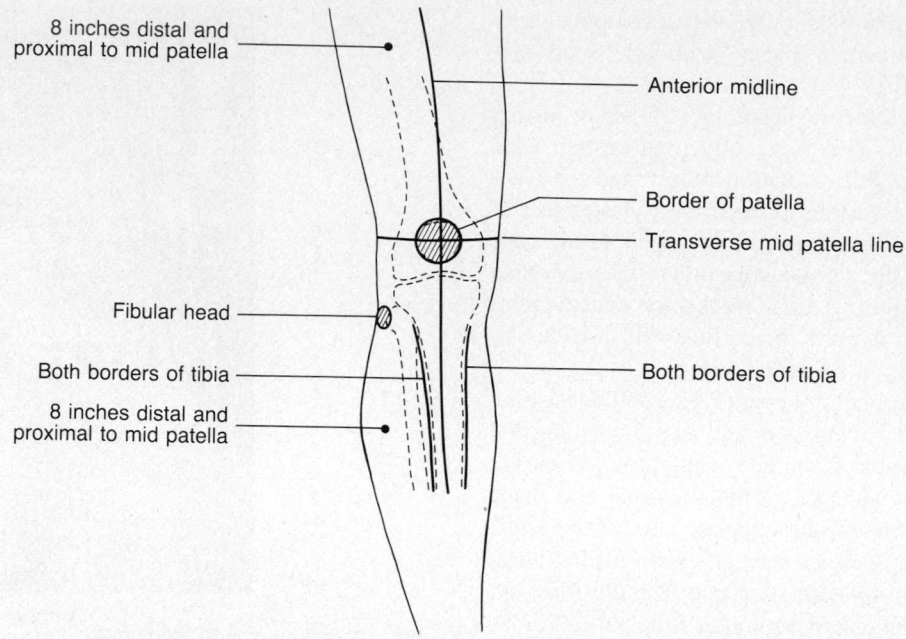

8 inches distal and proximal to mid patella

Anterior midline

Border of patella

Transverse mid patella line

Fibular head

Both borders of tibia

Both borders of tibia

8 inches distal and proximal to mid patella

Fig. 12-10. Anatomical tracings for Lenox Hill derotation brace.

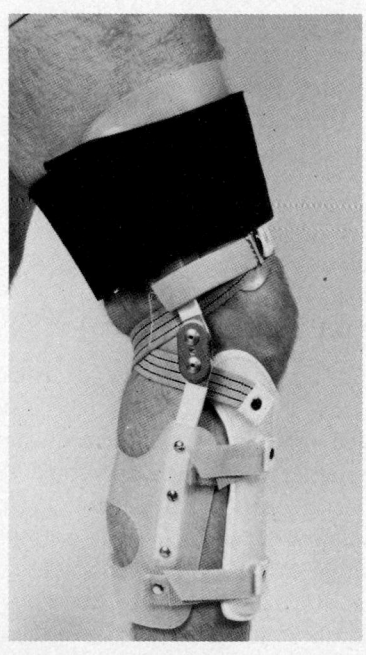

Fig. 12-11. Canadian-American (Can-Am) knee brace. (Courtesy Pro-Fit Orthotics, Inc, 85 Salem Street, Lynnfield, Ma 01940.)

direct lateral pressure appliance is also available in a wrap-around design. The lateral pad is stabilized by a proximal and distal strap that leaves the patella and popliteal spaces open.

An appliance to control patellar movement was initially described by Levine.[6] This consisted of a round padded support, approximately 2 cm in diameter, that attached posteriorly with a Velcro fastener. This was noted on radiographs to change the mechanics of the patella.[6]

The physical therapist should evaluate the patellar appliance on the individual. This is necessary to assess the effectiveness of the device in controlling unwanted patellar movement while allowing comfortable movement of the knee. This can be completed by having the client complete quadriceps exercises or stair climbing. There should be a decrease in the client's patellar discomfort with these activities.

PADS

Pads to protect an injured joint or to prevent a recurrence of an injury are being used more frequently in clinical practice. Perhaps the reason padding is not used more often to allow people to return to work, recreation, or sporting activities earlier is because many clinicians are unfamiliar with materials and techniques.

A protective pad is indicated whenever a client has a healing injury that might be reversed or halted by additional trauma to the area. Common examples include fractures, contusions, and myositis ossificans. Contraindications include undiagnosed conditions.

The liability for this type of treatment is minimal with proper medical clearance, correct selection of materials and techniques, good fit, and client education.

When considering a protective pad for a client, the clinician must decide on type, design, and fabrication technique. Pads may be stock or custom made. Design may be layered, donut, or cantilevered. The two fabrication techniques are free-form and positive model.

Stock pads. Stock pads are always desirable if they will adequately protect the client. Because they are already prepared and require no fabrication time from the clinician, the cost to the client is minimized.

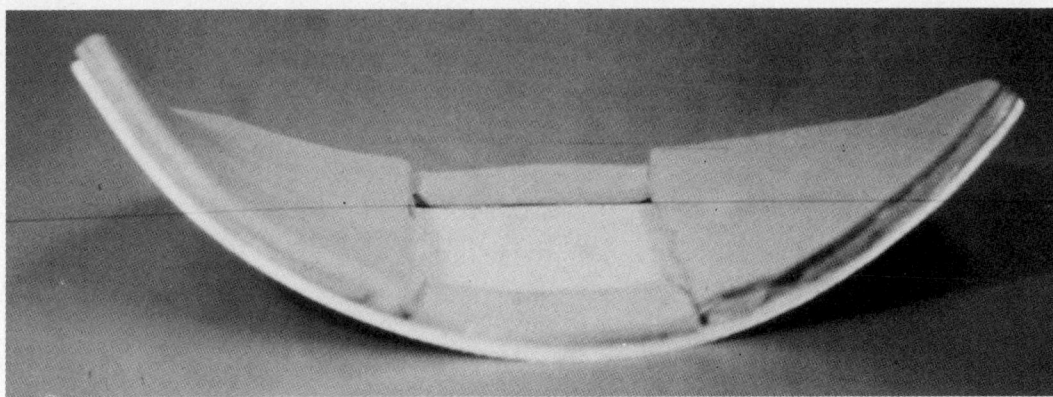

Fig. 12-12. Layered pad.

There are three basic designs of both stock and custom pads: layered, donut, and cantilever. The three different types of pads can be combined. As with all techniques, each type has advantages and disadvantages.

Layered pad. The layered pad consists of one or several layers of material to be placed over the injured area (Fig. 12-12). It requires minimal or no clinician time to cut and apply. This type of padding depends solely on the shock-absorbing properties of the material to provide adequate protection. For many conditions this type of padding will be ineffective (e.g., severe contusion or fracture). Whenever possible, the simplest (and most inexpensive) type of padding that will be effective should be used.

Donut pad. The donut pad has a cut over the injured area that will cause forces to be transferred around the injured area (Fig. 12-13). This is an effective technique if a small area is to be protected (e.g., foot-blister, metacarpophalangeal joint). If a larger area is involved (e.g., contusion on the anterior thigh), forces may be delivered to the injured area through the open area of the pad. The donut pad may be effective if placed under standard protective equipment, as under a football thigh pad. A disadvantage of this technique is that it requires additional time to plan, prepare, and apply.

Cantilever pad. The cantilever pad bridges the injured area with an elevated, firm protective covering (Fig. 12-14). These pads are used on many anatomical areas including anterior tibia, anterior thigh, iliac crest, rib, deltoid, acromioclavicular joint, and metacarpals. However, the cantilever pad is the most time-consuming to design, fabricate, and apply, making it more expensive than the other two types. Because of the expense, the cantilever pad should not be used unless the other types are ineffective. Materials and techniques are discussed in the box on p. 263.

Custom pads. The use of custom-made pads is sometimes mandated by the client's condition and/or activity level. Two fabrication techniques have been discussed: free-form and positive model. A custom-made protective pad can be fabricated using a free-form, positive mold technique to fit material directly to the client. A positive

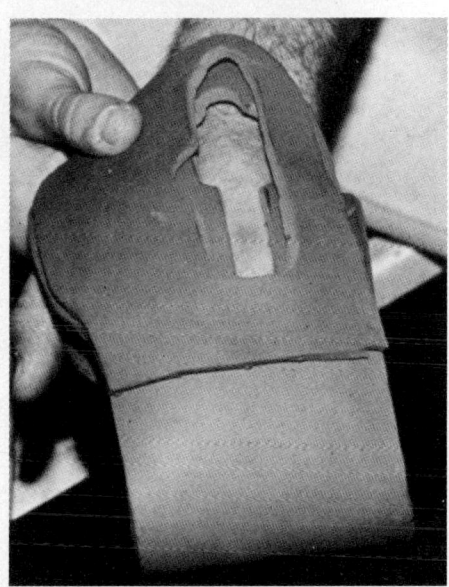

Fig. 12-13. Donut pad.

model technique requires casting the client, removing the cast, creating a positive model, and building the pad over the positive model (a protocol can be found in the box on p. 263). The free-form technique is much quicker but cannot always be used. The positive model is necessary when working with certain problems (e.g., metacarpal fracture) and some materials (silicone rubber, fiberglass).

Foot

Protective pads for the foot are designed to protect or support a specific area. The normal contour of the longitudinal or metatarsal arch may not be effectively supported following a sprain or strain to the supporting structures. These areas can be effectively supported with a longitudinal or metatarsal stock pad, which are available in multiple sizes and shapes (Fig. 12-15) and are constructed of felt or rubber. The physical therapist can construct a custom metatarsal or longitudinal pad if a stock pad is not available.

Protective pads are most commonly used on the foot to

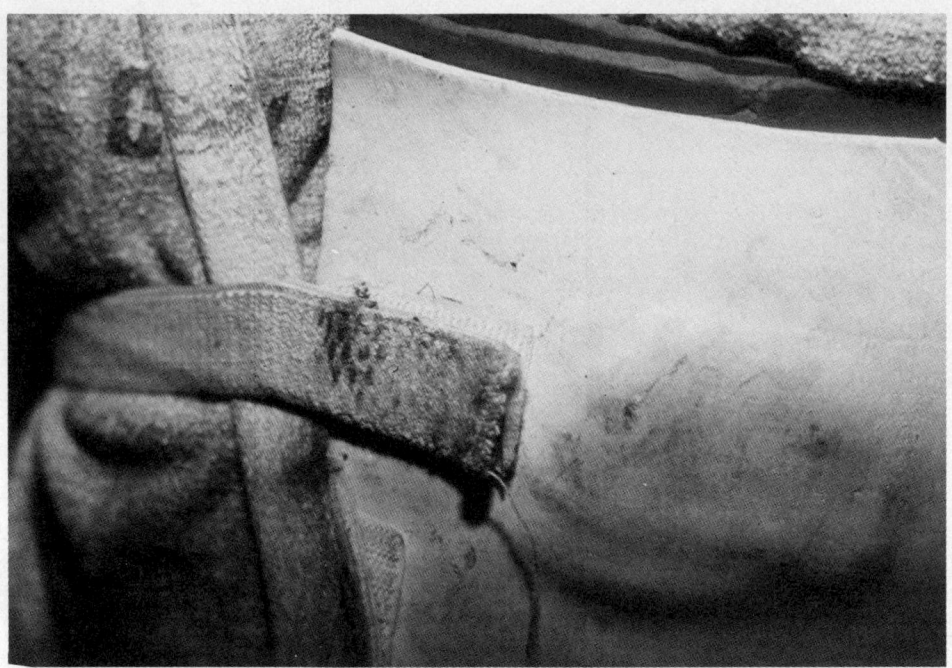

Fig. 12-14. Cantilever pad.

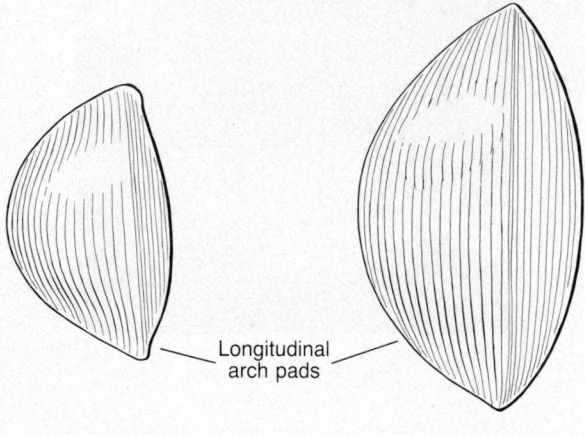

Longitudinal
arch pads

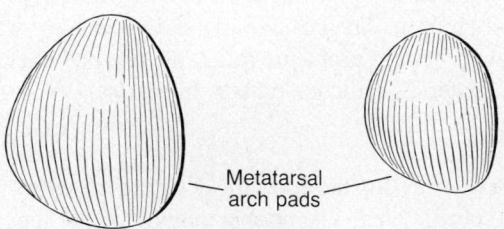

Metatarsal
arch pads

Fig. 12-15. Closed-cell pronatory pads.

protect blisters and corns. A donut pad is constructed of adhesive felt or moleskin. The opening must be wide enough to allow pressure to be directed to normal tissue. The donut must be thick enough to prevent forces from being directed on the blister but should also fit comfortably in the shoe. This donut can be filled with petroleum jelly and covered, allowing the athlete to comfortably return to participation.

Ankle

The most common injury to the ankle for which a protective pad is indicated is a contusion to the medial or lateral malleolus. The banjo pad (Fig. 12-16) provides protection while allowing movement. This pad is constructed of foam rubber or Plastizote* using the donut principle and can easily be made using the free-form method. Orthoplast is molded to cover the opening in the banjo pad. Once the banjo pad has been constructed, it is attached to the leg with an elastic wrap or elastic tape.

Shin

Protective pads have been designed for the shin in several sports because of the susceptibility of this area to injury. These provide varying degrees of protection for the entire anterior portion of the leg. The soccer shin pad provides the least amount of protection and covers only the anterior portion of the tibia. The Donzis shin guard† provides more protection but is also bulkier. Baseball and hockey pads are constructed with an extension from the shin guard that covers the patella.

A custom shin pad can be constructed with Orthoplast and foam rubber or Aliplast,* using the donut principle to protect the injured area. The soccer shin pad can easily be modified to provide more protection by adding foam rubber or Aliplast to enhance the donut effect.

*Alimed, 138 Prince Street, Boston, Mass 02113.

Protocol for thermoplastic orthotic fabrication

I. Materials
   A. Scissors
   B. Pen
   C. Materials—Plastizote*
   D. Positive model
   E. Elastic wraps or bicycle inner tube
   F. Toaster oven
   G. Grinder
II. Procedure
   A. Pattern
      1. Trace outline of foot from positive model onto orthotic materials.
      2. Leave extra ¼ inch on all sides.
      3. Cut along line so that no trace of pen marks remain.
      4. Cut out crescent-shaped longitudinal arch pad.
   B. Forming
      1. Place positive mold plantar surface on work area.
      2. Place materials (upper layer, lower layer, longitudinal arch pad) in toaster oven at 250°.
      3. Remove when materials are soft (3 to 5 minutes).
      4. Place soft materials on plantar aspect of model in following order:
         a. Top layer
         b. Bottom layer
         c. Long arch pad and/or post
      5. Press materials against mold with either elastic wraps or bicycle inner tube strips.
      6. Allow minimum of 20 minutes cooling time before removing from model.
   C. Grinding
      1. Shape to model.
         a. Length—to metatarsal heads
         b. Width—no wider than mold
      2. Grind bottom of device flat.
      3. Make wedge shaped with distal end paper thin.
      4. Grind center of plantar calcaneal aspect through.
      5. Place positive model under device to determine if foot balance has been achieved.

*Alimed, 138 Prince Street, Boston, Mass. 02113.

Protocol for leather orthotic application

I. Materials
   A. Scissors
   B. Pen
   C. Saran Wrap or Handi-wrap
   D. Leather
   E. Positive mold
   F. Elastic wraps or bicycle inner tube
II. Procedure
   A. Pattern
      1. Trace outline of foot from positive mold onto leather.
      2. Leave extra ¼ to ½ inch on all sides.
      3. Cut along line so that no trace of pen marks remain.
   B. Forming
      1. Place Saran Wrap or Handi-Wrap over plantar aspect of positive mold; remove wrinkles.
      2. Thoroughly wet leather cutout. Place on plantar aspect of positive mold over plastic wrap. (Be sure to place top surface against mold.)
      3. Press leather against mold with either elastic wrap or bicycle inner tube.
      4. Leather can be removed in approximately 24 hours. (NOTE: Leaving on longer than 24 hours can result in fungal mold growth on leather.)
   C. Application
      1. Apply Barge* cement to undersurface of leather and top of orthotic.
      2. Place leather and orthotic on positive mold (over plastic). Press with elastic wraps or bicycle inner tube.
      3. Allow to dry for 12 to 24 hours.
      4. Trim excess leather with scissors, scalpel, or grinder.

*Apex Foot Products, 200 Forest Avenue, Englewood, NJ 07631.

Donzis knee pad*—shock-absorbing foam covered with polyethylene plastic. These pads provide good protection when worn and kept in place.

The slip-on and wrestling knee pads can be modified depending on the area of injury. A donut pad can be inserted inside the pad to provide more shock absorption around the injury.

A protective pad for Osgood-Schlatter's disease has been described by Hanak.[5] This consists of an Orthoplast bubble inserted in a rubber knee sleeve to protect the tibial tuberosity.

Thigh and hip

Thigh and hip pads must be worn by football and hockey players to avoid serious contusions. Two types of stock pads are available for football players: (1) girdle pads—pads for the iliac crests and sacrum inserted into a pair of trunks, and (2) belt pads—hip and sacral pads at-

*Donzis Protective Equipment, P.O. Box 52849, Houston, Tex 77052.

The baseball shin protective pad is attached to the leg with elastic straps. The other shin pads are taped to the leg with adhesive or elastic tape.

Knee

Knee pads are routinely worn in sports where the athlete is susceptible to contusions and abrasions. There are four types of stock knee pads: (1) slip-on knee pad—rubber padding in an elastic sleeve; (2) wrestling knee pad—longer than the slip-on pad with the popliteal space open; (3) pad inserts—fitted into a pocket in football pants; (4)

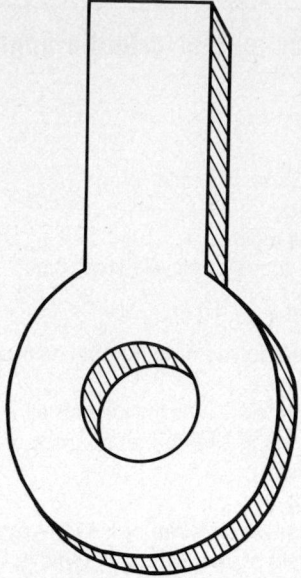

Fig. 12-16. Banjo pad.

Protocol for fabrication of fiberglass protective pads

1. Take a negative plaster mold of body part and construct a positive mold.
2. Outline area to be protected. A ¼ - to ½-inch layer of foam rubber is placed over this area if a bubble pad is being made. Coat with petrolatum to facilitate removal of fiberglass.
3. Outline total pad area, allowing minimum of 1½ to 2 inches of overlap over protected area.
4. Cut four pieces of fiberglass* according to total pad size.
5. Mix plastic resin† in proper proportions and impregnate each layer of fiberglass thoroughly.
6. Place on each layer of fiberglass individually and smooth out carefully. Allow to dry overnight.
7. Remove fiberglass and cut or sand to desired size.
8. Glue a minimum of ¼ inch layer of foam rubber to overlapping inside edge and entire outside of fiberglass.
9. Allow to dry and secure this pad to the client/athlete with an elastic wrap or elastic tape.

---

*Fiberglass weight #162.
†Ortho-Bond Resin, Vernon-Benshaff Co, Albany, NY, 12201. Use 4 parts A to 1 part B.

tached by a belt. Many football players like to wear knee pad inserts for hip pads. However, these provide much less protection to the iliac crests. Hip and sacral pads are built into hockey pants.

Thigh boards are inserted in all football pants to prevent contusions of the quadriceps muscle. These are constructed of press board and Insulite using a cantilever design. These pads are also available in shock-absorbing form covered with polyethylene plastic in different styles.

Thigh and hip pads can be custom made following an injury to provide more specific protection. These can be constructed of Orthoplast and foam rubber using a combination donut-bubble technique. Fiberglass pads can be custom made to provide greater protection,[16] but they are more difficult to construct. The protocol for fiberglass pads can be found in the box.

SUMMARY

Appliances and pads for support and protection of various body parts form a useful adjunct to primary intervention in musculoskeletal injuries. If potential areas of difficulty can be identified through adequate screening, supports and pads can be used preventively. In postinjury rehabilitation appliances and pads can be used to protect the area from further trauma as well as for movement guidance. When rehabilitation has been effective enough to allow resumption of activity, some bracing, wrapping, and pad use can be an effective deterrent to future injuries.

A knowledge of the materials available and fabrication techniques is an important part of the total rehabilitation scheme.

REFERENCES

1. Anderson G, Zeman SC, and Rosenfeld RT: The Anderson knee stabler, Physician Sportsmed 7(6):125, 1979.
2. Ferguson AB: The case against ankle taping, Am J Sports Med 1:46, 1973.
3. Fumich RM et al: The measured effect of taping on combined foot and ankle motion before and after exercise, Am J Sports Med 9(3): 1981.
4. Gardner L: For the problem knee, slip on a sleeve, Physician Sportsmed 3(5):111, 1975.
5. Hanak MP: Protective orthoplast "bubble" pad for Osgood-Schlatter's disease, Athletic Training 16:267, 1981.
6. Levine J: A new brace for chondromalacia patellae and kindred conditions, Am J Sports Med 6:137, 1978.
7. Malina RM: Effects of exercise upon the measurable supportive strength of cloth and tape ankle wraps, Res Q 34:158, 1963.
8. Ober FR: Recurrent dislocation of the patella, Am J Surg 43:497, 1939.
9. Palumbo PM: Dynamic patellar brace: A new orthosis in the management of patellofemoral disorders, Am J Sports Med 9:45, 1981.
10. Rarick JG and Regus RK: Role of external support in the prevention of ankle sprains, Med Sci Sports Exerc 5:200, 1973.
11. Rarick GL et al: The measurable support of the ankle joint by conventional methods of taping, J Bone Joint Surg (Am) 44:1183, 1962.
12. Rees D: Personal communication, Goteborg, Sweden, May, 1982.
13. Rees D: Personal communication, Swedish Society Sports Medicine Annual Meeting, Ronneby, Sweden, May 1982.
14. Richardson CD: Lenox Hill derotation brace, Bull Sports Med Sec APTA 3(1):8, 1977.
15. Roser LA: Effects of taping and bracing on the unstable knee, NW Med 70:544, 1971.
16. Rylander CR: Custom-made protective pads and heel caps, Athletic Training 8:183, 1973.
17. Simon JE: Study of the comparative effectiveness of ankle taping and ankle wrapping on the prevention of ankle injuries, J Nat Athletic Trainers Assoc 4:6, 1969.
18. Wells J: The incidence of knee injuries in relation to ankle taping, J Nat Athletic Trainers Assoc 4:16, 1969.

Chapter 13

SPINAL IMMOBILITY: BRACES AND CORSETS

Dennis L. Hart

Spinal bracing has existed for centuries to fulfill the specific needs of clients with spinal dysfunction. However, if the student of spinal orthotics compares the multitude of signs and symptoms that clients with spinal pain exhibit to the variety of appliances made available by creative practitioners of the past and present, he/she is confronted with a confusing array of orthoses that are devoid of specific criteria for their use. This confusion exists not only because the appliances have not been organized by their restrictive characteristics, but also because spinal pain frequently eludes a specific diagnosis. Further complicating the confusion is a diversity of terminology resulting from centuries of experimentation. Classifications and descriptions of appliances historically bore the name of the inventor or town from whence they came. Designs were modified regularly at different institutes as well. Unfortunately, many identical or similar braces were labeled with several different names. Fortunately, a new standardized nomenclature has been developed to provide a universal terminology for brace descriptions.[11] The new descriptions may seem clumsy at first, but they are logical in their anatomical correlations (i.e., cervicothoracic, thoracolumbosacral). It is hoped that future appliance modifications will be only briefly described by authors and inventors and will be allowed to bear the same functional nomenclature.

The literature contains only a few investigative studies that have analyzed the effectiveness of each appliance. These studies will be discussed in this chapter and their results and conclusions related to the arbitrary term *effectiveness*. For the most part, effectiveness can be defined as the ability to immobilize intervertebral segments as demonstrated by radiographic studies. The term will be used in this sense throughout the chapter. However, intervertebral immobility, although significant in the treatment of neurovascular and life-threatening disorders or trauma, may be irrelevant to the treatment of symptoms of muscle spasm or low-back pain. Indeed, all therapists have seen clients who are convinced of an appliance's ability to relieve their pain and provide adequate joint stability when there is no radiographic evidence that the orthosis offers any intervertebral segment immobility. Furthermore, most investigative studies on the effectiveness of various appliances have collected data from an unrealistically modified environment (i.e., volunteer normal subjects are used instead of clients with varying diagnoses). This, for the most part, is fortunate since modern medicine has not been able to corroborate diagnoses with scientific evidence for the majority of spinal pain syndromes. Research done by scientific investigative groups (i.e., the International Society for the Study of the Lumbar Spine, individual institutions, and individuals interested in the study of spinal problems) may help to shed light on the precise diagnosis of spinal pain syndromes. Only then, when precise diagnoses can be made, will appropriate treatments and their efficacy be confirmed according to the specific disorder to be treated.

FUNCTIONS OF SPINAL ORTHOSES
Immobilization

Spinal braces are clinically applied to treat a variety of diseases, signs, symptoms, and psychological disorders. Occasionally they are even applied because of the clinician's desire to "do something" for the client. For the most part, the appliances are prescribed to immobilize the affected part, particularly in the case of the postsurgical client. Indeed, rigid immobilization is necessary in the presence of serious instability to help prevent irreversible neurological damage secondary to bony impingement on vital neural structures. However, such cases of severe instability are not the common clinical entity. Although the goal of providing adequate intervertebral immobility has stimulated research projects that offer quantification for the effectiveness of orthoses,* no controlled studies have been published that compare bracing to any other treatment.

Support

In addition to providing the function of intervertebral segment immobilization, orthoses have other clinically useful purposes. Braces furnish an alternative to weak or denervated muscles or lax connective tissue structures by supplementing their support. The application of an abdominal or lumbosacral corset, for example, will reinforce or replace stretched and weakened abdominal muscles resulting from spinal cord injury. Although ligamentous laxity is difficult and dangerous to accurately assess in the spine, an analogy can be drawn between the athlete with torn medial knee ligaments and a client with a hyperflexed cervical whiplash injury and possible posterior element disruption. Orthotic devices can offer support while the insulted tissues heal yet cannot replace their functions adequately.

Rest

Braces also offer a method of rest. Although published research on altered electromyographic (EMG) activity during orthosis use is scant, it is still presumed that the application of the brace reduces the myoelectric output of the underlying muscles. To clarify this hypothesis, Waters and Morris[27] made an initial study of EMG activity during brace wearing by normal subjects. In that study the muscle activity of 10 normal young adults was examined while they wore a metal chairback (Knight) brace or a lumbosacral corset. The EMG activity of the abdominal and selected back muscles was studied with the subjects standing, walking at 4.39 and 5.29 km/hour on a level treadmill, and walking at 4.29 km/hour up a 5-degree incline, with and without an appliance. A variety of patterns occurred. While the subject was standing, both the brace and the corset either decreased or had no effect on the EMG activity of the back muscles. When the client walked slowly (4.39 km/hour), neither appliance altered the usual EMG activity. However, when walking at a faster speed (5.29 km/hour), subjects wearing the chairback brace had increased EMG activity. Apparently, the normal trunk rotation that occurs during regular walking is unaffected by either orthosis, but the back muscles begin to resist the restrictive qualities of the rigid appliance during trunk rotation when the subject walks at a faster speed.

On the other hand, EMG activity of the abdominal muscles either decreased or was unaltered during brace wearing when the client was standing or walking at a slower speed. Since the flexible anterior supports of both appliances offered assistance to the abdominal muscles, the need for these muscles to support the abdomen and maintain intraabdominal pressure was reduced. Similar studies need to be pursued on other appliances to describe muscular alterations occurring in clients with differing disorders.[27]

Protection

Another function of spinal bracing is protection of incompetent structures that result from trauma, surgery, or a disease process. For example, even though reported incidents of atlantooccipital joint trauma in clients suffering from advanced rheumatoid arthritis are infrequent, degeneration of the alar and transverse ligaments of the axis can produce potentially dangerous situations during upper cervical flexion. Appliances could provide protection to these two structures by restricting flexion.

Correction

The last, and probably the most studied, function of bracing is correction. Spinal deformity was the main catalyst that stimulated many inventors to produce a variety of braces in all shapes and materials. Ambrose Paré (1510-1590) was one of the early orthotic pioneers to use a metal corset. Lorenz Heister (1683-1758), a student of Nicholas Andry (1709-1756), is credited with the first spinal brace, known as the *iron cross*. In its crude way the iron cross was the first *halo orthoses* because the head was stabilized by a noninvasive attachment to the trunk. The era that fol-

*See references 8, 14, 16-18, and 23.

lowed produced a wide variety of orthotic designs that gave current clinicians many spinal orthoses that have not drastically changed from the original devices.

Recently, however, corrective devices have undergone considerable modification. For instance, a current popular corrective appliance is the Milwaukee brace.[2] As one of the more sophisticated spinal orthoses, the Milwaukee brace combines the simple concepts of three-point fixation and axial distraction to correct complicated side bending and rotation of the scoliotic curve. However, because of the unsightly appearance of the Milwaukee brace and the advances made in plastic molding techniques, the Boston brace has begun to replace it as the brace of choice for treating scoliosis.

Psychological reasons

Although bracing for psychological reasons exists, the merits of doing so can be debated. This type of bracing as a primary rationale for treatment will not be discussed in this Chapter. Instead, since current treatment is practical and goal-oriented, several different techniques or appliances that are available for treating similar disorders will be discussed.

BIOMECHANICAL FACTORS AFFECTING ORTHOSIS CHOICE

The spine is not directly accessible for bracing. The orthotist cannot apply a simple three-point fixation device directly to the spine since the trunk, abdominal contents, skull, and pelvis interfere. Therefore a more complicated, indirect approach is necessary. This means of fixation must apply stabilizing or corrective forces to the spine via the surrounding integument, viscera, muscle, and connective tissue, including bone. The properties of these structures must be assessed.

Direct animal models are not readily available for comparison to the human spine, and in vivo investigations of the spine are almost nonexistent. Therefore analogies must be drawn from those studies most directly applicable.

Connective tissue properties

Bone. Bone is a rigid form of connective tissue composed of cells and an intercellular matrix of organic and inorganic substances.[5] Although considered rigid, bone continuously remodels under stress. The remodeling process is related to many factors, including age, nutrition, hormonal influences, and the type of loading applied.[10] Studies describing the adaptability of vertebrae to stress as compared to long bones are limited. However, pilot studies suggest that cyclical loading of the lower extremities may initiate vertebral cortical remodeling.[3]

Laboratory studies and clinical experience have demonstrated that vertebrae can withstand large amounts of compressive loading. The compressive resistance strength is much greater in the lumbar region than in the thoracic and more in the thoracic region than the cervical.[28] However, as a person ages, the relationship between osseous tissue and vertebral strength changes. A 25% decrease in the osseous tissue of vertebrae causes a 50% decrease in vertebral strength. This change then translates to the load-carrying capacity of the vertical and horizontal trabeculae in the vertebral body.[28] The neural arch and facets also bear weight, and their load-carrying properties change. However, studies of the types of loads (i.e., distractive and shear stress) seen in the most common spinal orthoses are practically nonexistent.

Intervertebral disk. The various biomechanical properties of the intervertebral disk, a fibrocartilaginous connective tissue, have been well studied. The disk, primarily the lumbar, has been pounded, pulled, rotated, and sheared. In most instances the disk has responded well, even to the point of attempting to heal itself following puncture wounds. Of clinical significance to bracing, however, is the fact that there are no studies describing the disk's reaction in vivo to complex loads, particularly stress, placed on it while in a brace.[28] However, cadaveric disks studied responded to offset loading by bulging radially on the compressed side and by straightening under a tensile tangential strain on the opposite side.[26] Displacement of the nuclear cavity away from the radial bulge was identified but not quantified. This quantification is currently under study.[12]

Posterior elements. Facet joints and capsules also respond to spinal loading by contributing to the restriction of compression and torsion.[7,8,28] Functioning along with the facets are ligamentous structures and disks. A hypothesis regarding degeneration of this three-joint complex has been proposed by Farfan.[7] He suggests that an alteration in the normal symmetrical movement pattern of any one of the three joints initiates a progressive pathological process, which in turn applies tension to the connective tissue surrounding the muscle fascicle. That, in turn, applies tension to the muscle tendon. By no means are internal and external tensions the same under weak contractions. When a passive stretch is applied to a muscle via a brace, for instance, all of the externally applied tension does not go to the sarcomere. The connective tissue sheaths and tendons are also affected. The internal tension, referred to as *muscle tone,* must be overcome, preferably by relaxation not force, before muscle may attain its most lengthened position. Only then will the muscle fiber be stretched.

Properties of muscle

When a muscle is not taken through its normal range of motion regularly (while maintaining normal or increased tone), the connective tissue shortens. In fact, if a muscle becomes nonfunctional because of bracing, the number of sarcomeres decreases. However, during training that requires stretching of a muscle or increased muscular tension, sarcomeres are added at the terminal ends of the muscle, increasing their length and strength.

For the most part, braces and corsets are not used specifically to support weak or tight muscles. However, during the progression of a disease that alters posture, muscle and connective tissue changes occur. In the course of treating such diseases, muscles and connective tissues can also be treated, many times fortuitously, although the effects may be either positive or negative.

For example, clients with low back pain from mechanical derangement or disease processes may use a lumbosacral corset or chairback (Knight) brace. Evidence supports the theory that with these appliances EMG activity of the back muscles and the internal and external oblique muscles either is unaltered or decreased when the client is standing, and EMG activity of the abdominal muscles is unaltered or decreased when the client walks at a fast speed (4.39 km/hour).[27] Only when the client walks at a fast speed (5.29 km/hour) do the abdominal and back muscles become as active as they would be without the supports. Clinically, then, clients wearing back braces could expect muscular degradation, which would reduce the abdominal muscles' ability to support the lumbar spine, if they do not either exercise regularly or walk vigorously (i.e., faster than 5 km/hour). In a response to a questionnaire one unidentified clinician stated that he "never prescribes support without a plan to eliminate it."[24]

Muscle, theoretically, could be used to correct structural deformities with success similar to that achievable with the Milwaukee brace. Kinesiological studies of the posterior thoracic muscles, as described by serial cross-sectional analysis, show that they can generate, via electrical muscle stimulation, lateral bending moments of the same magnitude as the Milwaukee brace. However, current techniques cannot cause continuous muscle contraction nor can any one muscle provide pure lateral bending or the rotary force necessary to correct the rotational component of scoliosis. Most back muscles under increased tension would, in fact, exaggerate the lumbar lordosis.[25] It remains necessary, then, to determine if posterior spinal muscles may be able to be trained with specific techniques that could allow the muscles to generate enough force to actively assist in the correction of some deformities while within a passive constraint appliance.

Finally, coordinated activity of abdominal and erector spinal muscles is altered in clients with back pain.[15] Therefore the addition of an orthosis may not improve the condition but may enhance abnormal patterns simply by not allowing normal movement to occur.

Properties of skin

Unless skeletal fixation is used, braces will apply forces directly to the skin. The skin responds by becoming abraded or by necrosing as a result of the compression of blood vessels in the capillary beds. The potential, however, does exist for biomechanical adaptation to occur in skin following prolonged application of forces. For example, the hardness of the skin increases under the pelvic band of a Milwaukee brace with prolonged exposure.[28]

Sensibility of the skin is critical for proper adaptation to bracing appliances. Without sensation, protective mechanisms will not allow the client to actively reduce the pressure on the skin when necessary, thereby increasing the possibility of necrosis. Bony prominences are the primary sites of concern because they will break down faster than areas protected by adipose tissue.

Viscoelastic linkages

The preceding discussion has emphasized the biomechanical factors of the various tissues and structures involved in spinal bracing. The following discussion will focus on interrelations of those structures when forces are applied to them.

A decrease in spinal movement is frequently the goal of the clinician using orthoses. To attain this goal the clinician applies forces to anatomical structures known as low-stiffness viscoelastic transmitters, which in turn apply a force to the vertebral bodies.

Mechanically, the vertebrae are semirigid bodies in series, separated by disks and ligaments, or viscoelastic linkages (Fig. 13-1). A viscoelastic transmitter displays both the properties of a viscous and an elastic body. The viscous body is composed of cells and the intercellular matrix of organic and inorganic connective tissue, which is predominantly fluid in character. The elastic structure is represented by the elastic connective tissue within some of the spinal structures as well as by the ability of individual structures to absorb and generate tension following the application of a load to that structure.

The dashpot experimentally represents a viscous body (see Fig. 13-1). If a load is applied to the plunger, the plunger moves at a velocity that is dependent on the viscosity of the fluid. If the fluid is not viscid, as in the case of water, the plunger moves quickly. If the fluid is viscid, as in the case of cold oil, the plunger moves slowly. Following the release of the load, the plunger does not return to its original position since the dashpot is nonelastic. The resistance provided by the fluid is directly related to the rate of loading. It has been hypothesized but not corroborated by research that the nucleus pulposus responds as a dashpot with fluid moving away from the side of the applied compressive load.[26]

The arrangement of collagen and elastic fibers in various structures of the spine offers some elasticity. A good example of an elastic structure is a loaded spring. A load on the spring causes immediate deformation. Removal of the load allows the spring to return to its original position. The ligamentum flavum, specifically, represents an elastic structure.

Viscoelasticity results when there is a combination of a

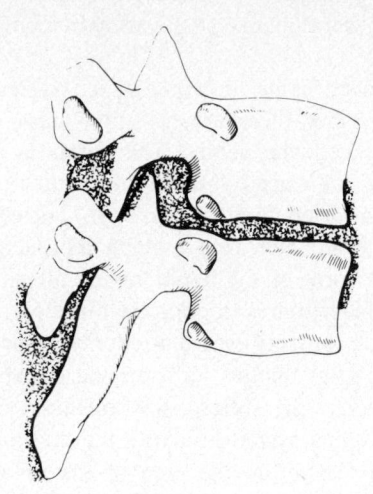
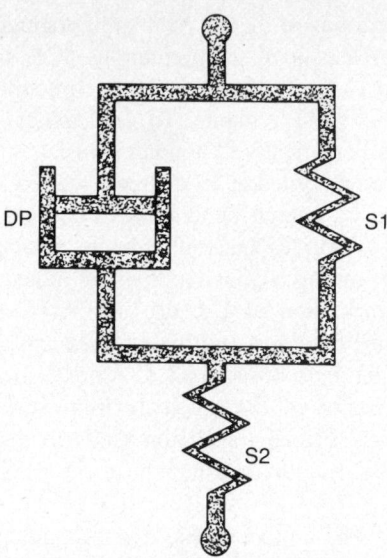

Fig. 13-1. Functional unit consists of two adjacent vertebrae and ligamentous structures connecting them. These ligamentous structures may be considered viscoelastic linkages. Three-element model of a dashpot *(DP)* and a spring *(S1)* in parallel are connected to a second spring *(S2)* in series. (Modified from White AA and Panjabi MM: Clinical biomechanics of the spine, Philadelphia, 1978, JB Lippincott Co, p. 348.)

viscous element and elastic element in parallel. When a force or load is applied to the system, an immediate strain, or change in length of the system, occurs. The total strain or deformation depends on the length of the spring or elastic structure, while the maximal rate of strain depends on the viscosity of the fluid.

The spine is basically a viscoelastic structure. Clinically, the system allows for load absorption and transmission through a series of elastic and viscoelastic structures. The ultimate load reaching a specific anatomical structure is therefore less than the force applied. During spinal bracing this system of viscoelastic linkages offers a complicated biomechanical problem for specific force application.

The viscoelastic linkages involve structures of various stiffness surrounded by a variety of other low-stiffness viscoelastic transmitters. For example, the cervical spine is surrounded mostly by muscle. The thoracic spine is surrounded by muscles, ribs, and air-filled lungs. The lumbar spine is surrounded by muscles, air, viscera, and fluid. Fat and skin also play a role of varying importance in each region. The ribs increase the stiffness or resistance of the thoracic spine to bending by 200%.[1] All the other structures have reduced stiffness. Combined, all these structures offer diverse, complex viscoelastic linkages of varying elasticity and viscosity that together complicate the process of applying forces directly to a specific intervertebral segment.

General kinematics

Before analyzing a clinical problem, the clinician needs to understand the normal motion available at each spinal area. Therefore an abbreviated review of normal kinematics in each portion of the spine will be given. Specific kinematic considerations include: (1) total range of motion available in three planes; (2) specific considerations altering the general motion available, such as C-1–C-2 rotation; (3) junctional considerations (i.e., in the cervicothoracic area) and (4) the coupling of various movements in specific areas.

Cervical spine. The cervical spine is the most mobile spinal region. Johnson et al[16] measured 136.5 degrees of flexion-extension between the occiput and T-1. Approximately 50% of that motion was flexion or extension from a neutral position. Since the starting position varies, actual amounts of flexion and extension may vary. However, the segments between C-4 and C-7 contribute 45% of all cervical flexion and extension. In this region the orientation of the facet joints facilitates sagittal plane movement, which is considered physiological motion.

Rotation and lateral bending are much more difficult to quantify. Fifty percent of the entire rotation of the spine occurs at C-1 to C-2. The articular processes are oriented appropriately to allow this motion. However, the articular surfaces of the rest of the spine are not properly oriented to provide smooth rotation or lateral bending separately. These movements therefore are considered nonphysiological in that they must be accompanied by additional components of flexion, extension, rotation, lateral bending, or translation. The combination of movements is called *coupling*. In the lower cervical spine lateral bending is coupled with rotation to the same side.[19] The amount of axial rotation per degree of lateral bending decreases caudally between C-2 and C-7.

Specific considerations in the cervical spine include the occiput to C-1 and C-1 to C-2 articulations. Combined with the occiput to C-1 articulations, the occipitoatlanto-axial joints are the most complex of the spine, both anatomically and kinematically. Flexion-extension at occiput to C-1 has been recorded at 19 degrees, while C-1 to C-2 was 14 degrees.[16] Lateral bending of 8 degrees and axial rotation of 47 degrees have also been reported.[28] However, most important is the coupling of axial rotation and vertical translation of C-1 on C-2. As C-1 rotates from a midline position (normal anatomical position, which is the highest position of C-1 on C-2), C-1 moves caudally because of the biconvex joint surfaces. Therefore the vertical caudal translation tends to distract the cervical spine during axial rotation if the client is braced.

Thoracic spine. The thoracic spine is not as mobile as the cervical and lumbar spines and has not been studied in vivo for normal mobility as extensively as the cervical spine because of difficulties in radiographic techniques. White and Panjabi[28] reported a total representative value of 64 degrees of flexion-extension between T-1 and T-12, with a segmental median of 4 degrees in the upper, 6 degrees in the middle, and 12 degrees in the lower thoracic region. Lateral bending totaled 7 degrees and rotation 72 degrees. Lateral bending increased from 6 to 9 degrees, and rotation decreased from 9 to 2 degrees cephalocaudally.

Coupling characteristics are not consistent and are not as important in the thoracic spine as they are in the cervical spine. First, in the upper thoracic spine lateral bending is coupled with axial rotation to the same side. In the middle and lower thoracic spines the pattern is variable.[28] Second, the rib cage decreases mobility by making the whole area more rigid and decreasing the clinical importance of coupled movements.

Lumbar spine. The arthrokinematic transition from a rather immobile thoracic to a more mobile lumbar spine may occur anywhere between T-9 and T-12. Change in facet-joint inclination, however, is consistently evident in the T-12 to L-1 intervertebral area when the plane of the facets is approximately vertical but angled 45 degrees anteriorly from the frontal plane. The latter angle decreases toward L-5 to S-1. Therefore there is little axial rotation (2 degrees) until the L-5 to S-1 level, where there is a 5-degree rotation. Lateral bending ranges between 3 to 8 degrees, with the most flexibility (8 degrees) at L-3 to L-4. Flexion-extension motion is the primary motion of the lumbar spine with approximately 12 to 20 degrees of motion per level. L-4 to L-5 and L-5 to S-1 exhibit the greatest movement.[28]

Lumbar spine coupling is opposite to cervical spine coupling because lateral bending is coupled with axial rotation to the opposite side. This movement is complicated by the position of the sacrum. However, as with most of the above movements, the measurements are open to controversy and possible clinical misrepresentation since the figures were obtained by various techniques, some not in vivo.[28]

Lumbar spine movement is particularly difficult to control since there are no good areas of purchase for a brace except the pelvis. The pelvis is a mobile structure heavily influenced by the mechanical advantage of the long lower-extremity lever arm and the weight of the trunk, head, and arms, which the sacrum must support. Weight borne on the lumbar spine forces the spine into lordosis and requires abdominal muscle strength to equalize the load. Any orthosis that applies anterior pressure to the lumbar spine applies its force via the abdominal contents, which offer the softest, low-stiffness viscoelastic linkage of the spinal system, making the goal of spinal restriction elusive. Therefore the area of the greatest sagittal plane movement and most frequent insult, the L-4 to S-1 intervertebral area, is probably the most difficult area to control orthotically.

PRINCIPLES OF SPINAL ORTHOSES[28]
Balanced horizontal forces

Horizontal forces in the form of a three-point loading system are used by several braces (Figs. 13-2 and 13-3). The horizontal forces are effective in providing bending moments for the correction of lateral bending and rotation as well as immobilization.

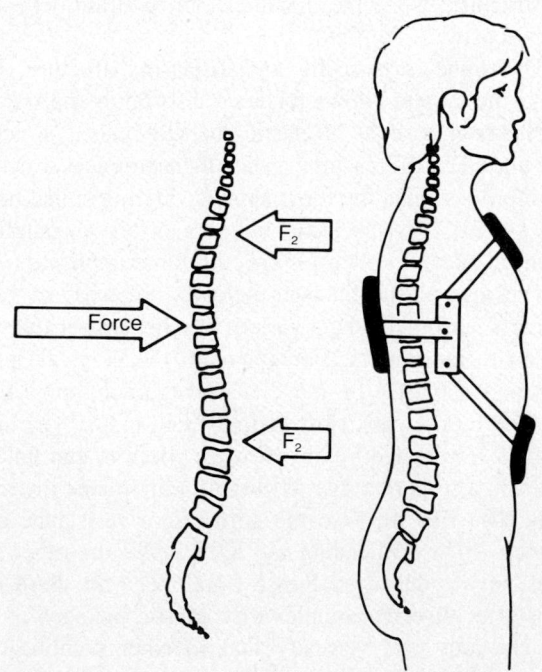

Fig. 13-2. Schematic representation of a Jewett brace. Forces represent three-point fixation that allows the Jewett brace to extend the thoracic spine. Biomechanically, each anterior force will be equal to one-half the posterior force if posterior force is midway between the two anterior forces. (Modified from White AA and Panjabi MM: Clinical biomechanics of the spine, Philadelphia, 1978, JB Lippincott Co, p. 354.)

The mechanical application of three horizontal forces is a relatively straightforward use of static equilibrium, which means that all the forces and their bending moments must add up to zero. In this system two forces are applied in one direction and a third is applied in a direction opposite the first two. Mathematically, these points are related and chosen, theoretically, for the maximal correction prescribed. For example, in Fig. 13-4, $F_A - F_B - F_C = 0$ and $F_B D_B - F_C D_C = 0$. Solving for F_B and F_C:

$$F_B = \frac{F_A \cdot D_C}{D_B + D_C}$$

and

$$F_C = \frac{F_A \cdot D_B}{D_B + D_C}$$

Referring further to Fig. 13-4,

$$F_B = \frac{2F_A}{3}$$

and

$$F_C = \frac{F_A}{3}$$

which means that, given a force, F_A, and distances, D_B and D_C, the forces at B and C need to be two thirds and one third, respectively, of the magnitude of the force at A if the system is to be in equilibrium.

In addition to appropriately locating the pads for specific correction of a spinal deformity, another point of clinical significance in this mathematical computation is determining the relationship of the pressure on the skin and the area of the skin pad. To reduce the potential for skin degradation, the pressure on the skin pads must be minimized. If a brace applies forces similar to the forces in Figs. 13-2 and 13-4 and equal skin pressure for each pad is desired, the areas for pads at points A, B, and C would need to be in a ratio of $3:2:1$. The optimal size of the pads should be clarified by clinical appropriateness.

Of primary importance in the force system is the bending moment produced by each force since that moment is ultimately responsible for the angular correction. In the three-point system the moment varies at different intervertebral spaces. In Fig. 13-4, the moment from F_A is maximal at point A and decreases to zero at points B and C. Maximal correction will be obtained then if F_A is placed at the apex of the curve and F_B and F_C are placed as far from F_A as possible.

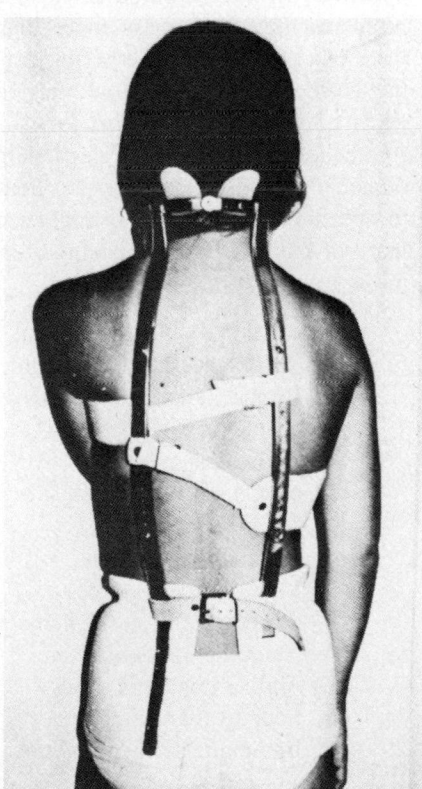

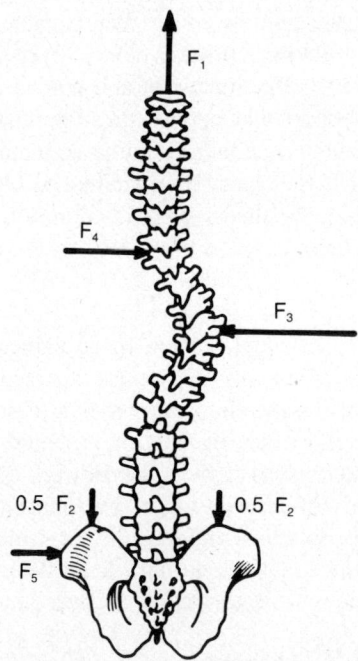

Fig. 13-3. Forces of the Milwaukee brace allow for axial tension in conjunction with lateral correction. Force F_3 represents the thoracic pad, F_4 represents the axillary sling, and F_5 represents the pelvic girdle. These forces represent a three-point force system. Maximum bending moment is applied at the level of F_3. (Modified from White AA and Panjabi MM: Clinical biomechanics of the spine, Philadelphia, 1978, JB Lippincott Co, p. 363.)

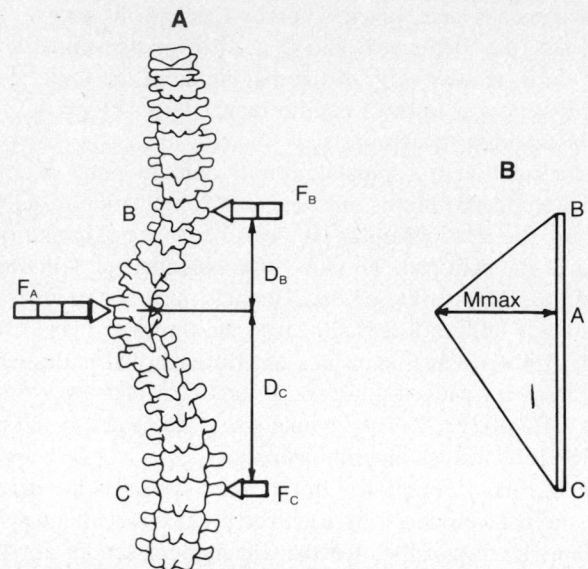

Fig. 13-4. A, A three-point force system. Magnitude of each horizontal force depends on the distance separating force *B* and force *C* from force *A*. **B,** Maximum bending moment is represented by this three-point force system. Maximum force for correction is applied at *A*. (Modified from White AA and Panjabi MM: Clinical biomechanics of the spine, Philadelphia, 1978, JB Lippincott Co, p. 353.)

Fluid compression

Compressing a fluid-filled container increases the pressure within the container. Plant turgidity is a good example. The tension within the fluid or cell is then capable of applying support to a structure. Orthotic devices take advantage of this principle to effectively rest and unload the spine by providing a support that applies pressure to the abdominal contents. Although neither common abdominal corsets nor lumbosacral braces have been studied to measure any pressure changes, the theory of fluid compression is generally accepted by clinicians.

Distraction

The distractive ability of axial tension to straighten a spine is well known by clinicians. However, distraction also increases the stability of the spine and renders it more capable of resisting a lateral force. Distraction probably alters the movement characteristics of the spine as well. This was discovered in a study of cervical braces by Johnson et al.[16] The cervical spine, within a rigid metal cervicothoracic-style brace and hale, "snaked" during forced flexion-extension trials, even though the cervical spine was not as mobile.

Sleeve principle

The sleeve principle implies the application of at least a pair of semicircular fixation points, one above the other, with rigid uprights between that act as a splint, distractor,

or attachments for various accessory devices. If one pair of the semicircular fixation points is used anteriorly and one pair posteriorly, the client is essentially placed in a "cage" that can be used effectively to apply forces anywhere.

Skeletal fixation

Skeletal fixation via metal pins is the only true means to effectively immobilize certain intervertebral segments.[16] Forces thus bypass the low-stiffness viscoelastic transmitters and are applied directly to bone. However, the halo traction system, with or without pelvic pins, is not a conventional but rather an invasive orthosis, and although it is more effective, it carries more risk than conventional braces.

REGIONAL REVIEW OF SPINAL ORTHOSES
Plan of analysis

The appropriate selection of a spinal orthosis should follow a consistent plan of analysis, similar to any other analysis of a clinical problem. Following the confirmation of a working diagnosis, the specific problems secondary to the diagnosis should be enumerated. The problems can be grouped into categories similar to the following: (1) pathological arthrokinematics or biomechanics, (2) muscular disorders or complications, (3) ligamentous or capsular disorders, or (4) neurological disorders. Several clinical problems may encompass more than one or even all of these categories. Once the pertinent problems are clarified, the goals of treatment should be determined. The basic goals of spinal support (rest, assistance), immobilization (protection), or correction need delineation. Finally, the clinician should match specific client problems and goals to specific qualities of the appliances available. A summary of the process of choosing a spinal orthosis is given in the following outline:

A. Establish a working diagnosis
B. Delineate specific client problems
  1. Biomechanical deficiencies
    a. Flexion
    b. Extension
    c. Lateral bending
    d. Axial rotation
    e. Axial distraction
  2. Muscular deficiencies
  3. Connective tissue deficiencies
  4. Neurological deficiencies
C. Determine treatment goals
  1. Support (rest, assist)
  2. Immobilization (protection)
  3. Correction
D. Match client problems and treatment goals to orthotic qualities

Diagnosis of a spinal problem is not simple and frequently requires time to monitor patterns of signs and symptoms in order to corroborate a working diagnosis. Second, analysis of a client's problem may be difficult since many testing procedures that determine which specific tissues are implicated are dangerous and unwarranted during the acute phase of an injury or disease process. Finally, there are few quantitative reports explaining the specific qualities of the currently available appliances. There are many elaborate descriptions but scanty analyses of the effectiveness of various braces.

Therefore it is important to review the goals, research available, and orthoses commonly used for problems in the three major areas of the spine: cervical, thoracic, and lumbosacral. Since research is limited, clinical experience and descriptive literature will have to prevail.

Cervical region

Bracing goals for the cervical spine should emphasize spinal support and immobilization and deemphasize correction. Biomechanical derangement—whether secondary to osteoarthritis or trauma to the posterior connective tissue elements or muscles—may represent a potentially serious neurological problem. Or indeed, the neurological dysfunction may be the primary problem. In that case surgical intervention is usually warranted. In biomechanical derangement, which is by far more common than primary neurological dysfunction, there are several anatomical features to consider in choosing an appropriate spinal orthosis. Through the contact on the mandible/occiput and thorax, there is some axial traction applied to the cervical spine that relieves the cervical lordosis. Therefore any brachial plexus irritation or temporomandibular joint disorder warrants careful monitoring during orthosis wearing.

Cervical orthoses are commonly classified into two categories: conventional and nonconventional. In the conventional category are cervical collars and the poster-style and cervicothoracic-style orthoses. In the nonconventional class is the halo traction system. This is considered a nonconventional orthotic device since it requires the invasive technique of skeletal pinning.

Investigations of the braced cervical spine in vivo em-

phasize studies in normal individuals,* with only one brief analysis of clients in halo-skeletal fixation systems.[16] Most of these studies use measurement techniques based either on plain radiographic investigation or cineradiography. Plain radiographs are superior in their resolution of fine bony detail but do not allow the clinician to examine movement at each instant during the motion. Cineradiography does not allow refined detail of bony anatomy but allows the investigator to view the movement patterns of the various structures throughout the entire range. Goniometry has also been used to effectively measure spinal movement but does not allow the reviewer to interpret intervertebral segment motion.

One of the first studies evaluating the effectiveness of various cervical orthoses was done by Jones.[18] In his study 22 clients wore collars of plastic, leather, or felt stockinette and two wore chin-occiput braces. The specific diagnoses of each client were not included. Each client, except one with a fusion, was studied cineradiographically with and without the collar by standard views of flexion and extension. The results of the study emphasized that the motion of the cervical segments was influenced by the collars. However, quantification was not given. The collars were reported to only slightly limit rotation of the upper segments, while the chin-occiput braces offered more restriction. Restriction in flexion or extension was related to the position of initiation of the movement. With initial head flexion and concomitant neck extension, the lower segments were not limited by the collars. However, if the head was extended first, a general restriction was noticed. Restriction of flexion and extension also increased when higher anterior collar sections were used. Also, as the height increased, anterior translation of the disks increased and facet-joint expansion and compression decreased.

In 1973 Colachis, Strohm, and Ganter[4] did a study of 11 normal young women who wore three different collars: soft-sponge, chin-piece, and Queen Anne. Nine lateral radiographs were taken to define sagittal plane motion of C-

*See references 4, 9, 14, and 16-18.

Table 13-1. Approximate percentage restriction of range of motion (C-1–C-7)

Orthoses	Motion picture			Cineradiograph		
	Flexion/extension	Lateral bending	Axial rotation	Flexion/extension	Lateral bending	Axial rotation
Soft cervical collar	5-10	5-10	0	0	0	0
Thomas hard plastic collar	75	75	50	75	75	50
Four-poster collar	80-85	80-85	60	85	85	60
Long two-poster collar	95	90	90	90	90	90
Guilford two-poster collar	90-95	90-95	90-95	90	90-95	90
Halo device			(Essentially no motion)			

Data modified from Hartman JT, Palumbo F, and Hill BJ: Cineradiography of the braced normal cervical spine, Clin Orthop 109:97, 1975, and White A and Panjabi M: Clinical biomechanics of the spine, Philadelphia, 1978, JB Lippincott Co, p. 355.

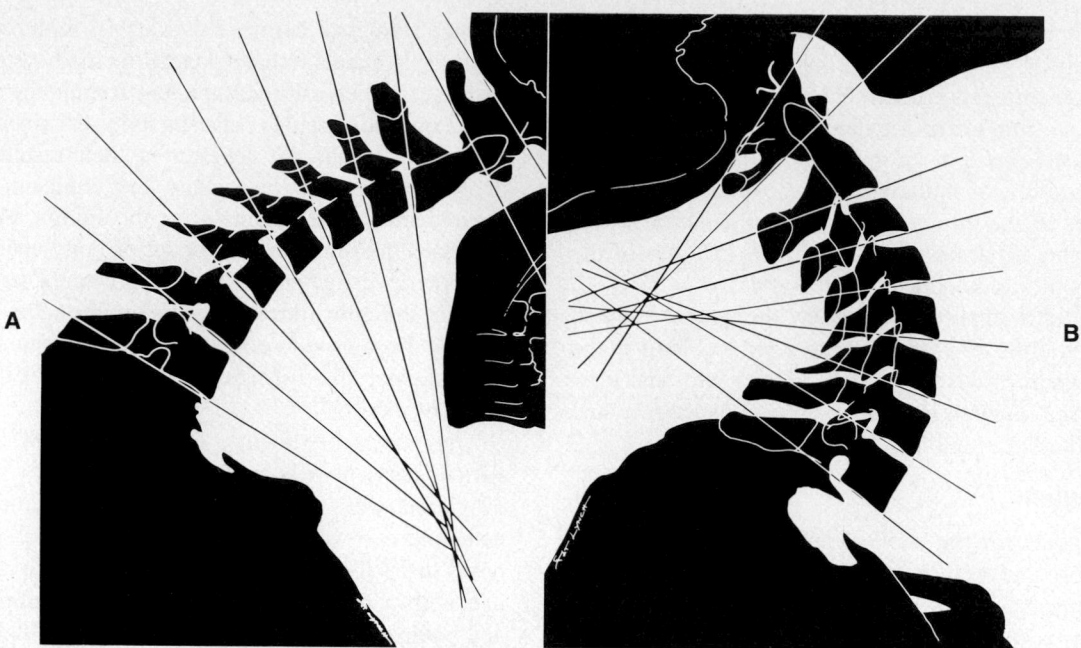

Fig. 13-5. The cervical spine in flexion **(A)** and extension **(B).** Reference lines were constructed tangentially to base of skull at foramen magnum and basioocciput, along inferior aspect of ring of atlas and through inferior lips of each vertebral body below this level. Lines were extended to form angles at their points of intersection, which were used to measure the angles in flexion and extension. (Modified from Johnson RM et al: J Bone Joint Surg (Am) 59[3]:332, 1977.)

2 to T-1 with and without the collars. Millimeter displacements were recorded instead of degress of motion to emphasize transverse translation. The soft collar did not restrict movement in either flexion or extension. The chinpiece collar, however, straightened the upper cervical spine with limitation at that level. Flexion of the lower levels was limited. The Queen Anne collar limited extension, particularly in the upper cervical spine, and straightened the spine.

In 1975 Hartman, Palumbo, and Hill[14] studied a combination of five students and clients with relatively similar, normal cervical spines as determined by cinefluoroscopy. Each subject wore five different braces and was studied by film and cineradiography. Emphasis was placed on the meticulous fit of mandibular and occipital pieces, designed specifically for restriction of rotation. The results are summarized in Table 13-1. The soft cervical collar offered little immobilization. The firmer the appliance, the better the restriction.

Fisher et al[9] studied 10 normal subjects who wore four different braces: (1) the polyethylene Camp plastic collar, (2) the polyethylene Philadelphia collar, (3) the four-poster collar, and (4) the sternal occipital mandibular immobilization (SOMI) collar. Lateral radiographs were taken of the subjects both with and without each brace in the neutral, flexion, and extension positions. Distortion forces applied to the chin and occipital pieces were standardized for each

trial. The results of the study were similar to those reached in a study by Johnson et al[16] on 44 normal subjects wearing three of the four braces in question. In the Johnson study each subject was measured with and without the three different braces. Plain lateral radiographs were taken in neutral, maximal flexion, and maximal extension positions. Anteroposterior radiographs were taken of neutral and maximal lateral bending. Axial photographs were taken of rotation (Figs. 13-5 to 13-7). The effectiveness of the halo with a plastic body vest was also studied on seven clients. Ultimately, as a result of their research, Johnson and the other investigators designed a new brace called the Yale cervical orthosis (Fig. 13-8).[29]

The results of the Johnson study are listed in Tables 13-2 to 13-6. The overall conclusion was that no orthosis eliminates all intervertebral motion, not even the halo. In general, increasing the rigidity of the appliance improved its ability to restrict intervertebral motion. However, lateral bending and rotation over the entire cervical spine as well as flexion and extension at the upper levels were not well controlled by any of the conventional orthoses.

Fixation to the chest and the addition of rigid connections between the anterior and posterior components, as in the cervicothoracic brace, improve the control of rotation and flexion in the lower part of the cervical spine, but restricting lateral bending and sagittal plane motion of the upper part of the spine is not improved. The standard or-

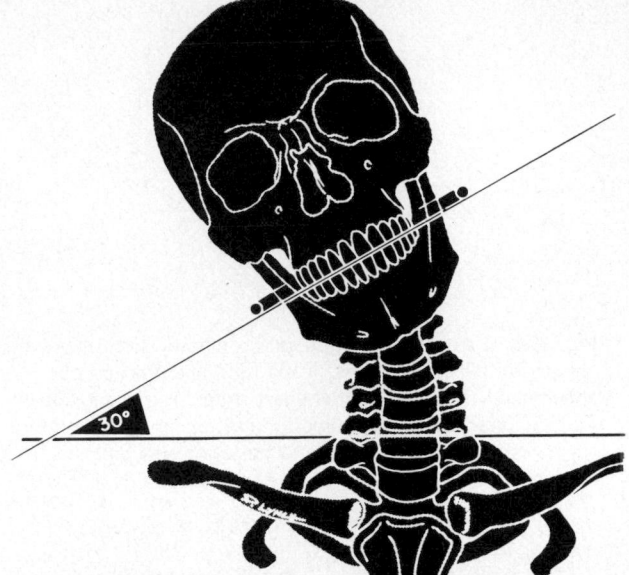

Fig. 13-6. Total lateral bending of the cervical spine measured on anteroposterior radiographs at extremes of motion. A reference line representing position of skull intersects a reference line from superior margins of transverse processess of T1. (Modified from Johnson RM et al: J Bone Joint Surg (Am) 59[3]:332, 1977.)

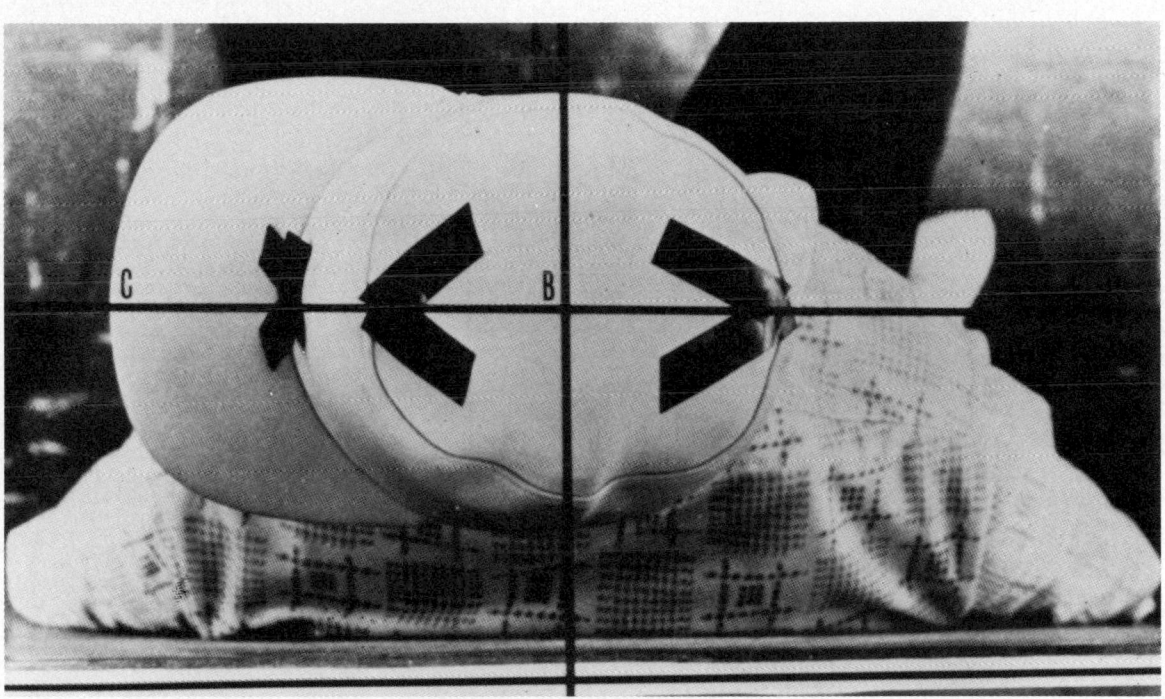

Fig. 13-7. Axial rotation measured using overhead photographs of head and shoulders made with subject wearing tight-fitting cap equipped with reference marks to delineate position of head. Subject sat with shoulders pressed firmly against perpendicular flat frame. Angle between head and plane of shoulders was measured with subject rotating maximally to right and to left. Two resulting angles are averaged to give a value for amount of rotation from midline. (Modified from Johnson RM et al: J Bone Joint Surg (Am) 59[3]:332, 1977.)

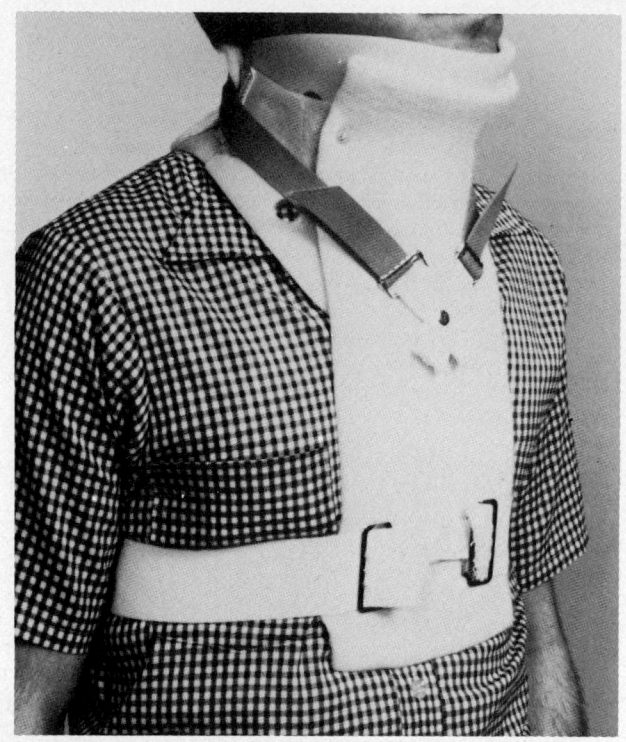

Fig. 13-8. Yale cervical orthosis is a modification of polyethylene collar (Philadelphia collar), using rigid anterior and posterior attachments. Circumferential chest straps restrict movement of rigid thoracic attachments and superior attachments reduce inferior and superior gliding of anterior and posterior attachments. (Modified from Johnson RM et al: J Bone Joint Surg (Am) 59[3]:332, 1977.)

Table 13-2. Normal motion allowed from the occiput to the first thoracic vertebra (mean percentage and 95% confidence limits of the mean)

Test situation	Number of subjects (male/female)	Mean age (years)	Mean percent of normal motion allowed					
			Flexion-extension	Significance*	Rotation	Significance*	Lateral bending	Significance*
Normal, unrestricted (all subjects)	44 19/25	25.8 (20-36)	100		100		100	
Soft collar	20 10/10	26.2 (20-36)	74.2 ± 7.2	0.001	82.6 ± 4.6	0.001	92.3 ± 8.0	0.057,NS
Philadelphia collar	17 9/8	25.8 (20-34)	28.9 ± 4.7	0.001	43.7 ± 6.7	0.001	66.4 ± 10.7	0.001
SOMI brace	22 7/15	25.0 (21-31)	27.7 ± 6.6	0.772,NS	33.6 ± 6.4	0.05	65.6 ± 9.4	0.899,NS
Four-poster brace	27 11/16	25.9 (21-36)	20.6 ± 5.4	0.05	27.1 ± 3.9	0.05	45.9 ± 7.5	0.001
Cervicothoracic brace	27 11/16	25.9 (21-36)	12.8 ± 3.0	0.05	18.2 ± 3.2	0.001	50.5 ± 7.1	0.063,NS
Halo with plastic body vest	7 6/1	40.0 (20-48)	4		1		4	

Modified from Johnson RM, Hart DL, et al: Cervical orthoses: a study comparing their effectiveness in restricting cervical motion in normal subjects, J Bone Joint Surg (Am) 59(3):332, 1977.

*Significance recorded is the probability value of one brace or collar varying significantly compared with the test situation listed above, using the paired t-test. For example, flexion-extension in a soft collar was significantly different from normal unrestricted motion (P < 0.001). The Philadelphia collar was significantly better in restricting flexion-extension than the soft collar (P = 0.772).

Table 13-3. Flexion and extension allowed at each segmental level (mean degrees and 95% confidence limits of the mean)

Test situation	Motion	Occ.–C-1	C-1–C-2	C-2–C-3	C-3–C-4	C-4–C-5	C-5–C-6	C-6–C-7	C-7–T-1
Normal,	Flexion	0.7 ± 0.5	7.7 ± 1.2	7.2 ± 0.9	9.8 ± 1.0	10.3 ± 1.0	11.4 ± 1.0	12.5 ± 1.0	9.0 ± 1.1
unrestricted	Extension	18.1 ± 2.1	6.0 ± 1.2	4.8 ± 0.8	7.8 ± 1.1	9.8 ± 1.2	10.5 ± 1.3	8.2 ± 1.2	2.7 ± 0.7
Soft collar	Flexion	1.3 ± 1.3	5.1 ± 1.9	4.5 ± 1.2	7.4 ± 1.5	8.4 ± 2.4	9.9 ± 1.7	9.7 ± 0.9	7.7 ± 2.5
	Extension	13.7 ± 3.5	1.9 ± 1.4	3.9 ± 1.0	5.8 ± 1.7	6.8 ± 1.6	7.8 ± 1.2	7.4 ± 1.4	2.8 ± 1.9
Philadelphia	Flexion	0.9 ± 1.0	4.0 ± 1.8	1.6 ± 1.0	3.1 ± 1.1	4.6 ± 1.8	6.2 ± 1.9	6.2 ± 1.6	5.5 ± 1.8
collar	Extension	6.8 ± 2.2	4.5 ± 1.5	1.8 ± 0.9	3.4 ± 1.0	5.8 ± 1.2	5.9 ± 1.2	5.8 ± 2.0	1.3 ± 0.9
SOMI brace	Flexion	3.6 ± 1.8	2.7 ± 1.8	0.9 ± 0.7	1.6 ± 1.1	1.9 ± 0.8	2.8 ± 1.2	2.9 ± 1.6	3.1 ± 1.8
	Extension	9.1 ± 2.6	5.4 ± 1.9	4.4 ± 1.1	6.3 ± 1.4	6.0 ± 1.8	6.0 ± 2.0	5.6 ± 1.8	2.1 ± 1.1
Four-poster	Flexion	2.9 ± 2.0	4.4 ± 2.1	1.6 ± 1.0	2.1 ± 1.1	1.8 ± 0.9	3.0 ± 1.2	3.9 ± 1.6	2.8 ± 1.4
brace	Extension	9.3 ± 2.2	3.2 ± 1.4	2.0 ± 0.7	3.2 ± 1.2	3.4 ± 1.3	2.9 ± 0.9	3.1 ± 1.5	1.6 ± 0.8
Cervicothoracic	Flexion	1.3 ± 0.9	5.0 ± 1.9	1.8 ± 0.8	2.9 ± 1.2	2.8 ± 0.7	1.6 ± 0.8	0.7 ± 0.6	2.4 ± 1.0
brace	Extension	8.4 ± 2.1	2.5 ± 0.8	2.1 ± 0.7	1.6 ± 0.7	2.2 ± 0.9	2.8 ± 0.9	3.4 ± 1.1	1.7 ± 0.8

Modified from Johnson RM, Hart DL, et al: Cervical orthoses: a study comparing their effectiveness in restricting cervical motion in normal subjects, J Bone Joint Surg (Am) 59(3):332, 1977.

Table 13-4. Mean percentage of normal flexion-extension restricted at each segmental level of the cervical spine (mean percentage flexion-extension and 95% confidence limits of mean percentage)

Orthosis or collar	O–C-1	C-1–C-2	C-2–C-3	C-3–C-4	C-4–C-5	C-5–C-6	C-6–C-7	C-7–T-1
Yale	53.7 ± 15.6	28.5 ± 23.6	70.8 ± 7.5	75.0 ± 5.7	69.6 ± 7.5	72.1 ± 6.9	68.4 ± 9.7	64.4 ± 14.5
Cervicothoracic	50.5 + 11.8	47.4 + 11.8	68.3 + 5.9	75.0 + 5.7	76.6 + 4.0	80.4 + 4.1	81.1 + 5.4	67.8 + 6.8
Four-poster	37.2 ± 12.4	48.2 ± 16.2	69.2 ± 7.5	69.3 ± 7.4	74.1 ± 7.0	73.1 ± 6.4	66.0 ± 7.3	64.4 ± 12.0
SOMI brace	31.9 ± 14.5	40.9 ± 18.4	55.8 ± 10.1	55.1 ± 10.3	61.2 ± 8.0	59.4 ± 9.2	58.7 ± 11.7	55.9 ± 17.1
Philadelphia	59.6 ± 10.8	38.0 ± 14.0	71.7 ± 8.4	63.6 ± 8.0	48.3 ± 9.9	44.7 ± 8.7	41.3 ± 13.1	42.4 ± 13.7

Modified from Johnson RM, Hart DL, et al: The Yale cervical orthosis: an evaluation of its effectiveness in restricting cervical motion in normal subjects and a comparison with other cervical orthoses; reprinted from *Physical Therapy* 58(7):865, 1978 with the permission of the American Physical Therapy Association.

Table 13-5. Mean percentage of normal flexion restricted at each segmental level of the cervical spine (mean percentage flexion and 95% confidence limits of mean percentage)

Orthosis or collar	0–C-1*	C-1–C-2	C-2–C-3	C-3–C-4	C-4–C-5	C-5–C-6	C-6–C-7	C-7–T-1
Yale	—	18.2 ± 30.6	73.6 ± 15.5	83.7 ± 10.3	80.6 ± 15.7	83.3 ± 9.7	79.2 ± 11.3	64.4 ± 18.1
Cervicothoracic	—	35.1 ± 25.3	75.0 ± 11.3	70.4 ± 12.3	72.8 ± 6.9	86.0 ± 7.1	94.4 ± 4.8	77.4 ± 11.3
Four-poster	—	42.9 ± 28.0	77.8 ± 14.1	78.6 ± 11.3	82.5 ± 8.8	73.7 ± 10.6	68.8 ± 12.9	68.9 ± 15.8
SOMI brace	—	64.9 ± 24.0	87.5 ± 9.9	83.7 ± 11.3	81.5 ± 7.8	75.4 ± 10.6	76.8 ± 12.9	65.6 ± 20.3
Philadelphia	—	48.0 ± 24.0	77.8 ± 14.1	68.4 ± 11.3	55.3 ± 17.6	45.6 ± 16.8	50.4 ± 12.9	38.9 ± 20.3

Modified from Johnson RM, Hart DL, et al: The Yale cervical orthosis: an evaluation of its effectiveness in restricting cervical motion in normal subjects and a comparison with other cervical orthoses; reprinted from *Physical Therapy* 58(7):865, 1978 with the permission of the American Physical Therapy Association.

*Measurements exceeded normal motion and are not considered reliable at this level.

thoses with mandibular and occipital supports are not well suited for controlling lateral bending or sagittal plane motion of the head and upper cervical spine. Extending these supports laterally and adding an upright and a circumferential band about the head may improve this control. However, there is a limit to the extent that motions of the head can be controlled by skin-contact devices. Certain clinical situations require skeletal fixation through a halo to control lateral bending, rotation, or sagittal plane motion in the upper part of the cervical spine or to control very unstable areas elsewhere. A review of cervical appliances available offers other functional considerations.[13,16]

The popularity of the soft cervical collar (Fig. 13-9), commonly used by the medical profession, is perpetuated by its ease of donning and great degree of client comfort. The theory that the soft cervical collar actually immobi-

Table 13-6. Mean percentage of normal extension restricted at each segmental level of the cervical spine (mean percentage extension and 95% confidence limits of mean percentage)

Orthosis or collar	0–C-1	C-1–C-2	C-2–C-3	C-3–C-4	C-4–C-5	C-5–C-6	C-6–C-7	C-7–T-1
Yale	59.7 ± 15.7	41.7 ± 27.8	66.7 ± 17.1	64.1 ± 15.7	58.2 ± 13.5	60.9 ± 15.5	52.4 ± 19.9	63.0 ± 43.7
Cervicothoracic	53.5 ± 11.8	58.3 ± 13.9	56.2 ± 15.0	79.5 ± 9.2	77.5 ± 9.3	73.3 ± 8.7	58.5 ± 13.7	37.0 ± 31.8
Four-poster	48.6 ± 12.3	46.7 ± 24.3	58.3 ± 15.0	59.0 ± 15.7	65.3 ± 13.5	72.4 ± 8.7	62.2 ± 18.7	40.7 ± 31.8
SOMI brace	49.7 ± 14.6	10.0 ± 33.0	8.3 ± 23.6	19.2 ± 18.3	38.8 ± 18.7	42.9 ± 19.3	31.7 ± 22.4	22.2 ± 43.7
Philadelphia	62.5 ± 12.3	25.0 ± 26.0	62.5 ± 19.3	56.4 ± 13.1	40.8 ± 12.4	43.8 ± 11.6	29.3 ± 24.9	51.8 ± 35.7

Modified from Johnson RM, Hart DL, et al: The Yale cervical orthosis: an evaluation of its effectiveness in restricting cervical motion in normal subjects and a comparison with other cervical orthoses; reprinted from *Physical Therapy* 58(7):865, 1978 with the permission of the American Physical Therapy Association.

lizes the cervical spine has not been confirmed.[16] If the appropriate size is chosen, however, the soft collar affords some vertical support of the cervical spine by reducing the amount of weight borne directly by the spine. The soft cervical collar—acting somewhat like a turtleneck sweater—simply reminds the client to keep the spine immobile voluntarily until the symptoms have disappeared. Clinically, if there is minor muscle spasm or pain in the cervical area and intervertebral immobility is not warranted, the soft cervical collar should be used.

The Philadelphia collar (Fig. 13-10) is similar to the soft collar with regard to comfort and ease of donning, but it offers more variability in available standard sizes and in the mixing of different sizes to establish a desired angle of head and neck position. In addition, the Philadelphia collar is more rigid than the soft cervical collar and thus affords more stability to the cervical spine.

The four-poster orthosis (Fig. 13-11) is also comfortable and easily donned. Adjustment is more complicated than with the soft collar and the Philadelphia collar but easier than with the cervicothoracic orthosis. Offering increased rigidity, the four-poster orthosis provides more control of the cervical spine than any of the collars discussed previously. The ease with which an orthotist can apply the four-poster collar to a client in standing, sitting, or supine positions, combined with its increased stability, allows the four-poster orthosis to be used on clients who need a great deal of stability.

The SOMI orthoses (Fig. 13-12) is comfortable, easily donned, and quick and simple to adjust. Johnson et al[16] found the SOMI collar effective for restricting flexion of the upper cervical segments but inadequate for restricting extension at all levels. Because this orthosis restricts flexion motion well and is remarkably easy to apply when the client is in the supine position, the SOMI collar is valuable for treating problems of flexion instability in the cervical spine.

The cervicothoracic orthosis (Fig. 13-13) is less comfortable than any of the other orthoses and much more difficult to don and adjust. The cervicothoracic orthosis, however, restricts motion more than do the other orthoses.

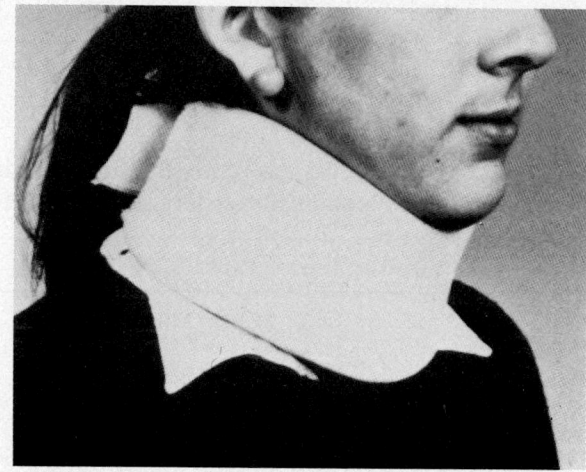

Fig. 13-9. Soft cervical collars are prefabricated pieces of foam rubber covered by stockinette and commonly fastened posteriorly. (Reprinted from *Physical Therapy* 58[7]:857, 1978 with the permission of the American Physical Therapy Association.)

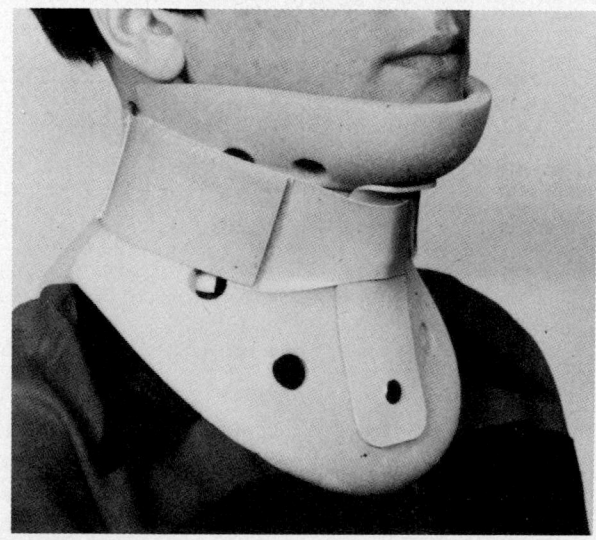

Fig. 13-10. Philadelphia collar is a prefabricated lightweight polyethylene foam collar with semirigid anterior and posterior plastic stays. (Reprinted from *Physical Therapy* 58:[7]:857, 1978 with the permission of the American Physical Therapy Association.)

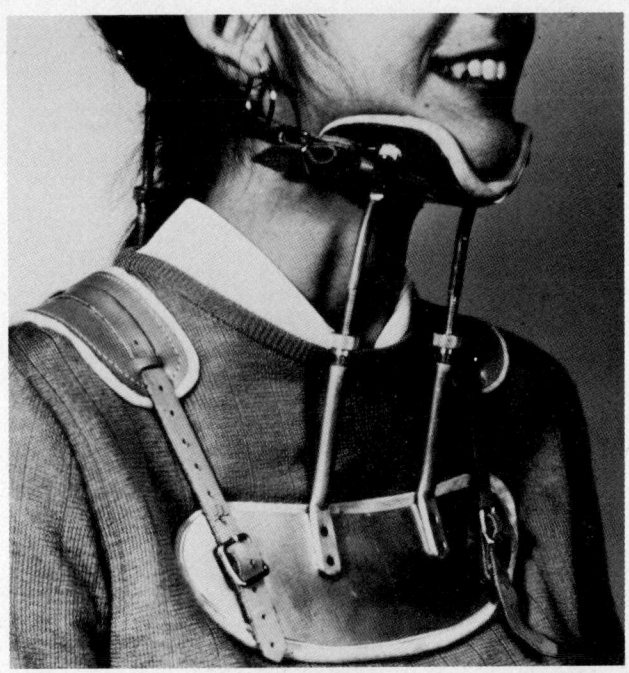

Fig. 13-11. Four-poster metal orthosis is adjustable in height with flexible leather straps connecting anterior and posterior sections. (Reprinted from *Physical Therapy* 58:[7]:857, 1978 with the permission of the American Physical Therapy Association.)

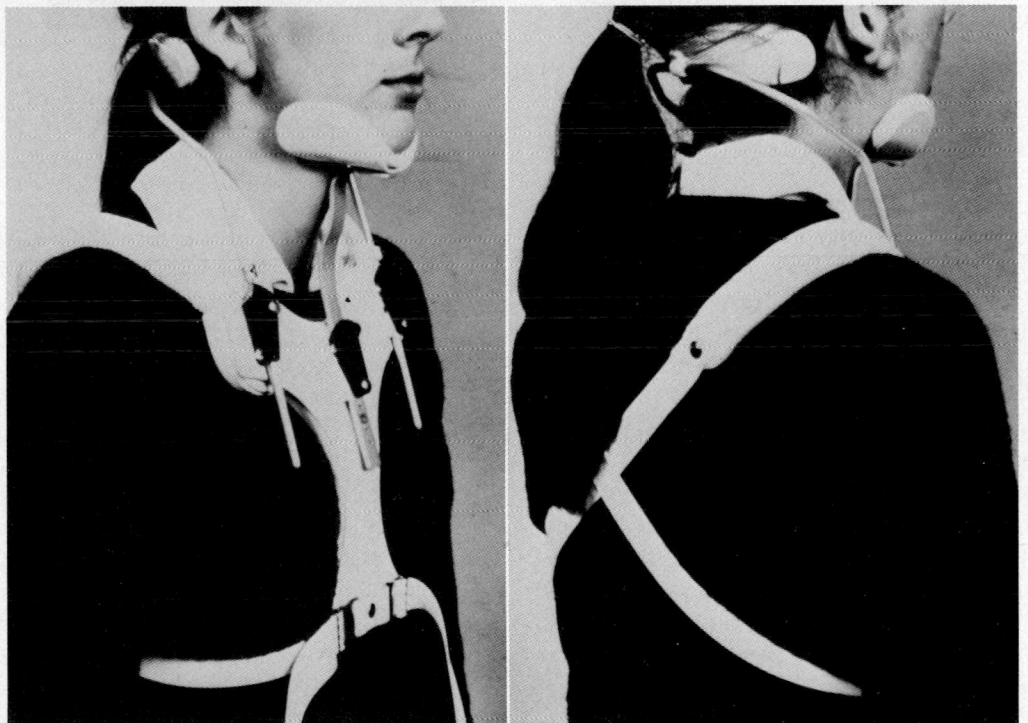

Fig. 13-12. SOMI orthosis is a prefabricated orthosis with a rigid mandibular support and a flexible posterior occipital support. The orthosis may also be ordered with leather straps connecting occipital and mandibular supports. (Reprinted from *Physical Therapy* 58[7]:857, 1978 with the permission of the American Physical Therapy Association.)

If an orthotist is available to do the fabrication, donning, and adjustments and the client is in need of increased intervertebral control of motion, then the cervicothoracic orthosis should be used.

The last spinal orthosis to be considered is the halo body jacket (Fig. 13-14). A word of caution is warranted in using this device. It should be applied only by an orthopaedic surgeon for most severe problems of cervical instability. If applied properly, the greatest intervertebral immobility will result, particularly in the upper cervical

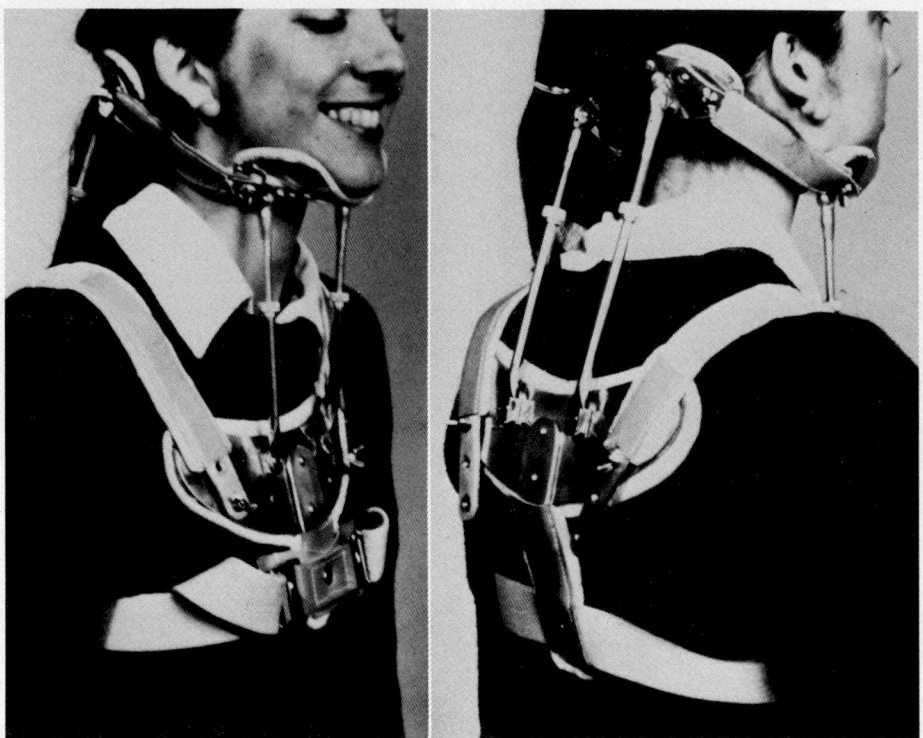

Fig. 13-13. Cervicothoracic orthosis is custom-fabricated metal orthosis similar to four-poster orthosis but with rigid anterior-posterior connections with a circumferential chest strap. (Reprinted from *Physical Therapy* 58[7]:857, 1978 with the permission of the American Physical Therapy association.)

spine. Surprisingly, clients wearing halo traction systems are remarkably comfortable. Minor adjustment may be performed by skilled allied health professionals, but fitting should be done only by an orthopaedic surgeon.

Thoracic region

Two major kinematic differences distinguish the thoracic region as compared to either the cervical or lumbar spine: (1) decreased intervertebral motion and (2) the immobilizing influence of the rib cage. Although the thoracic spine is mobile, facet-joint placement and the rib cage decrease rotation (caudally), lateral bending, and flexion and extension as compared to the cervical spine.[28] The rib cage, in addition to increasing the rigidity of the thoracic spine, provides stiffer viscoelastic transmitters so forces can be applied more directly to the intervertebral segments.

Of primary importance in treating thoracic spine disorders is prevention of and/or care for compression fractures of vertebral bodies as well as correction of scoliotic and kyphotic curves. Research appears to be minimal in the area of orthosis evaluation for both these problems, although many clinical studies have been conducted to evaluate the effectiveness of the Milwaukee brace for scoliosis.[2,6,20]

There are two primary orthoses for the care of compression fractures of the vertebral bodies: the Jewett or Griswald brace (see Fig. 13-2) and the Taylor thoracolumbar brace (Fig. 13-15). Both basically use the same biomechanical principle of three-point fixation to place the load-carrying capacity of the spine on the posterior elements of the thoracic vertebrae, therefore relieving weight on the anterior vertebral bodies (see Fig. 13-2). The Jewett brace affords more precise localization of stabilization because the three parts of the brace can be accurately positioned. Thus better immobilization of the particular region of the thoracolumbar spine is attainable. Restriction of lateral bending and rotation are not as effective as vertical stabilization, although none of the motions have been measured.

The Taylor brace controls the thoracolumbar spine through a pelvic band, abdominal pad, and posterior thoracic uprights with bilateral anterior shoulder-girdle straps. The sleeve principle is used for a "splinting effect."[28] Mobile axillary straps do not restrict rotation and lateral bending, and flexion appears to be more controlled than extension. Modifications offer better control for lateral bending and rotation. Again, no measurements have been made of the effectiveness of the brace.

The development of the Milwaukee brace was a major breakthrough for the treatment of the lateral and rotatory scoliotic curve (Fig. 13-3). However, accurate application of forces requires precise fitting and adjustment. Of particular importance is the molding of the pelvic band. Once

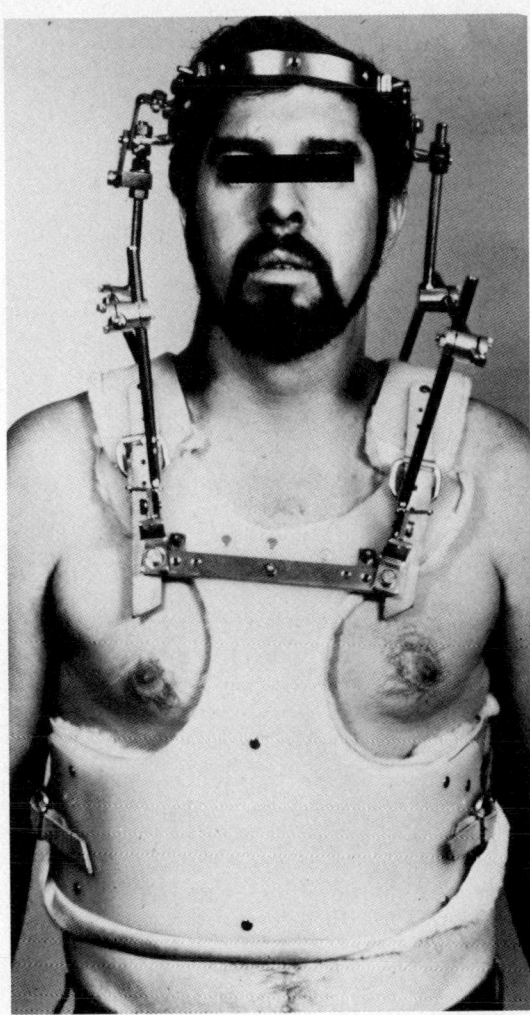

Fig. 13-14. Halo fixation is obtained by metal pins fixed to skull. An adjustable metal frame is bolted to a plastic body jacket. (Reprinted from *Physical Therapy* 58[7]:857, 1978 with the permission of the American Physical Therapy Association.)

molded, effective placement of the lateral pads is determined by radiographic localization of the apex of the curve. However, controversy surrounds the exact placement of the pads, which requires further investigation. Distraction may be applied via turn-buckles, screw placement, and springs between the pelvic mold and the mandibular and occipital pads.[28] Although the following description of how the brace operates is very simplified, the Milwaukee brace represents a high degree of sophistication in the art of bracing. Specifically, the brace and the spine form a complex three-dimensional structure that is subject to both passive and active loads. The correctional effect is on a long-term basis and involves not only immediate mechanical effects but also biological adaptation. Any mechanical analysis and optimization of such a system is extremely complex. The complexities include elements as divergent as the variability of the stiffness of the spine and

the equilibrium of the enthusiasm between the therapist and the patient.

To gain some understanding of the mechanics involved in the Milwaukee brace, the spine system may be studied in the grossly simplified manner shown in Fig. 13-3. The real situation is modeled as a plane curved bar subjected to a set of forces. Forces F_1 and F_2 are the mandibular-occipital pads and the pelvic support forces, which seem to correct the spine deformity by stretching. (Actually the angular correction is obtained by producing bending moments in the scoliotic spine.) Forces F_3 (thoracic pad), F_4 (axillary sling), and F_5 (pelvic support) form a neat three-part force system. The purpose of these three forces is to bend the spine into a curvature opposite to that of the scoliotic curve and thus correct it. The two force systems may be applied separately or together. In the combined situation they are interdependent.[28]

A variety of modifications of the Milwaukee brace are available to the orthotist and clinician. For example, the Boston brace has replaced the Milwaukee brace in many clinics because it is superior in cosmetic qualities and similar in corrective properties (Fig. 13-16).

Clinical investigations of the forces of the lateral pads, axial distraction, and other activities that can be achieved with the brace are available.[28] However, of more clinical importance are studies on the clinical outcomes of the use of the Milwaukee brace.

Mellencamp, Blount, and Anderson[20] reported that the use of the Milwaukee brace improves and maintains the immature scoliotic spine for several years. However, the results were quite variable and can be grouped into four distinct responses:

1. Following bracing of the immature spine, correction and subsequent maintenance of the correction were gratifying up to a skeletal age of 18 years.
2. For a similar type of client there was rapid correction initially but considerable loss of correction with "weaning off" the brace, and continued correction loss was noted until stabilization occurred between skeletal ages of 20 to 29 years.
3. More commonly, with similar client limitations, good early correction occurred with minimal relapses before age 18 years, although, after discharge, moderate loss of correction occurred until skeletal maturation was achieved between ages 20 to 29 years.
4. Rare "malignant" or rapidly progressing curves did not respond to bracing and required surgical intervention.

A follow-up study was performed on clients treated with the Milwaukee brace.[6] The study concluded that the Milwaukee brace was rarely as effective as surgery. However, progression of small- or medium-sized curves (60 degrees or less) was routinely halted. Unfortunately, loss

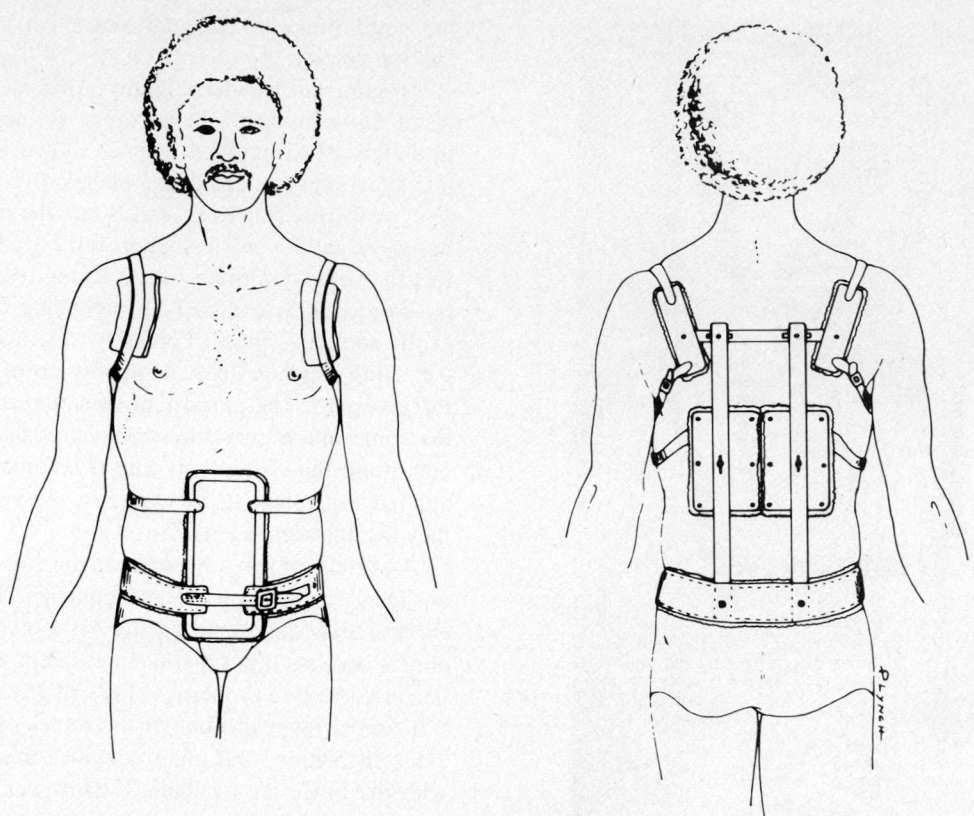

Fig. 13-15. Taylor thoracolumbar brace provides another form of three-point fixation emphasizing thoracic extension. This brace is similar to Jewett brace in function. (Modified from White AA and Panjabi MM: Clinical biomechanics of the spine, Philadelphia, 1978, JB Lippincott Co, p. 360.)

of improvement appeared gradually and almost uniformly following brace cessation. The Milwaukee brace was concluded to be effective only for the skeletally immature with small, flexible, nondeforming curves.

Therefore in treating the thoracic spine, as with the cervical spine, the most precise control demands skeletal fixations via the halo apparatus. The entire spine can be more effectively controlled with pelvic and cranioskeletal pins.

Lumbar region

Treatment of clients with disorders producing low-back pain continues to be one of the most costly enigmas in medicine. Since the majority of clients with low-back pain lack a definitive diagnosis with consistent corroborative evidence, goals for treatment usually emphasize the reduction of symptomatology, not the alleviation of pathological disorders. To that end, back braces represent "a valiant effort among the many attempts to treat a formidable clinical problem."[28] Fortunately, as a result of the proliferation of short courses for all disciplines emphasizing evaluation skills, normal arthrokinematics, and the basic sciences (as well as the chartering of the International Society for the Study of the Lumbar Spine), the scientific approach to clients with low-back pain is experiencing a growth in inter-

est, both clinically and investigatively. Consequently, clinicians should recognize the need to be open to continued efforts to help low-back pain sufferers since evidence exists neither to refute nor to confirm various unproven treatment techniques. The catalyst to spur sound investigation, however, should be the statement that, for the majority of clients with low-back pain "very few, if any, treatments presently available are superior to nature's own course."[22] No one would care to be the individual with low-back pain who was offered no treatment at all.

Spinal pain of lumbar origin commonly does not include disorders requiring surgical intervention. (Spondylolisthesis and other mechanical abnormalities, however, are exceptions.) Therefore the goals of lumbosacral bracing should be: (1) to serve as a reminder to the client to voluntarily restrict movement that may not be beneficial, (2) to act as a support via increased abdominal pressure to unload the lumbar spine and reduce the need for abdominal muscle contraction, and (3) to orthotically immobilize the thoracolumbar and lumbosacral spines in a specific treatment position.

Unfortunately, research is minimal in the evaluation of most appliances used for the lumbar spine. However, there have been several studies of interest. Perry[24] collected in-

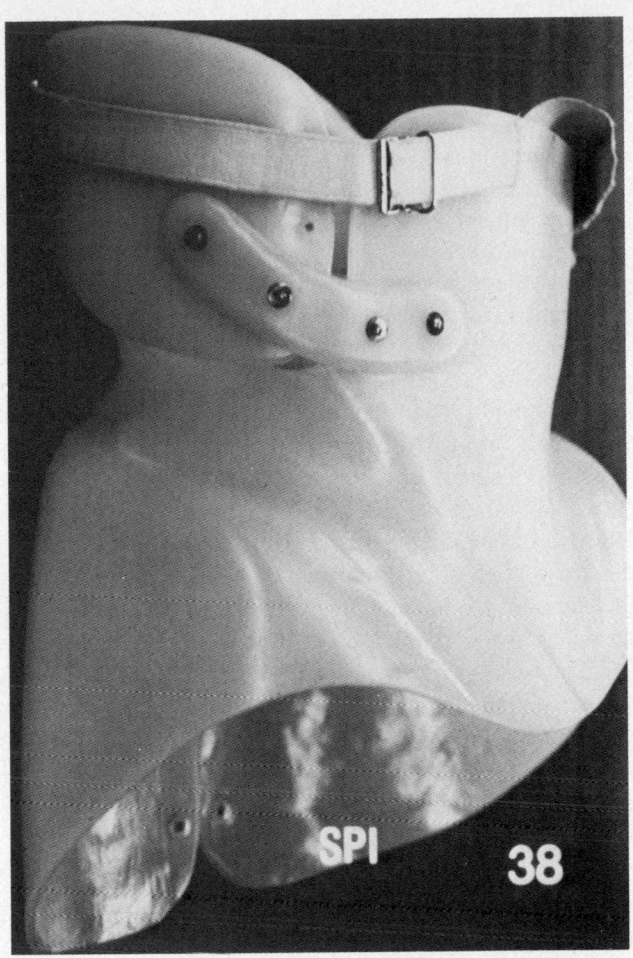

Fig. 13-16. Boston brace is commonly fabricated from moldable plastic and affords axial tension with lateral correction for clients with scoliosis. (Courtesy Crawford AH: The syllabus: pediatric orthopedic surgery, Science Image Communications, 2301 North San Fernandino Boulevard, Burbank, Calif 91504.)

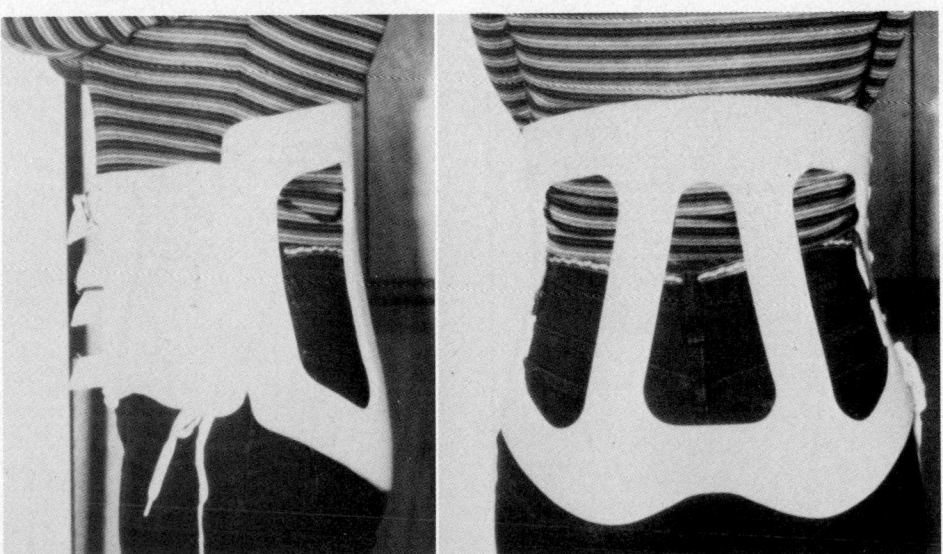

Fig. 13-17. Chairback (Knight) brace is a prefabricated orthosis of metal and leather with an adjustable anterior pad. (Courtesy Parlsey GM, CPO, Para-Med Corporation, 1212 Van Voorhis Road, Morgantown, WV 26505.)

formation from 3410 orthopaedic surgeons in a questionnaire study designed to determine how many physicians were using the commonly available braces and why. The appliances included the chairback (Knight) brace; the Williams, Norton-Brown, Goldthwait, and Bennett braces; the lumbosacral and sacroiliac corsets; and the flexion and body casts as well as the body cast with one leg (Figs. 13-17 to 13-21). The results of the study are summarized in Tables 13-7 and 13-8.

The lumbosacral corset was prescribed more often than any other appliance, with the chairback (Knight) brace second. External support was rarely used for an acute strain, a postoperative disk condition, or for an obese person with pain. However, the majority of physicians prescribed a brace for external support postoperatively for fusions, spondylolisthesis, or a pseudarthrosis. Most orthopaedists sought restriction of lumbosacral motion, abdominal support, postural correction, or unloading of the disk as goals of their orthotic treatment. However, the physicians used casts for restriction of motion or correction of posture. Even then, seldom did physicians believe that a cast, other than the flexion cast, actually immobilized the spine.

The influence of a few specific braces on the EMG ac-

tivity of back and abdominal muscles has already been discussed in this chapter.[27] However, a further explanation of the function of the trunk musculature during various conditions of trunk-loading would assist in understanding the role of these muscles when a client is wearing an orthosis. Morris, Lucas, and Bressler[21] investigated the question of how the lumbar vertebrae and the disk are able to withstand the load that is applied to them during lifting. Of particular interest were studies involving an inflatable corset meant to simulate either a tight-fitting corset, a brace with an abdominal pad that can be tightened, or a snug plaster body jacket. The corset first was inflated to the limit of comfort, and then the subjects performed various activities. During forced flexion, the resting abdominal pressure elevated further than during flexion without the corset. Intrathoracic pressure was virtually unchanged. However, maximal pressures generated in static loading of the spine were quite comparable to those obtained during the same loading without the corset. The EMG activity of the internal and external oblique muscles and rectus abdominis muscle was markedly decreased when the corset was worn, despite the fact that the intraabdominal pressures during static loading with and without the corset were the same. The conclusion then is that increased abdominal

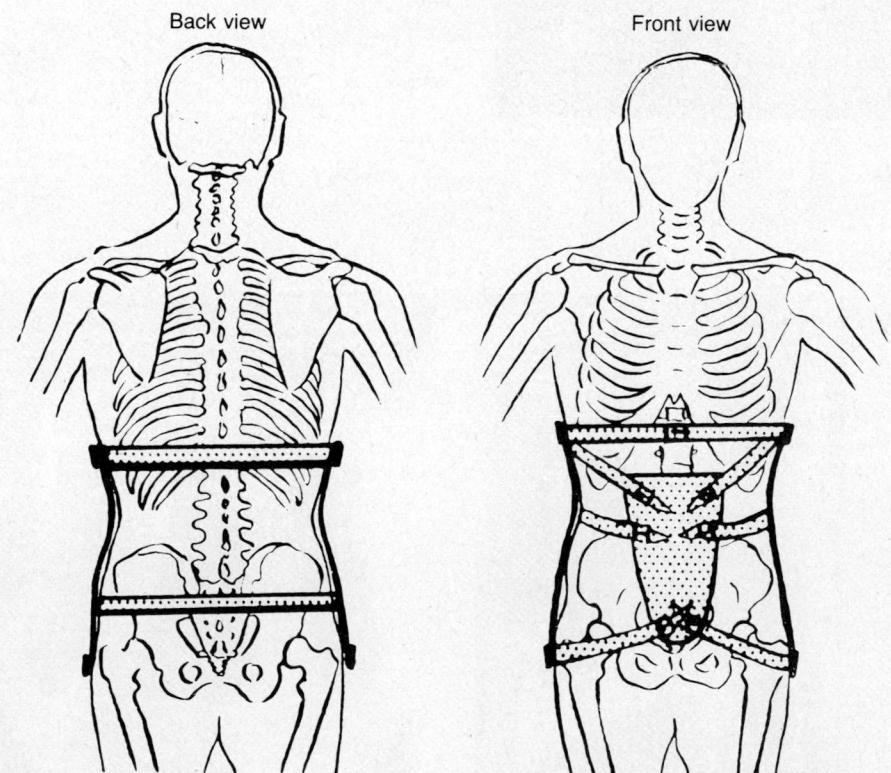

Back view   Front view

Fig. 13-18. Norton-Brown brace exemplifies an experimentally designed brace. Brace emphasizes forces applied in region of posterior superior iliac spine and over bony prominences of greater trochanters. These two forces effectively reduce motion of lumbosacral area as well as reducing abdominal pad shift during various flexion maneuvers. (Modified from Norton PL and Brown T: J Bone Joint Surg (Am) 39[1]:111, 1957.)

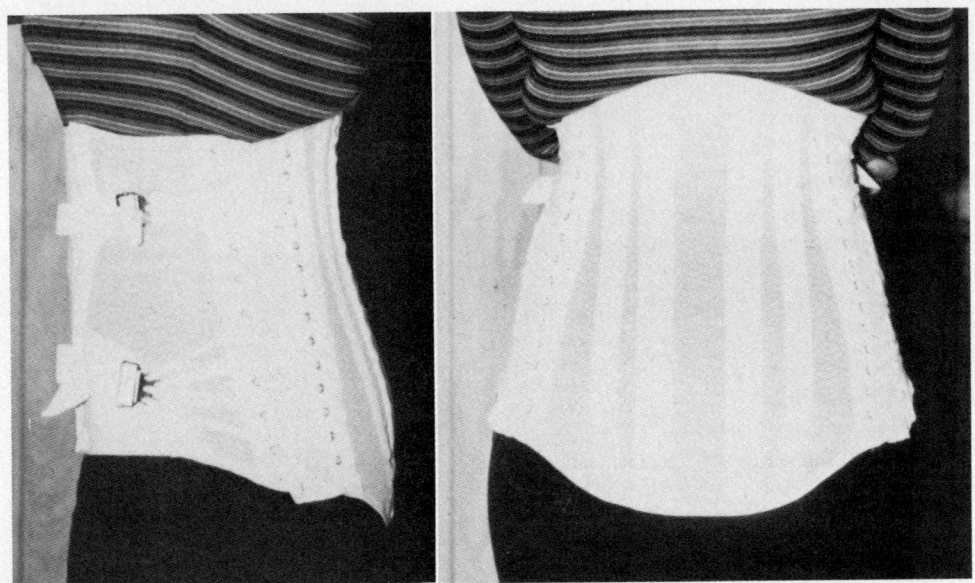

Fig. 13-19. Lumbosacral corset is a prefabricated fabric appliance commonly containing rigid posterior metal stays that can be molded to the contour of the lumbar spine with adequate anterior adjustments. (Courtesy Parlsey GM, CPO, Para-Med Corporation, 1212 Van Voorhis Road, Morgantown, WV 26505.)

Table 13-7. External support preference by clinical entity

| Clinical situation | Total Number | Percent | Frequency of use | | Support preference | | Cast (percent) |
			Rarely (percent)	Usually (percent)	Brace (percent)	Corset (percent)	
Postoperative fusion	3590	100	16	84	51	20	29
Spondylolisthesis	3472	100	30	70	59	33	28
Pseudarthrosis	2784	100	34	66	57	28	15
Preoperative trial	2523	100	46	54	37	25	38
Disk syndrome	3164	100	49	51	34	51	15
Chronic low-back pain	2635	100	52	48	29	67	4
Postoperative disk	1677	100	72	28	31	65	4
Obesity and pain	1453	100	81	19	13	84	2
Acute strain	1552	100	83	17	14	77	9

Modified from Perry J: The use of external support in the treatment of low-back pain, J Bone Joint Surg (Am) 52(7):1440, 1970.

pressures during static loading are not altered by the addition of a tight corset, but the necessary muscular support is decreased. Further, the increased intraabdominal pressure allows the vertebrae and disks to withstand pressures of lifting that would usually crush a vertebral segment in the laboratory.

The study of primary clinical significance for lumbar bracing is Norton and Brown's evaluation[23] of the immobility efficiency of selected back braces. Photographs, films, and radiographs were taken of various activities while normal subjects wore each of several braces. Kirschner wires were inserted into the spinous processes of several lumbar vertebrae and one of the posterior superior iliac spines to assist in the measurement of various activities (a procedure probably never to be repeated).

Several important conclusions were drawn. If a brace was adequately fixed to the chest but inadequately attached to the pelvis, forces during flexion were concentrated in the lumbar and thoracolumbar regions. At the same time, the appliance lifted off the pelvis, leaving the lumbosacral region unsupported during flexion. This was seen with the Taylor and Arnold-Abbot braces and the plaster jackets. In contrast, the Goldthwait and chairback braces and corset incorporated little fixation to the chest but relatively better pelvic fixation. During flexion activities these appliances pulled away from the pelvis less and maintained more pressure on the lumbosacral junction. Radiographically, some braces were observed to actually increase lumbosacral motion. Apparently, this was a compensatory motion following a decrease in motion at other spinal levels.

The sitting posture had a profound effect on the amount of flexion recorded. A slumped or erect client with a brace experienced a substantial amount of flexion at the L-4 to L-5 intervertebral level. The slumped position actually increased the amount of L-4 to L-5 flexion as compared to the maximal forward-bending position. Therefore, to immobilize the lower lumbar segments, the client either should not sit or one thigh as well as the lumbar spine must be immobilized.

Since Norton and Brown[23] believed that (1) none of the braces actually "immobilized" the lumbar spine, (2) the restrictive qualities of a brace were more related to the discomfort they produced, and (3) most forces were not localized low enough on the spine, they developed a new brace. Longer lateral uprights were used instead of the paraspinal uprights, and the brace applied a force to the

Table 13-8. Support preference

Support	By individual physicians (percent response)	For all clinical indications (percent response)
Lumbosacral corset	28.5	44.2
Chairback (Knight) brace	21.11	22.4
Williams brace	9.9	8.3
Body cast	9.2	6.3
Flexion cast	8.4	5.0
Body cast and one leg	6.0	2.6
Other braces*	11.6	8.3
Other corsets	3.9	2.5
Other casts	1.2	0.5
Total	99.8	100.1

Modified from Perry J: The use of external support in the treatment of low-back pain, J Bone Joint Surg (Am) 52(7):1440, 1970.
*Braces include Goldthwait, Bennett, Norton-Brown, and others not mentioned.

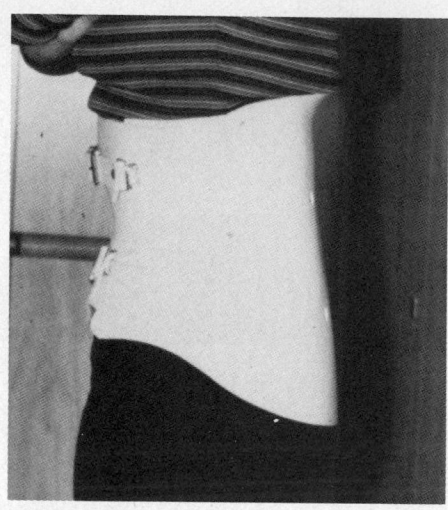

Fig. 13-20. Flexion jacket is fabricated out of any rigid material. Three-point fixation is applied via a concavity anteriorly and an extended posterior aspect of brace. Three-point fixation can be compared to the Jewett brace since the two braces have the three-point fixation in opposite directions. (Courtesy Parlsey GM, CPO, Para-Med Corporation, 1212 Van Voorhis Road, Morgantown, WV 26505.)

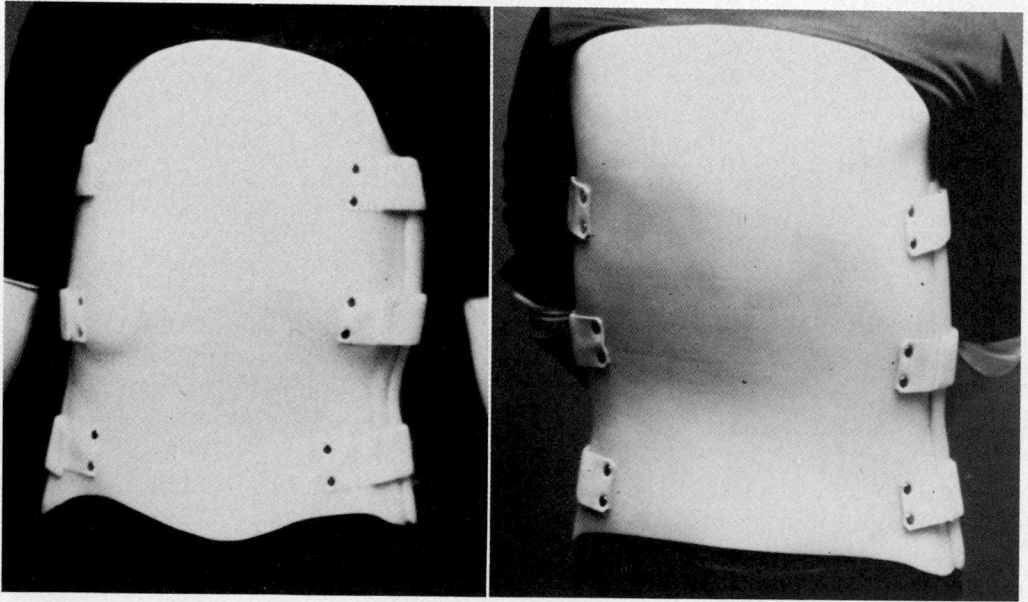

Fig. 13-21. Ranee body cast is made from any rigid material. The cast, made of two pieces of plastic, anterior and posterior, is fastened via Velcro straps. Spine can be held in any position, depending on what is required. (Courtesy Parlsey GM, CPO, Para-Med Corporation, 1212 Van Voorhis Road, Morgantown, WV 26505.)

Table 13-9. Treatment choices involving orthoses

Orthosis	Spinal region	Degrees of freedom controlled	Effectiveness of control
Soft cervical collar	Cervical	FE, LB*	Min*
Hard plastic collar (Thomas)	Cervical	FE, LB, (AR)	Int.
Philadelphia collar	Cervical	FE, LB, (AR)	Int.
Four-poster collar	Cervical	FE, LB, AR	Int.
Long two-poster collar (Guilford, Duke)	Cervical	FE, LB, AR	Int. (high)
Minerva cast	Cervical	FE, LB, AR	Most
Halo collar	Cervical	FE, LB, AR	Most (high)
Long thoracic corsets	Thoracic	FE, LB	Min.
Three-point corsets (Jewett, Griswold)	Thoracic	FE	Int.
Taylor corset	Thoracic, thoracolumbar	FE	Int.
Taylor corset (with lateral uprights)	Thoracic	FE, LB, AR	Int.
Use of clavicle pads	Thoracic	AR	Int.
Milwaukee brace (tightly worn)	Thoracic, thoracolumbar	FE, LB, (AR) Kyphosis correction	Most
Risser plaster jacket	Thoracic, thoracolumbar	FE, LB, AR	Most
Milwaukee brace (loosely worn)	Thoracic, thoracolumbar	Scoliosis correction	Most
Halo pelvic device	Thoracic, thoracolumbar	FE, LB, AR	Most (high)
Lumbar corsets	Lumbar	FE, LB	Min.
Williams brace	Lumbar (except L-4 to L-5)	FE, LB	Int.
Chairback (Knight) brace	Lumbar (except L-4 to L-5)	FE, (LB)	Int.
MacAusland brace	Lumbar (except L-4 to L-5)	FE, (LB)	Int.
Taylor brace	Lumbar (except L-4 to L-5)	FE, LB, AR	Int.
Norton and Brown experimental brace	Lumbar (except L-4 to L-5)	FE, LB	Int. (high)
Taylor brace (with thigh attachment)	Lumbar	FE, LB, AR	Most
Molded plaster jacket	Lumbar (except L4 to L5)	FE, LB, AR	Most
Molded plaster jacket (thigh included)	Lumbar	FE, LB, AR	Most
Halo pelvic device	Lumbar	FE, LB, AR	Most (high)

Modified from White AA and Panjabi MM: Clinical biomechanics of the spine, Philadelphia, 1978, JB Lippincott Co., p. 371.
*FE: Flexion-extension   Int.: Intermediate
LB: Lateral bending   Most: Most effective
AR: Axial rotation   (x-axis rotation)
( ) Slightly less controlled   (z-axis rotation)
Min.: Minimal   (y-axis rotation)

lumbosacral region by means of a crossbar. A painful stimulus was then felt when more movement than was desirable occurred. Therefore control of lateral bending and flexion of the lower intervertebral spaces in the sitting position were improved.

A final treatment approach involving either flexion or extension for a client with a painful lumbar spine should be considered. Several devices already mentioned, as well as the Ranee flexion brace (see Fig. 13-21), can be used to hold a client in the desired position of either flexion or extension. However, the merits of either flexion or extension await controlled studies.

SUMMARY

The application of orthoses for clients with spinal dysfunction offers a variable choice of treatment (Table 13-9). However, the limitations and strengths of the appliances and modern medicine's ability to adequately diagnose a painful back syndrome all influence the functional approach to clients, particularly those with low-back pain. Therefore the clinician must be honest with each client regarding the possible success of treatment and the potential for changes in therapy if the condition does not improve. A brace, if part of a treatment regime, should be approached for a majority of clients as a temporary appliance, and from the beginning of treatment the plan should include modalities that are geared to the ultimate elimination of the brace.

REFERENCES

1. Andriacchi T et al: A model for studies of mechanical interactions between human spine and rib cage, J Biomech 7:497, 1974.
2. Blount WP and Moore JH: The Milwaukee brace, Baltimore, 1973, Williams & Wilkins.
3. Burr D, Martin P, and Martin R: Lower extremity loads stimulate bone formation in the vertical column: implications for osteoporosis, Spine 8(7):681, 1983.

4. Colachis SC, Strohm BR, and Ganter EL: Cervical spine motion in normal women: radiographic study of the effect of cervical collars, Arch Phys Med Rehabil 54:161, 1973.

5. Coppenhaver WM, Kelly DE, and Wood RL: Bailey's textbook of histology, ed 17, Baltimore, 1978, Williams & Wilkins.

6. Edmonson AS and Morris JT: Followup study of Milwaukee brace treatment in patients with idiopathic scoliosis, Clin Orthop 126:58, 1977.

7. Farfan HF: Mechanical disorders of the low back, Philadelphia, 1973, Lea & Febiger.

8. Farfan HF: The pathological anatomy of degenerative spondylolisthesis, a cadaver study, Spine 5(5):412, 1980.

9. Fisher SV et al: Cervical orthoses effect on cervical spine motion: roentgenographic and goniometric method of study, Arch Phys Med Rehabil 58:109, 1977.

10. Frankel VH and Nordin M: Basic biomechanics of the skeletal system, Philadelphia, 1980, Lea & Febiger.

11. Harris EE: A new orthotics terminology, Ortho Prosthet 27(2):6, 1973.

12. Hart DL, Burr D, and Marano G: Nucleus pulposus movement, Unpublished data, 1982.

13. Hart DL et al: Review of cervical orthoses, Phys Ther 58(7):857, 1978.

14. Hartman JT, Palumbo F, and Hill BJ: Cineradiography of the braced normal cervical spine, Clin Orthop 109:97, 1975.

15. Janda V: Muscles, central nervous motor regulation and back problems. In Korr IM, editor: The neurobiologic mechanisms in manipulative therapy, New York, 1978, Plenum Publishing Corp, pp. 27-41.

16. Johnson RM et al: Cervical orthoses: a study comparing their effectiveness in restricting cervical motion in normal subjects, J Bone Joint Surg (Am) 59(3):323, 1977.

17. Johnson RM et al: The Yale cervical orthosis: an evaluation of its effectiveness in restricting cervical motion in normal subjects and a comparison with other cervical orthoses, Phys Ther 58(7):865, 1978.

18. Jones MD: Cineroentgenographic studies of the collar-immobilized cervical spine, J Neurosurg 17:633, 1960.

19. Lysell E: Motion in the cervical spine, Acta Orthop Scand (Suppl), 123, 1969.

20. Mellencamp DD, Blount WP, and Anderson AJ: Milwaukee brace treatment of idiopathic scoliosis: late results, Clin Orthop 126:47, 1977.

21. Morris J, Lucas D, and Bressler B: Role of the trunk in stability of the spine, J Bone Joint Surg (Am) 43(3):327, 1961.

22. Nachemson AL: The lumbar spine: an orthopedic challenge, Spine 1(1):59, 1976.

23. Norton PL, and Brown T: The immobilizing efficiency of back braces, J Bone Joint Surg (Am) 39(1):111, 1957.

24. Perry J: The use of external support in the treatment of low-back pain, J Bone Joint Surg (Am) 52(7):1440, 1970.

25. Rab GT: Muscle forces in the posterior thoracic spine, Clin Orthop 139:28, 1979.

26. Shah JS, Hampson WGJ, and Jayson MN: The distribution of surface strain in the cadaveric lumbar spine, J Bone Joint Surg (Br) 60(2):246, 1980.

27. Waters RL and Morris JM: Effect of spinal supports on the electrical activity of muscles of the trunk, J Bone Joint Surg (Am) 5(1):51, 1970.

28. White AA and Panjabi MM: Clinical biomechanics of the spine, Philadelphia, 1978, JB Lippincott Co.

29. Zeleznik R et al: Yale cervical orthosis: fabrication, Phys Ther 58(7):861, 1978.

ADDITIONAL READINGS

Abrahams, D and Shrosbree RD: Stabilization of the cervical spine using a Bio-Con collar, Paraplegia 17(2):192, 1979.

Ahlgren SA and Hansen T: The use of lumbosacral corsets prescribed for low-back pain, Prosthet Orthot Int 2(2):101, 1978.

American Academy of Orthopaedic Surgeons: Orthopaedic appliances atlas, vol 1, Chicago, 1952, The Academy.

American Academy of Orthopaedic Surgeons: Atlas of orthotics: biomechanical principles and application, St. Louis, 1975, The CV Mosby Co.

Bhalla SK and Simmons EH: Normal ranges of intervertebral-joint motion of the cervical spine, Can J Surg 12:181, 1969.

Bloomberg M: Orthopedic braces: rationale, classification and prescription, Philadelphia, 1964, JB Lippincott Co.

Buck CA et al: Study or normal range of motion in the neck utilizing a bubble goniometer, Arch Phys Med Rehabil 40:390, 1959.

Bunch W and Keagy R: Principles of orthotic treatment, St. Louis, 1976, The CV Mosby Co.

Carr WA: Treatment of idiopathic scoliosis in the Milwaukee brace, J Bone Joint Surg (Am) 62(4):599, 1980.

Compton J: New plastics for forming directly on the patient, Prosthet Orthot Int 2(1):43, 1978.

Costelvi A: Treatment of thoracolumbar scoliosis with a thoracolumbar sacral orthosis (TLSO) alternative to Milwaukee brace treatment, J Fla Med Assoc 66(1):71, 1979.

Dommisse QP: The lumbar disc brace, S Afr Med J 53(26):1064, 1978.

Drennan JC, Renshaw TS, and Curtis BH: The thoracic suspension orthosis, Clin Orthop 139:33, 1979.

Fielding JW: Cineroentgenography of the normal cervical spine, J Bone Joint Surg (Am) 39:1280, 1957.

Fisher SV: Proper fitting of the cervical orthosis, Arch Phys Med Rehabil 59(11):505, 1978.

Jayson M: The lumbar spine and back pain, New York, 1976, Grune & Stratton, Inc.

Jones MD: Cineradiographic studies of the normal cervical spine, Cal Med 93:293, 1960.

Jorday HH: Orthopedic appliances: the principles and practice of brace construction, Springfield, 1963, Charles C Thomas, Publisher.

Kottke FJ and Mundale MO: Range of mobility of the cervical spine, Arch Phys Med Rehabil 40:379, 1959.

Licht S, editor: Orthotics etcetera, New Haven, 1966, Elizabeth Licht.

Micheli LJ, Hall JE, and Miller ME: Use of modified Boston brace for back injuries in athletes, Am J Sports Med 8(5)351, 1980.

Miyasaki RA: Immediate influence of the thoracic flexion exercise of vertebral position in Milwaukee brace wearers, Phys Ther 60(8):1005, 1980.

Mulcahy T et al: A followup study of forces acting on the Milwaukee brace in patients undergoing treatment for idiopathic scoliosis, Clin Orthop 93:53, 1973.

Nash CL: Current concepts review: scoliosis bracing, J Bone Joint Surg (Am) 62(5):848, 1980.

Park J et al: A modified brace (Prenyl) for scoliosis, Clin Orthop 126:67, 1977.

Perry J: The halo in spinal abnormalities: practical factors and avoidance of complications, Orthop Clin North Am 3:69, 1972.

Piggot H: Management of structural scoliosis, Surg Ann 11:267, 1979.

Schweigel JF: Halo-thoracic brace management of odontoid fractures, Spine 4(3):192, 1979.

Sutcliffe BJ: Thermoplastic collar survey, Physiotherapy 62(2):65, 1976.

Taylor AN: An inflatable neck support, Clin Orthop 81:87, 1971.

Tohen H: Manual of mechanical orthopaedics, Springfield, 1972, Charles C Thomas, Publisher.

Watts HG: Bracing in spinal deformities, Orthop Clin North Am 10(4):769, 1979.

Watts HG, Hall JE, and Stanish W: The Boston brace system for the treatment of low thoracic and lumbar scoliosis by the use of a girdle without superstructure, Clin Orthop 126:87, 1977.

Wharton GW: Stabilization of spinal injuries for early mobilization, Orthop Clin North Am 9(2):271, 1978.

White AA: Kinematics of the normal spine as related to scoliosis, J Biomech 4:405, 1971.

White AA et al: Biomechanical analysis of clinical stability in the cervical spine, Clin Orthop 109:85, 1975.

Winter RB and Carlson JM: Modern orthotics for spinal deformities, Clin Orthop 126:74, 1977.

Yettram AL and Jackman MJ: Equilibrium analysis for the forces in the human spinal column and its musculature, Spine 5(5):402, 1980.

Part Four

REGIONAL CONSIDERATIONS

Chapter 14:

THE FOOT AND ANKLE: BIOMECHANICAL EVALUATION AND TREATMENT

Thomas G. McPoil, Jr.
Ronald Steven Brocato

The ability of the foot to function properly is essential for normal gait activity. During the stance phase of gait the foot must act as a loose adapter, a rigid lever, a system for shock absorption, and a mechanism for absorbing lower limb rotation. A traumatic event or overuse injury could prevent or delay any one of these functions from occurring in normal synchronization, thus leading to foot or lower extremity symptoms.

The physical therapist treating the client with suspected foot dysfunction must not only use standard therapeutic procedures (i.e., modalities, mobilization, exercise) but must also possess the ability to evaluate the various joints of the foot to determine if biomechanical management is required for an effective result. As with any joint in the body, proper evaluation of the foot and ankle requires a firm knowledge of anatomy and normal biomechanics. Unfortunately, for many health professionals instruction in anatomy and biomechanics ends at the ankle joint.

The purpose of this chapter is to explain the normal biomechanical activity necessary for proper foot function during gait. It will discuss the various abnormalities that can disrupt the normal gait sequence and lead to symptoms, either in the foot itself or referred to the proximal joints throughout the lower extremity. Techniques will be presented to allow the physical therapist to continue lower extremity examination into the foot to evaluate biomechanical function both statically and dynamically. Finally, various kinds of biomechanical treatment for the foot will be discussed, including illustration of functional orthotic fabrication.

ANATOMY

The foot is composed of 26 bones and 30 major synovial joints.[32] Of the numerous articulations only three play a major role in the biomechanical function of the foot. These joints are the talocrural or ankle joint, the subtalar joint, and the transtarsal joint, also referred to as the midtarsal or Chopart's joint.

While the detailed anatomical characteristics of the foot and ankle will not be discussed, the important components comprising these three joints will be explained.

Osseous components

The talocrural joint is composed of the distal articulating surface of the tibia with its malleolus and the lateral malleolus of the fibula, both of which form the ankle mortise that articulates with the trochlea of the talus.

The posterior or true subtalar joint is the articulation between the concave posterior facet on the inferior surface of the talus and the convex posterior facet on the superior surface of the calcaneus. Because the talus is an integral component of both the talocrural and subtalar joints, it is often referred to as the *keystone* of the ankle joint complex.[7]

The midtarsal or transverse tarsal joint is comprised of two separate joints: the talocalcaneonavicular and the calcaneocuboid. The talocalcaneonavicular joint is the articulation between the head of the talus and the posterior facet of the navicular bone as well as the middle and anterior facets of the talus and calcaneus. The talocalcaneonavicular joint capsule is completely independent from the joint capsule of the true subtalar joint. The calcaneocuboid joint is the articulation between the anterior facet of the calcaneus and the posterior facet of the cuboid bone.

Ligamentous components

Lateral structures. The lateral collateral ligaments of the ankle joint form three distinct structures: the anterotalofibular ligament, the calcaneofibular ligament, and the posterotalofibular ligament. A lateral view of the foot and ankle clearly shows the anterotalofibular ligament and calcaneofibular ligament, but the posterotalofibular ligament is hidden by the lateral malleolus.[22] Inman[22] reported that the average angle between the anterotalofibular and calcaneofibular ligaments is approximately 105 degrees in the sagittal plane. Of all three ligaments only the calcaneofibular ligament provides support to both the talocrural and subtalar joints.

Medial structures. The primary collateral ligament on the medial aspect of the ankle is the deltoid ligament. This triangular-shaped structure offers support to both the talocrural and subtalar joints. Turek[51] states that a rupture of this ligament is rare because of its strength, and injury to the medial ankle joint more commonly results in malleolar avulsion.

Subtalar structures. The true subtalar joint is supported by two major ligaments: the interosseous talocalcaneal and the cervical. The interosseous talocalcaneal ligament is a thick quadrilateral ligament that originates in the sulcus calcanei near the capsule of the posterior subtalar joint.[41] The fibers travel upward and medially to insert on the sulcus tali. The inner fibers are shorter than the outer fibers, with the medial fibers becoming taut during subtalar joint pronation. The cervical ligament is the strongest of the ligaments connecting the talus and the calcaneus.[41] The origin of the cervical ligament is the anteromedial aspect of the sinus tarsi near the insertion of the extensor digitorum brevis. The fibers travel upward and medially to attach on the inferior, medial aspect of the neck of the talus. The cervical ligament becomes taut during supination of the subtalar joint.[41]

Plantar structures. There are numerous ligamentous structures on the plantar aspect of the foot. However, three of these structures are more commonly referred to in the literature and will be reviewed. The *long plantar ligament*—the longest ligament in the foot—arises from the calcaneus, progresses anteriorly to attach to the cuboid bone, and then continues forward to insert into the third, fourth, and fifth metatarsal bases and, on occasion, into the second.[41] The long plantar ligament forms a tunnel from the cuboid bone to the bases of the metatarsals for the peroneus longus tendon as it traverses the plantar aspect of the foot to insert into the first ray. Directly beneath the long plantar ligament lies the plantar calcaneocuboid ligament, more commonly known as the *short plantar ligament*. Located medially to the long plantar ligament is the plantar calcaneonavicular ligament, more commonly referred to as the *spring ligament*.

NORMAL BIOMECHANICS

Efficient biomechanical function of the foot depends on its ability to act as a loose adapter, a shock absorber, a torque converter, and a rigid lever during the gait cycle.[11] Normal gait biomechanical activity can be explained by concentrating on the three major contributing joints: the talocrural, the subtalar, and the transtarsal. Consideration of the joint axes and ranges of motion available in each joint can assist in illustrating normal biomechanical function in the foot.

Terminology

A discussion of the joint axes requires a brief discussion of the three body planes to accurately describe the motions occurring within the articulations. The three planes of the body are the sagittal, the frontal, and the transverse. The *sagittal plane* divides the body into left and right halves, the *frontal plane* segments the body into anterior and posterior aspects, and the *transverse plane* creates superior and inferior divisions. If these means of division are related to the hip joint, which has an axis found in all three planes, kinesiologically, the hip joint has 3 degrees freedom of motion.[5] Thus flexion and extension occur in the sagittal plane, abduction and adduction in the frontal plane, and rotation in the transverse plane. This description of hip joint movement is helpful in explaining the motions that occur in the subtalar joint.

A final aspect to be discussed under terminology is the functional segments of the foot. The anterior portion of the foot, composed of the five metatarsals and the phalanges, is referred to as the *forefoot*. The *midfoot* is formed by the three cuneiform bones and the navicular and cuboid bones. The talus and the calcaneus are referred to as the *rearfoot*. Thus, when discussing the rearfoot and the forefoot, reference will be made to the position of the calcaneus and talus in relation to the position of the five metatarsal heads.

Joint axes and ranges of motion

Talocrural joint. Although commonly thought to be horizontal, the axis of the talocrural joint runs in an oblique direction between the distal ends of the malleoli. Investigations have demonstrated the obliquity of the joint axis to be approximately 82 degrees from the vertical bisection of the tibia.[22] Researchers have attempted to demonstrate that the talocrural joint axis is not a single axis but a variable axis that depends on the position of the articular surfaces.[17,40] Inman[22] has explained that, although there can be variability, in approximately 80% of all cases the

talocrural articulation can be considered to be a single-axis joint.[22] The degree of motion for the talocrural joint can range from 20 degrees of dorsiflexion to 50 degrees of plantar flexion, depending on the individual.[1] However, while marked variation may occur in these ranges of motion for a given population, biomechanically, normal foot function requires 20 degrees of plantar flexion and 10 degrees of dorsiflexion when the knee is extended and the foot is in a neutral position.[39] While few persons lack the necessary plantar flexion, many individuals lack the 10 degrees of dorsiflexion needed for normal gait. (During the gait cycle, immediately after midstance, with the knee extended and the foot in a neutral or slightly supinated position, the tibia moves anteriorly approximately 10 degrees over the trochlea of the talus. If this necessary dorsiflexion is not available, some form of compensation, such as early heel-off and/or subtalar joint pronation, will occur, leading to a pathomechanical problem.)

Subtalar joint. The axis of the subtalar joint increases the complexity of this articular structure. Manter,[26] Root et al[38] and Green, Whitney, and Walters[16] have all described the inclination angle of the subtalar joint axis as 42 degrees from the transverse plane and 16 degrees from the sagittal plane (Fig. 14-1). The subtalar joint axis extends in an oblique direction from a posterolateral plantar aspect to an anteromedial dorsal aspect. Functionally the subtalar

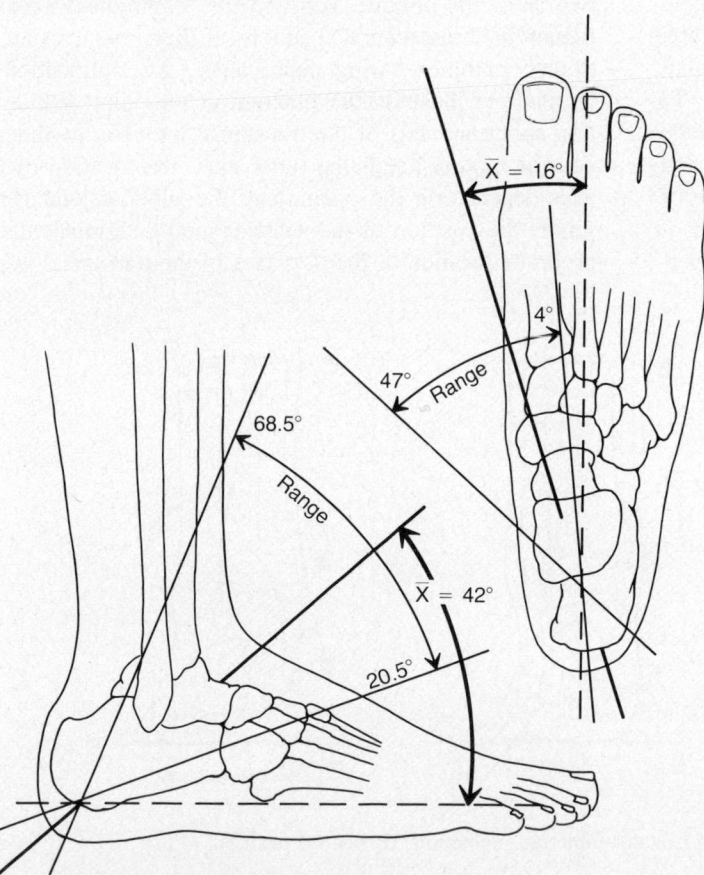

Fig. 14-1. Variations in angle of axis of subtalar joint.

joint is a simple single-axis joint that acts as a mitered oblique hinge.[22]

To understand the motions that occur via the subtalar joint, the term triplane motion must first be explained. *Triplane motion* refers to movement occurring simultaneously in the three body planes with concomitant motion about a single axis. (As previously mentioned, the hip joint has an axis with subsequent motion located within each body plane and can be described as having 3 degrees freedom of motion.) In the case of subtalar joint triplane motion (although only one joint axis exists because it travels in an oblique direction through all three body planes), as movement occurs about the axis, a component of motion occurs within each plane.[37,38]

The two motions of the subtalar joint are pronation and supination. *Pronation* can be defined as triplane motion consisting of simultaneous movement of the calcaneus and the foot in the direction of calcaneal eversion (frontal plane), abduction (transverse plane), and dorsiflexion (sagittal plane).[44] *Supination* is reverse triplane motion with calc aneal inversion (frontal plane), adduction (transverse plane), and plantar flexion (sagittal plane).[44] It should be emphasized that these motions exist only in a non–weight-bearing situation (an open kinetic chain), with the talus remaining stationary in the joint mortise. (This occurs when a person supinates and pronates the foot while dangling the lower leg off a table.)

In contrast, during the weight-bearing portion of gait, or stance phase, friction and reactive ground forces prevent the adduction-abduction and dorsiflexion-plantar-flexion elements of an open kinetic chain motion. To counteract these forces, the talus functions to maintain the transverse and sagittal plane components of supination and pronation. Thus closed kinetic chain supination consists of a calcaneal inversion with abduction and dorsiflexion of the talus, while similar pronation combines calcaneal ever-sion with adduction and plantar flexion of the talus (Fig. 14-2).[44] It is important to note, however, that even though the mechanical system necessary for supination and pronation is altered from open to closed kinetic chain motion, calcaneal eversion and inversion are not affected. Therefore evaluative measurements taken in a non–weight-bearing position would also be applicable to weight-bearing conditions.

The main function of the subtalar joint is to permit rotation of the leg in the transverse plane during the stance phase of gait.[21] This important relationship between the subtalar joint and the lower extremity can be easily demonstrated. If a person stands and externally rotates the left leg, the arch of the left foot will rise as the subtalar joint supinates (see Fig. 14-22). A posterior view of the lower extremity shows that the calcaneus will invert (as a component of supination) with external rotation. Conversely, if the left leg is internally rotated, pronation can be observed as the arch of the foot flattens with eversion of the calcaneus.

The range of motion of the subtalar joint has been estimated to be from 20 to 62 degrees.[22] However, it is of greater importance that supination be twice the value of pronation (i.e., 20 degrees supination to 10 degrees pronation).[48] It is also important to remember that for normal gait 4 to 6 degrees of pronation and 8 to 12 degrees of supination are required.[47]

Transtarsal joint. The transtarsal joint is composed of two axes: the oblique axis and the longitudinal axis. Although the biomechanical actions of these two axes are extremely complex during stance phase, a simplification can be made to illustrate the function of this joint. While motion about one axis of the transtarsal joint can be independent of motion about the other axis, the location of both axes depends on the position of the subtalar joint. In essence, the position of the subtalar joint determines the appropriate location of the two axes of the transtarsal joint.[47]

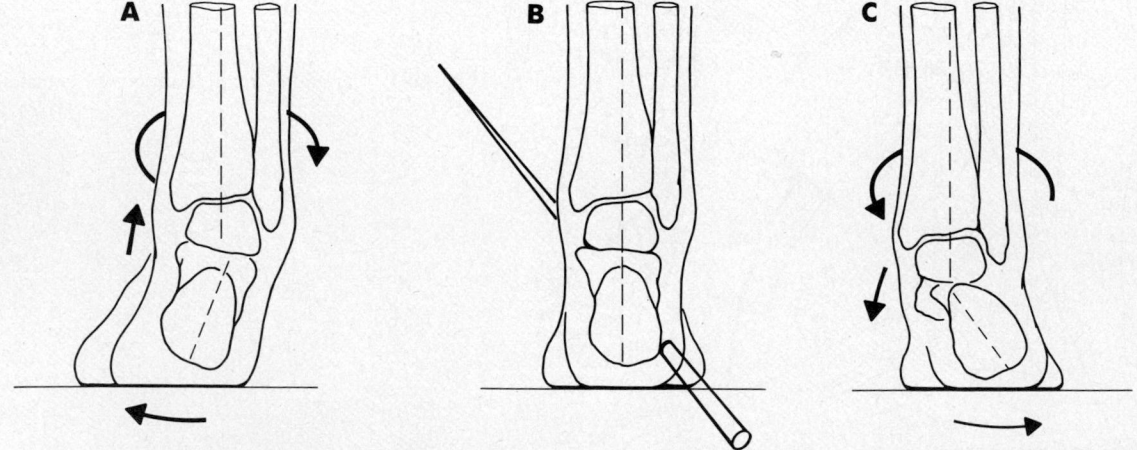

Fig. 14-2. Closed kinetic chain motion of subtalar joint: **A,** supination; **B,** neutral position; **C** pronation.

Thus dominance of the subtalar joint over the transtarsal joint is essential in achieving normal foot function.

If planes are drawn from the two axes of the transtarsal joint, they will become parallel as the subtalar joint pronates (Fig. 14-3, *A*). The resulting parallelism allows the foot to become a flexible, pliant structure.[49] As the subtalar joint moves from a pronated position to a neutral and then supinated one, the planes converge and the bones of the foot lock together, forming a rigid structure (Fig. 14-3, *B* and *C*).[47]

In summary, as the subtalar joint pronates, the transtarsal joint axes become parallel and the foot becomes flexible. As the subtalar joint moves from pronation into supination, the axes of the transtarsal joint converge and the foot becomes rigid and leverlike.

Normal gait

The foot is an extremely complex structure that must execute a series of important biomechanical functions, primarily during the stance phase of gait. The average length of the stance phase, only 0.63 second,[35] allows a minimal amount of time for these activities of occur.

The functions that the foot must provide during stance phase include providing (1) a base of support, (2) loose adaptation for accommodation to uneven terrain, (3) shock absorption, (4) rigid leverage for efficient propulsion, and (5) a mechanism for the absorption of transverse leg rotation. The synchronization of these significant functions is essential for normal gait.

Phases of gait. The normal gait cycle for each lower extremity consists of a swing phase (approximately 38% of the cycle) and a stance phase (approximately 62% of the cycle).[37]

Swing phase. The swing phase of gait is initiated by toe-off and is completed with heel strike.[37] Two important activities occur during the swing phase. First, momentarily after toe-off, the lower extremity begins to internally rotate throughout the entire period of swing phase.[48] Second, although the foot initially pronates to assist in toe clearance, during the last half of the swing phase the foot supinates so the calcaneus is inverted approximately 2 degrees at heel strike.[19,37]

Stance phase. During the stance phase several functions of the foot play an important role in the normal gait cycle. For the purpose of discussion, the stance phase can be divided into the contact period, the midstance period, and the propulsion period.

Contact period. The contact period initiates with heel strike and terminates with toe-off of the opposite leg.[34] This period constitutes the first 15% to 25% of the stance phase. Before heel strike the calcaneus is inverted approximately 2 degrees. At heel strike the lower extremity continues to internally rotate throughout the contact period. To allow the foot to maintain its line of progression, the subtalar joint pronates to absorb the internal rotation of the leg.[21] The pronation of the subtalar joint produces a simultaneous parallelism in the axes of the transtarsal joint and creates a pliant adaptation for accommodation to uneven terrain. The subtalar joint pronation has both a direct and an indirect effect on reducing the shock generated at heel strike. Pronation of the subtalar joint creates a shortening of the support leg that directly decreases impact forces.[37] Indirectly, pronation allows the tibia to internally rotate at a faster rate and farther than the femur.[37] Thus the knee joint can flex more rapidly to absorb shock force as a result of an entire lower limb shortening. At the end of contact the calcaneus everts approximately 4 to 6 degrees and pronation is complete.

Midstance period. The midstance period is initiated by the end of pronation of the subtalar joint. The lower extremity begins to externally rotate and the subtalar joint supinates to allow the foot to remain in its line of progres-

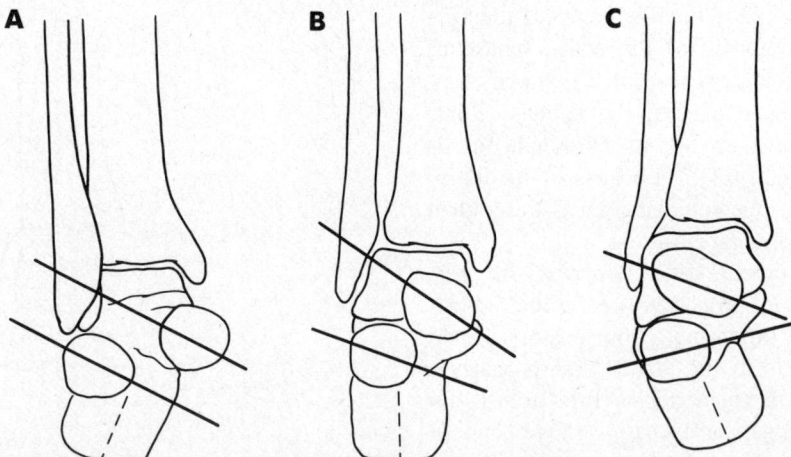

Fig. 14-3. Position of planes of the axes of transtarsal joint during **A,** pronation; **B,** neutral position; **C,** supination.

sion. As the subtalar joint supinates, the axes of the transtarsal joint converge and the foot is transformed from a flexible structure to a rigid lever for eventual propulsion.

At the midpoint of the midstance period (or approximately 50% to 60% into the stance phase), the calcaneus has moved from the everted position to a neutral position.[19] The *neutral position* can be described as congruency of the head of the talus within the mortise with a bisection of the calcaneus perpendicular to the floor. The five heads of the metatarsals should also be on a plane perpendicular to the bisection of the calcaneus.

During the last half of midstance, the subtalar joint continues to supinate and the calcaneus inverts approximately 2 degrees before heel-off. The continuing convergence of the transtarsal joint axes increases rigidity of the foot.

Propulsion period. The propulsive period of gait begins with heel-lift and concludes with toe-off.[37,48] This phase is a continuation of midstance with lower extremity external rotation, supination of the subtalar joint, and convergence of the transtarsal joint axes. At toe-off the calcaneus has inverted approximately 4 to 6 degrees.

To summarize, during stance phase the subtalar joint acts as a torque converter by absorbing lower extremity rotation while the foot maintains its line of progress.[11] Pronation and supination of the subtalar joint direct the planes of the axes of the transtarsal joint to be either parallel or convergant. Thus the foot is transformed from a pliant, accommodative structure at heel strike to a firm, rigid lever for effective propulsion at toe-off. Finally, a mechanism for shock absorption is produced through subtalar joint pronation by both a direct and an indirect effect.

Normally the foot is an efficient mechanism. However, any delay or extension of one of the three periods of the stance phase alters efficiency and creates an abnormal gait.

ABNORMAL FOOT TYPES AND CLINICAL PATHOMECHANICS

The abnormalities to be discussed in this section have one common causal factor—abnormal amounts of joint pronation during some component of the stance phase of gait. This abnormality occurs because of a compensatory movement about the triplane axis of the subtalar joint, which results in an alteration of normal alignment in another part of the foot (Fig. 14-4).[44] Because of its ability to move in a triplane area, the subtalar joint is the logical place to look for most foot compensation.

Normal compensatory pronation is a temporary or intermittent state of subtalar joint pronation (i.e., a foot adjusting to an uneven terrain). Abnormal compensatory pronation is constant and exists in the stance and propulsion phases. The consequence of this abnormal pronation is hypermobility, or the movement or excessive movements of a joint during stress or weight bearing when the joint should be stable or locked.[44] This instability will reduce the ability of the joint to properly transmit weight-bearing

forces and subsequently will create microtrauma to the soft tissue of the foot, metatarsal heads, and interphalangeal joints.[37]

The myriad of symptoms associated with hypermobility as a result of abnormal pronation include metatarsalgia, hyperkeratosis (shearing callus),[4] bunions,[37] heel spurs,[43] fasciitis, myositis (shin splints),[48] chondromalacia patellae,[3,6,48] and leg fatigue secondary to muscular overactivity.[24] All these symptoms are compounded with overuse and the additional stresses related to athletic competition. Lutter[25] reports that abnormal pronation accounts for 56% of the foot problems experienced by runners in a sports medicine clinic.

Five foot types cause compensation at the subtalar joint in the form of abnormal pronation: forefoot varus, forefoot valgus, subtalar varus, tibia vara, and equinus deformity.

Forefoot varus deformity

Clinical observation of this foot abnormality demonstrates a forefoot inverted to a bisection of the posterior aspect of the calcaneus when the subtalar joint is in a neutral position (Fig. 14-5, *A*). Hlavac[18] reports that this midtarsal joint abnormality probably results from failure of the head and neck of the talus to completely derotate from their original infantile position. This rotation is in the form of a valgus torsion, equal in adult life to a 35 to 40 degree valgus tilt of the head and neck of the talus in relation to the trochlea.[19]

Compensation, occurring about the triplane subtalar axis during weight bearing, permits the medial forefoot components to make contact with the ground. Compensation can occur only if an adequate amount of pronation is available, thus allowing the calcaneus to evert and permitting the entire plantar surface to become weight bearing (Fig. 14-5, *B*).

Clinically, compensated forefoot varus resembles a pes planus or flatfoot. Posteriorly, the calcaneus is everted.

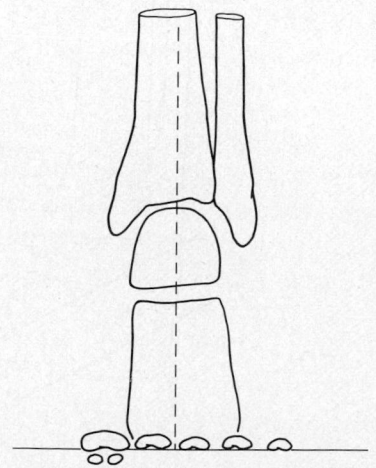

Fig. 14-4. Normal foot alignment.

Medially, the longitudinal arch is absent, with the head of the talus bulging proximal to the navicular tuberosity (adduction and plantar flexion of the talus on the calcaneus). On the plantar surface the callus pattern is concentrated under the second and third metatarsal heads. A hallux valgus deformity is often associated with this foot type, depending on the amount of compensatory pronation required and the chronicity of the problem.

If the necessary amount of subtalar joint pronation is not available, an uncompensated weight-bearing state will exist. During stance phase, because of the inability of the entire plantar surface to make contact with the ground,

ground reaction forces remain lateral, placing excessive pressure along the fourth and fifth metatarsal heads. Evidence of callus under the fifth metatarsal head is a good clinical indicator of this uncompensated state.

The forefoot varus deformity is a prime example of a foot type that maintains the subtalar joint in abnormal compensatory pronation during the stance phase of gait. This compensation occurs within the frontal plane, along the subtalar joint axis and the longitudinal axis of the midtarsal joint.[19,38,47] Instead of a normal 4 to 6 degrees of subtalar joint pronation occurring during the contact phase, increased ranges of pronation (allowed by the subtalar and

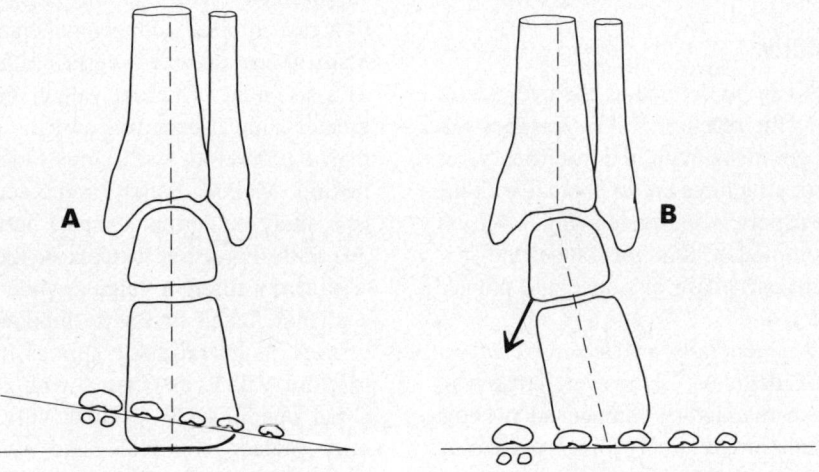

Fig. 14-5. A, Anterior view of uncompensated forefoot varus deformity. **B,** Compensated forefoot varus. Arrow defines adducted plantar-flexed position of talus. Note calcaneal eversion.

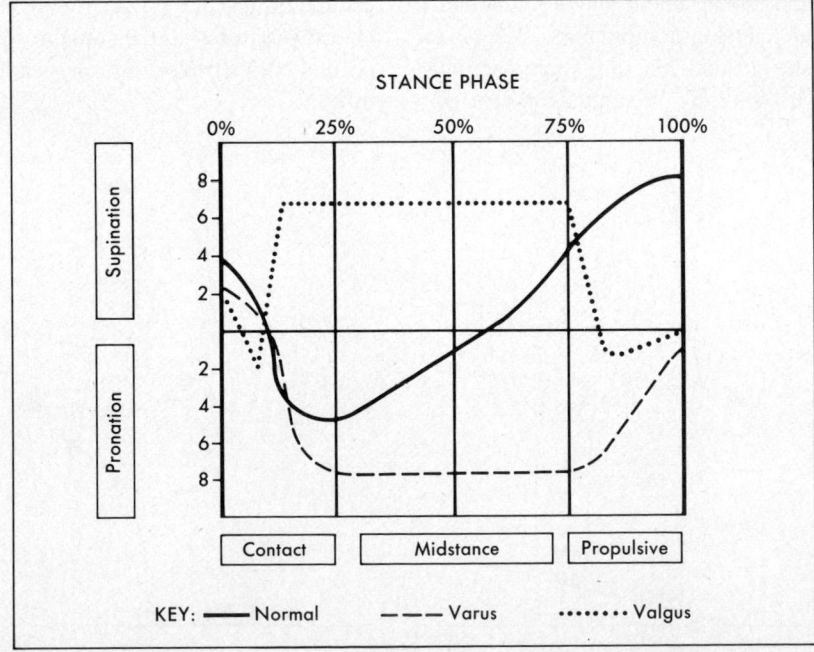

Fig. 14-6. Theoretical movement pattern for the subtalar joint for a normal forefoot to hindfoot alignment, a compensated forefoot varus deformity, and a forefoot valgus deformity.

midtarsal joints) continue into the midstance and propulsive phases. (Fig. 14-6).[37] This excessive pronation negates the rigid lever function of the foot that is essential for normal propulsion. Push-off is attempted on a loose bony articular complex. Because of this instability in both the rearfoot and the forefoot, abnormal shearing forces result between the metatarsal heads. Symptoms resulting from this foot type includes fasciitis, synovial inflammation, plantar callus, ligamentous stress, interdigital neuromas,[48] postural fatigue,[47] chondromalacia patella,[3] tendonitis, and shin splints.[37]

Conservative management of this abnormality includes the use of orthotic devices designed to balance the forefoot in relation to the rearfoot.

Forefoot valgus deformity

This foot abnormality can be defined as the eversion of the forefoot in relation to the rearfoot.[44] The forefoot valgus deformity directly contrasts with the forefoot varus type since the medial foot structures are in contact with the surface while the lateral aspect is suspended (Fig. 14-7). If the forefoot cannot accommodate this imbalance, the subtalar joint will supinate in one phase of stance and pronate during the next.

The midstance of gait is generally unaffected by a forefoot valgus of less than 6 degrees.[39] However, larger valgus variations will dictate mandatory compensation about the subtalar and midtarsal (longitudinal) joint axes during contact and the midstance portions of the walking cycle. It has been suggested that this supinatory compensation responds to lateral ground reaction forces that promote midtarsal joint pronation or locking against the rearfoot.[42] The unstable rearfoot will then invert about the longitudinal axis of the midtarsal joint, causing a supinatory rock (see Fig. 14-6). At heel-lift the ground reaction forces acting laterally will be extensive, resulting in subtalar joint pro-

nation during propulsion. This excessive pronation into the propulsive gait phase of the walking cycle can produce symptoms associated with hypermobility in the metatarsophalangeal and interphalangeal joints. These symptoms result in an unstable state during push-off.

A rigid forefoot valgus foot type resembles a typical cavus, or high-arched, foot. This abnormality may be associated with a rearfoot or subtalar varus and may be a causal factor leading to anterior tarsal tunnel syndrome. This foot type will be a poor shock absorber, thereby transmitting increased ground forces to the proximal joint structures.

Forefoot valgus can also be mistaken for another clinical problem involving the plantar-flexed position of the first ray complex (cuneonavicular-metatarsal articulation). Schoenhaus and Jay[42] describe the plantar-flexed first ray as a secondary forefoot valgus and suggest that there is a greater clinical occurrence of the forefoot valgus foot type than the forefoot varus foot type because of this plantar flexion. McPoil, Schuit, and Knecht[29] support this finding in a study of normal females between the ages of 19 and 30 years. Forty-five percent of the females surveyed demonstrated a forefoot valgus, while 15 percent demonstrated a plantar flexed first ray. Subotnick[48] reports a high percentage of lateral ankle sprains in athletes with increased forefoot valgus associated with a moderate heel varus.[48] Other conditions associated with a forefoot valgus deformity include iliotibial band syndrome,[45] sesmoiditis,[37] plantar fasciitis, and[48] leg and thigh pain.[53]

The treatment goal for this foot type is to support or balance the forefoot by posting or building up an orthotic device along the distal lateral aspect of the foot. This procedure brings the surface or ground up to the suspended lateral structures so the subtalar joint need not perform abnormal compensatory motion leading to general foot instability.

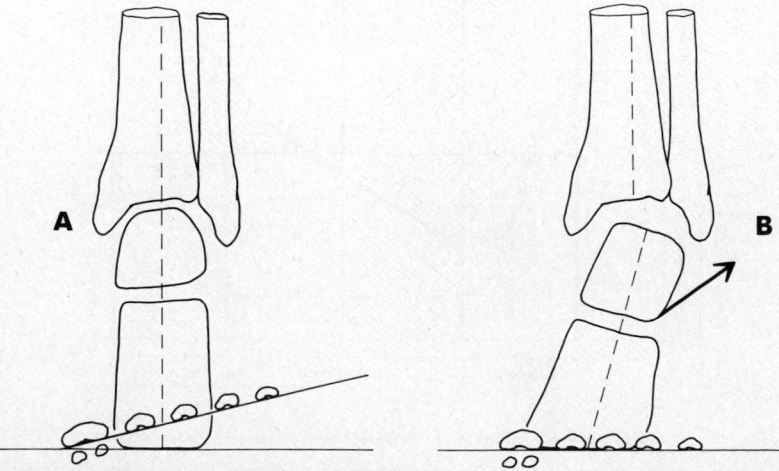

Fig. 14-7. A, Anterior view of uncompensated forefoot valgus. **B,** Compensated forefoot valgus. Arrow defines abducted-dorsiflexed position of talus. Note calcaneal inversion.

Rearfoot varus deformity

This deformity results from the failure of the posterior calcaneus to completely derotate from its original infantile position.[54] Evaluation of the rearfoot-forefoot relationship in non–weight-bearing position reveals an inverted calcaneus when the subtalar joint is neutral and the midtarsal joint is pronated (Fig. 14-8, *A*).

During weight bearing the rearfoot and the forefoot will be inverted relative to the ground, leaving the medial foot in non–weight-bearing position. Clinically, this uncompensated state is rare because the subtalar joint pronates to place the heel vertical to the ground and the forefoot in total contact with it (Fig. 14-8, *B*). Generally this vertically positioned calcaneus meets the requirements for additional pronation created by the varus deformity. Unlike the previously described foot abnormalities, compensatory pronation occurs only when the heel and foot have ground contact.[37] At heel-lift the subtalar joint is free to supinate and make partial to nearly full recovery during the propulsive phase.

Clinical evaluation of most feet reveals a moderate 2-degree to 3-degree rearfoot varus.[48] This deformity commonly occurs in combination with either a tibia vara or cavus foot. Subotnick[48] and Root et al[39] report minimal symptoms from this foot type during daily activities. However, during athletic training plantar tissue strains, spurs, shin splints, bursitis, patellar symptoms, and some hamstring muscle pulls occur because of the reduced shock-absorbing properties of the foot type.[48] Weil et al[53] also report in a study of high school and college basketball players that the rearfoot varus foot type is a significant contributor to lateral ankle sprains in the sport. These researchers discuss the need to acquire rearfoot measurements on athletes who have rearfoot varus as a predisposing factor of lateral ankle sprains. Since structural tibial varum is another etiological factor attributable to rearfoot varus,[48] the clinician must consider the summation of both measurements to determine the total amount of rearfoot varum deformity.

An orthosis with a medial heel wedge built to the number of degrees of the rearfoot varus and modified to allow normal amounts of subtalar joint pronation can be effective in reducing symptoms of rearfoot varus during athletic activity.

Tibia vara deformity

Unlike the previously discussed foot types that cause intrinsic pronation during the stance phase of gait, tibia vara is an extrinsic deformity, creating a deviation of the lower third of the tibia in the direction of inversion. The distal tibia will be closer to the midline of the body than the proximal portion, producing the common bow-legged deformity.

Evaluation of this condition in a non–weight-bearing position will generally reveal a normal rearfoot-forefoot relationship. However, during weight bearing influences of this deformity on the foot are similar to the rearfoot varus abnormality. During gait compensatory pronation occurs at the subtalar joint while the foot and heel are in contact with the ground. In the normal foot during heel strike the calcaneus becomes perpendicular to the walking surface. With a tibia vara deformity the subtalar joint must pronate more than 4 degrees to bring the heel to vertical position.[48]

As with rearfoot varus, this deformity can produce abrupt changes within the knee joint, creating stresses about the patellofemoral articulation during athletic or recreational endeavors.[6] This abnormality can be associated with some degree of rearfoot varus and has been reported as a component of the cavus foot type.[48]

Equinus deformity

Since a minimal range of 10 degrees dorsiflexion is required of the ankle joint during the stance phase of gait,

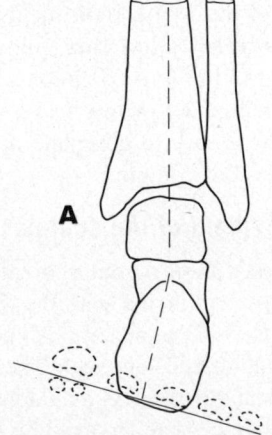
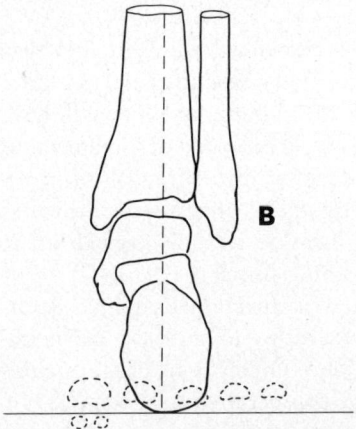

Fig. 14-8. A, Posterior view of uncompensated rearfoot varus. Observe inverted attitude of both rearfoot and forefoot. **B,** Compensated rearfoot varus. Note adducted, plantar-flexed position of talus used to bring calcaneus to vertical posture.

ankle joint equinus can be defined as a limitation of this minimal 10-degree range when the subtalar joint is in the neutral position, the midtarsal joint pronated, and the knee extended (Fig. 14-9, *A*).[39]

The cause of an equinus deformity in the athlete is primarily functional in nature. It occurs when the gastrocnemius or soleus muscle or both shorten as a result of muscular imbalance and the calf muscles overdevelop with associated shortening of these muscles.[3] Other causal factors include congenital and acquired osseous deformities of the ankle joints as well as congenital shortening of the gastrocnemius, hamstring, and iliopsoas muscles, which demand compensation from other lower extremity joints to complete locomotion requirements.[37]

Ankle dorsiflexion is required at the midstance of gait since the tibia must move 10 degrees over the talar dome before heel-lift. Limitation in this motion creates full compensatory pronation occurring about the subtalar joint axis just before heel-lift (Fig. 14-9, *B*).[37] The amount of compensatory pronation that is required is proportional to the amount of dorsiflexion limitation. If the subtalar joint range of motion cannot adequately compensate, the midtarsal joint will assist with movement about its oblique axis. Manter[26] and Elftman[14] report that the motion produced about this axis is dorsiflexion of the forefoot on the rearfoot, which can equal as much as 10 degrees. These compensatory motions create a hypermobile foot during the early propulsive phase, causing increased shear stress on the plantar aspect of the second, third, and fourth metatarsal heads.

Another form of compensation seen in the presence of an equinus deformity is a *bouncing gait.* [37] Clinical observation of this gait reveals premature heel-lift during midstance. Because heel-lift begins before knee flexion, the pelvis and trunk are elevated during midstance, giving the appearance of bouncing during gait. This early heel rise will also increase the duration of the propulsive phase of the walking cycle. Indeed, these forms of compensation are considered the greatest symptom producers in the human foot.[46]

Common foot symptoms associated with this foot type include medial arch pain, plantar fasciitis, and posterior leg fatigue.[48] McCluskey, Blackburn, and Lewis[28] have also reported an increased incidence of ligamentous sprains in athletes with this deformity as a result of inversion stresses caused by tightness of the gastrocnemius muscle. These symptoms must be strongly considered in any preseason athletic screening format.

Conservative treatment of a functional equinus deformity involves stretching exercises to increase the dorsiflexion range of the ankle joint. Other forms of the equinus deformity rarely respond to conservative treatment.

CLINICAL EVALUATION TECHNIQUES

The greatest error any evaluator can make in examining foot and ankle disorders is to concentrate on the specific

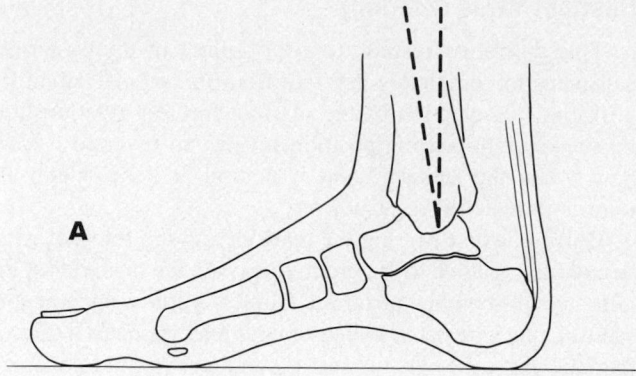

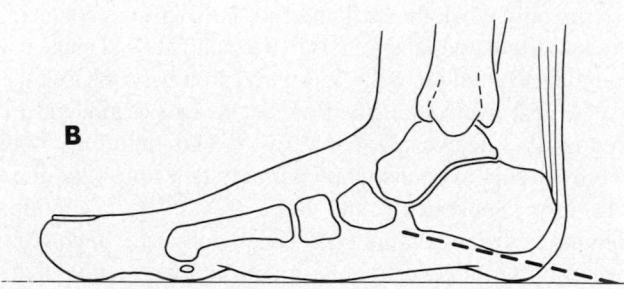

Fig. 14-9. A, Neutral foot position (medial view). Note tibial progression line depicting 10 degrees of tibial advancement over talar dome. **B,** Compensated forefoot caused by equinus deformity.

area of complaint without closely evaluating the entire extremity. Although the client's complaint may be localized to the foot, an entire examination of the lower extremity may be required to rule out involvement of proximal or distal joints.

The evaluation should begin with a complete history, including appropriate subjective data. The objective examination of the foot should include assessment of the ankle joint, subtalar joint, and musculoskeletal abnormalities proximal to the foot complex.

The remainder of this section will present clinical techniques necessary to complete an objective examination of the ankle-foot complex.

Measurement of the subtalar joint

Determination of range of motion of the subtalar joint provides the clinician with the degrees of motion available within this joint to accomplish normal foot functions, such as adaptation and leverage. These values can also be used to determine if there is available range within the subtalar joint to compensate for existing abnormalities either intrinsic or extrinsic to the foot complex.

Total range of motion for the joint is between 18 and 62 degrees with one third of the motion in the direction of pr-

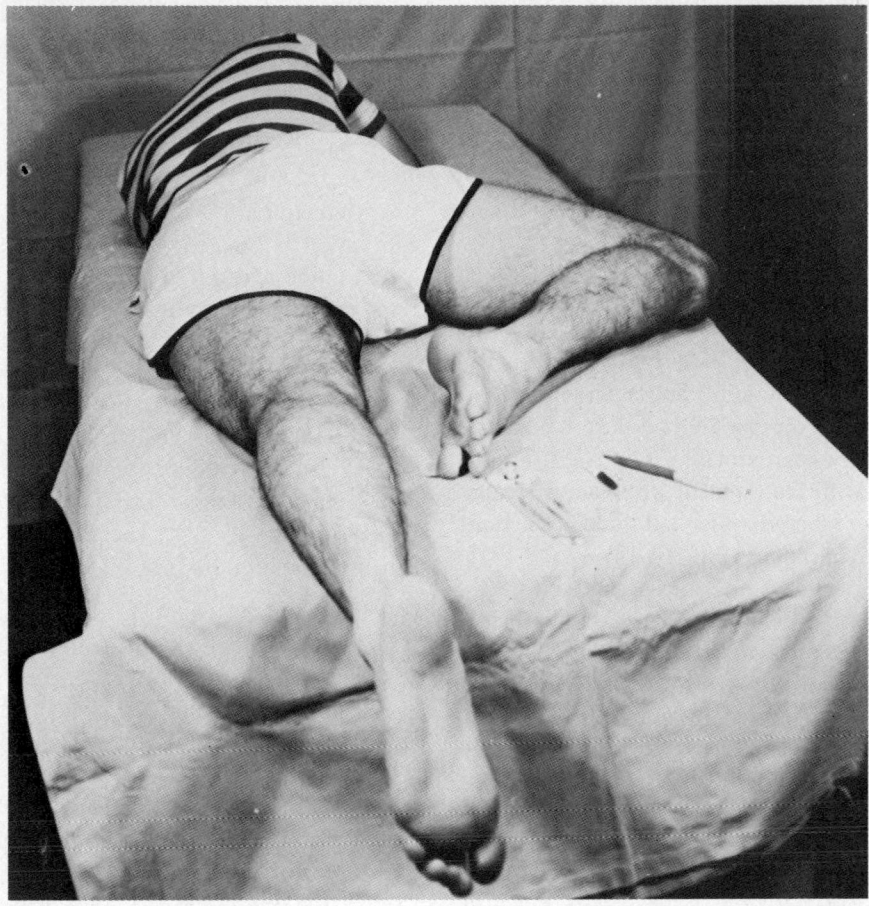

Fig. 14-10. Position of client in preparation for subtalar joint measurements.

onation (calcaneal eversion) and two thirds in the direction of supination (calcaneal inversion).[39]

Determination of subtalar joint range of motion. Subtalar motion can be analyzed by measuring the movement of the calcaneus in the frontal plane.[44] The following steps should be used by the therapist to determine the range of motion available in the subtalar joint:

1. Place the client in the prone position with the ankle and foot overhanging the end of the table. Place the calcaneus in the frontal plane by positioning the opposite extremity in hip flexion, abduction, and external rotation with knee flexion (Fig. 14-10). Generally this position will internally rotate the opposite limb to be measured, consequently placing the calcaneus in the correct position. The posterior surface of the calcaneus will be parallel to the ground.

2. Eye contact should be maintained on the perpendicular attitude of the calcaneus.

3. With a fine skin marker, bisect the middle one third of the posterior calcaneus (Fig. 14- 11). The midsection can be determined by palpating the medial and lateral calcaneal borders with the flexed proxi-

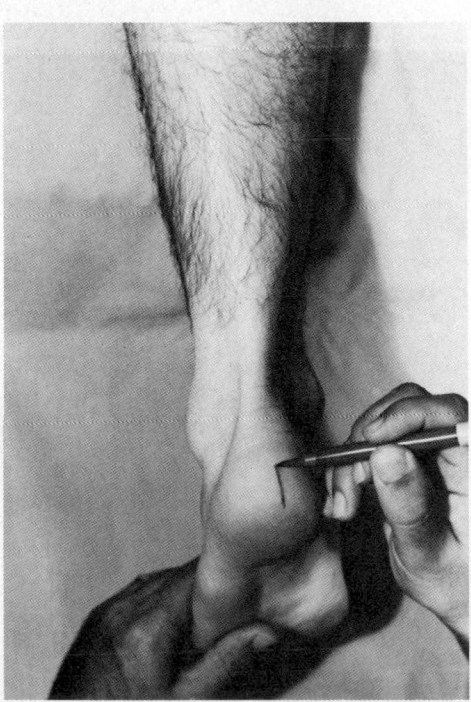

Fig. 14-11. Bisection of middle third of posterior calcaneus.

mal interphalangeal (PIP) joints of each index finger. Using the dorsal surface of the middle phalanx, stroke the medial and lateral sides of the calcaneus (Fig. 14-12) and observe for the ischemic response produced. Mark the bisection based on this response.

4. Extend the bisection line to the sole of the foot so that it can be used as a reference when observing forefoot measurement.[38]

5. Grasping the fourth and fifth metatarsal heads, maximally pronate the joint and extend the bisection line superiorly approximately 1 inch (Fig. 14- 13).

6. Maximally supinate the joint, and again extend the bisection line from the middle one third of the calcaneus superiorly approximately 1 inch. A Y form will develop, with the point of bifurcation located at the junction of the proximal and middle one third of the bisected calcaneus (Fig. 14-14).

7. Recheck the bisection before measuring.

8. Subtalar motion is measured relative to the bisection of the knee joint and the lower leg.[39] Bisect the distal one third of the lower extremity just proximal to the malleoli with a fine tip marker. Extension of this line superiorly should bisect the knee joint within the popliteal space.

9. Using a small goniometer or tractograph, place one arm of the device following the leg line and the other along the calcaneal line. The axis of the device should be placed between the malleoli within the frontal plane (Fig. 14- 15).

10. Maximally supinate the joint by again grasping the fourth and fifth metatarsal heads. Properly align the calcaneal arm, and read the number of degrees of calcaneal inversion.

11. Measure calcaneal eversion by pronating the joint in a similar fashion. Record the degrees of motion.

Determination of the subtalar joint neutral position. In order to clinically identify the relationship of the forefoot to the rearfoot, a technique for determining the subtalar joint neutral position must be acquired. Neutral position can be determined by appreciating the congruency of the head of the talus.[39,54] It should be remembered that during pronation the talus will adduct and plantar flex; therefore the talar head can be palpated medially. Conversely, during supination the talus will abduct and dorsiflex, thus becoming prominent laterally. The following steps can be used by the therapist to determine subtalar neutrality (Fig. 14-16):

1. Place the client in the identical position previously outlined (1, in preceding section on subtalar joint range of motion measurements).

2. Again maintain eye contact perpendicular to the posterior surface of the calcaneus.

3. On the medial side of the foot locate the navicular tuberosity, which is approximately 1 inch below and 1 inch distal to the medial malleolus. Lightly place the thumb just proximal to this tuberosity. Grasping the fourth and fifth metatarsal heads, pronate and supinate the foot. During pronation the head of the ta-

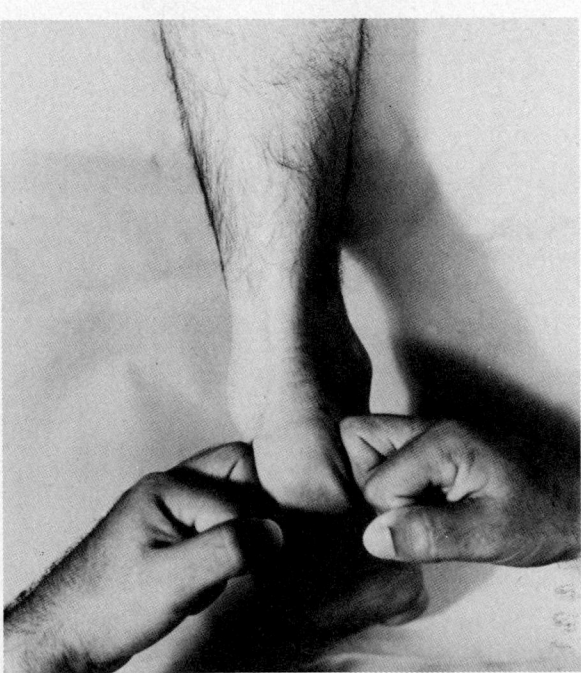

Fig. 14-12. Determining bisection of calcaneus.

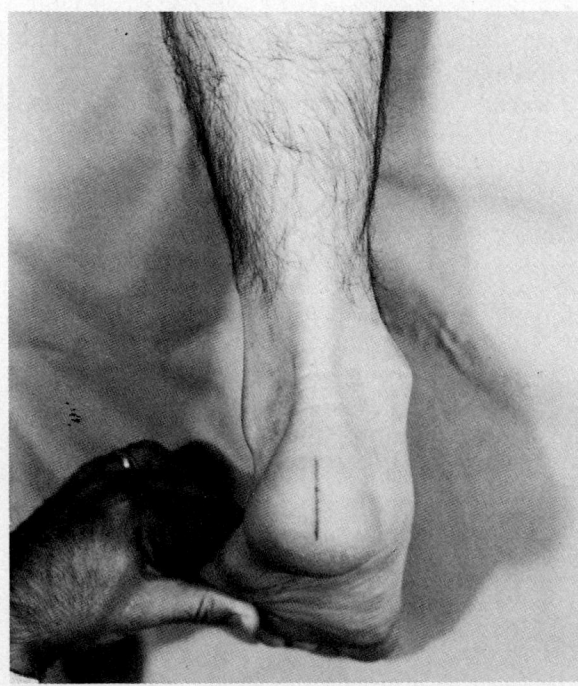

Fig. 14-13. Maximal calcaneal eversion with proximal extension of bisection line.

lus should contact the thumb, while during supination it should disappear.

4. During pronation observe the lateral aspect of the foot. A sulcus should be present that anatomically represents the sinus tarsi and the location of the talar head during supination. Place the index finger over this region, which is lateral and generally more anterior than the region of thumb placement. Again supinate and pronate the foot. The head of talus should be palpated during supination.

5. With the thumb and index fingers in place, supinate and pronate the joint until the medial and lateral sides of the talus are neither protruding nor depressed between the finger placement. At this point congruency of the subtalar joint, with resulting neutrality, has been achieved. One of the main clinical purposes of identifying subtalar joint neutrality is to capture the position of the foot in the most stable osseous position, which occurs approximately at the middle of midstance of gait. During this time the subtalar joint is in a neutral position, the ankle is dorsiflexed, and the midtarsal joint is pronated. Therefore, when subtalar joint neutrality has been identified, pronation of the midtarsal joints can be accomplished without disturbing the congruency of the talus.

6. With the thumb of one hand on the fourth and fifth metatarsal heads, gently dorsiflex the foot (not nec-

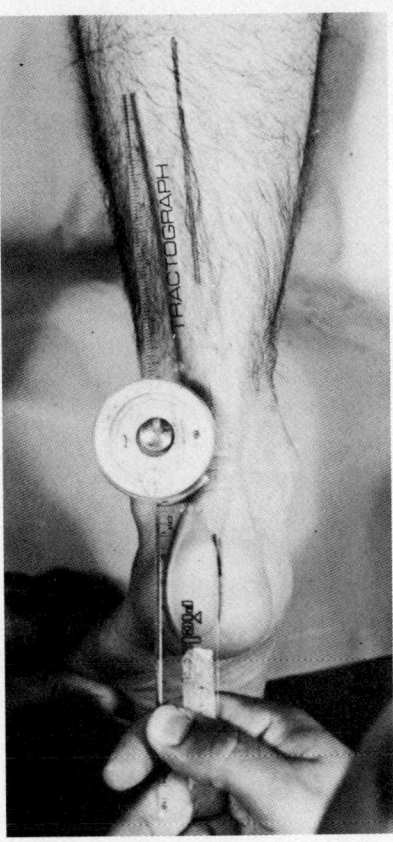

Fig. 14-15. Tractograph placement during measurement of calcaneal range of motion. Observe bisection of lower third of leg.

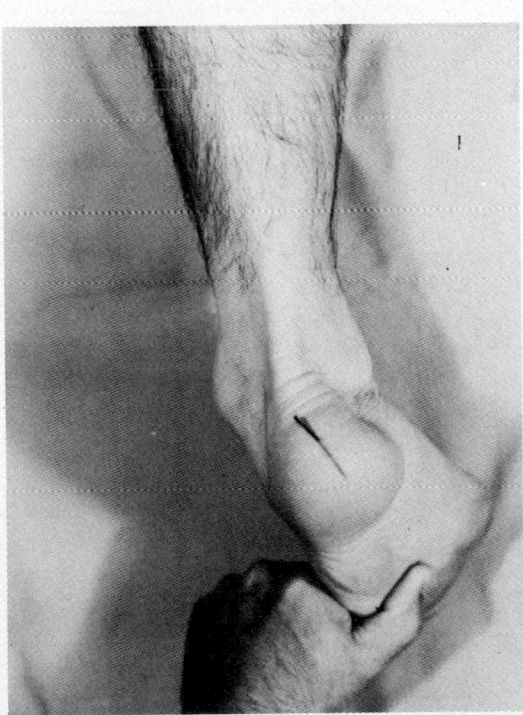

Fig. 14-14. Maximal calcaneal inversion with extension of bisection line proximally. Note the Y formation formed by two proximal bisections.

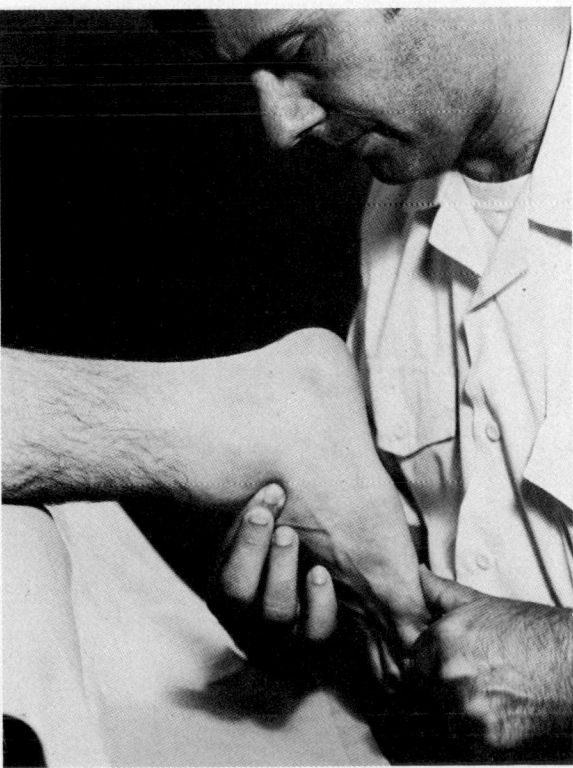

Fig. 14-16. Determining neutral subtalar joint position.

essarily to 90 degrees) until a slight resistance is felt.[39] Be sure not to pronate or supinate the subtalar joint. Maintain congruency of the talus.

7. With eye contact on the frontal plane or perpendicular to the posterior calcaneus, compare the relationship of the posterior calcaneal bisection to the plane of the forefoot, which includes the second, third, and fourth metatarsal heads. If the plane of the forefoot is perpendicular to the calcaneal bisection, there is no forefoot deviation. If the plane is either inverted or everted to the calcaneal line, there is forefoot varus or valgus, respectively. The calcaneal position, varus or valgus, can also be determined at this time.

Measurement of forefoot

We believe that accurately quantifiable forefoot measurements are clinically difficult to obtain and may be unreliable, whether a protractor, goniometer, or tractograph is used. The purpose of observation is qualitatively to determine the position of the forefoot relative to the rearfoot. The neutral position casting technique can capture any forefoot abnormality, which can then be objectively measured from the positive mold.

An approximately accurate forefoot measurement can be obtained by either of the following methods:

A. Protractor method
1. Determine the neutral subtalar position with midtarsal pronation as previously described.
2. Place the straight edge of the protractor along the plantar aspect of the heel, and align the straight edge with the plane of the forefoot.
3. Project an imaginary extension of the heel bisection over the protractor, and note the point of intersection.
4. The recording indicates the approximate amount of forefoot deviation.
B. Goniometer or tractograph method
1. Determine subtalar joint neutrality and metatarsal joint pronation.
2. Place one arm of the goniometer along posterior calcaneal bisection and the other arm along the plantar aspect of the heel. Align the latter arm with the plane of the forefoot, and read the degrees of forefoot deviation.

Measurement of ankle dorsiflexion

As previously mentioned, the ankle joint must have 10 degrees of dorsiflexion to satisfy gait requirements toward the middle and end of midstance. Measurement of this joint can be performed following subtalar measurement techniques since both are measured with the client in the prone position. (The supine position can also be used.)

1. Place the client in either a prone or supine position with the knee extended. Position the contralateral extremity as described for subtalar measurement. The posterior calcaneus will be maintained in this same plane.

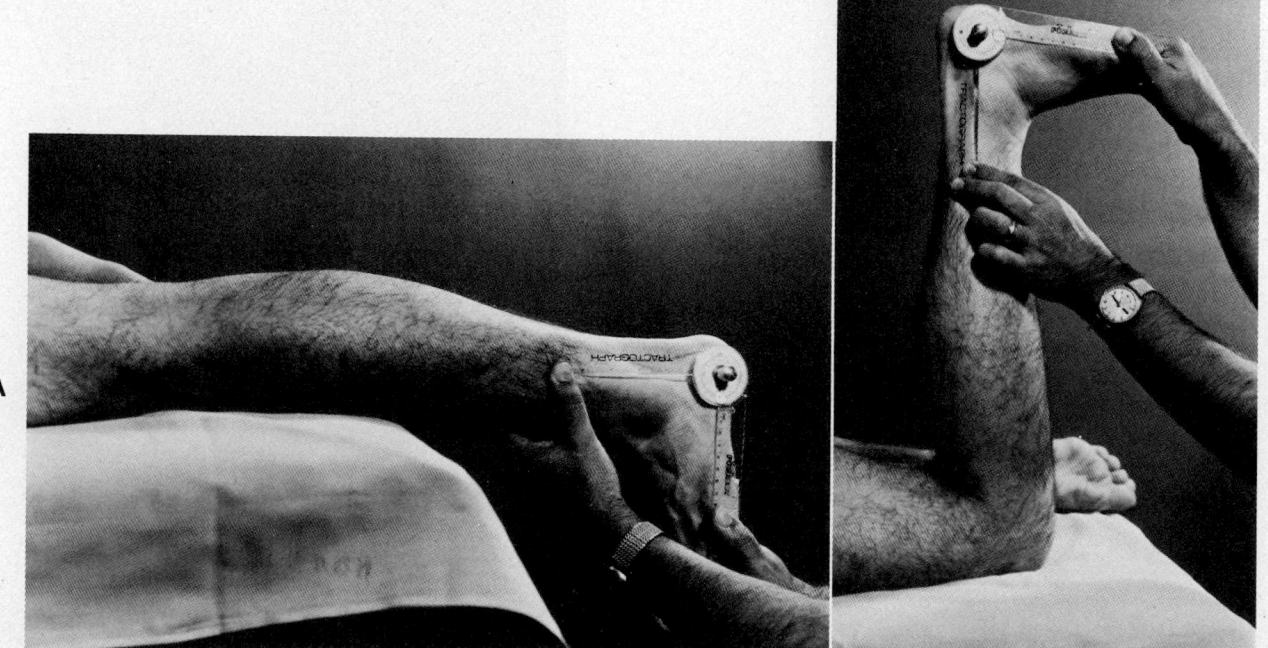

Fig. 14-17. Measurement of ankle dorsiflexion. **A,** With knee extended; **B,** with knee flexed.

2. Place the subtalar joint in neutral position.
3. Place the goniometer or tractograph as follows (Fig. 14-17, *A*):
   a. Have the distal arm run along an imaginary line from the plantar aspect of the calcaneus to the plantar aspect of the fifth metatarsal. Direct palpation can separate the plantar fascia from the posterior aspect of the fifth metatarsal, and the goniometer arm should be placed along this region.
   b. Position the axis along the lateral aspect of the calcaneus.
   c. Place the proximal arm of the goniometer along a lateral bisection of the lower third of the leg (which is generally located at the midmalleolus or just proximal to it).
4. Passively dorsiflex the foot to resistance while attempting to maintain the subtalar joint in neutral position. At this point the client should be able to actively dorsiflex the foot as long as the neutrality of the subtalar joint is maintained.
5. Perform ankle joint dorsiflexion while maintaining the subtalar joint in its neutral position. This prevents compensatory pronation by the subtalar and midtarsal joints in the presence of an equinus deformity—a common source of error in dorsiflexion measurement.
6. When less than 10 degrees of dorsiflexion is found with the knee extended, flex the knee to 90 degrees (Fig. 14-17, *B*). the 10-degree range becomes available, a gastrocnemius shortening is evident. Continued limitation in knee flexion represents either soleus muscle shortening or an intrinsic block at the ankle joint.

Measurement of tibia vara and neutral calcaneal stance

Measurements to determine tibia vara and neutral calcaneal stance should be done during weight bearing with the client positioned for individual angle and base of gait. The angle base of gait can be determined by observing the client's gait or having the client mark time standing in place. This position is needed to examine the foot in its normal midstance attitude.

A. Measurement of tibia vara
   1. Have the client stand in the normal angle and base of gait on a firm level surface, preferably at the examiner's eye level, while the examiner sits or kneels to observe the posterior calcaneus. The examiner should be positioned just medial to the foot being checked so that the line of vision is parallel to the posterior calcaneus.
   2. Place both of the client's feet in the neutral position by palpating for talar congruency (the talus should not protrude medially along the talonav-
icular articulation or laterally within the sinus tarsi). This can be accomplished by asking the client to rotate the trunk to the left and right, which allows the tibia to externally and internally rotate, thereby supinating and pronating the subtalar joint while the examiner is palpating with thumb and index fingers for talar congruency (Fig. 14-18).
   3. With both of the client's feet in the neutral position, recheck the bisections performed during subtalar joint range of motion measurements in a non–weight-bearing position. (Do not hesitate to recheck these bisections since they can change because of tissue movement.) When the bisections are acceptable, measure the frontal plane relationship of the tibia to the transverse plane (or level ground).
   4. Place the axis of the goniometer or tractograph along the posterior calcaneus. Have one arm of the goniometer resting on the ground, extending toward the lateral aspect of the ankle. Place the other arm parallel to the bisection of the distal third of the lower leg in the direction of the inversion (Fig. 14-19).
   5. The amount of deviation of the lower third of the leg from the vertical (90 degrees) is the amount of tibia vara. If the leg line is perpendicular to the ground, there is no tibia vara. Clinically, if the forefoot rises from the ground when the subtalar joint is in neutral position, tibia vara is present.

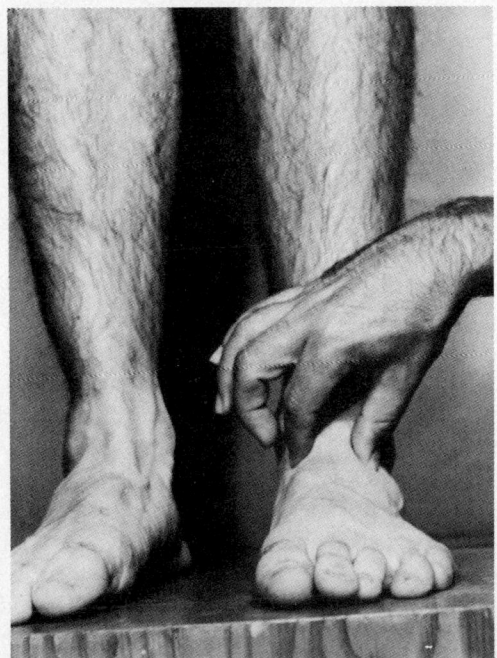

Fig. 14-18. Palpating subtalar congruency in weight bearing.

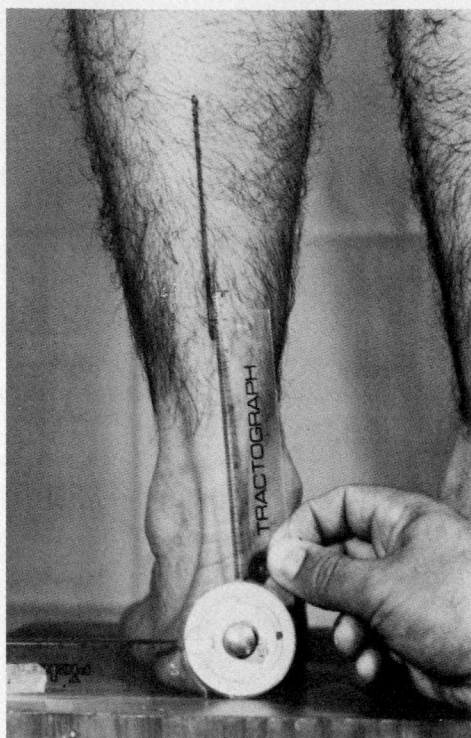

Fig. 14-19. Measurement of tibia vara.

B. Measurement of neutral calcaneal stance
 1. Have the client stand in a normal angle and base of gait. The neutral position is determined by a method similar to that described for measuring tibia vara.
 2. Using a protractor, place the straight edge along the supporting surface. The center of this straight edge is placed at the apex of the angle created by the calcaneal bisection and the supporting surface. The number of degrees is recorded from the top of the calcaneal bisection as it transverses the protractor.

Measurement of tibia vara and neutral calcaneal position during stance provides the examiner with the appropriate number of degrees the subtalar joint needs to compensate to accommodate any tibia vara or rearfoot deviation occurring during the midstance of gait. Measurement of relaxed calcaneal stance (which is recorded using the same technique as described for neutral calcaneal measurement except that the foot is allowed to assume a resting posture) will provide the examiner with the approximate number of compensated degrees moved by the subtalar joint to accommodate any proximal problem or foot deviation. McPoil, Schuit, and Knecht[31] have stated that if consistent measurement of tibial varum with repeated office visits are to be made, it is essential that the patient's dynamic angle and base of walking be determined and maintained for each visit. They also questioned the need for the

patient to maintain subtalar joint neutrality during the measurement of tibial varum if the dynamic angle and base is reliable between measurements.

Gait evaluation related to the foot and ankle

Thorough evaluation of the subtalar joint in both stance and non–weight-bearing position is essential to determine what will happen to the foot-ankle complex during gait. Awareness of the kinetic phases—neutral, supination, and pronation—is required, but to the untrained eye they cannot be truly appreciated in a clinical setting.

Five important factors of the foot and ankle can best be evaluated during gait:[54]

1. *The angle and base of gait.* Normally, this angle does not exceed 15 degrees from the midline of the body.[39] Any significant deviation from the distance between each heel bisection or the angulation of the foot from the midline could be a result of some existing lower extremity abnormality and should be noted during the gait evaluation.
2. *Point of heel contact.* The position of the calcaneus in either eversion or inversion during heel strike should be observed.
3. *The approximate time of pronation.* Normally, pronation will occur 15% to 20% into the contact phase of gait.[37,44] A prolongation of this triplane movement into other phases should be noted.
4. *The approximate time of supination.* Supination will occur in the last half of the stance cycle.[39,44] This motion provides osseous stability during propulsion.
5. *Adequate range of motion in ankle dorsiflexion and plantar flexion.* During midstance a minimum of 10 degrees of dorsiflexion is required for normal function, and at least 20 degrees of plantar flexion is necessary for propulsion.

Root, Orien, and Weed[37] offer some clinical observations to assist in the determination of joint positions or movement during gait analyses:

1. *Recognition of pronation.* Active calcaneal eversion always indicates ongoing pronation, as does internal rotation of the leg, especially when one is observing the patella and malleolli. As the talar head adducts and plantar flexes during pronation, a bulge can be seen medially. Also, along the lateral margin of the foot, a small indentation at the level of the calcaneocuboid articulation results from abduction of the forefoot in relation to the rearfoot.
2. *Neutral position observations.* In the posterior view of the foot the tissue just below the lateral malleolus is smooth and moderately concave in appearance when the three facets of the talocalcaneal joint are congruent. With pronation this concavity increases since the talus will adduct on the calcaneus. Con-

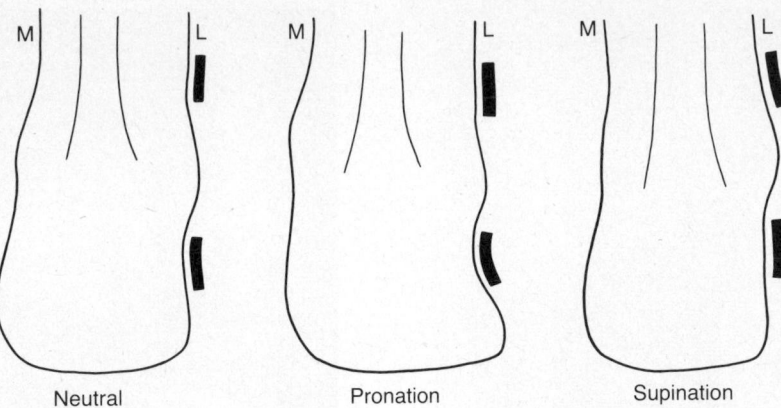

Fig. 14-20. Posterior views demonstrating lateral tissue configurations with different foot positions.

versely, a convex shape appears during supination when the talus abducts on the calcaneus (Fig. 14-20).

3. *Recognition of supination.* Active calcaneal inversion and lower extremity external rotation always indicate supination. The height of the medial longitudinal arch increases and the lateral indentation about the calcaneocuboid articulation disappears since the forefoot is adducting in relation to the rearfoot.

A very effective clinical tool can be easily constructed to appreciate subtalar joint motion as well as the translatory motion performed about the tibia during gait. The materials required include: two small rods, approximately ⅛ inch in diameter (the circumference of a clothes hanger); small amounts of splinting material, enough to contain each rod securely and be molded about the tibial tuberosity of the leg and the dorsum of the talus of the foot; two long pieces of the pile Velcro; and four small pieces of the hook Velcro. The hook Velcro will be glued onto the splinting material. The pile Velcro can then attach to both ends of the splinting material to encompass either the calf or midfoot. Some additional small moldable disks can be fixed along the top of each rod if desired. These tools should then be strapped to the extremity via the Velcro, and the client should attempt normal gait with the evaluator observing forward progression. During pronation the rods will move toward the midline of the body because of tibial internal rotation and talar adduction (Fig. 14-21) and away from the midline during supination or tibial external rotation and talar abduction (Fig. 14-22).

Obviously, this is not a quantitative measuring technique; however, by using it, the examiner can note if the subtalar joint fails to supinate during the midstance and propulsive phases of gait. The technique also demonstrates the clear translatory motions produced proximally as a result of subtalar movement. Such devices are also good teaching tools for any clinic involved with gait analyses.

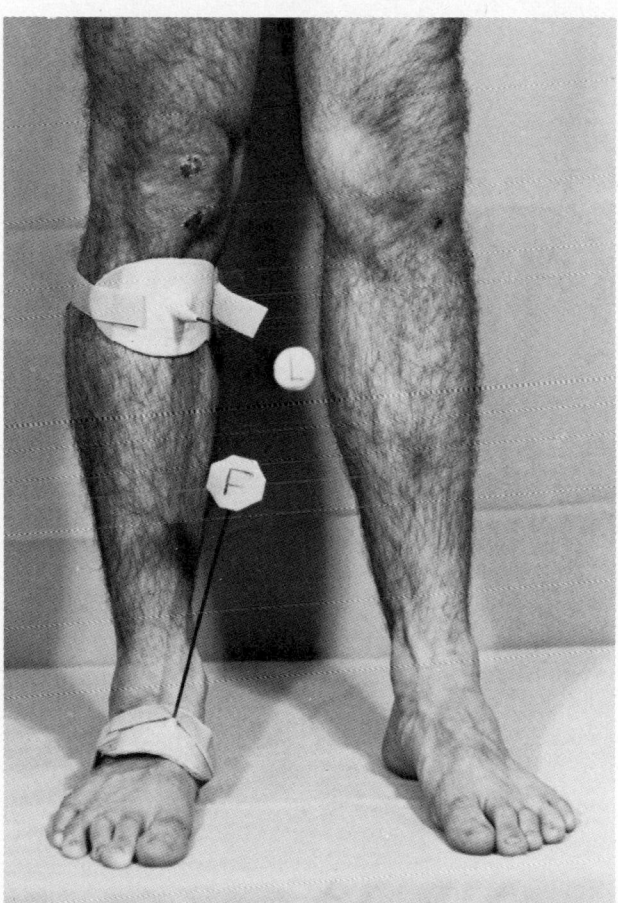

Fig. 14-21. Subtalar joint pronation with tibial internal rotation.

Radiographic characteristics determining foot position

This section will discuss the radiographic findings that describe the static foot positions during weight bearing. There are a wide variety of foot types, and total range of motion will vary. However, the static osseous structures

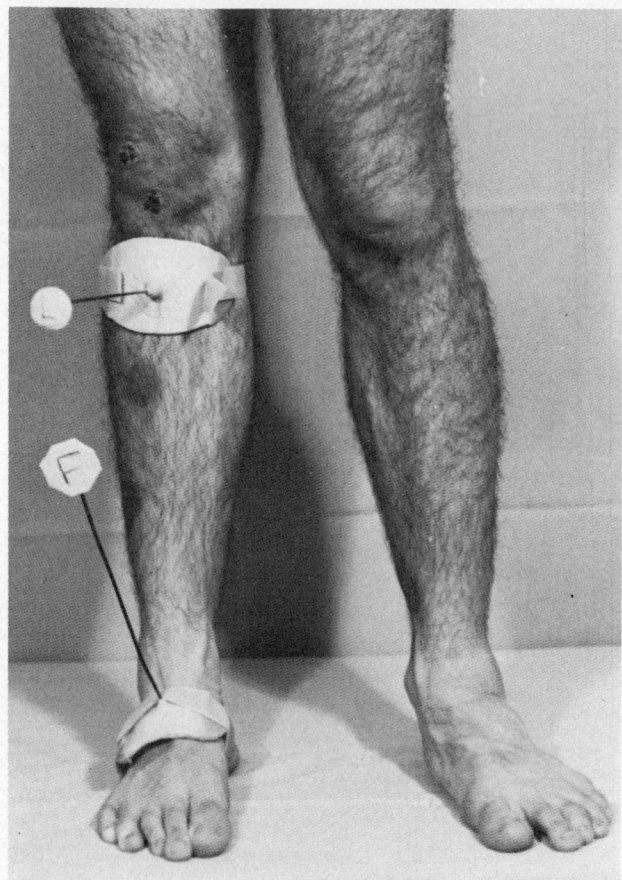

Fig. 14-22. Subtalar joint supination with tibial external rotation.

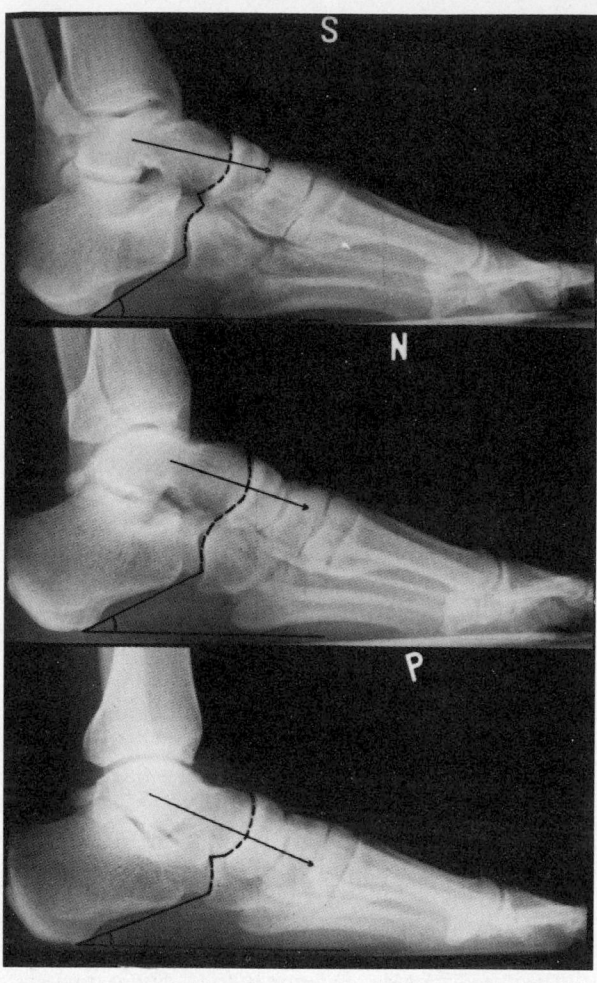

Fig. 14-23. Smooth S-shaped cyma line *(N)* demonstrating neutral subtalar position. Anterior break in cyma line *(P)* indicating subtalar joint pronation. Posterior break in cyma line *(S)* indicating subtalar joint supination.

will generally conform to a standard set of radiographic parameters.

A few of these parameters are visible in both anteroposterior and dorsoplantar and lateral views.

Lateral projection

The cyma line. This midtarsal joint line is formed by the talonavicular and calcaneocuboid joint surfaces.[15,20] Normally, if a line were drawn from the dorsum of the talonavicular joint down through the joint spaces to the base of the calcaneocuboid articulation, a smooth S curve would be formed depicting subtalar joint neutrality (Fig. 14-23, *N*). The term *broken cyma line* is used to denote incongruity between the joint surfaces.[15,44] A shift in this line either anteriorly or posteriorly represents motion or position of the subtalar joint. With pronation the talar head moves anteriorly as it adducts and plantar flexes, therefore creating an anterior break in the cyma line (Fig. 14-23, *P*). Conversely, with supination the talar head moves posteriorly as it abducts and dorsiflexes, creating a posterior break in the line (Fig. 14-23, *S*). This posterior break is not as evident on lateral views as is the anterior break. This broken line can be anterior or posterior with either the talonavicular or the calcaneocuboid articulations.

Talar declination angle. This angle is formed between the bisection of the head and neck of the talus and the weight-bearing surface (Fig. 14-23). The measurement provides an index of a decrease in pitch of the talus toward this weight-supporting surface.[20] Green, Sgarlato, and Wittenberg[15] report an average of 21 degrees for this angle. In pronation the head and neck of the talus move in a plantar direction. This bisection, when extended, will also move in a plantar direction in relation to the first metatarsal head, thereby increasing the talar declination angle (Fig. 14-23, *P*). Since the talar head and neck move dorsally with supination, the extended bisection of this osseous component will also move dorsally relative to the first metatarsal head, thereby decreasing the talar declination angle (Fig. 14-23, *S*).

Calcaneal inclination angle. This angle serves as an index of the pitch of the calcaneus above the weight-supporting plane.[20] The angle is measured from a line between the plantar aspect of the calcaneus and the plantar aspect of the fifth metatarsal head (Fig. 14-23). The aver-

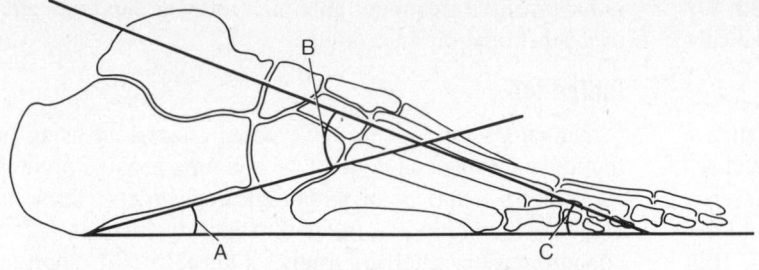

Fig. 14-24. Lateral talocalcaneal angle *(B)*, calcaneal inclination angle *(A)*, and talar declination angle *(C)*.

age angle ranges from 18 to 20 degrees.[15] Di Giovanni and Smith[12] report a larger average angle range of 17 to 32 degrees with a mean of 24.5 degrees. In pronation the inclination angle decreases since the body of the calcaneus will move toward the weight-bearing surface with eversion. Inversion shifts the calcaneal body upward, therefore increasing the pitch of the angle in relation to the weight-bearing surface. However, the significance of these angular changes associated with pronation and supination is challenged by Di Giovanni and Smith.[12] They report that the change in the calcaneal inclination angle is statistically insignificant and should not be used as the only index in the assessment of the flatfoot and/or cavus foot.

Lateral talocalcaneal angle. This angle is formed posteriorly by the intersection of a line bisecting the head and neck of the talus and a line extending from the plantar aspect of the calcaneus to its anteroinferior border (Fig. 14-24). This measurement is equal to the calcaneal inclination angle plus the talar declination angle.[12]

Hlavac[20] reports that this angle increases with pronation and decreases with supination. Mean calculated values for neutral, pronated, and supinated angles are 45.4, 50.3, and 41.8 degrees, respectively. These angular changes are directly related to the sagittal plane motion of the talus. The lateral talocalcaneal angle is considered to be an accurate parameter in assessing movement of the subtalar joint.

First ray complex (first metatarsal–first cuneiform articulation). The first ray complex will dorsiflex in relation to the navicular and talar segments during pronation. Conversely, it will plantar flex in relation to these same segments during supination. In the neutral weight-bearing position, the first ray will continue as a linear extension of the talonavicular articulation.

Anteroposterior or dorsoplantar projection

Longitudinal bisection of the lesser tarsus. Green, Sgarlato, and Wittenberg[15] measure this line by marking a point midway between the medial aspect of the first cuneonavicular articulation and the medial aspect of the talonavicular articulation. Another mark is placed midway between the lateral aspect of the calcaneocuboid articulation and the lateral aspect of the fifth metatarsocuboid articulation. These two points are connected, and a perpendicular line drawn to the midpoint of the base of the second metatarsal is the longitudinal bisection of the lesser tarsus (Fig. 14-25, *A*).

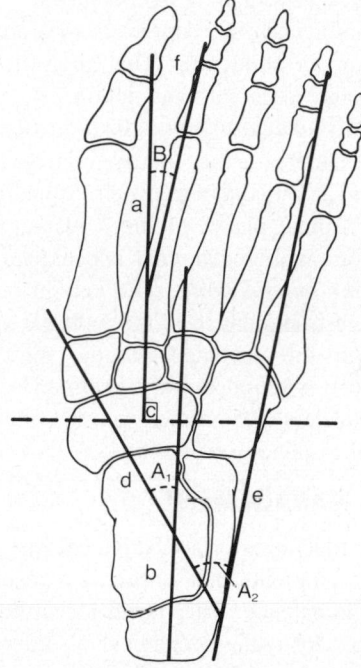

Fig. 14-25. Ninety-degree angle *(C)* formed by longitudinal bisection of lesser tarsus. Talocalcaneal angle *(A₁)* formed by intersection of long axis of calcaneus and talar head-neck bisection. Alternative measurement of the talocalcaneal angle *(A₂)* by Di Giovanni and Smith and metatarsus adductus angle *(B)*.

Long axis of the calcaneus. The long axis is formed by a line connecting the bisection of the posterior aspect of the calcaneus to the anteromedial dorsal aspect of the calcaneus (Fig. 14-25, *B*). The lines formed will now be used with additional bisections to form other positional angulations.

Talocalcaneal angle. The talocalcaneal angle is formed by the line bisecting the head and neck of the talus (Fig. 14-25, *D*) and the long axis of the calcaneus (angle A_1, Fig. 14-25, *B*). The average values for this angle range from 15 to 18 degrees.[15] With adduction and plantar flexion of the talus pronation, this angle will increase. Abduction and dorsiflexion of the talus during supination will decrease the angle. Di Giovanni and Smith[12] report that the longitudinal bisection of the rearfoot and the calcaneus is difficult to visualize in the dorsoplantar view. An alternative method is possible using an angle formed by the bisection of the head and neck of the talus (Fig. 14-25, *D*) and a line running parallel to the lateral surface of the calcaneus (angle A_2, Fig. 14-25, *E*).

Metatarsal angle. The metatarsal angle is formed between the long axis of the second metatarsal head (line *f* passing from the center of the base of the second metatarsal and extending through a point dividing the transverse distance across the neck of the second metatarsal) and the bisection of the lesser tarsus (angle *B*, Fig. 14-25, *A*). This angle generally favors adduction of 10 to 20 degrees in most feet, with an average of 14.5 degrees.[15,20] The metatarsus angle influences the degree of forefoot position in either abduction or adduction. This angle decreases with pronation and increases with supination.

Shape of the navicular bone. In pronation the navicular bone demonstrates a long rectangular appearance seen from the dorsal and medial aspects. In supination this bone rotates in the frontal plane, giving a plantar medial view and thus a short, wide rectangular appearance.

Shape of the cuboid bone. The cuboid bone becomes wider and more triangular in shape with the apex pointing distally when in the supinated attitude. With the foot pronated, the bone is rounded and less broad.

These parameters are outlined to assist the evaluator in biomechanical evaluation of the foot.

ORTHOTIC MANAGEMENT

The use of functional orthotics is necessary in the treatment of foot symptoms that occur as a result of biomechanical foot imbalance. The functional orthotic device is designed to control pathomechanical disorders in the foot and leg by maintaining the foot approximately in a neutral position. Bates et al[2] have demonstrated that orthotic devices create adjustments in the mechanical function of the foot, thus emulating normal gait activity.

The functional orthotic device should not be considered an arch support (or navicular pad) because control is maintained by applying pressure under the metatarsal shafts (proximal to the metatarsal heads) or under the calcaneus. In essence, the orthotic device transposes the floor to the plantar surface of the foot so that the neutral position can be maintained through prevention of compensatory pronation. James, Bates, and Osternig[23] have referred to the orthotic device as a "shim" positioned between the foot and the shoe. Thus the orthotic device, if properly fabricated, can act to increase the efficiency of foot mechanics during walking or running.

Commercially available appliances can prove useful if the client only requires a navicular and/or metatarsal pad or an antifriction component within the shoe. However, because commercially made devices are mass produced, they cannot be expected to correct a biomechanical imbalance within the foot (i.e., forefoot varus or forefoot valgus). If, after biomechanical evaluation, the client's symptoms can be identified as resulting from a biomechanical

imbalance, the treatment approach must be the fabrication of a functional orthotic device.

Indications

Numerous researchers have noted success in using orthotic devices as components of a comprehensive program for treating a variety of pathological disorders. These include back and hip pain related to foot dysfunction.[19,32,33] chondromalacia patellae,[6] runner's knee,[3,23,25,43] short-leg syndrome,[47] shin splints (posteromedial),[9,13,23] Morton's neuroma,[19,27,50] myofacial pain syndrome,[24] and anterotarsal syndrome.[8]

However, the only indication for a functional orthotic device is a structural foot imbalance (i.e., forefoot varus, forefoot valgus, or rearfoot varus), which in a majority of cases is the primary cause of the pathological conditions just mentioned.

Functional orthotic devices may also be indicated for the individual with a rigid pes cavus, or high-arched foot. These clients lack necessary shock absorption because of a limited range of pronation. While the use of rigid appliances has shown only limited success, the use of semirigid orthoses appears to be better tolerated by clients with this foot classification.[19,23]

Contraindications

Two main contraindications for dispensing an orthotic device are:

1. *Compensatory pronation secondary to a functional equinus disorder of the ankle joint.* In most cases the cause of an equinus deformity is decreased ankle-joint dorsiflexion, resulting from a reduction in the length of the gastrocnemius muscle. The treatment of choice in such clients is an intensive stretching program for the calf muscle group.
2. *An improperly performed biomechanical evaluation.* To attain any positive result from orthotic treatment, one must be certain that the evaluation is precise and that the neutral position cast of the foot is correct.

The following principles should also be considered when determining the proper orthotic prescription:

1. In general, clients with a supinatory foot type (i.e., rigid forefoot valgus or uncompensated rearfoot varus) do very poorly with rigid orthotic control. This group appears to do much better with a semirigid appliance that provides increased shock absorption.
2. The rigid orthotic device, with its narrow base (especially the medial border that bisects the shaft of the first metatarsal), provides less than favorable results in clients demonstrating an extreme forefoot varus or athletes participating in lateral movement sports (i.e., football, basketball, or volleyball). In

both cases the foot has a tendency to slide off the orthotic device during midstance because of the narrowed support base. In a majority of clients the semirigid orthotic device is more appropriate because its broadened medial and lateral flares can prevent the occurrence of sliding. Therefore foot control can be maintained comfortably at midstance.

Orthotic classification

Orthotic devices vary in their design, size, and shape. Additionally, variations exist as a result of the different types of material used in fabrication. The categorization of orthotic devices depends on the degree of rigidity as well as the process necessary for fabrication. The standard classifications for orthotic devices include soft (flexible), semirigid, and rigid (Fig. 14-26).[19]

Soft devices.   The soft insert is designed to provide accommodative support to the structures of the foot without biomechanical posting or balancing. No attempt is made to place the foot in the neutral position when casting is performed. Fabrication of this type of appliance can be done directly on the foot with heated materials or can be "cold molded" within the shoe. As would be expected, since softer substances are used in construction, these materials compress or "bottom out" after short intervals of time (3 to 6 months) and must be periodically replaced.

Semirigid devices.   The semirigid orthotic device incorporates softness while providing a rigid support for biomechanical control. This device is fabricated over a cast of the foot in a neutral position using various combinations of leather, cork, and thermoplastic substances for construction. The semirigid type of functional control is classified as extrinsic posting. *Extrinsic posting* differs from cast preparation for a rigid orthotic device in that no modifications are made on the neutral position cast. Rather, the rearfoot and forefoot posts are formed by the addition of materials under either the calcaneus or the metatarsal shifts. Since two or three layers of materials are required in fabrication, the placement of this type of orthosis into an oxford or athletic type shoe is rarely a problem. The advantage of extrinsic posting over intrinsic posting of the rigid orthosis is that modifications can be made by removing material once the semirigid device is completed.

Rigid devices.   The rigid orthotic device is the most unyielding of the three classifications discussed. The rigid device is usually fabricated from a single layer of heat-moldable plastic approximately ⅛ to ³⁄₁₆ inch in thickness. The strength of the plastic material allows for a rigid rearfoot or forefoot support with only a minimal amount of material. However, unlike the semirigid extrinsically posted device, the rigid orthosis requires extensive modification of the neutral position cast of the foot. The term *intrinsic posting* refers to the detailed plaster additions superimposed on the neutral foot cast. Thus functional control is achieved through the modification of the plaster cast rather than by increasing material as in the semirigid orthotic device. The intrinsic posting technique allows minimal marginal latitude for error in rigid orthotic fabrication. Any discrepancy in evaluation or in the neutral cast modifications will produce an unacceptable fit for the client.

In summary, the selection of the appropriate orthotic device depends on a number of contributing factors, including the client's foot type, sports participation, and age. Wide disagreement exists among professionals as to which type of orthosis is best to use. While each orthotic device has its advantages and disadvantages, the final decision should be based on evaluation of the individual.

FABRICATION OF ORTHOTIC DEVICES

A semirigid or rigid orthosis can provide effective functional control if properly fabricated. However, proper fabrication requires the following: (1) ability to perform a bi-

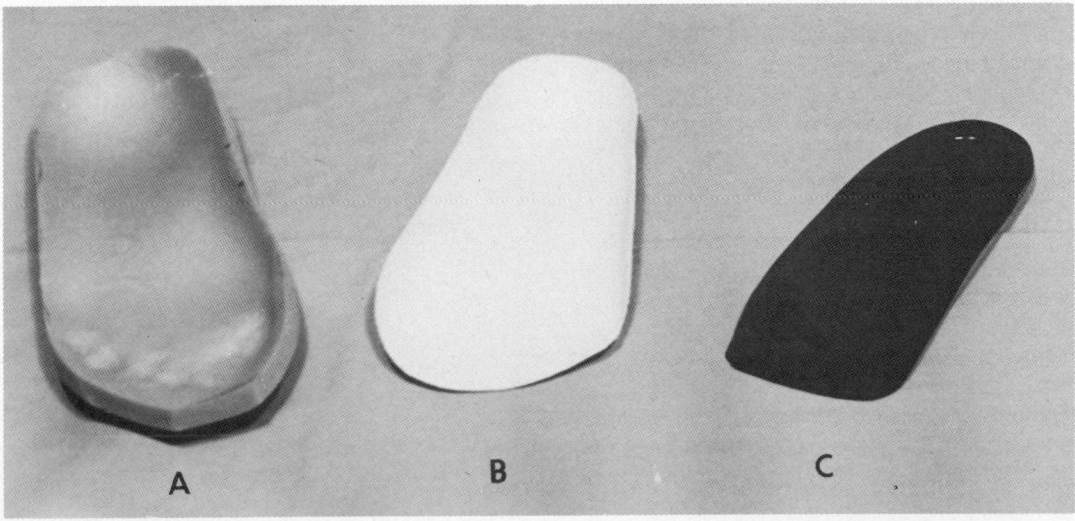

Fig. 14-26. Major classifications of orthotic devices; **A,** soft (flexible); **B,** semirigid; **C,** rigid.

omechanical evaluation and to correctly fabricate a molded plaster neutral cast (both of which require intensive practice for skill development); (2) experience in the use of various kinds of thermoplastic materials; (3) clinical time for fabrication (1½ hours for the experienced therapist to 3 hours for the novice); (4) initial capital outlay for materials and equipment (over $1200); and (5) a separate work space. These factors (especially appropriate neutral position casting and fabrication skills) preclude many clinics and practitioners from attempting the fabrication of a semirigid or rigid orthotic device.

Following is a description of the concepts of orthotic fabrication and construction procedures (including neutral casting) for a semirigid orthotic device (see box on page 316). However, caution must be observed since simply following illustrations or written directions may not necessarily lead to satisfactory results.

The second procedure described—the *immediate clinical orthotic device* or *cobra pad*—is offered as a realistic alternative for first attempts at orthotic construction (see box on page 318). Fabrication of the cobra pad requires no cast, minimal supplies, and a reduced fabrication time.

Semirigid orthotic device

Neutral cast technique. The fabrication of a semirigid orthotic device requires obtaining a neutral-position plaster impression of the foot. The application of an appropriate casting technique is essential in the production of a satisfactory, comfortable orthosis. The purpose of the neutral casting technique is to reproduce that position of the foot that should ideally occur at midstance (i.e., the neutral foot position).[36]

Numerous casting techniques have been developed to best capture the neutral foot position. These include sus-

---

Neutral casting: prone technique

Positioning

1. The client is placed in a prone position with the leg to be casted internally rotated to place the calcaneus in the frontal plane (see Fig. 14-10).
2. No plaster parting agent is used so the skin lines may be readily detected once the cast is removed.

Supplies

1. Two plaster of Paris splints, 5 × 30 inches, folded in half. Once wet, each 5 × 15 inch splint is again folded approximately ¼ inch on the proximal border to facilitate cast removal.

Cast preparation
Procedure

1. The first splint is placed in a U fashion over the calcaneus and the medial and lateral aspects of the foot. The plaster is molded smoothly along the plantar surface as well (Fig. 14- 27).
2. The second splint is also placed in a U fashion, starting from the tips of the toes and again encompassing the medial and lateral aspects of the foot (Fig. 14-28). Care must be taken not to compress the toes as the plaster is applied. The plaster should be carefully molded, especially over the plantar aspect of the foot, while it is still moist.
3. Once the two plaster splints are molded in place, the caster should grasp the fourth and fifth metatarsal heads, while at the same time palpating the head of the talus. When the neutral position of the subtalar joint is determined, the midtarsal joint is locked by dorsiflexing the foot till resistance is met. At the same time an abductory force is applied to prevent possible supination (Fig. 14-29). (*Note:* The caster must constantly palpate the head of the talus to maintain the neutral position of the subtalar joint.)

4. Precautions must be taken during the entire procedure to prevent extrinsic muscular contraction, especially of the anterior tibial muscle, which, if contracted, could produce a false forefoot varus impression.
5. When dry, the cast is removed by grasping the plaster over the calcaneus, pulling the cast off the heel, and finally gliding it over the toes.

Model preparation

1. The neutral position cast will now become the negative model for the positive mold of the foot (Fig. 14-30). Before pouring the positive mold, the neutral cast is lined with a plaster parting agent, either powder or liquid soap. The positive model is then poured and the plaster allowed to dry (approximately 24 hours).
2. Once hardened, the original neutral cast is removed, leaving a positive impression of the individual's foot.
3 The area of finger indentation over the fourth and fifth metatarsals is filled with plaster to provide a smooth level surface.
4. The positive model is then carefully and gently smoothed using sand-screen* or fine sandpaper. Only rough edges and skin lines should be removed to prevent model distortion.
5. Once smoothing is completed orthotic fabrication can be initiated.

---

*Fillauer Orthopedic, PO Box 1678, Chattanooga, Tenn 37401.

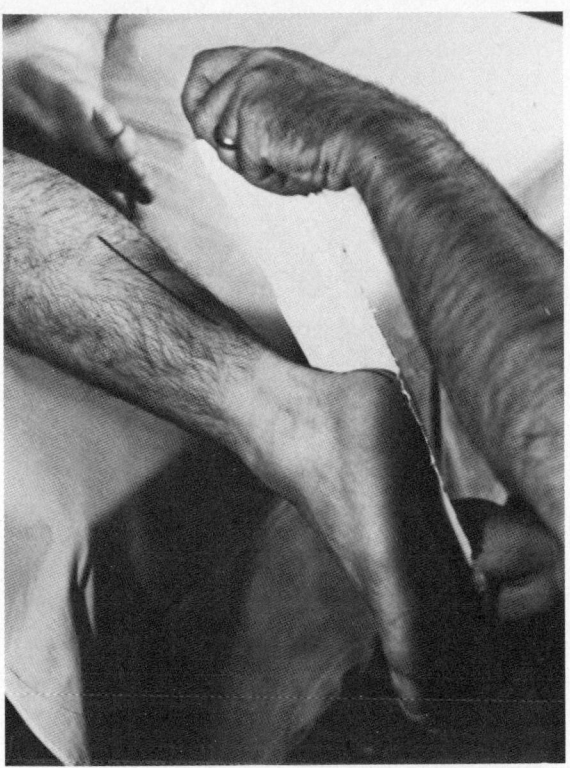

Fig. 14-27. Initial splint in neutral position cast technique, placed over calcaneus and molded smoothly over entire plantar surface.

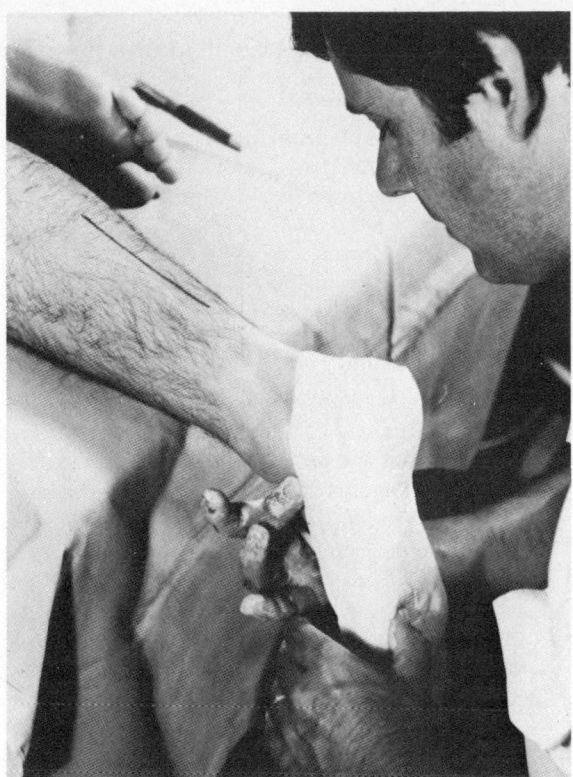

Fig. 14-29. Neutral position palpated and midtarsal joint locked once splints are appropriately placed.

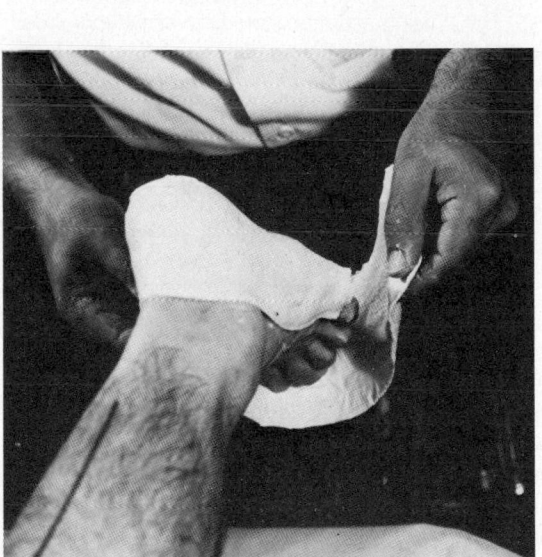

Fig. 14-28. Second splint started from toes and molded smoothly over medial, lateral, and plantar aspects of foot.

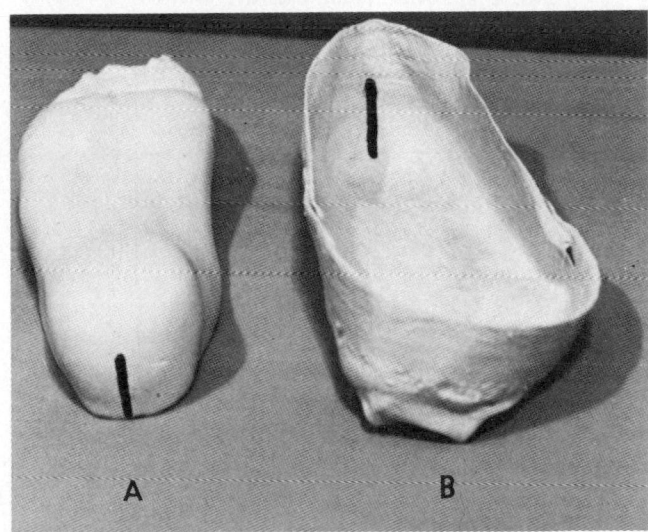

Fig. 14-30. A, Positive mold of foot derived from negative neutral position cast; **B,** Note calcaneal bisection visible in both.

pension, prone, and semi–weight-bearing techniques. Valmassy[52] has provided an excellent synopsis of the various casting techniques. Although all three techniques have their inherent advantages and disadvantages, only the prone technique will be outlined (see box on page 314). Recent research has indicated that the same forefoot to

hindfoot alignment can be obtained using either the suspension or prone casting techniques, but not with the semi–weight-bearing method.[30] However, the semi–weight-bearing technique would produce an acceptable foot model if the goal of treatment was an accommodative foot orthosis not designed to balance a forefoot deformity.

Semirigid orthotic device: construction technique

Supplies/fabrication needs

1. An oven capable of reaching a temperature of 138° C (280.4° F), a bench grinder for sanding, a form press,* and a knife or scissors (Fig. 14-31).
2. Aliplast 10* (⅛ inch)
3. Pelite firm* (³⁄₁₆ inch)
4. Thermocork† (¼ inch)
5. Rubber cement or Barge†

Fabrication technique

1. The neutral cast is positioned on the form press.
2. Aliplast 10 (15 × 27 cm) is used to form the first layer next to the cast and assist in reducing friction between the foot and the orthotic device. It is heated to the appropriate temperature, then placed over the cast and pressed into position until cool (approximately 30 seconds).
3. Once cooled, the Aliplast 10 is covered with rubber cement. The Pelite firm layer (15 × 27 cm), which provides shock absorption, is also coated with rubber cement, and when dry, is heated and bonded to the Aliplast 10 via the form press.
4. The Thermocork (12 × 20 cm), which provides the actual post in the orthosis, is the final layer to be bonded once the initial two layers have cooled (for approximately 3 to 5 minutes). The Pelite firm layer is coated with rubber cement while the Thermocork is placed in the oven. When pliable, the Thermocork is removed and placed over the Pelite firm. Before pressing, cellophane must be placed over the Thermocork to prevent it from sticking to the rubber bladder of the press.

5. After cooling, the cast with all three material layers is removed from the press and is allowed to set for 24 hours.
6. Grinding can begin at the end of 24 hours.

Grinding procedure

1. Before grinding, the calcaneus is bisected on the cast.
2. The first step involves grinding the medial and lateral sides of the orthotic device so they are parallel to the bisection of the calcaneus (Fig. 14-32).
3. The grinding procedure continues with the bisection of the calcaneus aligned perpendicularly to the sanding drum. While maintaining that position, the cork material is removed until a white spot (Pelite) appears under the calcaneus (Fig. 14-33).
4. Then, still maintaining the perpendicular attitude of the calcaneus in relationship to the grinder, Thermocork is removed from the forefoot. The amount of material removed depends on the deformity to be posted (i.e., in a forefoot varus, cork will remain under the medial aspect of the metatarsal shafts with the reverse true in a forefoot valgus deformity).
5. Before undertaking the final grind, a line must be drawn approximately 1 cm proximal to the heads of the first and fifth metatarsals. These lines, when connected on the material, indicate the maximum distal point for the post. The posting material should *never* extend under the heads of the metatarsals. Once this line is established, the remaining trim lines can be derived either through rough estimate or by placing the shoe insole over the bottom of the orthosis and outlining it (Fig. 14-34).

*Alimed, 138 Prince Street, Boston, Mass 02113.
†Apex Foot Products, 200 Forest Avenue, Englewood, NJ 07631.

The final selection of the most suitable casting technique is dependent on the treatment goals and individual preference.

Orthotic fitting. Just as in wearing new shoes, the orthoses should be broken in by having the client wear them 2 hours the first day and increasing wearing time 1 hour daily thereafter. Sports activity should not be attempted until the client is comfortably wearing the orthoses 6 to 8 hours per day. The client should be seen for at least one, and preferably two, follow-up visits to determine if there is any discomfort after the orthoses have been worn for 2 weeks.

The immediate clinical orthotic device

The immediate clinical orthotic device or cobra pad is a modification of a treatment technique originated by Hlavac[20] at the California college of Podiatric Medicine. The cobra pad can provide effective in-shoe management of foot problems, keeping the time required for fabrication

and the cost of supplies to a minimum. If doubt exists as to whether or not a semirigid or rigid orthotic device is indicated, the cobra pad can provide temporary biomechanical control to ascertain if there is any condition improvement. In many cases, especially if well-constructed oxford or athletic shoes are available, the cobra pad can provide effective foot control without the need for more definitive orthotic management.

Orthotic fitting. While a break-in period for the cobra pad is recommended, the duration suggested is not as stringent as that needed for the semirigid orthotic device.

The following case studies illustrate the use of a biomechanical approach in the treatment of foot and ankle dysfunction.

CASE STUDY 1

G.S., a 42-year-old female physical education instructor, after returning to full-time work, started to experience left heel pain. She saw a physician after the pain continued for 2 months. A

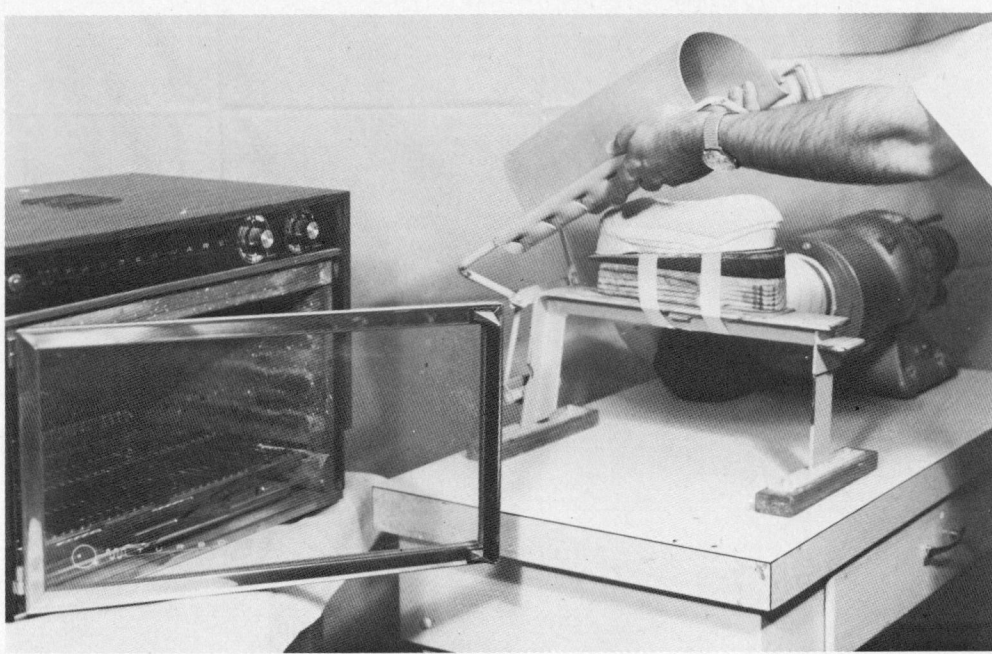

Fig. 14-31. Equipment required for semirigid orthosis fabrication includes oven, form press, and bench grinder for sanding.

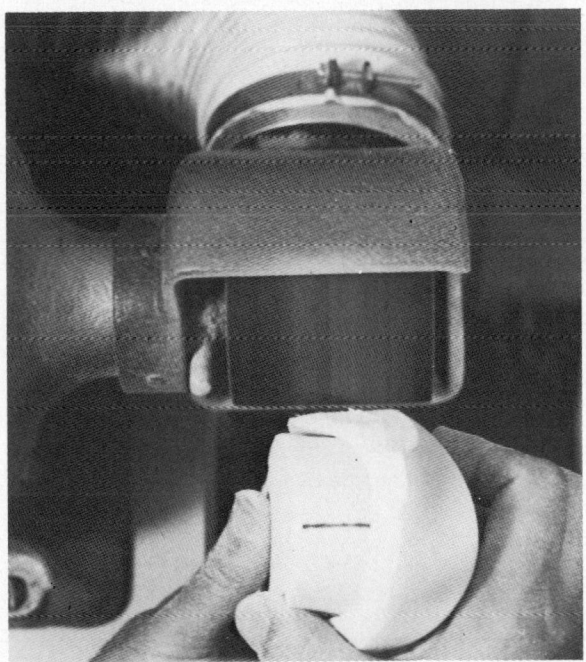

Fig. 14-32. Grinding of medial and lateral aspects of orthosis.

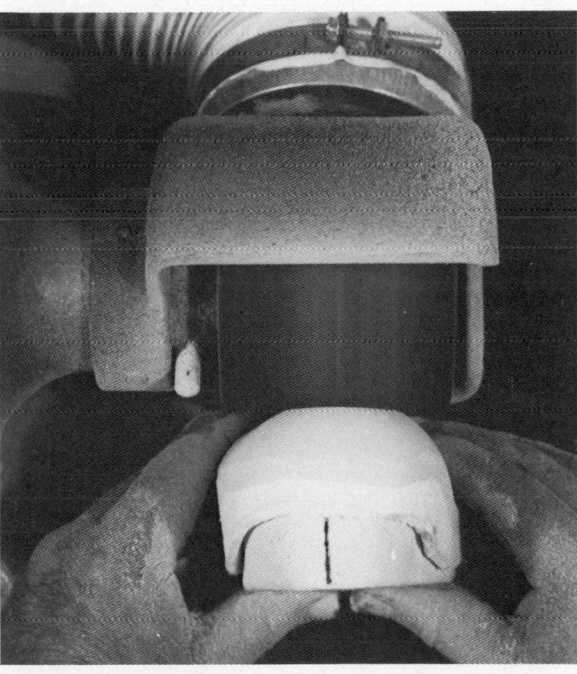

Fig. 14-33. Grinding of plantar surface of orthosis. Note calcaneal bisection is held perpendicular to sanding disk.

diagnosis of plantar fasciitis was made, and an oral antiinflammatory agent was prescribed. Although the medication gave moderate relief, symptoms reappeared as soon as the medication was discontinued. After reevaluation by a physician, the client was referred to physical therapy for foot evaluation.

At the time of initial evaluation, the client complained of constant heel pain while standing or active. Palpation of the left calcaneus revealed that the point of predominate tenderness was not on the plantar surface of the calcaneus but actually was located more anteriorly at the insertion of the plantar fascia. Biomechanical evaluation demonstrated normal findings in the hip, knee, and ankle joints.

A subtalar varus of 4 degrees was noted bilaterally with no tibia vara observed. However, an 8-degree forefoot varus was present on the left, while a 2-degree forefoot valgus was measured on the right. The gait evaluation demonstrated a greater

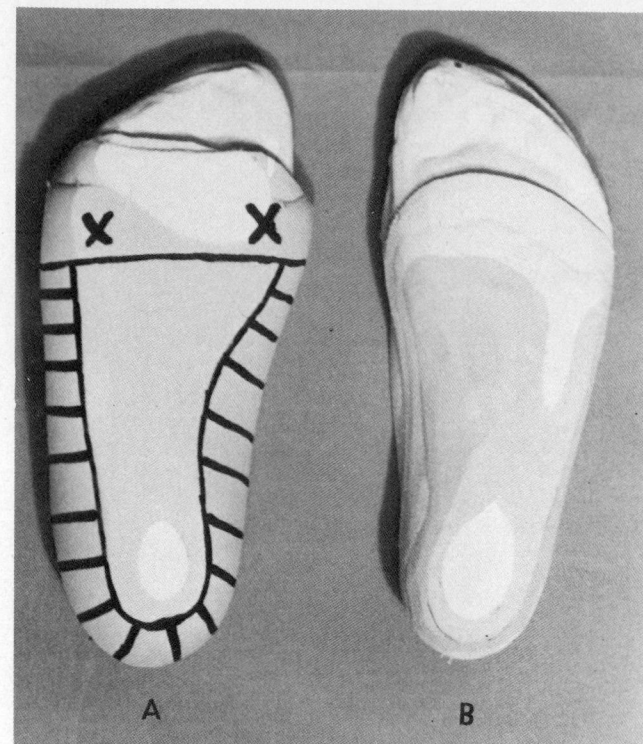

Fig. 14-34. A, Trim lines for final grind with crosses (Xs) representing first and fifth metatarsal heads. **B,** Finished product.

Cobra pad technique

Supplies

1. Spenco*
2. Adhesive felt or Pelite firm* layer (³⁄₁₆ inch)
3. Knife for skiving felt or grinder for Pelite
4. Rubber cement or Barge†

Fabrication procedure

1. Once the evaluation is completed, the client or athlete is placed in the long-sitting position on the plinth.
2. Spenco inlays are cut to fit the shape of the shoe last. If old insoles are present in the shoe, these can be removed and used as a template for cutting new inlays.
3. The inlays are then positioned over the client's foot and, using a broad-tipped felt pen, the posterior aspects of the first and second metatarsal heads are outlined (Fig. 14-35). This marking will serve to designate the farthest point for placement of the posting material.

4. Adhesive felt or Pelite is then cut to provide a post under the shafts of the first and second metatarsals as well as some degree of heel stabilization.
5. The felt or Pelite is then skived or sanded as in Fig. 14-36 to allow a smooth interface between the foot and shoe. These modifications are more easily performed if the felt or Pelite is attached to the Spenco.
6. When completed, the client should walk and then run to determine whether further modifications are necessary. (*Note:* The cobra pad fabrication procedure described is designed for a forefoot varus deformity. For a forefoot valgus classification, the pad design should be reversed.)

---

*Alimed, 138 Prince Street, Boston, Mass 02113.
†Apex Foot Products, 200 Forest Avenue, Englewood, NJ 07631.

---

amount of subtalar joint pronation on the left as compared to the right.

The impression from the evaluation was that the plantar fasciitis resulted from the excessive subtalar joint pronation present in the left foot. Semirigid orthoses were fabricated with forefoot posts to correct the deformities present.

On reevaluation after 4 weeks of wear, the client reported a 98% improvement in pain with a reduction noted in lower ex-

tremity fatigue. A 2-month followup revealed only a slight amount of heel pain after several hours of constant activity.

CASE STUDY **2**

N.J., a 39-year-old female distance runner, was referred by her physician for biomechanical evaluation and treatment. The chief complaint was left lateral knee pain with onset occurring 2

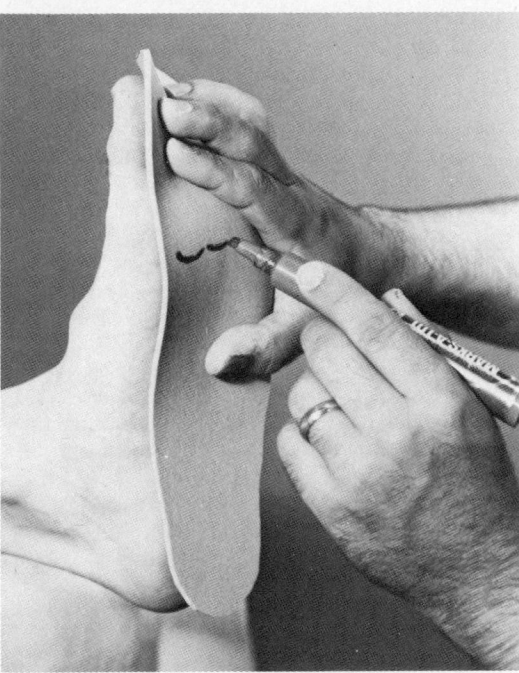

Fig. 14-35. Marking first and second metatarsal heads for determining farthest placement of posting material.

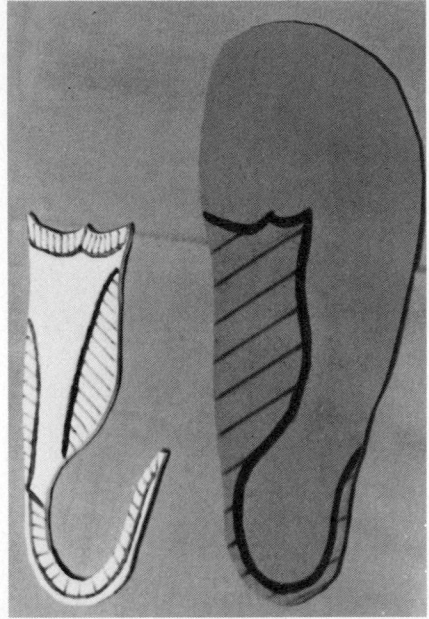

Fig. 14-36. Posting material sanded in those areas lined and then glued in place as outlined on Spenco.

miles into her workout. The client stated that the pain started 2 weeks after she increased her weekly mileage from 25 miles per week to 35 miles per week. At the time of initial evaluation, the symptoms had been present for 1 month. The client had undergone physical therapy, including ultrasound and cryotherapy, for 3 weeks with only a minimal reduction in symptoms.

Palpation demonstrated only minimal tenderness over the lateral aspect of the patellofemoral joint with normal patellar mobility. Knee joint instability and menisci tests proved negative. The biomechanical evaluation revealed normal range of motion throughout the entire lower extremity with excellent flexibility. No leg-length discrepancy was noted. Subtalar joint examination revealed a 5-degree subtalar varum on the left with 1 degree noted on the right. Six degrees of tibia vara were measured bilaterally. The evaluation of the midtarsal joint disclosed a 5-degree forefoot valgus bilaterally. Gait evaluation demonstrated inverted calcanei until immediately after midstance, when pronation occurred bilaterally with greater eversion of the left foot. Assessment of the results of the evaluation revealed the cause of the left lateral knee pain to be late, excessive pronation of the left foot.

Semirigid orthoses, with appropriate forefoot and rearfoot posts, were fabricated and given to the client. After the normal break-in period, the client reported a moderate reduction in symptoms during the first week of running. The client was asymptomatic after the second week of wear. After using the orthotic devices for 6 months, the client remained asymptomatic while running 30 to 40 miles per week.

SUMMARY

This chapter has introduced the concepts of biomechanical evaluation and treatment of the foot. It should be stressed that the foot is only one component in an entire closed kinetic chain and is by no means the key to all disorders affecting the lower extremity. However, abnormal pedal pathomechanics, caused by structural imbalances, can not only present symptoms in the foot but also in the proximal joints of the lower extremities.

The information presented in this chapter should provide a strong foundation for treatment, as well as an awareness of lower extremity dysfunction, for the physical therapist who is evaluating a dysfunction, whether the cause is related to an orthopaedic condition or sports activity. While there is no substitute for experience, it is hoped that this chapter will provide the stimulus for further study as well as improved clinical treatment of the foot and ankle.

REFERENCES

1. American Academy of Orthopaedic Surgeons: Joint motion: method of measuring and recording, Chicago, 1965.
2. Bates BT et al: Foot orthotic devices to modify selected aspects of lower extremity mechanics, Am J Sports Med 7:338, 1979.
3. Bogdan RJ, Jenkins D, and Hyland T: The runner's knee syndrome. In Rinaldi RR and Sabia M, editors: Sports medicine, Mount Kisco, NY, 1978, Futura Publishing Co, pp. 159- 177.
4. Bresnahan TP and Redmond CT: Injuries to the leg, J Am Podiatry Assoc 69:577, 1979.
5. Brunnstrom S: Clinical kinesiology, ed 3, Philadelphia, 1972, FA Davis Co.
6. Buchbinder MR, Napora NJ, and Biggs EW: The relationship of abnormal pronation to chondromalacia of the patella in distance running, J Am Podiatry Assoc 69:159, 1979.
7. Calliet R: Foot and ankle pain, Philadelphia, 1972, FA Davis Co.
8. Cangialosi CP and Schnall SJ: The biomechanical aspects of anterior tarsal tunnel syndrome, J Am Podiatry Assoc 70:291, 1980.
9. Clancy WG: Runner's injuries: evaluation and treatment of specific injuries, Am J Sports Med 8:287, 1980.
10. Coleman WC: Personal communication, 1980.
11. Demeter A and Gagea A: Biomechanics and physique. In Williams

JGP and Sperryn PN, editors: Sports medicine, ed 2, Baltimore, 1976, Williams & Wilkins.

12. Di Giovanni, JE and Smith SD: Normal biomechanics of the adult rearfoot: a radiographic analysis, J Am Podiatry Assoc 66:812, 1976.

13. Donovan JC et al: New England Deaconess Hospital podiatry service, J Am Podiatry Assoc 69:571, 1979.

14. Elftman H: The transverse tarsal joint and its control, Clin Ortho 61:423, 1971.

15. Green DR, Sgarlato TE, and Wittenberg M: Clinical biomechanical evaluation of the foot: a preliminary radiocinetographic study, J Am Podiatry Assoc 65:732, 1975.

16. Green DR, Whitney AK, and Walters P: Subtalar joint motion, J Am Podiatry Assoc 69:83, 1979.

17. Hicks JC: The mechanics of the foot: the joints, J Anat 87:345, 1953.

18. Hlavac HF: Differences in x-ray findings with varied positions of the foot, J Am Podiatry Assoc 57:465, 1967.

19. Hlavac HF: Compensated forefoot varus, J Am Podiatry Assoc 60:229, 1970.

20. Hlavac HF: The foot book, Mountain View, Calif, 1977, World Publications.

21. Inman VT: The human foot, Manitoba Med Rev 46:513, 1966.

22. Inman VT: The joints of the ankle, Baltimore, 1976, Williams & Wilkins.

23. James SL, Bates BT, and Osternig LR: Injuries to runners, Am J Sports Med 6:40, 1978.

24. Louis JM and Naftolin NH: Myofascial pain syndrome in the foot, J Am Podiatry Assoc 70:89, 1980.

25. Lutter L: Injuries in the runner and jogger, Minn Med 63:45, 1980.

26. Manter JT: Movements of the subtalar and transverse tarsal joints, Anat Rec 80:397, 1941.

27. Marshall RN: Foot mechanics and joggers' injuries, NZ Med J 88:288, 1978.

28. McCluskey GM, Blackburn TM, and Lewis T: Prevention of ankle sprains, Am J Sports Med 4:151, 1976.

29. McPoil T, Knecht H, and Schuit D: A survey of foot types in normal females between the ages of 18 to 30 years, J Orth Sports Phys Ther 9:406, 1988.

30. McPoil T, Schuit D, and Knecht H: A comparison of three neutral foot impression procedures in women 19 to 30 years of age, Phys Ther 69:448, 1989.

31. McPoil T, Schuit D, and Knecht H: A comparison of three positions used to evaluate tibial varum, J Am Podiatric Med Assoc 78:421-429, 1988.

32. Mennell JM: Foot pain, Boston, 1969, Little, Brown & Co.

33. Mirkin G and Hoffman M: The sports medicine book, Boston, 1978, Little, Brown & Co.

34. Morris JM: Biomechanics of the foot and ankle, Clin Orthop 122:10, 1977.

35. Murray MP, Drought AB, and Kory RC: Walking patterns in normal men, J Bone Joint Surg (Am) 46:335, 1964.

36. Root ML, Orien WP, and Weed JH: Neutral position casting techniques, Los Angeles, 1971, Clinical Biomechanics Corp.

37. Root ML, Orien WP, and Weed JH: Clinical biomechanics: normal and abnormal function of the foot, vol 2, Los Angeles, 1977, Clinical Biomechanics Corp.

38. Root ML et al: Axis of motion of the subtalar joint, J Am Podiatry Assoc 56:149, 1966.

39. Root ML et al: Biomechanical examination of the foot, vol 1, Los Angeles, 1971, Clinical Biomechanics Corp.

40. Sammarco GJ, Burstein AH, and Frankel VH: Biomechanics of the ankle: a kinematic study, Orthop Clin North Am 4:75, 1973.

41. Sarrafian SK: Anatomy of the foot and ankle, Philadelphia, 1983, JB Lippincott Co.

42. Schoenhaus HD and Jay RM: Cavus deformities: conservative management, J Am Podiatry Assoc 70:235, 1980.

43. Schuster RO: Podiatry and the foot of the athlete, J Am Podiatry Assoc 62:465, 1972.

44. Sgarlato TE: A compendium of podiatric biomechanics, San Francisco, 1971, California College of Podiatric Medicine Press.

45. Steindler A: Kinesiology of the human body under normal and pathological conditions, Springfield, Ill, 1970, Charles C Thomas, Publisher.

46. Subotnick SI: Equinus deformity as it affects the forefoot, J Am Podiatry Assoc 61:423, 1971.

47. Subotnick SI: Biomechanics of the subtalar and midtarsal joints, J Am Podiatry Assoc 65:756, 1975.

48. Subotnick SI: Podiatrics sports medicine, vol 4, Mount Kisco, NY, 1975, Futura Publishing Co, Inc.

49. Subotnick SI: Podiatric aspects of children in sports, J Am Podiatry Assoc 69:443, 1979.

50. Tate RO and Rusin JJ: Morton's neuroma: its ultrastructure, anatomy, and biomechanical etiology, J Am Podiatry Assoc 68:797, 1978.

51. Turek SL: Orthopaedics: principles and applications, ed 2, Philadelphia, 1967, JB Lippincott Co.

52. Valmassy RL: Advantages and disadvantages of various casting techniques, J Am Podiatry Assoc 69:707, 1979.

53. Weil LS et al: A biomechanical study of lateral ankle sprains in basketball, J Am Podiatry Assoc 69:687, 1979.

54. Wernick J and Langer S: A practical manual for a basic approach to biomechanics, Deer Park, NY, 1973, Langer Laboratories.

ADDITIONAL READINGS
Normal biomechanics and gait

Bates BT et al: Functional variability of the lower extremity during the support phase of running, Med Sci Sports Exerc 11:328, 1979.

Close JR et al: The function of the subtalar joint, Clin Orthop 50:159, 1967.

Elftman H: Dynamic structure of the human foot, Artif Limbs 13:49, 1969.

Gribbs RC and Boxer MC: The biomechanics of locomotion, J Dermatol Surg Oncol 6:252, 1980.

Hicks JH: The mechanics of the foot: the joints, J Anat 87:345, 1953.

Hicks JH: The mechanics of the foot: the plantar aponeurosis and arch, J Anat 88:25, 1954.

Hicks JH: The foot as a support, Acta Anat 25:34, 1955.

Inman VT: The influence of the foot-ankle complex on the proximal skeletal structures, Artif Limbs 13:59, 1969.

Jordan RP, Cooper M, and Schuster RO: Ankle dorsiflexion at the heel-off phase of gait, J Am Podiatry Assoc 69:40, 1979.

Mann RA: Surgical implications of the biomechanics of the foot and ankle, Clin Orthop 146:111, 1980.

Manter JT: Movements of the subtalar and transverse tarsal joints, Anat Rec 80:397, 1941.

Sanner WH et al: A study of ankle joint height changes with subtalar joint motion, J Am Podiatry Assoc 71:158, 1981.

Schoenhaus HD et al: Computerized analysis of gait, J Am Podiatry Assoc 69:11, 1979.

Pathomechanics and related injuries

Block P: A design to resolve the question of sports injury and foot type, J Am Podiatry Assoc 71:36, 1981.

Bodine KG: The subtalar joint and some related pathology, J Am Podiatry Assoc 60:205, 1970.

Botte RR: An interpretation of the pronation syndrome and foot types of patients with low back pain, J Am Podiatry Assoc 71:243, 1981.

Brody DM: Running injuries, Ciba Clinical Symposia 4:32, 1980.

Delacerda FG: The relationship of foot pronation, foot position, and electromyography of the anterior tibialis muscle in the subjects with different histories of shinsplints, J Orthop Sports Phys Ther 2:60, 1980.

Delacerda FG: A study of anatomical factors involved in shinsplints, J Orthop Sports Phys Ther 2:55, 1980.

Harris RI and Beath T: Hypermobile flatfoot with short tendo Achilles, J Bone Joint Surg (Am) 30:116, 1948.

Littetvedt J, Kreighbaum E, and Phillips RL: Analysis of selected alignment of the lower extremity related to the shinsplint syndrome, J Am Podiatry Assoc 69:211, 1979.

Massey EW and Pleet AB: Neuropathy in joggers, Am J Sports Med 6:209, 1978.

Mayfield GW: Popliteus tendon tenosynovitis, Am J Sports Med 5:31, 1977.

Miller BF and Buhr AJ: Pump bumps or knobbly heels, Nova Scotia Med Bull pp. 191-192, 1969.

Parlasca R, Shoji H, and D'Ambrosia, RD: Effects of ligamentous injury on ankle and subtalar joints: a kinematic study, Clin Orthop 140:266, 1979.

Renne JW: The iliotibial band friction syndrome, J Bone Joint Surg (Am) 57:1110, 1975.

Solcum DB: Overuse syndromes of the lower leg and foot in athletics, Am Acad Orthop Surg 17:359, 1960.

Solcum DB: The shinsplint syndrome, Am J Surg 114:875, 1967.

Subotnick SI: Orthotic foot control and the overuse syndrome, Phys Sports Med 3:75, 1975.

Tanz SS: The so-called tight heel cord, Clin Orthop 16:184, 1960.

Weiner BE, Ross AS, and Bogdan RJ: Biomechanical heel pain: a case study, J Am Podiatry Assoc 69:723, 1979.

Evaluation and management

Brown D and Smith C: Vacuum casting for foot orthoses, J Am Podiatry Assoc 66:582, 1976.

Burns MJ: Non–weight-bearing cast impressions for construction of orthotic devices, J Am Podiatry Assoc 67:790, 1977.

Donovan JC et al: New England Deaconess Hospital podiatry service: sports orthotic device, J Am Podiatry Assoc 69:571, 1979.

Keim HA and Ritchie GW: Weight-bearing roentgenograms in the evaluation of foot deformities, Clin Orthop 70:133, 1970.

MacLean KG: Photography of the plantar surface of the foot, Med Bio Illustr 27:141, 1977.

McGregor RR: The role of the podiatrist as first point practitioner in sports medicine, J Am Podiatry Assoc 70:54, 1980.

Subotnick SI: Case history of unilateral short leg with athletic overuse injury, J Am Podiatry Assoc 70:255, 1980.

Weed JH, Ratliff FD, and Ross SA: A biplanar grind for rear posts on functional orthoses, J Am Podiatry Assoc 68:35, 1978.

Chapter 15

THE KNEE

Lynn A. Wallace
Robert E. Mangine
Terry R. Malone

The frequency and severity of knee injuries in organized and recreational sports and in industry are well documented.[1,4,5] In American football, the knee is the most commonly injured joint.[5] Available data indicate that many of these injuries are preventable.[7,26,56] Many "overuse" knee injuries, which arc common in noncontact sports, are also predictable and preventable.[51] Unfortunately, many of these macro- and microtraumatic knee injuries tend to recur, indicating that optimal treatment was not rendered.[4] This chapter, which is concerned with rehabilitating knee injuries, addresses both cause and symptomatology.

Current physical therapy involvement is primarily directed toward achieving long-term goals, such as restoration of range of motion and strength. Physical therapy has had minimal involvement in the areas of prevention, recognition, realizing short-term goals (such as controlling inflammatory response), immobilization, minimizing loss of motion and strength, and achieving terminal goals (such as identifying and correcting causative factors). It is hoped that basic graduate and postgraduate education programs will increasingly prepare physical therapists for involvement in the areas of prevention, recognition, and provision of both acute and terminal care. In addition, therapists must continue to educate the medical community and public at large about the availability of these services.

ANATOMY
Osteology

The osseous structures that form articulations at the knee are the femur, the tibia, and the patella. These three bony structures form two separate articulations: the patel lofemoral and the tibiofemoral joints. Functionally, how-

323

ever, these two joints cannot always be considered separable, as there is a mechanical relationship between them. Evaluation of the client with an acute or chronic knee disorder demands thorough analysis of each articulation and its interrelated mechanics.

The proximal aspect of the knee consists of the distal femur. This is the longest bone in the body. It originates at the hip and courses in an inferior, medial, and distal direction as it descends distally. This combined direction of the shaft of the femur allows for the weight-bearing condyles of the bone to align with the axis of the lower extremity. In this alignment, a normal valgus angle is formed between the medially oriented femur and the slightly laterally oriented tibia as the two form the junction of the knee. Normal measurement of this angle is approximately 170 to 175 degrees. In women, generally, because of an increase in pelvic width, the angle tends to be less than 170 degrees, resulting in a tibia valga, or knock-kneed position. An angle greater than 175 degrees is referred to as *tibia vara,* or a bowlegged position.

The distal aspect of the femur flares into a pair of large condyles presenting an articulation with both the patella and the tibia. The articular condyles themselves are rather large and convex in both the sagittal and frontal planes. Anteriorly, the condyles are divided by a central sulcus that forms the articular surface for the patella. This sulcus is known as the *trochlear groove.* Posteriorly, the condyles are divided and separated by the intercondylar notch, which is filled by the cruciate ligaments. When the femur is viewed in the frontal plane with the knee in a flexed position, the configuration resembles a large horseshoe. This formation presents an articular arrangement with a closed anterosuperior surface and an open posteroinferior area. The condyles are covered by smooth hyaline cartilage that is very thick in order to withstand the extreme forces placed on the articular surfaces during weight bearing.

Adjacent to the articular condyles are the large epicondyles, which are convex surfaces pitted with vascular foramina. These highly vascular areas are the site of attachment for the capsular structures, ligaments, and tendons that surround the knee. The medial epicondylar region is easily distinguished by the adductor tubercle, which serves as a site of insertion for the adductor tendon and also serves as the origin of the tibial collateral ligament. The lateral epicondylar region can be easily palpated because of the extremely thin tissue covering it.

The lateral femoral condyle is more in line with the shaft of the femur, given that structure's oblique medial direction. In its anterior-to-posterior direction, the lateral condyle is somewhat flattened in configuration when compared to the medial femoral condyle. In a medial-to-lateral direction, the lateral condyle is convex as well as being slightly larger than the medial condyle in this plane. When viewed in a sagittal plane, the lateral condyle shows an in-

crease in height in the region of the trochlear groove. This accommodates the large lateral facet of the patella as well as preventing subluxation or dislocation during normal function.

The medial femoral condyle angles away from the shaft of the femur in comparison to the lateral side. This brings it into line with the mechanical axis of the lower limb. The medial femoral condyle's dimension is longer in its anterior-to-posterior direction and is convex in both the anteroposterior and the medial-lateral orientation. This longer distance allows for greater rolling to occur on this condyle, resulting in rotation, particularly during the terminal extension phase.

The distal portion of the femur shows one epiphyseal growth center at birth that remains active until fusing occurs with the main shaft of the femur. This occurs at approximately 18 years of age. This ossification center at the distal end of the femur transects the femur at the level of the adductor tubercle. The trabecular system of the distal femur shows a crisscrossing pattern within each condyle with long stress lines running up into the shaft. These lines of force run from the articular surface into the cortical bone. A second series of stress absorption lines forms in a transverse plane that serves to connect the two condyles.

The distal aspect of the knee consists of the proximal portion of the tibia, which is known as the *tibial plateau.* The tibial plateau is composed of two flattened shelves that anteriorly are even with the shaft of the tibia but posteriorly overhang the shaft. When viewed from the top, the tibial plateau resembles two round dishes that are, on first appearance, concave in both directions. The condylar surfaces are lined with hyaline cartilage, which drapes over the edge of the plateau by 2 or 3 mm. The capsule attachment falls along the edge of the periphery of the articular surface as well as being attached to the periphery of the menisci. The tibial plateau also has an epicondylar region that is adjacent to the condyles and is also pitted with vascular foramina.

The medial tibial plateau is an oval-shaped dish that is seen to be concave in both the sagittal and frontal planes. This condylar region is the larger of the two plateaus in the anterior-to-posterior direction and accommodates the larger medial femoral condyle. Its lateral border is recognized as the intercondylar area. When the tibia is viewed from the lateral side, the posterior portion of the medial condyle does not overhang the shaft of the tibia as much as does the lateral condyle. However, posteriorly, the tibia, because of the attachment of the capsule, is heavily pitted with vascular foramina just below the articular surface.

The lateral tibial plateau is circular in shape and also descends posteriorly, thus overhanging the shaft. Further flaring occurs in the posterior lateral corner to accommodate articulation with the fibular head. In the medial-to-lateral aspect, it is easy to see the concavity that forms on the inner surface of the plateau. When viewed from the lateral aspect, however, the anterior-posterior direction of the plateau tends to be flat. This shape facilitates rotation of the femoral condyle during movement.

The medial and lateral tibial plateaus are divided by the intercondylar region. However, there is a brief space anterior to this region where the medial and lateral tibial plateaus join, then follow the tibial shaft inferiorly to the tibial tubercle.

This intercondylar region is characterized by several features. The anterior region appears as a flattened depression separating the medial and lateral intercondylar eminences or tibial spines. This depression serves as the site of attachment for the anterior cruciate ligament. The medial and lateral tibial spines are found in the midregion of the tibial plateaus and can be observed as little mountains projecting upward between the plateaus. The shape of these spines is compact and linear. They project into the femoral intercondylar notch with flexion, during which time the greatest amount of rotation can occur.

Anterior-inferior to the tibial plateau along the shaft border lies the tibial tuberosity. This serves as the attachment for the patellar ligament (quadriceps tendon) that is the extension of the quadriceps mechanism. It also serves as the lowest border for attachment of the capsule as it overflows the anterior tibial plateaus following the patellar ligament. The space occupying this region is filled with the inferior patellar bursa and fat pad.

At birth, the femur, like the tibia, displays an ossification center in its proximal portion. This center remains active until fusion at 16 to 18 years of age. The tibial tuberosity region has two possible ossification mechanisms. First, ossification can occur as an extension of the proximal center itself, or it can occur as a separate ossification center that generally begins activity in about the twelfth year of life.

The trabecular systems of the tibia provide a similar model to those of the femur. Each condyle is represented as having crisscrossing stress lines that extend all the way from the articular surface to the underlying cortical bone. Overlying this system is a horizontal stress pattern that interconnects the two condyles for stress absorption in the transverse plane.

The patellofemoral articulation is formed by the anterior surface of the femur (trochlear groove) and the posterior facets of the patella. The patella is the largest sesamoid bone in the body and is interposed in the quadriceps mechanism. When viewed from a frontal plane, the patella appears as a large triangular bone with a broad superior border and a distal inferior apex. A transverse section of the patella also reveals a triangular pattern, with a broad superior border and a distal inferior apex, a broad superior apex (serving as the attachment site of the quadriceps extensor mechanism), and a posterior apex, which divides the articular surfaces into medial and lateral facets. The anterior surface of the patella is roughened and pitted with vascular foramina because of the extensive attachment of the femoral quadriceps muscle. Upon insertion over the broad superior border, the tendon continues inferiorly across the patellar surface, eventually narrowing into a tendinous band that extends into the inferior insertion on the tibial tuberosity. The region from the inferior apex of the patella to the tibial tuberosity is called the *patellar tendon,* or the *quadriceps tendon,* and/or the *patellar ligament.*

Posteriorly, the patella is divided by a vertical ridge into medial and lateral facet regions. Each side can further be subdivided into three facets: superior, middle, and inferior. These come into contact with the femur at various points in the range of motion. A seventh facet is also identified on the far medial aspect of the patella. This region, which comes into contact with the femur during extreme flexion, is identified as the flexion or "odd" facet. The patellar facets are convex in shape in order to accommodate the concave femoral surface. The lateral patellar facet is correspondingly wider to accommodate the femoral condyle. The medial facet also is characterized by an "odd" or flexion facet that is found on the extreme medial border. The articular cartilage on the posterior surface of the patella is the thickest in the human body, being approximately 5 mm in density.

At birth, the primary patella is composed of cartilage cells and is an easily palpable structure. Several separate ossification centers quickly fuse in about the sixth year of life. The trabecular system of the patella radiates in two directions. The first of these is parallel to the anterior surface, spanning in a horizontal pattern. The second system runs in a perpendicular direction, radiating from the articular surface and moving superiorly to the anterior surface.

Menisci

The geometric shape of the knee is, from a bony standpoint, poorly designed for stability. To enhance stabilization, a fibroelastic meniscal system lies on the tibial shelf, thus deepening the tibial plateaus. Two intraarticular fibroelastic menisci are arranged along the peripheral border of the tibial shelf. The medial and lateral menisci are attached to the peripheral plateau of the tibia by the strong coronary ligaments. Other functions of the menisci, in addition to increasing the integrity of the joint, are aiding in transmission of the weight-bearing forces, improving lubrication, and aiding in the rolling of the femoral condyles during motion. A sagittal view shows them to be wedge-shaped crescents with a rounded peripheral surface presenting a concave apex within the joint. The superior surfaces are concave to accept the shape of the femoral condyles but tend to be more flattened on the inferior or tibial surface. When viewed from above, the menisci follow the shape of the tibial surfaces on which they sit. The medial meniscus is semilunar in shape with a wide base of attachment at both the anterior and posterior regions.

These areas are termed the "horns" of the meniscus. Furthermore, the body of the medial meniscus flares posteriorly and is wider in this portion than it is in the lateral meniscus. The lateral meniscus is more oval-shaped with a narrow base of attachment at its anterior and posterior horns. This configuration results in a greater degree of mobility for the lateral meniscus than the medial meniscus during knee motion. The anterior horns of the menisci are connected by a transverse ligament.

The peripheral meniscal attachments are quite extensive and include both dynamic and static controlling features. As previously mentioned, the menisci receive a slip of the quadriceps expansion, thus allowing tension transfer, resulting in an anterior translation of the menisci. Further attachment of the anterior horn of the medial meniscus occurs along the ridge of the anterior cruciate ligament, blending into the medial tibial eminence. This attachment flares anteriorly from the depression along the anterior crest of the plateau. The midportion of the medial meniscus is attached to the deep capsular layer of the tibial collateral ligament. The extensive capsular attachment also brings with it a vascular supply to the outer third of the meniscus. The inner portion of the meniscus is avascular. Posteriorly, the medial meniscus receives a slip of the semimembranous tendon by way of the capsule. This results in a posterior displacement during flexion. The extensive insertion of the medial meniscus in the capsule and aponeurotic slips result in a decreased movement in the anterior-posterior direction. The medial meniscus is thus allowed only approximately 6 mm of motion in this plane.

The lateral meniscus receives the same anterior attachment of the quadriceps expansion from the patella, which results in an anterior translation of this structure. Along its midportion, however, the insertion of the ligament in the capsule is not as extensive. On its posterior border, it receives a slip of the popliteal tendon through the capsule, which can be visualized during arthroscopy. The muscular attachment allows posterior displacement of the meniscus during knee flexion. The posterior horn of the lateral meniscus can receive an attachment from one of three possible structures: the posterior cruciate ligament, the ligament of Wrisberg, or the ligament of Humphrey. An important function of these structures is to provide stabilization of the lateral meniscus during movement. The total movement of the meniscus in the anteroposterior direction is approximately 12 mm.

Knee capsule

The articular surfaces of the knee are encased in the most extensive capsule in the body. This capsule gains both static and dynamic support from the surrounding ligaments and musculotendinous structures. Attachment of the knee capsule follows the articular surface of the patellofemoral and tibiofemoral joints and inserts just peripherally to the articular margins. There are many distinguishable features about this capsule because of its immense size: it has a posterior recess that covers both the medial and lateral condyles, an indentation following the intercondylar notch of the femur, and a large superior patellar pouch. Further characteristics include capsular attachment of the menisci along the peripheral border of the tibia, thus holding the menisci to the articular surface. This peripheral attachment is referred to as the *coronary ligament*.

Anteriorly, the capsule descends in an inferior fashion over the crest of the tibia, following the patellar tendon and fanning outward to the medial and lateral areas in a V shape. This shape forms a small pocket that is filled by the inferior patellar fat pad and the infrapatellar bursa, thus reducing friction between the tendon and tibial crest. When the capsule dissects away from the patellar tendon either on the medial or lateral side, it gains support from the aponeurotic expansion of the quadriceps mechanism. In the aponeurotic expansion, several thicknesses of ligament appear to help stabilize the patella and place tension on the menisci. These thickenings have been termed the *meniscopatellar ligaments* and *patellofemoral ligaments*. The meniscopatellar ligaments extend from the superior-inferior lateral and medial border of the patella to the anterior one-third of the menisci. Tension is placed on the menisci by these ligaments when the quadriceps muscle contracts. The second expansion comes horizontally off the patella at about its midpoint and turn in a transverse direction, inserting into the lateral and medial epicondylar regions. These ligaments serve to provide stabilization of the patella as it glides through the trochlear groove. There is some question as to whether these bands form as a result of stress of the capsule or are evolutionary vestiges within it.

The midmedial portion of the capsule is reinforced by the tibial collateral ligament. The deep portion of the capsule in this region is referred to as the *short* or *deep collateral ligament* and is divided into two segments. This first is a band-shaped superior portion running from the anterior surface of the femoral condyle to a midpoint above the superior border of the medial meniscus. The second portion runs from the peripheral border of the medial meniscus to the tibial crest just inferior to the articular surface. This deep layer is covered by a second outer superficial layer that is approximately 2.54 cm in width and originates from a fan-shaped attachment just below the adductor tubercle on the medial femoral epicondyle. A ligament descends past the joint line to a point approximately 3 or 4 cm below the tibial plateau, inserting beneath the pes anserinus tendon, and is separated from that tendon by the pes anserine bursa. This superficial ligament is delta-shaped in appearance, going from a wide base of origin to a narrow base of attachment. The significance of this shape is that biomechanically a portion of the ligament remains taut throughout the range of motion, thus stabilizing the tibiofemoral joint against valgus stress. The greatest degree of tension, however, is seen in the extended position. Directly posterior to the tibial collateral ligament is the posteromedial corner of the capsule. This portion of the capsule inserts into the tibia along the roughened groove just inferior to the articular surface. It receives dynamic support from the tibial portion of the semimembranous muscle. Hughston[19] has named this corner the *posterior oblique ligament* and emphasizes its importance in stabilizing the knee against anteromedial instability. This structure is very important in supporting the capsule and preventing excessive tibial rotation.

Posteriorly, the capsule forms two pouches that cover the articular surfaces of the femoral condyle superiorly and the tibial plateaus inferiorly. This aspect of the capsule also invaginates into the intercondylar notch, forming a large horseshoe shape and leaving the cruciate ligaments external to it. These ligaments are considered to be extracapsular; yet each is covered by a synovial sheath and is therefore intrasynovial. Superficial to the posterior cruciate, the two femoral condyles are bridged by the oblique popliteal ligament. From a medial-to-lateral aspect, the popliteal ligament runs obliquely, superiorly, and transversely across the posterior cruciate, drawing dynamic support from the capsular arm of the semimembranous muscle. The semimembranous muscle, with its insertion in the oblique popliteal ligament as well as the posterior oblique ligament, can exert tension through the capsule to the medial meniscus. Contraction of that muscle during flexion results in a posterior glide of the corresponding meniscus, thus preventing impingement by the femoral condyle.

The posterior lateral aspect of the capsule is a complex of static and dynamic support structures. Capsular attachment follows the bulging lateral femoral condyle along its superior peripheral border. Support of this portion of the capsule is provided by the arcuate complex, the popliteal tendon, and the lateral head of the gastrocnemius muscle. The arcuate complex has an arching superior attachment originating on the oblique tendon, converging and inserting into the fibular head. The shape of the fibers upon cadaver dissection can be seen to be triangular with a broad superior border and an inferior apex. Further support of the capsule is provided by the popliteal tendon. Fibers of the tendon and muscle blend with the aponeurosis of the posterior lateral capsule, which has an attachment to the posterior portion of the lateral meniscus. As the popliteal tendon crosses posteriorly, it blends with the oblique popliteal ligament, thus preventing multidirectional fiber orientation. Further ligamentous support on the lateral and posterolateral aspects of the knee is provided by the fabellofibular ligament and the lateral collateral ligament. These three structures insert into the fibular styloid process and run in a superior (oblique) direction to the lateral femoral condyle, with the fabellofibular ligament being the most posterior and the lateral collateral ligament being the most superficial. The combined result of these structures is a posterolateral pillar, similar in function to the posterior oblique ligament of the medial aspect, with the common goal being the prevention of excessive rotation of the tibia.

Two structures of the knee that have received wide attention are the anterior and posterior cruciate ligaments. These structures lie in the intercondylar notch of the femur and are covered by their own synovial sheaths, separating them from the capsule of the knee joint. The term *cruciate* is descriptive in that the ligaments form a twisting pattern as the knee moves through a range of motion.

Recent work by Girgis, Marshall, and Almonajem[14] has further elucidated the anatomical shape and function of the cruciates. The anterior cruciate lies most anteriorly in the intercondylar notch, originating in the depression anterior to the medial tibial eminence. From this origin it turns in a superior, oblique, posterior direction to insert on the lateral femoral condyle in a semicircular pattern, giving it a twisted configuration. At its tibial origin, the anterior cruciate is seen to have a slip that runs and attaches to the anterior horn of the lateral meniscus. Girgis[14] has not found an attachment to the medial meniscus to be common. It is generally accepted that, by its mode of attachment, the anterior cruciate can be divided into two functional structures: the *anteromedial* and *posterior bands*. The anteromedial band is described as being taut in the flexed position because of its shortened anatomical dimension and its anterior position.

The posterior cruciate lies in the posterior region of the intercondylar notch. The femoral attachment site is on the posterolateral aspect of the medial femoral condyle forming a semicircular posterior pattern with the arch of the circle running adjacent to the femoral condylar articular surface. From this region, the posterior cruciate runs in a posterior, oblique, inferior direction to insert into the posterior depression between the tibial plateaus, continuing downward for approximately 1 cm, which gives it a very broad and convex configuration. Furthermore, the ligament sends a slip into the posterior horn of the lateral meniscus. The posterior ligament also can be divided into two functional structures: the anterolateral and posterior functional bands. Unlike the anterior cruciate, the posterior portion of the posterior cruciate ligament becomes taut in flexion, with the main bulk of the anterior portion being maximally stretched during extension. Both attachments in this ligament are posterior to the mechanical axis of the knee.

Two common but poorly understood posterior ligaments are the Wrisberg and Humphrey ligaments.[16] These ligaments are found in various combinations and are usually described as attaching on the posterior horn of the lateral meniscus and running in a medial direction to the medial femoral condyle. Gray[16] describes these structures as giving support to the rotational movement of the tibia.

Bursae

There are in excess of two dozen bursae located in the area of the human knee.[16] Each of these bursae functions to reduce friction, either between muscle and tendon, tendon and tendon, or tendon and bone. Four of these bursae are routinely seen to be involved in inflammatory states: the prepatellar, infrapatellar, suprapatellar, and the pes anserine bursae. The supra-, infra-, and prepatellar bursae are generally injured as a result of direct trauma. Football, soccer, wrestling, and baseball are sports in which injuries to these bursae are common. These three bursae are located on the anterior aspect of the knee. The pes anserine bursa, which is located just distal and medial to the medial joint space, is generally injured as a result of repetitive mechanical trauma. Such trauma might result if a long-distance runner participates in extremely long duration running.[14] The mechanical cause of inflammation to this particular bursa may be the result of incorrect technique and/or a biomechanical dysfunction, such as foot pronation.

Clinically, it is important to distinguish between swelling as a result of bursitis or swelling as a result of a primary joint effusion. Bursitis is localized and remains outside the knee capsule itself, while an effusion is an indication of a disordered status within the joint.

Musculature

The musculature about the knee plays an important role in both the normal functioning of the knee and in protection against injury.[2,47] The function of the musculature is to decrease the susceptibility of the knee to injury either directly (i.e., secondary to the ligamentous system) or indirectly (i.e., because of vastus medialis obliquus dysfunction causing patellar tracking problems).[27] A long list of references is available to support the importance of the thigh musculature in prevention of knee injuries, minimization of acute symptoms, and restoration of function to minimize future susceptibility.*

Anterior musculature. The anterior thigh musculature is dominated by the femoral quadriceps muscle group. The sartorius and the iliopsoas muscles are also included in the anterior group. The femoral quadriceps muscle group consists of the rectis femoris, vastus lateralis, vastus intermedius, and vastus medialis. Specifically, the vastus medialis obliquus must attach distally enough to allow for normal patellar tracking.[27] Much has been written in the literature regarding selective functions of different portions of the femoral quadriceps muscle group.[28] Visually observable atrophy of the vastus medialis is an indication of atrophy of the entire musculature.[29] Vastus medialis atrophy can occur because of the obliquity of its fibers, the distalness of its insertion, and its limited fascial covering.[29] Although attention in the literature primarily has been paid to weakness of the vastus medialis in relationship to the various patellar dysfunctions, there is some evidence that hypertonicity of the vastus lateralis muscle may also be a problem. We prefer to view the vastus medialis obliquus

*See references 4, 7, 11, 26, 27, and 37.

as a mirror of the femoral quadriceps musculature, meaning that the vastus medialis obliquus reflects the functional status of this structural group. The femoral quadriceps muscles can generate tremendous force in an athlete who through exercise has hypertrophied the group. It is not uncommon for athletic individuals to lift 40% of their body weight.

The iliopsoas muscles have also been identified as being related to certain lower-extremity disorders. Weakness of this muscle group is a common finding following injury. It is not uncommon for someone with a previous knee injury to be evaluated years later with no apparent deficits in quadriceps and hamstring musculature, but with a significant difference in hip flexor strength. It should be remembered that the anterior muscle groups are only one portion of the four-part muscle system surrounding the knee. All of these groups provide support for the knee, and proper attention to the posterior, lateral, and medial groups must be given for both prevention and rehabilitation of knee injuries.

Posterior musculature. The posterior thigh musculature includes the hamstrings group and the gastrocnemius and popliteal muscles. All three muscle groups provide posterior support for the knee; however, the hamstrings have an additional function. They have an indirect effect through their biarticular action upon the paired innominates. Weakness of this group can cause an anterior rotation of an innominate, and tightness can cause a posterior rotation of the innominate. The hamstrings also control rotatory movement of the tibia while the semimembranous muscle, through its attachment to the posterior horn of the medial meniscus, functions to retract that structure during knee flexion. The femoral biceps muscle serves as an external rotator of the tibia while the semimembranous muscle functions as an internal rotator.

The hamstring muscles normally do not produce as much force as the quadriceps. However, it should be kept in mind that during isokinetic testing at very high speeds, the force produced by the hamstrings will approximate that of the quadriceps. It should also be kept in mind that the normal testing position for these muscle groups allows gravity to assist the hamstrings, thus possibly accounting for a portion of this increase and the consequent functioning of the muscles at a relatively enhanced level. The importance of the hamstrings as knee stabilizers is not commonly emphasized in the literature; however, the hamstring muscles certainly are important in protecting the knee. The function of each of these muscles must be considered when rehabilitating knee injuries. This is especially true in rotatory instabilities and their rehabilitative protocol.

Lateral and medial musculature. Rarely is either the lateral or medial musculature mentioned as being important; however, one study indicates that both groups play an important role in stabilizing the knee as well as affecting the knee indirectly through their influence on the pelvis. Weak lateral musculature can cause an upward movement of the innominate, resulting in a functional limb-length difference. Weakness of the medial musculature can cause pubic movement that can refer pain to the lower extremity as well as creating a functional limb-length imbalance. The medial musculature also serves to stabilize the femur during activity, preventing rotation and thereby allowing normal function. Tightness of the iliotibial band, described as *excessive lateral compressive syndrome,* can be related to subluxation of the patella. All these possibilities emphasize that attention should be directed to the medial and lateral muscle groups rather than being concentrated purely on the anterior and posterior structures.

BIOMECHANICS/ARTHROKINEMATICS
Tibiofemoral joint

The complex movements of the tibiofemoral and patellofemoral joints are coordinated and guided by the action of the musculature and the ligamentous structures previously described.

The tibiofemoral joint is best described as a rolling, gliding, rotating hinge joint. The contribution of each of these actions is required if the tibiofemoral joint is to function in its normal state. The key tibiofemoral joint movement is described as *helicoid* or *spiral*.[16] This description allows us to visualize the tibia winding itself over the medial femoral condyle of the femur during flexion and extension. Studies of the movement of the tibia indicate that it is the axis of centroid that allows the rotation or axis point to change during flexion to extension. This distributes surface tension, thus allowing normal wear of the articular surfaces. Frankel and Nordin[13] have done extensive research into this phenomenon.

Patellofemoral joint

Mechanics of the patellofemoral joint is influenced significantly by the quadriceps muscle, the shape of the trochlear sulcus, the patellar shape, soft-tissue restraints, and biomechanics at the hip and foot.[23] The patella's role is to increase the distance from the joint axis, to provide a smooth articular surface (rather than allowing the quadriceps tendon to articulate), and to protect the anterior knee.[6] Normal function of the patella is to glide in the trochlear groove in a rhythmical pattern, increasing the leverage of the quadriceps muscle. However, to perform this activity, the patella must withstand shear and compressive forces placed on the articular surfaces.

In this extended position, the patella lies above the trochlear groove, resting on the suprapatellar fat pad and suprapatellar synovium. This position is slightly lateral because of the externally rotated end point of the tibia during extension and the physiological valgus of the knee. Even in the extended position, the patella can be felt to slide superiorly approximately 1 cm with quadriceps contraction.[44] The patella is pulled distally during flexion into the trochlear groove. This distal movement allows the patella to pass over the medial femoral condyle because of the unlocking of the tibiofemoral joint as it internally rotates. According to Outerbridge,[44] there occasionally develops a slight overgrowth of the osteochondral junction. Constant shearing of the patella over the ridge may lead to early medial-distal pull degeneration. At 20 to 30 degrees of flexion, the patella is well embedded in the trochlear groove and drifts to the lateral aspect, placing compressive forces across the medial and lateral facets. With further flexion, the pressure continues and the patellar articular surfaces segmentally come in contact with the trochlear groove, with the exception of the "odd" facet.[6] Continuation of flexion allows a smaller portion of the medial aspect of the patella to be contacted, with greater resultant pressure. With extreme flexion, the "odd" or flexion facet comes into contact with the inner margin of the medial femoral condyle in the region of the intercondylar groove. Lateral contact is of a similar nature and occurs in the extreme inner margin.

As flexion continues, the patella glides through the trochlear groove with increasing lateral pressure because of the tension of the lateral structures. Thus pressure is generated laterally during flexion; during extension, there is increasing medial pressure. Clinical observation of clients performing active progressive resistance exercises from a flexed to extended position shows that the medial facets are often the source of crepitus. Further observation demonstrates a slight lateral displacement of the patella as the knee nears terminal extension.

Arthrokinematically, the patella slides distally over the femoral trochlear groove, being pulled much like a glider being pulled through space. At the end of flexion, the patella tilts slightly laterally. This can be observed in clients performing resistive movements. In extension, the patella glides proximally, being pulled upward by the quadriceps mechanism. At the end of extension, a lateral displacement of the patella is again observed.

Patellar stabilization is provided by static and dynamic mechanisms. Active stability is provided through traction of the vastus medialis with an emphasis placed on the oblique fibers of this muscle. This muscle also provides a degree of static stability through its insertion and acts with other soft tissue structures on the medial side of the knee to assist in providing a degree of static stability. Further static stability is provided by the trochlear groove in conjunction with patellar size and type of patellar vertical orientation. Thus the function of the patellofemoral joint is intricately linked to movement of the tibiofemoral joint, and total knee function includes a dynamic relationship between all functional components.

Kinetic chain

The kinetic chain concept allows us to view the action of the total lower extremity as a functional relationship.

The open versus closed kinetic chain has a primary influence on knee injuries. The lower extremity is an open kinetic chain when the foot is off the ground and a closed kinetic chain when the foot is in contact with a supporting surface. The significance of this difference is that the closed kinetic chain is an encapsulated system prohibiting the function of one portion of the system (i.e., the foot) to the exclusion of the remaining parts (i.e., the knee and the hip). Forces, if abnormal, cannot be dispersed but must be absorbed into other tissues in the closed kinetic chain. The mandatory absorption of abnormal forces frequently leads to injury. Abnormal forces originating in the lower extremity, therefore, frequently have a profound effect upon the knee. Foot, pelvic, and soft tissue dysfunctions have the potential to produce these abnormal forces.

Abnormal foot function is not uncommon and causes a variety of knee ailments, including patellar tendonitis, lateral knee pain, and patellar pain.[49,51] For example, abnormal compensatory pronation will cause excessive internal tibial rotation, forcing musculature to contract longer and out of phase.[51] The musculature may become glycogen-depleted and may cease to function in its shock-absorbing capacity.

With pelvic involvement (i.e., posterior innominate), the resulting change in limb length will trigger a compensatory change in the foot (pronation, supination) or a change in the total extremity position (toe-out, toe-in).[36,44]

Soft tissue dynamics (flexibility, strength) also place stress on other tissues in the lower extremity kinetic chain. Abnormally tight hamstring muscles will produce an increase in passive resistance to knee extension, causing an increased workload on the quadriceps muscles.[55] Weak muscles (i.e., hip extensor weakness causing an anterior innominate) can also trigger changes in lower extremity mechanical balance.[36,44]

KNEE INJURIES
Mechanisms of injury

Microtrauma includes a series of inflammatory reactions to submaximal loading that eventually produces clinical signs and symptoms. Microtraumatic injuries can occur as a result of several mechanisms, including excessive normal forces, abnormal forces, or excessive abnormal forces. Our bodies can absorb normal forces daily without causing inflammatory responses. A normal force is absorbed by an individual who walks several miles during a 15-hour day. However, if this same individual were to hike 10 miles in a 5-hour period, an inflammatory condition would result from an excessive normal force. Excessive normal forces include either high-repetition activities with a low load or low-repetition activities with a high load.

Abnormal forces also cause microtraumatic injuries. A limb-length difference, pronatory problem, or a flexibility or strength deficit will necessitate compensatory changes in lower extremity kinetic chain loading and a diminished ability to absorb or disperse such forces, which can lead to tissue breakdown.

However, some individuals get along well with abnormal forces until these forces become excessive. People with limb-length differences as great as ¾ inch, gross pronation, and very tight, weak muscles may never have problems until they change or increase their activity level. This mechanism, which produces microtrauma, is referred to as *excessive abnormal force*. Individuals, unable to accommodate such forces, increasingly find their way to physicians' offices and thus to physical therapy as the fitness boom continues. The microtraumatically induced inflammatory process that results from excessive abnormal forces can be located in the ligament, tendon, contractile unit, capsule, articular cartilage, and/or bone. It is not uncommon for several tissues to be involved and for the client to have previously had pain in other anatomical locations. When pain first appears, the client can either curtail activity or attempt to compensate, with compensation being the rule. Compensation, however, will ultimately lead to pain in another area and the process will start anew. When the client can no longer compensate, he/she will seek medical attention.

When treating the microtraumatic injury, the cause of the injury must be addressed. Frequently, if only the symptoms are treated, there is a recurrence of symptoms when the activity is resumed. The pathomechanical causes of lower extremity microtraumatic injuries are usually the big three and/or the little one. The big three are limb-length difference, foot dysfunction, and flexibility deficits; the little one is strength deficiency/imbalance.

Macrotrauma is trauma resulting from an injury of a magnitude that causes immediate clinical signs and symptoms. Macrotrauma can disrupt the ligaments, muscle-tendon units, joint capsules, bones, nerves, and/or blood vessels. It is rare for macrotrauma to affect only one tissue. An individual can be predisposed to macrotraumatic injury. (Predisposing factors are discussed at the beginning of this chapter.) Macrotraumatic injuries can be a result of direct or indirect mechanisms. An example of direct injury to the knee joint occurs when varus force causes compression of the medial meniscus. An indirect injury occurs when a valgus force causes the medial joint space to open, thus applying traction forces to the medial collateral ligament and its attachment to the medial meniscus.

As with microtraumatic injury, in addition to treatment of the symptoms, the predisposing factors (causes) of the macrotraumatic injury must be identified and treated if successful management is to be achieved.

Prevention of knee injuries

The incidence and severity of knee injuries in sports mandate that more attention be paid to prevention. Abott[1] and Bender[4] have demonstrated that it is possible both to predict and to prevent knee injuries through appropriate intervention. Cahill and Griffin[7] have demonstrated that some types of knee injuries can be prevented at the high-school level as a result of appropriate exercise and pre-season conditioning programs. Nicholas[36] has shown that muscle weakness as a consequence of knee injuries can persist, thus increasing the likelihood of reinjury, if the injury is not thoroughly rehabilitated.

In addition Cameron and Davis[8] have discussed other factors, such as the type of foot gear worn, that are responsible for the incidence and severity of injuries. Klein[25] has pointed out that a limb-length difference can be responsible for both micro- and macrotraumatic injuries of the knee, and Blythe[5] indicates that the number and quality of coaches available in athletics have a direct effect upon the incidence and severity of injuries.

These existing facts must be recognized and used in preseason screening and for treating past as well as present and future injuries. Neither the lack of a definite program of treatment nor the lack of thorough and aggressive rehabilitation, once an injury has occurred, can be tolerated. These facts supporting intervention to prevent knee injuries should not be ignored. Furthermore, it is important that these facts be presented and made available to the medical community and the general public.

Structural predisposition

An individual's biomechanical structure can be responsible for a predisposition to knee injuries. Abnormal positioning of the patella, hypermobile joints, hormonal influences in women, inherited or acquired biomechanical problems of the foot, and/or limb-length differences are all examples of structural predisposition. These factors should be identified as part of a screening examination, and the individual should be counseled as to the types of sports that might be most beneficial to participate in as well as what remedial exercise programs and/or supportive devices might minimize the chances of injury.

Functional predisposition

An individual or athlete's gait pattern, such as a pronated or toed-out gait, can be a predisposing factor in many knee injuries. Additional factors include posture, genu recurvatum, an abnormally flexed knee, pes planus, and pes cavus.

Physical condition may also serve as a functional predisposition. Conditioning provides many benefits, such as increased tensile strength in the ligament when muscles around the joint are exercised.[52] Strength itself has been demonstrated to be a primary protective mechanism.[1,4,7] To be effective, this mechanism must have the ability to function repeatedly, thus emphasizing the need for endurance rather than just maximal muscular strength. Most epidemiological data collected indicate that the majority of injuries in most sports take place at the end of the day (as in skiing) and/or in the final periods of play (as in football).[12]

Previous injury

Previous injury is also a predisposing factor to knee disorders. Variables resulting from previous injury that may predispose the athlete to injury include:

1. Decreased strength, power, and endurance
2. Instability
3. Insufficient collagen maturation
4. Decreased range of motion and flexibility
5. Decreased reaction time and balance
6. Adhesions
7. Altered gait
8. Poor (or incorrect) diagnosis
9. Lack of (or insufficient) treatment

Muscular factors

Strength. The importance of muscular strength around joints for an athlete has been demonstrated many times. Exercising the muscles around the joint will increase the tensile strength of the ligaments and will also increase the strength of the ligament-bone interface. Exercise will also increase the bone circumference, which will provide further protection against bony injury.

Muscle groups that must be considered in relationship to knee injury include all of those of the lower extremity. Most frequently clinicians think only of the anterior compartment of the thigh because of the obvious importance of the quadriceps mechanism in maintaining the stability of the patella and in protection of the knee. One cannot deny the importance of this group, both in prevention of injury and the recurrence of injury, but the posterior muscular structures are equally important. The posterior muscle groups have a role to play in prevention of linear and rotatory instability. The medial and lateral structures of the knee also have been demonstrated to be of value in preventing knee injuries. Posteriorly and inferiorly the gastrocnemius muscle provides a support mechanism to the posterior aspect of the knee. Other muscle groups, such as the abdominals, hip rotators, and muscles of the leg that support the foot, indirectly influence the lower extremity kinetic chain and therefore can be responsible for applying abnormal stress to the knee if, in fact, they are not functioning optimally.

Evaluation of the strength of musculature around the knee demands the identification of parameters and normal values. Parameters that should be considered for these muscle groups include:

1. Strength of the group versus body weight
2. Right-versus-left ratio
3. Relationship of agonists and antagonists
4. Total leg strength (right to left)
5. Variations of these relationships with different speeds of testing

Power. Although the layman uses the terms *strength* and *power* synonymously, they are not interchangeable.

Strength refers to the amount of force that a muscle-tendon unit can generate, whereas *power* refers to the amount of force that can be generated per unit of time. The importance of the ability to generate force in a short period of time cannot be overemphasized. If an athlete needs 100 foot-pounds of strength to stabilize or protect the knee joint in $\frac{1}{10}$ second, but that individual requires $\frac{1}{5}$ second to generate that much force, the joint has already been injured and the amount of force produced has been of no value. Therefore power is a very significant aspect in both prevention and rehabilitation programs. Appropriate functional testing must be done to ensure that power requirements have been successfully met. We recommend the development of a functional progressive program to fit the needs of each individual undergoing rehabilitation. This involves the delineation of performance tasks and the organization of these tasks in a continuum from the most easily accomplished through a return to the desired activity.

Endurance. Endurance is another goal that must be considered and vigorously pursued. The ability of a muscle-tendon unit to produce strength and power is of no value if these cannot be successfully reproduced. Endurance must be adequately incorporated in a preventive program so that an athlete can avoid injury when he/she becomes fatigued. The development of adequate enzyme production, glycogen deposition, and oxygen utilization capabilities requires a significant period of time and specific stimuli.

Flexibility. Lack of flexibility in muscle-tendon units around the knee can be responsible for either direct or indirect joint injury. Nonflexible muscles are not as efficient and therefore may tire more quickly, causing opposing muscle groups likewise to tire more quickly since they must work to compensate for the passive resistance of a restricted or tight muscle. As muscle function increases, glycogen depletion takes place earlier, and the tired muscle is unable to complete the function of joint protection. Tight muscles may also cause abnormal stresses throughout the lower extremity kinetic chain, leading to knee disorders. For example, a tight gastrosoleus muscle group may cause an athlete to excessively pronate the foot, producing patellar tendonitis or chondromalacia of the knee.

Proprioception

Seldom are proprioceptive factors considered in a preventive program. However, through the work of Wyke,[58] the importance of this parameter has become increasingly clear. It should be obvious that an athlete with good balance and reaction time will be less susceptible to injury. The athlete should be better able to avoid injury-producing situations and should need to work less vigorously to restore body position after losing balance.

Balance can be tested with a modified Stork test timed with a stopwatch or with an objective testing mechanism, such as a mechanical balance evaluator. Use of the latter is particularly recommended for competitive athletes. Testing protocols and normative data are being developed for this area.

Shoes

Shoes can also be responsible for either micro- or macrotraumatic knee injuries. Cameron and Davis[8] have demonstrated that shoe design in football can make a difference in the incidence and severity of knee injuries. Other clinicians have reported that shoes can be a primary cause of microtraumatic (overuse) types of injuries about the knee. Design, construction, fit, and wear (asymmetrical and excessive) are all factors to be considered.

Environmental factors

Environmental factors, such as uneven ground and slippery and sticky surfaces, are also primary factors. Although environmental factors cannot always be controlled, they should be evaluated and minimized whenever possible.

PHYSICAL EXAMINATION OF THE KNEE
Evaluation form

We recommend the development of an evaluation form that establishes an encompassing, systematic format to be followed for each individual seen in the clinic. This form will allow standardization of the evaluation process and enhance reliability.

Subjective examination

Physical examination of the knee begins with the examiner assuming the posture of an investigator and starting the investigation with a subjective assessment of the client's complaints. The following questions should be routinely included in this subjective examination: How, when, and where did the injury take place? What was the immediate treatment? How rapidly did the knee swell (if swelling took place)? Has the knee "given way"? Does it catch or lock? Clarification of each of these questions and the importance assigned to them involves the length of time since the injury occurred. The client's description of how the injury occurred should include details such as the direction of forces, the position of the injured knee, whether the foot was planted, and the type of surface involved. Immediate treatment, including whether the individual continued with the activity or was unable to do so, is also extremely important to determine. Frequently clients know more about their knees and their injuries than clinicians can assess by examination.

Intraarticular disorders of the tibiofemoral joint range from isolated entities to complex rotatory injuries. Surgeons such as O'Donoghue,[43] Slocum,[46] Hughston,[19] Kennedy,[24] Noyes,[37-42] and Nicholas[36] have added new dimensions to injury recognition, surgical intervention, and time frames for healing. Furthermore, the advent and wide use of arthroscopy, allowing visualization of the injured structures, has helped advance surgical concepts.

Acute knee injuries, however, have created an aura of confusion among health care practitioners. Hughston,[19] for example, has attempted to classify injury mechanisms and resultant trauma. Smillie,[48] Slocum,[46] and O'Donoghue[43] have contributed significantly to the delineation of mechanisms of injury.

The importance of extracting subjective information in the orthopaedic examination is crucial if one does not see the injury occur. In clients with a chronic injury, it is necessary to have the individual attempt reenactment of the injury-producing situation—either verbally or by action—to help assess the direction of mechanical forces. Noyes[42] stresses the importance of understanding joint mechanics in soft tissues that stabilize the joint. This concept deals with primary and secondary restraints. The vast majority of clients' injuries occur in the loose-packed position, which provides only minimal stability of capsular and ligamentous structures.

Injuries can also occur at the extremes of range of motion. For instance, an individual who attempts to stand from a squatting position may, with tibial rotation, pinch the meniscus. Injuries in the extreme of extension, however, are uncommon as both maximal ligamentous tension and dynamic support are usually available in the close-packed position.

In the loose-packed position, many injuries occur with application of a rotational force. The most common force applied is external rotation of the tibia, resulting in an injury described by O'Donoghue[43] as *the unhappy triad:* damage to the medial collateral ligament, the medial meniscus, and the anterior cruciate ligament.

Other mechanisms of injury may include hyperextension, varus disorder, and internal rotation. Although none of these mechanisms is as common as those previously described, they can result in trauma equally significant to the anterior cruciate ligament, lateral collateral ligament, or lateral meniscus in the posterior lateral complex. When dealing with these mechanisms, one should not underestimate the significance of the injury.

In recording the client's subjective history, along with the mechanism of injury, the clinician should pay particular attention to the sequence of events following the injury. Many times the client will complain of a "popping" or "snapping" sensation, which can be the result of a tearing of the intraarticular structures (such as the ligaments, menisci, or osteochondral structures) or dislocation of the patella. An associated acute hemarthrosis within 2 to 24 hours can occur with significant clinical findings.

In clients with an acute hemarthrosis, arthroscopy is becoming a routine diagnostic tool. Noyes[40] found that 72% of acute hemarthroses show associated injury to the anterior cruciate ligament. This has led to increased numbers of primary repairs to the anterior cruciate ligament. Other associated disorders have been demonstrated through early arthroscopic examinations, including minimal involvement of associated ligamentous structures in 41% of treated cases and 62% of cases with meniscus lesions. Another condition that should be examined is a locked knee resulting either from meniscal displacement or hamstring muscle spasm. Locking can also be the result of effusion forcing the joint into a loose-packed position. The chief complaint then will be the inability to walk without a limp as the knee remains in a flexed position.

Clients with chronic knee disorders reveal a wide array of complaints. However, the clinician should not categorize complaints as always being evidence of a pathological disorder. A client's complaint of the knee "giving way" must be treated specifically, as this problem can occur while walking down steps, twisting, or decelerating, and may be the result of a wide range of problems. These problems can include subluxation of the patella, femoral quadriceps muscle weakness, meniscal pinching, ligamentous insufficiency, or effusion. Isokinetic documentation of quadriceps muscle weakness, in fact, has demonstrated that a significant decrease in strength occurs within weeks, and muscle output may be significantly decreased after one day. Often muscle weakness results in a sensation that the client's knee is going to "give way" or that the knee is very tired and the client feels he or she cannot continue to walk.

A second common complaint in the client with chronic knee disorders is locking, which can result from hamstring muscle spasm, true meniscal locking with joint blockage, or inflammation of the fat pad as a result of an original injury. Some clients will misinterpret the sensation of stiffness that often accompanies degenerative joint disease as a locking sensation. True locking, however, is the result of an injury associated with internal knee derangement, most commonly involving the meniscus.

Pain is one of the most common symptoms of which clients with chronic or acute knee disorders complain. Careful attention should be paid to the clients' description of the pain's location and intensity. The ability to reproduce this pain can assist the clinician in determining structural involvement and the extent of the injury. In a client with an acute knee injury, however, trauma or effusion-pressing on capsular joint receptors may lead to inaccurate physical examination because of client apprehension. It should be remembered that location and intensity of the pain vary widely with the specific injury. It is very important in a subjective history that the clinician identify the different types of pain, such as dull, aching, local, radiating, intermittent, or constant. Ability to reproduce the pain over palpable sites also allows the clinician to effectively delineate the involved tissues. However, with chronic internal derangement, pain may be referred to other structures.

Objective examination

Observation of the lower extremities. The next sequence in the examination is objective inspection or observation of the lower extremities. It is important in clients who complain of "giving way," stiffness, and an aching type of pain to do a total lower extremity examination, including evaluation of tibia valgus, tibia vara, internal tibial torsion, patellar alignment, and tibial rotation with active extension and flexion. In the client with acute knee injury, the primary emphasis should be on inspection for a locked-knee position, effusion, and the ability to ambulate, with or without a limp.

Examination of the tibiofemoral joint. Physical examination of the tibiofemoral joint will often be difficult in a client with an acutely injured or inflamed knee. Although the role of arthroscopy in assisting the diagnosis and treatment of acute problems is increasing, the physical portion of the examination should not be minimized. The importance and validity of the examination are enhanced if it is performed shortly after the injury. It is not unusual for a client to demonstrate significant instability initially, yet be unable to display instability 2 hours after the injury because of swelling. Internal derangement of the knee as a result of acute injury may include meniscal lesions, ligamentous lesions, lesions in the articular cartilage, and lesions of the synovium and/or capsule. Thorough evaluation is necessary in order to determine whether a primary or a secondary restraint is still functioning in the knee. As previously stated, the initial contact with the client should include a complete and accurate history followed by a systematic physical examination.

Palpation. With an acute injury, pain location is usually local and can be reproduced through palpation. Thus palpation allows localization of involvement. A classic case of needing to determine local involvement occurs when a person receives a direct blow to the medial collateral ligament, whereupon palpation can delineate the site of the injury as a femoral attachment injury, tibial attachment injury, or midsubstance tear.

Careful palpation for acute injury should include examination of the following structures:

1. The medial collateral ligament should be palpated from its distal attachment just below the adductor tubercle of the femur to its insertion approximately 2 to 3 inches below the joint line on the tibia. [However, careful delineation from the pes anserine bursa and tension at its tibial insertion is often difficult.]
2. The lateral collateral ligament should be palpated from the lateral femoral condyle to the fibular head. If pain and swelling permit, one may accentuate the palpation of the lateral collateral ligament by flexing and crossing the affected leg over the unaffected leg, thus allowing the hip to fall into external rotation. This is often referred to as the *figure 4* position.
3. The entire length of the joint line should be palpated on both the medial and lateral aspects. This is best performed by starting at the tibial tubercle and palpating up the patellar tendon until one hits a groove (the joint line), at which point the examiner should palpate medially and then laterally, pressing in an oblique inferior direction along the joint line. It is not uncommon in meniscal tears or coronary ligament involvement to have palpable tenderness at the joint line. Tenderness over the medial aspect of the joint line, however, is often compounded with meniscus or ligamentous injury.
4. Palpation of the patella and the surrounding capsule should be performed to assess capsular damage that may have occurred with acute subluxation or dislocation of the patella. Palpation should be done as low as the tibial tubercle since associated patellar tendon problems may also occur.
5. Pes anserine expansion palpation should be performed on the anteromedial aspect of the tibia where this tendon inserts superficially into the tibial attachment of the medial collateral ligaments and continues to the crest of the tibia. One must be somewhat cautious in this area when palpating the tendon, bursa, and/or tibial attachment on the medial collateral ligament. Pain in any of these structures may be the result of palpation in this area.
6. The lateral tibial crest is the site of the attachment of the iliotibial track. The lateral tubercle to which the iliotibial track is attached is known as Gerdy's tubercle.
7. Soft tissue palpation of the posteromedial and posterolateral aspects of the proximal tibia is important. Rotational instabilities often create tenderness of tissues located in these areas.
8. Palpation of the hamstring musculature for insertional pain to determine excessive tension is important as such tension can prevent full knee extension.
9. Palpation for joint effusion in an acute knee injury is usually simple to perform. First, a simple ballottement examination should be used. The examiner places one hand on the suprapatellar pouch and exerts a caudal pressure, thereby pushing the synovial fluid beneath the patella. Meanwhile the examiner's other hand is used to palpate the middle of the patella. A posterior force is exerted on the patella to determine whether it has been raised off the femoral condyle by excessive fluid. In a second type of effusion test (commonly called *milking*), the examiner palpates the suprapatellar pouch on the medial and lateral sides with both hands. The hands are then moved in a caudal direction, squeezing

the knee from a superior to inferior direction, forcing the fluid to move with the hands. Upon releasing the hands, an effusion can be seen returning in a rippling fashion into the suprapatellar pouch.

Accessory motion testing. The next section of the physical examination dealing with acute knee injury involves accessory motion testing. This is performed to establish the integrity of stabilizing structures about the joint.[15] The knee relies heavily on strong ligamentous and capsular expansions to provide the static stabilization necessary for normal motion. Stability examination, therefore, is important because primary repair of ligamentous injury is often thought to be crucial in successful return to full functional status. The extent of ligamentous injury has been classified many ways, including the classic orthopaedic terminology of *grade I, grade II,* and *grade III* (depending upon the degree of mobility as compared to the noninvolved extremity) and Hughston's[19] classification according to severity. Manual therapy recommends the use of a 0 to 6 grading scale in which the involved knee is rated in comparison to the opposite or noninvolved extremity. According to this scale, a grade of 3 is normal with the client serving as his or her own control. Regardless of the methodology of classification, adequate force must be used in order to provide relevant information. Noyes[37] points out that frequently traditional joint-stability tests are performed in a rather low-force environment, thus leading to potentially false-negative results. It has been advocated for years that examination of clients with acute injuries be performed while the clients are anesthetized, so as to make possible a more accurate assessment of stability.

It is important to assess both primary and secondary restraints available in the knee. Often, with injury to a primary restraint, the secondary static restraint or dynamic restraint may provide enough stability to cause a false-negative test result. Therefore, when performing joint-stability examinations, the clinician should follow four important rules.

1. Proper stabilization of both the proximal and distal segments is essential.
2. Proper clinician positioning is required for adequate palpation of the structure being tested.
3. When assessing accessory movement, it should be remembered that it is not only the degree of opening but also the end-feel achieved with testing that is important.
4. The clinician should always start by testing the opposite extremity to allow the client to feel how the test will be performed and to establish a baseline. Repeat or comparison testing is thus performed on the normal extremity.

Specific tests

Medial and lateral collateral ligament testing. Testing for the stability of these ligaments involves the following steps:

1. The client should be supine to ensure total relaxation while the clinician secures the ankle between his/her elbow and the trunk so that the hand and the clinician's arm can extend up the medial aspect of the tibia, thus placing the index finger or (preferably) the middle finger on the medial joint line. The clinician's opposite hand should be placed on the lateral aspect of the client's knee joint in a secure manner.
2. At this time, the knee is flexed 30 degrees, and a valgus force is applied by pushing the hand on the outside of the knee and rotating the trunk in the opposite direction. This will result in a gaping of the medial aspect of the tibia on the femur. This may be very obvious and palpable. As the clinician performs this task, a normal firm end-point should be felt. If any end-feel other than capsular is present, a disorder should be suspected. Upon relieving the pressure, the clinician may feel a reduction "clunk" of bony structures. This is often present in both normal and injured knees.
3. The test is then repeated with the knee in an extended position. Gaping occurring in both the extended and flexed positions indicates involvement of the posterior cruciate ligament as well as the collateral ligament.
4. To test the lateral aspect of the knee, the reverse of the above procedure is carried out, using a varus stress at the knee. Again, it is important that this test be performed in both 30-degree flexion and full extension to assess the stability of both primary and secondary restraints.

Anterior and posterior cruciate ligament testing. The anterior and posterior cruciate complexes provide stability for the knee to function in both planar and rotatory directions. These ligaments are found to be outside the joint capsule but within their own synovium. Classical testing of the anterior cruciate ligament involves the following procedures:

1. The client should be supine, hip flexed 45 degrees and knee flexed 90 degrees. (We suggest that one leg be tested at a time so as not to position the client where substitution will occur.)
2. The examiner's thumbs are placed on the anterior crest of the tibia along the joint line, with the index fingers placed posteriorly on the tibia to assess hamstring musculature. (A false-negative test is very common in clients who have dynamic hamstring support).

3. The test is performed simply by applying pressure in an anterior direction in an attempt to draw the tibia forward. In this position, an anterior displacement of 2 to 3 mm is considered normal. However, it is again necessary to check the opposite extremity as well as the end-feel achieved. It may be necessary to perform a ballistic movement in order to assess the desired end-feel.

4. In order to check the posterior cruciate, the clinician simply applies the force in the opposite direction. Again the amount and quality of movement and end-feel should be compared to the opposite side. (Often a false-positive anterior drawer will be assessed when in actuality the tibia has been posteriorly displaced). In order to assess this prior to performing the anterior and posterior drawer test, we advocate the use of the antigravity test. The client is placed in a supine position with the hips and knees flexed 90 degrees. The clinician holds the client's legs at the ankles, and a straight edge is applied across the crest of the tibia. This will allow assessment of a relative posterior displacement of the tibia. A positive antigravity test will show a valley appearance from the edge of the straight edge to the tibial tubercle.

Rotational examination. In association with drawer testing, Slocum[47] advocates the use of internal-external rotation of the tibia to detect rotational instability. External rotation of the tibia increases tension in the intact posterior medial structures, thereby reducing forward movement of the tibia even with involvement of the anterior cruciate ligament. With internal rotation, there is an increase in tension of the posterior lateral structures, thereby reducing the anterior displacement. However if in either instance the tibia continues to slide forward excessively, then an associated disorder is present in the structures. It is important to only slightly rotate the tibia on the femur because maximal rotation will tighten whatever portion of the structure is still intact, thereby decreasing the displacement present.

Hughston and others[19] have delineated the difference between straight and rotatory instabilities. These rotatory instabilities have been classified as *anterolateral, anteromedial,* and *posterolateral.* They are usually the result of selective structural damage, which has caused a change in the rotatory pattern of the tibia on the femur. The anterolateral rotatory instability is the most common. Further assessment of this rotatory instability has been proposed by Hughston and others[19] (the jerk test), MacIntosh (the pivot-shift test), Noyes[42] (the flexion-rotation drawer test), and Slocum[46] (the anterior drawer test with an internally rotated tibia). All of these tests are designed to detect subluxation of the tibia on the femur or reduction of the tibia on the femur.

It is important to assess throughout the range of motion the feeling perceived with the drawer test. Lachman[42] ad-

vocates a test for the anterior drawer in which the leg is held externally rotated, ending in 15 degrees of knee flexion. Torg[53] first described this positioning in 1976. The purpose of this position is to allow the posterior horns of the menisci to clear the femoral condyles. These structures may block movement in the traditional 90-degree knee flexion anterior drawer test. It should also be remembered that in the client with acute knee injury and effusion, flexion beyond the 45-degree position also results in a decreased joint movement. If the clinician lets the client assume a loose-packed position of approximately 15 to 20 degrees with an externally rotated leg and then applies an anterior force on the tibia, a much higher degree of accuracy in assessing the anterior cruciate ligament is seen. However, the clinician should not forget the importance of clinical end-feel and palpation of the relative joint movement.

The McMurray test was devised to detect posterior tears in the medial meniscus.[18] The medial meniscus, when damaged, may sublux in the intercondylar region of the knee joint. This examination combines the movement of flexion and extension with rotation of the knee. The examiner should palpate the joint lines in order to detect meniscal "popping" or "snapping" during the test if the test is positive. Occasionally, an audible "clicking" or "popping" can also be elicited with this maneuver.

The McMurray[18] test is performed with the client supine and the examiner grasping the bottom of the client's foot with one hand while palpating the joint line with the opposite hand. The knee is then flexed and placed into external rotation, after which the examiner applies a valgus force. The knee is then extended. A positive test elicits a "popping" or "snapping" sensation.

Appley's compression test for meniscal tearing is performed with the client in the prone position, knee flexed to 90 degrees.[18] The examiner grasps the plantar aspect of the client's foot and performs forceful compression through the foot to the knee joint. Simultaneously, the examiner performs internal-external rotation of the tibia, which may cause "catching" of the meniscus. A positive test again elicits "clicking," "snapping," or pain. (It should be noted that the client may need to have support under the thigh in order to prevent compression of the patella during this test maneuver. (This test should be done in different positions to duplicate function.)

Spring test. The spring test for tearing of the collateral ligaments is performed like the preceding tests. With the client in the supine position the examiner attempts to extend the client's knee. In a "locked" knee, forceful extension may be prohibited because of a displaced meniscus. This will result in a springy end-feel as the pressure is released from the inhibited range. The knee will "spring back" to the loose-packed position if impingement on the meniscus is minimal.

Functional assessment. The last portion of the objective examination for acute knee injury involves functional assessment. A systematic functional examination requires, first, that a client perform activities such as ambulating, ascending and descending stairs, making sudden movements, squatting, and hopping. The next step is to ask the individual to actually perform the specific movements required by his/her daily activities. This will allow the clinician to determine the client's ability to function in the presence of pain, limited motion, crepitus, and excessive motion. Functional stability, not just static stability, needs to be assessed because functional assessment is much more important than static assessment.

Foot examination. Following the basic knee examination, other tests should be done for foot posture and gait. All three are closely related in evaluating macro- and microtraumatic injuries of the knee.

Foot dysfunction can be either intrinsic or extrinsic. Intrinsic foot dysfunction can include either rearfoot or forefoot varus or valgus.[17,50,51] Extrinsic problems include limb-length differences and flexibility deficiencies.[36,54] If the foot dysfunction is extrinsic in origin, orthotic management normally will not provide a satisfactory result. Similarly, if the foot dysfunction is intrinsic, flexibility and strengthening exercises will yield poor results.

Static foot examination must include tests for both intrinsic and extrinsic problems. A quick test for intrinsic, biomechanical dysfunction of the foot is to place the client in a long-sitting position with the feet relaxed and passively hanging in a plantar-flexed position. This places the subtalar joint in a neutral position. An index card or business card is then held perpendicular to the rear foot, which allows identification of forefoot varus or valgus.[36] With the client in the same position, evaluation of dermatological response to forces should also be initiated. Common findings are that the client has callous formation on the medial aspect of the first metatarsal joint and the medial aspect of the first distal interphalangeal joint. Callous formation in either location is indicative of a pronated foot.[3] Asymmetrical pronation or supination can be evaluated in a functional (standing) position by measuring from the floor superiorly to the distal tip of the medial or lateral malleus with a business or index card, making a corresponding mark on the card.[3] If there is a right-left difference in terms of vertical dimension in measuring from the floor to the medial malleus, the side that is closest to the floor is probably in excessive pronation. The final portion of the preliminary foot examination should include analysis of shoe wear. Normal wear patterns are symmetrical and occur in normal areas. Wear should be on the posterior lateral aspect of the heel, and toe-off should not be at the metatarsal head but rather over the first toe.

An examination of the external forces affecting the foot should include flexibility and limb-length examinations. The flexibility examination should include assessment of the gastrocnemius and soleus muscle with the subtalar joint in a neutral position.[54] Hamstring muscles, hip rota-

tors, the iliotibial band, and hip flexors should also be tested for flexibility. We believe that limb-length assessment should be done in a functional position with measurement taking place from the anterior superior iliac spine (ASIS) to the distal tip of the lateral malleolus, accompanied by palpation of the iliac crest (ASIS) and the posterior superior iliac spine (PSIS). When assessing limb length, it is important to note whether dysfunction of the foot, recurvatum of the knee, or sacroiliac involvement affect limb length.

Posture. Client posture has a profound effect on forces affecting the knee. Clients should be evaluated for toeing-in and toeing-out, genu recurvatum, forward pelvis, forward shoulders, and excessive cervical flexion.[21] Many of these factors are interrelated and all must be resolved to rule out their involvement with the client's knee problems.

Gait evaluation. Gait evaluation serves as a final dynamic assessment of the client's lower extremity function. Initially, this examination should be done while the client is with walking normally; however, this can progress to jogging, jogging in place, or sprinting. Observation at fast speeds, of course, is very difficult, and a videotape and treadmill apparatus are desirable when available. Gait evaluation should follow a thorough static evaluation that can give clinicians an indication of what to look for.

Specifically, the clinician doing a gait evaluation should have the client do multiple circuits on the gait path while observation for only one dysfunction per circuit is made. It is recommended that the first and last strides be ignored.[3] The following specifics should be viewed during gait evaluation: toe-in/out, vertical calcaneus and heel position, patella alignment in relationship to the second toe, patella alignment in the frontal plane, the amount of knee extension, equality of heel flexion during the gait cycle, genu recurvatum, excessive medial roll of the navicular bone, and early heel-off.

Reexamination

Any tests that were suspiciously negative or that the clinician was unsure were conducted correctly should be repeated on future client visits. It is important to retest the knee since pain, swelling, and protective splinting can often lead to a false negative response. Repeating or expanding the examination process may be necessary if an initially minimum objective examination was performed on the client. It is not unusual to discover additional client problems at a later time during the treatment process. If a test is found to be positive once, then negative on recheck, it is reasonable to assume that a pathological condition exists.

Referral

If at any time the clinician is less than 100% certain of what tissues are involved or how severely they are affected, the client should be referred to another practitioner.

If there is any change that medical intervention is needed, the sooner the client is referred, the better. The only error that can be made by the clinician is a lack of prudence. Any errors should be made on the side of caution.

Medical practitioners can perform tests that are not available to the physical therapist to further differentiate the client's problem. Included in this testing battery are stress radiographs, arthrograms, arthroscopy, aspiration of joint fluid for culturing, and other blood and laboratory tests. It should be kept in mind that knee pain can often be of systemic origin or referred from other joints.

Specialized examination by physical therapists

In some situations, a minimal examination is all that is required. The rationale for a minimal examination is multifaceted. Frequently the clinician will be faced with time constraints, originating either from the client in question or from other causes. In this case doing a portion of the examination to allow commencement of the treatment is acceptable. A minimal examination can be defined as that which is required for client convenience, comfort, and safety.

Subjective examination. The subjective examination may allow for simplification of the objective examination—that is, common overuse injury may be more easily handled by a subjective examination than a traumatic football injury. In a client with the overuse injury, the knee may have just been examined by an orthopaedist who specializes in knee disorders. However, if important client information (such as type of surgery) is missing, extreme caution is required in the performance of stressful tests that may be indicated.

Minimal objective examination. A minimal objective examination may be acceptable if the clinician wants to save the most painful test until last and selects only those tests that will provide information that is necessary at a particular time.

The minimal objective examination that should be done on a client referred to physical therapy for rehabilitation should include range-of-motion testing; effusion, strength, and pain determination; and joint "clearing." The range-of-motion testing should include tests for accessory, passive physiological, and active physiological movements.[9,22,31]

The presence of a joint effusion is critical to determination of the rehabilitation program as it affects range of motion and strength.[11] In its presence, forcing range of motion and active exercise through the range of motion may be contraindicated. Tests that should be included are those involving palpation and objective measurement. (The ballottement[18] and "milking" tests that involve palpation have both been described previously.) Objective measurements should be recorded in metric terms presented in the record as right-to-left difference. We suggest using a measurement from the joint space (which is thus reproducible) and using distances of 9 cm above the joint space, 20 cm

above the joint space, and 15 cm below the joint space as reference points for objective testing.

Strength testing should be performed to determine the client's ability to contract the muscle, difficulty in maintaining the contraction, and/or any gross muscular deficiency. In the minimal examination, manual muscle testing is generally used as a timesaving measure. Other more objective tests can be used in the complete examination at a later time.

The assessment of pain is subjective; yet a measure of objectivity can be added by asking the client to place the degree of pain on a scale. The clinician can use either a 10- or 100-point scale, but in any case some type of continuum is necessary. The type of pain (burning, aching, shooting, constant, episodic) should be noted. Other key factors to note are whether there is pain with activity or only after activity and whether there is pain with active, passive, and/or resistive motions.

A "joint-clearing" examination should be performed on all joints that may refer pain or mechanically influence the knee. The foot, ankle, hip, sacroiliac complex, and lumbar spine should be "cleared." The "joint clearing" examination typically involves the use of over-pressure at the extreme range of motion.[18] A quick knee-screening examination consists of the spring test (collateral ligaments), drawer test (cruciate ligaments), and Lachman's test (anterior cruciate).

This minimal objective examination for the knee can be completed in less than 10 minutes and provides the clinician with a data base from which to initiate treatment.

ASSESSING AND TREATING RANGE-OF-MOTION DEFICIENCIES

Range-of-motion deficiencies are a common clinical problem. Unfortunately, the usual clinical approach is to resort to a simplistic approach of whirlpool treatments, forcing motion, weight-lifting, and hoping that the problem will resolve. A better approach is to systematically evaluate the deficiency and select specific treatment techniques. A four-part evaluation scheme and several specific treatment techniques are recommended.

The purpose of the evaluation scheme is to determine the tissue or tissues responsible for motion deficiency and their degree of involvement. After this has been done, selection of the appropriate treatment techniques can be clarified. The final portion of the scheme is designed to determine when it is appropriate to begin restoration of movement to the affected joint. The system consists of testing for capsular patterns, end-feels, glides, and pain-resistant sequences.

Testing for capsular patterns, first described by Cyriax,[10] refers to the fact that any joint with a capsular involvement will have a predictable loss of range of motion. The capsular pattern for a knee disorder is a slight limitation of extension and a gross limitation of flexion. The typical knee with a capsular involvement might exhibit a 15-degree loss of extension and a 60-degree loss of knee flexion.

End-feel, also described by Cyriax,[10] refers to the feeling imparted to the examiner's hands at the end of the range of motion. There are six types of end-feels (Table 15-1). However, only two indicate conditions treatable through physical therapy intervention. In particular, capsular and spasm end-feels may be rectifiable with capsular and muscle-tendon techniques.

The evaluation of joint glides has been emphasized by Kaltenborn.[22] *Physiological movement* refers to the joint movement that is under the client's active control. *Accessory movements* are movements necessary for normal joint function but which are not under the client's active control. An example would be the gliding movement of the tibia posteriorly on the femur with knee flexion. A tight posterior capsule would limit the ability of the tibia to glide posteriorly. A listing of accessory movements of the knee can be found in Table 15-2.

A pain-resistance sequence has been proposed by Cyriax[10] to determine if the joint is ready to have range of motion restored. The three possibilities of pain resistance are pain before resistance, pain with resistance, and resistance before pain. This system signals a red, yellow, or green light directing the therapist toward appropriate action. Table 15-3 provides additional information regarding this.

This four-part system for evaluating range-of-motion deficiencies can be completed in less than 1 minute and provides the therapist with the information necessary to proceed with a safe and efficient treatment approach.

TREATMENT

Treatment of knee injuries can be directed at either the capsule, the muscle-tendon unit, or, on occasion, both. Selection of proper treatment techniques will optimize results. Positive results can be measured as an increase in range of motion without a concomitant increase in pain or effusion.

Passive joint mobilization for capsular problems

Capsular restriction requires use of capsular treatment techniques, i.e., passive joint mobilization. Joint mobilization is directed at restoring accessory joint motion by selectively stretching the shortened tissues. Three principles serve as a basis for joint mobilization: hypomobility, the convex-concave principle, and the graded application of mobilization techniques.

Hypomobility of a joint during an accessory movement is evaluated by comparison to the opposite unaffected side. This evaluation can be classified by using the Paris scale (Table 15-4). The theory of convex versus concave joints simplifies the process of mobilization.[22] The knee joint is a concave joint because the concave bone (tibia) moves on the convex bone (femur). Concave joints are mobilized in the same direction; therefore, if knee flexion is restricted, the tibia would be mobilized posteriorly on the femur.

Maitland's gradation of movement allows the therapist to carefully control the force applied to the client.[11] If the system is followed carefully, the client should experience no discomfort and no damage should be done to a surgeon's work. Maitland's system consists of four movements (Table 15-5).

The therapist normally begins with a grade I movement and progresses according to client tolerance. At the end of the treatment, the therapist returns through the system, ending with a grade I. This reversal minimizes posttreatment discomfort.

Muscle-tendon techniques for noncapsular problems

The spasm end-feel and noncapsular patterns require muscle-tendon techniques. A large number of techniques are available. The wise clinician will select the best technique—that is, the technique that will produce results and that can be used most easily by the client. Heat, ice,

Table 15-1. Range-of-motion end-feels

Name	Description
Capsular	Leathery
	Example: normal glenohumeral external rotation
Spasm	Firm, contracting muscle
	Example: cramping muscle
Springy	Bounces back
	Example: Internal joint derangement, "loose" bodies, "bucket handle" meniscus tear
Bone-on-bone	Hard, solid, unmovable
	Example: normal elbow extension
Tissue approximation	Further range of motion (ROM) impeded by opposition of two tissues
	Example: maximum knee flexion (posterior leg touches posterior thigh)
Empty	Feels like more movement is there, but it is unobtainable
	Example: metastasis with referred pain

Modified from Cyriax J: Textbook of orthopaedic medicine, vol 1, Baltimore, 1975, Williams & Wilkins.

Table 15-2. Accessory movements at the knee

	Flexion	Extension
Patellar movement	Cephalic	Caudal
Tibial movement	Posterior internal rotation	Anterior external rotation

Modified from Kaltenborn F: Mobilization of the extremity joints, Oslo, Norway, 1976, Olaf Norbis Bokhandel.

Table 15-3. Pain-resistance sequence

Reaction to movement*	Joint status	Physical therapy action
Pain before resistance	Acute	Red light—no attempt should be made to gain ROM
Pain with resistance	Subacute	Yellow light—gentle attempt can be made to regain ROM, but should be done cautiously (vigorous attempts may revert joint to acute state)
Resistance before pain	Chronic	Green light—vigorous intervention may be necessary to restore ROM

Modified from Cyriax J: Textbook of orthopaedic medicine, vol 1, Baltimore, 1975, Williams & Wilkins.
*Refers to passive movement through physiological range.

Table 15-4. Classification of accessory movement

Classification	Status
0	Ankylosed
1	Very hypomobile
2	Slightly hypomobile
3	Normal
4	Slightly hypermobile
5	Very hypermobile
6	Unstable

Modified from Paris S: The spinal lesion, Christchurch, New Zealand, 1965, Pegasus Press Ltd.

Table 15-5. Maitland's grades of movement

Grade	Description*
I	Small-amplitude movement at the beginning of the accessory range
II	Large-amplitude movement within the available range but not to either limit
III	Large-amplitude movement beginning and extending up to the end of the accessory range
IV	Small-amplitude movement at the end of the accessory range
V	A manipulation (a high-velocity thrust)

Modified from Maitland GD: Vertebral manipulation, London, 1968, Butterworth Publishers.
*All movements take place within the accessory range.

spray-and-stretch, electricity, contract-relax, hold-relax, and active contractions are helpful techniques that can be used.

UNACCEPTABLE RESULTS

If treatment has not been initiated soon enough, or if inappropriate techniques have been used, improvement may not result. There should be improvement during each treatment session, and the client at the next clinic visit should possess an equal—if not increased—range of motion.

If a knee will not move, transverse friction massage[9] and prolonged mechanical stretching may be used.[36] It should be remembered that some clients' knees "can't move" because they are restricted by masses of adhesions. Two or three successive treatments without increase in range of movement should be considered a failure. Appropriate information should be conveyed to the referring physician and consultation should be sought.

Rehabilitation

Rehabilitation can be best viewed as a specified sequence of tasks performed to allow the accomplishment of desired activities. Therefore rehabilitation must be individualized to fit the needs of each client by merging the goals and aspirations of the client, the physician, and the therapist.[34] Frequently this merger is neglected and an unsuccessful outcome is the result. As stated previously, the sequence of activities should achieve functional progression and this development is the responsibility of the physical therapist. Such an approach means that instead of following a "cookbook" system of rehabilitation, the physical therapist should follow a framework of parameters and phases of rehabilitation that can be used specifically with the individual client.

Parameters of rehabilitation

Treating the total client. The client represents a complex entity that cannot be separated into distinct parts. Although it would be very convenient if a clinician could rehabilitate a torn meniscus without dealing with the total client, it is doubtful that the rehabilitation process would be complete or fulfilling. Because each client possesses individual goals and aspirations, goal-setting must involve examination and treatment of the total individual.

Psychological and physiological factors come together in this process to result in an acceptable social compromise. This compromise is an unwritten understanding of the intended outcome for treatment and rehabilitation. It is very effective to have a comprehensive plan of action outlining activities to allow accomplishment of the ultimate outcome. Monitoring of intermediate accomplishments allows quantification of progress and a reorientation of activity when appropriate. Rehabilitation should be monitored much like an employee evaluation; i.e., it should be results-oriented, rather than intention-controlled.

Psychological factors. Several psychological factors must be addressed during rehabilitation. Client motivation is of primary importance and should be assessed through verbal and nonverbal means. It is not uncommon for an in-

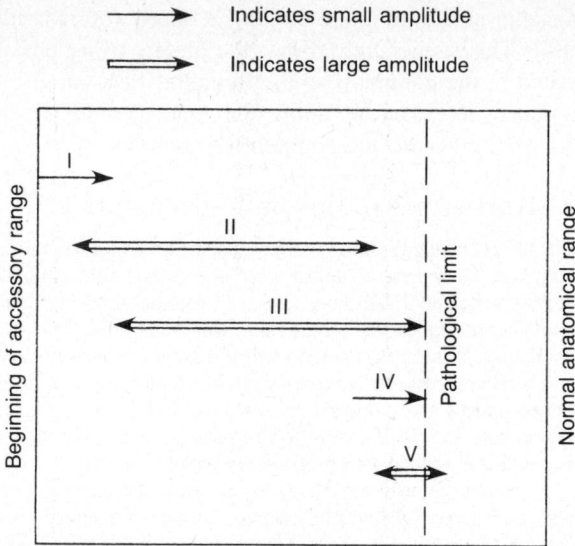

Indicates small amplitude

Indicates large amplitude

dividual client to "talk a good game" while being frightened and apprehensive about returning to a stressful environment. This is particularly true when persons are involved in competitive activities that require a high degree of skill but also possess potential for injury or reinjury. Secondary gains are always a possibility in clients dealing with a specific injury. Each segment of society has determined an role model that the individual undergoing rehabilitation is expected to emulate. When an individual does not conform to the model, psychological pressures may not allow rehabilitation to be successful.

Physiological concerns. Physiological concerns include range of motion, accessory joint motions, inflammation, and effusion considerations discussed before. Additional factors, such as tissue damage and healing, immobilization, articular cartilage maintenance, and musculotendinous maintenance and strengthening, are also of primary importance and must be addressed in the rehabilitation process.[30]

Phase concept. An effective method of integrating physiological factors with psychological parameters into a comprehensive rehabilitation protocol is to use a "phase" concept. Several different phase systems have been discussed in the recent literature.[20,32] We recommend a five-phase system that is comprehensive.

1. Phase 1 is termed the *maximum protection period* and includes treating inflammation, achieving primary tissue healing, and maintaining function.
2. Phase 2 is described as the *moderate protection period* and its primary concerns are tissue maturation, strengthening, endurance, and protected development.
3. Phase 3 is known as the *minimum protection phase* and consists of determining the time segment needed to deal with tissue maturation/reorientation, basic

light functional activity, and skill reacquisition/acquisition.

4. Phase 4 is the *advanced level of rehabilitation* and includes functional progression and a return to a skilled or demanding environment.
5. Phase 5 is referred to as the *maintenance period* and involves consistent effort to avoid the in-season/out-of-season trauma that is frequently seen with the "weekend warrior."

Exercise prescriptions. Exercise prescriptions must provide progressive stress on maturing tissues while also allowing a gradual increase in functional demands on non-involved structures.[34] A common mistake in rehabilitation is to deal only with the injury and not provide adequate protection or attention to other related structures. The ability of the musculotendinous unit to generate tension and to function repeatedly is dictated by the complex interaction of functional demands. It must be remembered that inactivity affects not only the articular, bony, and ligamentous tissues but also greatly decreases the contractile element capabilities. A too-rapid increase in activity during rehabilitation often results in problems with a contractile-related element rather than the feared articular or ligamentous tissue involvement. In knee rehabilitation, patellar tendonitis is frequently observed in clients who are moved too quickly into too demanding an activity.

Rehabilitation protocols. Incorporating all the previously discussed features of the rehabilitation process, the development of functional progression allows the therapist to truly individualize the rehabilitation program to fit the needs of the individual client.[56] Functional progression is ideal because it not only outlines for the therapist what is expected but also dictates what is expected of the client. Monitoring of the rehabilitation process is greatly facilitated by this process, as pain, swelling, and client apprehension are the parameters used to guide progression.

In order to describe the use of a functional progression in the rehabilitation of clients with different needs, two examples are presented.

CASE STUDY: REHABILITATION OF AN ATHLETE

J.J., a 21-year-old running back, sustained a second-degree sprain of the medial collateral complex. The treatment of choice was a 30-to-90 degree hinged cast to maintain adduction and internal rotation. J.J. was placed in a cast for 6 weeks and performed range-of-motion, isotonic, and isometric exercises for the total lower extremity during this time period. He was to maintain a non–weight-bearing position and a general maintenance program for cardiovascular and other nonrelated muscle groups was followed. Following cast removal, range-of-motion exercises, strengthening and endurance training, the use of an internal rotation brace, progressive weight-bearing, and specific work to the active stabilizers were performed. This phase lasted for approximately 2 to 4 weeks and incorporated the early portions of a functional progression. Two to 4 weeks of additional rehabilitation followed, involving a typical functional progression sequence including strengthening and endurance activities, specific activities of the sport, with an emphasis on the development of neuromuscular integrity.

A typical functional progression chart for this client would appear as follows:

1. Immobilization—primary healing
2. Range of motion—protected
3. Strengthening—endurance activities
4. Activities—progressive weight-bearing, balance activities, proprioceptive redevelopment, functional strengthening, walk-jog sequence, jog-run sequence, hopping-jumping sequence, cutting sequence, sprinting sequence, agility drills, specific activities related to the sport of football.
5. Return to sport

The typical sequencing for these activities should involve an increase in speed from approximately half speed through full speed. The athlete should participate at four or five of the levels in a functional progression at any one time. This means performing at half-speed a later portion of one phase of the sequence while performing at full speed at lower levels. The athlete should be able to perform the activity without an increase in symptoms if there is careful monitoring of pain and swelling. Client apprehension is another element that should always be monitored. It should be remembered that pain and swelling can be residual or acute.

Proprioceptive activities should commence as soon as weight bearing is permitted. These activities include weight bearing on both lower extremities, followed by individual extremity weight-bearing. Weight shifting and the incorporation of proprioceptive boards (multiplanar and uniplanar) should begin as soon as permitted. Proprioception should be performed with the eyes open and closed to more accurately simulate the environment in which the athlete may be participating.

Of primary importance to the rehabilitation of a running back is the cutting sequence. The cutting sequence begins with general figure-eight running with an increase in speed and a decrease in the size of the figure eights. The cutting sequence proper involves the athlete running to a predetermined position, planting, and then cutting with a crossover or normal cut. These cuts should be a half- to three-quarter speed and should increase until the individual is able to perform them at full speed. The final feature of these cutting sequences should involve the athlete cutting on command to either the right or the left. This much more closely simulates the environment to which the individual is attempting to return.

As the athlete proceeds through the sequence with increasing speed and effectiveness, protected activities can give way to a less protected environment. This less protected situation is typically termed the "dummy" activity and is often a portion of most football practice sessions. From the "dummy" activity, the athlete can proceed to a controlled scrimmage environment and finally to live scrimmage where teammates are the enemy! Although this is a game situation, there is still a degree of individual control. This sequencing allows the athlete to become acclimated to the competitive environment, thus gaining the confidence necessary to allow the final step in the process—safe return to the competitive sport.

CASE STUDY: REHABILITATION OF A NON-ATHLETE

H.H., a 21-year-old mail carrier, slipped on wet pavement and sprained the medial collateral complex of her right knee. The mode of treatment was very similar to that used on the running back, but the functional progression was quite different. The initial stages of the progression were the same, but the advanced levels differed greatly. She was treated during the hinged-cast phase exactly the same as the athlete. The early mobilization period saw emphasis placed on regaining range of motion and strength and on allowing progressive weight bearing.

In discussions with the client, the clinician should try to design a functional progression that involves balance activities, proprioception development, and functional strengthening, without placing emphasis on the advanced activities involved in a cutting sequence or sprinting. Thus the goals and aspirations of the client involve a return to the work environment, not to an athletic environment.

What follows is the functional progression outlined for the second client:

1. Immobilization—primary healing
2. Range of motion—protected
3. Strengthening—endurance activities
4. Progressive weight bearing
5. Activities—proprioceptive redevelopment, functional strengthening, walk-jog sequence, hopping-jumping sequence, return to work environment

Functional progression. The rehabilitative sequence for each and every client should be individualized to fulfill the needs of that client. As physical therapists attempt to develop rehabilitation protocols to meet specific pathological conditions or surgical procedures, the functional progression outline can be easily modified to fit those conditions. By integrating healing constraints, phases of rehabilitation, and individual goals and aspirations, a well-defined rehabilitation progression emerges. Discussion of individual conditions and procedures is beyond the scope of this chapter. The following guidelines are presented only as basic tenets to be used in any rehabilitation program. Individual conditions and modes of exercise are presented to provide a general clinical framework for physical therapy management of knee problems.

Conservative management. Conservative management means non-invasive management of a particular condition. It typically involves monitoring of inflammation, determining range of motion, tissue reaction, swelling, and general response of the client to treatment. It is important not to neglect the overall maintenance of physiological function in non-involved structures during conservative management. The therapist should attempt to develop a balance between external forces and internal forces during this period to allow appropriate resolution of the condition. It is important to remember that many of the concepts of conservative management are incorporated into follow-up care for surgical management. Thus the application of proper procedures and consistent monitoring of client progress are necessary in both conservative and surgical management. Conservative management is an outgrowth or continuation of surgical treatment.

Exercise. Three basic forms of exercise are incorporated in the vast majority of rehabilitation programs. Isometric contractions are familiar to physical therapists as an early mode of intervention. Isometrics can be used at various points in the range of motion, thus giving much more effective functional results, and can be used throughout the rehabilitation process rather than only during the acute or immobilization phases. Isotonic weight-lifting involves moving a weight through a range of motion at approximately 60 degrees per second. Its effectiveness has been well documented and its uses are obvious. Isokinetic rehabilitation has received great attention in the recent past. It allows much higher speeds of exercise (several hundred degrees per second), thus more closely approaching functional speed. We recommend that all forms of muscular activity be used in a rehabilitation program to allow a true integration of function. We further recommend that weight lifting follow a progression very similar to that which is compatible with fibrous healing. This means that the individual is not subjected to maximal stress but rather undertakes a sequence of lifting involving submaximal work. A limited range of motion is first used, progressing to full range of motion at submaximal levels, finally culminating in unrestricted range of motion with maximal effort. This sequence should obviously be modified according to the specific disorder treated, such as limiting terminal extension when dealing with certain cruciate instabilities.

Flexibility. In all clients with knee instability, it is important to maintain flexibility in related muscle groups. The gastrocnemius-soleus complex, the femoral quadriceps (rectus femoris), the hamstring musculature, the tensor fascia latae (IT band), hip rotators, hip adductors, and hip abductors are examples of muscle groups that must be of appropriate length for normal mobility. Flexibility exercises are incorporated in the functional progression that involves both a warm-up and a cool-down process. Static flexibility exercises are primarily used as a warm-up to involve affected muscle groups before heavy functional activity.

SURGICAL MANAGEMENT

Surgical intervention is necessary if there is a condition that will not resolve through physiological healing. Most orthopaedic surgeons will allow a conservative trial before surgical intervention in a large number of cases. If conservative management fails to resolve the condition, surgical treatment is indicated. One of the more exciting advances in surgical management of knee conditions has been the tremendous increase in the use of the arthroscope. The arthroscope allows a fairly benign comprehensive examina-tion of the interior of the knee joint in which some disorders can be arthroscopically corrected. The list of conditions treated by arthroscopic surgery continues to increase rapidly because of increasing surgeon awareness and skill acquisition.

Specific pathologies

Meniscus lesions. Meniscus lesions are typically corrected by surgery either arthroscopically or through an open arthrotomy. Initial care is dictated by the type of surgery and the specific details of the client's condition. The physical therapist should be aware of the client's general status before surgery, how much of the meniscus was removed or repaired, whether protection is needed or mobility is allowed, what levels of stress will be placed on the structure by the client, and what are the long-term goals for this particular individual.

As a therapist proceeds through a functional progression treating a client with a meniscus condition, it is important to minimize compressive loading of the tibia until adequate muscular protection and joint reorganization have been developed. This frequently means substituting jogging with more rapid running for shorter distances. We recommend mid-ROM work to minimize rotational stress. Or, early in the rehabilitation program, this type of loading can be minimized by substituting bicycling or swimming. It is important to make athletic individuals aware that the injured knee may develop a slight degree of swelling when heavy repetitive activities are performed. Typically, this is true for football players who practice 2 or 3 times a day. The athlete may complain of swelling occurring toward the end of the day during summer practice, with resolution of the condition seen as practices become less frequent.

Ligamentous repairs. Ligamentous repairs require rapid surgical intervention to reposition or stabilize damaged tissues. Rehabilitative constraints should be based upon the actual procedure done and the structure involved. The therapist must be aware of what tissues have been violated in reaching the involved structure and what activities can be used to minimize stress or to increase stress on the damaged but healing tissues. A similar process should be followed for a ligamentous reconstruction. Reconstructions are usually performed much later and involve the substitution of a different tissue for a damaged structure. Rehabilitative protocol must be based on the structure used and what is going to be demanded of that tissue. The same rationale for stressing the tissue or minimizing stress to the tissue will dictate the development of the program.

Key factors in rehabilitating ligamentous tissues involve biomechanically analyzing the stresses that will be placed on the joint and the developing tissues and designing a rehabilitation program to allow progressive stress. Progressive stresses will allow normalization (reorganization) or maturation along lines of stress, thus providing the strongest tissue possible. An example of this process involves emphasizing exercise of the hamstring muscles in anterior cruciate-deficient knee disorders. Anterior cruciate repairs or reconstructions typically demand a rehabilitation protocol that minimized quadriceps muscle activity that attempts to anteriorly translate the tibia. This involves using mid-range quadriceps muscle work, not using terminal extension, and emphasizing hamstring muscle strengthening to provide active stabilization.

Patellofemoral problems. Patellofemoral problems are often related to compressive syndromes of the articular surface of the patella. The overused term *chondromalacia patellae* has been used frequently to describe patellofemoral arthritis and patellofemoral compressive syndromes. To minimize compressive loading of the patella, it is recommended that terminal exercises, quadriceps-setting in extension, and straight-leg raises be used early in rehabilitation. As an individual improves, incorporation of weight loading (isometrics at specific points in the range of motion) and high-speed isokinetic exercises are often quite effective. An isokinetic progression should proceed from submaximal to maximal loading.

Tendonitis conditions. It must be remembered that the tendon is a portion of the musculotendinous unit. We have frequently seen patellar tendonitis in clients who have been asked to perform high-speed or high-resistance work before the tissue is ready for such stresses. Thus it is very important not to ask clients to perform high-repetitive stress activities, such as high-speed isokinetics, with maximal effort until the individual is physiologically capable of handling such activities. These activities should progress as gradual overload stresses on the client, while clinical signs and symptoms are continually reassessed.

Articular conditions. Articular cartilage represents a unique tissue that requires mobility for nourishment, yet is frequently damaged by compressive loading. Articular cartilage often responds quite positively to high-speed isokinetic exercise. This is typically performed at submaximal levels and probably is effective because of decreased compressive loading and improved nutrition. However, this view is speculative and represents only initial clinical judgement.

SUMMARY

It has been our intention to present a concept of phased rehabilitation, which develops into an all-encompassing progression of activity termed *functional progression*. Rehabilitation is a multifaceted activity that involves the individual aspirations of all parties involved. The meshing of these goals is required if rehabilitation is to be successful. Rehabilitation can thus be viewed as a progression into function.

REFERENCES

1. Abott HC and Kress JB: Preconditioning in the prevention of knee injuries, Physical Medicine and Rehabilitation Association (booklet), 1969.
2. Basmajian J: Muscles alive: Their functions, revised by electromyography, Baltimore, 1962, Williams & Wilkins.
3. Beckman S: Pronation syndrome. Paper presented at the Podiatric Physical Therapy Conference, La Crosse, Wisconsin, 1980.
4. Bender JA: Factors affecting the occurrence of knee injuries, J Am Phys Med Rehabil 18:537, 1964.
5. Blyth CS: Football injury survey. I, Phys Sports Med. 2(9), 1974.
6. Brattstrom H: Shape of the intercondylar groove normally and in recurrent dislocations of the patella, Acta Orthop Scand 8:226,1964.
7. Cahill BR and Griffin EH: Effect of pre-season conditioning on the incidence and severity of high school football knee injuries, Am J Sports Med 6:372, 1978.
8. Cameron B and Davis O: The swivel football shoe: a controlled study, Am J Sports Med 1:2, 1973.
9. Cyriax J: Textbook of orthopaedic medicine, vol 2, ed 8, Baltimore, 1974, Williams & Wilkins.
10. Cyriax J: Textbook of orthopaedic medicine, vol 1, ed 8, Baltimore, 1975, Williams & Wilkins.
11. De Andrade JR, Grant C, and Dixon SJ: Joint distension and reflex muscle inhibition in the knee, J Bone Joint Surg (Am) 47:313, 1965.
12. Ellison A, producer: Ski injuries, New Brunswick, NJ, 1972, Johnson & Johnson Co (film).
13. Frankel VH and Nordin M: Basic biomechanics of the skeletal system, Philadelphia, 1980, Lea & Febiger.
14. Girgis FG, Marshall JL, and Almonajem, RS: The cruciate ligaments of the knee joint: Anatomical, functional, and experimental analysis, Clin Orthop 106:216, 1975.
15. Gould J: Spinal evaluation and treatment; course taught at Cleveland State University, March, 1980.
16. Gray H: Gray's anatomy, Philadelphia, 1974, Lea & Febiger.
17. Hlavek H: The foot book, Mountain View, Calif, 1977, World Publications.
18. Hoppenfeld S: Physical examination of the spine and extremities, New York, 1976, Appleton-Century-Crofts.
19. Hughston JC, et al: Classification of knee ligament instabilities I and II, J Bone Joint Surg (Am) 58:159, 1976.
20. James A: Rehabilitation for anterior instability of the knee, J Orthop Sports Phys Ther 3:121, 1982.
21. James SC and Brubaker CE: Biomechanics of running, Orthop Clin North Am 4:3, July, 1973.
22. Kaltenborn F: Mobilization of the extremity joints, Oslo, Norway, 1976, Olaf Norlis Bokhandel.
23. Kaufer H: Mechanical function of the patella, J Bone Joint Surg (Am) 53:1153, 1971.
24. Kennedy JC, editor: The injured adolescent knee, Baltimore, 1979, Williams & Wilkins.
25. Klein K: Knee injuries. Paper presented at the Second Annual Physician-Therapist Conference, Chicago, December, 1981.
26. Klein K and Allman FC: The knee in sports, Austin, Texas, 1969, Jenkins Publishing.
27. Larson RL: Subluxation-dislocation of the patella. In Kennedy J, editor: The injured adolescent knee, Baltimore, 1962, Williams & Wilkins.
28. Lieb FJ and Perry J: An anatomical and mechanical study using amputated limbs, J Bone Joint Surg (Am) 50:1535, 1968.
29. Lieb FJ and Perry J: Quadriceps function: An EMG study under isometric conditions, J Bone Joint Surg (Am) 53:749, 1971.
30. Light K, Kuzik S, and Personius W: Low-load versus high-load brief stretch in treatment of knee contractures. Paper presented at the annual meeting of the American Physical Therapy Association, Anaheim, California, 1982.
31. Maitland GD: Vertebral manipulation, London, 1968, Butterworth Publishers.
32. Malek MM and Mangine RE: Patellofemoral pain syndromes: A comprehensive and conservative approach, J Orthop Sports Phys Ther 2:108, 1981.

33. McLaughlin R: Personal communication, March, 1975.

34. Mennell J: Joint pain, Boston, 1974, Little, Brown & Co.

35. Mitchell F, Moran P, and Pruzzo N: An evaluation and treatment manual of osteopathic muscle energy procedures, Valley Park, Mo, 1979, American Osteopathic Medicine Association.

36. Nicholas JA: A study of thigh muscle weakness in different pathological states of the lower extremity, Am J Sports Med 4:241, 1976.

37. Noyes FR: Functional properties of knee ligaments and alterations induced by immobilization: A correlative biomechanical and histological study in primates, Clin Orthop 123:210, 1977.

38. Noyes FR, Delucas JL, and Torvik PJ: Biomechanics of anterior cruciate ligament failure in primates, J Bone Joint Surg (Am) 56:236, 1974.

39. Noyes FR, Delucas JL, and Torvik PJ: Biomechanics of ligament failure II: An analysis of immobilization, exercise, and reconditioning effects in primates, J Bone Joint Surg (Am) 56:1406, 1974.

40. Noyes FR, et al: Effect of intra-articular corticosteroids on ligament properties: A biomechanical and histological study in rhesus knees, Clin Orthop 123:197, 1977.

41. Noyes FR, et al: Arthroscopy in acute traumatic hemarthrosis of the knee: Incidence of anterior cruciate tears and other injuries, J Bone Joint Surg (Am) 62:687, 1980.

42. Noyes FR, et al: Clinical biomechanics of the knee: Ligament restraints and functional stability. In Funk J, editor, American Academy of Orthopaedic Surgeons: symposium on the athlete's knee, St Louis, 1980, The CV Mosby Co.

43. O'Donoghue DH: Treatment of injuries to athletes, Philadelphia, 1976, WB Saunders Co.

44. Outerbridge RE: The etiology of chondromalacia patellae, J Bone Joint Surg. (Br) 44:752, 1961.

45. Paris S: The spinal lesion, Christchurch, New Zealand, 1965, Pegasus Press Ltd.

46. Slocum DB: Rotary instabilities of the knee. In Funk J, editor: American Academy of Orthopaedic Surgeons: Symposium on sports medicine, St Louis, 1969, The CV Mosby Co.

47. Slocum DB and Larson RF: Rotary instability of the knee, J Bone Joint Surg (Am) 50:211, 1968.

48. Smillie IS: Injuries of the knee joint, Edinburgh, 1970, Churchill Livingstone Inc.

49. Spencer A: Practical podiatric orthopaedic procedures, Cleveland, 1978, Ohio College of Podiatric Medicine.

50. Subotnick SL: Podiatric sports medicine, Mt Kisco, NY, 1975, Futura Publications.

51. Subotnick SL: Biomechanics of the ankle. Paper presented at the annual meeting of the American Physical Therapy Association, Phoenix, Ariz, June, 1980.

52. Tipton C, James SL, and Mergner W: Influence of exercise on the strength of the medial collateral ligaments of dogs, Am J Phys Med 218:894, 1970.

53. Torg JS, et al: Clinical diagnosis of anterior cruciate ligament instability in the athlete, Am J Sports Med 4:84, 1976.

54. Wallace L: Lower quarter pathomechanics. Paper presented at the Mississippi Sports Physical Therapy Association, Jackson, Miss, February, 1982.

55. Wallace L: Rehabilitation of patellofemoral problems. Paper presented at the annual meeting of the American Physical Therapy Association, annual meeting Anaheim, Calif, June, 1982.

56. Wallace L and Davies GJ: Knee rehabilitation, Am J Sports Med (in press).

57. Wallace L and McKitrick B: Balance testing as a prediction of knee injuries. Paper presented at the annual meeting of the American Physical Therapy Association, Anaheim, California, June, 1982.

58. Wyke B: The neurology of joints, Ann R Coll Surg Engl 41:25, 1967.

Chapter 16

THE HIP

Christine E. Saudek

The hip joint consists of the articulation of the head of the femur with the deep cuplike acetabulum of the pelvis. It is the best example of a multi-axial ball-and-socket joint in the body. Though its construction allows for mobility, it is not as mobile as the shoulder ball-and-socket joint, and its weight-bearing function makes it better known for stability. The function of the human hip, however, is not only to carry and distribute load but also to facilitate movement of the body through space with a pain-free, controlled motion between the thigh and the trunk. The rhythmical pattern with which this occurs is necessary for efficient movement. The mobility and stability of the hip joint allow us not only to move through space but also to fit comfortably into various types of seats, to bend over to perform daily household tasks, and to dress. Until the hip joint becomes stiff or causes some degree of discomfort, its stability and mobility are taken for granted. Since the hip joint is part of a closed kinetic chain, any abnormal stress on this joint will be transmitted superiorly to the trunk and inferiorly to the knee, ankle, and foot. In effect, a disorder of the hip can be responsible for creating asymmetries and discomfort from the foot to the neck.

The physical therapist is playing an increasingly important role in the evaluation and treatment of musculoskeletal disorders. This places a greater responsibility on the therapist to be knowledgeable of the detailed anatomy and biomechanics of each joint as well as of a wide spectrum of disorders and associated orthopaedic procedures. With this knowledge, a well-planned and thorough analysis can be performed, the cause of the problem can be assessed, and the treatment plan can follow logically. The scope of this chapter is to provide the physical therapist with the knowledge base necessary to thoroughly analyze and treat dysfunctions of the hip. This will include a thorough review of the anatomy of the hip, biomechanics of normal and abnormal hip movement, suggestions for examination of the hip, discussion of selected hip disorders and the conditions that may create them, and treatment.

ANATOMY
Comparison of hip and shoulder girdles

The hip joint and the shoulder joint are both ball-and-socket joints, and both provide three degrees of movement. Though parallels exist between the hip and the shoulder, the joints differ in four major aspects:

1. The shoulder girdle is capable of movement independent from the body axis. The hip girdle, however, because of its attachment to the body axis by the abdominal, erector spinae, and psoas muscles, as well as the muscles and ligaments of the sacro-iliac joint, cannot actively move independently of the body axis.
2. Because of the relatively flat articular surface of the shoulder girdle, it depends on muscles and ligaments for its articular stability. Although the ligaments contribute to the stability of the hip joint, the deep cuplike acetabulum makes the joint inherently stable during weight-bearing. The muscles of the hip are more involved in postural stability than in articular stability.
3. Because the *articular surfaces* of the hip joint must bear weight, they are more prone to wear and tear and thus to degenerative changes than those of the shoulder joint.
4. The range of motion of the hip is not as great as that of the shoulder because movement has been sacrificed for stability and strength.

Osteology

Femur. The femur is the longest and strongest bone in the body.[76] It consists of an upper portion made up of the head, the neck, and the two trochanters; the shaft; and the lower portion, which is divided into two large condyles. The head has been described by some as spherical[40,69,76] and by others as more ellipsoid, compressed in an anteroposterior direction.[62] The surface of the head is smooth, being completely coated with articular cartilage except for a slight ovoid depression called the *fovea centralis*. This

fovea allows for the attachment of the ligament of the head or the *ligamentum teres*. During embryonic development, the neck and shaft become angulated in two planes. The angle in the frontal plane, called *the angle of inclination*, is approximately 150 degrees in the newborn. Because of weight-bearing, this angle is found to decrease in the early years, and in the adult averages about 125 degrees (Fig. 16-1). In the elderly, it may be reduced to 120 degrees. When the angle of inclination is excessive, the condition is called *coxa valga;* when it is considerably less than 125 degrees, it is called *coxa vara*. The angulation created in the transverse plane between the neck and the shaft is called the *angle of torsion* or *anteversion*. This angle is determined by positioning the femur so that the femoral condyles are flush with a flat table surface. The angle of torsion is then measured between the surface of the table and the axis of the neck (Fig. 16-2). In vivo, this angle is measured using radiographs. Normally the head and neck rotate outward from the shaft, creating an average angle of torsion in the adult of 15 to 25 degrees. An increase in this angle creates *anteversion,* and a decreased angle is associated with *retroversion.*

The angle of inclination helps to move the abductor muscles laterally away from the axis of joint movement, which increases the lever arm for the abductors and therefore increases the torque they can generate. The angle of anteversion increases the lever arm of the gluteus maximus, thus increasing the torque of that muscle. Varying angles of torsion and inclination can be responsible for differences in gait pattern and muscular imbalances and are often related to numerous pathological conditions.

The neck of the femur is wider at its attachment with the shaft than at its attachment with the head. Its inferior, medial aspect gives rise to the lesser trochanter, which lies at the junction between the neck and the shaft. The wider part of the neck, which lies superiorly and laterally, gives

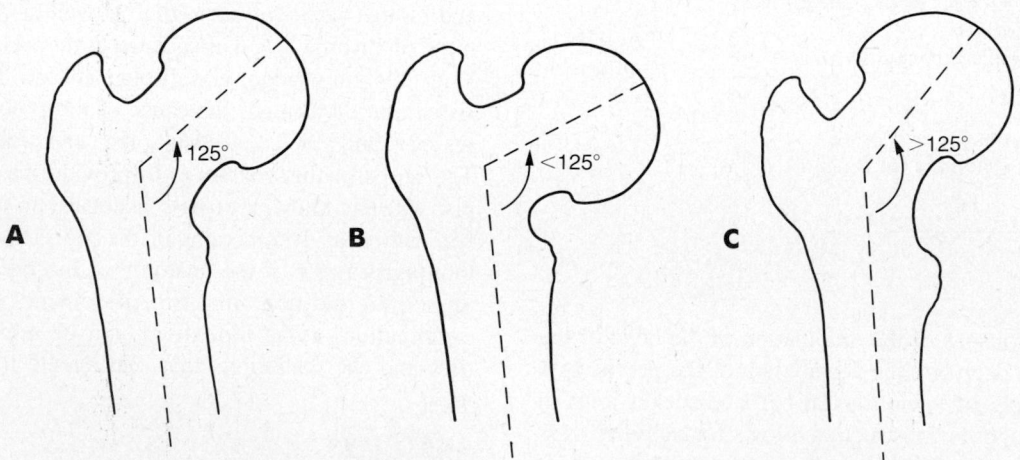

Fig. 16-1. Neck-shaft angle, angle of inclination. **A,** Normal: neck-shaft angle of 125 degrees. **B,** Coxa vara: neck-shaft angle of less than 125 degrees. **C,** Coxa valga: neck-shaft angle of greater than 125 degrees.

rise to the large quadrilateral eminence of the greater trochanter, which also joins the neck to the shaft. The greater and lesser trochanters are united in the front and back by the anterior and posterior intertrochanteric ridges. The posterior intertrochanteric crest forms a deep groove with the posterior aspect of the neck. Within this groove, just below the greater trochanter, lies the trochanteric fossa. Along this posterior intertrochanteric crest, approximately one-third of the way between the trochanters, lies the quadrate tubercle.

All of these crests and prominences serve as insertions for various muscles controlling hip movement. Impressions on the superior portion of the greater trochanter provide for the insertions of the piriformis, the obturator internus, and the two gemellus muscles. The greater trochanter also serves as the attachment for most of the gluteal muscles, including the gluteus minimus, the gluteus medius, and some of the deep fibers of the gluteus maximus. The external obturator muscle inserts into the trochanteric fossa and the quadrate tubercle receives the insertion of the quadratus femoris muscle. The lesser trochanter is the site of attachment for the psoas major muscle.

The femoral shaft is cylindrical in its upper half, tapers to its narrowest point in the middle, and becomes more oblong as it proceeds toward the condyles. Just above the femoral condyles, it is more triangular. The anterior aspect of the shaft is fairly smooth but, along with the lateral surface, provides for attachment of some of the knee extensor muscles. The posterior surface, however, has several crests and prominences. The lateral superior portion is roughened by the gluteal tuberosity, which receives some of the deeper fibers of the gluteus maximus. Just inferior to the lesser trochanter and above the spiral line, are found the insertions of the iliacus and pectineus muscles. The *linea aspera,* a prominence down the middle of the shaft, is important in the study of the hip because it provides for attachment of the adductor magnus, brevis, and longus muscles medially, and for the attachment of the short head of the biceps femoris muscle laterally. The medial supracondylar line runs into the adductor tubercle, which can be easily palpated and is an important part of the objective examination of the hip. The lower end of the femur at the femoral condyles is of most concern when examining the knee.

Architecture of the femur. The trabecular structure of the superior portion of the femur is divided into three main

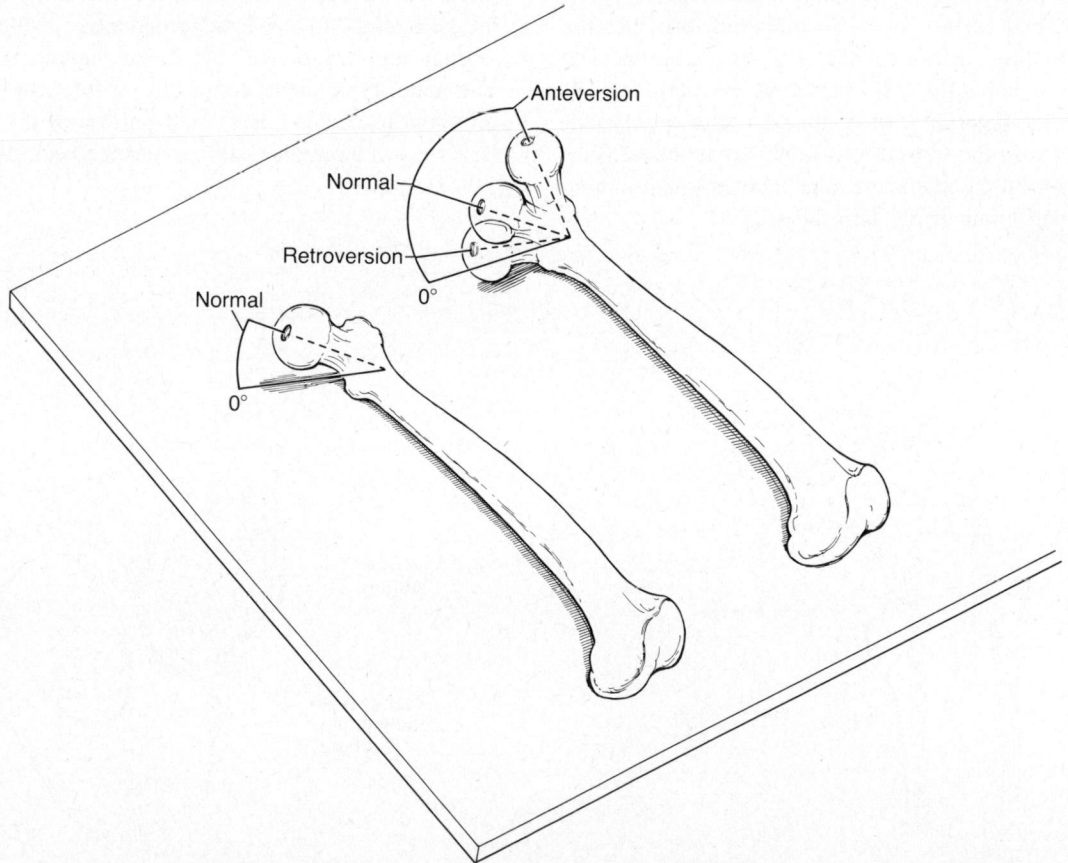

Fig. 16-2. Angle of torsion, showing a normal angle, anteversion, and retroversion. (Modified from Hoppenfeld S: Physical examination of the spine and extremities, New York, 1976, Appleton-Century-Crofts.)

systems designed to bear the necessary forces of tension and compression. In accordance with Wolf's law, these systems are disposed along the lines of greatest stress (Fig. 16-3). The strong arcuate system, resisting the forces of tension, runs along the thick lateral cortex and arches up to the inferior border of the head and neck of the femur. The relatively straight, strong medial system runs along the medial cortex of the neck of the femur to the superior surface of the head of the femur. This system helps resist the forces of compression. The weaker lateral system extends from the area of the lesser trochanter to the greater trochanter and just below, and resists weaker forces of tension and compression.

The shaft of the femur is formed of cortical bone with a large medullary cavity. The cortical bone walls of the cylindrical shaft are thickest in the middle third of the shaft where the bone is narrow. Above and below this, the bone is thinner and the medullary cavity is wider.

Acetabulum. The anterior and posterior walls of the acetabulum are formed by the ramus of the pubis and the body of the ischium, while the body of the ilium forms its superior wall. Inferiorly, the anterior and posterior walls end before they meet, forming the acetabular notch. The acetabulum is hemispherical to receive the global femoral head and opens laterally, inferiorly, and anteriorly. The half-moon-shaped surface of the acetabulum provides the smooth articulating surface for the head of the femur. The socket of the acetabulum is deepened by the peripheral fibrocartilaginous exterior called the *acetabular labrum,* which blends with the transverse acetabular ligament (Fig. 16-4). The labrum and the acetabular ligament help to hold the head of the femur firmly into the socket.

Several ridges, prominences, and fossae exist on the innominate and are significant for the attachments of the hip musculature. Of particular importance are the *ischial tuberosity* (the attachment for the common origin of the hamstring muscles), the *pubis* (important for its origin of the adductor muscles), and the *anterior inferior iliac spine* (AIIS) where the rectus femoris originates. The *iliac crest,* the *anterior superior iliac spine* (ASIS), and the *posterior superior iliac spine* (PSIS) are important points for palpation to determine asymmetries. The *obturator foramen,* which lies inferior and anterior to the acetabulum, is a large hole in the pelvis that provides an area of transit for the hip rotators on their way to attachments on the femur.

The sacrum cannot be neglected in a study of the hip because of its connection through the ilium. The sacroiliac joint must always be considered as a possible source for hip pain. The specific examination of the sacroiliac joint is discussed in Chapter 22.

Noncontractile soft tissue

Capsule. The capsule of the hip joint surrounds the neck of the femur and is attached anteriorly to the intertrochanteric line, posteriorly to the neck of the femur just above the trochanteric crest, superiorly to the medial surface of the greater trochanter, and inferiorly to the base of the neck close to the lesser trochanter. It blends with the labrum and transverse acetabular ligaments proximally. The majority of the fibers of the capsule run longitudinally proximal to distal, but a small portion of the zona orbicularis runs in a circular path around the neck of the femur at

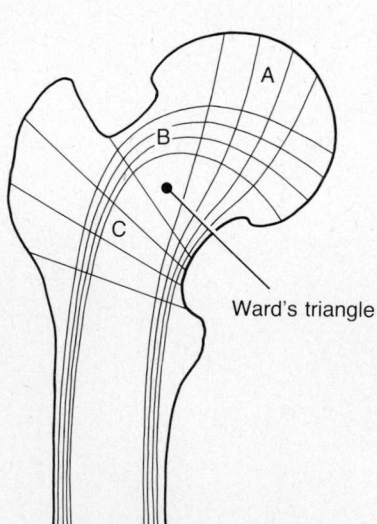

Fig. 16-3. Trabecular structure of proximal femur indicating *(A)* medial system; *(B)* arcuate system; *(C)* lateral system and the weak area of Ward's triangle. (Modified from Ramamurti C: In Tinker R, editor: Orthopaedics in primary care, Baltimore, 1979, Williams & Wilkins.)

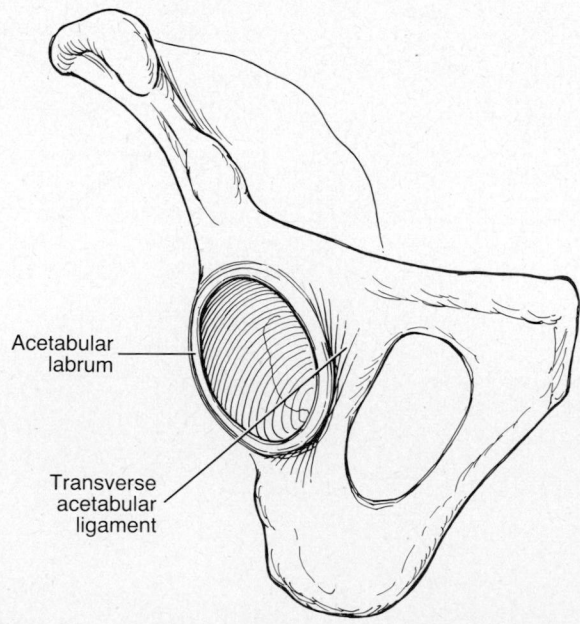

Fig. 16-4. Acetabulum deepened by acetabular and transverse acetabular ligaments. (Modified from Ramamurti C: In Tinker R, editor: Orthopaedics in primary care, Baltimore, 1979, Williams & Wilkins.)

the base. This circular portion is sometimes considered to be a ligament. The longitudinal fibers are reinforced by the iliofemoral ligament. The pubofemoral and ischiofemoral ligaments also reinforce the capsule, and the tendon of the psoas muscle blends intimately with the capsule. The capsule is thickest at the superior anterior part of the joint, where a large amount of resistance is required in stance and gait, and thin posteroinferiorly.

Synovium. The synovium lines the capsule and the acetabular fossa and covers the portion of the head and neck of the femur that is contained within the hip joint capsule. It also covers the two surfaces of the acetabular labrum and forms a sheath around the ligament of the head, as well as around the acetabular fat pad. It attaches around the edge of the fossa and the transverse acetabular labrum.

Ligaments. The ligaments of the hip can be divided into capsular and extracapsular ligaments. Within the capsule, the ligament of the head and the transverse acetabular ligaments can be found. The ligament of the head attaches to the fovea centralis, and two bands of it blend with the transverse ligament on each side of the acetabular notch (Fig. 16-5). This ligament is stressed when the limb is adducted and slightly flexed. Its mechanical role is minor; its main function is to carry blood vessels to the femoral head. The transverse acetabular ligament has been discussed previously.

The extracapsular ligaments, named for their attachments (iliofemoral, pubofemoral, and ischiofemoral), blend exteriorly with the capsule, thus reinforcing it. The *iliofemoral ligament* is the strongest ligament in the body and is the chief stabilizer of the hip in the erect position. It is also referred to as the Y ligament because it is shaped like an inverted Y. The anterior band, which has proximal attachment to the anterior surface of the body of the ilium and distal attachment to the intertrochanteric line, resists extension. The posterior portion rotates medially from its attachment on the posterior surface of the body of the ilium to the greater trochanter and resists internal rotation.

The *pubofemoral ligament* passes transversely from its attachment on the body of the pubis to blend with the capsule and the medial portion of the iliofemoral ligament. This ligament resists abduction and outward rotation.

The *ischiofemoral ligament* is a thin spiral ligament extending over the posteroinferior portion of the capsule. This ligament can be ruptured in a posterior dislocation of the hip.

Acetabular fat pad. The fat pad fills the acetabular fossa. It is covered with synovial membrane and serves as a means to increase the surface areas of the synovial membrane. It acts as a cushion and fills irregularities of the joint that are not filled with synovial fluid. The fat pad

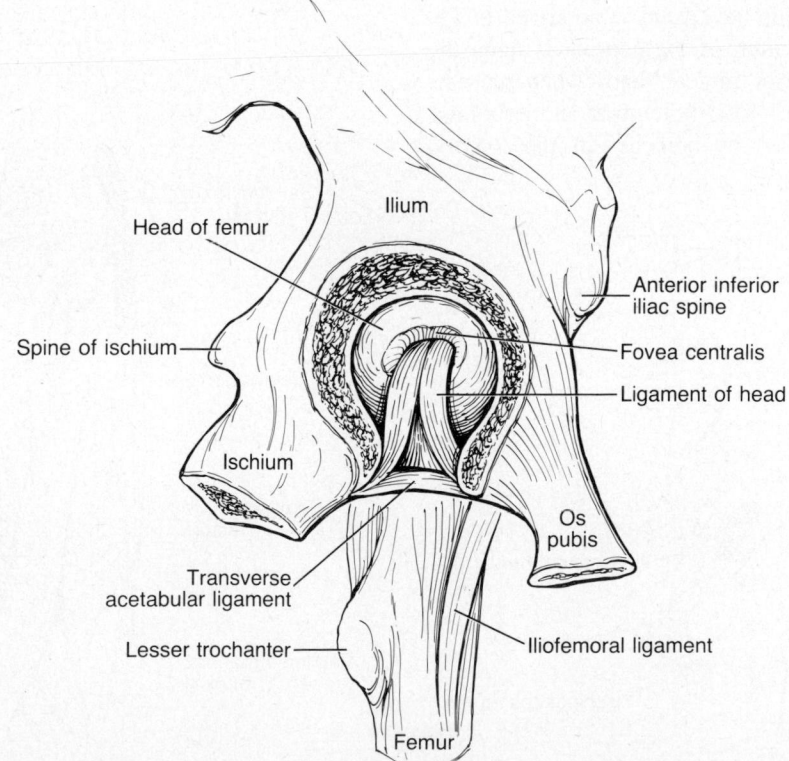

Fig. 16-5. Left hip joint, opened to illustrate ligament of head and its attachments to fovea and to transverse ligament. (Modified from Warwick R and Williams P, editors: Gray's anatomy, 35th British edition, Philadelphia, 1973, WB Saunders Co.)

promotes the better distribution of the synovial fluid within the joint.

Bursae of the hip joint. As in any joint, the bursae around the hip act as a means of reducing friction and protecting sensitive structures from excessive pressure. They become clinically important only if they have been irritated such that bursitis results and pain is produced. Their anatomical location provides important information needed to perform a complete hip evaluation (Fig. 16-6).

The trochanteric bursa is clinically the most important bursa in the region of the hip. It is located between the tendon of the gluteus maximus muscle and the posterolateral surface of the greater trochanter. The iliopectineal bursa lies deep to the iliopsoas tendon over the front of the hip joint. The ischiogluteal bursa is found between the tuberosity of the ischium and the gluteus maximus muscle. Inflammation of these three bursae is discussed later in this chapter.

Neurology

Structures of the hip joint that are innervated are (1) the muscles creating movement of the hip, (2) the articular cartilage and underlying bone, (3) the capsule and synovial membrane, and (4) the periosteum and intracapsular bone. Innervation of the hip is of clinical significance most frequently in the treatment of pain and is also of importance in the treatment of paralysis. The innervations to all the muscles surrounding the hip have been summarized in Table 16-1. Sensory innervation of the capsule is from the femoral, obturator, superior gluteal, and, when present, accessory obturator nerves. The iliofemoral and pubofemoral ligaments are supplied by branches of the femoral

nerve and accessory obturator nerve, the medial portion of the capsule by the articular branch of the obturator nerve, and the superior gluteal nerve. Branches of the sciatic nerve also supply the posterior aspect of the hip capsule.

Three nerves in particular should be singled out because of their frequent involvement in hip disorders: the *sciatic* nerve, the *obturator* nerve, and the *femoral* nerve. The sciatic nerve has the largest diameter of any nerve in the body. It is a continuation of the sacral plexus, passing out of the pelvis through the greater sciatic notch, between the piriformis and the obturator internus muscles. It then descends between the greater trochanter of the femur and the ischial tuberosity along the back of the thigh deep to the hamstring muscles (Fig. 16-7). Irritation of the sciatic nerve can frequently be responsible for hip pain. This is most often caused by a low-back problem but can also result from compression by a tight piriformis muscle, inflammation in the hamstring muscles caused by injury, or even by irritation from ischial bursitis. The sciatic nerve can also be crushed by a posterior dislocation of the femoral head.

The femoral nerve is the largest branch of the lumbar plexus. It descends through the thigh over the iliopsoas and pectineus muscles. Terminal branches of the femoral nerve supply muscles in the front of the thigh and the hip joint. The femoral nerve, in rare instances, is injured by

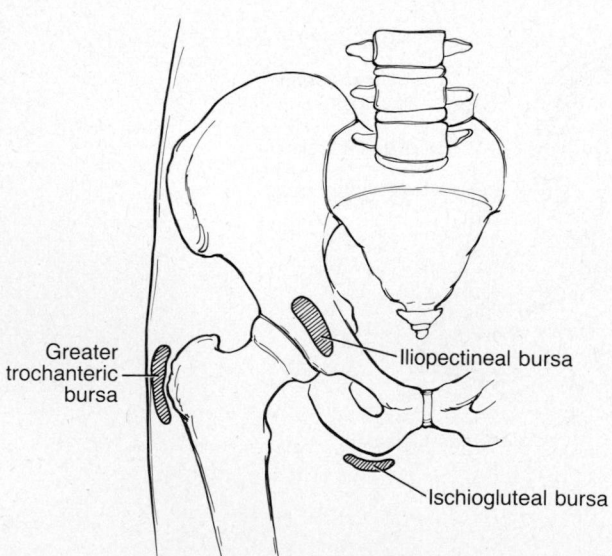

Fig. 16-6. Anterior view of the hip joint, showing bursae about the hip. (Modified from Raney R, Brashear H, and Shands A, editors: Shands' handbook of orthopaedic surgery, St. Louis, 1971, The CV Mosby Co.)

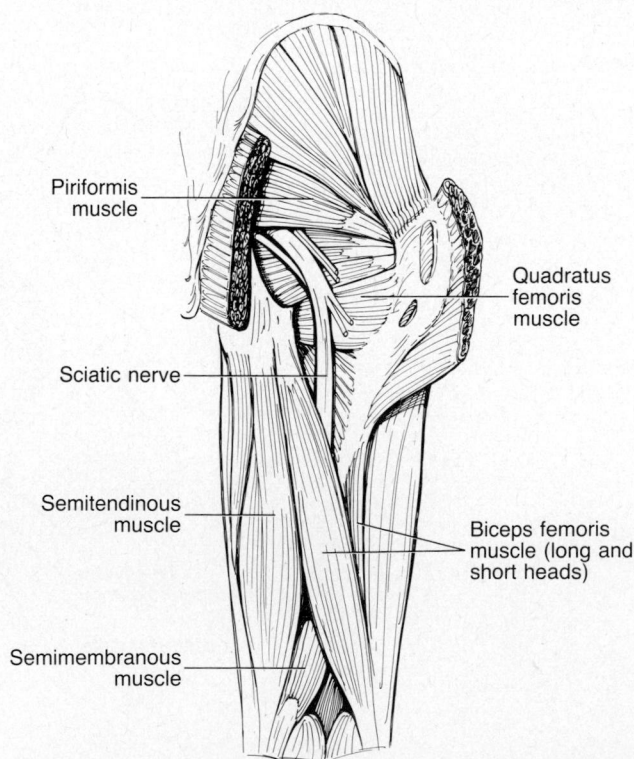

Fig. 16-7. Posterior view of sciatic nerve in relation to external rotators and hamstring muscles. (Modified from Warwick R and Williams P, editors: Gray's anatomy, 35th British edition, Philadelphia, 1973, WB Saunders Co.)

Table 16-1. Origin, insertion, and innervation of muscles acting on the hip (by action)

	Origin	Insertion	Innervation
Muscles producing flexion			
Psoas major	Transverse processes, bodies, and disks of T-12-L-5	Lesser trochanter	Branches of the femoral nerve L-1-L-4
Iliacus	Iliac crest, floor of iliac fossa, ala of sacrum	Lesser trochanter	Branches of femoral nerve L-2 and L-3
Sartorius	Anterior superior iliac spine	Medial, proximal tibia	Femoral nerve L-2, L-3
Rectus femoris	Two heads: straight head from the anterior iliac spine; reflected head from groove above the acetabulum	Patella via quadriceps tendon	Branches of femoral nerve L-2, L-3, L-4
Pectineus	Superior ramus of pubis	Pectineal line of femur	Femoral nerve L-2, L-3
Muscles producing adduction			
Gracilis	Inferior medial ramus of pubis	Proximal medial tibia	Obturator nerve L-2, L-3
Adductor brevis	Body and inferior ramus of pubis	Pectineal line and proximal linea aspera	Obturator nerve L-2, L-3, L-4
Adductor magnus	Inferior ramus of pubis, ramus of ischium, and ischial tuberosity	Medial femur and adductor tubercle	Obturator nerve L-2, L-3, L-4, tibial portion of sciatic nerve L-2, L-3, L-4
Adductor longus	Anterior and inferior superior ramus of pubis	Midmedial linea aspera	Obturator nerve L-2, L-3, L-4
Muscles producing abduction			
Gluteus medius	Anterior gluteal line	Greater trochanter	Superior gluteal nerve L-4, L-5, S-1
Tensor fasciae latae	Anterior outer lip of iliac crest and deep surface of fasciae latae	Proximal iliotibial tract	Superior gluteal nerve L-4, L-5
Gluteus minimus	External surface of ilium	Greater trochanter	Superior gluteal nerve L-4, L-5, S-1
Muscles producing extension			
Gluteus maximus	Posterior portion of ilium and dorsal surfaces of sacrum and coccyx	Proximal iliotibial tract and deep fibers to gluteal tuberosity of femur	Inferior gluteal nerve L-5, S-1, S-2
Semitendinosus	Ischial tuberosity	Medial flare of tibia	Tibial branches of sciatic nerve L-5, S-1, S-2
Semimembranosus	Ischial tuberosity	Posterior medial condyle of tibia	Tibial branch of sciatic nerve L-5, S-1, S-2
Biceps femoris (long head)	Ischial tuberosity	Head of fibula and lateral condyle of tibia	Tibial branch of sciatic nerve L-5, S-1, S-2
Muscles producing external rotation			
Piriformis	Anterior surface of sacrum	Greater trochanter	Sacral plexus L-5, S-1, S-2
Quadratus femoris	Lateral border of tuberosity of ischium	Quadrate line of femur	Sacral plexus L-4, L-5, S-1
Obturator internus	Internal surface of obturator membrane and margin of obturator foramen	Greater trochanter	Sacral plexus L-5, S-1, S-2, S-3
Obturator externus	Rami of pubis and ischium and external surface of obturator membrane	Trochanteric fossa of femur	Obturator nerve L-3, L-4
Gemellus superior	Spine of ischium	Greater trochanter	Sacral plexus L-5, S-1, S-2, S-3
Gemellus inferior	Tuberosity of ischium	Greater trochanter	Sacral plexus L-4, L-5, S-1, S-2
Muscles producing internal rotation (secondary function)			
Semitendinosus			
Semimembranosus			
Adductor magnus (posterior portion)			
Gracilis			
Gluteus minimus			
Gluteus medius			

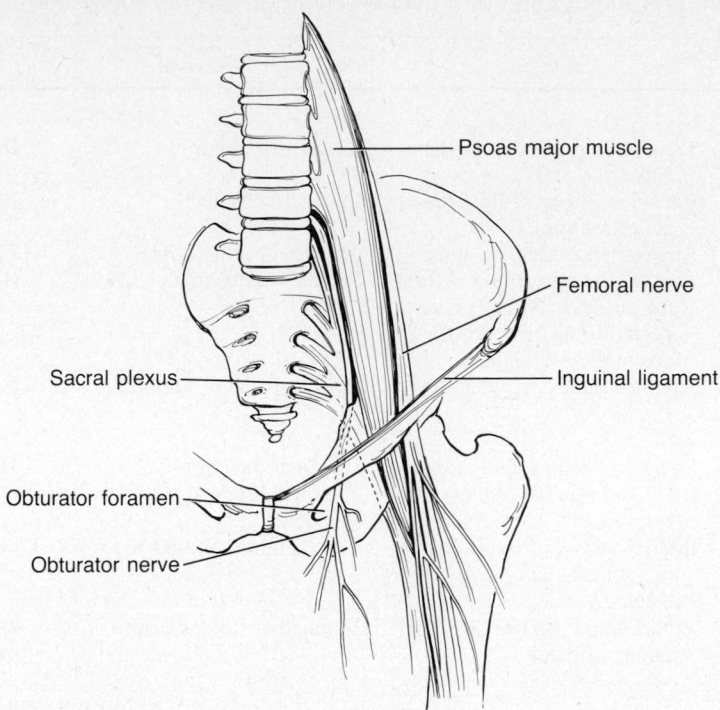

Fig. 16-8. Anterior hip, showing positions of related nerves and psoas major muscle.

wounds in the groin or thigh. The major effect of injury to the femoral nerve is paralysis of the quadriceps femoris and decreased cutaneous sensitivity on the anterior and medial aspects of the thigh.

The obturator nerve arises from the lumbar plexus and is formed in the substance of the psoas major muscle. It runs over the obturator internus muscle and then divides and leaves the pelvis via the obturator foramen (Fig. 16-8). Irritation of the obturator nerve is often responsible for referring hip pain to the medial thigh or the knee joint.

Angiology

A basic knowledge of the arterial anatomy of the hip is essential for understanding some of the diseases affecting the head of the femur and the acetabulum. According to Harty,[34] there are more vascular disorders in the human femoral head than in any other skeletal element. The medial and lateral circumflex arteries, branches of either the profunda femoris artery or the femoral artery, supply most of the head and neck of the femur (Fig. 16-9). Supplementary vessels found in the ligament of the head are usually derived from the obturator artery. A ring of arteries formed by large branches of the medial and lateral circumflex arteries surrounds the base of the femoral neck at the level of the capsular attachment at the hip. Branches from this arterial ring then enter the hip joint by passing through the capsule close to the bone. These retinacular arteries extend up the femoral neck, between the bone and its synovial lining, and form the main vascular source to the head of the femur. The greater and lesser trochanters are sup-

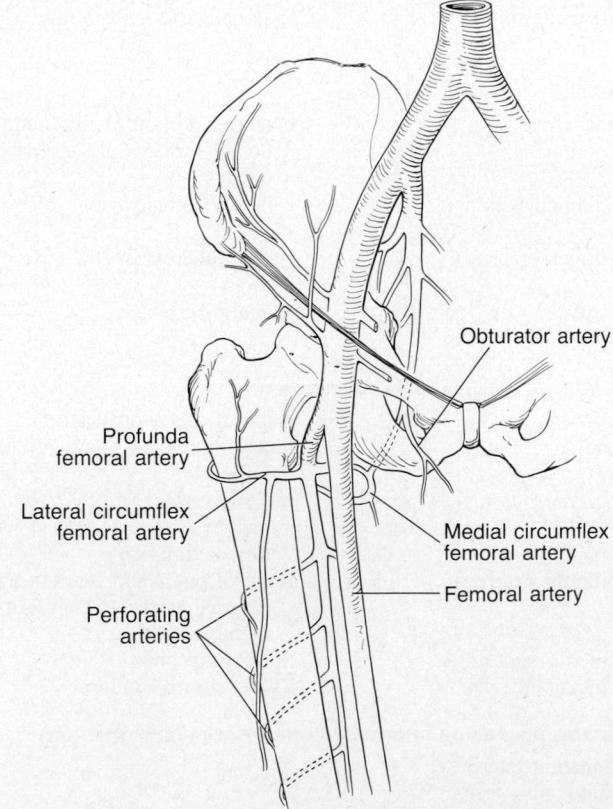

Fig. 16-9. Anterior view of lower limb, showing arterial supply. (Modified from Moore K: Clinically oriented anatomy, Baltimore, 1980, Williams & Wilkins.)

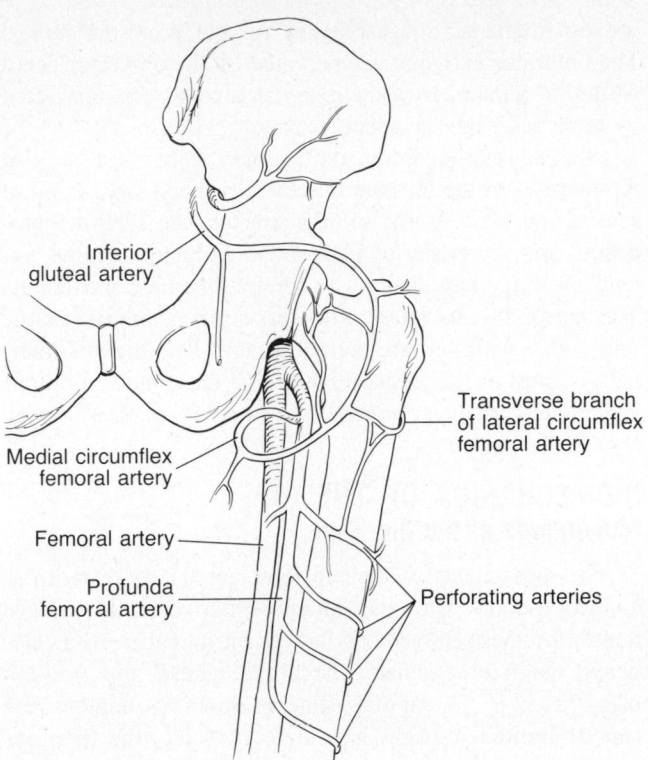

Fig. 16-10. Posterior view of limb, showing arterial supply. (Modified from Moore K: Clinically oriented anatomy, Baltimore, 1980, Williams & Wilkins.)

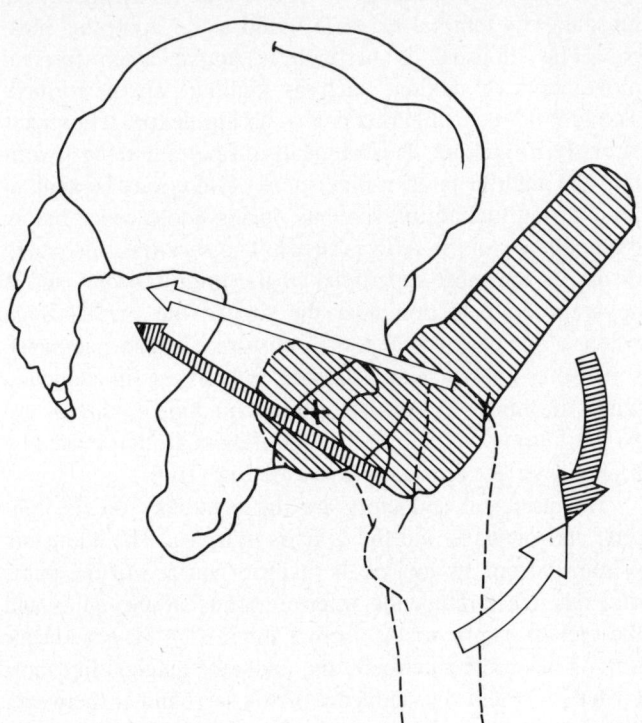

Fig. 16-11. When the hip is in the neutral position, the piriformis muscle produces lateral rotation, flexion, and abduction *(white arrow)*. When the hip is in exaggerated flexion, the piriformis muscle produces medial rotation, extension, and abduction *(shaded arrow)*. (Modified from Kapanji IA: Physiology of the joints, vol 2, Lower limb, New York, 1975, Churchill Livingstone, Inc.)

plied primarily by branches of the extracapsular ring formed by the medial and lateral circumflex arteries. The shaft of the femur is primarily supplied by perforating branches of the profunda femoris artery (Fig. 16-10).

Myology

Muscles completely surround the hip capsule and produce movement in three planes. The flexors and extensors provide movement in the sagittal plane and the abductors and adductors in the frontal plane; the hip rotators are responsible for movement in the transverse plane. The major muscles producing these movements and their origins, insertions, and innervations are summarized in Table 16-1. It should be noted however that Table 16-1 does not list the secondary functions of muscles. For example, the adductor muscles also have a role in flexion and extension depending on their origin. In the anatomically neutral position, if they arise from a position posterior to the frontal plane that runs through the axis of the joint, they contribute to extension (particularly the inferior fibers of the adductor magnus). If they arise from a position anterior to the frontal plane (pectineus, adductor brevis, and adductor longus, upper fibers of the adductor magnus and gracilis) they contribute to flexion.[44] The pectineus, because of its origin and insertion produces adduction, but acting alone it would also produce the additional movements of flexion and lateral rotation. In fact most muscles, because of the

fact that they do not run in a perfectly straight vertical direction, perform more than one movement when they contract.

A second limitation of Table 16-1 is related to what Kapandji terms *the inversion of muscular action*, which results in a change of direction of the muscle fibers when the position of the hip is other than anatomically neutral.[44] Depending on the position of the joint, the motor muscles will often change action. For example, when the hip is in the neutral position the piriformis produces lateral rotation, flexion, and abduction. However, when in a position of exaggerated flexion, it produces medial rotation, extension, and abduction (Fig. 16-11).

Though the following analysis of the muscles is divided according to their major actions the reader must always keep in mind that the actions of the muscles of a joint with 3 degrees of freedom often vary according to the position of the joint. This is why a very explicit knowledge of anatomy and kinesiology and not just an academic knowledge of the major actions of muscles is important in the analysis of normal and abnormal movement.

The strongest hip flexor is the iliopsoas, actually made up of the psoas minor and major and the iliacus muscles,[76] which crosses the hip joint just lateral to the pectineus muscle. The femoral nerve is found to lie upon this muscle. The iliopsoas is particularly active when forceful movements of flexion, such as kicking, are performed. Though the rectus femoris is a weak hip flexor, it contracts strongly in kicking. It is clinically important since its origin, the anterior inferior iliac spine (AIIS), may be avulsed with strong kicking movements during adolescence before the epiphysis of the AIIS is fused. The sartorius, also a hip flexor, is the most superficial of the thigh muscles and is apparent on palpation near the top of the medial thigh when a manual muscle test is performed. The pectineus, sometimes known as an adductor, only assists in adduction when the hip is flexed; its primary function is that of hip flexion during walking. All of the flexors are innervated by branches of the femoral nerve (see Fig. 16-8).

The principal adductors are the adductors brevis, longus, and magnus, and the gracilis muscles. The adductors originate from an area of the anterior surface of the pubis that extends through the inferior ramus of the pubis and the ischial ramus to the ischial tuberosity. The adductor longus lies most anteriorly, the adductor magnus lies most posteriorly, and the adductor brevis is found in between. They all insert into the posterior surface of the shaft of the femur, and the adductor magnus has a slip to the adductor tubercle. The gracilis is found medial to the three adductors and is the most medial muscle of the thigh. All the adductor muscles are innervated by the obturator nerve (see Fig. 16-8).

Abduction is primarily the action of the gluteus medius and minimus, both originating from the posterior portion of the ilium and inserting on the greater trochanter. The tensor fasciae latae, a small muscle that inserts into the iliotibial band, assists the pectineus in hip flexion during walking but also aids in abduction of the thigh. These three muscles are innervated by the superior gluteal nerve.

The extensors of the hip are primarily the three hamstring muscles (the semitendinosus, semimembranosus, and biceps femoris) and the gluteus maximus muscle. The hamstrings originate from the ischial tuberosity and take their insertions about the knee. They are innervated by the sciatic nerve. The gluteus maximus arises from the posterior ilium, sacrum, and coccyx to insert into the iliotibial band, merging with the fibers of the tensor fasciae latae. Some of the deep fibers insert into the lateral aspect of the posterior proximal femur. The gluteus maximus muscle is innervated by the inferior gluteal nerve. The posterior portion of the adductor magnus muscle assists the gluteus maximus muscle in its major function of extending the hip while a person is climbing stairs or getting up from sitting. It is also active with the hamstrings in walking.

The deep external rotators originate deep in the posterior portion of the hip joint on the sacrum or the ischium or, in the case of the obturator internus, from the inner surface of the obturator membrane. They all insert on the

greater trochanter or just below on the proximal femur. The obturator externus is innervated by the obturator nerve while the remainder of the external rotators are innervated by branches from the sacral plexus.

Internal rotation is not the primary function of any of the muscles of the hip, but is seen as a secondary action of several muscles. As the semitendinosus, the semimembranosus, and the posterior part of the adductor magnus extend the hip, they also act to internally rotate the femur. The tensor fasciae latae, when assisting in flexion of the thigh, also works as an internal rotator. The gracilis internally rotates as it adducts the hip, and the gluteus minimus and gluteus medius contribute to internal rotation as they abduct the hip.

BIOMECHANICS OF THE HIP
Movements of the hip joint

The movements of the hip joint are flexion-extension, abduction-adduction, and internal-external rotation. The norms for these movements are given in Table 16-2. Hyperextension or extension from the neutral hip position takes place in the sagittal plane to about 28 degrees and can be limited by tight hip flexor muscles, the iliopsoas and/or rectus femoris, and the iliofemoral ligament or anterior capsule. Adduction is most frequently limited by tightness of the tensor fasciae latae muscle and abduction by the adductors. Adduction in flexion, however, is often limited by the piriformis and other deep muscles of the buttocks. Flexion of the hip with the knee flexed is not a frequent limitation, whereas flexion with the knee extended occurs frequently because of tension in the hamstring muscles.

Accessory movements of distal and lateral glides occur in the hip joint and will be discussed in the portion of this chapter that deals with evaluation and treatment.

Mobility

Though the hip is more important for its function as a stable joint, mobility is very important for activities of daily living. A physical therapist should be aware of the degree of movement needed in the hip to perform certain

Table 16-2. Average ranges of joint motion for hip movements

	Degrees
Flexion (knee flexed)	0-113
Extension	0-28
Abduction	0-48
Adduction	0-31
External rotation	0-45
Internal rotation	0-45

Modified from American Academy of Orthopaedic Surgeons, Joint motion: Method of measuring and recording, Chicago, 1965, The Academy.

tasks when setting goals in the treatment of a hip disorder. The mean motion used during walking in normal men has been found to be 15 degrees extension, 37 degrees flexion, 7 degrees abduction, 5 degrees adduction, 4 degrees internal rotation, and 9 degrees external rotation.[40] In order to tie a shoe with the foot on the floor, a normal person uses an average of 129 degrees flexion, 18 degrees abduction, and 13 degrees external rotation. Stooping requires approximately 125 degrees flexion, 21 degrees abduction, and 15 degrees external rotation. The flexion normally used to climb up stairs is about 67 degrees and to go down stairs, about 36 degrees.[39] Of course many individuals who do not have these normal ranges are able to perform the mentioned tasks. For example, patients with only 100 degrees of passive hip flexion when measured supine will often be capable of tying their shoes. This is either because of the influence of the weight of the trunk when bending over or because of compensatory movements.

A lack of mobility can be attributed to numerous disorders and/or lack of flexibility. Surprisingly, the lack of mobility resulting from a unilateral arthrodesis of the hip in slight flexion is not obvious at very slow walking speeds.[29] At normal walking speeds and faster, compensation is accomplished by three major movements:[29] (1) a greater anteroposterior pelvic tilt (since an increased anterior pelvic tilt is needed in an attempt to extend the fused hip backward while the sound limb is in the swing phase),

(2) an increased transverse rotation of the pelvis (in an attempt to lengthen the step on the fused side), and (3) increased knee flexion on the side of fusion during stance (also possibly to increase the step length on the fused side). These same compensatory movements can be seen in clients with an insidious onset of stiffness in the hip. It may be postulated that some of these same compensations could also be seen in a runner with flexibility deficits, particularly of the hip flexors.

Though Table 16-2 lists what is considered "normal" ranges for the hip movements, it is important to know what is normal for the individual under examination. The normal for a patient who is a dancer or a gymnast may be well in excess of what is universally considered normal. In addition, variations are seen with age and sex. In the study by Ellis and Stowe[17] 200 subjects without known hip pathologies were tested to determine the active range of normalcy in ambulation and variation with age and sex. Particularly dramatic was the decrease in range of all subjects with age and most marked was the decrease in the movements of flexion and extension. For example, the mean flexion range for women dropped from 106 degrees in the 10 to 20 year age group to 72.1 degrees in the 70 to 80 year group. Extension in the same groups dropped from 24.7 degrees to 7.1 degrees. Extension showed the most marked reduction with age. For many of those tested in the 70 to 80 and 80+ groups, no

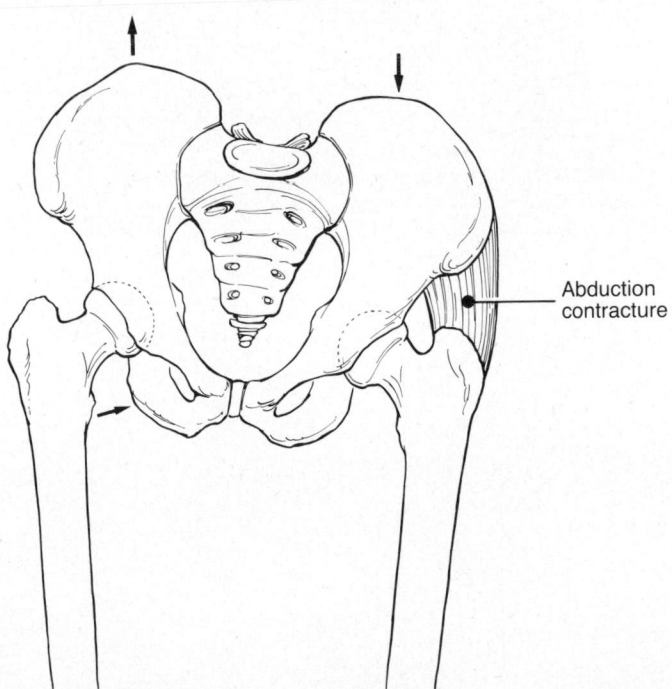

Fig. 16-12. Abduction contracture of hip and its effect on pelvis and hip joint. (Modified from Steindler A: Kinesiology of the human body under normal and pathological conditions, Springfield, Ill, 1955, Charles C Thomas, Publisher.)

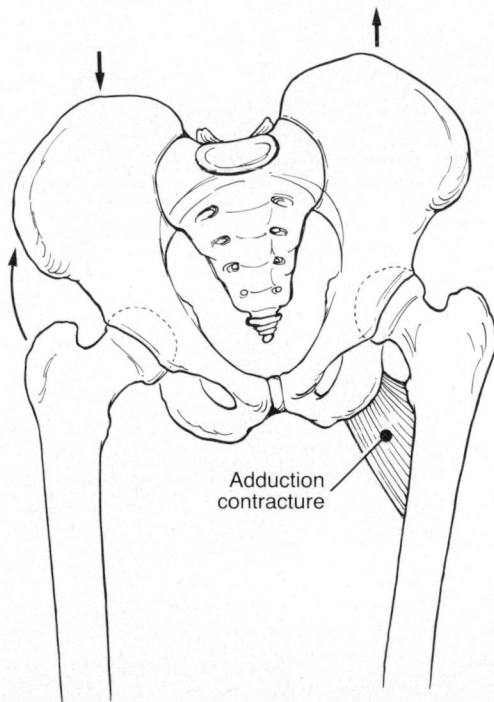

Fig. 16-13. Adduction contracture of hip and its effect on the pelvis and hip joint. (Modified from Steindler A: Kinesiology of the human body under normal and pathological conditions, Springfield, Ill, 1955, Charles C Thomas, Publisher.)

extension was possible and extension could not be increased when performed passively.

Stability

The hip joint is inherently stable because of its unique anatomy. The factors contributing to the innate stability of the hip joint include (1) its osseous structure with the deep acetabular socket and the tightly-fitting femoral head, (2) the vacuum effect of the ball-and-socket construction resisting distraction, (3) its thick articular joint capsule, which holds the head of the femur snugly into the acetabulum, (4) the ligamentous support around the articulation, and (5) the balance of the adjacent muscles about the joint. The position of greatest stability of the hip is that of complete extension because it puts the most tension on the ligaments and also causes the articular surfaces to become congruent. In flexion, however, all the ligaments and parts of the fibrous capsule are slack. This is the position of dislocation that most commonly occurs when there is a hard blow to the knee when the individual is seated.

The physical therapist is perhaps most often concerned directly with the balance of the adjacent muscles about the joint. This can be approached according to the balance created in the three planes of movement.

In the frontal plane, the adductors of one side of the hip work synergistically with the abductors of the opposite side. In a symmetrical position, the abductors and adduc-tors are under equal tension on both sides.[69] However, any disturbance in this equal tension will shift the pelvis to one side. For example, if there is a deficiency in either the abductors or the adductors in both legs, the individual may be able to stand evenly on both feet, but side movements become precarious. An abduction or adduction contracture will also cause the pelvis to assume an asymmetrical position (Figs. 16-12 and 16-13). An adduction contracture raises the pelvis on the affected side, thus creating an apparently shorter leg, while an abduction contracture creates an apparent longer leg.

Sagittal plane balance is generally performed by reciprocal contractions of the extensors and the flexors. An imbalance between the extensors and flexors can be seen when there is a bilateral paralysis of the gluteal muscles, such as in progressive muscular dystrophy. In this condition, the client must throw his or her body backward to avoid falling over from the unopposed action of the flexors. Another imbalance occurs in a bilateral hip flexion contracture where there is an increased lumbar lordosis found as compensation (Fig. 16-14).

Transverse plane balance depends on the inward and outward rotators. The power of the inward rotators is much less than that of the outward rotators. An imbalance caused by overpowering external rotators can cause excessive toeing-out. A unilateral external rotator contracture forces the backward rotation of the pelvis on the affected

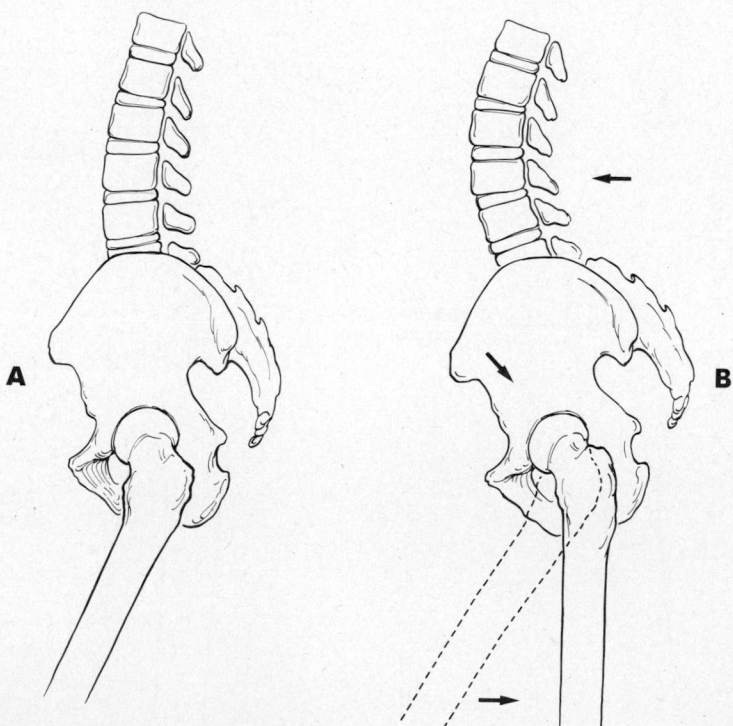

Fig. 16-14. A, Hip fixed in a flexed position. **B,** Compensation for **A** by lumbar lordosis. (Modified from Steindler A: Kinesiology of the human body under normal and pathological conditions, Springfield, Ill, 1955, Charles C Thomas, Publisher.)

side. This increases anterior and posterior movement in the other hip, which then tends to act as a pivot in walking.

Dynamic stability, as determined by electromyography, depends on the activity of the muscle groups during gait. Hip flexion is performed primarily by the iliopsoas muscle, which contracts at the beginning of the swing phase to initiate the movement.[36] The sartorius and the rectus femoris, which are weaker hip flexors, show a burst of activity at toe-off to aid in the swing-through phase.[2] The tensor fasciae latae muscle apparently also assists in hip flexion, showing a burst of activity simultaneous with the iliopsoas muscle.[36]

The hip extensors become active immediately after heel strike, assuming an elongated position that allows them to be the most forceful muscles in extending the hip.[36]

The abductor muscles are particularly important as stabilizers of the pelvis in the frontal plane. They prevent excessive downward movement of the pelvis on the weight-bearing side during single leg support.

The action of the adductors is most strongly seen at the beginning of the swing phase.[2] Since they do not create a great deal of adduction, it might be hypothesized from knowledge of their location that their activity aids more in flexion of the hip than in adduction.

The action of the internal and external rotators during the gait cycle has not been studied in detail, possibly because of (1) the deep location of the external rotators and (2) the fact that no muscles have internal rotation as their primary action.

Every gait cycle analysis performed consists of a study of the dynamic stability of the hip. The sequence of the movements in the hip during gait is summarized as follows. Hip flexion occurs just following heel-off and increases until or slightly before heel strike. Extension begins at heel strike and continues until the later stance phase. Abduction starts at the late stance phase and continues until just after toe-off. Adduction begins at midswing and increases until the late stance phase. External rotation starts at the midstance phase and continues until after toe-off, when internal rotation of the hip begins.[74]

In analyzing the dynamic stability provided at the hips in gait, the therapist must be aware that frequently one group of muscles acts to produce the movement for which another group is called on to provide stability. For example, while the muscles such as the iliacus, psoas, and rotators of the hip participate in the forward movement of the limb during swing, the same muscles of the opposite extremity as well as the abductors, adductors, and extensors are active to stabilize that extremity.

Forces imposed on the hip joint

In receiving super-incumbent load, the femur is subjected to pressure, bending, and shearing stresses. These stresses have a significance in the production of fractures as well as in the development of various disease processes.

The weight stress, however, is only one factor to take into account when looking at stresses sustained by the femur, particularly in the head and neck. Another equally important factor is the stresses transmitted by contraction of the hip muscles, especially the abductors.[35] Standing on one leg has been found create a force on the hip that is 2.5 times the body weight. This force is increased to 3 times the body weight when walking up stairs, while the dynamic effects of running create forces on the hip joint of 4.5 to 5 times the body weight.[62] Under normal circumstances, the femoral head can withstand a load of up to 12 to 15 times body weight before a fracture occurs.[62] This allows a considerable margin of safety in the normal hip.

As the body balances on one leg, the abductor muscles on the standing leg side must contract to stabilize the pelvis, creating considerable force on the hip joint (Fig. 16-15). In order to reduce this force, the person transfers his or her weight laterally by leaning to the side of the standing leg, thereby reducing the contraction of the abductors (Fig. 16-16). In walking, this motion results in a Trendelenburg lurch. If a client is asked to balance on the side of

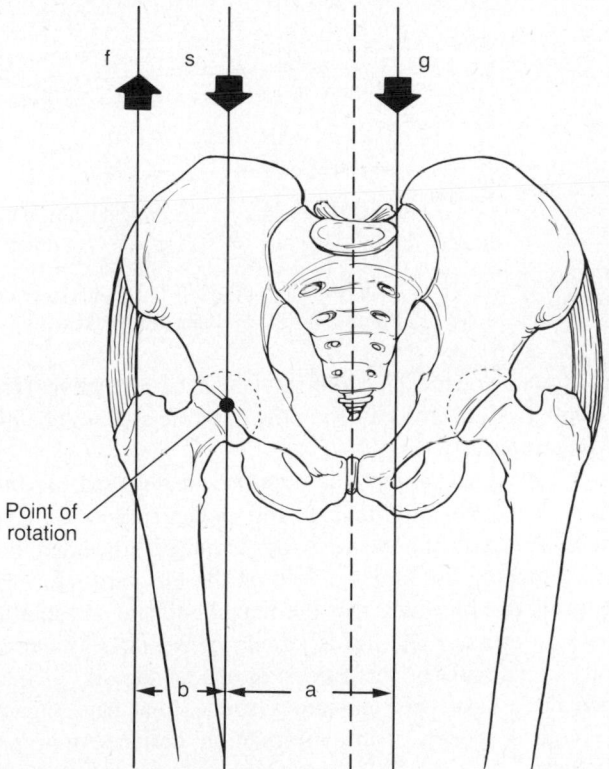

Fig. 16-15. Forces imposed on right hip joint during gait phase of single leg support on the right: the force of gravity (g) at a distance (a) from the point of rotation and the force of the abduction (f) working at a distance (b) from the point of rotation. fb = ga, and if g, which is the weight of the body, is 150 lb and a/b = 3/1, then f = g(a/b), which is 450 lb. The force (s) at the point of rotation is f + g = 600 lb. (Modified from Ramamurti C: In Tinker R, editor: Orthopaedics in primary care, Baltimore, 1979, Williams & Wilkins.)

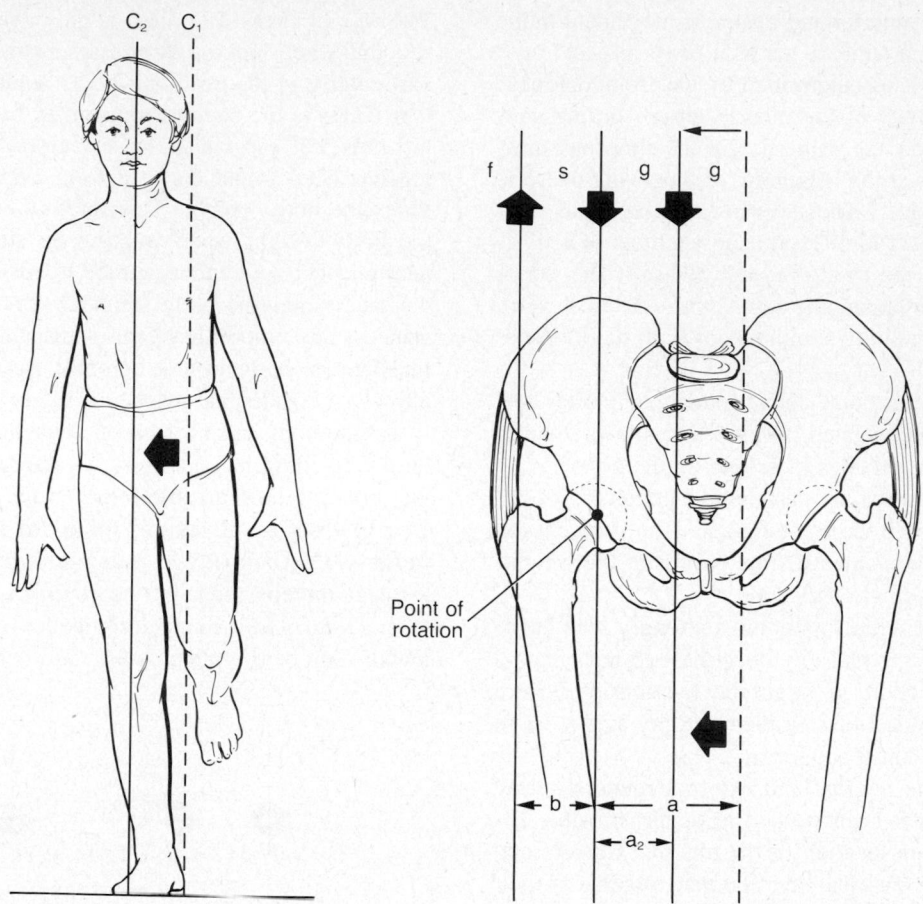

Fig. 16-16. Forces acting on right hip if the individual leans to the right during single right leg support. Now the force of gravity *(g)* moves a distance of a_2 from the point of rotation where $a_2 <$ a of Fig. 17-14. $fb = ga_2$ and, if $a_2/b = 1$, then for $g = 150$, $f = 150$. The force (s) is now $f +$ $g = 300$ lb. (Modified from Ramamurti C: In Tinker R, editor: Orthopaedics in primary care, Baltimore, 1979, Williams & Wilkins.)

weak abductor muscles, the result will be a positive Trendelenburg sign. The pelvis on the opposite side will be displaced inferiorly (Fig. 16-17).

A cane used on the side opposite an involved hip produces a movement similar to the abductor muscle movement, thus reducing the need for the muscle force and likewise reducing the forces placed on the hip joint.[3] In 1951 Pauwels demonstrated that the magnitude and direction of the load crossing the hip is largely determined by muscle forces, particularly the forces of the abductors.[59] Since then there have been numerous studies that have created theoretical models using information derived from gait analysis.[3,35,41,52,53,68,77] However, an interesting study was done more recently by Clark and Haynor who used computed tomography to look directly at the anatomy of the abductor muscle in normal live subjects.[14] They found a great variation in the inclination of the axis of the abductor muscles in both the frontal plane (17 to 29 degrees) and the sagittal plane (−2 to 14 degrees). They also observed marked differences in the size and locations of the separate muscles. They concluded that the capacity to map the

anatomy of any hip undergoing biomechanical analysis was important. Although this is a relatively new approach to biomechanical problems in the hip, the therapist should be aware of it and also of the fact that great variations occur between patients. Exercise may need to be adjusted accordingly.

The stresses applied to the hip joint result mostly from pressure.[40] Since pressure is defined as force per unit of area, it depends not only on the forces created primarily by the body weight and muscular contraction but also on the area over which this force is distributed. The joint is slightly incongruent with low loads, becoming more congruent for maximum surface contact with high loads. This serves to diminish the force per unit area or pressure of high loads.

Other stresses on the hip joint include those of bending, shearing, and torsion. Where and how movement occurs and the osseous formation of the femur determine where these three stresses are greatest. Shear stresses are greatest at the upper end of the femur, bending stress is maximal in the subtrochanteric region, and torsion stress is maximal

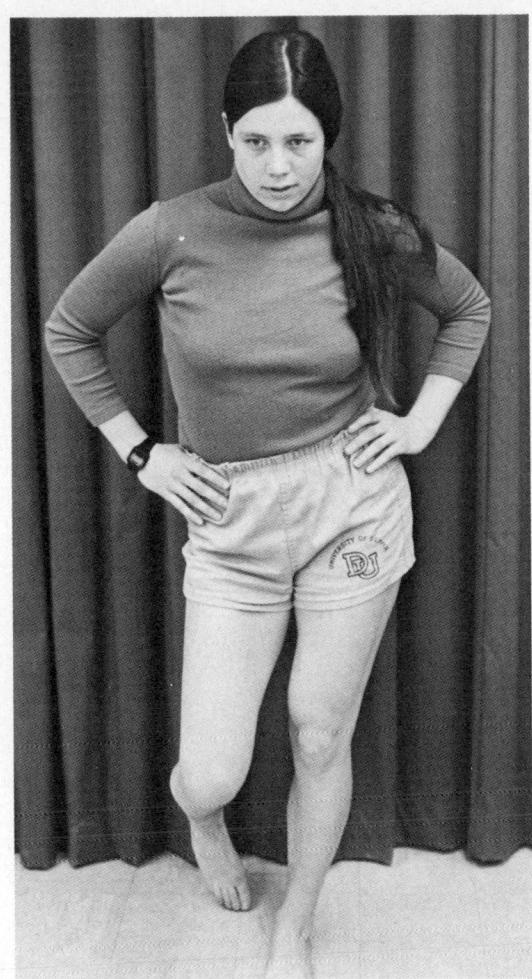

Fig. 16-17. Trendelenburg sign indicating weak abductors on left.

at the upper end of the femur, although applicable throughout the length of the femur.[8] A knowledge of these stresses is useful in understanding disease processes and the mechanism of fractures.

Coxalgic gait. The pathomechanics of deformities and disease processes will be discussed separately under each disorder. A factor in most hip problems, however, is pain, and coxalgic gait has certain common characteristics regardless of its cause. The painful hip is most often held in slight flexion, abduction, and external rotation. This is the position that ensures the least tension and the least irritation of the inflamed, sensitive synovial membrane.[69] Walking speed is notably slower for individuals with hip pain, and their steps are shorter and unequal. They will take longer steps with their painful limb than with the uninvolved limb in an attempt to prevent pressure on the painful side. When walking, the center of gravity is thrown over the affected side by the tilt of the body, producing a Trendelenburg lurch. Since a reflex response to hip pain is slight flexion, a compensating lordosis may be apparent in gait, particularly in those individuals who have

bilateral hip pain. An assistive device is often used by clients on the side opposite the hip pain because of its aid in substantially decreasing the force on the hip.

CAUSES OF PAIN IN THE HIP JOINT

In order to best evaluate the hip the various causes of hip pain should be well understood. No matter what the cause of joint disease, most of the pain arises from the joint lining and, in particular, from the synovium and the capsule of the joint. There is usually some degree of inflammatory change, called *synovitis,* in the lining of the hip joint. In synovitis, the pain arises from the stimulation of the sensory nerve endings in the synovium. It is usually dull in nature, often throbbing, and worse at night and when the patient is immobile. The patient will often awaken with a painful hip and require gentle movement until the pain subsides. This pain will vary in severity depending on the degree of inflammation present in the synovium.

Capsular pain is caused by stretching and compression of pain nerve endings between the collagen fibers. In osteoarthritis there is secondary capsular fibrosis due to recurrent synovitis. The capsular fibrosis leads to a shortening of the capsule around the joint with increasing deformity. The hip is pulled into a position of adduction, flexion, and external rotation to relax the capsular fibers. This is the characteristic position of the osteoarthritic hip. With capsular pain, active movement aggravates the condition because it stretches the capsular fibers, thus stimulating the pain nerve endings. This then leads to repeated contraction of the surrounding muscles.

Articular cartilage cannot in itself give rise to pain since it does not contain nerve endings. However, if the normal matrix of articular cartilage is destroyed, it is replaced by fibrocartilage, which is invaded by nerve endings. The result of this is pain on any weight bearing.

Bone pain also occurs on weight bearing and the greater the load, the more the pain. It can occur with abnormal loading in the case of loss of articular cartilage. This is relieved by rest.

The pain caused by inflammation of the tendons or the bursae is often the result of spreading capsular inflammation. This pain will therefore be felt on active movement and its exact location can be confirmed by palpation.

Whatever the cause of pain in the hip it inevitably causes stiffness, from capsular fibrosis, from contracture of the muscles, from inactivity due to pain or bedrest. Physicians may initially try to relieve pain with anti-inflammatory drugs without suggesting physical therapy. However, once stiffness is a factor, the patient is often referred to the physical therapist.

EVALUATION OF THE HIP

Thorough evaluation of any part of the body requires a systematic approach that will aid the therapist in efficient collection of relevant data. This requires considerable practice, but a well-thought-out form will facilitate the recording of important information. The essential aspects of a hip evaluation consist of two parts: subjective examination and objective examination. Though these parts are separated for recording purposes, they are intertwined throughout the evaluation process. Experience has shown that a client may share very pertinent subjective information with the therapist while the objective examination is being per-

formed. Also, although conducting the subjective examination, initial objective observations should be made while the client is sitting in the waiting room, rising from the seated position, and walking into the evaluation room. A clinical form for an evaluation of the hip is given in Fig. 16-18.

Subjective examination

The subjective examination will provide the therapist with an indication of the severity, irritability, and nature of

EVALUATION OF THE HIP

Date _____   # _____
Name _____ Age_____ Sex_____
Address_____ Occupation_____
Diagnosis or referral _____
Referring physician _____

A. SUBJECTIVE EXAMINATION OF THE HIP
1. Client's chief complaint_____
2. Location of symptoms _____

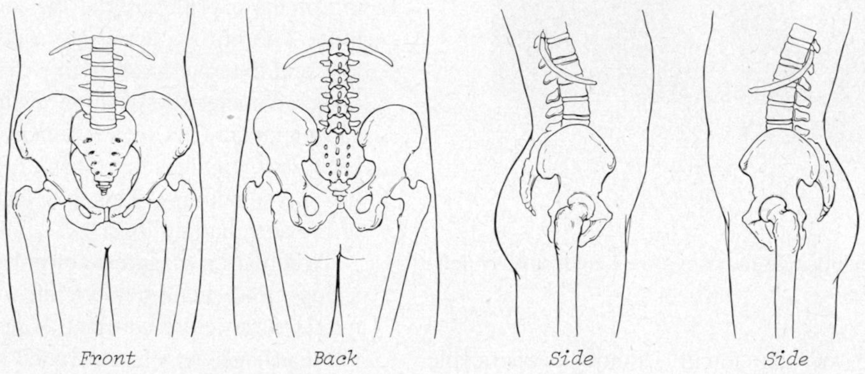

Front   *Back*   *Side*   *Side*

3. Onset of symptoms
    Date of injury/onset_____
    Nature and mechanism_____

4. Nature of symptoms_____
    _____
    Where did the symptoms start?_____
    Have they spread?_____Where?_____
    Is there any tingling or numbness?_____
    Is the pain sharp, a dull ache, deep, etc.?_____

5. Previous history
    First episode in detail_____
    _____
    Successive episodes
        How frequently?_____
        Ease of onset _____
        How long to recover?_____
        Previous treatment and results_____

Fig. 16-18. Evaluation of hip, clinical form.

the condition. The following are the essential aspects of the subjective examination:

1. Client's chief complaint
2. Location of symptoms; where did it originate and where did it spread?
3. Onset of symptoms
4. Nature of symptoms
5. Previous history

6. Behavior of symptoms, relation to rest, posture, activity and exertion
7. Previous treatment and results
8. Other medical history and family history
9. Hobbies and leisure activities

The subjective examination will set the tone for the objective examination and help determine the necessary special tests. For example, the objective examination of a 72-year-old sedentary woman with pain in the hip joint will

EVALUATION OF THE HIP—cont'd

6. Behavior of symptoms
   Constant or intermittent? _____
   What brings them on? _____
   What relieves them? _____
   What makes them worse? _____
   Is there associated stiffness? _____
   What is the effect of prolonged sitting? _____
   _____
   What is the effect of walking? _____
   _____

7. Previous treatment and results
   Treatment to date for present problem _____
   Effects? _____

8. Other medical history and family history
   Medications _____
   Radiographs _____
   Recent illnesses _____
   Family history _____
   General health _____

9. Hobbies and leisure-time activities _____
   Still able to do these activities? _____

B. OBJECTIVE EXAMINATION OF THE HIP
1. Initial observation
   Sitting posture _____
   Sitting to standing _____
   Gait _____
   Ease of movement _____

2. Standing
   Posture _____
   _____
   Detailed gait evaluation _____
   _____
   Balance
      Digital scale weight bearing   R_____ L_____
      Stork standing test: Standing on R leg_____ Standing on L leg_____
   Lumbar spine active movements
      Flexion _____
      Extension _____

Fig. 16-18, cont'd. Evaluation of hip, clinical form.

Lateral flexion R _____

Lateral flexion L _____

Squat _____

3. Sitting

Lumbar spine active movements

Rotation R_____ L_____

Active, passive, and resisted internal and external rotation

Internal rotation R_____ L_____

External rotation R_____ L_____

Active and resisted hip flexion R_____ L_____

Sartorius muscle test _____

Thomas test: R hip extended _____

L hip extended _____

4. Supine

Palpations of anterior aspect _____

Leg-length measurements R_____ L_____

SI joint compression and distraction _____

Fabere's test R_____ L_____

Scouring R_____ L_____

Distal and lateral traction R_____ L_____

90-90 straight-leg raise R_____ L_____

Knee clearing _____

Passive, active, and resisted hip movements

Flexion   R_____ L_____

Abduction R_____ L_____

Adduction R_____ L_____

5. Side-lying position

Palpations of lateral and posterior aspects _____

_____

Active, passive, and resisted hip movements

Extension R_____ L_____

Abduction R_____ L_____

Flexion   R_____ L_____

Adduction: Ober test (knee extended) R_____ L_____

Knee flexed R_____ L_____

Hip and knee flexed (piriformis tightness test) R_____ L_____

6. Prone

Palpations of posterior aspect _____

_____

Active, passive, and resisted hip movements

Hip extension: Knee extended R_____ L_____

Knee flexed   R_____ L_____

Internal rotation R_____ L_____

External rotation R_____ L_____

Prone knee bend (femoral nerve stretch) R_____ L_____

7. Miscellaneous

Other observations of tests _____

Subjective comments during objective examination _____

_____

_____

_____

8. Summary of findings

Fig. 16-18, cont'd. Evaluation of hip, clinical form.

be very different from an objective examination of a 16-year-old athlete with groin pain.

The onset of symptoms, including the mechanism of injury (if known), determines whether the condition is acute, subacute, or chronic. It can also indicate the type of disorder, such as muscle strain, degenerative joint disease, or bursitis. The nature of the symptoms is important for determining the type of pain present, whether the pain may be referred, or whether there are any associated neurological signs. The history of the present disorder will indicate the frequency and previous treatment of the condition. This will give the therapist an idea of whether the problem is a recurring one and the extent and success of previous treatment.

The severity and irritability of the symptoms are determined primarily by the response to questions concerning the behavior of the symptoms. Other medical history will provide information on the general health of the client, diseases that may be contributing factors, the predisposition to a disease process through family history, and any medications that may be influencing the disease process. Information about the client's hobbies and leisure activities will often help the therapist establish parameters for returning a client to activity. This information will influence the form of treatment, particularly in the case of an active person. Maintaining over-all body strength and cardiovascular fitness while rehabilitating an injured hip may be of foremost importance.

Objective examination

The objective examination consists of reproducible, measurable, and reliable data relating to the present disorder. It is particularly pertinent, in the case of a painful hip disorder, that a client be subjected to as little movement as possible, therefore the objective examination has been organized by position.

The following is the sequence of testing for the objective examination:

1. Initial observation
   a. Posture
   b. Gait evaluation
2. Standing
   a. Posture
   b. Detailed gait evaluation
   c. Balance
      (1) Digital scale weight bearing
      (2) Stork standing test
   d. Lumbar spine flexion, extension, and lateral flexion
   e. Squat
3. Sitting
   a. Lumbar spine rotation
   b. Active, passive, and resisted internal and external rotation

   c. Active and resisted hip flexion
   d. Sartorius muscle test
   e. Thomas test
4. Supine
   a. Palpations of anterior as well as lateral aspect such as the gluteus minimus and medius, and the trochanteric bursa
   b. Leg-length measurements
   c. Sacroiliac joint compression and distraction
   d. Fabere's test
   e. Scouring
   f. Distal and lateral traction
   g. 90-90 straight-leg raise
   h. Knee "clearing"
   i. Active, passive, and resisted hip flexion, abduction, and adduction
5. Side-lying position
   a. Palpations of lateral and posterior aspects
   b. Active, passive, and resisted extension, abduction, flexion, and adduction
      (1) Ober test
      (2) Piriformis tightness test
6. Prone
   a. Palpations of posterior aspect
   b. Active, passive, and resisted extension, internal and external rotation
   c. Prone knee bend (femoral nerve stretch)

The following demonstrates the organization of the examination by types of tests:

1. Initial observation
   a. Posture
   b. Gait evaluation
   c. Ease of movement
2. Balance
   a. Digital scale bilateral comparison
   b. Stork standing test
3. Peripheral "joint-clearing" tests
   a. Lumbar spine active movements
   b. Squat
   c. Sacroiliac compression and distraction
   d. Knee varus and valgus stress and bounce home test
4. Active movements of the hip
   a. Flexion
   b. Extension
   c. Abduction
   d. Adduction
   e. Internal rotation
   f. External rotation
5. Passive movements
   a. Physiological
      (1) Flexion
      (2) Extension
      (3) Abduction

(4) Adduction
(5) Internal rotation
(6) External rotation
b. Accessory
  (1) Distal traction
  (2) Lateral traction
6. Resisted movements
a. Internal rotators
b. External rotators
c. Flexors
d. Extensors
e. Abductors
f. Adductors
7. Palpation
a. Anterior aspect
  (1) Bony
    (a) Anterior superior iliac spine
    (b) Iliac crest
    (c) Iliac tubercle
    (d) Pubic tubercle
    (e) Adductor tubercle
  (2) Soft
    (a) Inguinal area
    (b) Femoral pulse
    (c) Site of iliopsoas and iliopectineal bursas
    (d) Sartorius muscle
    (e) Adductor longus
b. Anterolateral aspect
  (1) Bony
    (a) Greater trochanter
  (2) Soft
    (a) Gluteus minimus
    (b) Gluteus medius
    (c) Site of greater trochanteric bursa
c. Posterior aspect
  (1) Bony
    (a) Posterior superior iliac spine
    (b) Ischial tuberosity
    (c) Greater trochanter
    (d) Sacrum and coccyx
    (e) L-4, L-5
    (f) Sciatic notch
  (2) Soft
    (a) Sciatic nerve
    (b) Piriformis and other deep rotators
    (c) Site of ischial bursa
8. Special tests
a. Thomas test
b. Ober test
c. Fabere's test
d. Scouring
e. Femoral nerve stretch
f. 90-90 straight-leg raise
g. Piriformis tightness test

The form used for the objective examination of the hip is all-encompassing, but not every test can be performed for each client. Evaluation of a client who has just received a total hip replacement will include little more than subjective comments, some range-of-motion measurements, and observation of gait. Later assessments may include observation of posture, gait, active movements, and muscle and flexibility tests. The form given is intended to be a guide for a complete hip evaluation (see Fig. 16-18).

A thorough objective examination of the hip includes observation, balance testing, "clearing" of the lumbar spine, sacroiliac joints, and knee, active hip movements, passive hip movements (including accessory movements), manual muscle tests, palpations, and special tests for flexibility and stress to certain structures. Generally, passive physiological movements, active movements, and resisted movements are done in sequence.

For example, when evaluating hip abduction in the supine position, the limb should be passively taken through the range of motion; next, the client should perform the movement actively, and then resistance should be added (if appropriate). If the resistance indicates good muscle strength, technically the client would need to be retested in the side-lying position for proper documentation. If the resisted movements reproduce symptoms, and passive stretching of the same musculotendinous unit in the opposite direction also produces symptoms, then a contractile unit is implicated. If only passive movements around the hip reproduce symptoms, then a disorder involving the hip capsule is implicated.

Accessory movements are used to assess joint play and may later be used as treatment techniques. The special tests primarily involve assessing flexibility. Scouring is used to assess the condition of the joint surfaces, to reproduce pain, and to treat pain.

Standing. A careful postural examination should focus on the client's posture from head to foot. It should include analysis of the foot and alignment of the knees, weight-bearing leg-length measurements, bilateral comparison of the location of the anterior and posterior superior iliac spines and the iliac crests, and observation of any deviation of posture to one side and stooped posture possibly caused by hip-flexion contractures. Any asymmetry, such as unilateral atrophy of the gluteals, thighs, or calves, should be documented and measured when possible. A note of caution should be made as to the degree of accuracy of leg-length measurements. Although clinical methods may have been shown to be reliable,[13,27,56] Friberg points out that the observer error of 10 mm either way that has been found in several studies[13,22,55,56,57] should not be overlooked.[21] Consequently, Friberg suggests a standing roentgenogram method that differs from previous methods in exposing only the region of the hip joints and is regarded as free of any risk of radiation. Leg-length inequality is then measured as the difference between the heights of the highest articular points of the femoral heads. Since roentgenograms are often taken when the patient complains of hip pain, the therapist may have access to them and may wish to correlate their clinical findings with the method of measurement Friberg suggests.

Gait evaluation should include observation and documentation of stride-length differences, any listing or lurching to one side, an antalgic gait, the distance walked before fatigue, and abnormal movements of the hips. Gait patterns can show weaknesses, contractures, or limitations of range. This dynamic measure of functional activity should never be neglected.

A digital scale reading will indicate asymmetry in weight bearing, which will be diminished on the painful side. In the absence of a digital scale, two bathroom scales may be used. This measure is especially useful for future reference since a decrease in pain will normally result in more willingness to bear weight on the involved side. The stork standing test (Fig. 16-19) is used to evaluate balance

but may also indicate a gluteus medius weakness by a positive Trendelenburg sign (Fig. 16-17).

Both the lumbar spine active movements and the squat are considered to be peripheral "joint clearing" tests. It is not unusual that low lumbar spine problems refer pain into the buttocks region via the sciatic nerve. Infrequent disorders of L-1, L-2, or L-3 nerve roots may also refer pain into the lateral aspect of the hip or anterior thigh via the femoral nerve. The squat will not only help to "clear" the knees but also will indicate willingness to move in the hip and lumbar region. With all the active tests, the therapist is looking for a reproduction of symptoms in the hip region.

Sitting. When sitting, the client performs active lumbar rotation and external and internal rotation of the hip. The therapist should demonstrate the passive movement of internal or external rotation for the client. This is the position for normal, good, and fair muscle-testing grades for the hip rotators and hip flexors, so both active and resisted movements may be tested in this position. The sitting position may also be used to test the sartorius muscle (Fig. 16-20). Pain at the location of the anterior superior iliac spine may result if this muscle has been strained.

The Thomas test is a passive test for the length of the hip flexors. It is begun in the sitting position and the client is instructed to bring the knees to the chest and roll back to the supine position while holding the knees. Then one leg is held with the hip flexed and the other hip is extended with the knee bent. It is important to prevent any abduction or adduction of the thigh as it is extended. Normal flexibility of the hip flexors allows the posterior thigh of the extended hip to rest against the plinth. Fig. 16-21

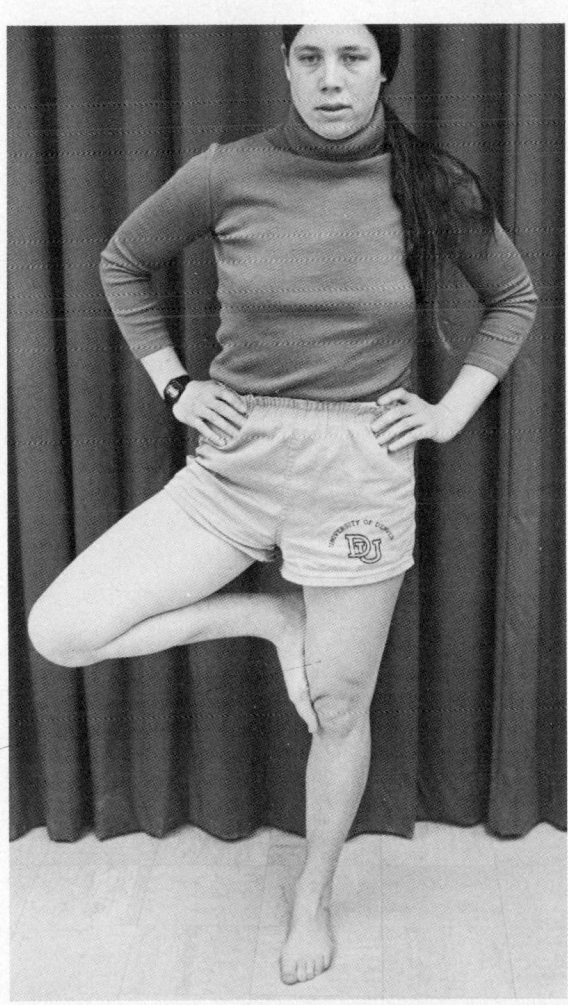

Fig. 16-19. Stork standing test.

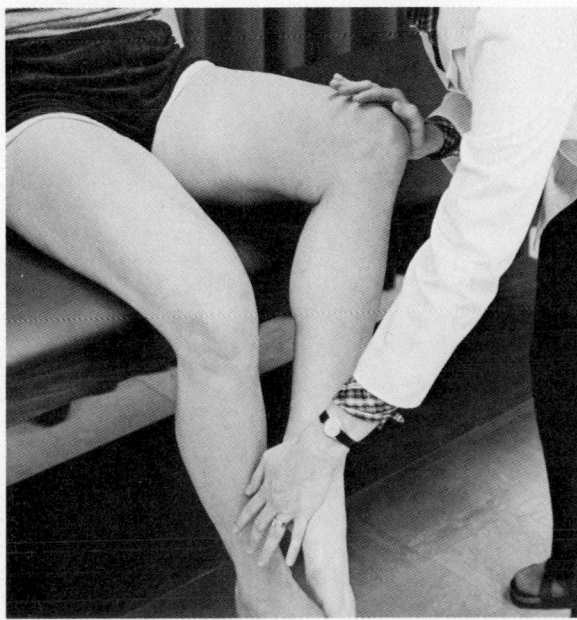

Fig. 16-20. Manual muscle test of sartorius muscle.

shows the Thomas test when hip flexor tightness restricts hip extension.

To further isolate the rectus femoris muscle from the iliopsoas muscle, the flexed hip is allowed to extend until the contralateral posterior thigh comes down to the plinth. When the knee is flexed back in this position, resistance indicates tightness of the rectus femoris muscle (Fig. 16-22). If the Thomas test is positive but the client's modification is negative, then the iliopsoas muscle is considered to be the cause for restriction of motion. This test might

also reproduce pain in the case of iliopectineal bursitis.

Supine. In the supine position, palpations should be done at the anterior superior iliac spine, iliac crests, iliac tubercles, greater trochanters, pubic tubercles, inguinal area, femoral pulse, sartorius muscle, adductor tubercle, and at the insertion of the adductor longus. A complete knowledge of anatomy is necessary to understand the reasons for pain in any of these areas. The adductor longus is the muscle most frequently involved in an adductor strain. Pain on palpation of the greater trochanter may be indica-

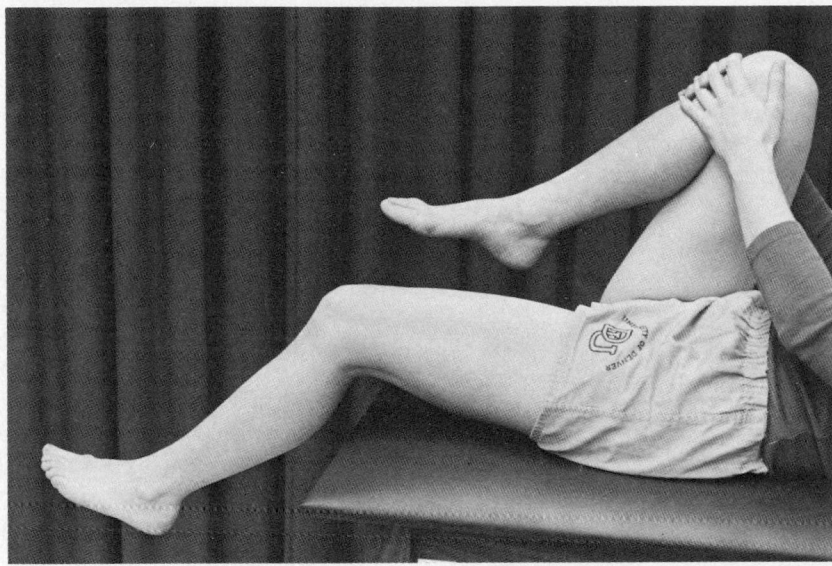

Fig. 16-21. Positive Thomas test illustrating hip flexor tightness.

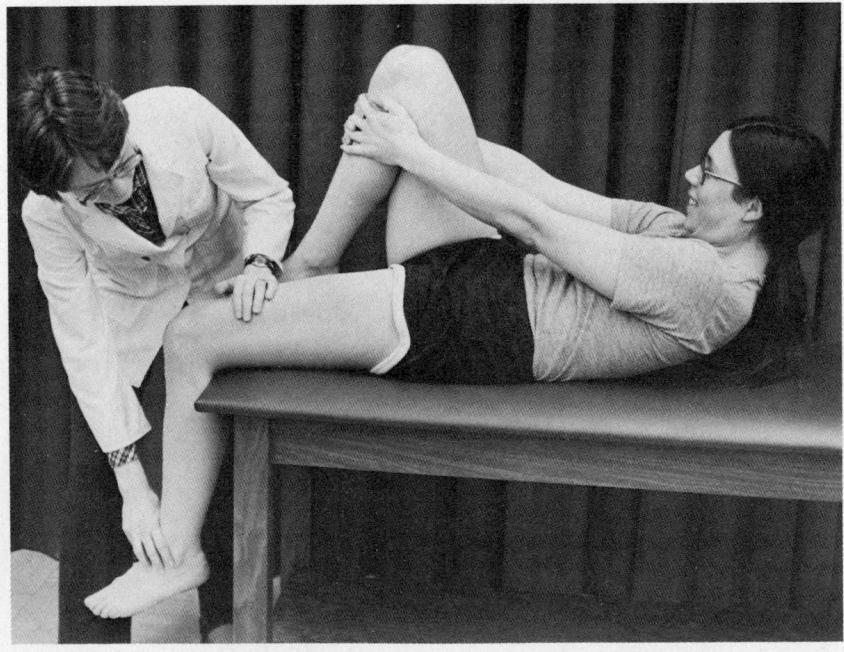

Fig. 16-22. Test for length of rectus femoris muscle.

tive of greater trochanteric bursitis, while pain on palpation of the pubic tubercles may indicate adductor strain. Non–weight-bearing leg-length measurements may be made in the supine position and compared with weight-bearing measurements. The sacroiliac joint is stressed in the compression and distraction tests as well as in Fabere's test (Fig. 16-23) and scouring (Fig. 16-24). A more thorough evaluation of the sacro-iliac joint should be done if these tests are positive for pain in that area. Fabere's test also stresses the anterior medial capsule of the hip. Scouring is used to stress the posterior and lateral hip capsule and will often elicit a grating sensation or sound in the

case of an osteoarthritic hip. The hip is flexed and adducted and a posterolateral force is applied through the joint as the femur is rotated in the acetabulum (see Fig. 16-24). Distal and lateral tractions of the hip are accessory movements to assess restrictions of hip movement (Figs. 16-25 and 16-26). The 90-90 straight-leg raise is a test for the flexibility of the hamstring muscles (Fig. 16-27). The client flexes the hip to 90 degrees and grasps behind the knee with both hands. The leg is then extended through the available range. A measurement of 20 degrees from full extension is within normal limits. Any measurement of larger magnitude would indicate a hamstring tightness.

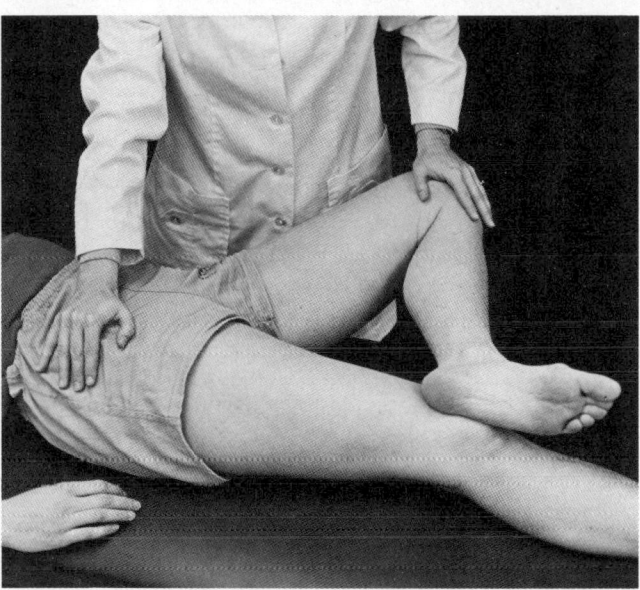

Fig. 16-23. Fabere's test.

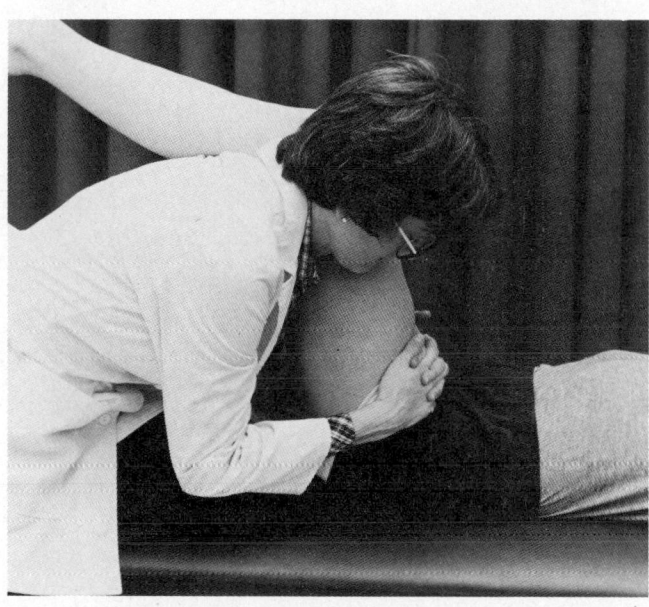

Fig. 16-25. Distal traction of hip.

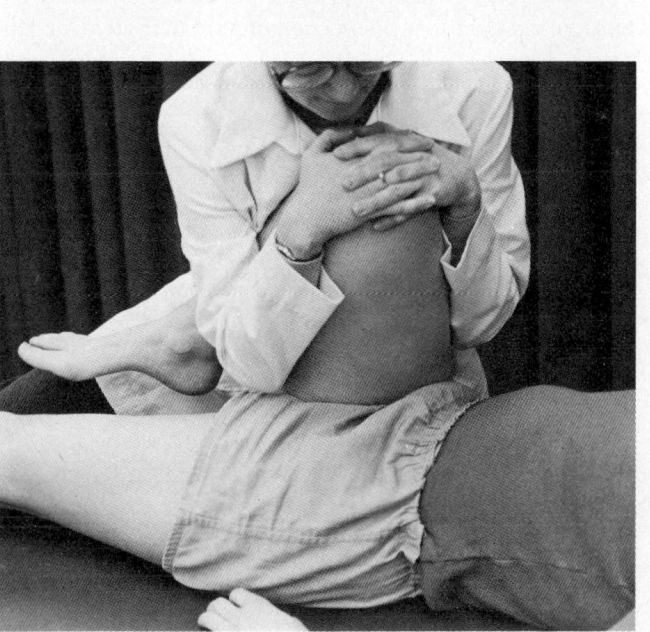

Fig. 16-24. Scouring of hip.

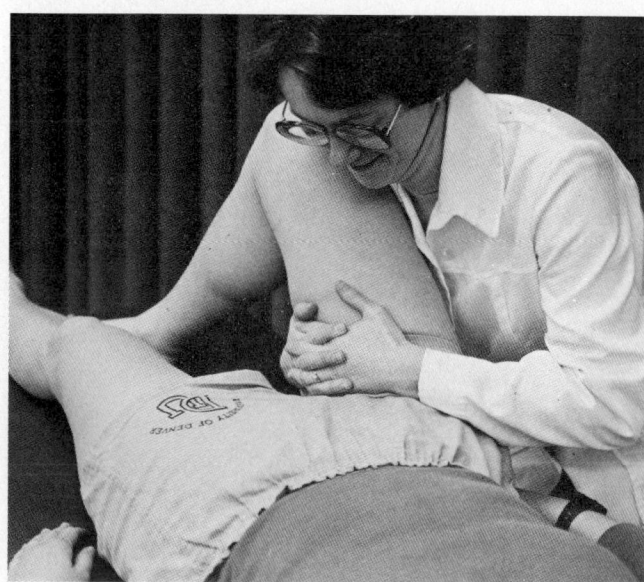

Fig. 16-26. Lateral traction of hip.

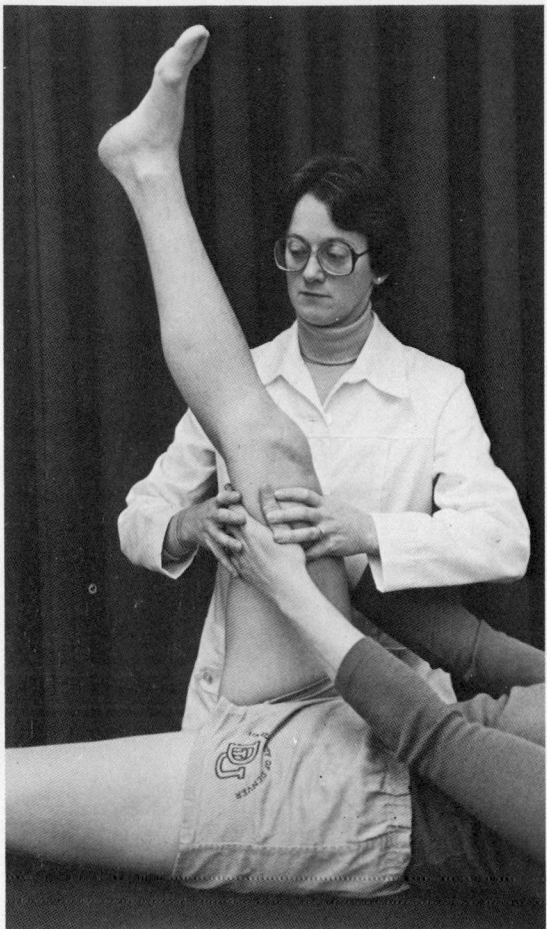

Fig. 16-27. 90-90 straight-leg raise.

Knee "clearing" tests are important since pain in the knee may be referred up to the hip via the obturator nerve. Valgus and varus stress tests and the bounce home test will clear the knee.

Hip flexion strength can be tested with the client in the supine as well as in the sitting position. The supine position is the preferred position for goniometric measurements of hip flexion and abduction, and adductor flexibility tests are also performed in this position. The examiner should stabilize the hip by placing one hand over the anterior superior iliac spine to prevent hip hiking and then passively abduct the hip, making sure not to allow external rotation (Fig. 16-28). To eliminate the influence of the gracilis muscle, the knee is bent at the end of range and the limb is moved further, if possible (Fig. 16-29). If the leg can be abducted further with the knee bent, the gracilis is the source of some limitation in abduction. During this test, pain in the region of the pubic tubercles may indicate an adductor strain.

The supine position may also be used for a poor or trace grade in manual muscle testing for hip abduction, adduction, and internal and external rotation, as well as for a poor or trace grade of the strength of the sartorius muscle.

Side-lying. The side-lying position is often uncomfortable for clients with lateral hip problems because of the adduction force imposed on the top limb by gravity. In this case, adaptations may need to be made. Palpations of the lateral aspect of the hip include the sciatic notch, the sciatic nerve, the ischial tuberosity, and the greater trochanter. If the sciatic nerve or the ischial bursa is irritated, palpations will indicate pain in those areas. The side-lying position is used for normal and good grade positioning of manual muscle tests for hip abduction and hip adduction. Poor and trace grades for manual muscletesting of hip extension and flexion is also done lying on the side. The ten-

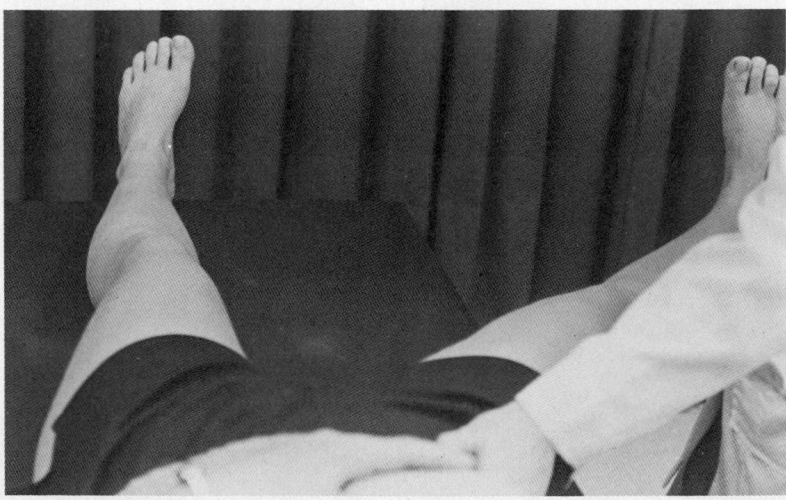

Fig. 16-28. Adductor flexibility test, knee extended.

sor fasciae latae is tested as an abductor with the hip flexed to about 45 degrees, and the gluteus medius is tested for strength with the hip in the neutral position.

A positive Ober test indicates a contraction of the iliotibial band (Fig. 16-30). It is performed in the side-lying position with the hip well stabilized to prevent a false negative test. With the knee extended, the top leg is slightly extended and dropped toward the plinth. In a negative test, the adducted leg should reach the level of the plinth. To put the iliotibial band on slack and test for the flexibility of the short fibers of the tensor fasciae latae muscle, the knee

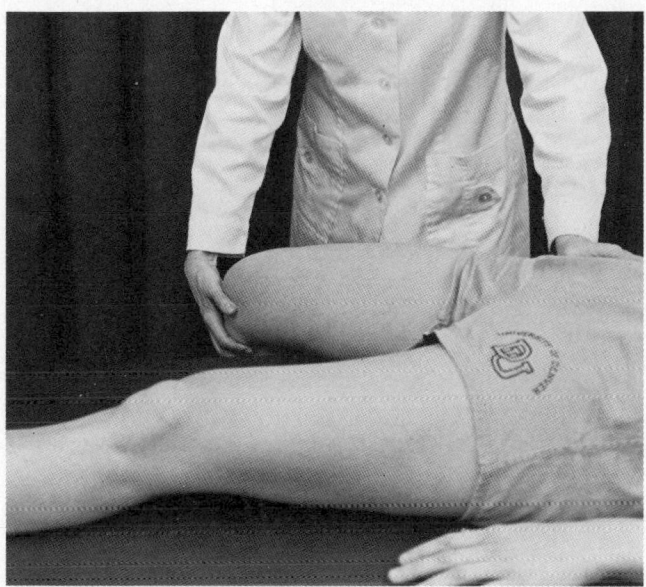

Fig. 16-29. Adductor flexibility test, knee bent to eliminate influence of gracilis muscle.

is bent and dropped down in a similar manner (Fig. 16-31). To test for external rotator tightness, particularly in the piriformis muscle, the hip is flexed to 90 degrees and the knee is flexed. The examiner places one hand on the hip for stabilization and applies pressure to the knee (Fig. 16-32). If a tight piriformis muscle is impinging on the sciatic nerve, this test will produce pain in the buttock region.

Prone. Palpation of the posterior aspect of the hip area includes the posterior superior iliac spine, coccyx, sacrum, and lumbar spine. Sometimes piriformis muscle tightness can be felt deep to the gluteus maximus muscle. A hip flexion contracture may also be apparent in this position and should be measured. The prone position is used for goniometric measurement of hip extension as well as for normal and good grades of hip extension. The prone position is also the preferred position for goniometric measurements of internal and external rotation of the hip.

The prone knee bend is performed with the hip extended and the knee flexed (Fig. 16-33). It stretches the femoral nerve, and pain on this test in the lateral hip or anterior thigh may indicate an impingement of L-1, L-2, or L-3 nerve roots.

Daniels and Worthingham[16] give details of specific muscle testing.

Summary of findings and plan

A concise and complete summary of a client's limitation should be used for purposes of communication with the physician or other therapists. All positive findings should be summarized, and correlations should be made to facilitate an assessment. The goals and plan will not only depend on the objective findings and assessment but will also be influenced by the age, level of physical activity,

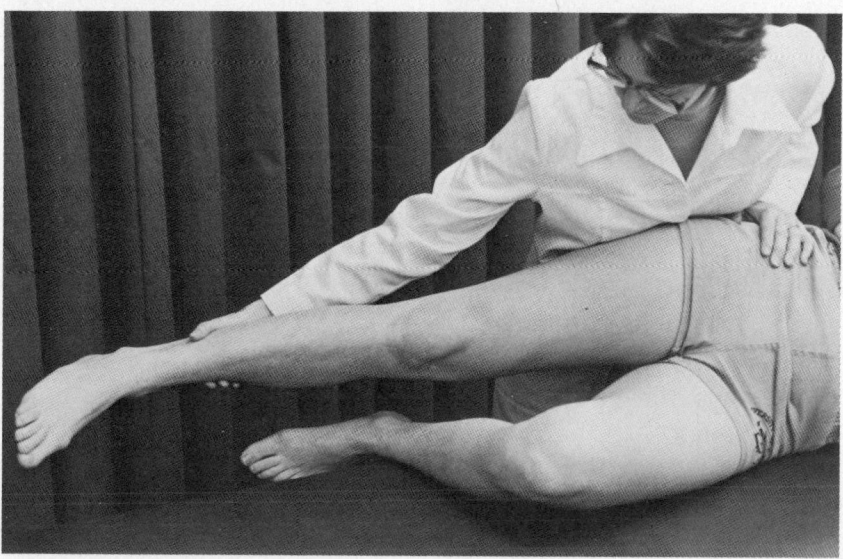

Fig. 16-30. Ober test for iliotibial band contraction.

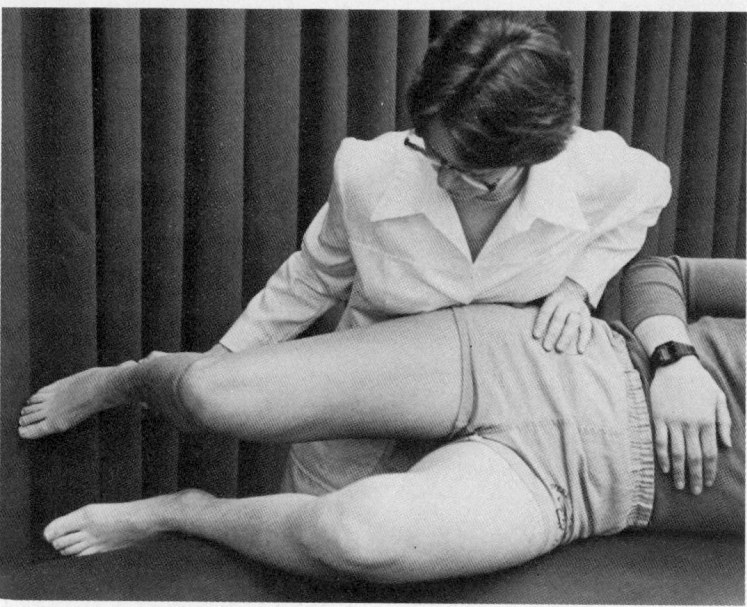

Fig. 16-31. Modified Ober test for tightness of short fibers of tensor fasciae latae muscle.

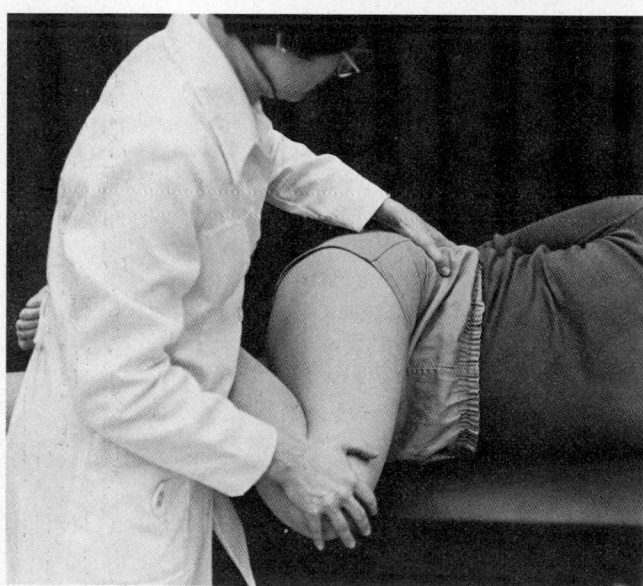

Fig. 16-32. Piriformis test for external rotator tightness.

life-style, and occupation of the client as well as other subjective findings.

CONDITIONS AND TREATMENT OF VARIOUS HIP DISORDERS
Osseous malformations of the hip

Coxa valga. *Coxa valga* is characterized by the persistence into adulthood of a neck-shaft angle that is greater than 130 degrees. The neck-shaft angle is usually 150 degrees at birth and decreases to 130 degrees by adulthood. Coxa valga can be congenital, caused by trauma, dislocation of the hip, diseases such as spastic paralysis, or the elimination of weight bearing in early childhood. From a mechanical point of view, the relative straightening of the neck on the shaft will increase pressure on the femoral head while decreasing the bending stress on the femoral neck.[59] The relative lengthening of the limb causes a pelvic obliquity that places the hip on the affected side in adduction (Fig. 16-34). The weight bearing of the head is transferred closer to the center of the head. The acetabulum has been noted to become elongated and oval, thus facilitating subluxation,[70] and the abnormal pressure of the head against the upper acetabular rim appears to flatten out the rim. The lever arm for the abductors is shortened in coxa valga and thus creates an unfavorable situation for abduction and contributes to the adduction of the affected side (Fig. 16-35).

Clinical findings. With moderate unilateral involvement, gait evaluation will reveal a gluteus medius limp that is often painless. A leg-length difference will be an objective finding with the longer leg on the involved side. An upward pelvic obliquity accompanied by adductor tightness will also be found on that side. A bilateral comparison of abductor strength will show a weakness on the side affected by coxa valga. Radiography must confirm the diagnosis.

Because of the altered mechanics of the pelvis, coxa valga may be the cause of back pain or sacro-iliac joint dysfunction.

Treatment. It is important to treat even asymptomatic coxa valga since, by causing a leg-length difference, it may be a predisposing factor in osteoarthritis[26] and/or a possible cause of back or sacroiliac pain.

If coxa valga is severe, causing repetitive dislocation and/or considerable leg-length difference, an osteotomy

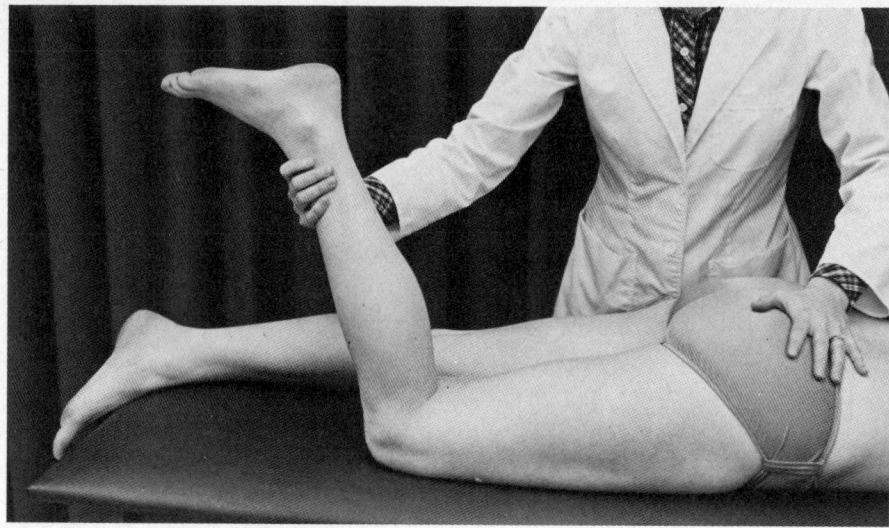

Fig. 16-33. Prone knee bend, femoral nerve stretch.

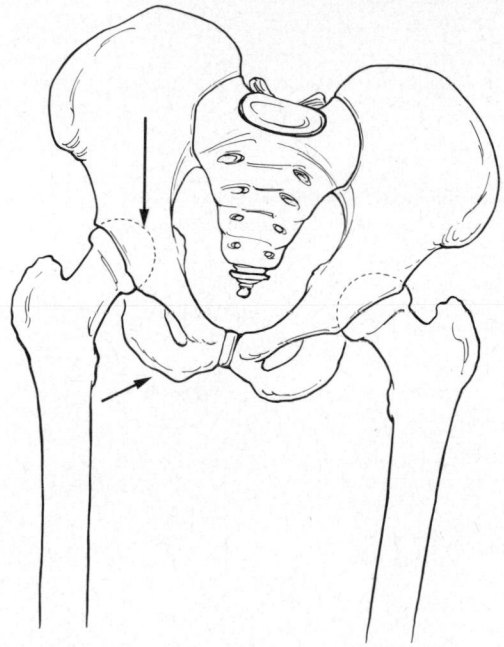

Fig. 16-34. Result of coxa valga is relative lengthening of limb, placing affected hip in adduction.

may be performed. Otherwise the main goal of treatment is to restore proper mechanics by equalizing leg length. Stretching exercises for the adductors on the involved side and strengthening exercises for the abductors of the same side are also essential aspects of a treatment program.

Coxa vara. *Coxa vara* is a deformity wherein the neck-shaft angle is decreased from the normal 125 degrees. It may be caused by several factors, including trauma, a slipped epiphysis, arthritis, and rickets, or it may be congenital. Congenital coxa vara is often bilateral.[28] The condition decreases the pressure on the femoral head while increasing the bending stress in the neck.[59]

This increased bending stress may lead to a greater predisposition to fracture of the neck of the femur. Of great importance is the stress that increases the shearing of the capital femoral epiphysis, enhancing the tendency for slipping of the epiphysis.[66] There will be a relative shortening of the limb, which will result in a pelvic obliquity with the pelvis dropped on the affected side. The weight-bearing area can be seen to shift more to a superior, lateral area of the head of the femur (Fig. 16-36). Whereas coxa valga is normal at birth and the neck-shaft angle usually normalizes with weight bearing, in coxa vara weight-bearing will often severely aggravate the condition. In severe cases of congenital coxa vara, an osteotomy is inevitable.

Clinical findings. Normally, the thighs can be crossed at about midfemur level. In severe coxa valga, there is noticeable widening of the hips, and the thighs can be crossed much higher up on the femurs. This indicates an increase beyond the normal range of adduction. With unilateral involvement, the gait evaluation will reveal a limp because of a relative shortening of the limb on the involved side. The pelvis on the affected side will be dropped on weight bearing, and there may be a restriction of abduction because of the impingement of the greater trochanter against the ilium. The high position of the greater trochanter also results in abductor inefficiency and contracture (Fig. 16-37), and a positive Trendelenburg sign will be found on the affected side. Back pain or sacroiliac dysfunction may initially be the chief complaint of an individual with coxa vara.

Treatment. Treatment must be of a preventive nature whenever possible. Coxa vara may be asymptomatic but, if discovered, should be treated to prevent future problems that may be as serious as osteoarthritis of the hip or spine. It is of great importance to equalize leg lengths as much as possible. The osseous obstruction on abduction is unavoid-

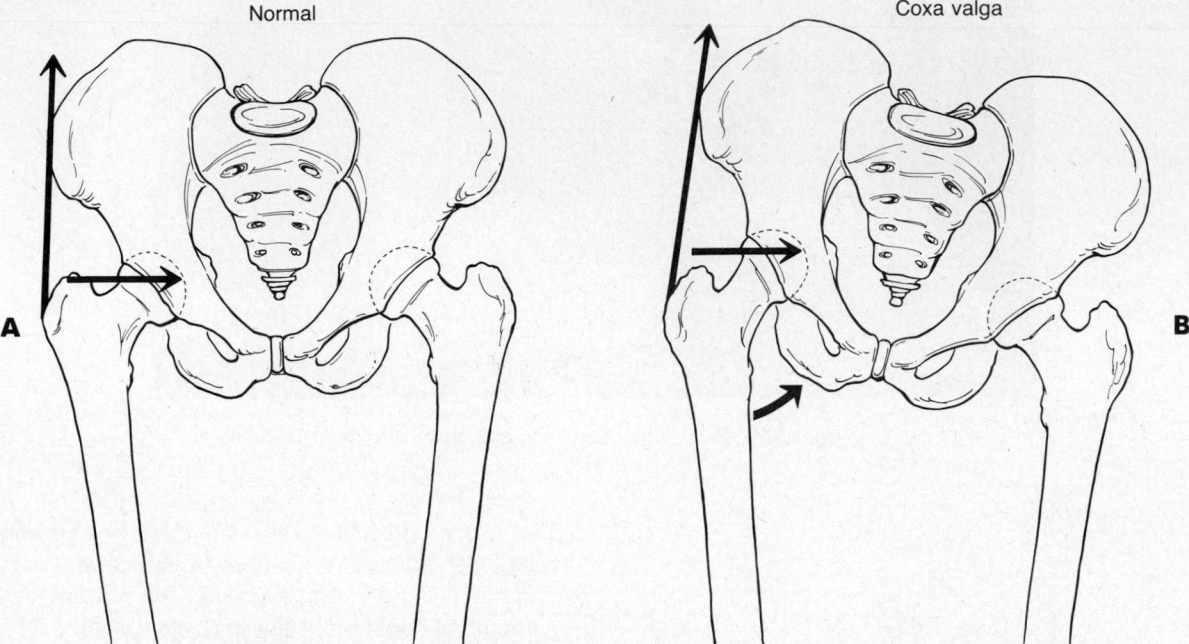

Normal

Coxa valga

A

B

Fig. 16-35. Lever arm for abductors is shortened in coxa valga and creates an unfavorable position for the abductors, which contributes to adduction of affected side. **A,** Normal. **B,** Shortened lever arm.

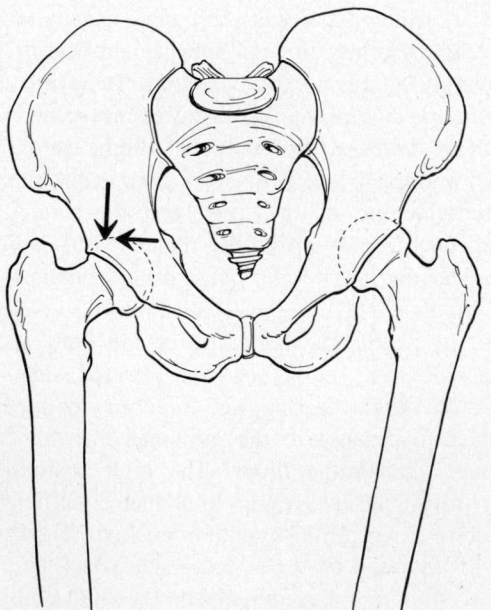

Fig. 16-36. Coxa vara condition illustrating weight-bearing area of femur to be more superior and lateral.

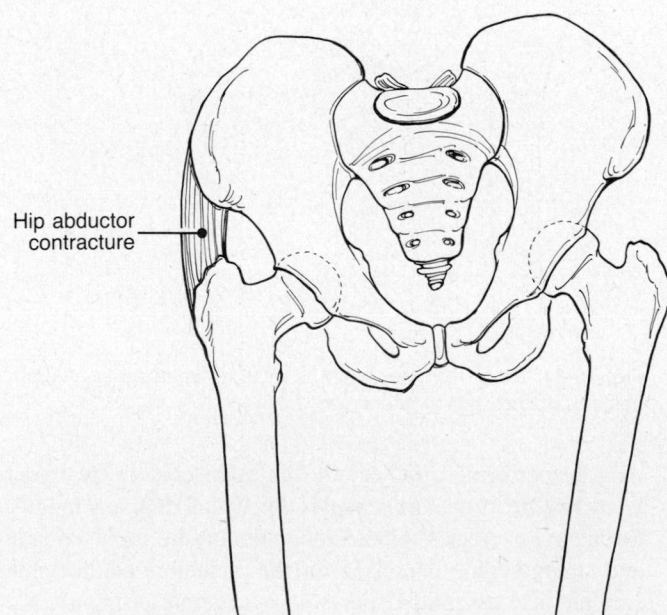

Hip abductor contracture

Fig. 16-37. Abductor contracture resulting from coxa vara.

able and cannot be treated with physical therapy; however, the abductors can be strengthened within the range available.

Anteversion. The angle of torsion in adults is normally about 150 degrees and an increase in this angle is considered to indicate femoral neck anteversion. It is often greater in children and may result in a toed-in gait. It has been speculated that persistent infantile femoral anteversion can contribute to osteoarthritis at a later age.[30] This may result from increased rotational wear, increased muscle forces across the hip joint to derotate the head, or decreased congruency leading to areas of increased pressure and/or areas of little or no pressure, all of which are discussed in the section on osteoarthritis. By allowing the head to put more pressure against the superior and anterior parts of the acetabulum, the increased angle may also cause dysplasia of the acetabulum.[69] A dysplasic acetabulum results in a greater potential for anterior dislocation of the femur.[51]

Clinical findings. Femoral anteversion will often be noticed by the physician during a normal physical examination or by the physical therapist when evaluating gait. It is characterized primarily by a toed-in gait, an increased Q-angle caused by an increased external tibial torsion, and pronated feet compensating for the torsion. There may be increased lumbar lordosis because of poor anterior femoral head coverage resulting in back problems. If the condition is unilateral, compensatory pronation would lead to an apparent leg-length difference, also possibly causing sacroiliac dysfunction or low-back pain.

Knee pain may also be the chief complaint of a client found to have femoral anteversion, since this may lead to patellar malalignment syndromes or patellar subluxations. Alternately the client with femoral anteversion may have foot pain caused by excessive pronation.

The most dramatic finding in anteversion directly related to the hip, however, is a dramatic increase in internal rotation to 60 to 90 degrees and a decrease in external rotation (Fig. 16-38). The feet of a client lying in a relaxed supine posture will often be seen in a neutral rotational position instead of in the normal toeing-out position of about 45 degrees (Fig. 16-39).

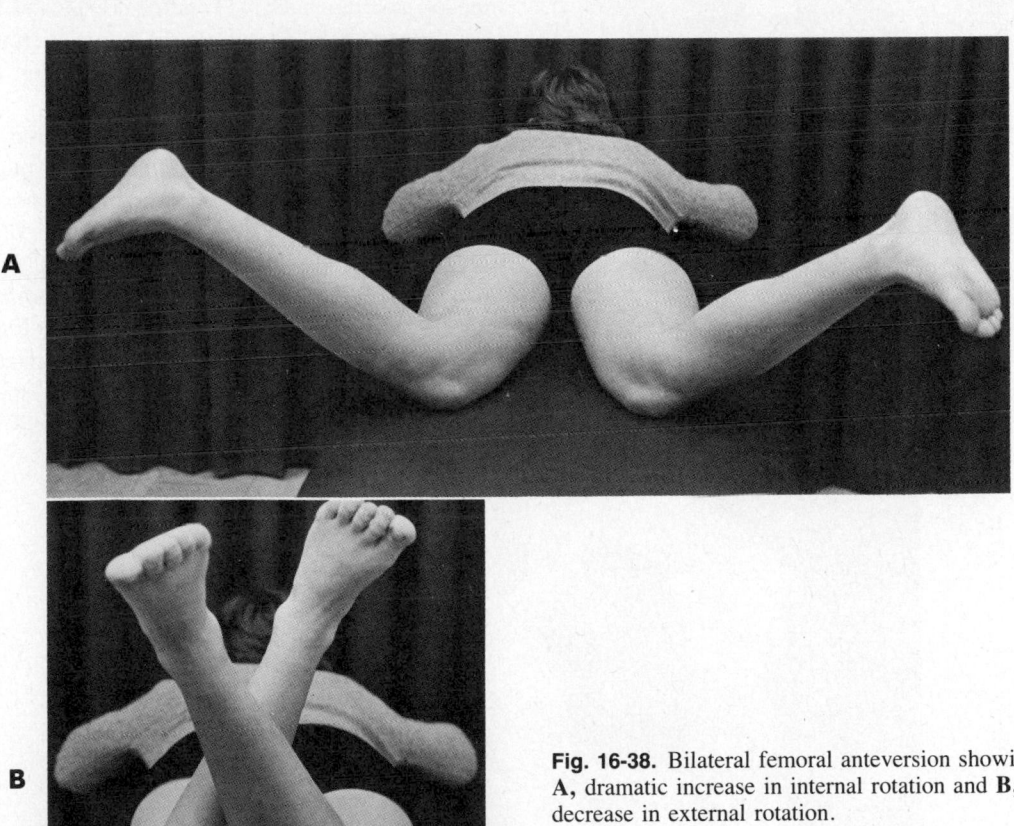

Fig. 16-38. Bilateral femoral anteversion showing **A,** dramatic increase in internal rotation and **B,** decrease in external rotation.

Treatment. Prevention of later hip disease or related disorders in the spine, knee, or foot and ankle calls for early and continued treatment of femoral anteversion. Physical therapy treatment at the hip would primarily involve incorporating exercises to increase external rotation into a home exercise program. Mobilization to increase external rotation could be used in the clinic (Fig. 16-40). Other treatment may also involve correcting the pathomechanics of the foot, knee, and spine, such as correcting leg-length differences, treatment aimed at increasing the strength of the vastus medialis obliquus (VMO) muscle, or correcting excessive lumbar lordosis.

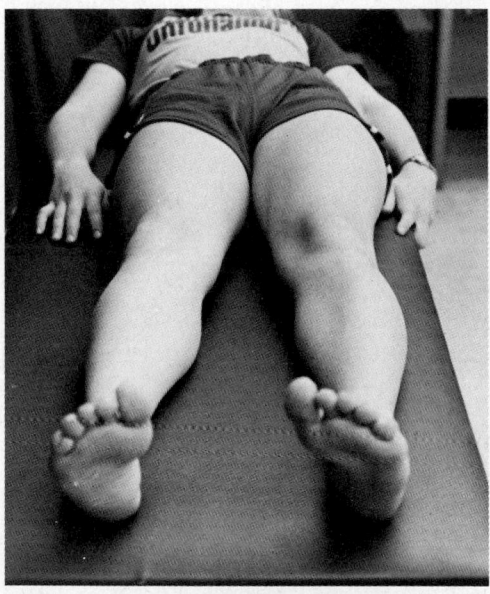

Fig. 16-39. Client with femoral anteversion in relaxed supine position showing neutral rotational position and lack of out-toeing.

Retroversion. When the angle between the neck and shaft in the transverse plane is dramatically decreased, retroversion results (see Fig. 16-2). A toed-out gait indicates the possibility of retroverted hips. Retroversion may also increase rotational wear and contribute to an increased internal tibial torsion and supinated feet. The increased forces on the hip (caused by the effort of the muscles to internally rotate the hip) will not have as great an effect as derotational forces in anteversion because of relatively weak internal rotators.

Clinical findings. The toed-out gait may be the first indication to the clinician that a femoral retroversion exists. An increased internal tibial torsion, decreased Q-angle, and/or supinated feet may also be noticed. Unilateral retroversion resulting in a unilateral increase in supination may lead to an apparent leg-length discrepancy. Compensations may cause pain from the lower back or sacro-iliac joint to the feet. An increased external rotation may be noted in the affected hip (Fig. 16-41).

Treatment. As in anteversion, the pathomechanics should be treated as much as possible. Direct treatment of the hip involves internal rotational exercises and stretching the tight external rotators in the home exercise program as well as mobilizations into internal rotation to be done in the clinic (Figs. 16-42 to 16-44).

Congenital dysplasia and dislocation of the hip. *Congenital dysplasia of the hip,* a term meaning malformation of the hip joint, is one of the more common congenital deformities.[5] It will be apparent in the case of subluxation or dislocation. However, acetabular dysplasia that does not result in subluxation or dislocation may not be apparent until it is later revealed by pathologic gait and/or radiographs. If any of these are not recognized and treated early, they can lead to osteoarthritis in adult life.[63]

Congenital dysplasia of the hip occurs six to eight times

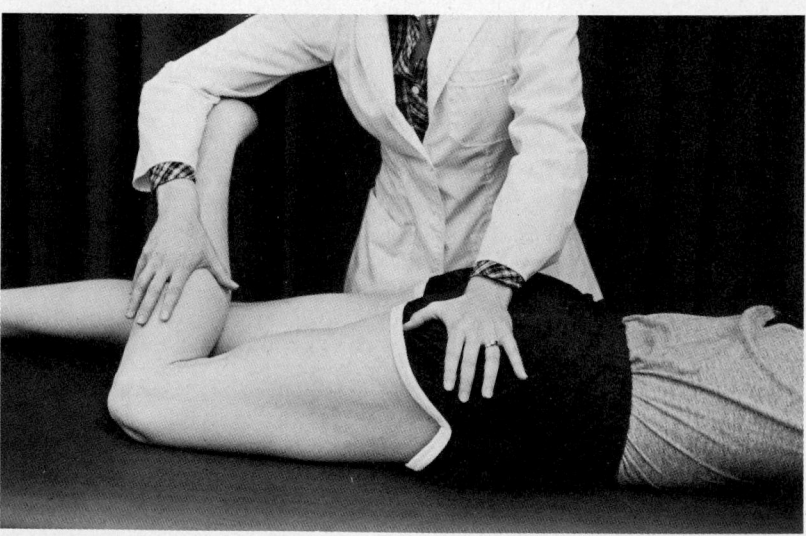

Fig. 16-40. External rotation mobilization technique. This can be done using oscillations or hold-relax techniques.

more frequently in girls than in boys, and its cause is unknown.[72] Its incidence in the United States has been reported to be 1.55:1000.[23] In acetabular dysplasia, which precedes nontraumatic subluxation or dislocation of the hip, the normal femoral anteversion is increased, and the acetabulum is misshapen and often shallow. Early diagnosis is extremely important since the changes occurring become progressively more difficult to correct. Subluxation occurs where the head rides on the ridge of the acetabu-

lum, and can result in a permanent dislocation. In a dislocation, the femoral head lies entirely outside the acetabulum. Although dislocation in infants born with acetabular or femoral head dysplasia may not be apparent immediately, dislocation is usually noted by 3 months of age.[72]

Clinical findings. One consistent positive finding in congenital dislocation is limited hip abduction.[33] There is a shortening of the affected leg since the head of the femur rides up and out of the acetabulum. The prominence of the

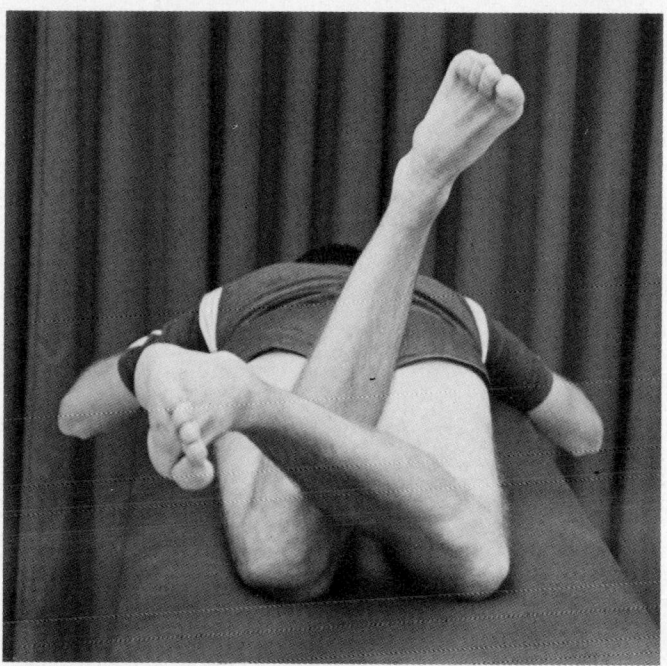

Fig. 16-41. Unilateral femoral retroversion showing an increased external rotation in the affected hip.

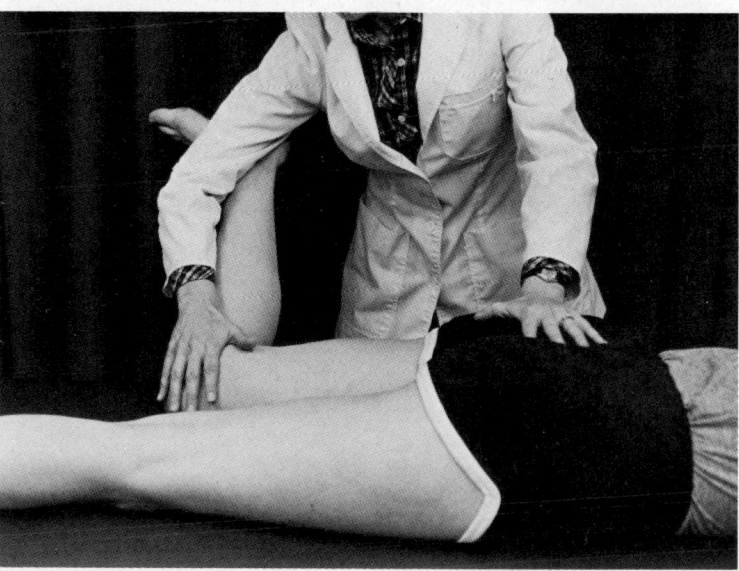

Fig. 16-42. Internal rotation mobilization technique. This can be done using oscillations or hold-relax techniques.

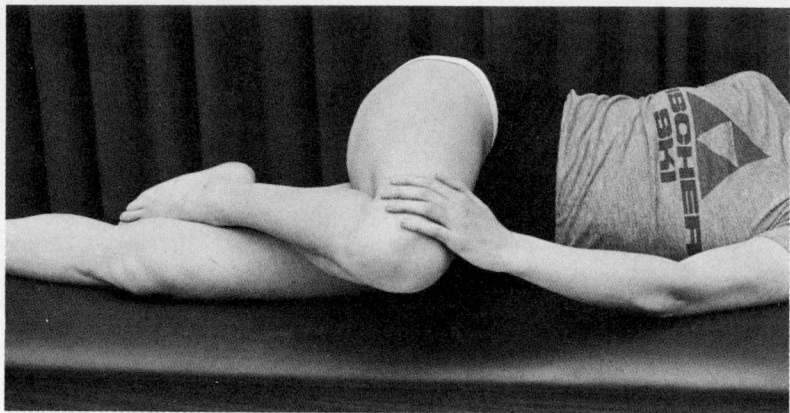

Fig. 16-43. Side-lying stretch for piriformis tightness.

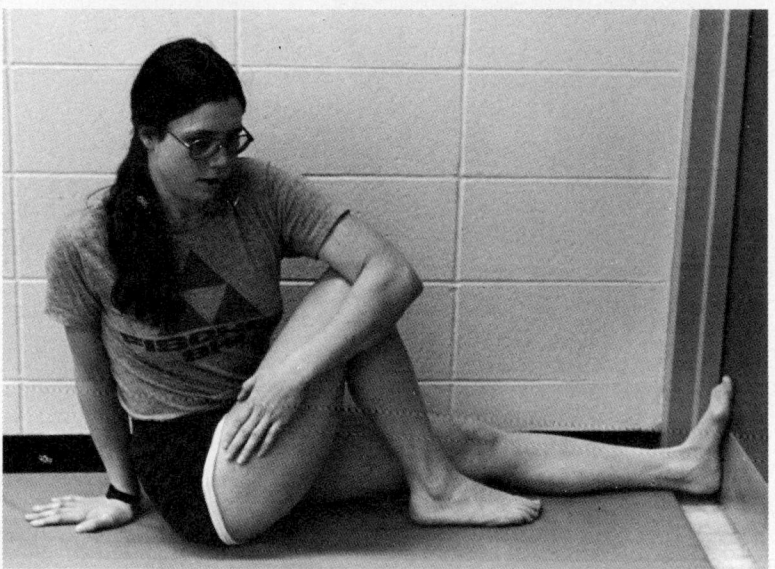

Fig. 16-44. Sitting stretch for piriformis tightness.

proximal femur is palpable in an abnormal posterosuperior position.

If congenital dislocation is not corrected, when the child begins to walk he/she will show a marked limp if the dislocation is unilateral and a waddle if it is bilateral. The weak hip abductors will cause a Trendelenburg lurch in walking and a Trendelenburg sign when an attempt is made to balance on the affected limb.

Treatment. Early diagnosis with orthopaedic treatment is essential in the case of congenital dislocation of the hip. Splinting in abduction is often done early and for several months to develop a normal acetabulum. Persistence of this condition—seen often in clients with spastic cerebral palsy—prevents use of the hip and produces pain with any movement. In the case of a child who has been treated conservatively with a splint or by surgery, a therapist may be called upon to provide range of motion, gait training, and stimulation of motor development. Joint approxima-

tion using a Swiss ball is useful and entertaining for the child. Swimming and biking, when appropriate, will also increase range of motion.

Legg-Calve-Perthes disease

Legg-Calve-Perthes disease, also called *coxa plana* and *juvenile osteochondrosis,* is a hip disorder that occurs in children between the ages of 3 to 12, with a peak incidence of 6 years.[19] Its estimated occurrence in the general population is 1:1200,[54] and it occurs most often in boys.[11,20,28] When it occurs in females, more extensive involvement of the epiphysis is typical.[65] The disease is characterized by avascular necrosis of the femoral head* resulting in a flattened femoral head. The cause of the avascular necrosis is unknown but may result from a chronic synovitis. If not treated, the disease process may

*See references 11, 20, 28, 65, and 72.

result in severely limited range, residual deformity, and osteoarthritis of the hip.[64] If treated, its prognosis seems to depend on the age of the client and the extent of involvement of the epiphysis.[10] Perhaps because younger children have a greater growth potential after healing, the prognosis is considerably better if the disease is treated at a young age.[11]

Clinical findings. The history generally indicates an insidious onset of intermittent pain. An antalgic gait (which is more apparent following exertion) and stiffness with internal rotation restriction are found. There is usually spasm of the adductor muscles on the affected side that restricts abduction. Atrophy of the thigh and buttocks on the involved side may also be observed. The location of pain is in the anterior groin, sometimes into the anterior thigh and knee.

Radiographic findings differentiate Legg-Calvé-Perthes disease from nonspecific synovitis and slipped capital femoral epiphysis. They show widening of the joint space and a flattening of the epiphysis and sometimes a change in the acetabular shape. In later stages, new bone formation will be evident around the head and neck of the femur. It takes approximately 2 to 4 years for the entire process of necrosis and reconstruction to run its course.

Treatment. Orthopaedic treatment generally consists of application of some form of abduction cast. Initially traction is used to reduce the adductor spasm and obtain 45 degrees of abduction and slight internal rotation, which is the position where the femoral head is best centered. The abduction brace allows for partial weight bearing and mobilization with crutches. However, in some hospitals children are kept recumbent on a skate board. When a skate board is used, the splint is removed daily for exercise, which most frequently involves pool therapy.

If the child is placed in a cast, it is removed periodically to mobilize the knee and ankle and to take a radiograph of the healing hip. The cast is then reapplied. This process is repeated every few months throughout the entire course of the disease until there is evidence of a round femoral head placed firmly in the acetabulum.

When the cast is removed only every few months, the child will also often participate in pool or whirlpool therapy, and good range of motion of the hip, knee, and ankle must be regained before the cast is reapplied. Movement may also be obtained using a bike and/or a Swiss ball. The therapist may be involved initially to assist in gait training with crutches.

Slipped capital femoral epiphysis

The epiphyseal plate at the head of the femur is especially subject to displacement before the adolescent years, when it fuses. Slipped capital femoral epiphysis usually occurs between the ages of 10 and 15 in a male-to-female ratio of 2:1.[38] The disorder can result from direct trauma but sometimes comes on suddenly with no history of

trauma. It is also bilateral in about 15% to 20% of cases, indicating that trauma is not the only cause.[11]

The exact cause of the disease remains unknown, but it has been associated with abnormal weakening of the bone.[46] Endocrine factors or pituitary dysfunction have also been suggested,[28,72] which could account for abnormal bone formation. Others have found the disease more prevalent among obese[46,72] or very slender children.[28,72]

Clinical findings. The child will show an antalgic gait and can have a history of trauma or violent exertion or no history of trauma, with a sudden onset of limping followed by pain. The pain is frequently only felt in the knee; thus the true cause at the hip may be overlooked. The importance of "clearing" a joint above and below the painful joint is particularly relevant in this case.

On evaluation, the hip shows limited motion into internal rotation, especially when flexed and abducted. It will take on an attitude of external rotation that is particularly noticeable in the supine position. The client may also walk with the affected limb externally rotated.

Radiographs in the anteroposterior and lateral views will reveal an inferior and posterior slippage of the capital epiphysis. If these views do not reveal a disorder that is highly suspected, a true lateral view may confirm the diagnosis.[72] With the slippage inferiorly and posteriorly, the hip takes on a coxa vara deformity.[28]

Treatment. Once the diagnosis has been confirmed, the treatment of a slipped capital femoral epiphysis is surgical plate-closure. This is the only method to guard against further slippage.[38] Postsurgically, the physical therapist will be rehabilitating the client in the same way as he/she would rehabilitate a client following a fracture. A general program of range-of-motion, gait training, and strengthening exercises should be creative and suited to the age and disposition of the client.

Avascular necrosis of the femoral head

Avascular necrosis of the femoral head is frequently a complication following fractures of the neck of the femur or dislocations of the head. It may occur at any time postoperatively, even up to 20 years later.[37] Its high incidence, reported to be between 12% and 35%, is caused by the fact that the head, when displaced, is often rendered avascular at the time of the trauma. Avascular necrosis could also result from vascular occlusion as a consequence of immobilization. The vulnerability of the medial and lateral femoral circumflex arteries as they circle closely around the head of the femur may explain the high incidence of avascular necrosis of the femoral head. It is more frequent among the elderly, since femoral neck fractures are rarely seen in the young. However, it may be seen in younger individuals following dislocations.

Clinical findings. The first sign of avascular necrosis of the femoral head may simply be unexplained aching in the hip joint. The client may be unable to sit for any length of time because of stiffness, may report a weak feeling in the hip, and will exhibit a limp. Radiographs may not show signs of the disease until it is somewhat advanced so that the femoral head has started to flatten and become irregularly shaped. Later signs reveal osteoarthritis and its characteristic clinical findings.

Treatment. The condition of avascular necrosis of the femoral head is more common and has a worse prognosis in older clients than in younger ones, who are still undergoing growth. In some cases, the condition is not severe enough to warrant further surgery, and the physical therapist may be called upon to provide a home program to maintain strength and mobility of the joint and to recommend an assistive device for protected weightbearing. If complete collapse of the head occurs and/or increasing pain is felt, a prosthetic replacement is usually performed. In this case, the treatment will follow that of a total hip replacement.

Osteoarthritis

Degenerative joint disease, commonly referred to as *osteoarthritis,* is the most common painful condition of the hip joint.[9] It has been estimated to occur in as much as 20% of people over the age of 55[45] and in a female-to-male ratio of 3:2.[42] In a study by Jorring,[42] it was observed that osteoarthritis in women was more painful and more limiting than in men.

Primary osteoarthritis is distinguished from secondary osteoarthritis by the elimination of predisposing factors and relevant pre-existing disease of the hip. Primary osteoarthritis is considered to be a result of aging alone, whereas *secondary osteoarthritis* is the term used when the condition follows previous damage by mechanical disorders. A few of these are congenital dislocation or dysplasia of the hip, Legg-Calve-Perthes disease, slipped capital femoral epiphysis, fractures, or traumatic dislocations.

The idea that osteoarthritis can actually result from some undetermined abnormality of the subchondral bone or cartilage, abnormally superimposed on normal growth and development of the hip (called *primary osteoarthritis*) is controversial. Harris[31] researched thousands of roentgenograms of adult patients who were diagnosed to have primary osteoarthritis of the hip. Where roentgenograms were available to make an assessment on the normality of the hip at the end of growth, he found that 90% of those diagnosed with primary or ideopathic osteoarthritis clearly showed previous abnormalities in the hip joint. Harris, in stating his belief that primary osteoarthritis may not in fact be an existing disease, or is a very rare one, identified metabolic abnormalities as also leading to osteoarthritis of the hip.

In any case, osteoarthritis is characterized by progressive degenerative changes in articular cartilage and the bones of the affected joint. The sequence of pathological events taking place in the disease process creates a vicious circle, beginning with changes in the articular surfaces and leading to further cartilaginous destruction. Cartilage is designed to withstand a great amount of wear and tear. It is composed mainly of cells, collagen fibers, and mucopolysaccharides. The first observable change in nontraumatic osteoarthritis is the loss of mucopolysaccharides from an area of articular cartilage.[12] The result is a loss of elasticity in the cartilage and a decrease in its ability to protect the cells by absorbing shock. Once this has occurred, minor stresses create fibrillation in the weakened area, thus creating further damage. The fragments of cartilage that become detached are absorbed by the synovial membrane, which causes synovial hyperplasia and subsequent capsular fibrosis. Synovitis also results from increased cartilage wear or capsular strain. When there is severe cartilage damage, an eburnated bone is laid down but not in such a way that the normal shape of the bone is restored. Radiographic evidence shows a flattening of the femoral head and acetabulum.[50] Lloyd-Roberts[50] reported that in clients who required surgery for osteoarthritis of the hip, the following observations were made:

1. The synovial membrane was abnormally congested and particularly villous for the age of the client.
2. The capsule and subsynovial connective tissue were fibrotic.
3. The articular debris fragments occurring in the diseased joint were directed to the area below the neck of the femur, where increased synovial congestion was apparent.

A narrowing of the joint space is also generally apparent.[42]

In one study, the greatest cartilage degeneration was shown to be in the upper quadrant of the femoral head, which is where the head contacts the acetabulum in a weight-bearing position or in moderate range during gait.[15] In a later study,[7] two areas of cartilage lesions on the head were found to be on (1) the perifoveal and inferior medial femoral head and (2) the anterior and superior peripheral area of the femoral head. Acetabular degenerative changes were seen on the roof at the base of the superior lip. In the study by Bullough, Goodfellow, and O'Connor,[7] a correlation was made between areas of habitual degeneration and areas of habitual disuse.

Two opposing hypotheses therefore exist as to the cause of initial changes in the articular cartilage, one being that of excessive wear and tear and the second that of habitual disuse. Although the hypothesis that primary osteoarthritis is simply a wear-and-tear phenomenon is the more popular one, it has never been proved. The coefficient of friction in joints is so low[49] that it would seem improbable that joints could wear out from rubbing. Many people who have done heavy work for most of their lives never experience the symptoms of osteoarthritis. Yet gross cartilage changes in rabbits' knees have been produced by subjecting them to an impulse load equal to their body weight at a rate of 60 times per minute 1 hour daily for 30 days.[60] The degree and type of force may be more significant to the process of joint wear than the actual total force.

Use and compression of cartilage are necessary to maintain its continual health, which suggests that mechanical forces are necessary for cartilage nutrition. This would support the hypothesis that a lack of pressure is a cause of cartilage degeneration. It has been suggested that a pumping action of alternate compression and rest is essential to ensure nourishment of the articular cartilage.[32] If the pressure is either absent or excessive in quantity or duration, adequate tissue-fluid exchange would be prevented and cartilage degeneration would be promoted. Therefore the opposing hypotheses may both be correct. It is certain, however, that excessive trauma will accelerate the degenerative process once it has begun.

Any alteration in the mechanics of weight bearing could impose disproportionate stress on the hip and contribute to the development of the degenerative changes in osteo-arthritis. Some of these have been mentioned earlier in the chapter. Another important one may be leg-length disparity. Although the leg on the side of an osteoarthritic hip shortens with the progression of the disease, it has been found to be the longer leg in most cases.[25,26] When the two limbs are not equal in length, the pelvis is adducted toward the longer leg and the hip on that side is subjected to greater-than-normal stress. Clients with leg-length discrepancies frequently complain of low-back pain. By elevating the short leg with a suitable lift, the physical therapist may not only cure the client's low-back pain but also inadvertently prevent later manifestations of osteoarthritis of the hip. In a study by Friberg,[22] in a group of patients with leg-length inequality of 5 mm or more, chronic pain and arthroses of the hip occured in 229 of 254 patients (89% of the cases) on the side of the longer extremity. The symptoms were interpreted to be caused or exacerbated by biomechanical responses to the lateral imbalance in the erect posture. When correcting the leg-length inequality with an adequate shoe lift, complete alleviation of the symptoms was accomplished in most cases.

Clinical findings. The progressive signs and symptoms of osteo-arthritis are at least partially the result of fibrosis, which interferes with the normal function of the joint capsule. The capsule is tightest in extension with some abduction and internal rotation, which is the position of greatest stability on weight bearing.[75] The fibrosis of the capsule causes shortening and deformity upon flexion, adduction, and external rotation, exposing the capsule to painful stretching in the weight-bearing position. This will, in turn, cause reflex guarding by the muscles supplied by the motor branches of sensory nerves to the inferior capsule. Fibrosis at the musculotendinous junction can follow,[70] causing permanent deformity.

Clients will generally seek medical advice because of the pain of osteoarthritis of the hip, which sometimes radi-

ates down the thigh and into the knee. In minor arthritis the pain is felt chiefly in the groin. As the disease progresses, the patient will generally complain of stiffness, particularly in the morning, painful weightbearing, easy fatigue in walking, pain that keeps them awake at night, and difficulty doing daily tasks because of a decreased range of motion. A characteristic Trendelenburg lurch over the affected hip is frequent. In bilateral osteoarthritis, the client will exhibit a waddling gait as his/her trunk lurches from side to side and the lower extremities externally rotate and adduct. Because of the assumed position of flexion, adduction, and external rotation, pain is caused by efforts to extend, abduct, and internally rotate. Evaluation will also reveal atrophy of adjacent musculature, flexion contractures, and subsequent shortening of the affected leg. Radiographs may show narrowing of the joint space, changes in the shape of the femur and/or acetabulum, and the presence of osteophytes.

Treatment. Treatment must consist of decreasing the forces on the hip. A cane used on the unaffected side can reduce the forces on the affected hip to just slightly more than the body weight.[62] Clients should attempt to reduce their walking and lose excess weight. Range-of-motion and strengthening exercises for all the hip musculature, but particularly for the abductors, should be performed. Some form of heat or massage can precede exercise. These treatments have an analgesic effect and also reduce muscle spasm, therefore increasing range of motion and decreasing pain. Biking and swimming are excellent treatments since they avoid excessive stress on the hip joint while maintaining fitness and range of motion. Mobilizations can be used in the case of osteoarthritis to loosen capsular adhesions. Distal traction will stretch the posterior inferior capsule and increase flexion (see Fig. 16-25). Lateral traction is effective to reduce any restriction of movement (see Fig. 16-26). The range of internal rotation and hip extension may also be increased by internal rotation mobilizations and hip extension mobilizations respectively (Fig. 16-45 and see Fig. 16-42). Scouring is also an effective pain-relieving treatment technique (see Fig. 16-24).

Total hip replacements

Total hip replacement is indicated in cases of severe osteo-arthritis, rheumatoid arthritis, fractures of the femoral neck and acetabulum (especially in the elderly), chronic dislocations of the femoral head, avascular necrosis of the head, and many other conditions. It has become a fairly common procedure on the hip.

Preoperative and postoperative treatment. Before performing a total hip replacement in the case where the surgery is elective and no trauma immediately precedes surgery, the therapist generally assesses gait, range of motion, activities of daily living, and muscle strength. Additional measurements that may be important are leg-length measurements and anthropometric measurements as well

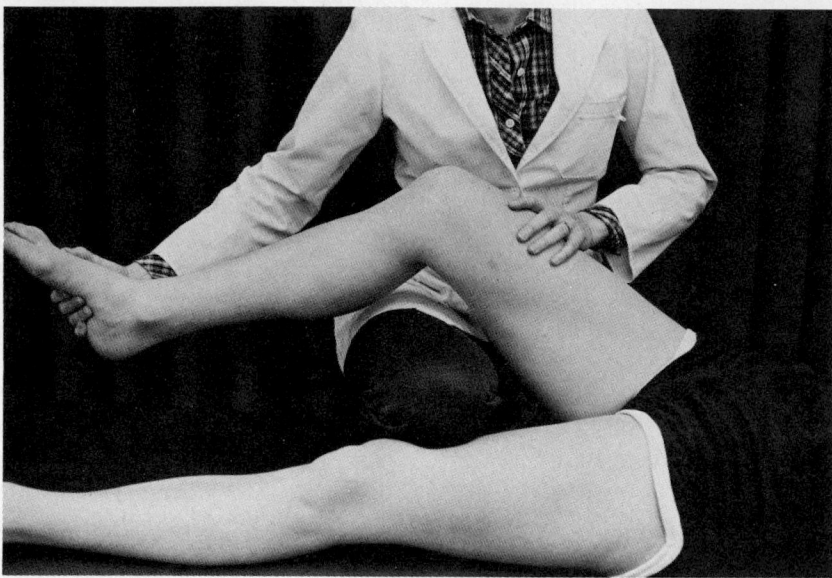

Fig. 16-45. Hip extension mobilization. This can be done using oscillations (hitting onto examiner's thigh) or using a hold-relax technique.

as some subjective measure of pain present. The client is instructed in the postoperative routine and is cautioned against flexion past 90 degrees, adduction past the body midline, external rotation, and unsupported dangling of the affected side.

Before beginning postoperative treatment of a total hip recipient, the therapist must check the surgical report for any complications or factors that may require special precautions. Communication with the physician regarding these is essential. The postoperative program usually begins on the afternoon of the surgery with isometric exercises to maintain muscle tone and increase circulation. The affected hip should be supported in the neutral position or in internal rotation by a trochanter roll with the client supine. When rolling the client to the side-lying position, the therapist must take extreme caution not to adduct the hip past the midline. Two pillows can be placed between the knees to prevent this while the client is side-lying. Getting in and out of bed is always done on the unaffected side to avoid active abduction.

Ambulation with a walker and weight-bearing as tolerated is usually begun the day after surgery, and active assistive exercises are performed for hip flexion, hip extension, and adduction from a passively abducted position. Generally the client progresses to active range of motion including abduction, weight-shifting exercises in sitting and standing, and ambulation with a cane. A mirror is an excellent tool for client feedback to indicate imbalances in walking or standing and how they can be improved. Prone-lying later in the postoperative program should not be neglected. Prone-lying is a good position to reduce hip flexion contractures and to work on hip extension exercises.

A stationary bicycle or restorator can be used to increase range of motion and maintain cardiovascular fitness. The seat height when using a stationary bicycle may be adjusted to the degree of hip flexion allowed. No resistance should be added initially but can be added as the client's strength increases. Exercises in a therapeutic pool provide the client with variety and can help increase the range of motion while decreasing pain. Before the client is discharged, leg lengths are measured by the physical therapist to determine whether a lift to level the pelvis is indicated. Precautions should be in effect for an extended period of time as specified by the physician, usually three months, following which the client can gradually resume daily activities as desired.

Dislocation is one of the postoperative complications of total hip replacement. Extreme caution should be used when transferring or working with a client. Any excessive flexion, internal rotation, and adduction will increase the possibility of dislocation after total hip replacement.

Fractures

Fractures can be caused as a result of macrotrauma or repetitive microtrauma. In the case of osteoporotic bone, the fracture may result from a simple movement. In the case of a stress fracture, repetitive microtrauma is generally the cause. In an avulsion fracture the mechanism of injury involves a violent muscle contraction. The treatment of fractures depends on the client's age and condition, the type of fracture, and the surgery (if surgery is performed).

Stress fractures. Stress fractures usually occur in young, active people as a result of repetitive microtrauma and, when protected, heal without difficulty. They are not common in the hip, although occasionally they do occur at the anterior iliac crest as a result of faulty running mechanics. Individuals will be observed to run swinging their arms across their body, causing a pull of the oblique abdominal muscles on the iliac crest.[6] Pinpoint tenderness and pain will be found in the area of the stress fracture, but initially the radiographs may appear normal. The history of the client, including activities and change in activities, as well as an analysis of movement, is essential for a diagnosis. As in the treatment of all stress fractures, the cause should be of utmost concern and must be treated. Stress fractures of the anterior iliac crest are initially treated by rest, by relieving weight bearing, and by avoiding stressful, non–weight-bearing positions.

Avulsion fractures. Avulsion fractures usually occur in the teenage years before the epiphyseal growth plates are completely closed. The anterior superior iliac spine can be avulsed by a forceful contraction of the sartorius muscle during running or jumping. The anterior inferior iliac spine is a more frequent location of avulsion fractures because of the role of the rectus femoris in hip flexion. Unusual muscular violence in kicking or running can cause an avulsion fracture at the proximal attachment of the rectus femoris muscle. Isolated avulsion of the greater trochanter from the pull of the abductor muscles or of the lesser trochanter from the pull of the iliopsoas muscle is also seen occasionally. Palpation will reveal point tenderness at the avulsion site and careful palpation may even reveal a displaced fragment of the bone. Active movement and passive stretch of the involved muscle will be painful. Radiographs will confirm a suspected diagnosis.

Avulsion fractures usually require internal fixation, but, when the avulsion is not complete, immobilization may be the treatment of choice. When fixation is obtained, the client may be crutch-walking and performing isometric exercises the day after surgery. While the cast is on, active exercise should be continued with the other leg and the upper body to maintain fitness and psychological well-being. Once the cast is removed, active rehabilitation is performed.

Traumatic fractures

Fracture of the femoral neck. Femoral neck fractures rarely occur in the young since they are usually associated with osteoporosis.[28,48,71] The forces that produce these fractures are often small and sometimes simply consist of a twisting action while weight bearing and trying to avoid a fall. The actual fall is often secondary to the fracture, and the delicacy of the bone is attributed to osteoporosis.[28,48,71] The femoral neck fracture is the most common hip fracture and occurs in 1 : 1000 women over 70 years of age.[43] The susceptibility of the femoral neck to fracture may to some extent be caused by the trabecular structure of the neck, which does not reinforce Ward's triangle (see Fig. 16-3). This area remains weak, especially to twisting and shear forces, and is the most vulnerable to

hip fracture.[72] A femoral neck fracture is an intracapsular fracture and thus disrupts the normal blood supply to the head of the femur. This disruption often results in avascular necrosis of the femoral head.

Intertrochanteric fractures. An intertrochanteric fracture usually occurs as the result of a fall, with both direct and indirect forces being responsible for the site of the fracture. The indirect forces are caused by the pull of the iliopsoas and abductor muscles on the lesser and greater trochanters, respectively. The direct forces act on the axis of the femur.[6] Intertrochanteric fractures are also found primarily among the elderly.

Subtrochanteric fractures. Subtrochanteric fractures are the least common among the three types of traumatic fractures mentioned. They are, however, the most difficult to treat because of the intense mechanical stress on this area of the femur.[18] They result from direct trauma of considerable force. Subtrochanteric fractures occur in a younger age-group than either femoral head fractures or intertrochanteric fractures.[6]

Treatment of traumatic fractures. Strong internal fixation devices have been developed for the treatment of hip fractures. In the case of a severely osteoporotic hip that has been fractured, a total hip replacement may be indicated, especially when the fracture is intracapsular. In either case, the treated hip must be protected from dislocation by proper positioning, as mentioned in the discussion on total hip replacements. Range-of-motion and muscle-strengthening exercises, and gait training will be the responsibility of the physical therapist following surgery. If osteoporosis is present, treatment must include goals to improve this condition. Exercise has been shown to increase bone density and reverse the rate of osteoporosis in some cases.[67] A special program of exercise following the healing of the fracture can be done, primarily while the client is seated. This will maintain strength and range of motion while minimally stressing the joint.

In a study of outcomes following hip fractures, Barnes and Dunovan[1] found that in 65 patients with a mean age of 79.8 years at the time of their fractures, 54 reached independent ambulation (i.e., could use an assistive device without needing the help of another person) at some time between the date of surgery and one year later. However, the surgical technique used to repair hip fractures proved to be significant in the speed with which a patient reached independent ambulation. Sixty days following surgery only 30% of the patients with pinned hips were independent ambulators, but 58% of those with hip prostheses were independent ambulators. Usually, however, limited weight-bearing is imposed following surgery for a period of time determined by the doctor for those patients with pinned hips. At one year those with pinned hips had essentially "caught up" with those patients with hip prostheses in terms of independence in ambulation. Therapists should be aware of the important difference between procedures for the treatment of traumatic hip fractures since expectations in rehabilitation should differ appropriately.

Bursitis

Greater trochanteric bursitis. The most common form of bursitis around the hip is greater trochanteric bursitis. The greater trochanteric bursa lies between the tendon of the gluteus maximus and the posterolateral surface of the greater trochanter. There are many possible causes for this bursitis; a major one relates to the iliotibial band into which the gluteus maximus muscle inserts. The iliotibial band moves anteriorly with flexion and posteriorly with extension. If its flexibility is compromised, the result may be irritation of the greater trochanteric bursa. If the habit of standing on one leg with the other leg adducted is followed repeatedly by an activity such as running, the result could be trochanteric bursitis on the side of the adducted leg. Similarly, an imbalance between the adductor and abductor muscles in a runner with a broad pelvis and increased Q-angle can cause a painful trochanteric bursa. Other possible causes of trochanteric bursitis related to running activities are excessive posterolateral heel wear on the shoe or running on a banked surface. Excessive posterolateral heel wear results in an increased supination at heel strike, which is transmitted proximally to the lateral side of the leg. This increased pull on the gluteus maximus muscle via the iliotibial band is a logical cause of trochanteric bursitis. Running with one foot on a lower surface than the other or running with a leg-length discrepancy causes an abnormal pelvic tilt and thus an imbalance that could irritate the greater trochanteric bursa. Even a repeated adduction of the limb, such as occurs in soccer, can create a similar result.

Clinical findings. This disorder produces pain over the lateral aspect of the hip and thigh, radiating down to the knee in some cases, and occasionally into the lower leg. The client will often report an insidious onset and complain of pain while walking and when attempting to cross the legs when seated or when lying on either side. The pain often increases gradually, especially if activity is not reduced at its onset. It is aggravated most in activities of daily life by ascending stairs, which results in a strong contraction of the gluteus maximus muscle and pressure on the aggravated bursa. Often patients will report that they are unable to lie on the affected side. Palpation reveals an area of increased temperature and tenderness over the greater trochanter. The position of palpation with the client side-lying on the uninvolved side may create discomfort because of the flexed and adducted position of the involved leg. Ober's test (see Figure 16-30) will usually be positive, and resisted abduction will increase the symptoms. The patient otherwise has normal active and passive range of motion and normal joint play. Resisted abduction and, occasionally, resisted extension will be painful.

Treatment. As in any case, discovering the cause is essential to the treatment of this syndrome. Treating the symptoms with the classical routine of ultrasound or diathermy with no regard for the cause is unacceptable. Gait, posture, flexibility, running patterns, and shoes must be carefully assessed. Treatment may include applying ice in the acute stages, the use of ultrasound or diathermy, as well as a stretching program or deep-tissue massage to increase the flexibility of the iliotibial band, a recommendation of new shoes or a new running pattern, or an orthosis to correct leg-length differences or faulty mechanics in gait.

Ischial bursitis. The ischial bursa, lying between the tuberosity of the ischium and the gluteus maximus, is most often inflamed in persons with occupations requiring prolonged sitting. It is often associated with or can be mistaken for hamstring strains when the origin of the muscle has been affected. Ischial bursitis is found much less frequently than greater trochanteric bursitis and is easier to treat.

Clinical findings. Tenderness is localized over the ischial tuberosity, which is easily palpated in the side-lying position with the hip flexed or in the prone position with the involved leg in the frog-leg position. Pain often radiates into the hamstring muscles. The client will report pain with walking, climbing stairs, and flexion of the hip or trunk. It will be painful to sit on the affected side, and the common practice of carrying a wallet in the back pocket may aggravate the symptoms.

Treatment. Often the best treatment for ischial bursitis is to suggest chair padding or appropriate positioning to prevent aggravation of the ischial bursa. To relieve pain, ice or heat may be used effectively. If it is suspected that the problem is related to a compromised flexibility of the hamstrings, a stretching program should be recommended.

Iliopectineal bursitis. The iliopectineal bursa lies deep to the tendon of the iliopsoas muscle over the front of the hip joint. A common cause of iliopectineal bursitis is osteoarthritis of the hip. It may also be caused by a tight iliopsoas muscle.

Clinical findings. Pain is caused by tensing the iliopsoas muscle during forced flexion or stretching it during hip extension. The patient may present with a flexion deformity of the hip. Point tenderness will be found on palpation in the inguinal area. Referred pain into the anterior thigh and knee sometimes occurs and may be caused by inflammation resulting in irritation of the nearby femoral nerve.

Treatment. Diathermy may be used to reduce pain. The treatment of osteoarthritis has been discussed; if this is found to be a possible cause, treatment of the original condition is important. The iliopsoas muscle should be stretched if it is found to be contracted and a possible cause of the bursitis.

Muscle strains

The muscles of the thigh are under considerable stress since they function to propel the body through space and aid in kicking, jumping, and running activities. Muscle strains around the hip often develop into chronic problems because of prolonged self-treatment and/or continued activity in spite of pain. A muscle strain that causes tissue injury will result in inflammation and pain; if activity is continued, there will be additional tissue injury. The final result is a vicious cycle of continuous pain and injury.

The most commonly strained muscles around the hip are the hamstrings, adductor longus, iliopsoas, and rectus femoris.[61] A first-degree strain will often resolve itself without treatment and no disability will result. A second-degree strain is most frequently seen in the clinic and will reduce the the muscle's ability to function. All these muscle strains are frequent in active sports.

Mechanisms of injury. The mechanism of injury, as in any muscle strain, may be insidious or traumatic. In the case of an insidious onset, clients should be carefully questioned about any changes in activities or patterns of running or stretching. If the injury has been traumatic, a complete description of the position in which the injury occurred and of anything clients felt or heard should be requested. Excessive loading of the muscle during an intensive training period is often the cause of injury. Injury of the iliopsoas or rectus femoris occurs through repeated flexing movements, forced flexion against resistance, or excessive hip extension. The adductor longus is strained when forced external rotation and abduction occur or by repeated forceful adduction, such as in soccer. Running with a pelvic imbalance can also cause repetitive trauma to the adductor longus. A hamstring strain occurs frequently in runners, skiers, bikers, and jumpers. A typical ski injury where the skier falls in a position where the leg is straight at the knee, the hip is flexed and exaggeratedly abducted can result in a combined hamstring and adductor strain. An excessive stretch into hip flexion while the knee remains extended, or repeated hip extension will often result in a hamstring strain.

Clinical findings. A typical client who has incurred a muscle strain has localized pain at the muscle belly, the point of origin and/or insertion of the muscle, and increased stiffness. The pain and stiffness may decrease during exercise but return after exercise, often with greater intensity. Active or resisted movement in the direction of the muscle action will reproduce pain and often weakness. Passive stretching in the opposite direction will also be painful. Palpation may not only reach painful areas but may also reveal some apparent hardening or knotting in the muscle belly or at the point of origin or insertion. A history of recurrence of the disability is not uncommon. An individual will often reduce or halt his/her activity until the pain has subsided but then return to the same activity too soon and incur repeated injury. A radiograph will rule out fractures if they are suspected.

Treatment. Though a risk of intramuscular hemorrhage has been a concern of some authors who caution nothing but rest 5 to 7 days following an injury,[47] some clinicians feel that immediate massage will decrease swelling and stiffness and that early stretching is essential.[73] Immediately following the injury, frequent application of ice, elevation, and pressure from an elastic wrap are useful. Rest is essential, and an elastic wrap applied from the knee to the groin will protect the muscles during walking. There is no set time when cryotherapy should be changed to heat treatments. Ice should be used as long as it is effective. After this, heat may prove to be valuable in treatment. To prevent a random alignment of new collagen fibers, ultrasound and/or cross-friction massage and stretching should be used. Once the resistance to stretching has decreased and a full painless range is achieved, the client may start with submaximal isometric exercises. Immobility, which is sometimes recommended by the doctor, has actually been found to be detrimental to healing. Zarins and Ciullo stated that immobilization decreases the rate of healing by causing a vascular reabsorption of collagen.[78] Parker[58] describes the effect of immobilization as a decrease of protein synthesis resulting in muscular atrophy. Booth and Gould[4] also showed an increase in collagen concentration with exercise. Pain-free exercise early in the rehabilitation process also helps in the formation of scar tissue along the lines of force instead of randomly.[78] On about the third day after injury, or sooner if the exercises are pain-free, the client should start with submaximal isometric exercises, progressing to isometrics with increasing load. Short-arc active exercises with resistance followed by more aggressive training of an isotonic exercise program or isokinetics can be added over time. Continued stretching should be emphasized as the client moves into a specialized training program. If at any time in the exercise program movements are very painful, they should be postponed until they can be performed with minimal pain. Pool therapy is excellent to encourage active movement.

Prevention of strains is the best treatment and is accomplished by proper stretching. Suggestions of exercises to stretch the adductor group muscles, the hamstrings, the rectus femoris, and the iliopsoas are shown in Figs. 16-46 to 16-55. Stretching should be performed for an extended period of time, such as a minimum of 2 minutes, for optimal results. Some excellent static stretching techniques for increasing hip flexion and extension range of motion done in the clinic have been described by Godges et al.[25]

It should be noted that muscle strains in muscles of the hip other than those mentioned above can certainly occur. When discomfort is reported in the buttocks region that extends down into the hamstring muscle, with differential tests ruling out involvement of the lumbar spine and sacro-

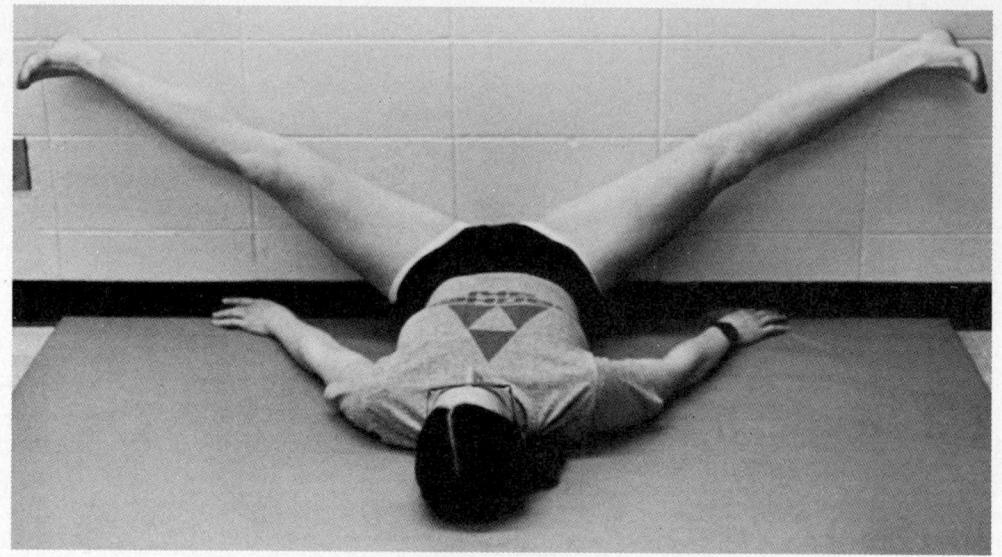

Fig. 16-46. Exercise to stretch adductor muscles.

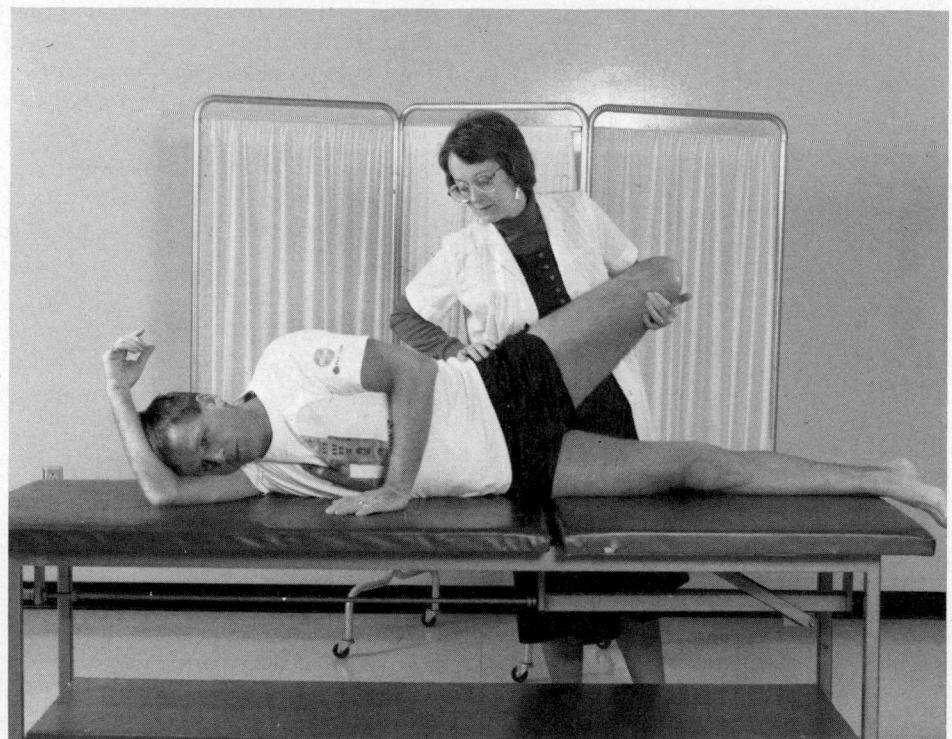

Fig. 16-47. Therapist assisted adductor stretch emphasizing the adductor magnus.

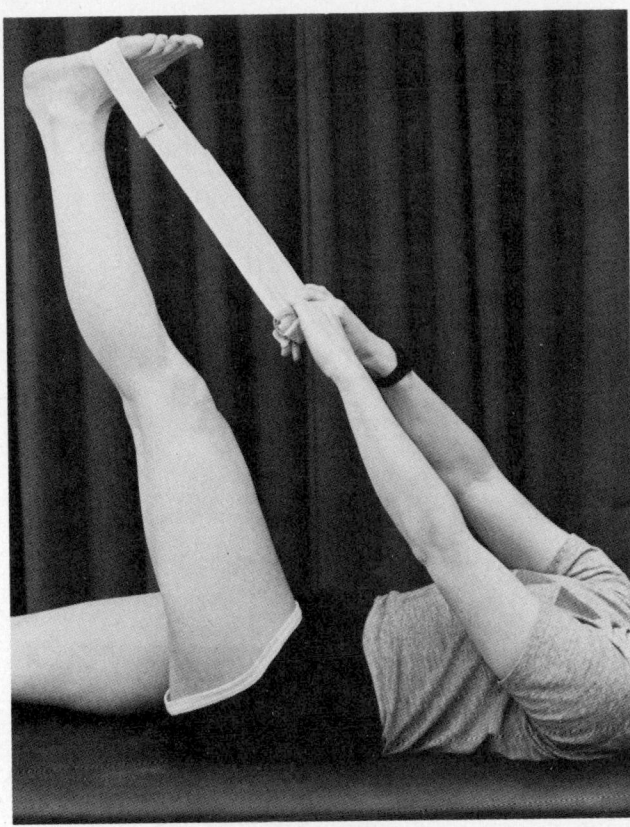

Fig. 16-48. Supine stretch for the hamstring muscles. Note that while stretching the left leg, the right leg should be in the neutral position and remain straight to stabilize the pelvis.

iliac region, the clinician might suspect some deeper muscles of the gluteal region. The external rotators can be the victims of repeated microtrauma that often goes unrecognized or that is misdiagnosed as sacroiliac dysfunction. These muscles can be carefully palpated in the frog leg position (see Fig. 16-59) and deep cross-transverse friction massage can also be performed in this position when hardening or tightness is found. The tightness frequently found in the piriformis muscle is called the *piriformis syndrome*.

Piriformis syndrome

The piriformis syndrome is irritation of the sciatic nerve as it passes underneath or through the piriformis muscle. In most cases, the sciatic nerve passes entirely underneath the piriformis muscles, but in 15% of the population the nerve cuts through and separates the muscle into two parts.[9] The piriformis syndrome occurs about six times as frequently in women as in men[9] and can cause chronic pain. It may occur as a result of compression of the sciatic nerve by a tight piriformis muscle.

Clinical findings. The client with piriformis syndrome complains of deep localized pain in the posterior aspect of the hip near the sciatic notch. There may also be numbness and tingling down into the leg and low-back pain indicating sciatica. A thorough examination of the low-back and

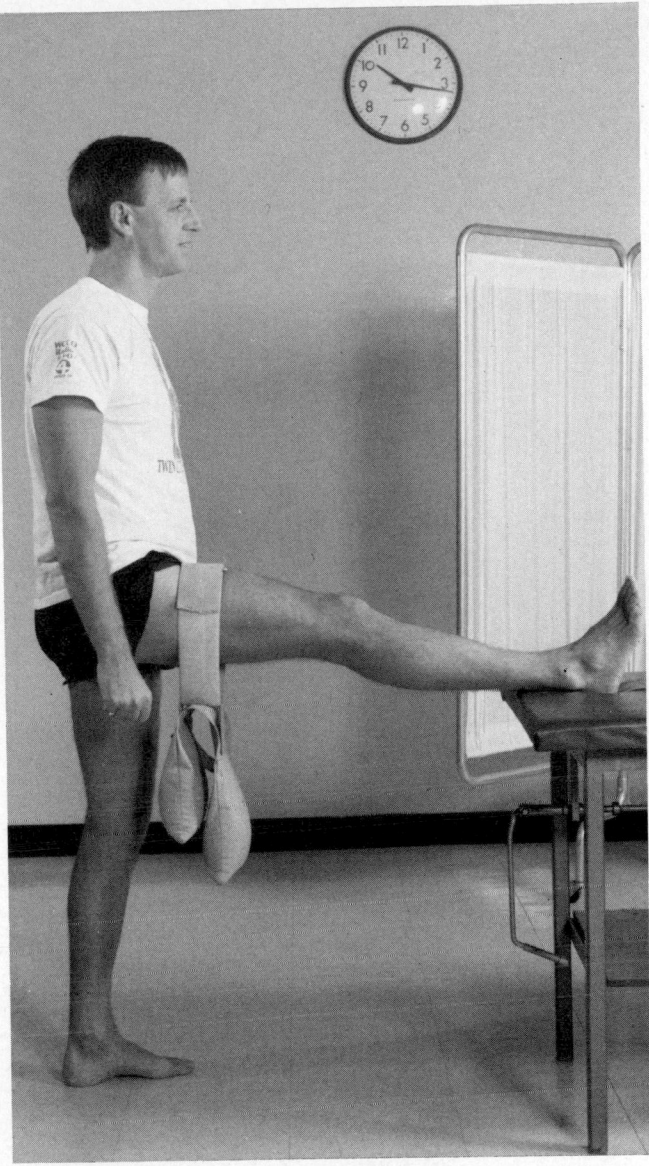

Fig. 16-49. Standing stretch for the hamstrings. Note that while stretching the right leg the left leg should not externally rotate and should remain straight to stabilize the pelvis.

sacroiliac joint should rule these out as sources of the problem. However, one should be alert to the fact that a pelvic imbalance may be responsible for an imbalance between the internal and external rotators.

The most significant finding implicating the piriformis muscle will be if both active external rotation with resistance and a passive stretch into internal rotation produce pain. As mentioned previously, the deep external rotators may be palpated with the client lying prone in the frog-leg position (see Fig. 16-59). Then the tightness will be felt and pain will result from palpation.

Treatment. If the sciatic nerve is very irritable and inflamed, the initial treatment may be ice, rest, and aspirin. Mild stretching can later be performed from a side-lying or

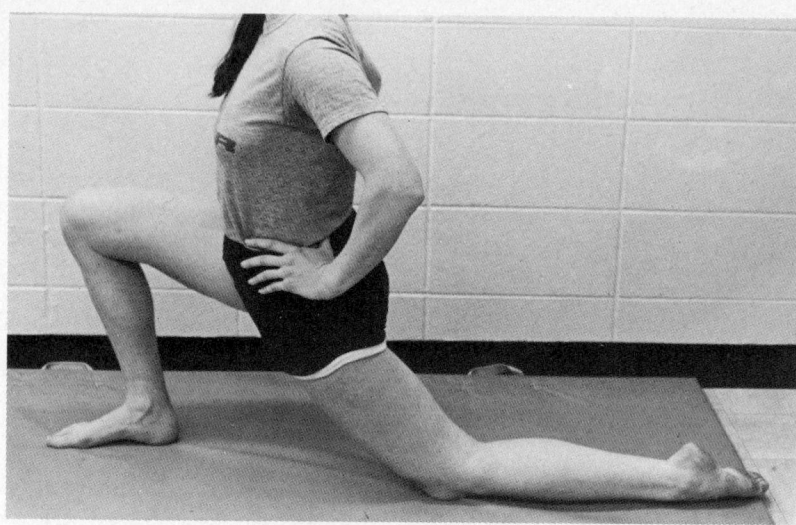

Fig. 16-50. Exercise to stretch iliopsoas muscle.

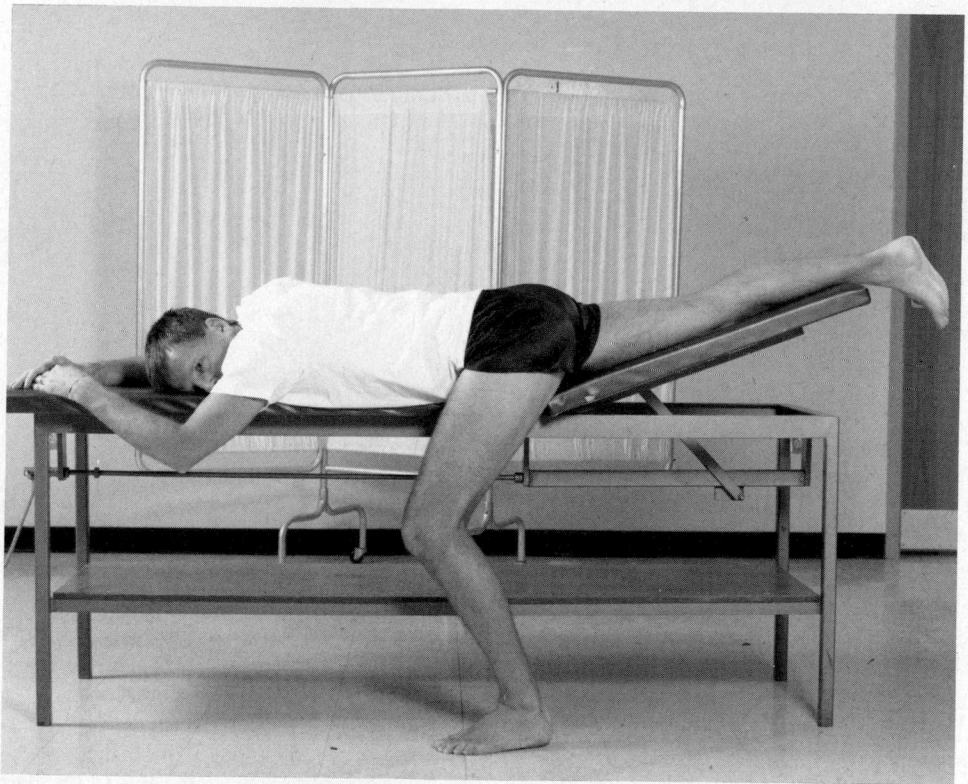

Fig. 16-51. Stretch for the iliopsoas.

sitting position (see Figs. 16-43 and 16-44). Contract-relax exercises performed in the side-lying position (see Fig. 16-32) should also prove to be effective to help stretch the piriformis muscle. Self-stretches of all the deep rotators and the piriformis can be seen in the positions shown in Fig. 16-56 to 16-58. Also effective in the treatment of tight piriformis muscles is deep cross transverse friction massage performed in the position shown in Fig. 16-59.

SUMMARY

The accurate diagnosis and treatment of hip disorders depend on the knowledge and experience of the therapist. The necessary knowledge base, including the anatomy and biomechanics of the hip, has been presented in this chapter. A systematic approach for an evaluation has been suggested, and various disorders and treatments of the hip have been discussed.

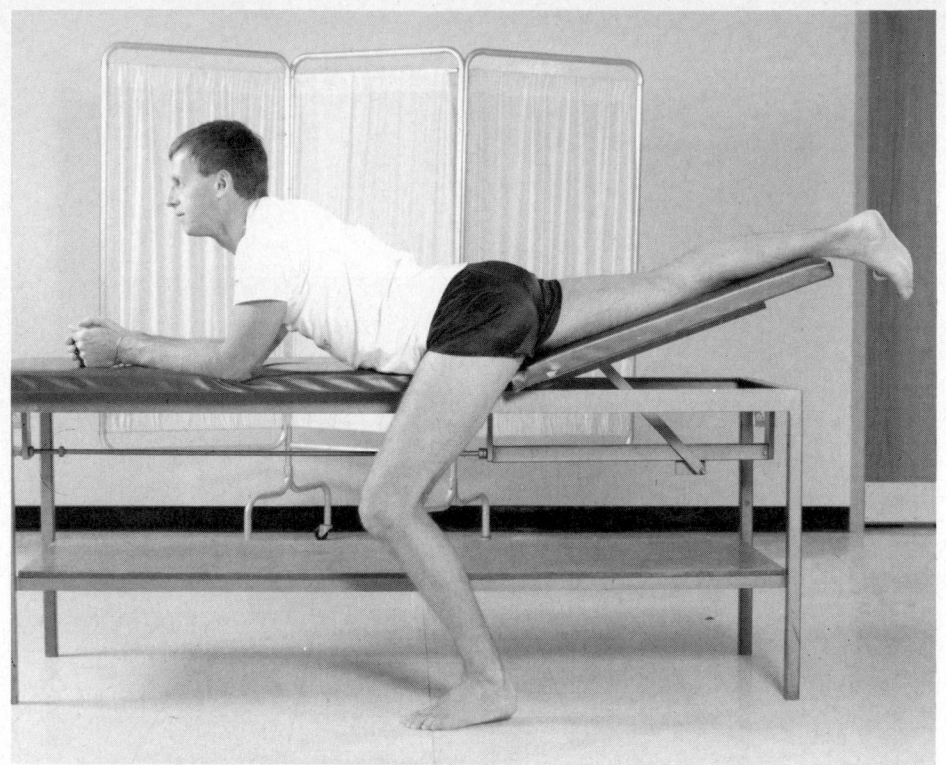

Fig. 16-52. Stretch for the iliopsoas with emphasis on the iliacus.

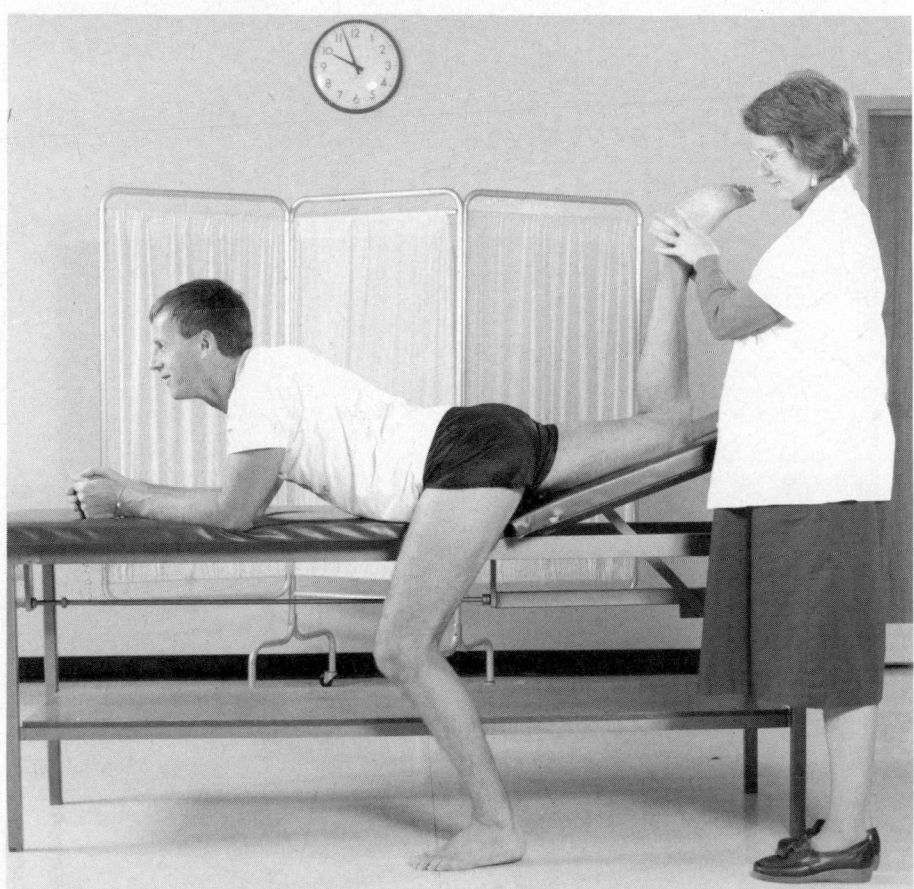

Fig. 16-53. Stretch for the iliopsoas and rectus femoris with emphasis on the rectus femoris.

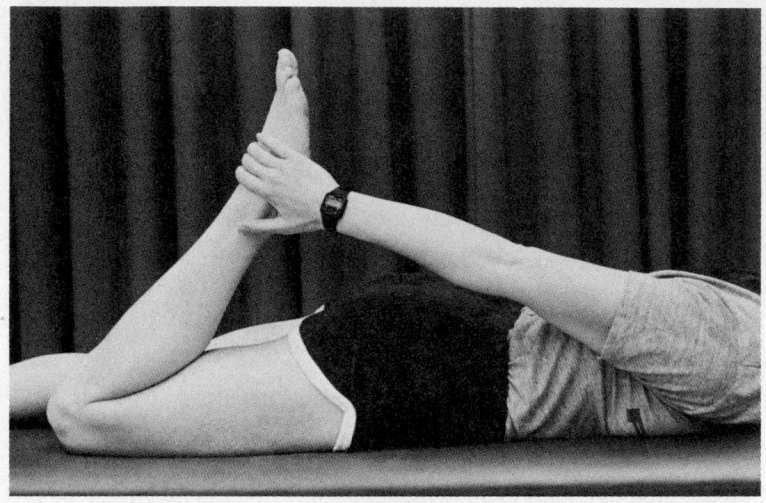

Fig. 16-54. Exercise to stretch rectus femoris muscle.

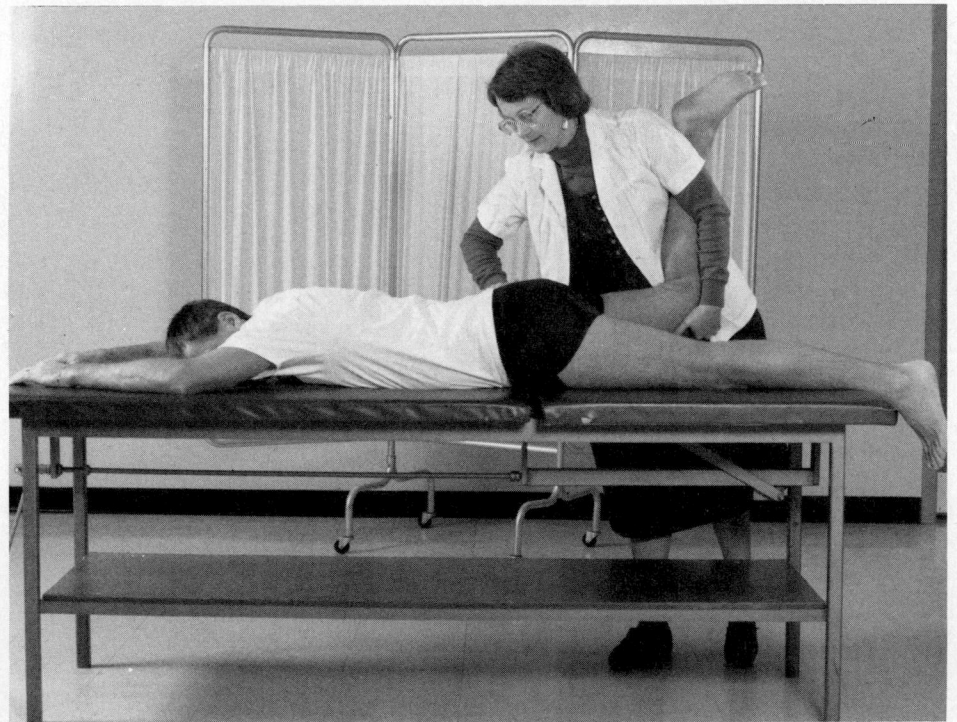

Fig. 16-55. Therapist assisted stretch of the rectus femoris.

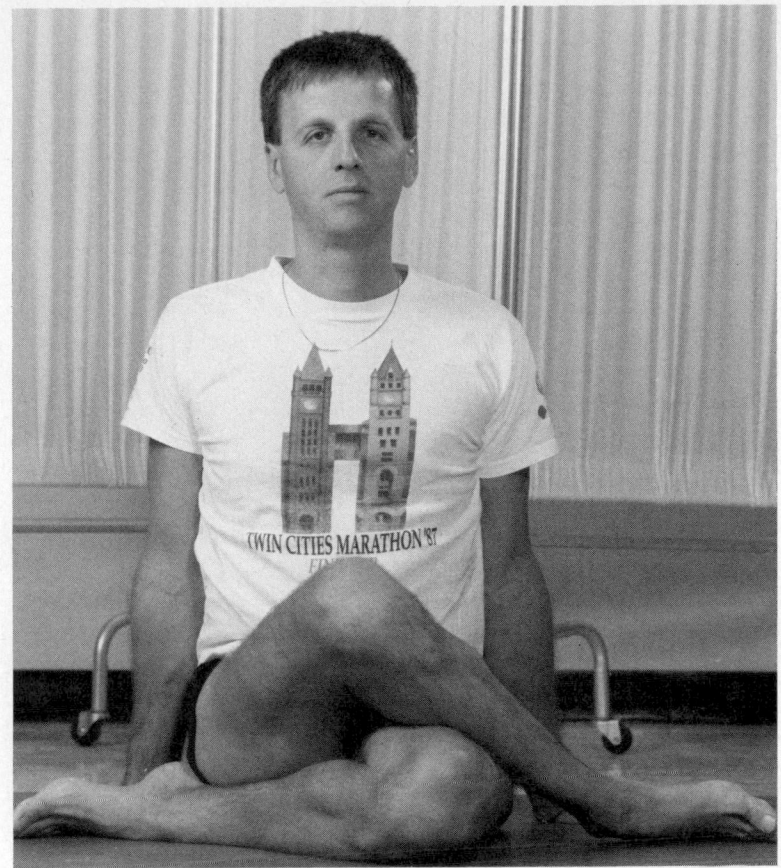

Fig. 16-56. Stretch for the right piriformis.

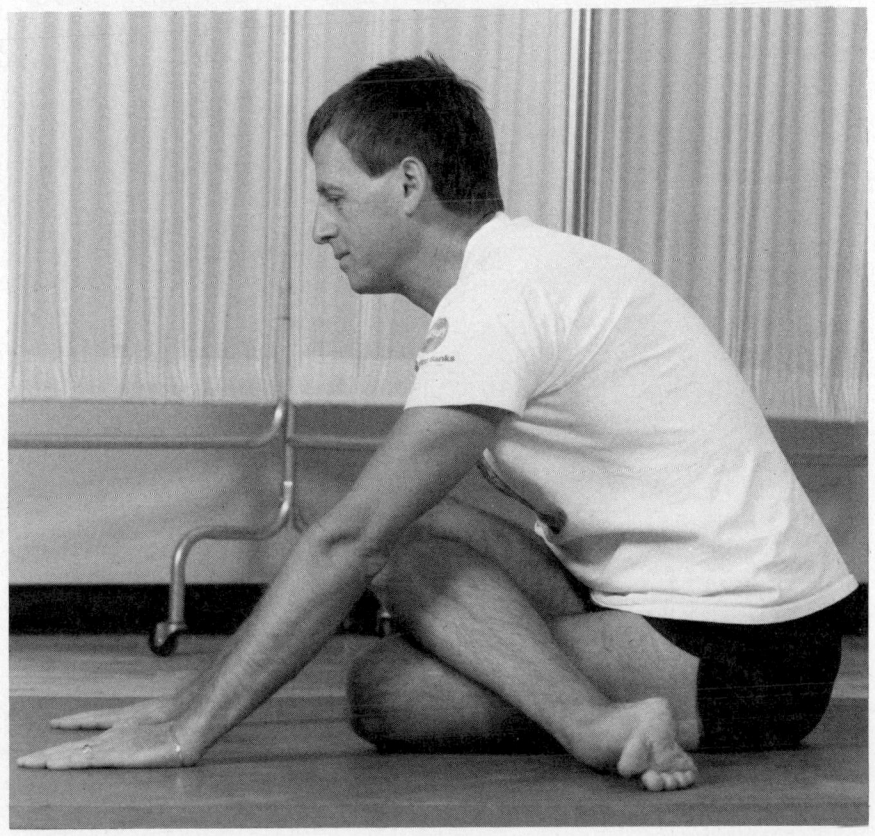

Fig. 16-57. Client moving forward to increase the stretch on the piriformis seen in Fig. 16-56.

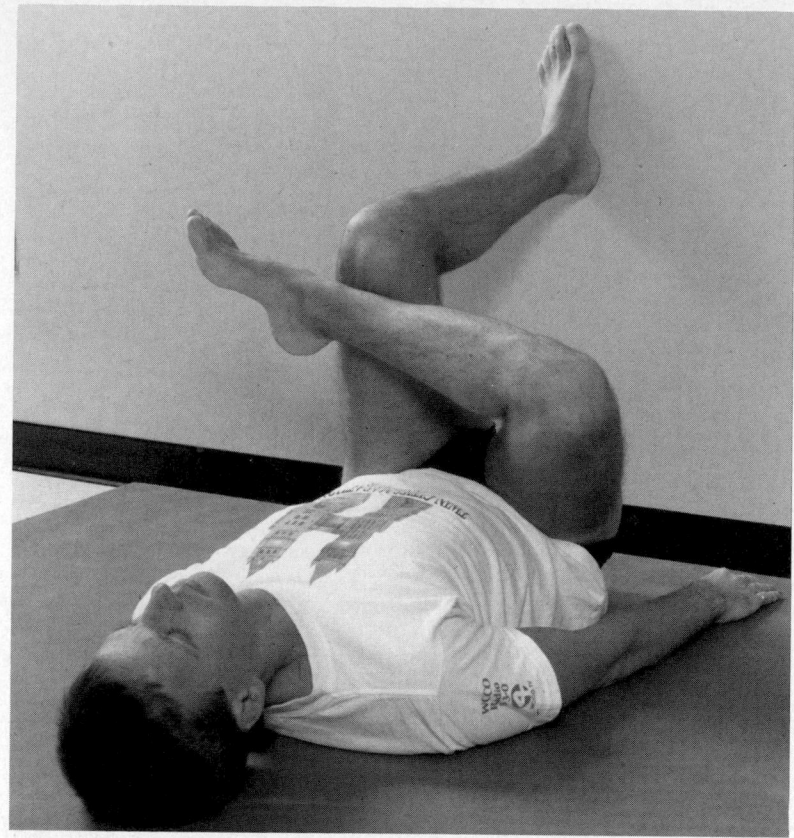

Fig. 16-58. Stretch of the deep rotators on the right.

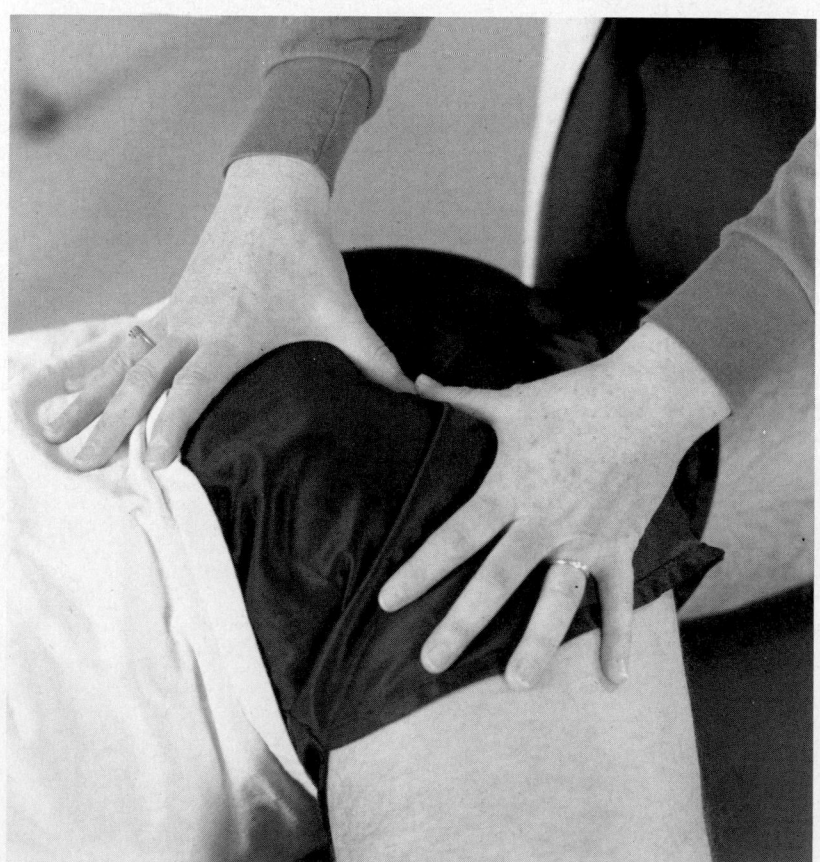

Fig. 16-59. Position used for cross transverse friction massage of the piriformis and other external rotators.

REFERENCES

1. Barnes B and Dunovan K: Functional outcomes after hip fracture, Phys Ther 67(11):1675, 1987.
2. Basmajian JV: The human bicycle in biomechanics V-A. In Komi PV, editor: Biomechanics V-A: Proceedings of the Fifth International Congress on Biomechanics, Jyvaskla, Finland, Baltimore, 1976, University Park Press.
3. Blount W: Don't throw away the cane, Presidential Address, Annual Meeting, Academy of Orthopaedic Surgeons, J Bone Joint Surg (Am) 38:695, 1956.
4. Booth F and Gould E: Effect of training and disuse on connective tissue. In Wilmore J and Keough J editors: Exercise and Sports Sciences Review, p 105, New York, 1975, Academic Press.
5. Brashear HR and Raney RB: Handbook of orthopaedic surgery, St. Louis, 1986, The CV Mosby Co.
6. Brody D: Running injuries, Ciba Clin Symp 32:29, 1980.
7. Bullough P, Goodfellow J, and O'Connor, J: The relationship between degenerative changes and loadbearing in the human hip, J Bone Joint Surg (Br) 55:746, 1973.
8. Byers P, Contepomi C, and Farkas T: A post mortem study of the hip joint, Ann Rheum Dis 29:15, 1970.
9. Cailliet R: Soft tissue pain and disability, Philadelphia, 1977, FA Davis Co.
10. Cattell A: The natural history of Perthes disease, J Bone Joint Surg (Br) 53:37, 1971.
11. Catterall A: Coxa plana, Mod Trends Orthop 6:122, 1972.
12. Chrisman O: Biomechanical aspects of degenerative joint disease, Clin Orthop 64:77, 1969.
13. Clark G: Unequal leg length: An accurate method of detection and some clinical results, Rheum Phys Med 11:385, 1972.
14. Clark J and Haynor D: Anatomy of the abductor muscles of the hip as studied by computed tomography. J Bone Joint Surg (Am) 69(7):1021, 1987.
15. Collins D: The pathology of articular and spinal disease, London, 1949, Edward Arnold & Co.
16. Daniels L and Worthingham C: Muscle testing, Philadelphia, 1980, WB Saunders Co.
17. Ellis MI and Stowe J: The hip, Clin Rheum Dis 8:655, 1982.
18. Fielding WJ and Cochran G: Subtrochanteric fractures. In American Academy of Orthopaedic Surgeons: Instructional course lectures, vol 23, St Louis, 1974, The CV Mosby Co.
19. Fisher R: An epidemiological study of Legg-Perthes disease, J Bone Joint Surg (Am) 54:769, 1972.
20. Fisher F: Legg-Perthes: I. Characteristic features and etiology. In American Academy of Orthopaedic Surgeons: Instructional course lectures, vol 22, St Louis, 1973, The CV Mosby Co.
21. Friberg O: Length asymmetry of lower extremities: An etiological factor of stress fractures. Ann Med Milit Fenn 55:149-154, 1980.
22. Friberg O: Clinical symptoms and biomechanics of lumbar spine and hip joint in leg length inequality, Spine 8(6):643, 1983.
23. Gartland J: Fundamentals of orthopaedics, Philadelphia, 1974, WB Saunders Co.
24. Godges J, et al: The effects of two stretching procedures on hip range of motion and gait economy, J Orth Sports Ther 10(9):350, 1989.
25. Gofton J: Studies in osteoarthritis of the hip: II. Osteoarthritis of the hip and leg-length disparity, Can Med Assoc J 104:791, 1971.
26. Gofton J and Trueman G: Unilateral idiopathic osteoarthritis of the hip, Can Med Assoc J 97:1129, 1967.
27. Gogia P and Braatz J: Validity and reliability of leg length measurements, J Orthop Sports Phys Ther 8(4):185, 1986.
28. Gordon EJ: Diagnosis and treatment of common hip disorders, Med Trial Tech Q 28:(4):443, 1981.
29. Gore D, et al: Walking patterns of men with unilateral surgical hip fusion, J Bone Joint Surg (Am) 57:759, 1975.
30. Halpern A, Tanner J, and Rinsky L: Does persistent femoral anteversion contribute to osteoarthritis? Clin Orthop 145:213, 1979.
31. Harris W: Etiology of osteoarthritis of the hip. Clin Orthop 213:20, 1986.
32. Harrison M, Schajowica F, and Trueta J: Osteoarthritis of the hip: A study of the nature and evolution of the disease, J Bone Joint Surg (Br) 35:598, 1953.
33. Hart V: Congenital dysplasia of the hip joint and sequelae, Springfield, Ill, 1952, Charles C Thomas, Publisher.
34. Harty M: The anatomy of the hip joint. In Tronzo, R, editor: Surgery of the hip joint, Philadelphia, 1973, Lea & Febiger.
35. Inman V: Functional aspects of the abductor muscles of the hip, J Bone Joint Surg (Am) 29:607, 1947.
36. Inman V, Ralston H, and Todd F: Human walking, Baltimore, 1981, Williams & Wilkins.
37. Iversen L and Clawson D: Manual of acute orthopaedic therapeutics, Boston, 1982, Little, Brown and Co.
38. Jacobs B: Diagnosis and history of slipped capital femoral epiphysis. In American Academy of Orthopaedic Surgeons: Instructional course lectures, vol 21, St Louis, 1972, The CV Mosby Co.
39. Johnston R: Hip motion measurements for selected activities of daily living, Clin Orthop 72:202, 1970.
40. Johnston R: Mechanical considerations of the hip joint, Arch Surg 107:411, 1973.
41. Johnston R, Brand R, and Crowninshield R: Reconstruction of the hip: A mathematical approach to determine optimum geometric relationships, J Bone Joint Surg 61A:639, 1979.
42. Jorring K: Osteoarthritis of the hip, Acta Orthop Scand. 51:523, 1980.
43. Jowsey J: Osteoporosis and its relationship to femoral neck fractures. In The Hip Society: The hip, St Louis, 1977, The CV Mosby Co.
44. Kapandji IA: Physiology of the joints, vol 2, Lower limb, New York, 1975, Churchill Livingstone.
45. Kellegren J: Osteoarthritis in patients and populations, Br Med J 2:1, 1961.
46. Kelsey J and Southwick W: Etiology, mechanism, and incidence of slipped capital femoral epiphysis. In American Academy of Orthopaedic Surgeons: Instructional course lectures, vol 21, St Louis, 1972, The CV Mosby Co.
47. Krejci V and Koch P: Muscle and tendon injuries in athletes, Chicago, 1979, Year Book Medical Publishers.
48. Lewinnek G et al: The significance and comparison analysis of the epidemiology of hip fractures, Clin Orthop 152:35, 1980.
49. Linn F: Lubrication of animal joints, J Bone Joint Surg (Am) 49:1079, 1967.
50. Lloyd-Roberts G: Osteoarthritis of the hip, J Bone Joint Surg (Br) 37:8, 1955.
51. Massie W and Howorth M: Congenital dislocation of the hip, J Bone Joint Surg (Am) 32:519, 1950.
52. McLeish RD: Abduction forces in the one legged stance, J Biomech 3:191, 1970.
53. Merchant AC: Hip abductor muscle force: An experimental study of the influence of hip position with particular reference to rotation, J Bone Joint Surg 47A:462, 1965.
54. Molley M and MacMahon B: Birthweight and Legg-Perthes disease, J Bone Joint Surg (Am) 49:498, 1967.
55. Morscher E: Etiology and pathogenesis in leg length discrepancies, Progr Orthop Surg 1:9, 1977.
56. Morscher E and Figner G: Measurement of leg length, Progr Orthop Surg 1:21, 1977.
57. Nichols P and Bailey, N: The accuracy of measuring leg length differences: An "observer error" experiment, Br Med J 2:1247, 1955.
58. Parker M: Characteristics of skeletal muscle during rehabilitation: Quadriceps femoris. Athl Training 18:122, 1981.
59. Pauwels F: Biomechanics of the normal and diseased hip, New York, 1976, Springer-Verlag.

60. Radin E et al: Response of joints to impact loading. III, J Biomech. 6:51, 1973.

61. Renstrom P and Peterson L: Groin injuries in athletes, Br J Sports Med 14:30, 1980.

62. Rydell N: Biomechanics of the hip joint, Clin Orthop 92:6, 1973.

63. Salter R: Textbook of disorders and injuries of the musculoskeletal system, Baltimore, 1970, Williams & Wilkins.

64. Salter R: Legg-Perthes disease. V. Treatment by innominate osteotomy. In American Academy of Orthopaedic Surgeons: Instructional course lectures, vol 22, St Louis, 1973, The CV Mosby Co.

65. Savastano A: Clinical review of Legg-Perthes disease, Int Surv 59:96, 1974.

66. Singleton R and LeVeau B: The hip joint: Structure, stability and stress, Phys Ther 55:957, 1975.

67. Smith E: Exercise for prevention of osteoporosis: A review, Phys Sports Med 10:72, 1982.

68. Soderberg G and Dostal W: Electromyographic study of three parts of the gluteus medius muscle during functional activities, Phys Ther 58:691, 1978.

69. Steindler A: Kinesiology of the human body under normal and pathological conditions, Springfield, Ill, 1955, Charles C Thomas, Publisher.

70. Steindler A: Postgraduate lectures on orthopaedic diagnosis and indications, Springfield, Ill, 1957, Charles C Thomas, Publisher.

71. Stevens J et al: The incidence of osteoporosis in patients with femoral neck fractures, J Bone Joint Surg (Br) 44:520, 1962.

72. Tinker R, editor: Ramamurti's orthopaedics in primary care, Baltimore, 1979, Williams & Wilkins.

73. Tsujii Y: Personal communication, Nagoya University, College of Medical Technology, Nagoya, Japan, 1988.

74. Wadsworth J, Smidt G, and Johnston R: Gait characteristics of subjects with hip disease, Phys Ther 52:829, 1972.

75. Walmsley T: The articular mechanism of the diarthroses, J Bone Joint Surg (Am) 10:40, 1928.

76. Warwick R and Williams P, editors: Gray's anatomy, ed 35, Philadelphia, 1973, WB Saunders Co.

77. Williams J and Svensson N: A force analysis of the hip joint, BioMed Eng. 3:365, 1968.

78. Zarins B and Ciullo J: Acute muscle and tendon injuries in athletes, Clin Sports Med 2:167, 1983.

ADDITIONAL READINGS

American Academy of Orthopaedic Surgeons: Joint motion, method of measuring and recording, Chicago, 1965, The Academy.

Hoppenfeld S: Physical examination of the spine and extremities, New York, 1976, Appleton-Century-Crofts.

Kendall H and Kendall F.: Muscles, testing and function, Baltimore, 1971, Williams & Wilkins Co.

Moore K: Clinically oriented anatomy, Baltimore, 1980, Williams & Wilkins Co.

Steindler A: Mechanics of normal and pathological locomotion in man, Springfield, Ill, 1955, Charles C Thomas, Publisher.

Wells, K.: Kinesiology, Philadelphia, 1966, WB Saunders Co.

Chapter 17

EXAMINATION OF LOWER-EXTREMITY DYSFUNCTION

Gary C. Hunt

Efficient performance of any multijointed structure depends on balanced mechanical relationships. When these mechanical relationships are altered, compensatory mechanisms work to re-establish an equilibrium. Increased interest in regular sports activities has resulted in a variety of neuromusculoskeletal problems that have frustrated both client and clinician. The study of the kinematics and kinetics of human locomotion is essential if rational and realistic management approaches are to develop.

The ability to identify specific occurrences during gait is absolutely necessary, but the simultaneous movement of body segments can present a confusing picture. The im-

portance of visualizing and analyzing segment and joint movement is necessary if clinicians are to successfully manage lower-extremity problems. Considerable anatomical variations exist,[24,26] but in spite of these variations people generally function adequately. The key to successful management is the determination of optimal functional strength and motion for a particular individual and the establishment of a program to approach a balanced state. Therefore a systematic evaluation of the lower extremity is essential in order to help the individual with his/her problem. The goal of this chapter is to present practical examination of management approaches to lower-extremity dysfunction by including discussions on gait analysis with an emphasis on the foot, static examination, pathomechanics, and treatment approaches.

DYNAMIC CLINICAL GAIT EVALUATION

One basic objective of human locomotion is minimal energy expenditure. The ability to ambulate efficiently results from a smooth biomechanical integration of numerous body segments starting with the foot. The walking gait cycle is divided into a *stance phase* and a *swing phase*. The stance phase takes approximately 62% of the cycle, and it is this phase that will be emphasized in the following discussion. In order to ambulate efficiently, the foot must function in at least four ways during stance: (1) as a base of support, (2) as a shock absorber, (3) as a mobile adapter, and (4) as a rigid lever. The first requirement is met simply by making contact with the ground. However, the next three functions occur in a timely sequence. The stance phase, which lasts approximately 0.60 to 0.69 seconds[25,38,42,49] is composed of three periods: (1) contact (heel or rearfoot strike to footflat), (2) midstance, and (3)

Written in author's private capacity. No official support or endorsement by the United States Department of Health and Human Services is intended or should be inferred.

roll-off (heel rise to toe-off).[23] The following discussion includes a description of these periods with an emphasis on how the foot changes function in free speed walking. One must consider that as walking speed increases, initial contact may occur at the midfoot or the forefoot.

Contact phase

As one observes the gait cycle from the posterior view, the position of the calcaneus should be identified relative to the supporting surface (Fig. 17-1). Just before initial contact, the calcaneus should be slightly inverted.

At heel contact, the subtalar joint begins to rapidly pronate as indicated by calcaneal eversion and continues until the foot is flat at approximately 20% to 25% of the stance phase, as illustrated in Fig. 17-2. Subtalar joint pronation is initiated by internal rotation of the lower extremity and pelvis.[11,57] The total amount of subtalar joint pronation necessary has been measured to be from 8 to 12 degrees, depending on the orientation of the subtalar joint axis.[24,54,57]

The importance of the subtalar joint complex cannot be overemphasized.[27,30] Inman's[24] description of the subtalar joint as a mitered hinge demonstrates the rotational interrelationship between the leg and foot. As the lower extremity rotates internally, pronation occurs around the subtalar joint axis and, as external rotation occurs, so does supination. This interrelationship is demonstrated in Figs. 17-3 and 17-4.

The average horizontal inclination of the subtalar joint axis has been measured to be approximately 45 degrees and allows 1 degree of leg rotation for every degree of subtalar rotation.[24,34] However, the inclination of the axis in the sagittal plane varies from 21 to 69 degrees.[24] A logical question arises: how does function vary when subtalar joint axes are at the extremes? If the axis angle is 20 degrees from the horizontal, the amount of subtalar rotation will be greater than 1 degree for every degree of leg rotation. The opposite would be true for an axis angle of 70 degrees. Functionally, a low-inclination axis angle would be found with foot structures described as *pes planus* and a high inclined axis with *pes cavus*. Fig. 17-5 demonstrates the variation of motion as seen in a 45-degree, 20-degree, and 70-degree axis angle within the sagittal plane.

Pronation allows the foot to become a loose adapter and a shock absorber. The impact shock at heel strike is thus dampened by calcaneal eversion, ankle plantar flexion, and knee flexion, all of which are facilitated by subtalar joint pronation. During this motion, the talus adducts and the plantar flexes, and the leg moves forward more quickly, resulting in knee flexion.[11,40] The key event to observe during heel contact is whether the calcaneus strikes the ground inverted, perpendicularly, or everted. Figs. 17-6 and 17-7 depict normal and abnormal heel contact.

The absorption of impact shock is facilitated by the movement of the calcaneus from an inverted to an everted position. This can be illustrated by the example of falling. If one does not roll when falling, the impact force is greater. If the calcaneus does not evert during heel contact, then an increase in impact shock may occur, potentially causing excessive proximal trauma. In addition, if one lands with the calcaneus excessively inverted, then a potential for lateral instability may result with lateral ankle strains and sprains.

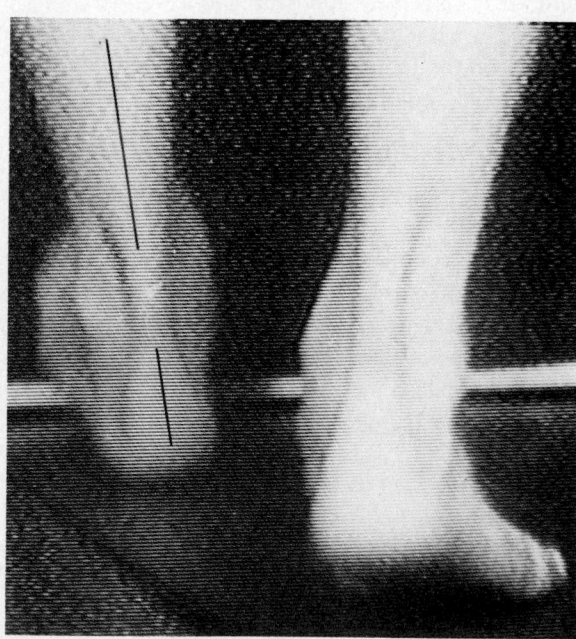

Fig. 17-1. Left heel contact.

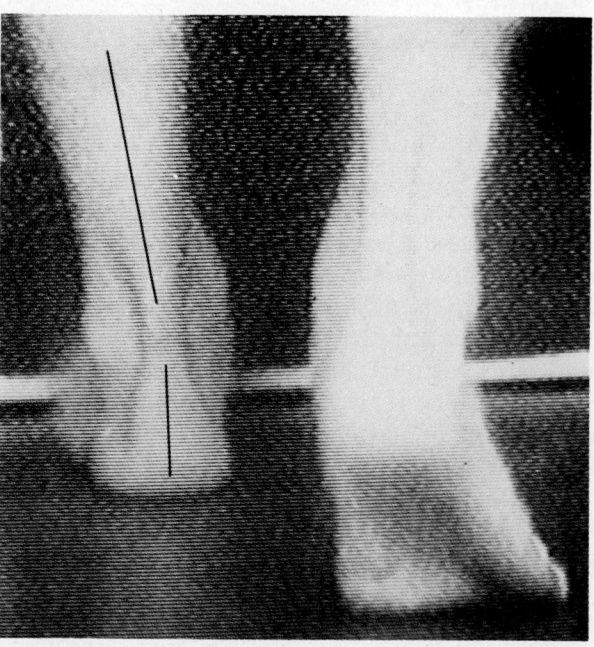

Fig. 17-2. Left footflat.

Footflat occurs rapidly and includes that period of time from heel contact to contact of the forefoot with the ground. In a free walking gait, this time takes approximately 0.10 to 0.15 seconds.[44,49] During this short interval, rapid pronation occurs, which is primarily a passive movement. To observe the calcaneus evert during this interval without the use of slow motion analysis is difficult, and to differentiate the pathological from the physiological may not be easy.

Muscular activity occurring from heel contact to footflat involves the pretibial group, and authorities agree that this prevents a footslap.[14,33,51] It is during this part of stance

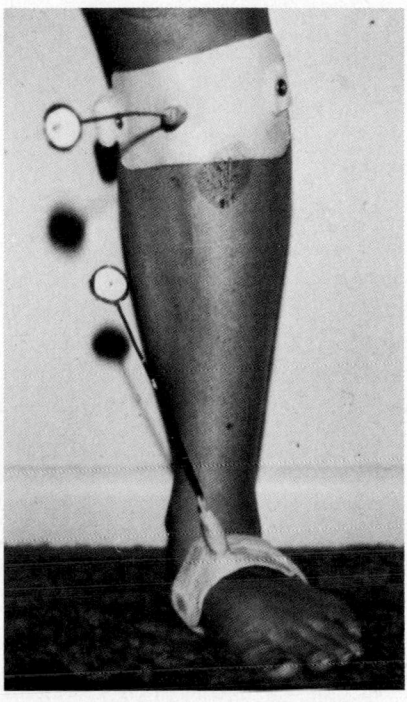

Fig. 17-3. Internal rotation with pronation.

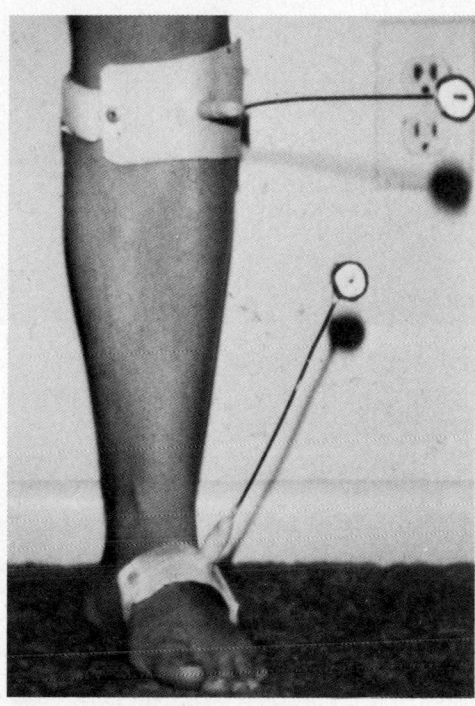

Fig. 17-4. External rotation with supination.

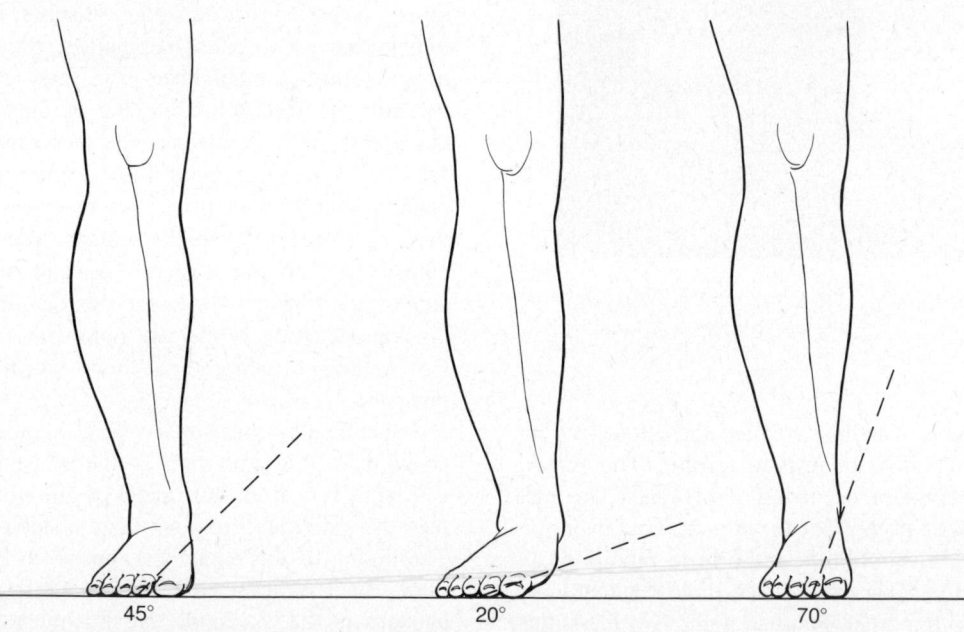

Fig. 17-5. Note equal rotation in 45-degree angle as compared with 20-degree angle (where there is greater pronation) and with the 70-degree angle (where there is less pronation).

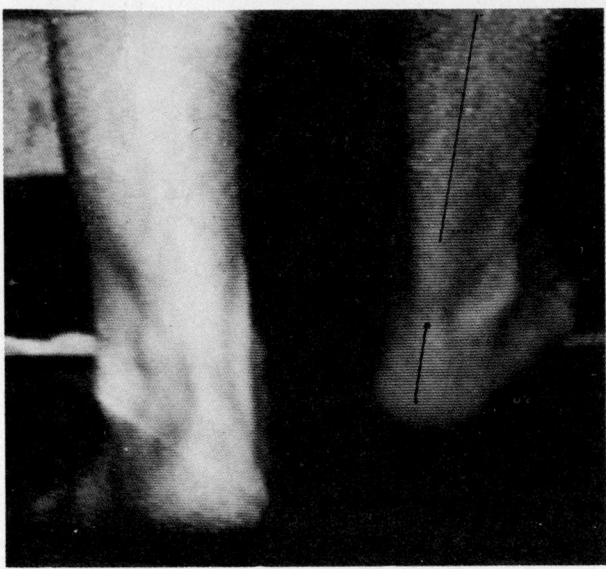

Fig. 17-6. Normal right heel contact.

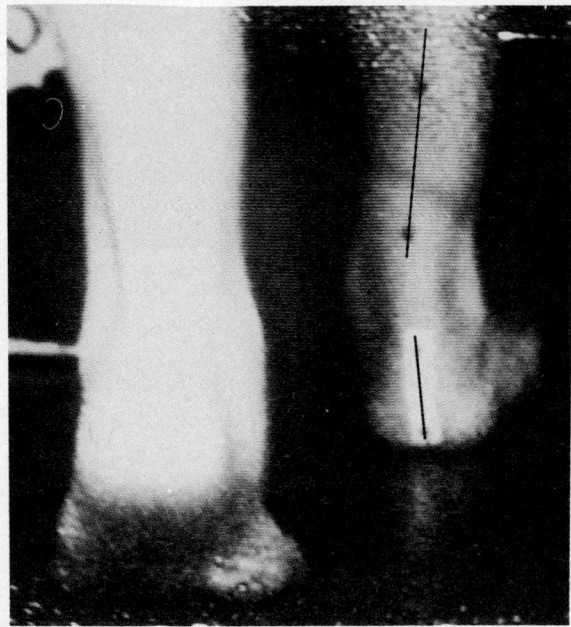

Fig. 17-7. Abnormally everted heel contact on right.

that the foot becomes a mobile adapter and allows the individual to accommodate to uneven terrain. The importance of subtalar pronation occurring at this phase becomes evident as it allows the midfoot to unlock. This event allows further shock absorption in addition to mobile adaptation of the forefoot. The occurrence of lower extremity internal rotation is important because without it the subtalar joint would be unable to pronate and thus prevent the expected shock absorption and mobile adaptation. One can

start to appreciate what might happen if an individual's lower extremity internally rotates insufficiently or excessively during this period of time.

The first posterior leg muscle to function during this phase is the tibialis posterior. If one agrees that the tibialis posterior is a supinator of the midfoot and hindfoot, then one can understand that this muscle is working eccentrically to control subtalar joint pronation and in certain instances could be subject to excessive force and overuse. The other posterior leg muscles (i.e., the peroneus longus, soleus, and gastrocnemius) function shortly thereafter in that order.[25,45]

Midstance phase

The midstance period begins at footflat and ends with ipsilateral heel-off and takes approximately 0.24 seconds.[49] During this phase the foot must make its transition from a mobile adapting shock-absorber to a rigid lever for roll-off. Supination begins approximately at the beginning of midstance and continues through the remainder of the stance phase.[45] Supination is accomplished by a combination of calf muscular activity and external rotation of the lower extremity and pelvis. This external rotation is relative to the plane of progression and is not necessarily femur to pelvis. As the subtalar joint supinates, the midtarsal joint axes become progressively more oblique and thus the midfoot becomes rigid for roll-off.[7,54] Fig. 17-8 demonstrates the midtarsal joint axes as influenced by the subtalar joint position.

The leg muscular activity in this stage includes the previously mentioned posterior muscles plus the flexor digitorum longus, peroneus brevis, and flexor hallucis longus in that order. The line of pull of the gastrocnemius/soleus, tibialis posterior, flexor hallucis longus, and flexor digitorum longus act to cause supination. Meanwhile the peroneus longus plantar-flexes the first ray and actually pronates the forefoot while the peroneus brevis tightens the lateral midfoot to make the foot more stable for roll-off.[3,44,48] Often confusion may result from the terms "pronation" and "supination." As discussed in Chapter 14, these terms refer to triplane motion. The subtalar and specifically the oblique axis of the midtarsal joint produce similar movements of plantar flexion/dorsiflexion and abduction/adduction while the dominant movement around the midtarsal longitudinal axis is forefoot eversion/inversion.[45]

Functionally, the subtalar joint should be near neutral position by the latter part of the midstance phase. If the calcaneus is still in an everted position during this period, then the individual may not have a stable foot for roll-off. The timing of this sequence appears to be critical. To review, the foot must first become loose and flexible; this happens in 0.15 seconds. Next it must rapidly become a rigid lever by 0.40 seconds into the stance phase.[45,49]

If the individual's foot for any reason is excessively pr-

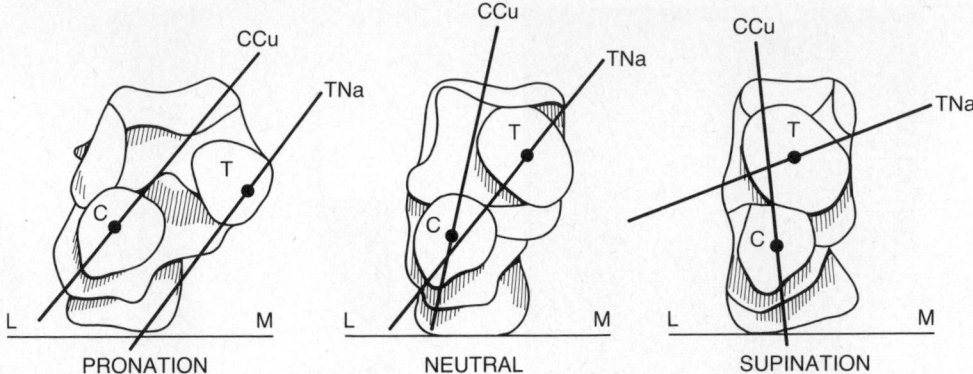

Fig. 17-8. Midtarsal joint axes with subtalar influence—pronation, neutral, supination. *L*, lateral; *M*, medial; *C*, calcaneus; *T*, talus; *CCu*, calcaneal-cuboid line; *TNa*, talonavicular line. (From Elftman H: Clin. Orthop. 16:41, 1960; and Hunt GC: Subtalar joint pronation: influence of balanced insoles, unpublished MA thesis, College Park, 1980, University of Maryland.)

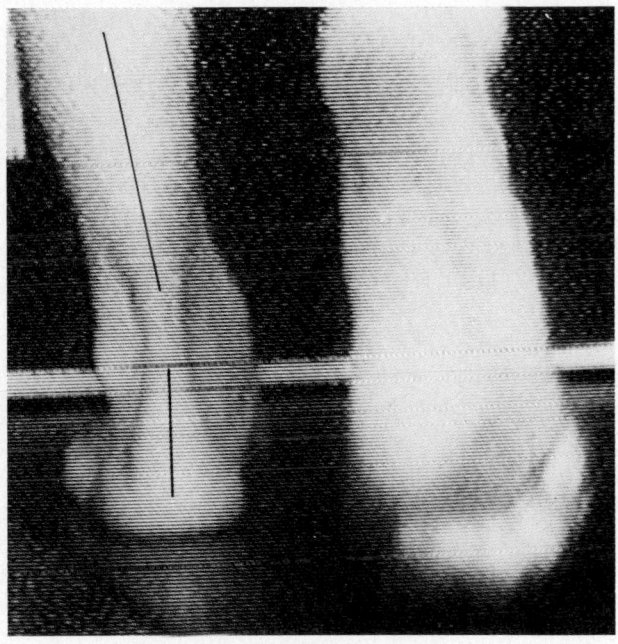

Fig. 17-9. Normal left midstance.

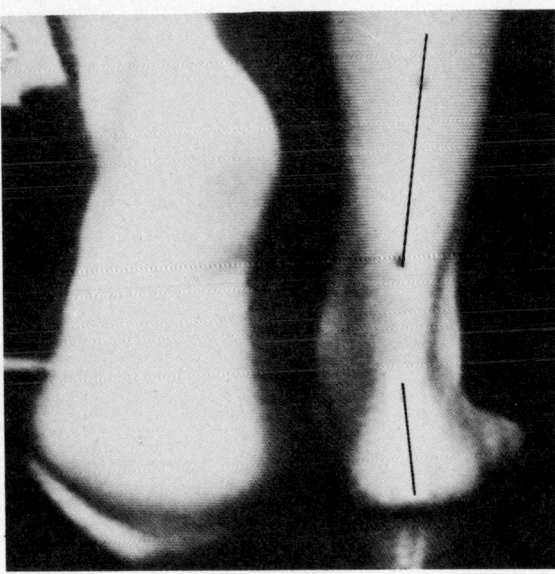

Fig. 17-10. Excessive right pronation at midstance.

onated at midstance, then he/she may have insufficient time to resupinate to make the foot rigid, in spite of adequate muscle strength. Reasons for excessive pronation could result from femoral anteversion, tight medial hamstrings, forefoot or rearfoot varus, or decreased flexibility of the gastrocnemius/soleus muscles and Achilles' tendon. Figs. 17-9 and 17-10 demonstrate the normal and excessively pronated midtarsal and subtalar joints during midstance.

Roll-off phase

The roll-off phase comprises the period from heel rise to toe-off and takes approximately 0.2 seconds.[49] During this period the subtalar joint continues to supinate with the heel progressively inverting and adducting as the foot leaves the ground. Figs 17-11 and 17-12 demonstrate this phase.

For efficient toe-off the toes must be held firmly against the ground, which can be accomplished only when the metatarsals are stable. This stability depends on locking the midtarsal joints before heel-off.[3,17,18,45] As mentioned earlier, the most stable foot is one with the rearfoot supinated and the forefoot pronated. Functioning of the toes in providing stability has been discussed in the literature and is still open to question, but what must be considered is the speed of walking and various foot types.[48]

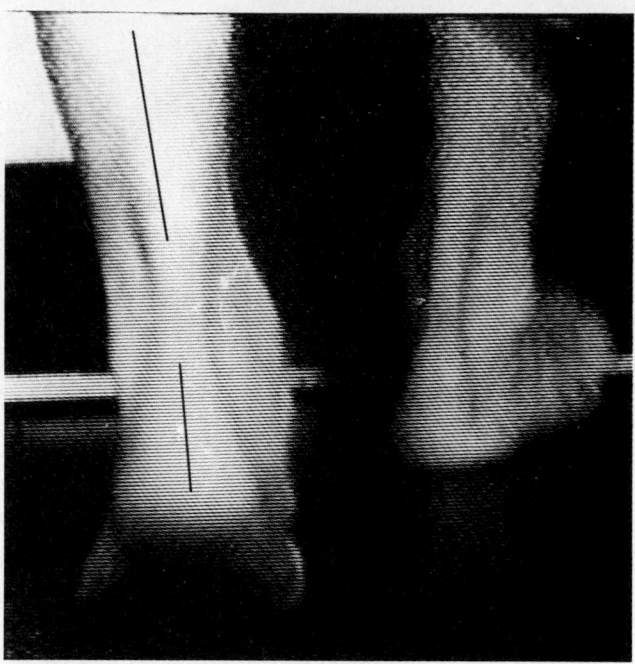

Fig. 17-11. Initial left heel-off.

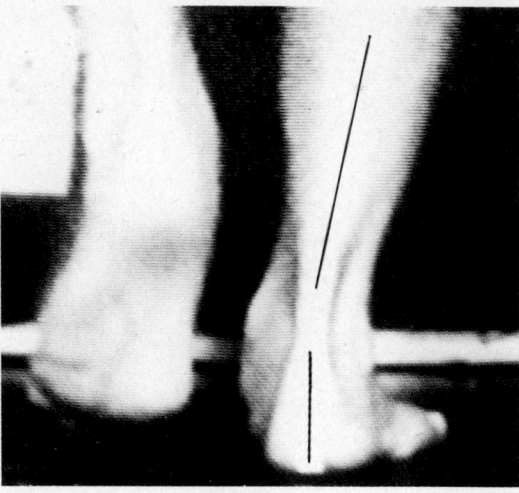

Fig. 17-13. Limited calcaneal eversion with excessive midtarsal joint pronation.

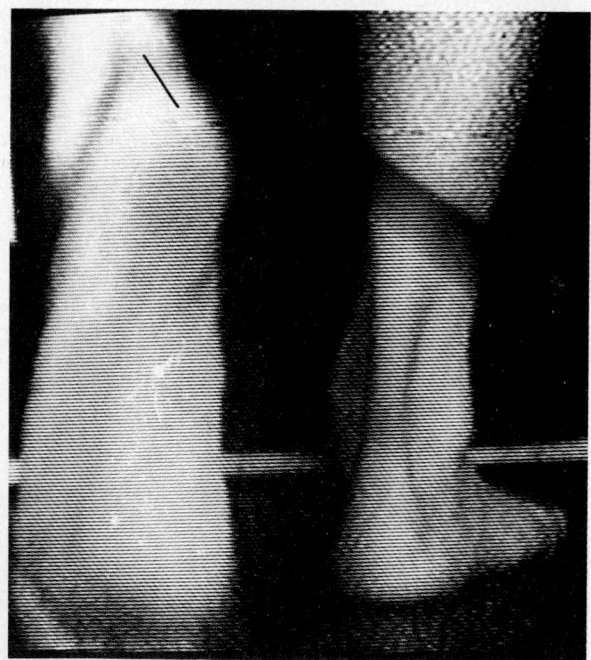

Fig. 17-12. Terminal left heel-off.

Discussion

Pronation during stance appears to be a passive movement. Electromyographic studies of gait have indicated that the only significant muscular activity distal to the knee from heel strike to 25% of stance comes from the anterior tibial muscles.[14,33,51] As mentioned earlier, this function appears to prevent footslap during ambulation. The elec-

tromyographic findings compared with the timed sequence of subtalar joint pronation in stance suggests that the movement is passive. From 25% of stance to toe-off, the electromyographic activity of leg and foot muscles significantly increases, which indicates that supination during gait is an active muscular event.[33] For further information on muscle function and gait, the reader is referred to other sources.*

Electromyographic gait studies have revealed that leg and foot intrinsic musculature generally are active for a greater part of the gait cycle in the pronated foot.[14,51] Mann and Inman[33] found that in the normal foot, stabilization of the midfoot begins at approximately 35% of the gait cycle, whereas in the pronated foot stabilization begins at 0% to 26% of the cycle. Their results suggest that the pronated foot requires greater intrinsic muscular activity in an attempt to stabilize the midtarsal and subtalar joints.

So far, descriptions of gait analysis have included rearfoot functional assessment, which is observed best from the posterior aspect. In certain instances, signs of excessive pronation may not be clear by viewing the calcaneus alone. For example, if an individual has limited subtalar pronation, the calcaneus will not demonstrate an everted position relative to the floor even when the subtalar joint is fully pronated. In this case, signs of excessive pronation may result from movement around the oblique axis of the midtarsal joint and will be identified as a medial bulge or prominence of the midfoot during midstance. Midfoot pronation or collapse may be observed in this situation and is demonstrated in Fig. 17- 13.

Another anatomical landmark to follow is the patella. Normally the patella should deviate internally only slightly

*See references 2, 5, 16, 31, and 45.

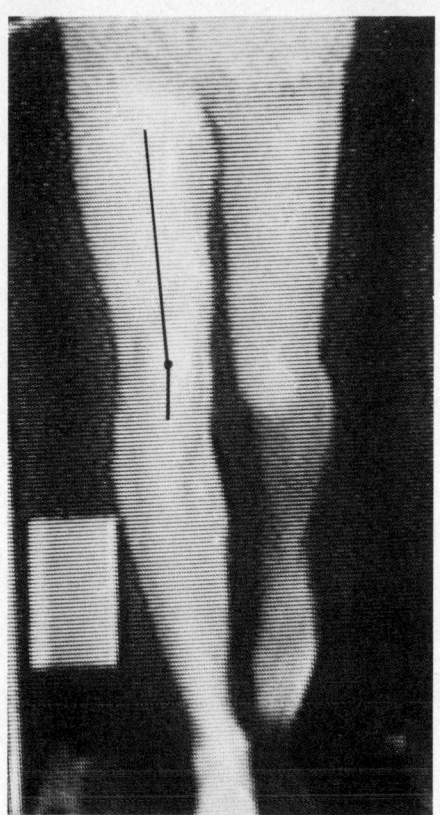

Fig. 17-14. Right lower extremity during midstance—normal.

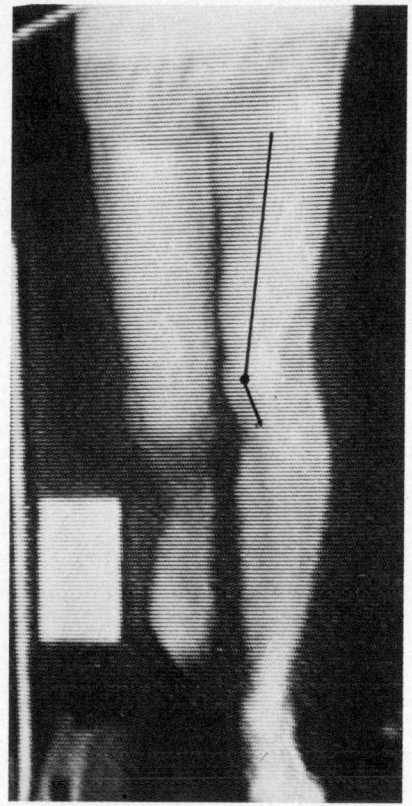

Fig. 17-15. Left lower extremity during midstance—abnormal internal rotation.

from heel contact to midstance (Fig. 17-14). With excessive internal lower-extremity rotation, the patella will rotate more medially and produce the "squinting" appearance illustrated in Fig. 17-15. The opposite may result if the lower extremity does not internally rotate.

Movements in the sagittal plane should also be viewed to detect the amount of hip flexion/extension, knee flexion/extension, ankle plantar flexion and dorsiflexion, and stride length. For further explanation of proximal movement patterns in gait, the reader is referred to other sources.*

Asymmetry should be looked for in all views. Excessive pronation on one side may be identified by increased calcaneal eversion, medial midfoot bulging with abduction of the forefoot, or increased internal hip rotation.

Summary

For the foot, the critical periods to identify during gait include the following:

1. Contact (heel or rearfoot strike to footflat)
2. Midstance
3. Roll-off (heel rise to toe-off)

Fig. 17-16 illustrates a comparison of critical events oc-

*See references 25, 37, 39, 42, and 47.

curring in stance for normal and excessive pronation. One should compare the events of heel/foot contact (HC), midstance (MS), and heel rise (HR). (It should be emphasized that the position of the calcaneus as observed from the posterior view is made relative to the floor.)

• • •

To avoid confusion, one anatomical area should be observed and evaluated at a time. The tendency to look at all moving parts simultaneously tends to produce frustration. Videotape or film analysis with slow motion, if available, is an excellent tool to sharpen gait evaluation skills. Videotape is also invaluable in client education as well as staff education. Fig. 17-17 demonstrates a dynamic analysis evaluation protocol that may assist the clinician.

The use of a treadmill to evaluate gait has been discussed in the literature.[4] According to Brandel and Williams,[4] differences between treadmill and over-ground parameters (velocity, stride length, and cadence) were found to be statistically insignificant, particularly between 2.5 and 3.2 miles per hour. As a result, they concluded that the treadmill was a valid tool in the evaluation of most limb motion data. However, it should be noted that individuals with slow gaits or significant gait disturbances have great difficulty on the treadmill and in those cases

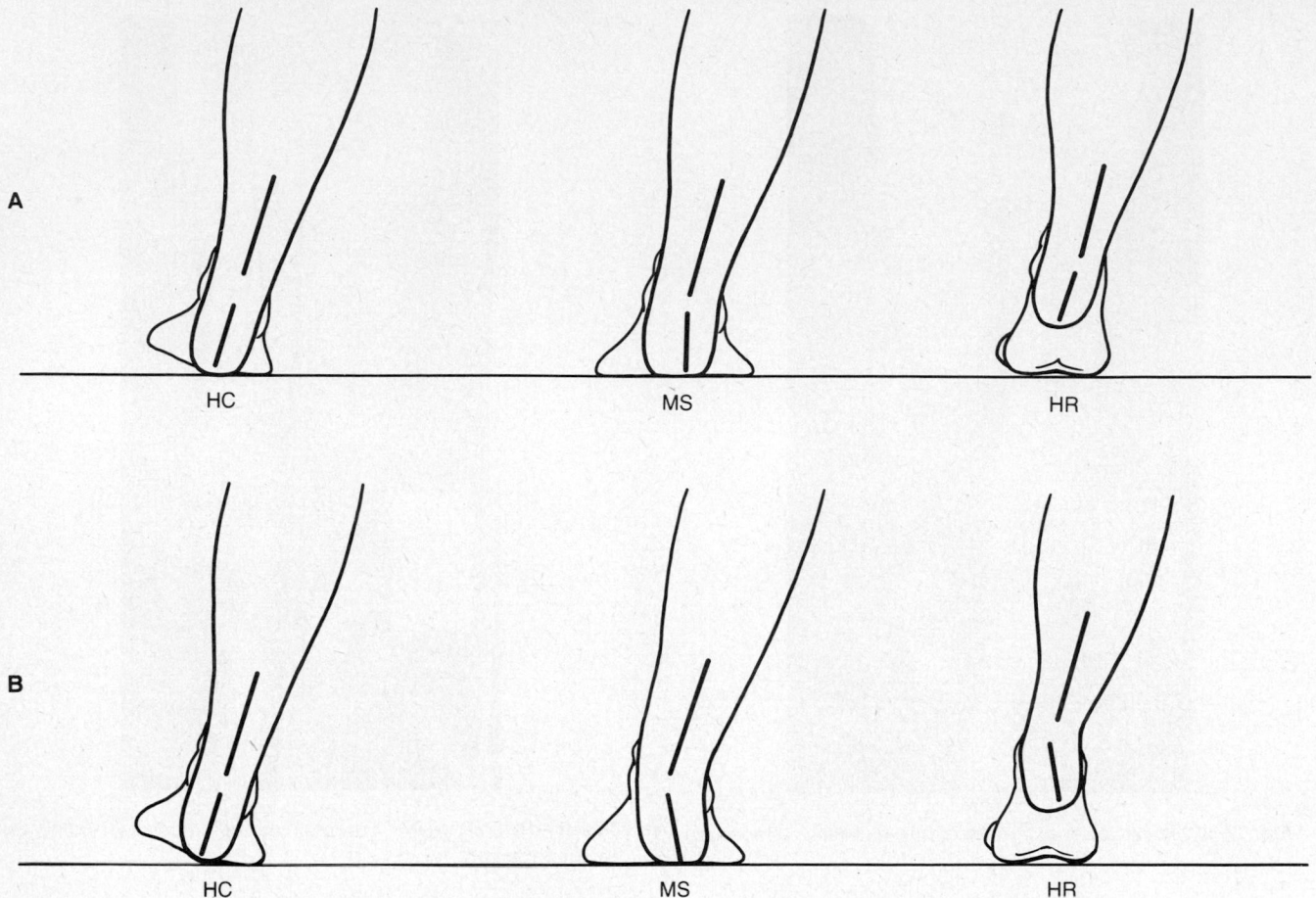

Fig. 17-16. A, Normal gait, and **B,** excessive, pronated gaits. Shown is foot in heel contact *(HC)*, midstance *(MS),* and heel rise *(HR).*

over-ground assessment is essential. If the subject is able to walk on the treadmill safely, adequate time should be allowed for practice in order to attain a natural gait rhythm for analysis. The practical advantage of a treadmill is the control of speed and lighting for video or film analysis. Fig. 17-18 depicts a gait analysis system that allows simultaneous observation of all three gait views: anterior, posterior, and side.

STATIC CLINICAL EXAMINATION

In order to more fully understand the functional occurrences during gait, one must be able to identify static relationships in the lower extremities. Fig. 17-19 displays an example of a clinical evaluation form, based on the SOAP format. The following discussion of the form includes a description of the testing procedures cited with examples to clarify its use. Only the static part of the evaluation is discussed.

Pulses

Palpation of the dorsalis pedis and posterior tibial pulses should be noted with some designation meaningful

to the evaluator. Various qualitative descriptions that are adequate have been described, such as the multiple (+) system with 1 + indicating the weakest to 4 (+) the strongest. Weakened or absent pulses may lead one to suspect vascular insufficiency if there are complaints of arch pain or cramping of the intrinsic foot muscles. Asymmetry of pulse strength is the important factor to consider, since wide variation can exist.

Range of motion or position

Ankle joint. The measurement of ankle joint dorsiflexion can be misleading if care is not taken to avoid subtalar joint pronation. One must remember that dorsiflexion is one component of pronation occurring at both the subtalar and oblique axis of the midtarsal joints. Thus a composite measurement would result if pronation were not controlled while dorsiflexion is measured.

Limited ankle joint dorsiflexion is a common cause of excessive pronation during midstance. If observed during this period of gait, the calcaneus would remain in an everted or valgus posture when it should be nearly perpendicular to the floor. Most authorities note that an angle of

DYNAMIC GAIT EVALUATION

Date_____   #_____
Name_____ Age_____ Sex_____ Weight_____
Walking_____ Jogging_____ Running_____ Barefoot_____ Shoes_____ Orthotics_____
==

POSTERIOR OBSERVATION: Symmetrical_____ Asymmetrical_____

	L	R
Head tilt (frontal plane)	___	___
Shoulder level (frontal plane)	___	___
Pelvic level (frontal plane)	___	___
Base of gait	_____	

	Initial contact		Midstance		Roll-off		Swing	
	Left	Right	Left	Right	Left	Right	Left	Right
Rearfoot								
Midfoot								
Forefoot								

==

ANTERIOR OBSERVATION: Symmetrical_____ Asymmetrical_____

	Initial contact		Midstance		Roll-off		Swing	
	Left	Right	Left	Right	Left	Right	Left	Right
Knee motion Transverse								
Frontal								
Midfoot								
Forefoot								

==

SIDE OBSERVATION: Symmetrical_____ Asymmetrical_____

	Initial contact		Midstance		Roll-off		Swing	
Arm swing	Left	Right	Left	Right	Left	Right	Left	Right
Pelvic tilt (sagittal)								
Hip Flexion								
Extension								
Knee Flexion								
Extension								
Ankle Flexion								
Extension								

==

Key:
- ↑ = high
- ↓ = low
- R = right
- L = left
- I = inverted
- E = everted
- ⊥ = perpendicular
- P = pronated
- S = supinated
- Ab = abducted
- Ad = adducted
- MHW = medial heel whip
- IR = internal rotation
- ER = external rotation
- > = excessive
- < = insufficient
- At = anterior
- Pt = posterior
- N = normal

SUMMARY

Fig. 17-17. Dynamic gait evaluation protocol.

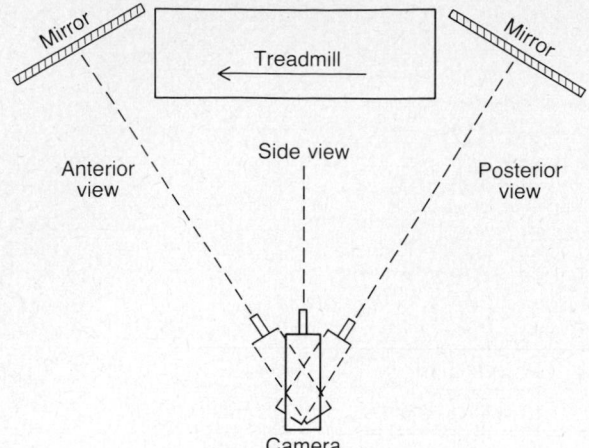

Fig. 17-18. Video gait analysis system.

10 degrees of dorsiflexion is necessary for a normal walking gait. However, multiple variables exist, such as limb length, stride length, and speed of gait, that might be expected to require different degrees of motion.[52] The individual who takes a longer stride or who increases the speed of walking needs greater dorsiflexion. For instance, Scranton and others[48] in a study comparing walking, jogging, and running found that during jogging 35 degrees of dorsiflexion was recorded during late midstance. Consequently, it seems reasonable that individuals have different needs for their particular morphology and varied gait circumstances. The amount of motion largely depends on a number of factors previously mentioned. The amount of functional plantar flexion has been recorded to be 25 to 30 degrees and again depends on individual need.

Subtalar joint. Pronation and supination cannot be measured because they are triplane movements; therefore calcaneal eversion and inversion are measured to reflect subtalar joint motion. The frontal plane movement of the calcaneus occurs as influenced only by the subtalar joint and thus is reasonable to measure. The technique is described in Chapter 15. The necessary amount of subtalar motion depends on other key anatomical relationships, which will be discussed.

Tibial frontal plane position. Tibia vara as it relates to calcaneal eversion is a significant measurement. The degree of tibia vara is measured using the distal third of the leg and is the same reference line when calcaneal eversion or inversion is measured. The angle of the tibia is measured relative to the supporting surface. This measurement is made while the individual stands with his/her weight shifted over the leg being measured in order to approach the functional lower-leg position. This is important because the vara attitude of the tibia increases as one walks and is reflected in a narrower base of gait as compared with static standing. Figs. 17-20 and 17-21 demonstrate these two measurement techniques.

Functionally, calcaneal eversion should at least equal the tibia vara measurement. If calcaneal eversion does not equal tibia vara, the individual may have difficulty with more strenuous ambulation. If tibia vara is excessive in this situation, then lateral ankle and foot instability may occur. Excessive pronation with rearfoot varus occurs during the heel contact phase of stance and often is difficult to distinguish from a normal pattern. An important principle to remember is that an individual's foot in this situation will be completely pronated at the subtalar joint and yet not have heel valgus. Therefore one must correlate the static examination with the gait evaluation to determine the degree to which the individual is compensating.

Great toe extension. For the force on the great toe to be well distributed at heel-off, sufficient extension at the first metatarsophalangeal joint must occur. If sufficient motion is unavailable, increased stress will be placed on the distal aspect of the great toe. In an individual with insensitivity, such as a person with diabetes mellitus, the end result may be ulceration under the distal aspect of the great toe, whereas in a person with normal sensation, it may mean pain either in the distal great toe or first metatarsophalangeal joint. The limitation of motion may also affect other physiological joint movements in the foot.

The measurement can be made while the individual is standing. The great toe is extended actively and assisted passively without dorsiflexing the first ray. Minimal values are difficult to state because of different functional requirements, but an angle of 45 degrees has been found to be adequate for walking velocities.[32] Fig. 17-22 demonstrates this measurement technique.

Forefoot and rearfoot relationships. The ability to identify static relationships of the forefoot and rearfoot depends on the ability to determine the neutral position of the subtalar joint. This position is determined by palpating the medial and lateral margins of the talar head for congruency while simultaneously applying an abduction and dorsiflexion force on the fourth and fifth metatarsal heads. In this position, the subtalar joint is in neutral with the midfoot locked on the rearfoot. The forefoot plane can then be identified as it relates to the calcaneal bisection. Ideally it should be perpendicular, but variations either in a varus or valgus position may be present and are discussed more specifically elsewhere in this text.

Forefoot varus is a significant deviation because it can cause excessive pronation during midstance. This excessive midstance pronation during gait cannot be distinguished from midstance pronation caused by limited ankle joint dorsiflexion. Therefore the importance of the static examination is paramount, since the treatment approach will be quite different. With forefoot varus, the treatment may include an orthotic device to support the forefoot deviation, whereas the approach for limited dorsiflexion would be directed toward increasing functional dorsiflexion through stretching or heel lifts. Orthotic devices to

LOWER EXTREMITY EVALUATION

Date _____   # _____

Name _____ Age _____ Sex _____ Weight _____

SUBJECTIVE EXAMINATION:

GAIT ASSESSMENT (SIGNIFICANT ABNORMALITIES):

STATIC EXAMINATION:

1. Pulses   R   L

    Dorsalis pedis   ____   ____
    Posterior tibial   ____   ____

2. Range of motion/position   R   L   R   L

    Dorsiflexion: knees extended   ____   ____   Tibial torsion   ____   ____
                   knees flexed   ____   ____   Hip: internal rotation   ____   ____
    Plantar flexion   ____   ____   external rotation   ____   ____
    Calcaneal inversion   ____   ____   Hamstring length   ____   ____
    Calcaneal eversion   ____   ____   Hip flexor length   ____   ____
    Tibia vara   ____   ____   Rectus femoris length   ____   ____
    Great toe extension   ____   ____   Hip abductor length   ____   ____
    Forefoot position   ____   ____   Limb length   ____   ____
    Rearfoot position   ____   ____

3. Skin stress patterns

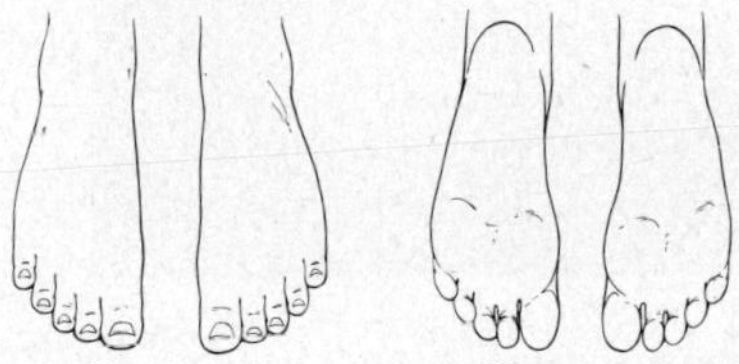

            R   L   L   R

4. Footwear

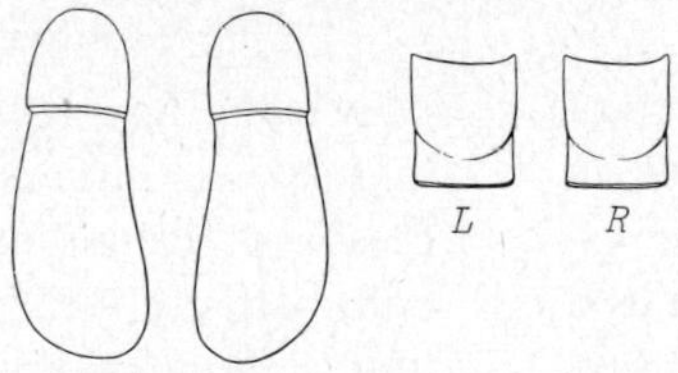

            L   R   L   R

5. Strength assessment (significant deficits)

ASSESSMENT:

PLAN:

Fig. 17- 19. Lower extremity evaluation form based on SOAP format.

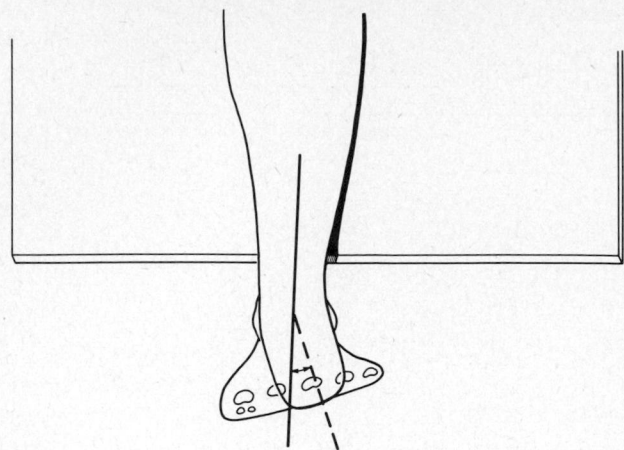

Fig. 17-20. Calcaneal eversion measurement made from prone position.

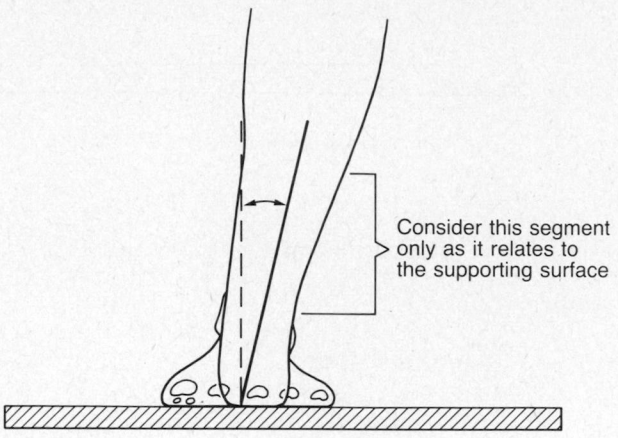

Consider this segment only as it relates to the supporting surface

Fig. 17-21. Tibia vara measurement made from standing position.

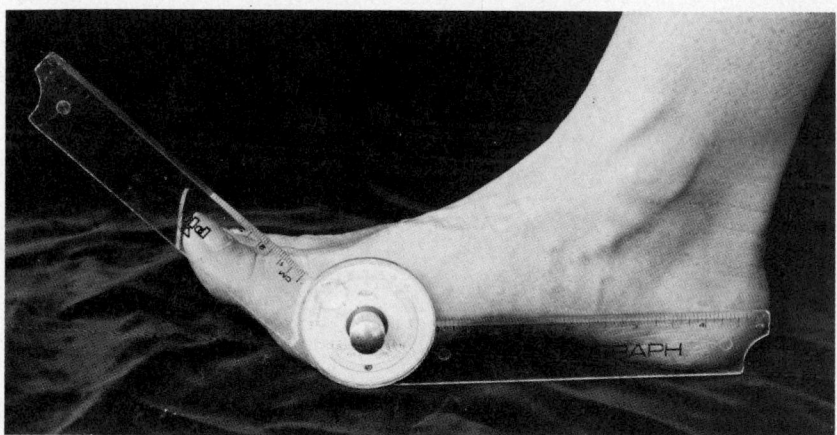

Fig. 17-22. Dorsiflexion of first metatarsophalangeal joint.

control pronation as a result of causes other than forefoot or rearfoot deviations have not been as effective and in some cases have increased the individual's symptoms.

Rearfoot position is a relationship between the distal third of the leg and the calcaneal bisection. This position should reflect a calcaneal bisection that is parallel or continuous with the distal third of the leg bisector. A slight varus position of the heel is commonly observed and may not have any malfunctional significance if the tibia vara measurement is small.

Transverse anatomical relationships and rotation have not received the same attention as those in the sagittal or frontal plane.[36] Deviations in either direction may have a significant influence on the timing sequence in gait. For example, with increased internal rotation of the lower extremity, the individual may pronate excessively, resulting in an abduction component of subtalar joint, thus straightening the foot. This compensation could result from any number of factors causing toed-in gait, such as internal tib-

ial torsion, femoral anteversion, or tight medial hamstring muscles. As discussed previously, various reasons for excessive pronation may exist, and observing this during gait only partially identifies the problem. The static examination in conjunction with dynamic analysis allows the clinician to identify the source of the problem more clearly.

Tibial torsion. Average tibial or malleolar torsion has been measured to be approximately 15 degrees external.[45] This assessment can be made with the individual sitting over the edge of a plinth. A qualitative evaluation of tibial torsion—or more appropriately, malleolar torsion—is made while the knee axis is in the frontal plane. The relationship of lateral malleolus to medial malleolus is observed with the examiner placing one thumb just anterior to the lateral malleolus and the other thumb on the apex of the medial malleolus. By visually connecting a line between the thumbs, one can assess whether the malleolar torsion is internally or externally rotated. This procedure is not quantitative but does allow the examiner to gain a feeling for this transverse relationship. Fig. 17-23 illustrates excessive internal tibial torsion.

Hip transverse rotation. Internal and external rotation is measured with the hip extended and may be compared with motion as measured with hips flexed. Forty-five degrees of internal and external rotation is considered within normal limits. If the range of motion is the same for both the flexed and extended positions, then soft-tissue limitation is usually not a consideration. As described earlier, increased internal rotation of the femur may cause excessive pronation around the subtalar joint. An increased internal femoral rotation may be caused by tightness of soft tissues around the joint or femoral anteversion. One might anticipate that limitation caused by soft-tissue tightness could be stretched out while a femoral anteversion would not change with exercise. Fig. 17-24 demonstrates hip rotation measured with the hip extended. Measurement with the hip flexed is made while the individual is sitting down.

Hamstring muscle flexibility is determined by placing the individual supine on a plinth with the hips extended and the knees flexed to 90 degrees. One hip is then flexed to 90 degrees, and the knee is extended. A measurement of knee extension can be determined by the number of degrees to vertical (see Figs. 17-23 and 17-24). To test the tightness of the medial hamstring muscle, the hip is externally rotated completely and the knee is then extended as before. If the knee extends less than when the hip was in the original test position, the medial hamstring group is tight. The same procedure can be performed for the lateral hamstring muscle except that this time the hip should be internally rotated. Figs. 17-25 and 17-26 demonstrate the procedure for testing hamstring muscle flexibility.

A tight medial hamstring muscle can cause excessive internal thigh rotation with a toeing-in gait that results in excessive subtalar joint pronation. The reason for a toeing-in gait, therefore, must be evaluated to decide whether it is a result of internal tibial torsion, femoral anteversion, femoral rotation, or tight medial hamstring muscles.

Hip flexor tightness is checked using the Thomas test position. In addition to causing sagittal plane limitations, tight hip flexors influence transverse rotation. Since the hip flexors externally rotate the thigh, tightness will limit internal rotation of the femur, possibly causing an increased compensatory transverse rotation of the pelvis. This limitation may be noted when hip transverse rotation is measured. If tight hip flexors exist, greater internal hip rotation will be possible with the femur flexed to 90 degrees. In gait an individual with a tight right hip flexor might demonstrate a right medial heel whip during late midstance on the right. This individual could possibly also have an increased lumbar lordotic curve and a left pelvic lead in swing.

Rectus femoris tightness can be assessed with the indi-

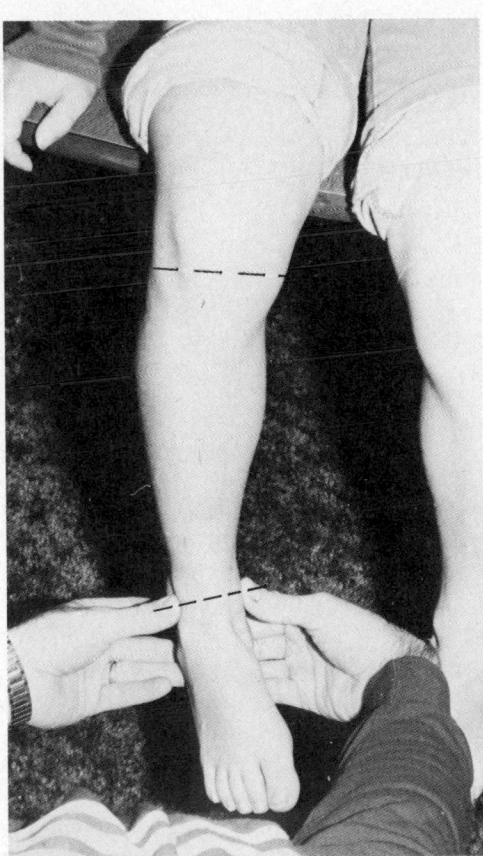

Fig. 17-23. Clinical assessment of tibial torsion demonstrating excessive internal torsion.

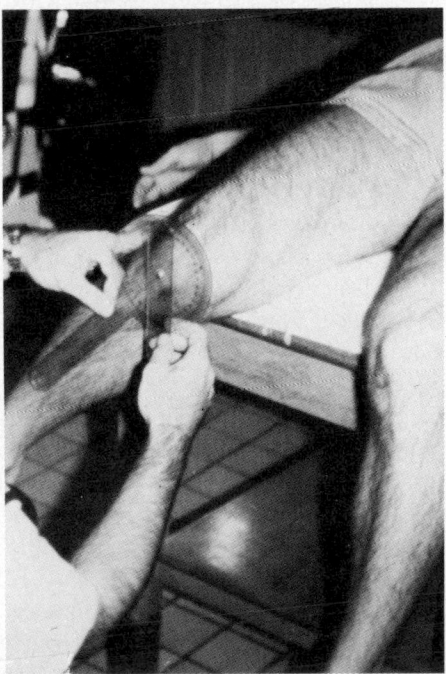

Fig. 17-24. Hip rotation measurement.

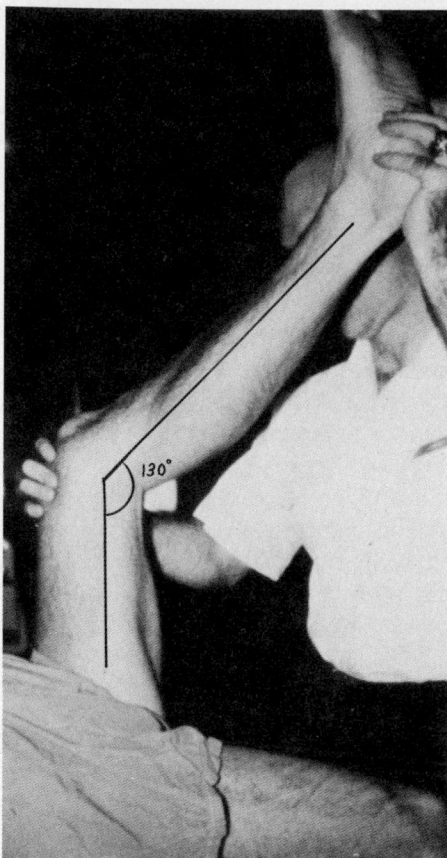

Fig. 17-25. Limited hamstring flexibility with hip externally rotated at 130 degrees of knee extension.

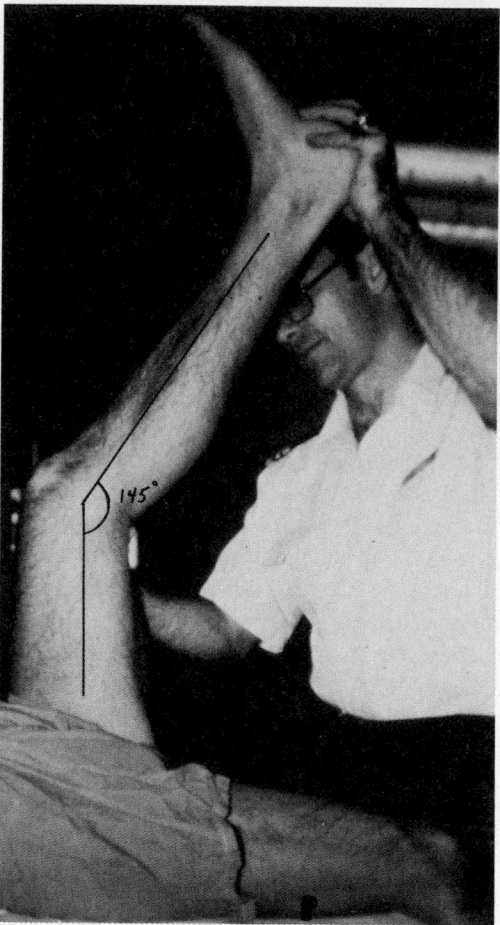

Fig. 17-26. Hamstring flexibility with hip in neutral rotation at 145 degrees of knee extension, indicating medial hamstring tightness.

vidual in the supine Thomas test position with the knees flexed to the chest at the edge of a plinth. While one hip is held flexed to about 120 degrees and the opposite leg is lowered to the table, the lowered thigh should comfortably rest on the plinth with the knee at approximately 80- degrees flexion.[29]

Hip abduction. The Ober test can be used to test this muscle group. In assessing the length of the hip abduction and the tensor fascia latae, the clinician must pay close attention to hip stabilization, otherwise erroneous judgements can be made. Further explanation can be found in Kendall and McCreary[29] and Williams and Worthingham.[56]

Limb length. With the individual lying supine while a gentle traction force is applied on the legs at the ankles, one can check leg length. The inferior margin of the medial malleoli can be identified by the examining thumbs. By having the individual come to a long-sitting position, influence of pelvic rotation can be identified. Pelvic rotation and its influence on leg length should be carefully evaluated to rule out a true anatomical leg-length discrepancy versus an abnormal rotation within the pelvic region (see Chapter 22). While the individual is weight bearing, the relationship of the anterior superior iliac spine (ASIS)

to the ipsilateral posterior superior iliac spine (PSIS) can help identify leg-length inequality as a result of pelvic imbalance. For example, if the ASIS and PSIS are lower on the same side when the individual is evaluated in the standing position, an anatomical shortening may be suspected. If, however, the ASIS is higher and the PSIS is lower on the same side, then a posteriorly rotated ilium may be suspected. The opposite relationship would suggest an anteriorly rotated ilium. With the latter situation, the anterior rotation would lengthen the lower extremity, thus causing the inequality. Thorough evaluation to determine the cause of leg-length inequality is important because inappropriate treatment should be avoided.[9,12] For a true anatomically short leg, a shoe lift would be the treatment of choice, whereas with a pelvic rotational imbalance, stretching the soft tissues and mobilization may be the treatment of choice. Figs. 17-27 and 17-28 demonstrate the assessment of limb length and pelvic rotation.

Q angle. This angular measurement represents the pull of the quadriceps muscle on the patella and its influence on patella tracking. Consideration of this measurement should

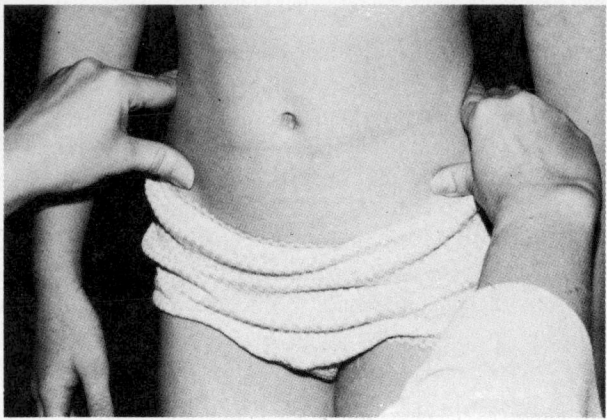

Fig. 17-27. ASIS measurement.

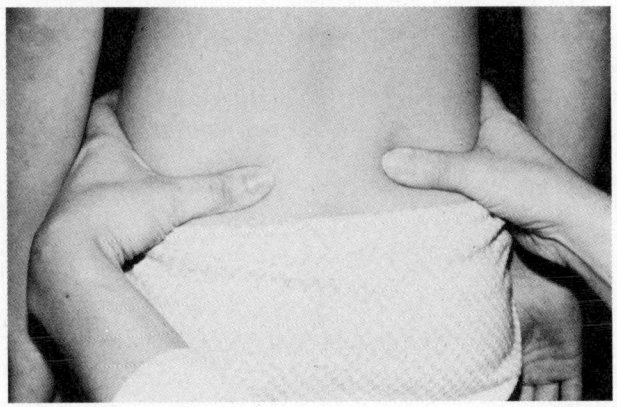

Fig. 17-28. PSIS measurement.

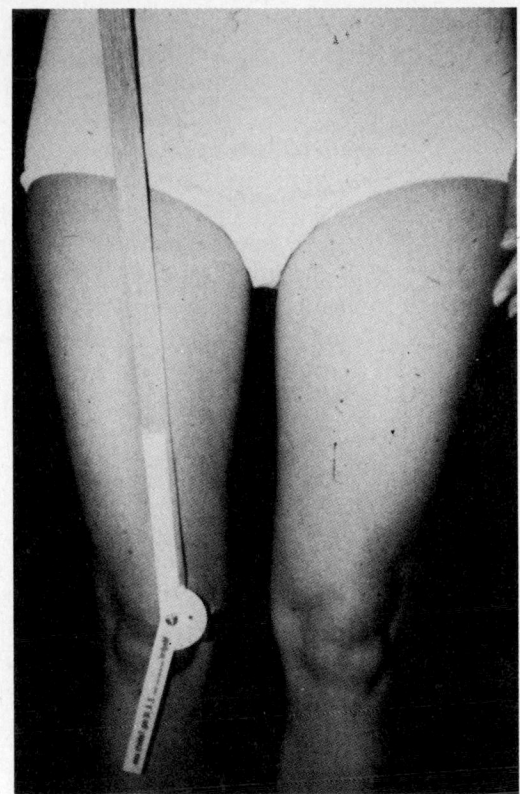

Fig. 17-29. Q angle measurement.

include taking it while the individual stands in his/her angle and base of gait to ensure functional significance. Fig. 17-29 demonstrates a modified goniometer.

Callous pattern. Friction and shearing forces produce hypertrophy of tissues. Characteristic callous patterns can be found to correlate with general foot types. In a flexible foot that excessively pronates, calluses will generally be found under the second and third metatarsal heads and medial great toe. The callous pattern under the second and third and sometimes fourth metatarsal heads is usually elongated and results from the lengthening of the foot with excessive pronation while the medial great toe callus results from pinching against the shoe. In a more rigid foot that has insufficient calcaneal eversion, the callus results from pinching against the shoe. In a more rigid foot that has insufficient calcaneal eversion, the callus will usually be found over the first and fifth metatarsal heads with minimal, if any, callus under the central heads. Callus on the medial great toe has also been found in this rigid foot type if there is medial push-off.

Footwear. It is helpful to correlate an assessment of external and internal footwear patterns to static and dynamic information. Shoe construction is an important consideration. In certain instances, a shoe that is worn excessively or has insufficient stability can aggravate a biomechanical imbalance.

Summary

The importance of systematically evaluating static postural relationships and correlating that information with dynamic gait analysis is important in understanding an individual's problem. Since various gait deviations may be caused by different circumstances, it is important for the clinician to have all available information that will help rule out possibilities in setting up an appropriate management program.

MECHANISMS INFLUENCING GAIT DEVIATION

Pain in the lower extremity resulting from weight bearing and ambulation may occur from any one or a combination of three factors: (1) improper footwear, (2) biomechanical imbalances, or (3) increased activity level.

A common cause of foot and leg pain is an improperly fitted shoe. If an individual starts a jogging program while wearing basketball or tennis sneakers, he/she may very well develop calf problems as a result of overstretching the posterior soft tissues. The running shoe, having an elevated heel, is designed to relieve posterior calf strain. Another individual may wear a thin, hard-soled shoe in a job that requires long periods of standing and walking and may have metatarsal head pain. Relief for this person can be obtained by changing to a softer, thicker-soled shoe that would protect the forefoot. Therefore, in some cases, simply changing the shoe may solve the problem.

However, at times individuals may develop problems even if they are wearing appropriate shoes. Biomechanical imbalances throughout the lower extremity may cause excessive stress in a number of structures. For example, forefoot varus can cause the foot to excessively pronate during midstance when supination should occur. This chronic situation might produce a variety of symptoms ranging from posterolateral calf discomfort, forefoot pain, and mediodistal tibial pain to knee pain. Treatment considerations with this particular deviation should include an attempt to allow the foot to function close to its neutral position. The treatment could involve the application of an orthotic device to accommodate the forefoot position and an exercise program to strengthen any muscular imbalance. In the case of any biomechanical imbalance, the treatment approach must attempt to rebalance the lower extremity.

In spite of proper shoes and appropriately treated biomechanical imbalances, individuals may still develop problems that most likely relate to their activity level. For example, a runner in training may decide to increase his/her weekly mileage from 30 to 50 miles in 1 week. In most cases, the body will be unable to adjust to this increase and an overuse syndrome may develop. In another example an individual might change to a job that necessitates more standing and ambulation. The result again may be an overuse syndrome.

In arriving at a reasonable management program, all three of the factors just discussed must be considered. Two people may have the same biomechanical imbalance with inappropriate footwear, but only one may be symptomatic. The difference is probably caused by an increased activity level and, as a result, only the symptomatic person may be treated. Therefore one must closely evaluate the treatment approach because functional needs may vary for two individuals of similar morphological structure.

Norms for measuring gait deviation

Traditionally clinicians have tried to establish norms for motion requirements of each joint. Values have been identified but it is debatable whether these values are functionally meaningful. For example, the importance of tibia vara is evident if one must measure the amount of calcaneal eversion. By definition, tibia vara is the angle of the supporting surface and the bisection of the distal third of the leg while the individual stands with his/her weight shifted on the leg being measured. The amount of calcaneal eversion as measured prone is determined by the angle produced by the bisection of the distal third of the leg and the

calcaneus after the rearfoot has been maximally pronated. For example, if an individual has 5 degrees of tibia vara and 10 degrees of calcaneal eversion, the calcaneus can be expected to be perpendicular to the supporting surface while the person is standing and still have 5 degrees of eversion remaining (Fig. 17-30). However, in another individual with the same tibia vara position of 5 degrees but with only 5 degrees of calcaneal eversion (Fig. 17-31), the calcaneus may also be perpendicular to the supporting surface, but the person would have no additional eversion available. In this second situation, even though the calcaneus is perpendicular to the floor, the subtalar joint is maximally pronated. This concept differs from the more traditional explanation of pronation with heel valgus. The important point to remember, however, is that an individual does not have to have a valgus heel to indicate pronation.

The degree of forefoot varus will also influence the frontal plane position of the calcaneus. For instance, when an individual with 5 degrees of forefoot varus (Fig. 17-32) stands, the calcaneus will be fully pronated and will measure 5 degrees valgus. The explanation for this is that the

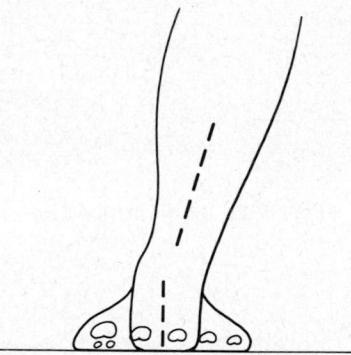

Fig. 17-30. Calcaneal eversion 10 degrees, tibia vara 5 degrees, and balanced forefoot with 5 degrees of calcaneal eversion remaining.

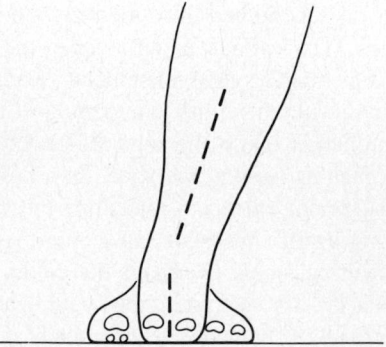

Fig. 17-31. Calcaneal eversion 5 degrees, tibia vara 5 degrees, and balanced forefoot with 0 degrees of calcaneal eversion remaining.

subtalar joint compensates for the tibia vara and forefoot varus by pronating until the medial forefoot rests completely on the floor, which then places the calcaneus in 5 degrees of valgus. However, if another individual with the same static relationship but who has only 5 degrees of calcaneal eversion stands, the calcaneus will be perpendicular to the floor with the medial side of the forefoot elevated off the floor. This individual is unable to compensate completely at the subtalar and midtarsal joints and thus may plantar flex the first ray or adduct the knee in order to obtain medial/lateral stability (Fig. 17-33, *A* and *B*). Therefore, in order to fully appreciate the biomechanical function of the foot, one must be able to relate lower-extremity posture to joint motion.

Mechanical devices for control of gait deviation

Numerous mechanical devices have been used for the conservative management of the foot with excessive subtalar joint pronation. Most are constructed of metal, leather, or plastic and include a variety of modifications to fit individual needs.[33,46,58]

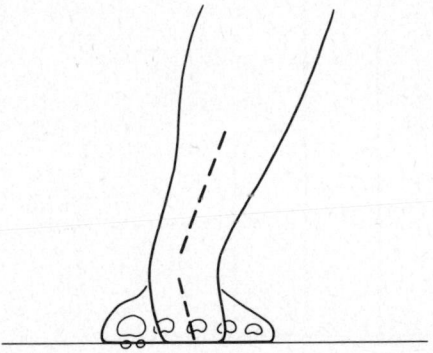

Fig. 17-32. Calcaneal eversion 10 degrees, tibia vara 5 degrees, and forefoot varus 5 degrees with 0 degrees of calcaneal eversion remaining with the calcaneus in 5 degrees valgus.

Earlier concepts of producing a medial longitudinal arch by direct pressure have been tempered by more realistic techniques that include heel control. Attempts to restore the medial longitudinal arch in a low-profile foot are fundamentally unachievable.[41] Numerous investigators have discussed the importance of heel control in managing the pronated subtalar joint.* Internal control has been considered more effective than external shoe modifications.[46]

Current philosophy on the management of a pronated subtalar joint caused by forefoot varus deformity recommends balancing the forefoot to the rearfoot. This is accomplished by a device that supports or accommodates the forefoot varus posture such that the subtalar joint can function closer to the neutral position in midstance, thus negating unnecessary compensation.[22]

Fig. 17-34, *A* demonstrates the valgus position of the calcaneus as a result of forefoot varus. In Fig. 17-34, *B* the forefoot has been balanced with a medial wedge or post and thus the calcaneus is perpendicular to the supporting surface.

Subtalar joint pronation: influence of orthotic devices. Although few studies have investigated the use of foot orthotic devices, this author has evaluated the effect of balancing the forefoot to the rearfoot, using electromyography.[23]

Thirty feet demonstrating subtalar joint pronation resulting from forefoot varus of at least 4 degrees were studied. Quantitative electromyography[8,10] was used to evaluate the effectiveness of a balanced orthotic device on leg muscular activity in static stance. The peroneus longus, tibialis anterior, and lateral soleus muscles were monitored using surface electromyography.

The results indicated that the balanced orthotic device significantly decreased the amount of muscular activity in

*See references 6, 35, 43, and 46.

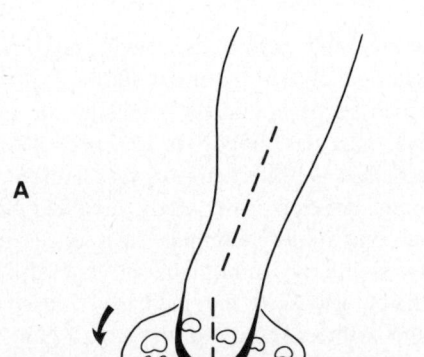
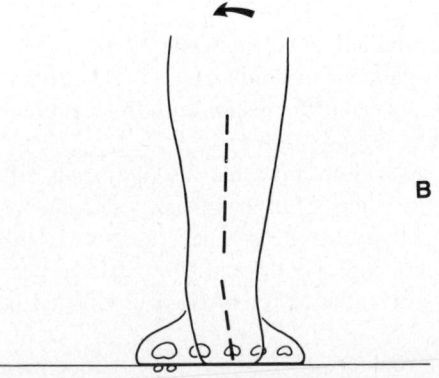

Fig. 17-33. A, Calcaneal eversion 5 degrees, tibia vara 5 degrees, and forefoot vara 5 degrees with −5 degrees of calcaneal eversion for compensation. In **A** compensation is achieved by plantar-flexed first ray and in **B** by adducting tibia. The latter is usually associated with internal femoral rotation.

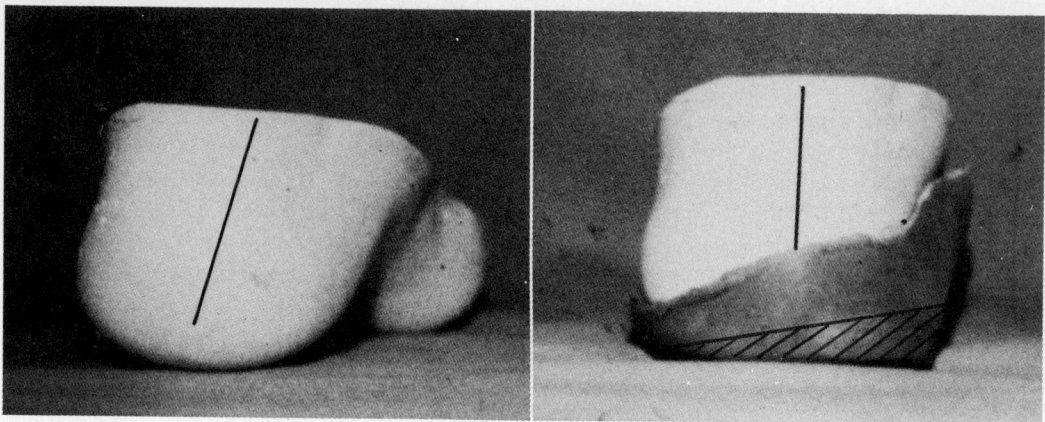

Fig. 17-34. Effect of balancing forefoot varus.

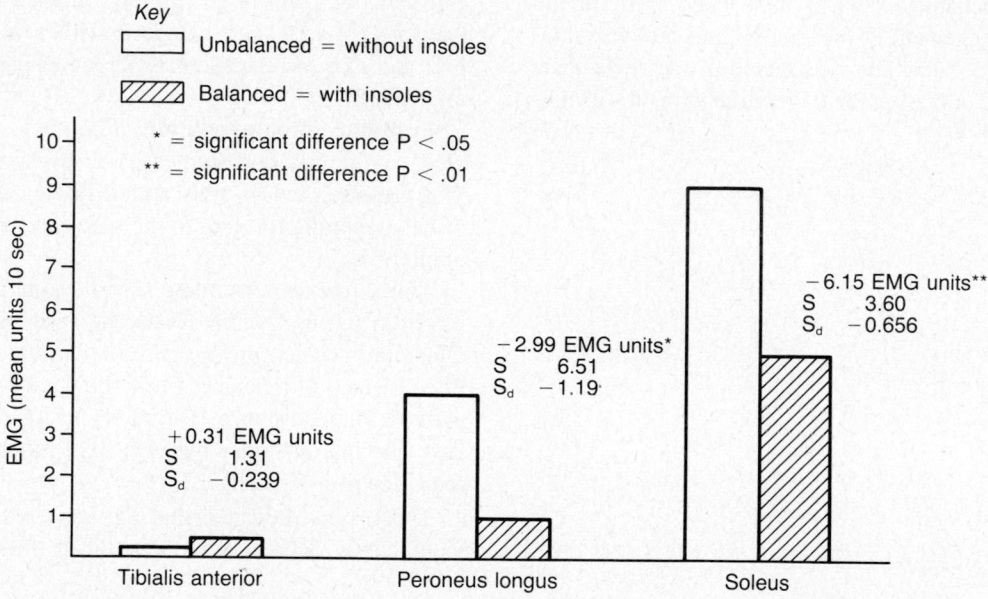

Fig. 17-35. Effect of balanced insole on muscle activity; $n = 30$. (From Hunt GC: Subtalar joint pronation: influence of balanced insoles, unpublished MA thesis, College Park, 1980, University of Maryland.)

the peroneus longus and lateral soleus while the tibialis anterior revealed no significant change. Fig. 17-35 demonstrates the EMG activity and the response to the rigid balanced orthotic device.

Analysis of variance tests indicated no significant difference for the tibialis anterior but significant reductions of electromyographic activity for the peroneus longus and the lateral soleus muscles at $P < .05$ and $P < .01$, respectively. The analysis of variance for EMG data is listed in Table 17-1.

The presence of foot or leg fatigue without foot pain seems consistent with the existence of increased muscular activity in the posterolateral leg. All the subjects related that the symptoms developed after prolonged weight-bearing and were relieved with rest. There was decreased electrical activity with the addition of the balanced insole, which suggests that by balancing the foot, the role of active muscular support is lessened. The conclusion is that with less muscle activity, less muscular strain or fatigue might develop. This study involved only static standing, but one might anticipate that excessive muscular activity would be minimized in gait also. Previous investigators discussed the increased muscular activity in persons with excessive pronation in gait, but they neglected to evaluate the means of controlling this excessive motion.[14,33,51]

Specific comparisons of this study to previous studies are difficult because of inadequate descriptions of foot

Table 17-1. Analysis of variance for EMG data (2 × 2 factorial)

Source	df	Tibialis anterior muscle				Peroneus longus muscle			Soleus muscle		
		SS	MS	F		S	MS	F	SS	MS	F
Subject	14	51.44	3.67	5.32*		387.35	26.67	1.27	1479.46	105.68	10.25*
Treatment	1	1.34	1.34	1.94		133.77	133.77	6.13†	244.22	244.22	23.69*
Leg	1	0.86	0.86	1.25		3.95	3.95	0.18	6.49	6.49	0.63
Treatment and leg	1	0.57	0.57	0.83		7.58	7.58	0.35	2.27	2.27	0.22
Error	42	28.92	0.69			915.86	21.81		433.20	10.31	

From Hunt GC: Subtalar joint pronation: influence of balanced insoles, unpublished MA thesis, College Park, 1980, University of Maryland.
*$P < .01$.
†$P < .05$.
df = degrees of freedom.
ss = sums of squares.
ms = means of squares.
F = "F" ratio.

types. Few studies have clearly defined the foot type under investigation. Gray[15] investigated the role of the tibialis anterior, peroneus longus, tibialis posterior, and the soleus in 27 individuals with flat feet and six with normal feet. He did not, however, classify his flatfoot population according to cause of the condition. In spite of this, he concluded that the leg muscles attempt to control the subtalar and midtarsal joints in subjects with a pronated foot. Given the deep origin of the tibialis posterior, one may question whether Gray actually recorded from this muscle. Smith,[52] Basmajian and Bentzon,[1] Close et al.,[7] Joseph,[28] and O'Connell[39] have suggested that the increased activity of the soleus is the result of postural (anterior/posterior) control. Since the insertion of the Achilles tendon is such that it causes inversion of the calcaneus, the activity of the soleus might also increase as a result of an eversion moment in the pronated foot.

The functional significance of the peroneus longus has been discussed by numerous investigators.[13,44,54] As one looks at the anatomical course of the peroneus longus and its action on the first ray and the midtarsal joints, it becomes clearer why it may be more active in the pronated foot. Gray[14] stated that the peroneus longus is in part responsible for returning the foot to neutral and maintaining it there at midstance. However, since the midfoot and first ray are less stable with subtalar pronation, the peroneus longus is at a disadvantage and must work harder to achieve frontal plane balance. The importance of first ray stability in stance and in the roll-off phase of gait has been well documented.* The peroneus longus might then be more active since it is working at this mechanical disadvantage.

Common to many of the studies on subtalar joint pronation is the lack of quantification of EMG data in studying

*See references 19, 20, 34, 44, and 50.

muscular activity. Gray[15] used a grading system that including the following:

1. Nil—no spikes
2. Slight—a few low-voltage spikes
3. Marked—many spikes displayed, including those of intermediate voltage.

Basmajian and Bentzon[1] reported studies using similar qualitative methods. However, the influence of subjectivity with resultant difficulty in duplicating such studies makes this method of reporting questionable. A need for greater sensitivity of equipment and more objective quantification of data is thus needed.

Summary

Pain and dysfunction in the lower extremity may result from any one or a combination of factors: (1) improper footwear, (2) biomechanical imbalances, or (3) increased activity levels. The management program should be influenced by a consideration of all three factors.

As clinicians become more sensitive to functional demands, the value of establishing absolute degrees of motion is less important. For example, the amount of calcaneal eversion necessary for gait would depend on the frontal plane position of the tibia. Since the amount of tibia vara will vary among individuals, so will the degree of necessary calcaneal eversion.

A variety of orthotic devices have been developed to manage the pronated foot. More current concepts of orthotic control have been discussed and supported by clinical investigation and research. From the data collected the following conclusions may be justified:

1. The symptom complex of the individual with excessive subtalar joint pronation as a result of forefoot varus appears related mainly to mechanical imbalances.

2. Balancing the forefoot to rearfoot has a beneficial effect by reducing excessive muscular activity that appears to cause fatigue and discomfort in the posterior leg.

In the final analysis, thorough biomechanical evaluation of the lower extremity is necessary to better understand symptoms related to gait deviations.

CASE STUDIES

The following examples will help clarify dynamic and static evaluation principles.

CASE STUDY 1

E.H., a 22-year-old male long-distance runner, had a history of chronic left medial knee pain resulting in a partial medial meniscectomy with arthroscopic surgery. Following an uneventful postoperative rehabilitation program with return of muscle strength, the individual noted an increase in original symptoms after increasing his mileage to 70 miles per week. The biomechanical evaluation is listed below:

Dynamic

Increased left foot pronation and internal lower extremity rotation were observed during midstance.

Static

	Right	Left
Dorsiflexion with knees extended	10[o]	10[o]
Dorsiflexion with knees flexed	14[o]	14[o]
Calcaneal eversion	5[o]	5[o]
Tibia vara	8[o]	14[o]
Forefoot	Slight plantar-flexed first ray	Forefoot varus, including second through fifth metatarsal with plantar-flexed first ray
Tibial torsion	Normal	Normal
Hips		
Internal rotation	30[o]	30[o]
External rotation	35[o]	40[o]
Hamstring length	Normal	Normal
Flexor length	Normal	Normal
Rectus femoris length	Normal	Normal
Abductor length	Normal	Normal
Limb length		¼ inch longer crest

Comments

The combination of left forefoot varus with a high degree of tibia vara and insufficient calcaneal eversion causes greater internal lower-extremity rotation with excessive pronation and medial knee strain. In this case, minimal calcaneal eversion was present on posterior gait observation. The most obvious gait deviation was noted from the anterior view as illustrated in Figs. 17-36 and 17-37.

The management approach included prescription of an or-

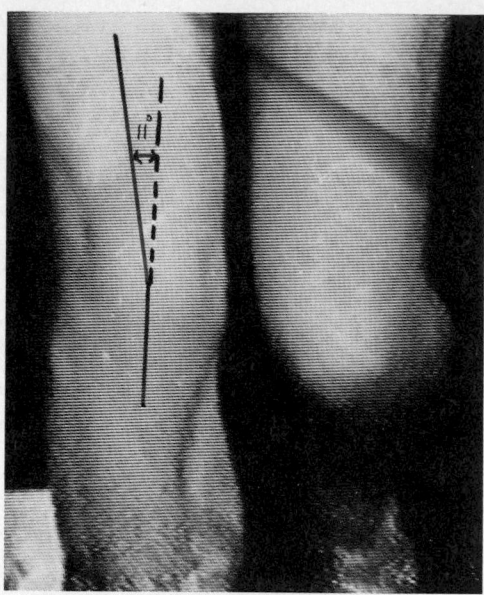

Fig. 17-36. Right Q angle measures 11 degrees with a balanced alignment.

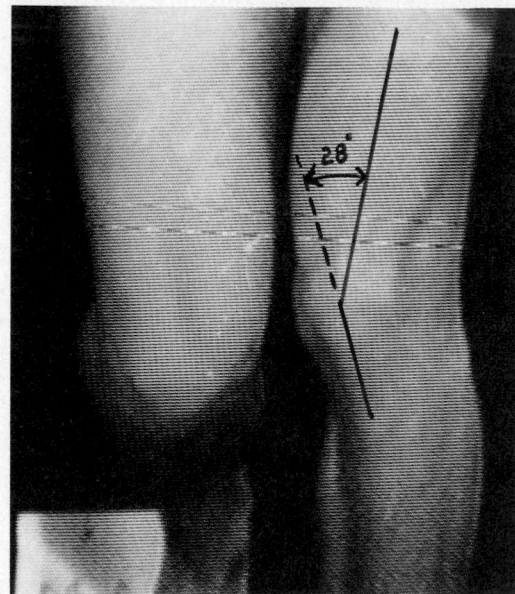

Fig. 17-37. Excessive left internal rotation with a 28-degree Q angle produces excessive torque at knee.

thotic device to balance the forefoot and rearfoot varus deviations and a ¼-inch right heel lift. Stretching exercises for hip rotation were also included. Fig. 17-38 demonstrates the Q angle with balanced orthotics.

CASE STUDY 2

J.B., a 22-year-old male runner, noticed an increase in pain located posterior and medial to the right medial malleolus since he started using a new softer shoe. The biomechanical evaluation is listed below:

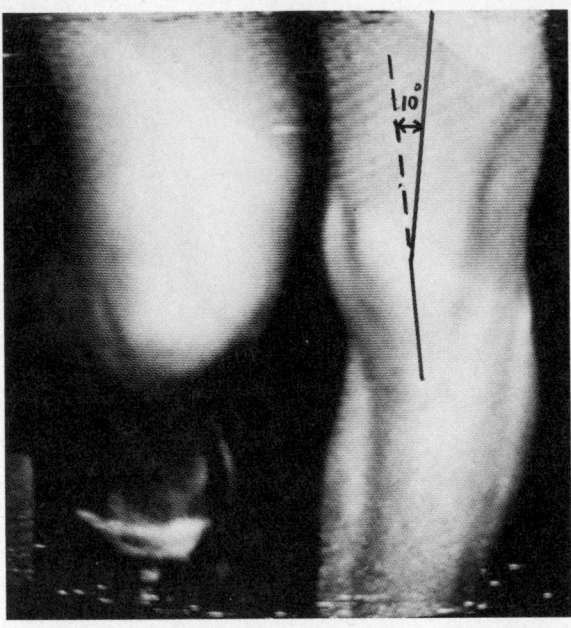

Fig. 17-38. Improved Q angle with balanced orthotic device.

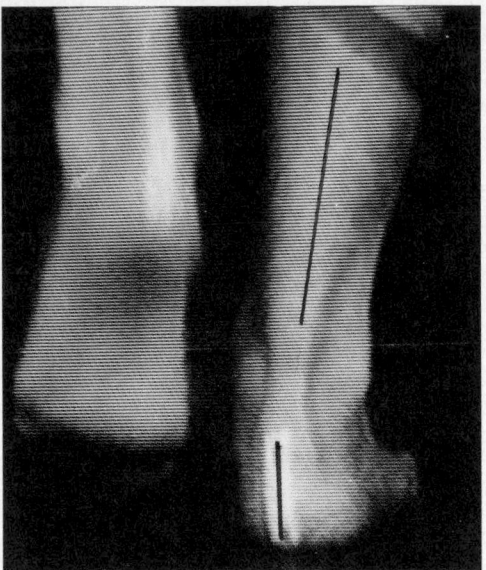

Fig. 17-39. Midstance with slight pronation.

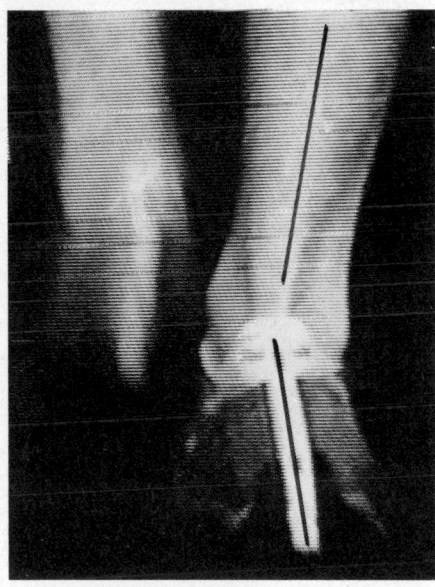

Fig. 17-40. Accentuated pronation with softer shoe.

Dynamic

Bilateral slight midfoot pronation, which was accentuated with shoes and observed during late midstance. A right medial heel whip occurred during early propulsion.

Static

	Right	Left
Dorsiflexion with knees extended	0[o]	0[o]
Dorsiflexion with knees flexed	10[o]	10[o]
Calcaneal inversion	15[o]	10[o]
Calcaneal eversion	10[o]	10[o]
Tibia vara	10[o]	10[o]
Forefoot	Perpendicular	Perpendicular
Rearfoot	Normal	Normal
Tibial torsion	Normal	Normal
Hip		
Internal rotation	25[o]	40[o]
External rotation	50[o]	40[o]
Hip flexor length	Tight	Tight
Rectus femoris length	Normal	Normal
Abductor length	Normal	Normal
Limb length	Equal	

Comments

The significant findings included decreased ankle joint dorsiflexion and decreased right hip internal rotation. The increased pronation with the soft flexible shoe most likely occurred as a result of subtalar and midtarsal joint compensation for the decreased ankle joint dorsiflexion. This compensatory pronation was probably responsible for the posterior medial stress and pain. The medial heel whip on the right during propulsion seemed to result from decreased hip internal rotation and hip extension. Figs. 17-39 and 17-40 demonstrate the effect of the soft shoe in accentuating the pronation. Management included a change to a more stable shoe with ¼ -inch heel lifts. The individual was also given stretching exercises for the plantar flexors and right hip external rotators.

CASE STUDY 3

S.H., a 29-year-old man, was seen in the physical therapy clinic with complaints of lateral anterior left knee pain. Significant past medical history included a fracture of the right femoral shaft 13 years previously in an automobile accident. Treatment included a closed reduction using traction. Following healing, he was noted to have a 1½ -inch shortening of the right lower extremity that was corrected for his shoes. Being an active, athletic individual, 2 years ago he trained and ran in a marathon, after which time he noted pain in his left lateral anterior knee. He had tried rest and various physical agents with limited results. He had no pain as long as he did not run. The biomechanical evaluation follows:

Dynamic

Minimal, if any, subtalar pronation occurred during midstance; however, the left side demonstrated slightly more midfoot pronation. The right side demonstrated early heel-off and decreased hip flexion with a fully extended knee on heel contact. The left side revealed increased hip and knee flexion at heel contact.

Static

A summary of the static evaluation included adequate ankle dorsiflexion bilaterally, limited calcaneal eversion when compared with tibia vara, rearfoot varus bilaterally, and plantar-flexed first rays bilaterally. The right hip displayed decreased internal rotation, whereas left hip internal and external rotations were equal. The right lower extremity was 1½ -inches shorter than the left. Callus appeared on the fifth and first metatarsal heads and medial great toes bilaterally.

Comments

The individual compensated extremely well at the hip, knee, and ankle joints for his leg-length discrepancy. Minimal calcaneal eversion was observed from the limited eversion available. The left knee pain seemed to exist as a result of the prolonged flexed position associated with increased patellofemoral compression. The subject noted no pain when not running, and since his running shoes did not have the correction for length, he was advised to have his right shoe corrected by ¾ inch. Figs. 17-41 to 17- 44 demonstrate the compensations occurring for this individual.

CASE STUDY 4

S.K., a 20-year-old female collegiate middle-distance runner, had a history of bilateral knee and posterior medial ankle pain. A tendon sheath release was performed on the right posterior tibial tendon 7 months before this evaluation with equivocal results. The biomechanical evaluation follows:

Dynamic

Both sides demonstrated limited calcaneal eversion at heel contact, with the right worse than the left. Increased internal femoral rotation was present along with genu valgum bilaterally.

Static

	Right	Left
Dorsiflexion with knees extended	2[o]	2[o]
Dorsiflexion with knees flexed	5[o]	8[o]
Calcaneal inversion	20[o]	15[o]
Calcaneal eversion	5[o]	8[o]
Tibia vara	8[o]	8[o]
Forefoot	Perpendicular	Perpendicular
Rearfoot	Slight varus	Normal
Tibial torsion	Normal	Normal
Hip		
Internal rotation	55[o]	55[o]
External rotation	25[o]	25[o]
Rectus femoris	Tight	Normal
Hamstring, hip flexor, and abductor lengths	Normal	Normal
Limb length	Equal	

Comments

Limited ankle dorsiflexion and greater hip internal rotation were two explanations for the stress occurring at the medial ankles and knees. With limited subtalar joint pronation, compensation occurred at the knee resulting in a valgus stress. Had this individual sufficient flexibility of the first ray to plantar- flex or enough eversion of the longitudinal midtarsal joint axis, then stress on the knee might have been less. Management included stretching the plantar flexors and hip internal rotators and

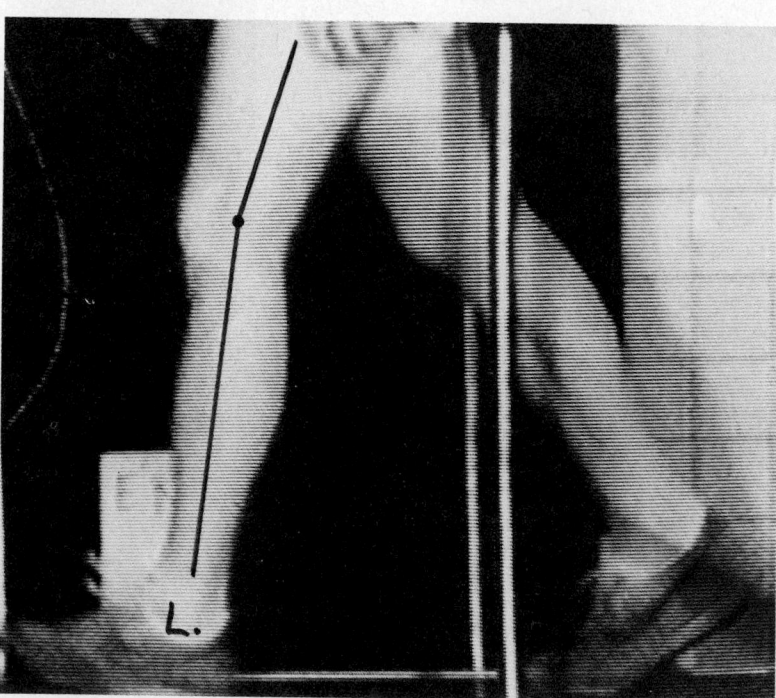

Fig. 17-41. Left heel contact notes 12-degree flexed knee.

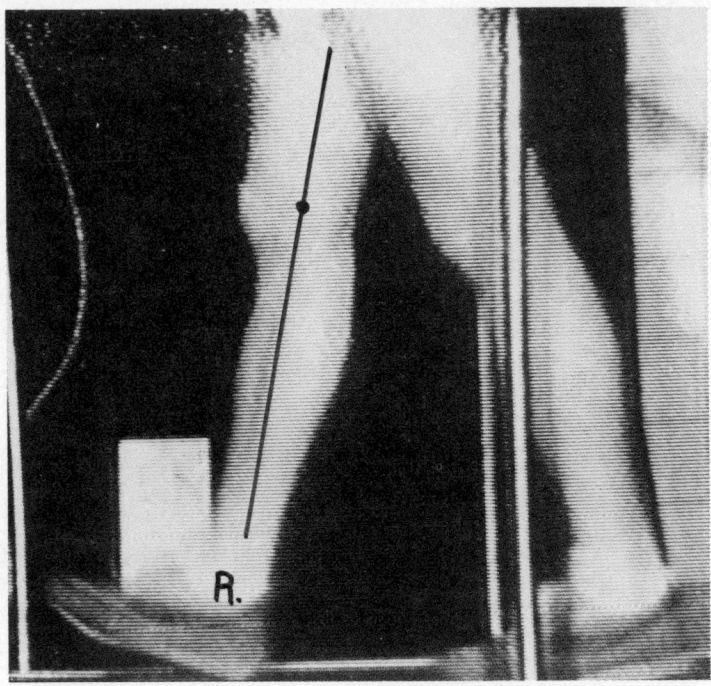

Fig. 17-42. Right heel contact notes 0-degree extended knee.

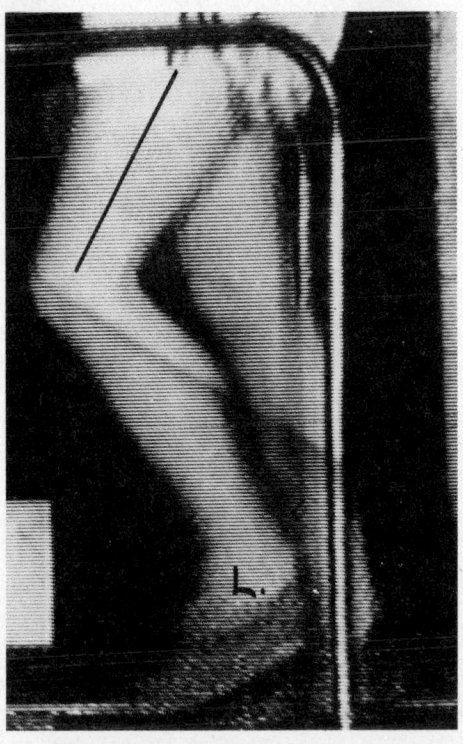

Fig. 17-43. Left hip flexion.

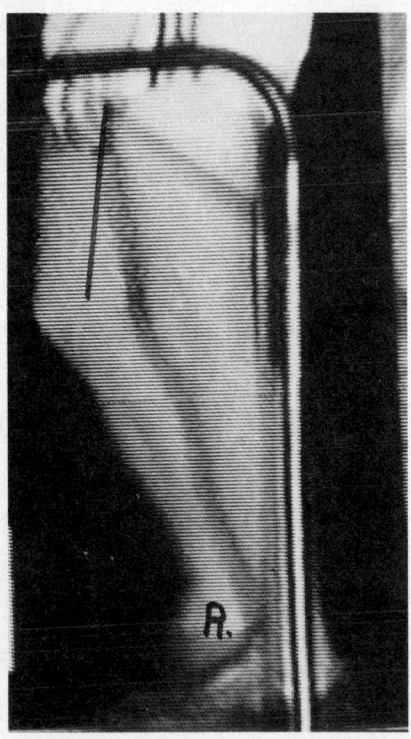

Fig. 17-44. Right hip flexion.

strengthening the external hip rotators and internal tibial rotators. Shoe modification included lateral heel counter reinforcement and shock-absorbing insoles with mild varus heel wedges. Figs. 17-45 and 17-46 illustrate the valgus knee stress as a result of internal femoral rotation.

CASE STUDY **5**

G.S., a 16-year-old male high school 1-mile and 2-mile runner, had calf and foot discomfort aggravated by running. The right side was more symptomatic. The biomechanical evaluation follows:

Dynamic

Both heels were everted at heel contact with the right worse than the left. During midstance the right pronated excessively, resulting in an apropulsive gait.

Static

	Right	*Left*
Dorsiflexion with knees extended	8[o]	8[o]
Dorsiflexion with knees flexed	18[o]	18[o]
Calcaneal inversion	20[o]	20[o]
Calcaneal eversion	8[o]	10[o]
Tibia vara	5[o]	5[o]
Forefoot	Varus	Perpendicular
Rearfoot	Varus	Varus
Tibial torsion	Normal	Normal

Hips		
Internal rotation	45[o]	40[o]
External rotation	40[o]	45[o]
Hamstring length	Tight (medial)	Tight (medial)
Abductor, hip flexor, and rectus femoris length	Normal	Normal
Limb length	Equal	

Comments

The greater pronation, with heel valgus, on the right side was a result of forefoot varus. The amount of eversion was greater than tibia vara, and thus heel valgus was possible. The tight medial hamstrings were also contributing to the excessive pronation. Management included orthotic devices to balance the feet and stretching exercises for the hamstrings, particularly the medial group. Figs. 17-47 and 17-48 illustrate the gait deviation and correction.

CASE STUDY **6**

A.S., a 20-year-old female collegiate sprinter, had a 4-month history of pain in the area of the right posterior medial malleolus that started during the indoor track season. On physical examination, she exhibited tenderness posterior to the medial malleolus with resistance to the flexor hallucis longus but not to the tibialis posterior or flexor digitorum longus. The biomechanical evaluation follows:

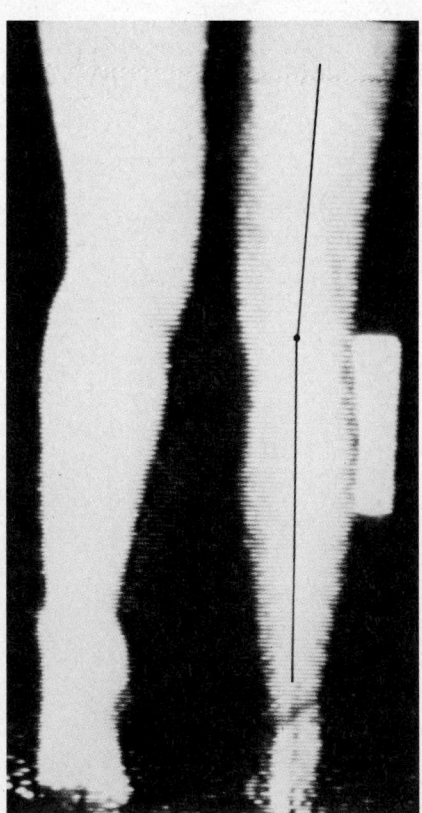

Fig. 17-45. Three degrees genu valgus at early midstance on right.

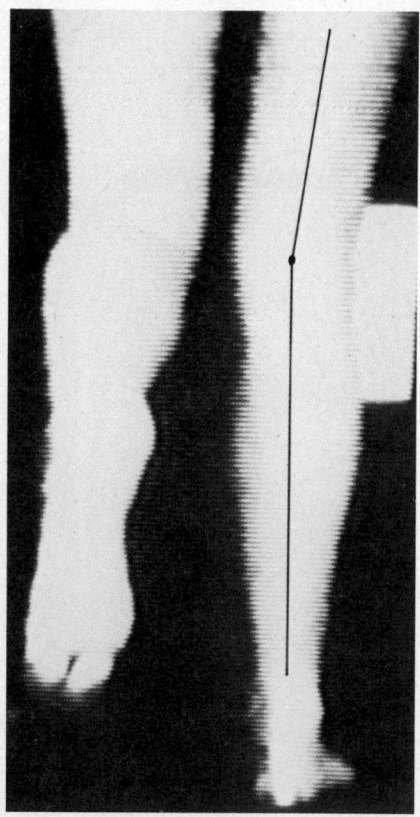

Fig. 17-46. Valgus angle increases to 10 degrees at late midstance.

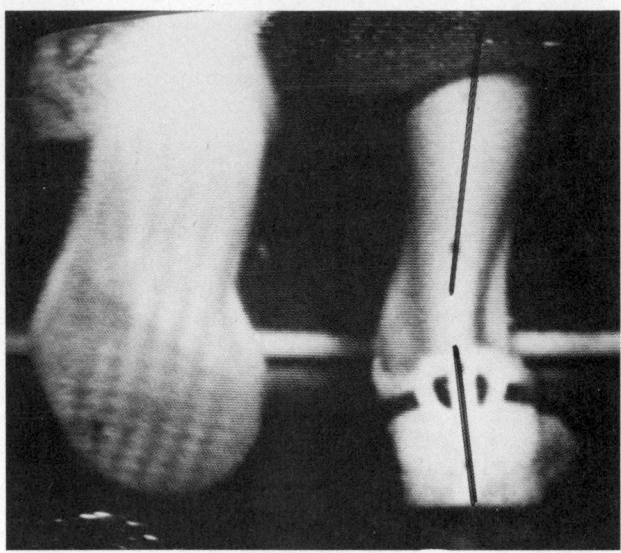

Fig. 17-47. Excessive calcaneal eversion with medial ankle bulge at midstance.

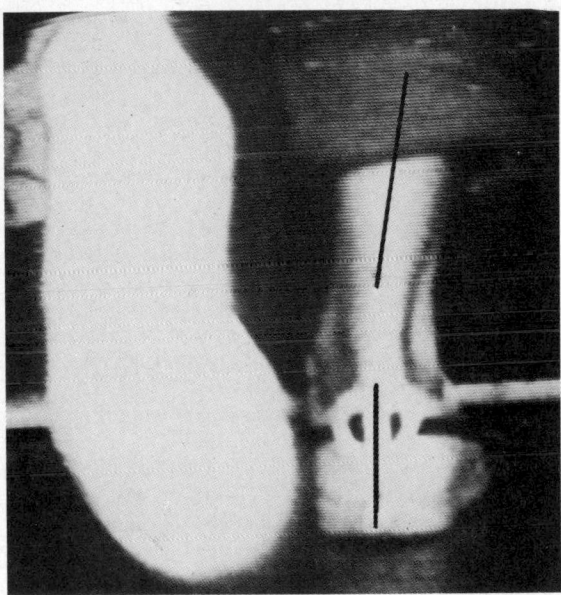

Fig. 17-48. Improved calcaneal position with balanced orthotic device at midstance.

Dynamic

Increased pronation was observed during late midstance associated with an exaggerated midfoot collapse at heel rise; the right was more pronounced.

Static

	Right	Left
Dorsiflexion with knees extended	5[o]	5[o]
Dorsiflexion with knees flexed	10[o]	10[o]
Calcaneal inversion	20[o]	20[o]

Calcaneal eversion	8[o]	10[o]
Tibia vara	12[o]	12[o]
Forefoot	Slight forefoot varus	Perpendicular
Rearfoot	Normal	Normal
Hips		
Internal rotation	55[o]	55[o]
External rotation	30[o]	30[o]

Comments

Right forefoot varus and excessive tibia vara resulting in excessive pronation around the oblique axis of the midtarsal joint were causing excessive stress to the flexor hallucis longus. Overuse of the flexor hallucis longus was more logical than the tibialis posterior because she was a sprinter and did not land on her heels. (An individual who is a heel striker in this same situation would most likely have tibialis posterior stress). Individually testing each muscle for pain is important because it helps to identify the inflamed tissue. This midfoot problem was difficult to manage with an orthotic device because the individual was a forefoot striker. Another explanation for its management difficulty may be that the oblique midtarsal joint axis was more vertical than usual, resulting in excessive transverse rotation with a midfoot collapse. Transverse abnormalities are difficult to control with orthotic devices. A more stable shoe was prescribed with a balanced orthotic device with only fair results. Figure 17-49 illustrates the pronation during late midstance.

SUMMARY

The importance of identifying specific occurrences in gait is fundamental to understanding human locomotion, but the correlation of the dynamic and static examination is ultimately the most critical. The purpose of this chapter was to demonstrate the integration of the dynamic and static analyses.

Sequences of the walking gait cycle should be identified

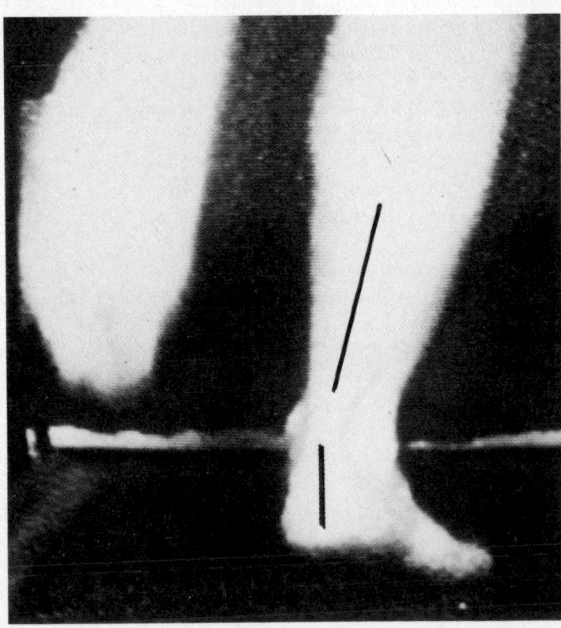

Fig. 17-49. Right pronation during late midstance.

and correlated with basic kinematic principles. Problems in terminology should be discussed and clarified with particular reference to the subtalar joint complex. Slow-motion videotape analysis can be used as an aid to improving clinical expertise in this area. A guide to gait analysis should include observations from anterior, posterior, and side views.

Various gait deviations may be caused by different anatomical variants, and treatment approaches should be based on identifying and treating the primary anatomical problem.

Mechanisms influencing gait deviation can include improper footwear, biomechanical imbalances, or increased physical activity. The consideration of all three areas is important in understanding the individual's problem. The relationships between limb position and joint motion should be examined along with the possibilities for orthotic application. Case studies demonstrate the evaluation procedures and the development of management approaches.

In conclusion, the positive results of any treatment program will depend largely on a cooperative client and a clinician who is willing to systematically evaluate the entire kinetic chain. Failure to do so will be met only with continued frustration by all concerned.

REFERENCES

1. Basmajian JV and Bentzon JW: An electromyographic study of certain muscles of the leg and foot in the standing position, Surg Gynecol Obstet 98:662, 1954.
2. Basmajian JV and Stecko G: The role of muscles in arch support of the foot, J Bone Joint Surg (Am) 45:1184, 1963.
3. Bowden REM: The functional anatomy of the foot, Physiotherapy 53:120, 1967.
4. Brandell BK and Williams K: An analysis of cinematographic and electromyographic recordings of human gait. In Nelson R and Morehouse C, editors: Biomechanics IV, Baltimore, 1974, University Park Press.
5. Bruce J and Walmsley R: Some observations on the arches of the foot and flat-foot, Lancet 235:656, 1938.
6. Cinzio JR: Retarded osseous development as a primary factor in weakfoot, J Am Podiatry Assoc 51:183, 1961.
7. Close JR et al: The function of the subtalar joint, Clin Orthop 50:159, 1967.
8. Currier DP: Maximal isometric tension of the elbow extensors at varied positions. II. Assessment of extensor components by quantitative electromyography, J Am Phys Ther Assoc 52:1265, 1973.
9. Dontigny RL: Dysfunction of the sacroiliac joint and its treatment, J Orthop Sports Phys Ther 1:23, 1979.
10. DeVries HA: Muscle tonus in postural muscles, Am J Phys Med 44:275, 1965.
11. Elftman H: The transverse tarsal joint and its control, Clin Orthop 16:41, 1960.
12. Erhard R and Bowling R: The recognition and management of the pelvic component of low back and sciatic pain, Bull Orthop Sect APTA, 2:4, 1977.
13. Ferciot CF: The etiology of developmental flat-foot, Clin Orthop 85:7, 1972.
14. Gray EG and Basmajian JV: Electromyography and cinematography of leg and foot (normal and flat) during walking, Anat Rec 161:1, 1968.
15. Gray ER: The role of leg muscles in variations of the arches in normal and flat feet, J Am Phys Ther Assoc 49:1084, 1969.
16. Hagy JL et al: Normal angular and force measurement data and normal electromyographic data, San Francisco, 1973, Shriners' Hospital for Crippled Children Publication.
17. Hicks JH: The mechanics of the foot. I. The joints, J Anat 87:345, 1953.
18. Hicks JH: The mechanics of the foot. II. The plantar aponeurosis and the arch, J Anat 88:25, 1954.
19. Hicks JH: The foot as a support, Acta Anat 25:34, 1955.
20. Hicks JH: The mechanics of the foot. IV. The action of muscles on the foot in standing, Acta Anat 27:180, 1956.
21. Hlavac HF: Compensated forefoot varus, J Am Podiatry Assoc 60:229, 1970.
22. Hlavac HF: The foot book, Mountain View, Calif, 1977, World Publications.
23. Hunt GC: Subtalar joint pronation: Influence of balanced insoles, unpublished master's thesis, College Park, 1980, University of Maryland.
24. Inman VT: The joints of the ankle, Baltimore, 1976, Williams & Wilkins.
25. Inman VT et al: Human walking, Baltimore, 1981, Williams & Wilkins.
26. Isman RE and Inman VT: Anthropometric studies of the human foot and ankle, Bull Prosthet Res Spring, 1969.
27. Jones RL: The functional significance of the declination of the axis of the subtalar joint, Anat Rec 93:151, 1945.
28. Joseph J: Electromyography of posture on gait in man, Bull Am Assoc EMG Electrodiagnosis 12:24, 1965.
29. Kendall FP and McCreary EK: Muscle-testing and function, Baltimore, 1983, Williams & Wilkins.
30. Lapidus PW: Kinesiology and mechanical anatomy of the tarsal joints, Clin Orthop 30:20, 1963.
31. Manley MT: Biomechanics of the foot. In Helfet AJ and Gruebel Lee DM, editors: Disorders of the foot, Philadelphia, 1980, JB Lippincott Co.
32. Mann RA and Hagy JL: Running, jogging and walking: A comparative electromyographic and biomechanical study. In Bateman JE and Trott AW, editors: The foot and ankle, New York, 1980, BC Decker Inc.
33. Mann RA and Inman VT: Phasic activity of intrinsic muscles of the foot, J Bone Joint Surg (Am) 46:469, 1964.
34. Manter JT: Movements of the subtalar and transverse tarsal joints, Anat Rec 80:397, 1941.
35. Mereday C et al: Evaluation of The University of California Biomechanics Laboratory shoe insert in "flexible" pes planus, Clin Orthop 82:45, 1972.
36. Merrifield HH: Influence of gait patterns on hip rotation and foot deviation, J Am Podiatry Assoc 60:345, 1970.
37. Murray MP: Gait as a total pattern of movement, Am J Phys Med 46:290, 1967.
38. Murray MP et al: Walking patterns of normal men, J Bone Joint Surg (Am) 46:335, 1964.
39. Murray MP et al: Walking patterns of normal women, Arch Phys Med Rehab 51:637, 1970.
40. O'Connell AL: Electromyographic study of certain leg muscles during movements of the free foot and during standing, Am J Phys Med 37:289, 1958.
41. Pepin WA and Lauritsen WH: The genicular effects of the imbalanced foot, J Am Podiatry Assoc 55:518, 1965.
42. Perry J: The mechanics of walking, J Am Phys Ther Assoc 47:9, 1967.
43. Risser JC: Cause and management of the pronated foot, Ind Med Surg 37:197, 1968.
44. Root ML et al: Axis of motion of the subtalar joint, J Am Podiatry Assoc 56:149, 1966.

45. Root ML et al: Normal and abnormal function of the foot: Clinical biomechanics, vol 2, Los Angeles, 1977, Clinical Biomechanics Corp.

46. Rose GK: Correction of the pronated foot, J Bone Joint Surg (Br) 44:642, 1962.

47. Saunders JB et al: The major determinants in normal and pathological gait, J Bone Joint Surg 35A:543, 1953.

48. Scranton PE et al: Forces under the foot: A study of walking, jogging, and sprinting: Force distribution under normal and abnormal feet. In Bateman JE and Troot AW, editors: The foot and ankle, New York, 1980, BC Decker Inc.

49. Scranton PE et al: Support phase kinematics of the foot. In Bateman JE and Trott AW, editors: The foot and ankle, New York, 1980, BC Decker Inc.

50. Sgarlato TE: A compendium of podiatric biomechanics, San Fransciso, 1971, California College of Podiatric Medicine.

51. Sheffield FJ et al: Electromyographic study of the muscles of the foot in normal walking, Am J Phys Med 35:223, 1956.

52. Slocum DB and James SL: Biomechanics of running, JAMA 205:97, 1968.

53. Smith JW: Muscular control of the arches of the foot in standing: An electromyographic assessment, J Anat 88:152, 1954.

54. Subotnick SI: Biomechanics of the subtalar and midtarsal joints, J Am Podiatry Assoc 65:756, 1975.

55. Sutherland DH: An electromyographic study of the plantar flexors of the ankle in normal walking on the level, J Bone Joint Surg (Am) 48:66, 1966.

56. Williams M and Worthingham C: Therapeutic exercise, Philadelphia, 1957, WB Saunders Co.

57. Wright DG et al: Action of the subtalar and ankle-joint complex during the stance phase of walking, J Bone Joint Surg (Am) 46:361, 1964.

58. Zamosky I: Shoe modifications in lower-extremity orthotics, Bull Prosthet Res Fall, 1964, p. 54.

Chapter 18

THE WRIST AND HAND

Carolyn Thaxton Wadsworth

Restoration of the disabled wrist and hand requires a knowledge of the essentials of anatomy, mechanics, and pathokinesiology, with emphasis on the structure and function of parts that commonly limit motion. This chapter provides such essential information along with a systematic evaluation format and a synopsis of the pathology and management of common hand and wrist disorders.[1]

CLINICAL ANATOMY AND MECHANICS OF THE WRIST AND HAND
Osteology

The radius, ulna, and 27 bones of the hand proper (excluding sesamoids) comprise the wrist and hand skeleton

The information in this chapter is a compilation of much the author has learned from clients, instructors, colleagues, and students—to all of whom gratitude is expressed for making this work possible.

(Fig. 18-1). The distal radius displays a wide articular surface, marked by shallow depressions where it contacts the scaphoid and lunate bones. Laterally, the radial styloid process projects distally, and medially, the ulnar notch indents the radius. Posteriorly, Lister's tubercle is prominent on the distal radius.

The ulna is slightly enlarged at the wrist, where the ulnar head provides an articular surface and the ulnar styloid process projects distally on its medial border. The ulnar styloid is ½ inch shorter than the radial styloid, thus permitting range of motion in ulnar deviation that exceeds radial deviation.

Anatomists commonly classify the bones of the hand into three parts, the phalanges, metacarpus, and carpus, according to similarities in structure and function (see Fig. 18-1). The 14 *phalanges* resemble miniature long bones, with shafts and expanded ends. The concave proximal ends, the bases, display two shallow depressions that fit the corresponding pulley-shaped heads of adjacent phalanges. The heads, with their distinct condyles, form the convex partner of the interphalangeal (IP) joints. The close congruency of these hinge surfaces contributes greatly to finger joint stability. (The bases of proximal phalanges two through five are modified to articulate with the rounded metacarpal heads and thus possess biconcave surfaces.)

Five bones, also characterized by elongated shafts and expanded ends, comprise the *metacarpus*. The metacarpal bases articulate with the distal row of carpal bones in the common carpometacarpal joint. The bases of metacarpals two through five also articulate with one another. The convex distal metacarpal heads are rounded rather than pulley-shaped like the phalanges. The configuration of the biaxial metacarpophalangeal (MP) joints allows for a great amount of mobility, with inherently less bony stability than the IP joints. The first metacarpal differs in that its head is pulley-shaped and its base is separate from the common joint formed by the others.

The bones of the *carpus* form two transverse rows, with four bones to a row. The distal row includes (lateral to medial) the trapezium, trapezoid, capitate, and hamate, and the proximal row contains the scaphoid, lunate, triquetrum, and pisiform. The trapezium is distinguished by a tubercle for the attachment of the flexor retinaculum, a groove for the flexor carpi radialis tendon, and a saddle-shaped facet for articulation with the first metacarpal. The trapezoid is the smallest bone in the distal row. The capitate, the largest and most centrally located carpal, articulates with seven other bones, and most of the intercarpal ligaments radiate from it. The hamate is easily identified

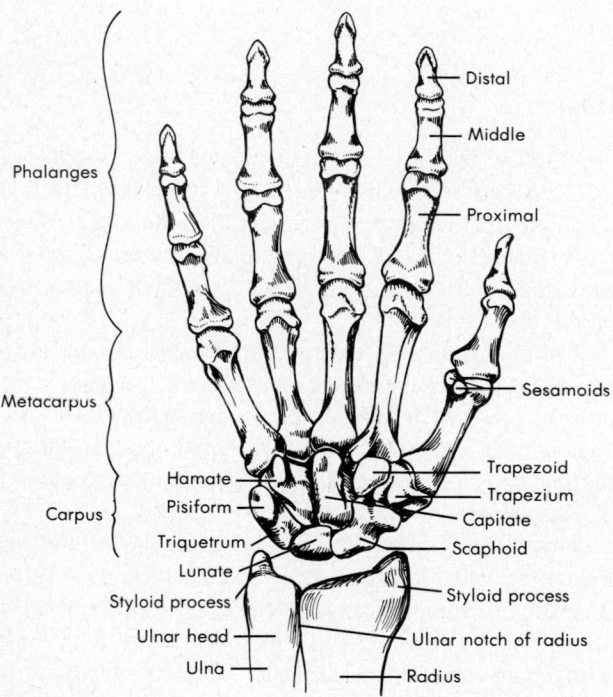

Fig. 18-1. Volar view of hand skeleton.

by its hooklike hamulus, which offers protection for the ulnar artery and nerve and a site of attachment for the flexor retinaculum. The scaphoid occupies the proximal row of carpals but actually bridges the joint between the two rows. It receives forces transmitted through the radius when the body weight is supported by the arm and is thus commonly fractured in falls. Because the proximal pole of the scaphoid is without its own blood supply in about 30% of the population, a fracture through the waist of the scaphoid often results in avascular necrosis or delayed union.[1] The scaphoid displays a prominent tubercle to which the flexor retinaculum attaches. The lunate, named for its semilunar shape, is the most commonly dislocated carpal, an injury that has potentially serious consequences if unreduced because of the bone's proximity to the median nerve. The triquetrum is three-sided and possesses a facet for articulation with the pisiform. The pea-shaped pisiform is the smallest carpal but has multiple attachments, including the flexor and extensor retinacula, pisohamate and pisometacarpal ligaments, and tendons of the flexor carpi ulnaris and abductor digiti minimi muscles.

Three volarly concave arches emerge from the arrangement of the wrist and hand bones to enhance prehensile function. The *longitudinal arch* spans the hand lengthwise, and two lateral arches run transversely, one at the level of the metacarpal heads and the other at the carpus. The flexible *metacarpal arch* is controlled by action of the intrinsic muscles, particularly the thenar and hypothenar muscles; it assists grasping and pinching functions. The relatively stable *carpal arch* forms a base for finger motion as well as the floor of the carpal tunnel, which provides support and protection of the finger flexor tendons and the median nerve (Fig. 18-2).

When the hand is viewed from the radial side, the volar projections of the scaphoid and trapezium tubercles are prominent. They form the lateral boundary of the osseous carpal tunnel and in addition provide a supporting base for the thumb in a plane that allows it to oppose the rest of the hand. The importance of thumb opposition to the grasping

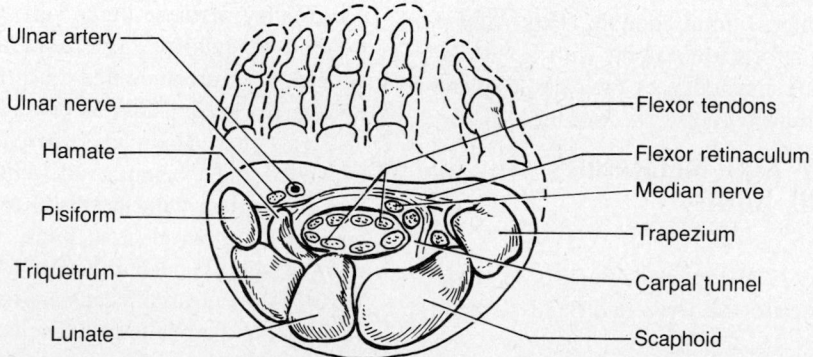

Fig. 18-2. Carpal tunnel boundaries include carpus dorsally and flexor retinaculum volarly; carpal tunnel is occupied by median nerve and flexor tendons of fingers and thumb.

ability of the hand cannot be overemphasized. Disability compensation schemes attribute 50% of the value of the hand to the thumb.[11]

An ulnar view reveals the anterior projections of the pisiform and hamulus, which form the medial boundary of the carpal tunnel. Another tunnel, the distal ulnar tunnel, conveys the ulnar artery and nerve and may be a site of compression injury. The flexor retinaculum, pisohamate ligament, and pisometacarpal ligament form its floor; the palmar (volar) carpal ligament, palmaris brevis muscle, and the palmar aponeurosis form its roof.

Arthrology

Distal radioulnar joint. The distal radioulnar joint participates in both wrist and forearm function (Fig. 18-3). It is a double pivot type of joint, connecting the distal ulna and radius and the ulna and articular disk. During forearm rotation the concave ulnar notch of the radius sweeps around the convex ulnar head. In an anatomical position, with the forearm supinated, the radius lies lateral and parallel to the ulna. During pronation the radius crosses the ulna, bringing its distal end into a medial position, while the proximal end remains lateral. During pronation and supination the ulna also moves slightly, opposite to the direction of the radius (i.e., during pronation, the ulna moves in a posterolateral and distal direction).[22] In conjunction with the proximal radioulnar joint, the distal radioulnar joint permits up to 170 degrees of forearm rotation. Joint play movements include anterior and posterior glide of the radius and ulna on one another.

The articular disk, or triangular fibrocartilage complex, unites the radius to the ulna and is reinforced by fibrous bands that extend into the anterior and posterior radioulnar capsule. The base of the disk attaches to the medial radial margin and its apex to the ulnar styloid process. It is thicker peripherally than centrally and may become perforated in older persons. The bioconcave disk articulates proximally with the ulna and distally with the proximal carpal row, primarily the triquetrum.

An articular capsule encloses the distal radioulnar joint, preventing communication with the radiocarpal joint. It is quite loose and does not provide support to the joint or limit its movement.[3] The synovial cavity lies adjacent to the distal ulnar head and extends proximally between the bones, assuming an L-shaped configuration in longitudinal section. The proximal end forms a pouch, the recessus sacciformis, that is frequently inflamed in rheumatoid arthritis.

Carpal joints. The carpal bones are firmly bound together on the dorsal and palmar surfaces by short intercarpal ligaments. Many are also attached individually by deeper interosseous ligaments. They articulate with one another in synovial joints and can be passively moved in relation to each other. Joint capsules and interosseous ligaments divide the synovial cavity into the separate joints described below (Fig. 18-3).

The radiocarpal joint is the articulation between the convex proximal row of carpal bones and the concave radius and disk. The midcarpal joint lies between the proximal and distal rows of carpals; it may be described as a *compound articulation* in which each row acts as a unit and each has both a convex and concave articulating portion. Together, the radiocarpal and midcarpal joints produce the movements that occur at the biaxial wrist joint: flexion, extension, radial deviation, and ulnar deviation. The common carpometacarpal joint is an irregular combination of plane articulations between the distal row of carpals and the bases of metacarpals two through five. It al-

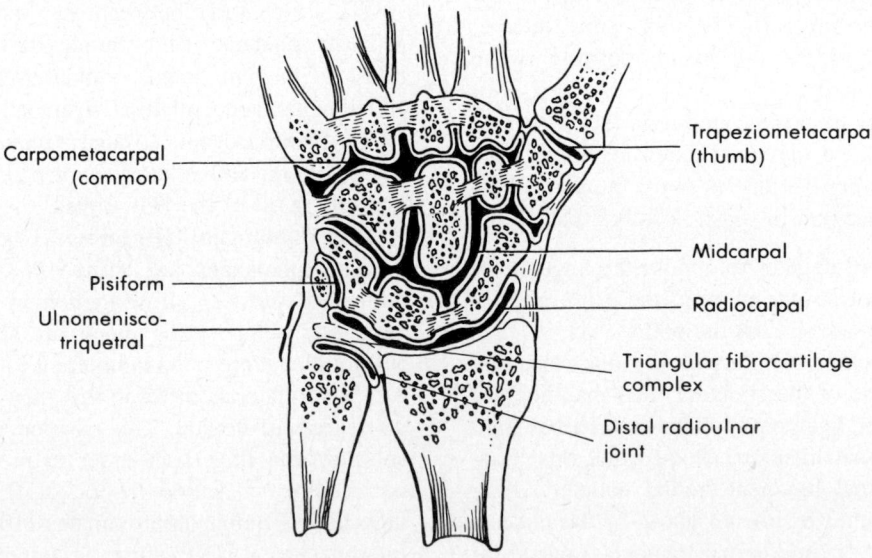

Carpometacarpal (common)

Pisiform

Ulnomenisco-triquetral

Trapeziometacarpal (thumb)

Midcarpal

Radiocarpal

Triangular fibrocartilage complex

Distal radioulnar joint

Fig. 18-3. Joints of carpus.

lows slight gliding and becomes more mobile toward the fifth metacarpal, making cupping of the palm possible.

The trapeziometacarpal joint is a saddle-shaped articulation between the trapezium and first metacarpal, which, with its exceptional mobility, is often referred to as the *key joint* of the hand. Its wide range of motion includes pure movements of flexion, extension, abduction, adduction, and combinations of movements producing opposition and circumduction. During abduction and adduction the convex metacarpal surface moves on the concave trapezium, while in flexion and extension the concave metacarpal surface moves on the convex trapezium. By definition, motions of the thumb occur in a plane perpendicular to the plane of the same movement in the digits (i.e., thumb flexion occurs in a frontal plane, which is perpendicular to the sagittal plane in which finger flexion occurs). The pisiform-triquetral joint is a small plane joint that has its own separate synovial cavity; it allows only a small amount of gliding. The ulnomeniscotriquetral joint is the articulation between the ulna, disk, and triquetrum and should be termed a *clinical joint* because it has no capsule and no separate synovial cavity; however, it becomes functionally important by providing component gliding, which accompanies supination and pronation.[8] Joint play movements occur in all of these carpal joints in response to traction, gliding, and rotary forces.

The approximate ranges of motion for the wrist are 70 to 80 degrees of extension, 75 to 85 degrees of flexion, 15 to 20 degrees of radial deviation, and 30 to 40 degrees of ulnar deviation. However, these ranges may be influenced by the position of the finger joints (or vice versa) through the constant length of the extrinsic finger flexor and extensor muscles. For example, wrist flexion is greater with the fingers extended. This property has important clinical ramifications, such as the following:

1. The need for maintaining a constant position of the other joints when any particular joint is measured
2. The need for identifying hand position when strength is measured
3. The need for incorporating tenodesis into treatment planning, such as using wrist extension to enhance grasp in a C-6 cord injury or wrist flexion to enhance finger extension in spastic cerebral palsy.

The thumb rotates 90 degrees to oppose the fingers, abducts 65 to 80 degrees from the plane of the palm, and extends 65 to 80 degrees away from the palm.

The ligaments attaching the carpals are often not distinct entities (like those of the shoulder) and may be hard to identify. The major ligaments of the radiocarpal joint are the volar radiocarpal ligament, volar ulnocarpal ligament, dorsal radiocarpal ligament, radial collateral ligament, and ulnar collateral ligament. Those of the midcarpal joint include the volar intercarpal ligaments, dorsal in-

tercarpal ligaments, and the interosseous ligaments. Ligaments of the common carpometacarpal joint are the volar carpometacarpal ligaments, dorsal carpometacarpal ligaments, and the intermetacarpal ligaments. The trapeziometacarpal joint is attached by the lateral ligaments, the volar ligament, and the dorsal oblique ligament (Fig. 18-4).

Metacarpophalangeal (MP) joints. The articulations formed by metacarpals two through five and the respective proximal phalanges are biaxial joints. The joint capsules are reinforced (or replaced) dorsally by the dorsal hood apparatus and volarly by the volar plates. The distal portion of the volar plate is cartilaginous and firmly fixed to the phalanx, whereas the proximal portion is membranous and loosely attached to the metacarpal. Adhesions may form between the membranous surfaces, which fold on themselves when immobilized in flexion.[34] On their palmar surface the plates are grooved to receive and pad the flexor tendons of the finger (see Fig. 18-4).

Laterally, the joints are supported by the collateral ligaments, which are strong cords that run obliquely from the dorsum of the metacarpals to the ventral aspect of the base of the phalanges (see Fig. 18-4). Because of their eccentric placement and the camlike action of the metacarpal head, which becomes larger palmarly and transversely, the collateral ligaments become taut as flexion increases.[11] Contractures of these ligaments contribute to loss of MP joint flexion. In order to prevent their shortening during immobilization, the fingers should be splinted with the MP joints in 70 to 90 degrees of flexion. The metacarpal heads are connected to one another by superficial and deep transverse metacarpal ligaments, which offer indirect support for the joints. Active movement increases progressively from the second to the fifth MP joint but is approximately 90 degrees flexion to 25 degrees extension and 20 degrees abduction to 0 degrees adduction.

The articulation between the first metacarpal and the proximal phalanx of the thumb is a hinge joint. Bony stability is inherent in its configuration and is enhanced by added volar and collateral ligamentous support (see Fig. 18-4). Flexion occurs to approximately 50 degrees. Traction, gliding, and rotatory joint play movements are also possible in all of the MP joints.

Interphalangeal (IP) joints. The articulations between adjacent phalanges are termed *hinge joints* because the pulleylike surfaces allow motion in only one plane. The volar and collateral ligaments are similar to those of the MP joints but are not as important to stability (see Fig. 18-4). The collaterals differ in that they are most taut at 15 to 20 degrees of flexion. This position, therefore, is ideal for splinting the fingers in order to prevent IP joint flexion contractures.[29] Active flexion at the proximal interphalangeal (PIP) joints approximates 110 degrees, at the distal interphalangeal (DIP) joints 90 degrees, and at the thumb

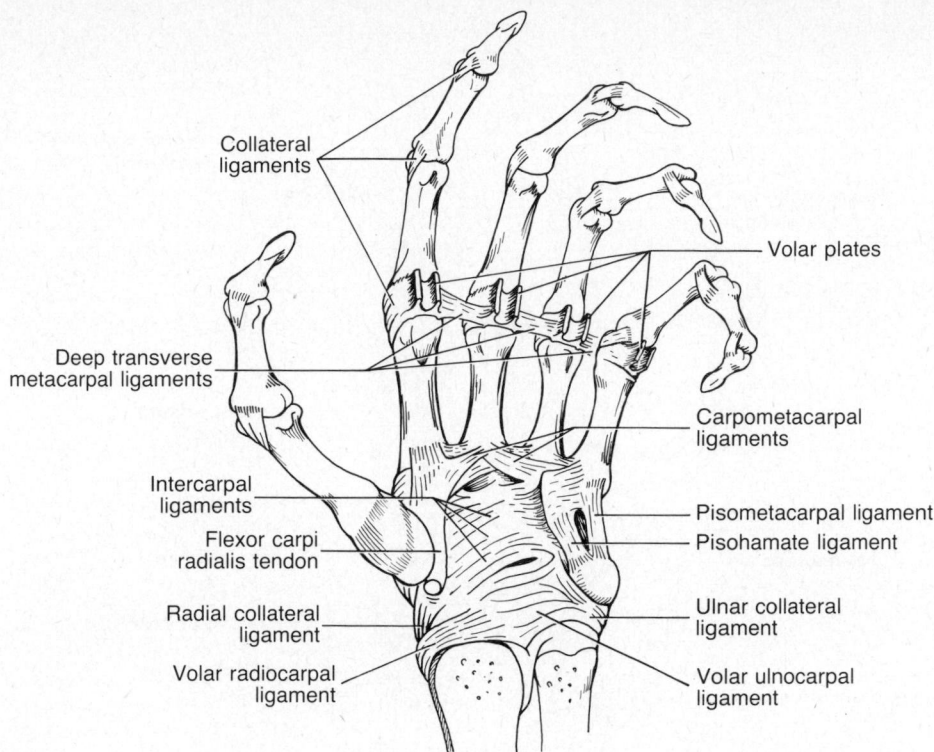

Fig. 18-4. Ligaments of wrist and hand.

interphalangeal joint 90 degrees. Traction, gliding, and joint play movements are also possible at the IP joints.

Soft tissue relationships and mechanics

The physical therapist frequently treats disorders of the hand stemming from pathological conditions of soft tissue. Some of the most common structures, their interrelationships, and disorders are discussed in this section.

The subcutaneous tissue of the dorsum of the hand is structurally quite different from the tissue of the palm. The dorsal areolar tissue is thin and elastic to permit stretching as a fist is made. Its loose attachment and preponderance of lymphatic vessels and veins account for swelling that is manifested predominantly on the dorsal surface, although the source of the problem often lies elsewhere in the hand.[16] In the palm many strong, fibrous fasciculi connect the skin tightly to the adjacent palmar aponeurosis, permitting relatively little sliding of the skin and enhancing secure grasp.

The palmar aponeurosis, just deep to the subcutaneous tissue, is composed of dense fibrous tissue. It is continuous with the palmaris longus tendon and fascia covering the thenar and hypothenar muscles and extends distally into the transverse metacarpal ligaments and flexor tendon sheaths. It provides protection for the ulnar artery and nerves and digital vessels and nerves and may transmit a weak flexion force from the palmaris longus tendon into the fingers (Fig. 18-5). Nodule formation or scarring in this structure produces the clinical entity known as Dupuytren's contracture, which may eventually result in flexion contractures of the digits.

The flexor retinaculum (transverse carpal ligament), deep to the palmar aponeurosis, spans the area between the pisiform, hamate, scaphoid, and trapezium. It forms the roof of the carpal tunnel, which transmits some of the tendons, vessels, and nerves of the hand. The retinaculum offers attachment for the thenar and hypothenar muscles, helps maintain the transverse carpal arch, prevents bowstringing of the extrinsic flexor tendons, and protects the median nerve (see Fig. 18-5). The median nerve is subject to compression in this relatively unyielding space, a condition known as carpal tunnel syndrome.

Muscles acting on the hand are referred to as extrinsic when their origin lies outside the hand and intrinsic when originating within the hand. The extrinsic and intrinsic muscles are listed in the accompanying box. A thorough review of muscle origins, insertions, and actions is recommended but, because of comprehensive coverage elsewhere,[20,33] is not included in this text. Instead the pathokinesiology of the moving soft tissues will be described.

Operation of the hand is notably enhanced by its large number of muscles. The design of the extrinsics, the muscle bellies of which are located in the forearm but taper into tendons proximal to the wrist, allows the action of many muscles without inordinate bulkiness. The extrinsic

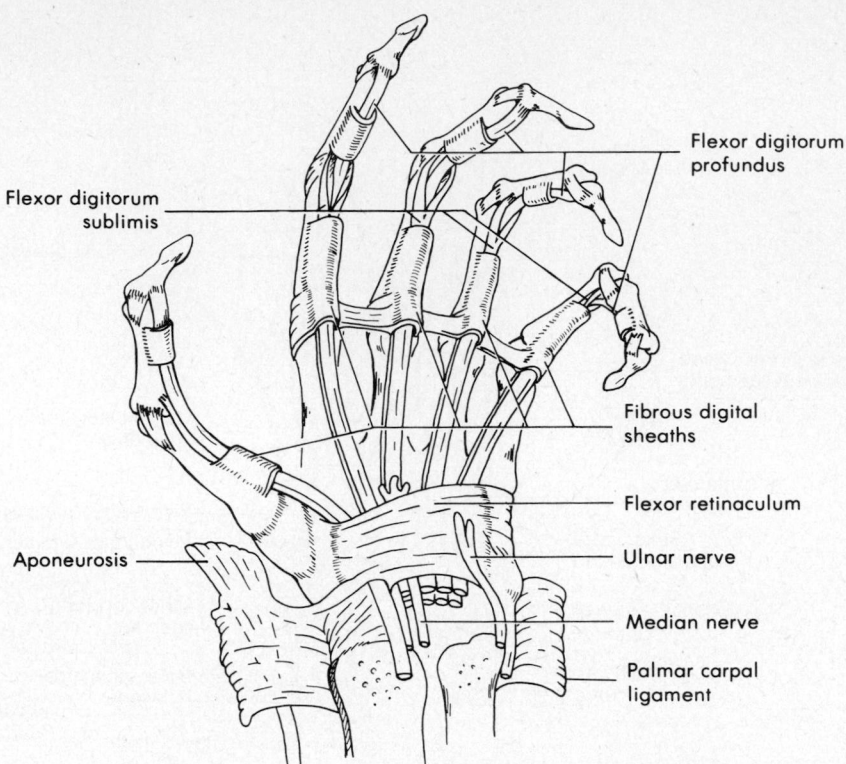

Fig. 18-5. Volar soft tissue relationships in wrist and hand.

muscle tendons en route to the fingers cross the wrist and serve to enhance its stability by forcing the hand proximally into the concave radial surface during cocontraction (see Fig. 18-5). The muscles acting on the wrist itself also contribute to wrist stability by achieving a balance of flexor and extensor forces through their attachment to corresponding surfaces of the stable metacarpal bases.[14]

Extrinsic and intrinsic muscles of hand

Extrinsic muslces	Intrinsic muscles
Extensor carpi radialis, longus, and brevis	Lumbricals
Extensor carpi ulnaris	Dorsal and palmar interossei
Flexor carpi radialis	Adductor pollicis
Flexor carpi ulnaris	Flexor pollicis brevis
Palmaris longus	Abductor pollicis brevis
Extensor pollicis longus and brevis	Opponens pollicis
Abductor pollicis longus	Flexor digiti minimi
Extensor indicis	Abductor digiti minimi
Extensor digiti minimi	Opponens digiti minimi
Extensor digitorum communis	Palmaris brevis
Flexor digitorum sublimis	
Flexor digitorum profundus	
Flexor pollicis longus	

The extrinsic flexor muscle tendons of the fingers pass into the hand deep to the flexor retinaculum. The flexor digitorum sublimis, which primarily flexes the PIP joints and secondarily assists MP joint flexion, divides into tendons that are capable of relatively independent action at each finger. The flexor digitorum profundus, which alone flexes the DIP joints and assists in flexion of the PIP and MP joints, also supplies tendons for each finger, but unlike the flexor digitorum sublimis, the tendons cannot operate independently. Therefore if one wishes to isolate the function of these two muscles in flexion of the PIP joint, one holds the finger(s) to the side(s) of the finger being tested in extension to pull the profundus distally. This position inactivates the profundus and allows the sublimis to act alone at the PIP joint (Fig. 18-6).[13]

The flexor tendons are tethered to the fingers by fibrous sheaths between the distal palmar crease and the PIP joint. This area is referred to as "no man's land" because of the difficulty of primary repair of severed tendons lying within this rigid fibroosseous space.

The dorsal extensor tendons are retained at the wrist by the extensor retinaculum. Toward the distal ends of the metacarpals the four tendons of the extensor digitorum communis (EDC) are interconnected by juncturae tendinum, limiting their independent motion (Fig. 18-7). Extension of the ring finger MP joint is hindered by flexion of the middle and little fingers because the juncturae tendinae pull the ring finger extensor distally, rendering it lax. Con-

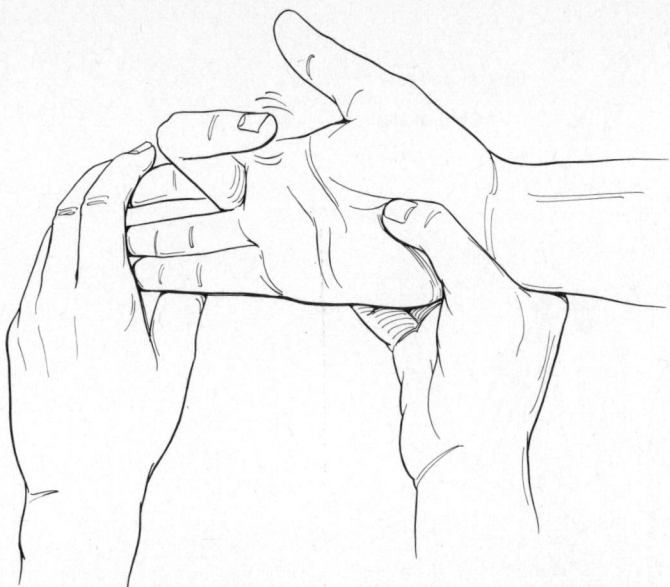

Fig. 18-6. Flexor digitorum sublimis is tested while adjacent digits are passively maintained in extension to tether flexor digitorum profundus. (Modified from Hoppenfeld S: Physical examination of the spine and extremities, New York, 1976, Appleton-Century-Crofts.)

versely, extension of the ring finger exerts an extensor force on its neighbors, so that they can be actively extended even if the middle and little extensor tendons are severed proximal to the juncturae.[26]

As the EDC tendons cross the region of the MP joints, their main connection to the proximal phalanx is through the sagittal bands, which pass palmarward to attach to the volar plates (Fig. 18-8). The primary function of the sagittal bands is to transmit the extension force of the EDC, thus extending the MP joint, but they also prevent bowstringing of the extensor tendon dorsally.[12,26,32] When hyperextension of the MP joint is not prevented, all of the force of the EDC will be transmitted to the proximal phalanx, extending the MP joint. In this situation excursion of the more distal attachments of the EDC is blocked, so consequently any IP joint extension that is to occur must be produced by the intrinsic muscles alone.[12,26,33] Thus a test to differentiate function of the extrinsic and intrinsic extensors involves maintaining full active extension of the MP joints and then attempting IP joint extension, an action that would only be possible if the intrinsics were operating.

Between the MP and PIP joints the EDC tendons divide into three parts: the central slip, which inserts into the base of the middle phalanx, and two lateral bands (see Fig. 18-7). These lateral bands eventually rejoin into a terminal tendon, which inserts into the base of the distal phalanx. Rupture of this terminal tendon produces a mallet finger, in which the DIP joint drops into flexion. Fibers from the

lumbricals and interossei join the EDC tendons over the proximal phalanx, contributing to the dorsal hood apparatus. These intrinsic muscle tendons pass volarly to the MP joint axis, thus exerting a flexion force on these joints, whereas both the intrinsic and extrinsic tendons pass dorsally to the PIP and DIP joint axes, exerting an extension force on these joints.

The lateral bands formed by the continuation of both extrinsic and intrinsic extensor tendons are prevented from dislocating dorsally by the transverse retinacular ligaments, which link them to the volar plates of the PIP joints (see Fig. 18-7). Stretching or laxity of these ligaments allows bowstringing of the bands, which transmits excessive extension force to the PIP joint from the intrinsics. This abnormal tension—combined with a volar plate rupture or the joint laxity characteristic of rheumatoid arthritis—contributes to hyperextension deformity of the PIP joint. Terminal phalangeal flexion commonly results from the taut profundus tendon in the presence of weakened DIP joint extension. This is referred to as *swan neck* (Fig. 18-9).[26]

The oblique retinacular ligament (Landsmeer's ligament) also contributes to interdependence of interphalangeal joint movement. It is attached between the PIP volar plate, where it is volar to the PIP joint axis, and the terminal tendon, where it is dorsal to the DIP joint axis (see Fig. 18-7). When the PIP joint is extended, it exerts a passive extensor force on the DIP joint, and when the PIP joint flexes, it allows the DIP joint to flex. In the normal hand the function of the oblique retinacular ligament is essentially nonexistent. However, if it becomes contracted after burns or trauma, it produces a tenodesis effect: that is, when the PIP joint is extended, the DIP joint will be brought into fixed extension by this ligament.[12]

When the PIP joint is flexed, the lateral bands slip volarly, decreasing the excursion required for full DIP joint flexion. If the PIP joint is fully flexed passively, the extensor mechanism is held distally by the central slip and is thus checkreined. The lateral bands become completely lax, thus permitting only weak and limited distal joint extension.[12,16] If, on the other hand, the central slip is ruptured from its insertion, the extensor mechanism is pulled proximally, rendering the lateral bands taut. The PIP joint is pulled into flexion by the unopposed flexor digitorum sublimis, and the lateral bands, which now lie volar to the PIP joint axis, function as flexors. The force of the intrinsic muscles and the EDC is transmitted directly to the distal phalanx, extending it and producing a *boutonniere deformity* (Fig. 18-10).[26,27,32] When the DIP joint is evaluated in cases of PIP joint contracture, these interrelationships must be considered.

The lumbrical muscles originate from the flexor digitorum profundus tendons and insert into the dorsal apparatus. During contraction they pull the profundus tendons distally, thus possessing the unique ability to relax their own antagonist.[26] In instances of lumbrical spasm or contrac-

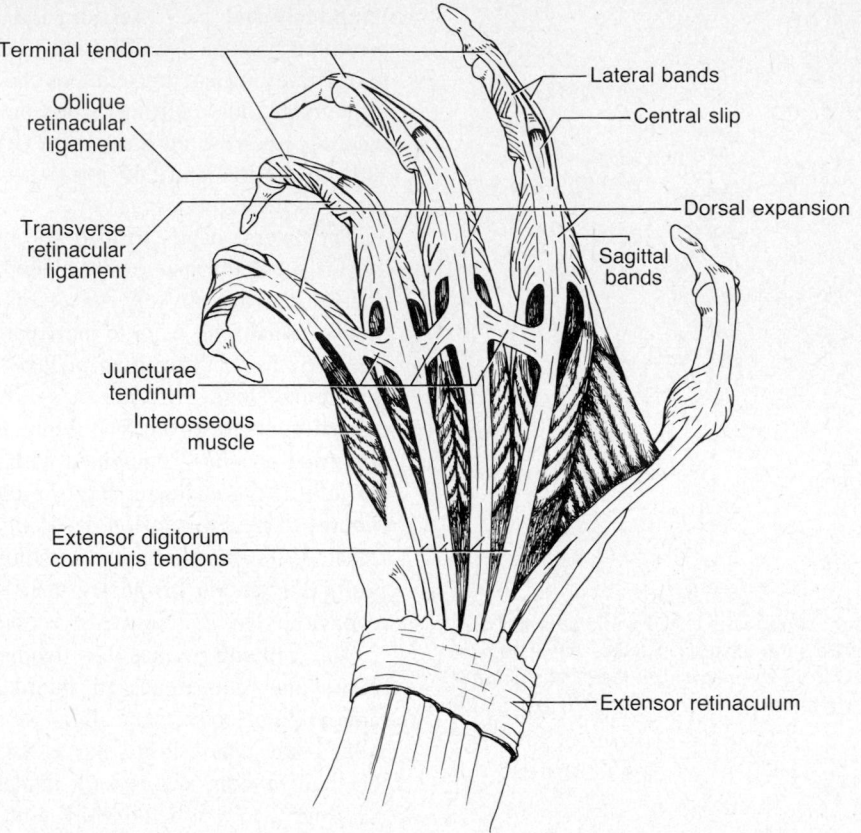

Terminal tendon

Oblique retinacular ligament

Transverse retinacular ligament

Juncturae tendinum

Interosseous muscle

Extensor digitorum communis tendons

Lateral bands

Central slip

Dorsal expansion

Sagittal bands

Extensor retinaculum

Fig. 18-7. Dorsal hood apparatus, extensor tendons, and ligaments of fingers.

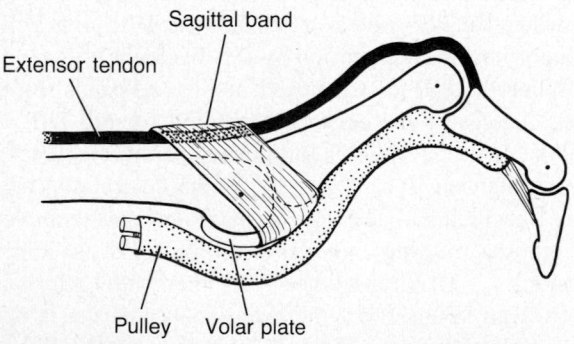

Sagittal band

Extensor tendon

Pulley Volar plate

Fig. 18-8. Sagittal bands extend proximal phalanx, rendering distal attachments of extensor digitorum communis lax. (Modified from Smith RJ: Clin Orthop 104:92, 1974.)

ture, as in rheumatoid arthritis, attempts to flex the fingers via the profundus result in transmission of force through the lumbricals into the extensor apparatus, contributing to IP extension rather than flexion. This may result in a lumbrical-plus deformity—that is, MP joint flexion and IP joint extension. The lumbrical muscles serve as a primary organ of feedback in the hand. They are ideally suited to link position and movement of the hand and finger joints because they were shown by Rabischong to contain more annulospiral endings per unit length than any other muscle in the body.[35]

Neurology

Motor innervation. Clinical evaluation of neurological damage is made difficult by the numerous muscles controlling the digits, the considerable substitution, and the sometimes varying nerve supplies of these muscles. Following is a general summary of the major nerves and the corresponding loss of function following their injury.

The median nerve in its passage along the forearm supplies the following muscles: pronator teres, flexor carpi radialis, palmaris longus, and flexor digitorum sublimis. The anterior interosseous branch of the median nerve innervates the flexor pollicis longus, pronator quadratus, and flexor digitorum profundus (to the index, the middle, and sometimes the ring fingers). The median nerve then passes under the flexor retinaculum and enters the palm, splitting into a sensory branch and a motor branch. The latter supplies the abductor pollicis brevis, opponens pollicis, flexor pollicis brevis, and first and second lumbrical muscles.

Impairment resulting from median nerve paralysis in-

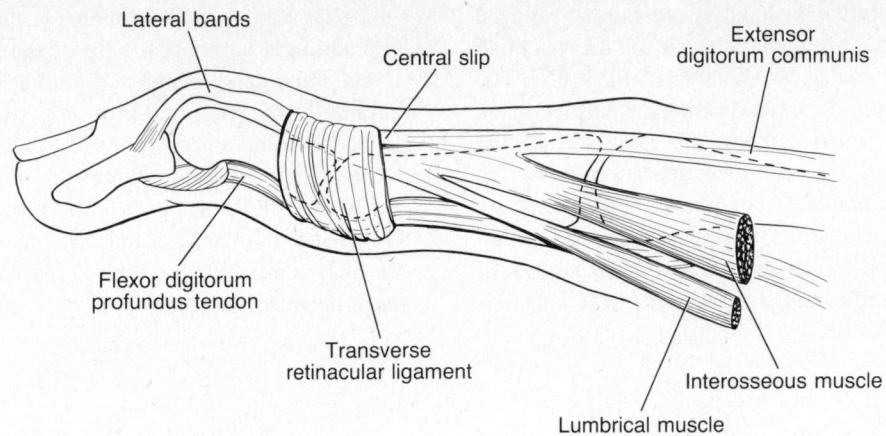

Fig. 18-9. Swan neck deformity, demonstrating laxity of transverse retinacular ligament. (Modified from Smith RJ: Clin Orthop 104:92, 1974.)

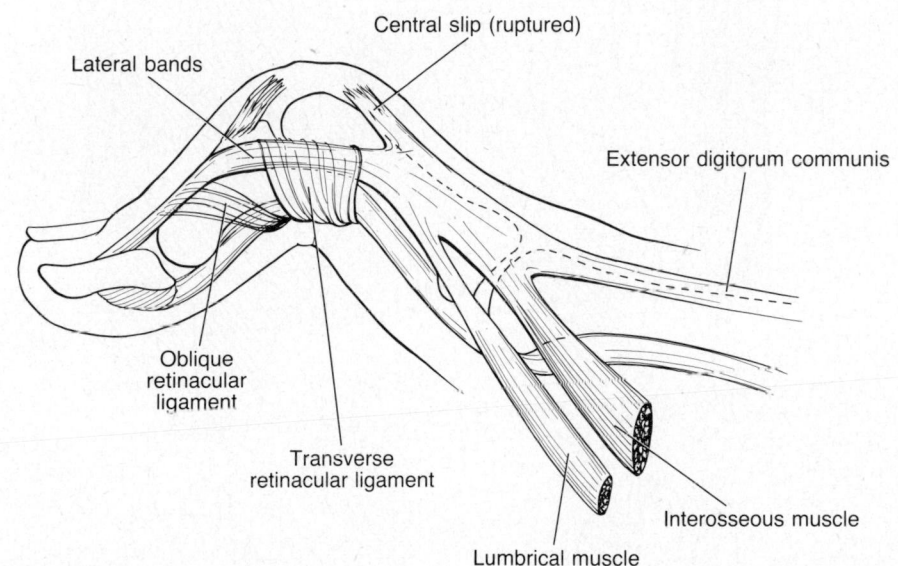

Fig. 18-10. Boutonniere deformity, demonstrating rupture of central slip. (Modified from Souter WA: Clin Orthop 104:116, 1974.)

cludes the inability to oppose the thumb, flex the IP joint of the thumb, and flex the first two fingers, resulting in a *benediction attitude*. Loss of the above functions severely hinders the ability to perform precision maneuvers.[17]

The ulnar nerve supplies the following muscles in the forearm: flexor carpi ulnaris and flexor digitorum profundus (to the little and sometimes the ring fingers). In the hand the muscles it innervates are the flexor digiti minimi, abductor digiti minimi, opponens digiti minimi, adductor pollicis, palmaris brevis, third and fourth lumbricals, and the interossei.

Paralysis of the ulnar nerve produces loss of thumb adduction (lateral pinch), weakness in power grip,[17] finger spreading, and inability to perform coordinated activities, such as piano playing. An ulnar claw hand deformity, also

called an *intrinsic minus* hand with MP joint extension and IP joint flexion, often results. This deformity is more severe in lesions distal to innervation of the flexor digitorum profundus.

The motor supply of the radial nerve is confined to the forearm, where branches are given to these muscles: extensor carpi radialis longus and brevis, extensor carpi ulnaris, supinator, extensor digitorum communis, abductor pollicis longus, extensor pollicis longus and brevis, extensor indicis, and extensor digiti minimi.

Radial nerve paralysis prevents extension of the wrist and MP joints of the fingers. Since wrist extension provides synergistic and stabilizing functions, this loss can significantly hamper hand function. The ability to extend and abduct the thumb is also lost.

Sensory innervation. The hand is sometimes referred to as a sensory organ because 24% of all the pacinian (touch) corpuscles in the body are located therein.[11] The motor system absolutely depends on the constant feedback it receives from the sensory receptors. Branches of the three major peripheral nerves carry sensation from the hand in the following manner:

The median nerve transmits sensation from the lateral portion of the palm and thenar surface and the volar part of the thumb, index, middle, and lateral half of the ring fin-gers, extending over the dorsum of the terminal phalanges; innervation is purest at the tip of the index finger.

The ulnar nerve supplies the ulnar side of the hand, medial half of the ring, and little finger (both dorsal and volar surfaces); innervation is purest at the tip of the little finger.

The radial nerve innervates the dorsum of the hand lateral to the fourth metacarpal and the dorsal surfaces of the thumb and the first two and one-half digits as far distal as the DIP joints; innervation is purest at the dorsal web space between the thumb and index finger (Fig. 18-11).

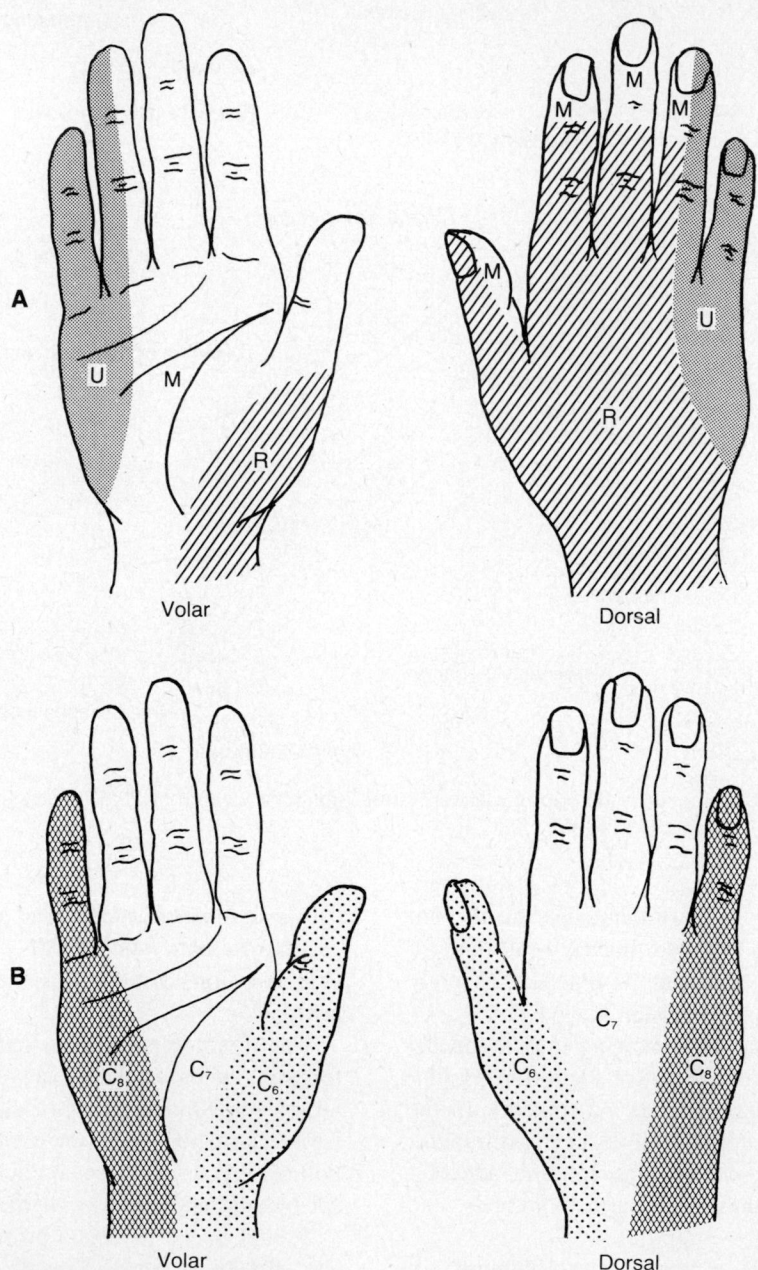

Volar   Dorsal

Volar   Dorsal

Fig. 18-11. A, Delineation of peripheral cutaneous sensation supplied by radial *(R)*, median *(M)*, and ulnar *(U)* nerves. **B,** Delineation of sensation derived from cervical root levels C6, C7, and C8. (Modified from Cailliet R: Hand pain and impairment, ed 2, Philadelphia, 1975, FA Davis Co.)

Sensory changes produced by cervical root pressure are commonly experienced in the most distal areas of the dermatomes, of which C-6, C-7, and C-8 extend into the hand. When the hand is evaluated, knowledge of the dermatomal distribution helps differentiate between nerve root and peripheral nerve lesions. Root level representation includes C-6 to the thenar area and thumb, C-7 to the mid-palm and dorsal areas and index, middle, and ring fingers, and C-8 to the hypothenar area and little finger (see Fig. 18-11).[7] Because of the similar patterns of C-8 and ulnar nerve sensory distribution, additional motor tests may be necessary to make a differential diagnosis.

Angiology

Arteries. The hand receives its blood from the radial and ulnar arteries. The radial artery courses along the lateral side of the forearm to the wrist, where its pulse is palpable just lateral to the flexor carpi radialis tendon. After giving off the superficial palmar branch, it winds laterally around the dorsum of the wrist and enters the palm between the first and second metacarpals, where it forms the deep palmar arch by uniting with the deep branch of the ulnar artery. The radial artery gives off a superficial palmar branch proximal to the scaphoid, which anastomoses with the corresponding ulnar branch, forming the superficial palmar arch. This arch is larger and more significant than the deep arch.

The ulnar artery crosses the wrist medially, where it is superficial to the flexor retinaculum. Just distal to the pisiform, it divides into a superficial branch (which continues across the palm as the superficial palmar arch) and a deep branch (which anastomoses with the radial artery, completing the deep arch).

From the deep palmar arch arise the palmar metacarpal arteries, which join the palmar digital arteries from the superficial arch. They extend into the fingers as digital arteries.

Veins. The hand is drained by a plexus of superficial and deep veins, of which the superficial is most significant.

The superficial system is better developed over the dorsal surface of the hand and becomes increasingly prominent with age. At the level of the wrist this system converges into the cephalic vein laterally and the basilic vein medially, both of which ascend superficially up the forearm.

The deep veins of the hand travel in pairs with the arteries (vena comitantes). They ascend from the digits to the palmar arches to the radial and ulnar arteries.

• • •

Given an understanding of these anatomical and pathokinesiological concepts, the clinician has a sound foundation to proceed with the evaluation of the client with hand dysfunction. Evaluation, in many respects, is the application of anatomy and kinesiology because the affected part is often identified by comparison of its aberrant structure and function with the norm.

EXAMINATION OF THE WRIST AND HAND

The rehabilitation goal of any client with hand disability—whether it is caused by birth defect, injury, or disease—is to obtain adequate hand and wrist function and cosmetic appearance and return to his/her former life-style in the shortest amount of time and at the least expense possible. To accomplish this goal, teamwork is essential. Health professionals as well as the client must join efforts in promoting the comprehensive care needed to achieve optimal results.

Accurate evaluation of the client's condition is a critical element in the rehabilitative process and the responsibility of all members of the team. The evaluative results provide information for establishing a diagnosis, setting realistic goals, planning a program of treatment and management, and determining a baseline for measuring progress. Also, the evaluation establishes functional impairment and cosmetic defects and informs insurance companies and law courts of the client's status. The rehabilitation team members may assume responsibility for different parts of the evaluation to accommodate their individual areas of expertise, but the overall process should yield a compilation of clear, precise, factual data that will be of subsequent use to multiple parties.

Following is a synopsis of procedures and techniques of importance to the orthopaedic physical therapist examining the hand. The examination requires thoroughness and accuracy, and the tests used should be objective, valid, and reliable. Methods for recording history and measuring anatomical, functional, and cosmetic deficits should be standardized, routine, and facilitated by the use of a form for listing the required information in an orderly fashion.[31] Because it is often difficult to visualize the relationship and extent of involvement of the numerous structures of the hand, a photographic record is also helpful in portraying the condition.

Before the examination the therapist should organize all testing equipment, forms, and materials he/she anticipates using. The examination area should also be prepared and should offer privacy and comfort to the client. Proper attire should be made available to the client in accordance with the needs of the examination.

The examination comprises two major areas: the client's history and the physical examination. The history provides relevant information about the site, nature, and behavior of current symptoms, as well as related background data. The content of the history, in conjunction with the provisional diagnosis if available, dictates the scope of the physical examination that follows. The physical examination is an objective means of revealing abnormalities in structure and function. After obtaining both subjective and objective data, the therapist proceeds to develop a problem list and plan for further testing, treatment, and management.

The format for an organized and sequential examination is described here. For convenience this process is also condensed into a wrist and hand examination form, which is easily adapted to most clinical settings. To determine the extent of the hand dysfunction, it is advisable to first perform a general assessment of the cervical spine and upper extremities. This ensures that referred pain or multiple lesions are recognized and their effect on the hand appreciated. The hand's location as the most distal member of the extremity often makes it the recipient of pain that is commonly referred from a proximal cause. Details of the examination of the cervical spine and other areas of the upper extremity are found in Chapters 19, 20, and 21.

History

When the client's history is obtained, it is important that certain questions are asked (Fig. 18-12). The evaluation form includes blanks for recording the identifying data (i.e., name, age, sex, and date). The provisional diagnosis and the precautions to be taken by the examiner based on the client's status or information found in the medical record, if available, should be listed on the evaluation form. The *chief complaint* is the client's brief description of the primary disturbance for which help is being sought.

Hand dominance is indicated. The condition of the hand before the onset of current symptoms should be noted; this is useful in delineating future expectations for the extremity.

Description of the present illness is a very important part of the history. The date of injury should be indicated if the disorder results from trauma; the date of onset should be indicated when the disorder is insidious (rheumatoid arthritis) or abrupt (localized infection). If the client required hospitalization, the dates should be included. The duration of incapacity should be stated. Note that the duration of incapacity may differ from the time elapsed since injury or onset; that is, a client may have suffered a hand burn in June (date of injury) but did not experience incapacity until hypertrophic scarring became severe in December (beginning of incapacity). It has often been observed that the longer a client has been incapacitated, the less likely it is that he/she will make a full recovery.

In the event of trauma, details are needed regarding the nature, mechanism, and ensuing results of the injury. For example, understanding how the finger was positioned when it was struck will help the therapist determine which structures were stressed and possibly damaged. Audible sounds at the time of injury are also helpful in distinguishing the structure injured. Deformity (i.e., interruption of bone, joint, or tendon continuity) should be described. If the client suffered disability following the incident, the

---

WRIST AND HAND EXAMINATION FORM

A. HISTORY

   1. Identifying data

      Name _____ Age _____ Sex _____ Date _____

      Provisional diagnosis _____ Precautions _____

      Chief complaint _____

      Dominant hand   R _____ L _____ Prior condition of hand _____

   2. Present illness

      Date of injury/onset _____ Insidious _____ Abrupt _____

      Dates of hospitalization _____ Duration of incapacity _____

      Nature and mechanism of injury _____

      _____

      Audible sounds at time of injury _____

      Results of injury

         Deformity _____ Corrected _____

         Disability: Type _____ Reason _____

         Time sequence _____

         Loss of motion (specify) _____ Time sequence _____

         Loss of strength (specify) _____ Time sequence _____

         Swelling: Immediate _____ After 24 hours _____

         Bleeding: Location _____ Amount _____

      Treatments, dates, and results _____

      _____

      _____

Fig. 18-12. Wrist and hand examination form: history, including identifying data and present illness through treatments.

type (e.g., restricted motion) and the reason (pain or bony block) should be detailed. The time sequence of disability also needs to be described. For example, a fall on the dorsiflexed wrist produces immediate pain from lunate dislocation but later produces symptoms of median nerve compression.

Loss of motion and strength should be determined; in both instances it is important to know the type of motion (e.g., MP flexion) or strength (lateral pinch) involved as well as the time sequence of development. The loss may be immediate, such as in rupture of a contractile structure, or slowly progressive, resulting from the effect of effusion within a joint or within an unyielding space occupied by nerves and vessels susceptible to compression.

Swelling around the traumatized area should be de-

scribed. It may result from bleeding, which will be obvious in 2 to 4 hours, or synovial joint effusion, which may take 12 to 24 hours to accumulate to a notable amount. If external bleeding occurs from a laceration or compound fracture, the location and amount may have important implications in emergency proceedings. The treatment(s) received by the client for the current condition, including the dates and results, should be described thoroughly. This provides information regarding the prior response of the client to, and efficacy or ineffectiveness of, specific regimens.

The present status of the condition should be assessed (Fig. 18-13). The client should be asked to judge whether the condition is acute, chronic, or intermittent and whether the symptoms are static or becoming better or worse. A

WRIST AND HAND EXAMINATION FORM—cont'd

Present status of condition: acute_____ chronic_____ intermittent_____ static_____
    better_____ worse_____
Musculoskeletal structure behavior
    Joint: catches_____ locks_____ grates_____ clicks_____ swells_____ dislocates_____
    Muscle: spasm_____ weak_____ increased tone_____ decreased tone_____
    Other: _____
Description of symptoms
    Location (code)
        Key: //// = pain
                ==== = paresthesia
                oooo = numbness
                xxxx = other 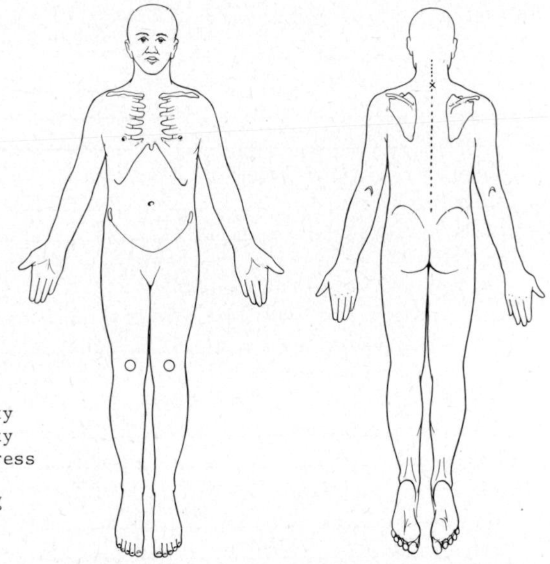
    Severity
        Scale: 1 = best
                  10 = worst

        0————————————————10

    Impairment
        Scale: 0%-25%   = annoying
                  25%-50%   = interferes with
                               activity
                  50%-75%   = prevents activity
                  75%-100% = prevents activity
                               and causes distress

        0%————————————————100%

    Nature
        Ache_____ Stab_____
        Throb_____ Twinge_____
        Burn_____ Tingle_____
        Other_____
    Constancy
        Constant_____ Varies in intensity_____
        When occurs_____ What elicits_____
        What worsens_____
        What improves_____
        How long lasting_____
        Morning stiffness_____ Duration_____

Fig. 18-13. Wrist and hand examination form: history, including present illness from present status through description of symptoms.

description of the behavior of the affected musculoskeletal structure should be requested; for example, does a joint catch, swell, or dislocate, or does a muscle display spasm or weakness? The client should be asked to describe the symptoms, delineating their location on a body chart. The severity of the condition and the impairment it imposes should be subjectively assessed according to given scales. A description of the nature of the symptoms should also be obtained from the client. It should be determined if the symptoms are constant; if they are, but vary in intensity, the client should be asked what makes them worse and what improves them. If they are not constant, the client should be asked when they occur, what elicits them, and what improves them. The presence and duration of morning stiffness should be ascertained; rheumatoid arthritis typically produces stiffness lasting 30 minutes or more after rising, whereas degenerative types of arthritis produce stiffness of shorter duration. The effects of rest and exercise may give a clue to the origin of symptoms; most acute disorders of the musculoskeletal system improve with rest and are aggravated by activity. Chronic types of disorders may become stiff with rest and improve with exercise in moderation. Disorders of visceral origin are generally not affected by rest or exercise.

To determine the relevant past history, a similar condition suffered in the past should be noted, including dates, nature, and treatment. Previous injury or preexisting pain may also alter a patient's ability or unwillingness to perform particular exercises. If other areas of the body are affected in addition to the hand, it is feasible to investigate for the presence of congenital anomalies or systemic disorders. Other relevant illnesses and general health status should then be summarized (Fig. 18-14).

A family history should include health problems of immediate family members and the presence of any familial diseases. A life-style summary should include the occupation, habits, living conditions, and physical activities of the client. What the client does to promote wellness may give some indication of the responsibility he/she will be likely to assume in a rehabilitation program. The client's concept of the cause of the complaint should be elicited. After all, the process of history taking is the examiner's opportunity to listen to the client. Also the client's description of functional and cosmetic deficits produced by the

WRIST AND HAND EXAMINATION FORM—cont'd

3. Relevant past history
    History of similar condition: Dates _____ Nature _____
    _____
    Treatment _____
    Other body parts affected _____
    Other relevant illnesses _____
    General health status _____

4. Family history
    Health problems of immediate family _____
    Familial diseases _____

5. Life-style
    Occupation _____ Habits _____
    Living conditions _____
    Regular (3 times/week) physical activities requiring:
        Strength _____ Agility _____
        Endurance _____ Flexibility _____
        Other _____
    What client does to promote wellness _____
    Client's concept of cause of condition _____
    Client's concept of functional deficit _____
    Client's concept of cosmetic deficit _____
    Anticipated life-style and goals _____

6. Other considerations
    Current medications _____
    Recent radiographs _____

Fig. 18-14. Wrist and hand examination form: history, including relevant past history, family history, life-style, and other considerations.

condition, as well as anticipated life-style, goals, and treatment expectations, are important in assessing the overall severity of the case and in planning for future management. Other considerations, including a listing of current medications and the interpretation of recent radiographs, completes the client's history (see Fig. 18-14).

Physical examination

Based on the interpretation of information obtained from the client history, a plan for the physical examination is formulated. The examiner selects the method, technique, and procedures that are appropriate to the purpose, body part, and client's status and that have a high potential for providing reliable baseline or comparative data. The comprehensiveness, focus, and detail of the physical examination are determined by the data base and client's response and are continuously modified so that they remain consistent with emerging data. Before the examination is initiated it may be necessary to take a quick pause to ensure that the needed equipment, forms, and materials are on hand.

The physical examination begins with inspection, during which the client is essentially untouched but is observed by the examiner. Inspection begins with the initial handshake and continues throughout the history taking: the general attitude of the extremity and positions of various joints should be noticed without the client's awareness. Next the appearance and posture of the hand should be noted (Fig. 18-15). The attitude of the hand at rest often portrays common deformities, such as ulnar deviation, volar subluxation of the MP joints, swan neck, clawing, and Dupuytren's contracture. The hand might also demonstrate collapse of the normal longitudinal or transverse arch framework—invariably affecting function—which can result from skeletal malalignment, muscle imbalance, or joint instability.

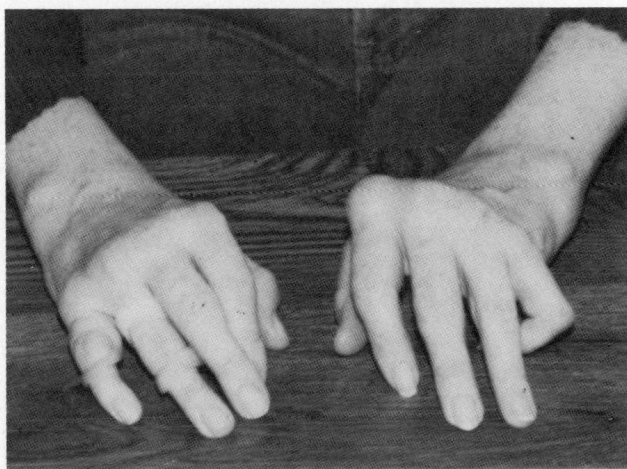

Fig. 18-15. Inspection of rheumatoid hands.

Next the shape of the hand should be described. Changes in contour should be noted, which may result from protuberances or nodules (such as ganglia or Heberden's nodes), loss of arches, absence of digits, narrowed web spaces, deviations in length and alignment, and swelling or atrophy. Circumferential measurements should be made at designated anatomical sites as described by Fess et al[10]: 7 cm proximal to the elbow flexion crease (arm), 11 cm proximal to the distal wrist flexion crease (forearm), at the distal wrist flexion crease (wrist), and at the distal palmar flexion crease (hand). Peripheral neuropathies typically produce atrophy of thenar and hypothenar eminences and guttering over the area of the interossei. Median nerve damage also can affect the thenar eminence with a type of atrophy commonly noted in carpal tunnel syndrome. Ulnar nerve loss is reflected by hypothenar and interossei atrophy. Generalized atrophy may also be associated with immobilization, but one should be alert to the fact that it can be masked by edema. A volumetric measurement is often indicated in cases of generalized edema, in which a volumeter is used for applying the principle of water displacement. Bilateral comparison helps identify subtle abnormalities. The clinical evaluation form is devised so that a number of deviations in shape can be easily charted on a diagram of the hand by means of a code (Fig. 18-16).

Use of the hand may be inspected as the client moves about and prepares for examination (e.g., when removing necessary clothing). Is the hand used in an effortless, coordinated manner, or are movements labored, jerky, stiff, protected, or compensated for? Unwillingness to put weight on the wrist when pushing up from a chair may be indicative of a painful arthritic condition or sprain of the carpal ligaments. Reflex sympathetic dystrophy is often associated with a painful edematous hand that the client protects and uses reluctantly if at all. Jerky, uncoordinated movements may stem from a neurological disorder.

The skin should be inspected for scars, lesions, color, texture, hair patterns, and nail changes. Trophic changes of the skin are common in peripheral vascular disease, diabetes mellitus, reflex sympathetic dystrophy, and Raynaud's disease. Clubbing and cyanosis of the nails are displayed in conjunction with pulmonary dysfunction. Again, use of a hand sketch facilitates localization of skin defects (Fig. 18-17).

Inspection ends with review and description of external aids worn by the client. The intended purpose of the aid should also be listed (e.g., a cock-up wrist splint worn to alleviate symptoms of carpal tunnel syndrome or "outrigger" flexor orthosis worn to prevent active finger flexion during healing of flexor tendon repair).

The next part of the physical examination deals with the assessment of movement. Because of the detail encompassed in this area, it is probably one of the most important contributions of the therapist to the overall evaluation

WRIST AND HAND EXAMINATION FORM—cont'd

B. PHYSICAL EXAMINATION

    1. Inspection

        a. Posture _____

           General appearance of extremity _____

           Joints affected: shoulder _____ elbow _____ wrist _____ thumb _____

               fingers I _____ M _____ R _____ L _____

           Hand posture/attitude at rest _____

           Integrity of arches _____

        b. Shape

           Key: X = missing digit

                   At = atrophy

                   S = swelling

                   D = deviation

                   θ = lacks web

                   An = ankylosis

                   SN = swan neck

                   B = boutonniere

               D/S = dislocation/subluxation

                   M = mallet finger

                   Z = collapse deformity

                   N = nodule

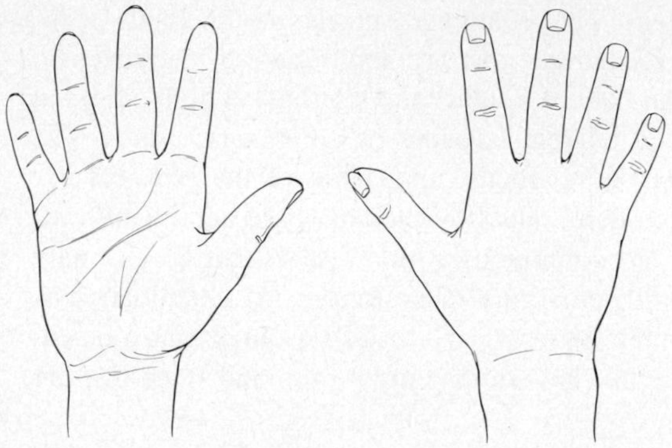

Circumferential measurements: arm _____ forearm _____ wrist _____ hand _____

Volumetric measurement: involved hand _____ ml displaced

                             uninvolved hand _____ ml displaced

Symmetry of extremities: yes _____ no _____ (explain) _____

Fig. 18-16. Wrist and hand examination form: physical examination, including inspection from posture through shape.

WRIST AND HAND EXAMINATION FORM—cont'd

        c. Use

           Hand protected/use restricted _____

           Handles clothing: independently _____ minimum assistance _____ maximum assistance _____

           Movement: jerky _____ stiff _____ uncoordinated _____ limited by pain _____

        d. Skin

           Key: C = cyanotic

                   R = reddened

                   W = whitened

                   S = scar

                   L = lesion

                   F = fixation

                  Na = nail deformity

                   T = texture changed

                  Ne = necrosis

                   H = abnormal hair pattern

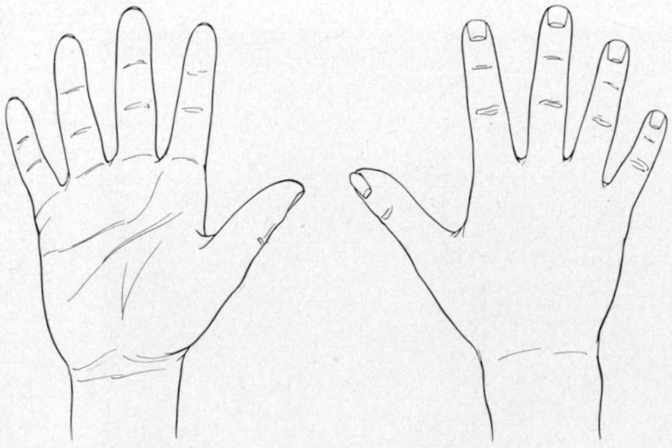

        e. Aids: sling _____ splint _____ orthosis _____ other _____

           Description _____

           Purpose _____

Fig. 18-17. Wrist and hand examination form: physical examination, including use, skin, and aids.

WRIST AND HAND EXAMINATION FORM—cont'd

2. Movement
   a. Functional active movements

   Power grip_____ (hammer)   Key: C = completes task
   Precision grip_____ (writing)   D = completes task with difficulty/discomfort
   Hook grip_____ (suitcase)   N = not able to complete task
   Lateral pinch_____ (key)
   Cylinder grasp_____ (2.5-cm cylinder)
   Spherical grasp_____ (5-cm ball)

Gross range of motion

Distance (cm)	I	M	R	L
Fingertips to PP crease				
Fingertips to MP crease				
Fingertips to dorsal plane				

Ability (yes or no)

Pulp-to-pulp pinch				
Lateral (key) pinch				

Gross grip and pinch strength

   Grip (Jaymar dynamometer) _____kg   handle position_____
   Grip, alternative (sphygmomanometer) _____mm Hg
   Pinch (pinch meter)
       Key (lateral) _____g
       Pulp _____g I_____g M_____g R_____g L_____g

Special tests

	+	-	Comments
Finklestein			
Bunnel-Littler			
Oblique retinacular ligament			
Weight bearing on extended wrist			

Fig. 18-18. Wrist and hand examination form: physical examination, including functional active movements and special tests.

process. Movements are divided into two groups, functional and physiological, for testing purposes. Functional active movements include the various types of grips, grasps, and pinches, which are assessed according to the ease with which the client completes the task (Fig. 18-18). A therapist may relate how well a client performs these maneuvers through handling of common objects, standardized tools, such as the Jebsen Hand Function test, or computerized devices, such as the BTE Work Simulator.*

Gross range of motion and strength tests are performed in functional positions. Maximal finger flexion incorporat-

ing all three joints is measured simply by determining the distance the fingertip lacks in touching the proximal palmar crease (Fig. 18-19, A), whereas to measure only the IP joints, the distance from the MP crease is determined. The same technique is applied to measuring gross extension, which is done by determining the distance the fingertip lacks in touching a flat surface extending from the plane of the dorsum of the hand (Fig. 18-19, B).

Pulp and lateral pinch ability are first determined by having the client attempt to oppose the thumb to each successive finger using a pulp pinch and then a lateral pinch. The ability to accomplish this feat is recorded simply as affirmative or negative. Gross grip strength is measured by

*Baltimore Therapeutic Equipment Co.

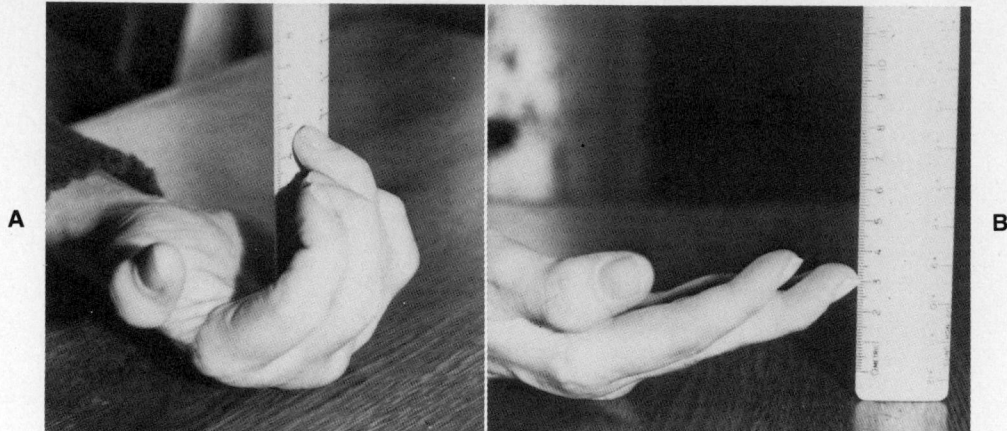

Fig. 18-19. A, Gross flexion is measured as distance between fingertips and proximal palmar crease. **B,** Gross extension is measured as distance between fingertips and dorsal plane.

a Jaymar dynamometer. Force generated by a normal man is about 46 kg and by a normal woman about 23 kg.[31,35] Four kilograms of force is required to perform 90% of daily living activities.[31] If the client is unable to grasp the dynamometer with the handle in the standard second position, adjustments are noted. If the client is not able to grip the dynamometer, a sphygmomanometer may be used. The attached blood pressure cuff is rolled to a 5 cm diameter and inflated to 50 mm Hg; as the cuff is squeezed, the change from 50 is recorded as the grip strength.[31] The normal grip strength of a man is usually greater than 300 mm, while the grip strength of a woman is about 200 mm. A pinch meter is used in testing pinch strength. It is held between the thumb pulp and lateral side of the middle phalanx of the index finger for lateral (key) pinch and the pulps of successive fingers for pulp pinch (see Fig. 18-18). The average pinch strengths for men and women are listed in Table 18-1.

Special tests include the Finkelstein test for tenosynovitis of the extensor pollicis brevis and abductor pollicis longus, in which the thumb is flexed and the wrist adducted to produce maximal tension on the involved musculotendinous structures. A positive test produces sharp pain over the radial aspect of the wrist and is often indicative of de Quervain's disease.

The Bunnel-Littler test is performed to ascertain intrinsic tightness. If the PIP joint lacks flexion, the problem could be caused by tightness of the intrinsic muscles, extrinsic extensor muscles, or joint capsule. To distinguish the structure involved, the MP joint is passively extended to tense the intrinsics and the PIP joint is passively flexed; then the MP joint is passively flexed, and if PIP joint flexion increases, the intrinsic muscle is at fault (Fig. 18-20, A). A test for shortening of the oblique retinacular ligament is based on the same principle: if DIP joint flexion is limited, the problem could be caused by either shortening of the ligament or capsular tightness. To distinguish the

Table 18-1. Average pinch strengths for men and women

	Men (g)	Women (g)
Lateral (key) pinch	7.3	4.8
Pulp pinch (index)	5.1	3.5
Pulp pinch (middle)	5.7	3.6
Pulp pinch (ring)	3.7	2.5
Pulp pinch (little)	2.3	1.7

From Swanson AB, Gorän-Hagert C, and Swanson G: Evaluation of impairment of hand function. In Hunter JM et al, editors: Rehabilitation of the hand, ed 2, St. Louis, 1983, The CV Mosby Co; and from Wynn Parry CB: Rehabilitation of the hand, ed 3, Sussex, 1973, Butterworth Publishers.

cause, the PIP joint is passively extended to tense the ligament and the DIP joint flexion is passively flexed; then the PIP joint is passively flexed, and if DIP joint flexion increases, the ligament is at fault (Fig. 18-20, B).

The client is asked to support his/her weight on the extended wrist, as in raising himself/herself from a chair. Pain produced in this manner is a positive test for injury or inflammation of the carpal joint ligaments, capsule, or synovium.

Physiological movements are assessed using traditional techniques for measuring individual joint range of motion and for testing the strength of isolated muscles. Precise measurements of active and passive joint range of motion are obtained through appropriate goniometric procedures. Selection of the instrument size is dictated by the joint being measured, and finger goniometers are available for the MP and IP joints (Fig. 18-21). Use of the neutral zero method (all motions measured from a zero starting position) is recommended by the American Academy of Orthopaedic Surgeons. Also, proximal joints should be in a neutral position when distal joints are measured to standardize the influence of tendon excursion.

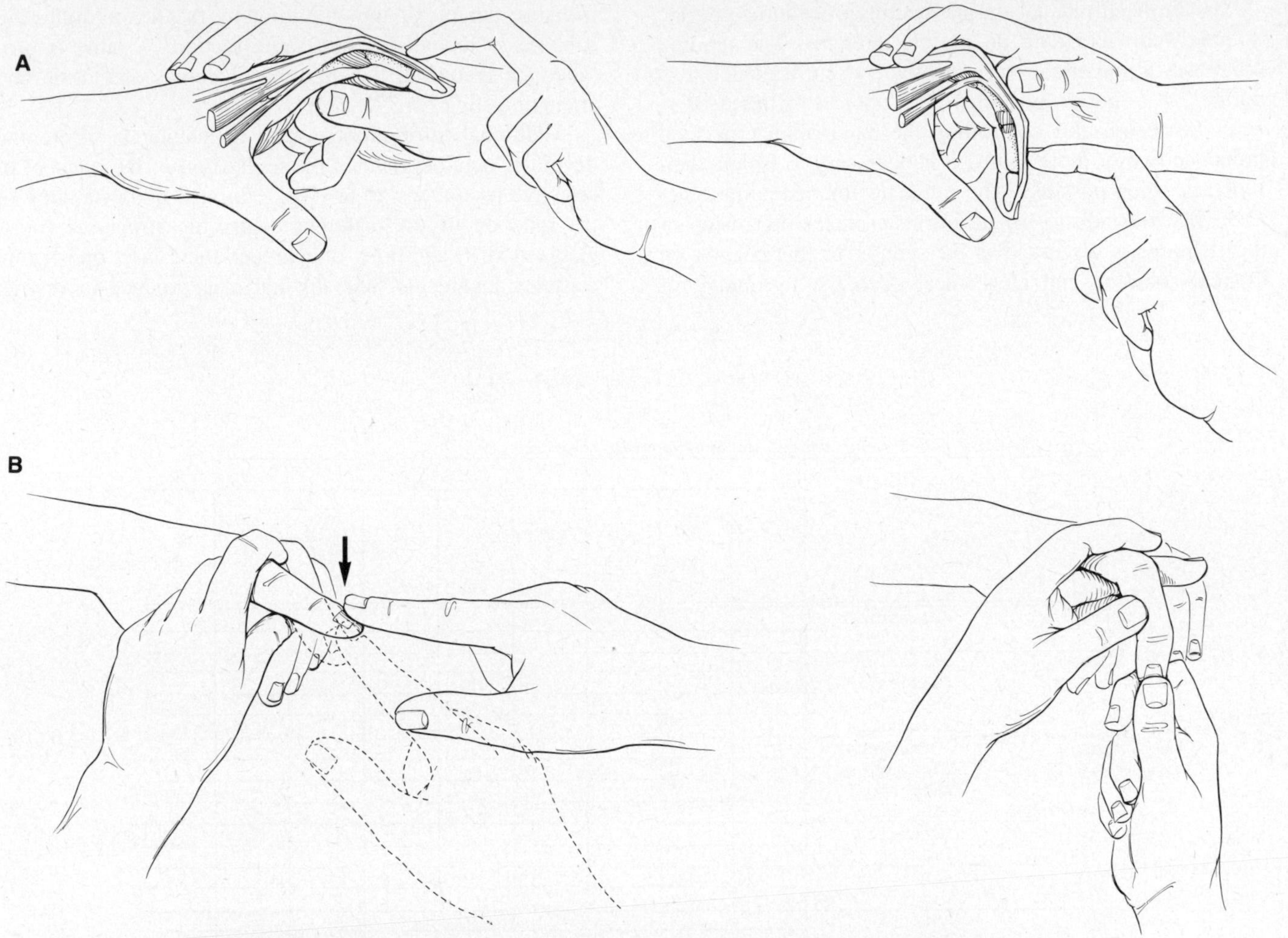

A

B

Fig. 18-20. **A,** Bunnel-Littler test for intrinsic tightness is performed by comparing amount of PIP joint flexion possible with MP joint extended versus flexed. **B,** Retinacular ligament test is performed by comparing amount of DIP joint flexion possible with PIP joint extended versus flexed. (Modified from Hoppenfeld S: Physical examination of the spine and extremities, New York, 1976, Appleton-Century-Crofts.)

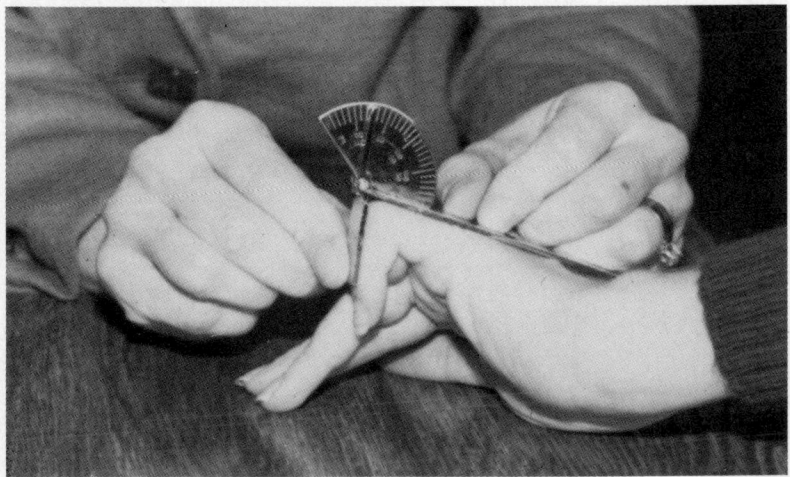

Fig. 18-21. Use of finger goniometer to measure range of motion in digit.

Standardized manual muscle testing procedures provide reliable and valid data on muscle strength. The grading scale uses a numerical or descriptive system in which 5 = normal, 4 = good, 3 = fair, 2 = poor, 1 = trace, 0 = zero. Since muscles controlling the hand often cross and influence two or more joints, it is necessary to isolate their function when possible. The rationale for maintaining active MP extension to isolate intrinsic muscle extension of the IP joints is discussed in the section of this chapter on clinical anatomy and mechanics. Also the technique for isolating flexion of the PIP joint by the flexor digitorum sublimis is included in the same section. A table is provided for recording the multiple outcomes of motion and strength testing (Fig. 18-22).

Additional information useful in making a differential diagnosis may be gleaned by application of the concept of selective tissue tension testing.[8] Through understanding of the function of the different contractile structures (muscles, tendons, and bony attachments) and inert ones (joint capsules, ligaments, bursae) that may produce or restrict

WRIST AND HAND EXAMINATION FORM—cont'd

b/c/d. Physiological movements: active/passive/resistive

			Active			Passive				Resistive	
			Degrees	Symptoms	Quality	Degrees	Symptoms	End-feel	Limiting structures	Strength	Symptoms
Forearm		supination									
		pronation									
Wrist		extension									
		flexion									
		abduction									
		adduction									
Thumb	CM	extension									
		flexion									
		abduction									
		adduction									
	MP	extension									
		flexion									
	IP	extension									
		flexion									
Index	MP	extension									
		flexion									
		abduction									
		adduction									
	PIP	extension									
		flexion									
	DIP	extension									
		flexion									
Middle	MP	extension									
		flexion									
		abduction									
		adduction									
	PIP	extension									
		flexion									
	DIP	extension									
		flexion									
Ring	MP	extension									
		flexion									
		abduction									
		adduction									
	PIP	extension									
		flexion									
	DIP	extension									
		flexion									
Little	MP	extension									
		flexion									
		abduction									
		adduction									
	PIP	extension									
		flexion									
	DIP	extension									
		flexion									

Fig. 18-22. Wrist and hand examination form: physical examination, including physiological movements.

movement, tension can be selectively applied to each. In this way, if the client's symptoms can be reproduced, the examiner can identify structures at fault. Active movements test the client's general ability and willingness to perform movement and demonstrate the degree of joint or soft tissue irritability. The extent, symptoms, and quality (ability to perform deftly without deviations or substitution) are recorded. Passive movements apply tension to the inert structures that normally limit and guide movement and maintain joint integrity. Passive movement may also be used to stress a contractile structure by applying force in a direction opposite to that in which the muscle moves the part. With the client totally relaxed, the examiner documents the range of passive motion permitted in each joint, as well as the symptoms and end-feel (bony block, spasm, capsular, empty) elicited by the test. The structure responsible for limiting motion is also noted (e.g., "intrinsic muscle contracture limits PIP joint flexion" or "collateral ligament contracture limits MP joint flexion").

An examiner should also pay close attention to the end-feel of the joint, as well as the sequence of pain and passive limitation in order to assess the irritability of a lesion.

The *constant length phenomenon* is a useful concept for isolating the site of range of motion restriction when the process of elimination involves soft tissue that spans two or more joints. For example, Dypuytren's contracture of the palmar subcutaneous tissue limits the excursion of the fibrous extensions into the fingers. The constant length of this tissue allows the MP joint to be extended only when the PIP joint is flexed or permits the PIP joint to be extended only when the MP joint is flexed. An examiner applies this same principle when testing the intrinsic muscles (Bunnell-Littler test) and extrinsic finger tendons as described earlier. Resisted movements test the contractile structures' ability to develop and sustain tension. An isometric contraction is desired to minimize the involvement of inert structures. The examiner records the strength and symptoms resulting from specific motions.

To conclude the assessment of movement, joint play movements are applied to the wrist and hand joints at which such movements are feasible (Fig. 18-23). The joint mobility is graded and elicitation of symptoms noted based on the following: 0 = ankylosis, 1 = extremely hypomobile, 2 = slightly hypomobile, 3 = normal, 4 = slightly

WRIST AND HAND EXAMINATION FORM—cont'd

e. Joint play movements

		Mobility (grade 0-6)	Symptoms
Radiocarpal and midcarpal joints	dorsal glide		
	volar glide		
	radial glide		
	ulnar glide		
Ulnomeniscotriquetral "joint"			
Intercarpal joints	scaphoid		
	lunate		
	triquetrum		
	pisiform		
	trapezium		
	trapezoid		
	capitate		
	hamate		
Carpometacarpal joints	1st		
	4th		
	5th		
Intermetacarpal joints	2-3		
	3-4		
	4-5		
Metacarpophalangeal joints	1		
	2		
	3		
	4		
	5		
Proximal interphalangeal joints	1		
	2		
	3		
	4		
	5		
Distal interphalangeal joints	2		
	3		
	4		
	5		

Fig. 18-23. Wrist and hand examination form: physical examination, including joint play movements.

WRIST AND HAND EXAMINATION FORM—cont'd

3. Palpation (note location and nature of abnormality)
    a. Skin and subcutaneous tissues: tenderness_____ temperature_____ swelling_____
        moisture_____ decreased mobility_____
    b. Muscles and tendons: tenderness_____ loss of continuity_____ loss of mobility_____
        other_____
    c. Tendon sheaths and bursae: tenderness_____ swelling_____
    d. Bones and joints: tenderness_____ swelling_____ prominences_____ instability_____
        deformity_____
    e. Arteries and nerves: radial artery pulse_____ ulnar artery pulse_____
        Allen test_____ Tinel's sign_____ Phalen's test_____

Fig. 18-24. Wrist and hand examination form: physical examination, including palpation.

hypermobile, 5 = extremely hypermobile, 6 = unstable.

Palpation is the next procedure undertaken in the examination sequence. This technique allows the examiner to identify the nature and location of physically detectable structural abnormalities (Fig. 18-24). The examiner first palpates the skin and subcutaneous tissues, the most superficial layers, to detect tenderness, temperature change, swelling, moisture, or decreased mobility. The dorsal tissues are normally thin and loosely attached, allowing for a 30% increase in length from the wrist to fingertips during hand flexion. The lack of fascial attachments may permit the collection of edematous fluid over the dorsum of the hand. By contrast, the palmar tissue should feel thick when palpated and have relative lack of mobility. The signs of inflammation readily detectable on palpation include heat and swelling. Sympathetic changes that occur after nerve injury include vasomotor alterations (i.e., skin is warm initially but later becomes cool) and sudomotor alterations (i.e., usually there is less sweating, but occasionally excessive moisture occurs). Profuse sweating may also suggest neurosis or vasomotor instability. In the early phases of reflex sympathetic dystrophy the skin feels dry, rough, and warm; later it becomes smooth, glossy, cold, and lacks mobility because of interstitial fibrosis.

Palpation of muscles and tendons may reveal tenderness, loss of continuity, or loss of mobility. Intrinsic muscle bellies are distinguishable in the hand, and most of the extrinsic muscle tendons can be felt beneath the skin when movement is resisted. Testing to determine if a tendon is severed, adherent, or not gliding smoothly within its sheath is necessary. The extensor pollicis longus tendon is especially subject to irritation at the dorsal radial (Lister's) tubercle, around which it makes a 45-degree turn. Tendon sheaths and bursae may be tender or swollen.

Bones and joints are palpated for the presence of tenderness, swelling, prominences, instability, or deformity. The carpus may be palpated systematically, beginning with the styloid processes as landmarks. The ulnar styloid marks the level of the radiocarpal joint. Just distal to it lies the triquetrum, which is felt easily on radial deviation. The pisiform is readily located resting on the triquetrum. Its position coincides with the distal skin crease of the wrist. To locate the hamate, the examiner places his/her thumb in the direction of the client's web space with his/her IP joint over the client's pisiform; the hamulus will lie directly under the pulp of the examiner's thumb.

Radially, the *anatomical snuffbox* lies just dorsal and distal to the radial styloid and is outlined by the extensor pollicis longus and brevis tendons. Tenderness in this area is found with a scaphoid fracture. The tubercle of the scaphoid is prominent volarly under the distal wrist skin crease. Just distal to the scaphoid but proximal to the thenar eminence is the trapezium, and its articulation with the first metacarpal is easily felt when the thumb is moved. Adjacent to the ulnar border of the trapezium is the trapezoid. The adjacent lunate and capitate are best palpated dorsally; the dorsal radial tubercle and base of the third metacarpal are connected by a line that also bisects the lunate proximally and the capitate distally. In the neutral wrist position the prominence of the capitate is felt, but the lunate lies in a depression. When the wrist is flexed, the lunate will slip out from underneath the capitate and fill out the depression.

The joints have been initially inspected for deformity and changes in shape. Palpation may reveal additional information regarding the site of tenderness and instability of the joints. Ligaments are normally not sensitive to pressure or stretch, so pain elicited by palpation may be indicative of injury or disease. A normal joint capsule cannot usually be felt. Synovial proliferation, however, can render it accessible and perhaps painful to palpation.

Palpation is applied in the assessment of certain qualities of arteries and nerves. The pulse of the ulnar artery can be felt just proximal to the pisiform by pressing the artery against the ulna. The radial pulse is easily palpated lateral to the flexor carpi radialis and medial to the radial styloid process. The Allen test is performed to determine patency of the radial, ulnar, and digital arteries: the client

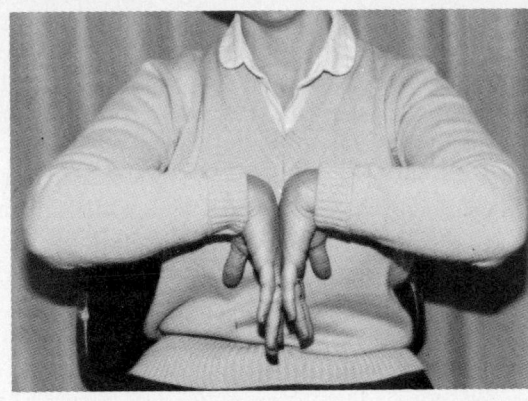

Fig. 18-25. Phalen's test for carpal tunnel syndrome is performed by maintaining maximal wrist flexion for 60 seconds in attempt to reproduce symptoms.

is requested to pump the blood out of the hand by clenching a fist several times and then maintaining a fist while the examiner occludes both arteries at the wrist; when the hand is opened, it will appear white, and arterial filling on the respective side can be observed as pressure is released from one artery at a time. The same maneuver is applied to the digital arteries by applying pressure to occlude flow at the base of the fingers.

In 1915 Tinel described a tingling sensation produced by pressure to an injured nerve.[28] This test, known as Tinel's sign, is used today to identify regeneration of sensory neurons. The affected nerve is gently tapped, starting at the site of injury and moving distally. Resulting paresthesias in the nerve's distribution are a positive indication of regeneration of that nerve. The level at which the sensations are felt by the client should be noted. The best prognosis is rapid progression of the distal sensation, with concurrent diminution of tingling at the injured site.[28] Tapping over the flexor retinaculum is commonly performed in the hand to test for median nerve compression within the carpal tunnel.

Phalen's test is performed to detect signs of median nerve compression within the carpal tunnel. A positive test is obtained when wrist flexion, maintained for 60 seconds, reproduces sensory changes in the median nerve distribution (Fig. 18-25).

The neurological portion of the examination reveals abnormalities in the conduction of neurological impulses that may be responsible for the client's signs and symptoms. Sensory disturbance, aberrant deep tendon reflexes, and motor control or coordination weakness, reveal neurological dysfunction. When attempting to identify the specific site of a lesion, a therapist should consider that there are overlaps and anomalies of musculoskeletal innervation. Therefore, for the therapist to make a definitive assessment of the dysfunction, an investigation of a combination of the results of several tests is sometimes required. Involvement of both the cervical nerve roots and peripheral nerves may affect both muscle strength and sensation in the upper extremity. The level of root involvement, if present, may be determined without testing every muscle by identifying a *key muscle* or joint action that is representative of a given root level. The key muscles acting on the hand include the extensor carpi radialis longus and brevis (representing C-6), extensor digitorum communis (representing C-7), flexor digitorum sublimis and profundus (representing C-8), and interossei (representing T1).[13]

Sensibility evaluation is performed to localize the area of a potential nerve lesion as well as assess hand function. When the area of involvement is localized, dermatomal versus peripheral patterns of aberrant sensation must be identified. Also, in a case involving nerve regeneration, it is important to determine the most distal level of return. Loss is indicated on a hand figure according to a code for specification of the sensory modality involved. The examiner should avoid leading questions and proceed by demonstrating the test. Then the client should be asked, with eyes closed, to report the tactile sensation that is felt. Stimuli should be applied to both radial and ulnar aspects of each digit to differentiate isolated digital nerve involvement.

Numerous tests have been described to evaluate the various sensory modalities. The four primary types of cutaneous sensibility are touch, pain, heat, and cold.[5] Light touch is commonly measured by a cotton wisp; a more sophisticated method uses von Frey hairs to determine cutaneous pressure thresholds. Pain may be elicited simply by pinprick or more objectively by an algesiometer. Tests for heat and cold use test tubes filled with tap water applied to the hand one at a time for 3 to 5 seconds; the normal hand can discriminate between 1° and 5° C.[2]

Sudomotor, or sympathetic, activity correlates with sweating in the palm and is assessed by the Ninhydrin sweat test. This test uses the reaction of amino acids in the sweat with Ninhydrin to form a colored tracing of perspiring areas. Although this may be the only objective measure of sensory function, its practical use in assessing hand function is debatable.

Evaluation of pain, temperature, and sudomotor activity may assist lesion identification but is not reliable in predicting functional recovery. After nerve repair, pain and temperature discrimination and sweating usually recover but function may not.[9] When functional assessment is the objective of examination, the classic Weber two-point discrimination test provides more accurate information.[5,9,10] The test measures the peripheral innervation density of the slowly adapting fiber/receptor system. It is performed by lightly applying two blunt ends to the skin about 15 mm apart, then decreasing the distance until only one point is felt; the digits should be supported to minimize sensory interference and to avoid proprioceptive input. Seven out of 10 correct responses are required to confirm appropriate perception. Normal discrimination averages about 3 mm in the fingertips; values for other areas of the hand, as well as functional correlations of results over 3 mm, are discussed in other sources.[9,35]

Dellon[9] states that, although the Weber test correlates with the hand's ability to perform static grip, this ability does not always parallel hand function. The essence of function—the ability to recognize objects (tactile gnosis)—requires discrimination of movement. Tactile gnosis depends on the quickly adapting fiber/receptor system and can be tested only by the moving two-point discrimination test.[9] This test is administered by moving two blunt points parallel to the long axis of the limb or digit, proximal to distal. One and two points are alternated randomly, while the interprong distance is progressively narrowed until a two-point limit is reached.[9] Seven out of 10 correct responses are required to verify tactile gnosis. The capacity for moving touch is recovered before constant touch. The normal hand is able to discriminate a 2 mm distance at the fingertip.[9]

The same nerve fibers belonging to the quickly adapting fiber group that mediates a vibratory stimulus also mediate moving touch. Thus the clinical evaluation of vibratory perception tests the same neural system as moving touch and correlates well with hand function.[9] Vibratory threshold measurements are easily tested with a tuning fork, which has the advantages of being accurate, easily administered, and noninvasive and rates a high level of client acceptance.[9] The 30 cycles per second (cps) tuning fork best measures the Meissner afferents located in the superficial dermis, and the 256 cps tuning fork best measures the pacinian afferents in the deep dermis and subcutis.[9] To perform the test, the tuning fork is applied alternately to involved and noninvolved areas, and the client is asked whether the feeling is the same; if a difference is noted, the client is asked to describe it.

The status of the motor system is described in terms of spasticity, flaccidity, rigidity, clonicity, and muscle spasm. This provides information regarding an overlying central nervous system (CNS) disorder versus involvement

WRIST AND HAND EXAMINATION FORM—cont'd

4. Neurological evaluation
   a. Key muscles (grades 0-5)
      C_6: ECRL and ECRB_____
      C_7: EDC_____
      C_8: FDS and FDP_____
      T_1: Dorsal interossei_____
   b. Sensibility

      Key: Lacking A = light touch sensation
              B = pinprick sensation
              C = temperature discrimination
              D = sweating (ninhydrin test)
              E = two-point discrimination (constant)
              F = two-point discrimination (moving)
              G = 30 cps vibratory perception
              H = 256 cps vibratory perception (moving)

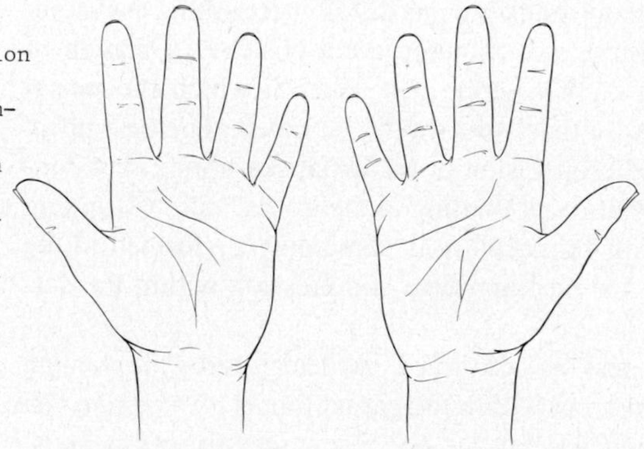

   c. Motor function: spastic_____ flaccid_____ rigid_____ clonic_____ spasm_____
   d. Coordination

      Trace a diagram_____   *Key:* N = completes with normal speed and coordination
      Button a button_____   CD = completes slowly with minimal coordination difficulty
      Tie a bow_____   SM = completes with searching movements
                                      U = unable to complete

5. Other tests recommended
   Radiography
   Laboratory
   Electrodiagnostic
   Arthroscopy/arthrography
   Other

Fig. 18-26. Wrist and hand examination form: physical examination, including neurological evaluation and other tests.

of a local muscle or nerve. Coordination is easily tested by performance of certain activities, such as tracing a diagram, buttoning, and tying a bow. A code on the examination form relates the client's competence in carrying out the designated activities (Fig. 18-26). Standardized tests, such as the O'Conner dexterity test or a Jebsen hand function test, are available for more detailed evaluation of manual dexterity and coordination.[10]

Other tests may be requested if the therapist feels that they are indicated by the results of the examination thus far. Clients are commonly referred for radiography, laboratory work, electrodiagnostic studies, arthroscopy, arthrography, or other necessary tests. Information from these tests may be needed by the therapist for the conclusive correlation and interpretation of data.

After the examination is completed and all the necessary data have been obtained, the therapist faces the task of interpretation. Irrelevant data must be recognized and dismissed. Patterns and trends recognized among the information lead to defining the client's status in terms of specific problems, structure(s) at fault, and baseline functional impairment (including rate and direction of change relative to the predicted course for similar types of impairment). The overall outcome will thus determine the functional capacity of the client.

The examination is successfully concluded when the following standards are satisfied: (1) the consistency of the client's status with the provisional diagnosis is ascertained; (2) data are provided for arriving at a definitive diagnosis; (3) data are provided for recommending client disposition (including physical therapy intervention); and (4) the need for additional data is determined. If physical therapy treatment is indicated, the therapist can then proceed with program planning and implementation.

COMMON DISORDERS

The orthopaedic physical therapist may be requested to consult on or treat a myriad of hand disorders. The pathology and management of the more frequently encountered conditions are discussed.

Rheumatoid hand

Rheumatoid arthritis is a chronic systemic disease characterized by inflammatory changes in numerous tissues. The synovial tissue of diarthrodial joints and tendon sheaths is typically attacked, imparting severe disability to the involved joints. Rheumatoid disease often affects the hand, producing pain, joint disorganization, and deformity. Because of the disease's chronicity and potentially devastating effects, proper management should be instituted as early as possible.

The pathological elements that lead to deformity include synovial inflammation and hypertrophy with exuberation of granulation tissue that extends across the joint surface as pannus. The pannus contains hydrolytic enzymes capable of eroding articular cartilage, subchondral bone, ligaments, and tendons. Joint capsules and supporting structures, weakened and distended by the inflamed tissue, yield under external forces, rendering the joints susceptible to the development of laxity and instability. Tendons, likewise, undergo fibrous dissolution, lengthening, and eventual rupture.

Atrophy and shortening occur in both intrinsic and extrinsic muscle bellies, but the exact mechanism that produces pathological changes is not understood. Myositis has been found to be associated with the rheumatoid process, but it is not believed to be the cause of the muscle changes that occur; nor is spasm believed to be a primary factor in the production of contractures.[11] It has been proposed that disuse of painfully inhibited muscles is the main cause of the atrophy and muscle shortening that develop.[32]

The events just described act in combination to destroy the delicate balance between the muscles, tendons, and bones of the hand. Characteristic deformities develop in involved joints. Both evaluation and treatment of the rheumatoid hand are based on a clear understanding of the pathomechanics underlying the classic deformities. Following is a description of the mechanisms of common deformities.

Rheumatoid arthritis commonly afflicts the distal radioulnar and wrist joints. Since these joints comprise a link system between the forearm and hand, their collapse may severely compromise hand function. Hand placement and stability are hindered by restriction at these more proximal joints. Also the functional length of the finger muscles and their ability to generate force are directly related to wrist position. Therefore wrist mobility is more critical to the hand with limited digital function, as is often the case in the client with rheumatoid arthritis.

The common positions of wrist deformity are flexion, radial deviation, and palmar subluxation. Spontaneous fusion may occur with the wrist in flexion. This would severely limit the excursion and power of the digital flexor muscles. The distal radioulnar joint is disrupted typically by dorsal subluxation of the ulnar head. The extensor carpi ulnaris tendon insertion is thus displaced palmarly and no longer affords ulnar stability during wrist extension, thumb abduction, and finger flexion. Ankylosis occurs within the intercarpal and carpometacarpal joints as well, destroying the transverse arch framework and the cupping ability of the hand.

Rheumatoid arthritis is a common cause of MP joint deformity, namely, ulnar deviation and palmar subluxation. This pathological condition may be partially explained by the normal anatomy of the MP joints. Unlike the IP joints, the MP joints lack inherent bony stability opposing varus and valgus forces; their integrity depends instead on the joint capsule, ligaments, and intrinsic muscles (structures that are prime targets of the rheumatoid process). Also, ulnar deviation and rotation naturally accompany MP flexion

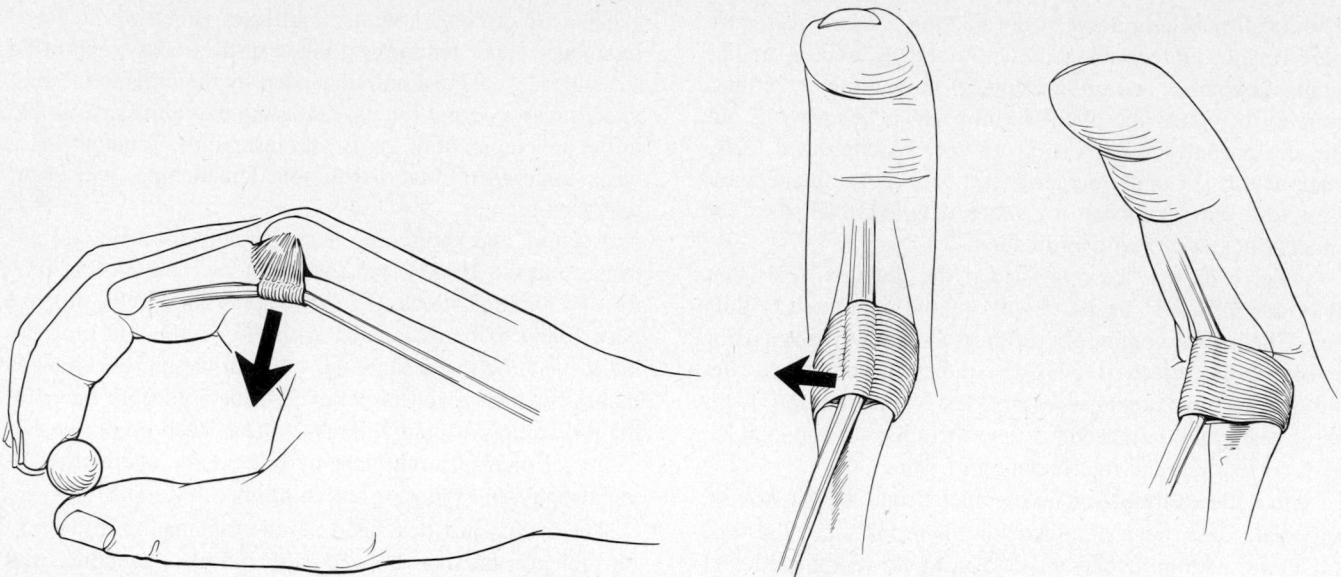

Fig. 18-27. Normal flexor tendon forces contribute to ulnar drift and volar subluxation of MP joint when supporting structures are weakened. (Modified from Flatt AE: Care of the arthritic hand, ed 4, St Louis, 1983, The CV Mosby Co.)

in most hand activities and are made possible by asymmetry of the collateral ligaments and the ulnar slope of the metacarpal heads. The hand demonstrates ulnar inclination of the phalanges at rest as well.

The disease process accentuates the normal ulnar deviation by weakening the supporting structures. This leaves the MP joint vulnerable to the propagation of deformity by the forces involved in the use of the hand.[11] During pinch and grasp activities a force having ulnar and palmar components is produced by the extrinsic flexor tendons (Fig. 18-27). This may have an adverse stretching effect on the anatomically weaker radial collateral ligaments, which along with the tendon sheaths may be undergoing attrition as a result of disease. The bases of the proximal phalanges are displaced ulnarly and palmarly, which allows bowstringing of the flexor tendons and further produces dislocating forces.

Likewise, the pathological stretching of the dorsal hood and synovial bulging on the radial side allow the extrinsic extensor tendons to shift from the dorsum to the ulnar sulcus adjacent to the MP joint. In this position they lie volar to the axis of flexion and lose their extensor ability. Thus the aberrant forces become self-perpetuating since the extensor tendons now contribute to flexion as well as ulnar deviation.

The intrinsic muscles also become deforming elements following lengthening of supporting structures. The normal mechanical advantage of the ulnar intrinsics is exaggerated by ulnar shift of the dorsal hood. The first dorsal interosseous muscle attaches to a broad area of the MP joint capsule; overstretching of the capsule allows the insertion of this muscle to move toward the palm, and it

loses its ability to abduct the index finger as it becomes an MP joint flexor.

The radial deviation of the wrist and carpometacarpal joints may produce a corresponding ulnar deviation of the fingers. This collapse deformity provides a mechanism for maintaining alignment of the fingers with the forearm.

The PIP joint is often involved in swan-neck or boutonniere deformities, which involve zigzag of an intercalated phalanx (middle) in the direction of greatest shortening within an unstable system. The swan-neck deformity, represented by hyperextension of the PIP joint and flexion of the DIP joint, results from imbalance of flexor and extensor forces to which joint laxity may be a compounding factor. If flexion of the PIP joint is restricted by synovitis of the flexor tendon, pain, or mechanical factors, the flexor force will be concentrated on the MP joint. The MP joint flexion, which may progress to MP joint volar subluxation, enhances the mechanical advantage of the intrinsics and promotes an extension imbalance at the PIP joint. As the transverse retinacular ligament becomes stretched, the lateral bands bowstring over the PIP joint and the deformity progresses (see Fig. 18-9). Exaggerated DIP joint flexion is generated by the flexor digitorum profundus, which is inadequately balanced by the lateral bands.

The boutonniere deformity, characterized by PIP joint flexion and DIP joint extension, commonly results when the central slip of the EDC tendon is weakened or ruptured in the disease process. PIP joint flexion is then essentially unopposed. Flexion is further accentuated by the lateral bands, which dislocate and come to lie volar to the joint axis; they become PIP joint flexors, while increased tension on the terminal tendon extends the DIP joint (see Fig.

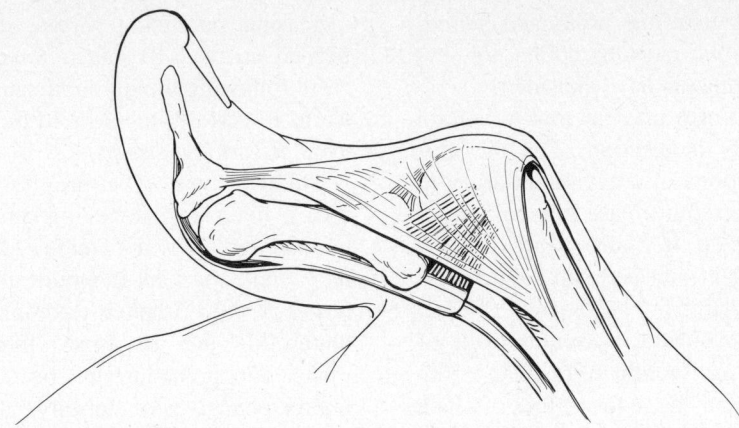

Fig. 18-28. Boutonniere deformity of thumb. (Modified from Flatt AE: Care of the arthritic hand, ed 4, St Louis, 1983, The CV Mosby Co.)

18-10). Extension of the DIP joint is unopposed by the flexor digitorum profundus because PIP joint flexion limits the range the profundus can mechanically shorten. Therefore the distal phalanx is pulled into hyperextension.

Dysfunction of the thumb in rheumatoid arthritis is a common occurrence. The thumb is the most important digit of the hand, and its impairment can impose severe restriction on prehension and strength. The most common deformity is the boutonniere, in which the MP joint is flexed and the IP joint is extended (Fig. 18-28). It is initiated by synovitis at the MP joint; stretching of the capsule and extensor apparatus follows, and the extensor pollicis longus tendon and adductor pollicis are displaced ulnarly. The extensor pollicis brevis becomes elongated with resultant loss of MP extension (*extrinsic minus* thumb). The power of the extensor mechanism is concentrated distally, producing hyperextension of the distal phalanx (*intrinsic plus* thumb). Attempts to use the thumb in pinch activities aggravate the deformity by exaggerating the collapse into MP joint flexion and IP joint extension.

A swan-neck deformity, in which the MP joint is extended and the IP joint flexed, may also occur at the thumb. Destructive changes at the trapeziometacarpal joint lead to radial subluxation of the metacarpal and contracture of adductor pollicis. The MP joint becomes hyperextended in response to the stretch forces applied during pinch. The IP joint is passively flexed by tension on the flexor pollicis longus.

Treatment and management of the rheumatoid hand involves close interaction of all members of the rehabilitation team. In the acute phase of the disease and during subsequent exacerbations, the hand should be protected until movement is relatively pain free.[11] During rest the hand should be properly positioned with a splint designed to meet the specific immobilization needs of the client.

Splinting can help relieve pain and swelling, maintain proper alignment of joints, and aid in prevention of defor-

mity during the early stages of the disease.[24] Common types of passive immobilization splints include the wrist cock-up, which supports the wrist while allowing finger movement; the resting hand shell, which protects both wrist and fingers; the ulnar deviation splint, which maintains joint alignment and allows function in the corrected position; the tripoint finger splint, which corrects developing flexion or extension deformities; and the thumb stabilizer, which is used for one or more involved joints.

During acute flare-ups exercise is limited to isometric muscle contraction and gentle range of motion activities. Excessive stretching, which only increases the pain and tissue damage already present, must be avoided. Application of local heat through use of a paraffin bath, whirlpool, or underwater ultrasound is helpful in stimulating circulation, reducing pain, and increasing mobility. Cryotherapy also provides benefit to clients with acute inflammation as well as those with postoperative swelling and pain.

As acute inflammation and spasm subside, joint movement will be less painful to the client. Periods of immobilization may be interrupted for carefully controlled activity. Active assistive exercise is useful in preventing joint stiffness and tendon adhesions. Isotonic exercises will enhance both strength and joint mobility. Finger extension is emphasized, even in the absence of flexion contractures, because extension force is generally weakened by tendon subluxation. Functional activities are built into the client's rehabilitation program to make the transition back to self-care and performance of daily tasks easier. Resistive exercises are usually discouraged in the client with rheumatoid arthritis because of the disruptive forces they impart on weakened and mechanically deranged tissues.

Fatigue must be considered during the treatment program. Inflammation and other factors in the disease may cause the client to tire easily. To prevent undue strain on the joints, rest periods should be incorporated as part of the overall program. Brief sessions of exercise interspersed throughout the day are better than one prolonged period. The client should continue to wear resting splints for several weeks after all acute symptoms have subsided.

During this phase the physician may attempt to control the effects of the disease by medication. The therapist should be aware of the functions of the various drugs to distinguish between drug-effected decrease in pain and inflammation versus true remission. If vigorous movement is initiated too early, considerable joint and soft tissue damage can occur.

After contractures have developed, a vicious cycle of increasing malfunction develops: contractures lead to decreased use of the hand, which leads to stiffness, which leads to further contracture.[11] This problem is dealt with by encouraging activity and using remedial splints, which alter joint position and direct muscle action. Splints commonly employed in this case are knuckle-bends, reverse knuckle-benders, and a dynamic splint designed to counteract wrist flexion contracture.

Often, surgery is required to alleviate symptoms, correct deformities, and restore function. It is recognized, however, that surgical techniques will not completely restore normal anatomical function; nor will they provide permanent correction. Surgery is not used in isolation but requires therapeutic management both in preoperative and postoperative phases. Therapy is administered preoperatively with the objective of decreasing the extent of surgery necessary by increasing mobility and muscle strength and by altering alignment through splinting. The postoperative therapy objective is to restore function necessary for the client to resume independence. This is accomplished through a combination of modalities, exercise, splinting, client education, environmental adaptation, and possibly vocational rehabilitation.

Surgery should not be postponed until total joint destruction has occurred. Prophylactic synovectomies are advocated to remove the diseased synovium before secondary changes occur in the adjacent structures. Intrinsic contractures are released by excision of the distal insertion of the intrinsic muscles before the development of MP subluxation, ulnar deviation, and swan-neck deformities. Portions of diseased tendons may be excised and repaired by end-to-end apposition in small areas or free tendon grafts in larger areas of involvement. Where tendon damage is extensive, tendon transfers may be required; an extensive program of muscle reeducation should follow to ensure that the client makes optimal use of the new motor ability.

Joint reconstruction procedures generally fall into three categories: arthrodesis, arthroplasty, and prosthetic replacement. Arthrodesis is reserved for those joints where stability is judged necessary for function based on the overall condition of the rest of the hand. Some joints chosen for fusion include the wrist, the thumb trapeziometacarpal, MP and IP joints, and the finger PIP joints. Arthroplasty involves realigning joint surfaces and tendons and

increasing stabilizing forces; it is most commonly performed on the MP joints. Supervised exercises are indicated following the immobilization period so that the client learns to perform the desired movement in the joint and to avoid deforming strains.

Another type of arthroplasty initiated by Swanson[30] uses a flexible silicone implant following resection. The implant serves as a dynamic spacer and maintains alignment while the joint is rebuilt through the body's *encapsulation process*. Implant arthroplasty is used for finger and thumb MP and IP joints, intercarpal joints, and wrist joints. This procedure has been found effective in satisfying the objectives of stability, mobility, durability, retrievability, and pain alleviation. Following surgery, early motion is encouraged to reduce edema, prevent soft tissue contractures and adhesions between gliding surfaces, and maintain strength. It is important that movement be carefully controlled to allow healing. At the same time, however, the joint must maintain enough volar and dorsal capsular laxity to permit flexion and extension while stabilizing against lateral motion. A dynamic brace is recommended as an adjunct to the exercise program to control motion in the desired plane and range and to assist flexor and extensor power. As healing progresses, the client is instructed in joint protection principles, such as prevention of deforming positions, substituting pulp-to-pulp pinch for lateral pinch, building up small-handled utensils, employing proper body mechanics in all activities, specifically choosing and arranging equipment, and using adaptive/assistive devices to meet individual needs.

Joint replacement has also been used successfully in the hand to restore motion, provide stability, correct deformity, and reduce pain. Prosthetic substitution for the rheumatoid joint is often functionally superior to fusion; however, the life of the prosthesis and its ability to remain seated within bone may be limited. Following joint replacement, active hand movement is started when the dressings are removed a few days after surgery. Strengthening of the extensor digitorum communis is especially emphasized. The therapist should be aware of the limitations inherent in the design of the prosthesis so that digits are exercised in the appropriate plane and degree of motion (i.e., a uniaxial prosthetic replacement of the MP joint should not permit abduction and adduction). Following MP joint replacement, *outrigger* splints to assist extension and radial deviation provide a useful adjunct to exercise.

Home programs for continuation of therapeutic measures are beneficial to clients with rheumatoid arthritis, whether they are undergoing conservative treatment or surgical management. The client should be thoroughly educated regarding the nature and course of the disease, signs and symptoms warning of impending flare-ups, increasing inflammation and joint damage, and techniques of treatment and joint protection that can be administered at home. The paraffin bath is a good modality for applying local heat to joints and can easily be adapted to home use. Passive, active, and resistive exercises can be adequately performed by the client in response to the changing status of the musculoskeletal structures. Energy-conserving devices should be considered whenever feasible.

Soft tissue syndromes

Carpal tunnel syndrome. The carpal tunnel syndrome is the most common and significant of all nerve entrapment syndromes.[23] Any pathological condition that decreases the area of the carpal tunnel or increases the volume of its contents may compress the median nerve. Examples of conditions associated with the cause of this syndrome include synovial hypertrophy, tenosynovitis, ganglia, fracture callus, and tumors. The pathogenesis involves fibrosis or thickening of the flexor synovialis within the carpal tunnel, the cause of which is not completely understood.

The typical history reveals a gradual onset of numbness and paresthesia in the median nerve distribution, burning pain that often awakens the client at night, predominance in women 40 to 60 years of age, and associated disease, such as rheumatoid arthritis and diabetes mellitus. The symptoms may be aggravated by vigorous use of the hand, which may produce venous engorgement within an already crowded space, but it is not the primary cause of the syndrome. According to Phalen's study of 598 cases, the predominant clinical finding was sensory disturbance (83%), including hypocsthesia, decreased sensation, hyperesthesia, and paresthesia. Other positive findings were Phalen's test (80%), Tinel's sign (60%), thenar atrophy (36%), decreased nerve conduction velocity (24%), and swelling over the volar aspect of the wrist (21%).[23]

Treatment of carpal tunnel syndrome involves eliminating the original cause, if possible, such as management of fluid retention with diuretics. Conservative management is often beneficial and may simply require restriction of activity and use of resting splints at night. Steroid injection around the flexor tendons within the carpal tunnel may also afford relief. Surgery is indicated for cases with thenar atrophy and progressive loss of function. After surgical division of the flexor retinaculum, a bulky compression dressing is applied and the hand is maintained in elevation for 3 to 4 days. Active exercises may then be initiated, with splint protection for the resting hand until the seventh postoperative day.

De Quervain's disease. De Quervain's disease is inflammation of the synovial sheath surrounding the abductor pollicis longus and extensor pollicis brevis tendons at the wrist. This condition may be elicited either by direct trauma to the tendon sheath or by repetitive minor irritation. It produces tenderness over the radial styloid, aggravated by active abduction of the thumb. A passive stretch produced by thumb adduction and wrist ulnar deviation is also painful (Finkelstein's test). The recommended treatment is heat and immobilization, hydrocortisone injection, with surgical release of the tendon sheath as a last resort.

Dupuytren's contracture. Dupuytren's contracture is a progressive fibrosis of the palmar aponeurosis of unknown cause. It is found to be more common in men over 40 and persons with alcoholism, epilepsy, or gout. This painless condition may be limited to nodule formation in the area of the proximal palmar crease or may be so extensive that it produces a fixed flexion contracture of one or more digits. Milder cases are treated conservatively by attempting to prevent secondary joint contractures through exercise and increasing fascial extensibility with ultrasound. In severe cases surgical excision of the abnormal tissue may be required. Following fasciectomy, active range of motion exercises may be initiated on the first postoperative day. All thumb, finger, and wrist movements are carried out regularly and are modified until full range of motion is obtained. A splint to maintain finger extension may be worn in conjunction with the exercise program.

Traumatic hand injuries

Sprains and dislocations

Lunate. A fall on the outstretched hand is the mechanism that produces most wrist injuries. The wrist is forced into extension with resultant ligamentous damage, dislocation, fracture, or combinations of these injuries. The most common type of dislocation involves an anterior dislocation of the lunate or a dorsal dislocation of the rest of the carpus relative to the lunate (perilunate dislocation). Occasionally the scaphoid is also fractured, in which case the proximal fragment is displaced with the lunate. The volar radiocarpal ligament remains intact and thus preserves blood supply to the lunate.[1,19] Because of the proximity of the median nerve, either lunate or perilunate dislocation has the potential of producing a severe compression syndrome if not corrected. These injuries may cause constriction of the flexor tendons within the carpal tunnel as well. Clinically, the volar projection of the lunate disrupts the normal surface configuration of the wrist and helps confirm the diagnosis.

Closed reduction followed by cast immobilization is the treatment of choice for lunate dislocation. However, if dislocation is not recognized until 2 or more weeks after the injury, open reduction is usually necessary. An exercise program is initiated while the client is casted to maintain shoulder, elbow, and finger function. After removal of the cast, active thumb and wrist exercises are added to the program. Attempts to restore motion lost because of immobilization must not stress the ligaments damaged by the initial injury. If complications, such as median nerve palsy and flexor tendon constrictions, occur, they must be treated accordingly.

First MP joint. Forceful hyperextension or abduction of the first MP joint (thumb) is a common injury sustained in sports. The membranous insertion of the volar plate or the ulnar collateral ligament may be torn. In cases of complete rupture or dislocation, gross clinical instability and pain, along with the mechanism of injury, make diagnosis relatively straightforward. If the dislocation can be reduced without interposition of soft tissue, it is accomplished through closed means; otherwise, open reduction is indicated. Immobilization is required for 2 to 6 weeks until stability and range of motion have returned.[1,19] Thereafter, protected range of motion and strengthening exercises are instituted, with stability taking precedence over mobility.

Second through fifth MP joints. The second through fifth MP joints are commonly injured by hyperextension, which, in extreme cases, forces the metacarpal head volarly between the lumbrical muscle and extrinsic flexor tendons. Reduction is best performed by open means. After successful reduction the joint is relatively stable, and early motion may be encouraged with the following restrictions: the joint is splinted in 30 degrees of flexion during the inflammatory phase and active flexion is begun from this position; further extension is avoided for about 5 weeks.[19]

Second through fifth PIP joints. The small hinged PIP joints are the most commonly injured joints in the hand and rank second to the wrist in incidence of all upper extremity trauma.[29] They are particularly vulnerable to injury because they have only one plane of motion, and the distal and middle phalanges serve as a long lever arm in transmitting bending and rotatory forces from the fingertip. The most common injury is a hyperextension sprain, which usually occurs when a person catches a ball or when the finger is jammed into a solid surface. Damage to the capsule, transverse retinacular ligaments, or collateral ligaments may occur. A more forceful injury may produce subluxation or dislocation with disruption of the volar plate.

Clinical characteristics of PIP joint injury include acute pain, localized swelling, and aberrant motion. The degree of instability will give the examiner an indication of the severity of the injury. If reduction is necessary, closed manipulation is usually satisfactory. The PIP joint is immobilized following strict protocol with regard to position and duration. The PIP joint is most vulnerable to flexion contracture. Experimental testing reported by Sprague[29] confirms that the PIP joint must be diligently splinted in 15 to 20 degrees of flexion; any further flexion allows shortening of the collateral ligaments, capsule, and the volar supporting structures, which become more redundant as flexion increases. Immobilization should be maintained for no longer than 3 weeks so that adhesions are not formed between the gliding tissue planes surrounding the flexor and extensor tendons. Active exercises are initiated 3 weeks after the injury. The healing digit may be taped to an adjacent finger for additional protection as well as an assistive exercise. Restoration of full pain-free motion may take as long as 6 to 9 months.

Fractures

Radius. The distal radius is more commonly fractured than any other bone in the body. As one attempts to break a fall with the arm, the hand is fixed on the ground so that the force is transmitted up through the forearm. In addition, a supination moment is created between the pronator quadratus and brachioradialis muscles, producing maximal stress at the junction of cortical and cancellous bone in the distal radial metaphysis.

Fracture of the distal radius 1 to 2 inches above the carpal extremity was first described by Abraham Colles, an Irish surgeon.[20] The term *Colles fracture* is currently applied to most dorsally angulated fractures of the distal 2 inches of the radius, with or without accompanying ulnar fracture. A similar fracture with a volarly angulated distal fragment is referred to as *Smith's fracture*.[19] A fracture through the dorsal articular area of the radius with dorsal and proximal displacement is termed *Barton's fracture*.[19]

Treatment of a Colles fracture consists of closed manipulation, which may require anesthesia, followed by immobilization in an above-elbow plaster cast. Perfect anatomical reduction may be difficult to obtain and maintain but is often functionally insignificant. The plaster should hold the wrist in a neutral position and not extend beyond the distal palmar crease to allow full MP joint motion. During immobilization it is extremely important to stress full range of motion of noninvolved joints and muscle strengthening exercises. When the cast is removed in 6 to 8 weeks, active and passive forearm, wrist, and thumb movements are initiated, often in conjunction with other modalities to reduce pain and enhance mobility. Complications may include malunion, subluxation of the distal radioulnar joint, joint stiffness anywhere in the upper extremity, and rupture of the extensor pollicis longus tendon where it contacts the roughened fracture site. Each complication is treated accordingly.

Scaphoid. When a young athletic individual falls on the outstretched hand, a scaphoid fracture is more common than a wrist fracture. Several unique features of this type of fracture make diagnosis difficult and yet necessitate adequate treatment to minimize serious late complications. The fracture, which often occurs transversely through the waist of the bone, is not easily recognized on initial radiographs. Pain and swelling, which are particularly localized in the "anatomical snuffbox," are good indications that a fracture has occurred even if there is no immediate radiographic evidence of such.

Treatment of scaphoid fractures requires plaster immobilization extending to the IP joint of the thumb and incorporating about two thirds of the forearm. Even when the diagnosis is uncertain, the area should be immobilized until a fracture can be ruled out or confirmed by bone resorption, which occurs about 2 weeks after injury. A scaphoid fracture inaccurately diagnosed as a wrist sprain, which is not immobilized, has a higher incidence of nonunion. The fact that the blood supply is confined to the distal pole in some cases also increases the healing time and the incidence of nonunion, avascular necrosis, and degenerative changes over time; 9 to 12 weeks may be required for healing. The high incidence of complications includes delayed union, nonunion, avascular necrosis of the proximal fragment, and osteoarthritis. When healing does not occur following prolonged immobilization, a bone graft may be required. Prosthetic scaphoid implants have been successfully employed in cases of nonunion and avascular necrosis. A young client is usually able to regain hand function by activity alone; thus extensive rehabilitation is not necessary.

Metacarpals and phalanges. The incidence of fractures of the metacarpals and phalanges varies; these fractures are often the result of a direct blow or forces similar to those producing the dislocations previously described. They are generally manually reduced and immobilized in plaster or by a splint. When immobilization is removed in about 4 to 6 weeks, active and passive exercises are often necessary to restore wrist and finger motion.

Tendon injuries. The goal of repairing tendon severance is to achieve full pain-free excursion without loss of power. Optimal results, however, are often precluded by the manner in which tendon healing occurs. Because the tendon's main vascular source is from vessels in the surrounding soft tissues and within the tendon sheath, revascularization following injury must occur from without. Trauma to structures surrounding the tendon creates a fibroblastic response, and tendon adhesion to adjacent tissues is inevitable. Differential wound healing is critical to the outcome; the severed tendon ends must remodel with strength sufficient to transmit muscular forces, whereas the collagen between the tendon and adjacent tissues must remain randomly oriented and elastic to permit tendon gliding.[1]

When these biological concepts of healing are applied to rehabilitation of a hand with severed tendons, the timing of a program of graduated motion becomes critical. A repaired tendon must be protected from disruption until tensile strength has developed in the wound, and yet passive gliding of the tendon is required to prevent total adherence to adjacent tissues. Generally, the repair is immobilized for 24 to 48 hours postoperatively to decrease excessive bleeding and tissue reaction. Afterward dynamic splinting is used to prevent stress on the healing tendon while allowing passive movement of the tendon in the desired direction. For example, following repair of flexor tendons in the palm, a dorsal splint is fabricated to maintain the wrist and fingers in moderate flexion; rubber band traction allows active extension of the fingers but enforces passive flexion to protect the repair (Fig. 18-29).[15] After 3 to 4 weeks the splint is usually removed to allow controlled active exercise. The client continues a program of graded exercise under supervision until maximal success is achieved.

The area of tendon injury and the type of repair elected

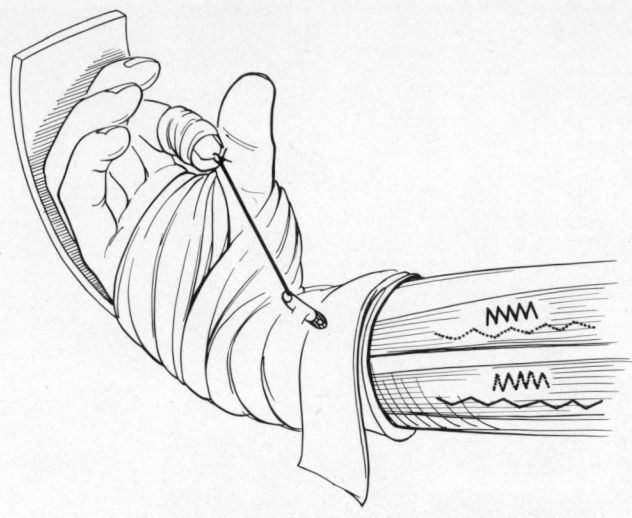

Fig. 18-29. Dynamic splint used after flexor tendon repair to allow full active extension of digits while removing tension from flexor tendons. (Modified from Kleinert HE and Meares A: Clin Orthop 104:23, 1974.)

also have an impact on the outcome. Damage to tendons with close continuity to other structures, such as dual injury of the extrinsic finger flexors within the digital sheath ("no man's land") or flexor tendon injury within the carpal tunnel, has a higher incidence of adhesion than does tendon injury in the forearm or over the dorsum of the hand. Primary tendon repair is most often elected when surgery is possible within 6 hours following injury and there has not been massive damage or wound contamination. A secondary repair is preferred when there is evidence of early wound infection, severe crush, or inadequate skin coverage. A free tendon autograft is preferred by some surgeons to traverse the area of maximal tissue damage and elect a more optimal site for anastomosis and subsequent healing.

A majority of hand injuries occur in laborers, most of whom plan to return to the work force. For many a work capacity evaluation and a work hardening program are indicated. In this manner an individualized program can assist a client in developing sufficient strength, endurance, and coordination to return to his/her former occupation or a satisfactory alternate occupation. Use of a work-oriented treatment program with a productivity-based outcome is a cost-effective and timesaving link between medical rehabilitation and returning to work.[18]

Graded activities may be planned according to a client's specific job demands. For example, at the lowest level of resistance (0 to 1 lb) he/she may begin with sorting objects (e.g., varied sizes of nuts and bolts), picking up and placing blocks or items in designeated spaces, or macrame. Progressing to more resistance (1 to 3 lbs), he may perform activities such as molding clay, assembling plumbing parts with or without tools (Fig. 18-30), leather work, and weight-resisted or mechanically resisted exercise. At a higher level (greater than 3 lb) he can train at prehension

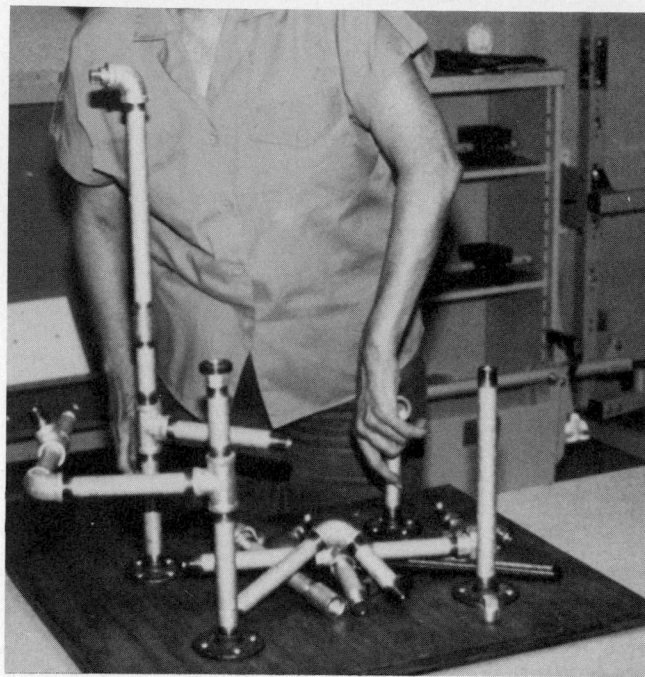

Fig. 18-30. An assortment of plumbing connectors, elbows, and pipes provides functional hand exercise for increasing strength, endurance, range of motion, and manipulative skills.

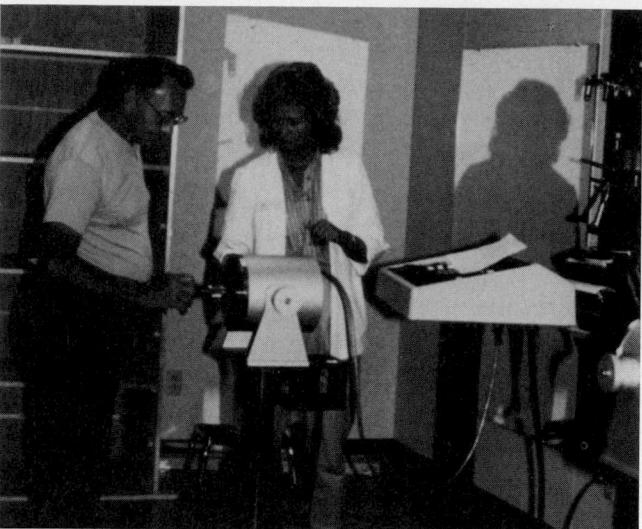

Fig. 18-31. The BTE Work Simulator records objective data for evaluating upper extremity function, and offers a variety of attachments for training at job-simulated tasks.

tasks requiring speed, accuracy, strength, and sustained grip, such as woodworking, lifting and carrying boxes, progressive resistive exercise, and actual job-simulated activity. Equipment such as the BTE Work Simulater* helps by reproducing job tasks and daily functions in a controlled clinical setting and provides feedback on the amount of torque generated and work performed (Fig. 18-31).

Advancing through these levels of activities allows a client to improve work tolerance, speed, and proficiency. Through instruction and supervision he/she learns appropriate techniques of pain mastery, body mechanics, and use of assistive or adaptive devices. Working toward an eventual goal of maximizing employability, a client should ultimately reach his/her work tolerance level or plateau, at which time he/she is discharged from the program and advised regarding acceptable levels of performance. In the event that he/she demonstrates inability to return to work, the program helps resolve the client's status in an unequivocal manner that may lead to justified pursuit of disability awards.[18]

Burned hand

Hands are the most commonly burned areas of the body according to numerous sources, including admission data from the Brooke Army Medical Center.[6] This is likely because of their exposed position and their use in protecting

*Baltimore Therapeutic Equipment Co, 7455-L New Ridge Road, Hanover, MD 21076.

the face when attempting to extinguish a fire. Not only are hand burns a major cosmetic concern, but also they may cause severe pain, deformity, and loss of function and skin sensitivity. The objective of therapeutic management, therefore, is to restore appearance, mobility, and function, with ultimate concern for the long-term results.

In the first hours following injury the client's life is threatened by burn shock. This necessitates administration of large amounts of lactated Ringer's solution. The added fluid in combination with the inflammatory response at the burn site contributes to massive edema, which reaches its peak about 2 days after a burn. Escharotomy and fasciotomy may be required at this time to release pressure and restore circulation. To combat edema the hands must remain elevated; this is usually best accomplished through use of a soft sling at the elbow that maintains the upper extremity above the head, with shoulder abduction and elbow extension to facilitate lymphaticovenous return.

Dorsal swelling and a position of comfort sought by the client contribute to wrist flexion and clawing deformities. These contractures can be explained by the fact that wrist flexion produces extension of the MP joint through tenodesis of the extensor digitorum communis; the MP joint collateral ligaments are lax and shorten to produce a fixed MP joint extension contracture. The action of the central slip may be lost at the PIP joint either by fixation of the sagittal bands at the MP joint, by burn scar, or by direct disruption of the dorsal hood by the burn; PIP joint flexion contracture develops from constant tension of the unopposed flexor digitorum sublimis.

The hand should be splinted at the onset of treatment in an antideformity position, which is 0 to 30 degrees of wrist extension, 70 to 90 degrees of MP joint flexion, and

IP joint extension and abduction.[25] Extra compression or padding is often necessary to maintain the web spaces. As the edema subsides, the splints are revised to maintain optimal position. Care should be taken that the splints are always placed and maintained in their correct position, or they may contribute to, rather than alleviate, deformity. Splints are to be worn at all times, except during periods of exercise and when they interfere with functional use of the hands.

Passive, active-assistive, and active motions are initiated early with the goal of reducing edema, maintaining strength, and preventing capsular and ligamentous contractures and tendon adherence. Tendon adherence is common because the abundance of protein-rich exudate in the burned hand renders it especially susceptible to fibrotic changes, especially when immobilized.[4] A custom-designed exercise program should be written and carefully instructed for the client, family, and health team members. The program should be supervised twice daily by the therapist and additionally performed every 2 hours by the client. Exercises using overhead pulleys, a wand, and wall pushups are beneficial for the entire upper extremity. Specific hand exercises include wrist circumduction, finger extension and abduction, thumb opposition, and cupping of the palm. Since dorsal burns are likely to involve the superficial dorsal hood, mass flexion of all joints should be avoided; when one attempts to increase flexion of any particular joint, the other joints of the same digit should be blocked in extension. The client should become involved in self-care and activities of daily living as soon as possible. These tasks exercise the hands and contribute to independence.

Rapid wound closure is a major goal when treating the acutely-burned hand. Many partial thickness burns are allowed to heal naturally, whereas full thickness burns require early removal of dead tissue and appropriate skin replacement. Following skin grafting, the immediate site must be immobilized for 5 days. During this time the immobilized parts can be used to perform isometric exercises, while other areas of the body may be used to continue their regular program. Active exercise is reinitiated after the first dressing change, or in about 5 days, and the client progresses as indicated. When healing is advanced, therapeutic putty is a good means of self-exercise for increasing strength and motion.

In addition to maintaining hand position and mobility, the therapist is involved in other objectives of burn care, such as preventing infection and achieving healing. Daily whirlpool treatments are indicated for most burns to assist wound cleansing and débridement, increase eschar pliability, and facilitate exercise. Topical antibacterial agents or dressings are applied after whirlpooling to reduce the incidence of infection and pain.

Custom-fitted pressure garments are beneficial in preventing postburn hypertrophic scarring. The therapist measures and fits the client when skin coverage is nearly complete, before discharge from the hospital. The garments are worn continuously up to 18 months after discharge because this length of time is required for scar maturation. While at home the client must also continue with exercises—and splinting if indicated—to ensure maximal recovery. Regular physical therapy follow-up is extremely important in order to objectively reassess progress, to revise exercises, splints, and garments as needed, and to encourage the client toward maximal function.

Peripheral nerve injuries

The status of motor and sensory innervation is the single most important factor determining the recovery of hand function.[1] Recovery from nerve injury is influenced by the client's age, type and extent of injury, precision of surgical repair, and rehabilitation program.

Peripheral nerve injuries fit into three groups: neurapraxia, which connotes contusion without Wallerian degeneration and complete functional recovery from paralysis within 6 weeks; axonotmesis, referring to axonal disruption by blunt trauma without disruption of Schwann tubes, allowing Wallerian regeneration to be completed through the original tube in about 6 months; and neurotomesis, in which the nerve is completely disrupted by laceration or traction, requiring precise surgical approximation with unpredictable recovery.

Following an injury producing complete nerve disruption, the hand should be examined to determine the level and extent of damage. In addition to motor and sensory loss, there will be loss of sudomotor activity (sweating) in the distribution of the sensory nerve caused by the loss of its accompanying sympathetic nerve. Subsequent dryness and diminished palmar papillary ridges are noticeable after a few weeks.[1]

Surgical repair is ideally performed within a few weeks of nerve injury. This procedure takes advantage of the increase in metabolic activity of the nerve cell body in preparation for producing new axoplasm, which must be extruded distally into the Schwann tube. The precise alignment of fascicles enhances the prognosis, although functional recovery is never complete. The repair must be protected from tension for 3 to 4 weeks. This is accomplished by flexing the joints that the nerve crosses only enough to relieve stretch; immobilization in excessive flexion increases the difficulty of obtaining full extension later.

The regeneration of sensory axons is ascertained by a positive Tinel sign. This positive Tinel sign may also be used as a criterion for regeneration of a mixed nerve, which contains both sensory and motor axons. Tinel's sign will be present when paresthesias in a distal cutaneous region are produced by percussion over the edge of the regenerating nerve. By this method axonal regrowth can be charted, which usually occurs at a rate of 1 to 3 mm per day. This sign is used in conjunction with manual muscle testing and a battery of sensory tests to measure the client's recovery. Most clients under 30 years of age recover protective sensibility for heat and cold, pain, position, movement, and deep pressure following repair of a single peripheral cutaneous nerve.[21]

Rehabilitation is initiated by efforts to reduce edema and fibrosis. This may be accomplished through elevation, massage, and movement through a range of motion that does not traumatize the repair. Strengthening exercises for noninvolved muscles should continue throughout the course of treatment. When tissue healing is sufficient, the client begins passive range of motion exercises for the involved part(s). Goal-directed functional use of the extremity is encouraged, with adaptive devices used when indicated. The client should be alerted to problems such as insensitivity and trophic changes.[34]

Splinting following nerve loss may be useful in maintaining a functional hand position and preventing deformities resulting from muscle imbalance. Although splint requirements differ according to individual needs, some generalizations can be made. Median nerve involvement requires a splint that at least maintains thumb abduction. Ulnar nerve loss typically produces clawing from loss of the intrinsic muscles in the fourth and fifth digits, so hyperextension of the MP joint should be counteracted by splinting. When radial nerve lesions are splinted, prevention of wrist drop is often all that is required to allow the fingers more normal function.

Sensory reeducation is used to enhance recovery of sensory modalities. This technique requires cortical correlation of sensory impulses with known stimuli. The sequence of sensory modality recovery usually occurs in the following pattern: pain, 30 cps vibration, moving touch, constant touch, and 256 cps vibration.[9] When the client can perceive 30 cps vibration, moving touch is relearned by heavy tracing of objects from proximal to distal areas. As client recognition improves, the heavy stimulus is gradually replaced by lighter materials. Direction of movement is acquired by tracing numerals on the involved surface. Next, constant touch is learned by feeling or handling objects until they can be recognized without visual input.

Two-point discrimination is used to qualify the level of return and is possible only after light constant touch is regained.[2] Most young adults do not acquire better than 15 mm two-point discrimination following repair of nerve injury.[21] Often motor function, such as picking up and handling objects, is used in conjunction with sensory reeducation and is useful in developing movement patterns. Therapy sessions may be required for a period of months, with the goal of gradually turning the program over to the responsible client.

TREATMENT CONSIDERATIONS AND CASE STUDY

Joint mobilization, a form of passive movement, can be used successfully as a treatment in selected cases of hand dysfunction. Joint mobilization assists in pain relief, de-

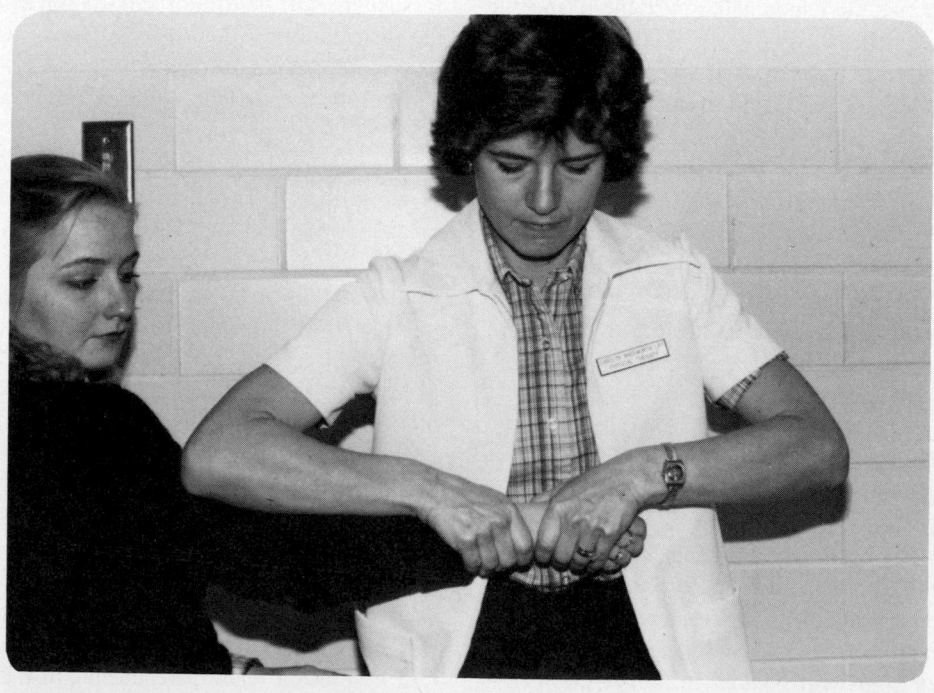

Fig. 18-32. Distal traction or carpus. Client's arm is stabilized against therapist's body with therapist holding close to the joint surfaces; mobilization force is parallel to long axis of extremity, moving carpus distally.

creasing muscle guarding and lengthening tissue (especially joint capsule and ligament). The therapist should perform a given technique in a controlled, reproducible manner at a grade and position appropriate for treating stiffness, pain, and/or spasm. Continual reassessment of the patient's response to treatment is always necessary. The direction of a technique is usually that which relieves pain or spasm in acute, irritable lesions, and that which increases mobility in chronic lesions. Often the most effective direction correlates with the kinematic principle that states: move a concave articular surface on a convex surface in the *same* direction as the osteokinematic (distal limb segment) movement desired; move a convex articular surface on a concave surface in the *opposite* direction as the osteokinematic movement desired. If this procedure increases a client's symptoms, however, one may apply techniques in the opposite direction. Chapter 9 discusses the specific grades of joint mobilization and the indications and contraindications for using these mobilization techniques.

When mobilization of the wrist is indicated, a trial treatment of traction is performed. Traction is applied by moving the carpus distal to the radius in a direction perpendicular to the plane of the joint (Fig. 18-32). The available joint play slack is taken up and the position held for approximately 10 seconds. This first treatment consists of 5 to 10 repetitions of traction; then the client is asked to report the response of the joint over the next 24 hours. If inflammation did not increase and increased pain did not

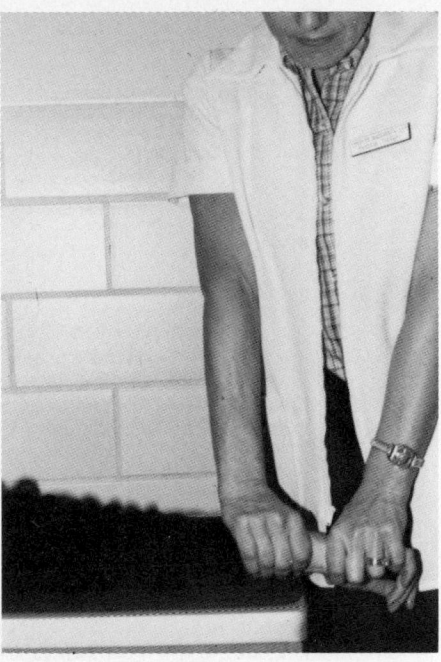

Fig. 18-34. Volar glide of carpus. Volar surface of client's forearm is stabilized against table; mobilization force moves carpus volarly perpendicular to long axis of extremity (distal traction is placed on carpus before and during mobilization).

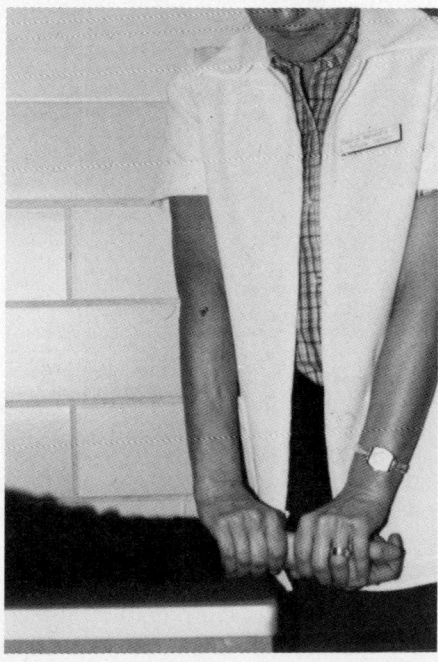

Fig. 18-33. Dorsal glide of carpus. Dorsal surface of client's forearm is stabilized against table; mobilization force moves carpus dorsally, perpendicular to the long axis of the extremity (distal traction is placed on carpus before and during mobilization).

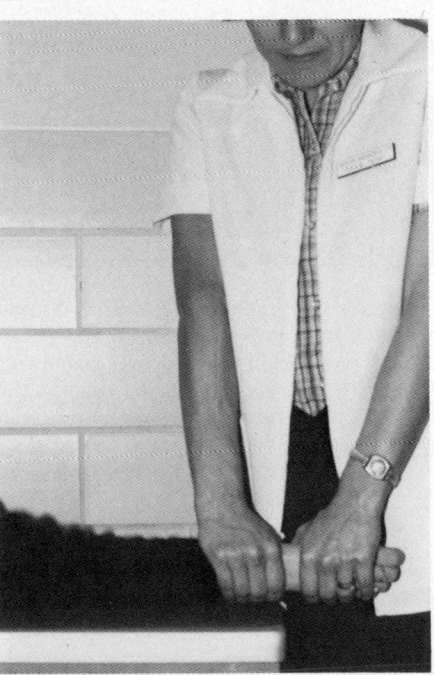

Fig. 18-35. Ulnar or radial glide of carpus. Ulnar (or radial) surface of client's forearm is stabilized against table; mobilization force moves carpus ulnarly (or radially) perpendicular to long axis of extremity (distal traction is placed on the carpus before and during mobilization).

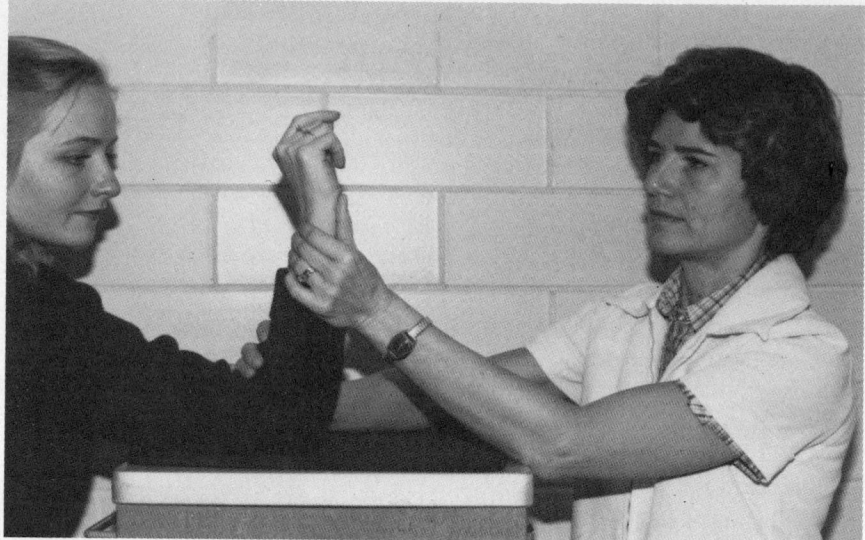

Fig. 18-36. Dorsal/volar glide of meniscus and triquetrum on ulna. Client sits with elbow supported on table and forearm stabilized by therapist; mobilization force is produced by therapist's thumb against client's pisiform, moving triquetrum dorsally relative to ulna, which is stabilized by therapist's index finger.

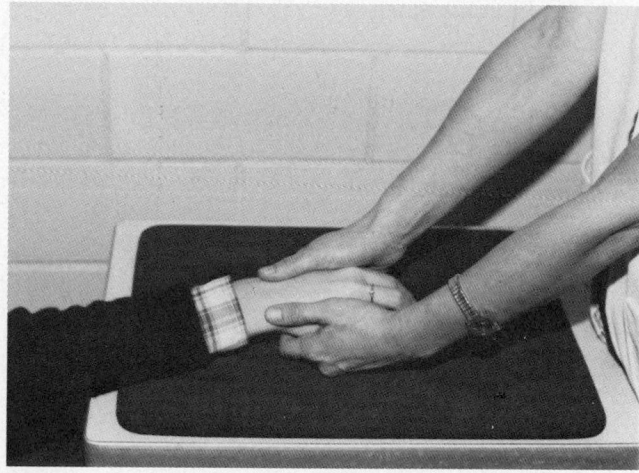

Fig. 18-37. Dorsal/volar glide of metacarpals: Volar surface of client's forearm is supported against table and metacarpals are stabilized by one hand of therapist; mobilization force moves metacarpals dorsally and volarly upon one another. (Each metacarpal may be moved individually for a specific mobilization, or all metacarpals may be moved together in a general mobilization to increase concavity of palm.)

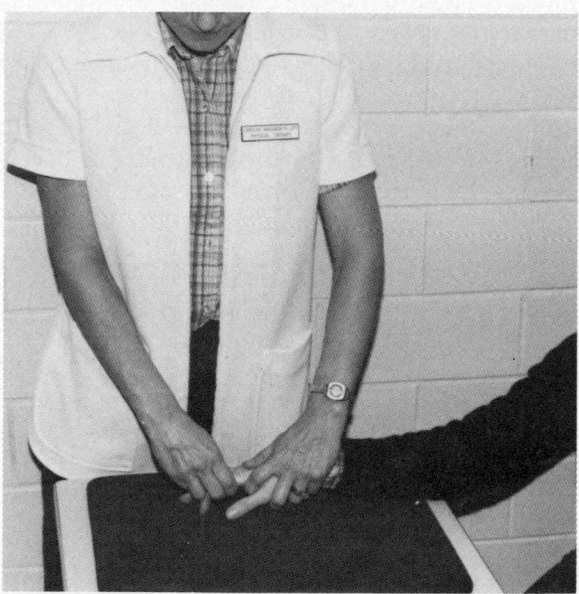

Fig. 18-38. Traction or glide of MP (or IP) joint. Volar surface of client's forearm and palm are supported against table and metacarpals are stabilized by therapist holding close to joint surface; mobilization force moves proximal (or middle or distal) phalanx distally for traction or volarly (or dorsally, radially, or ulnarly) for specific gliding mobilizations.

persist for more than 2 hours, the therapist may continue with mobilization treatment. It is best to add only one new technique at a time to avoid confusion as to the effects of each. A typical treatment of a joint may include three or four mobilization sessions lasting 30 seconds each, using 1 to 3 oscillations per second. Traction is used as a general procedure to relieve hypomobility in any direction of joint movement. Dorsal glide is a specific technique whereby the convex carpus is moved dorsally on the concave sur-

face formed by the radius and disk to increase wrist flexion (Fig. 18-33). Volar glide of the carpus is used to increase wrist extension (Fig. 18-34). Radial glide of the carpus is used to increase ulnar deviation, and ulnar glide of the carpus is used to increase radial deviation (Fig. 18-35). The ulnomeniscotriquetral joint is mobilized to increase supina-

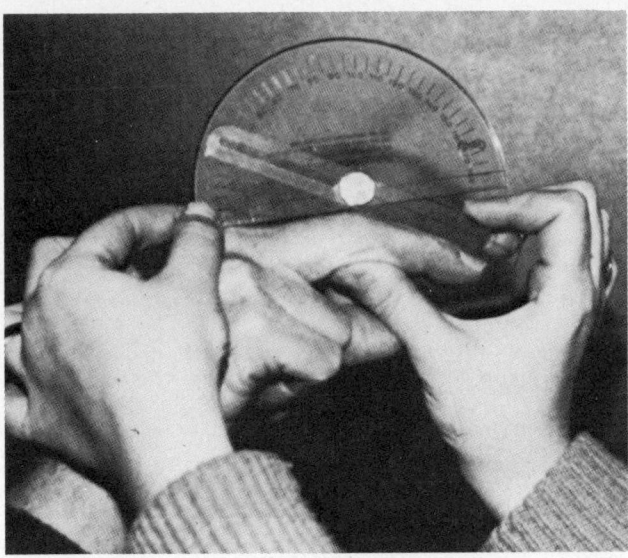

Fig. 18-39. Passive range of motion at initiation of treatment 2 months following traumatic PIP joint injury was 0 to 30 degrees flexion.

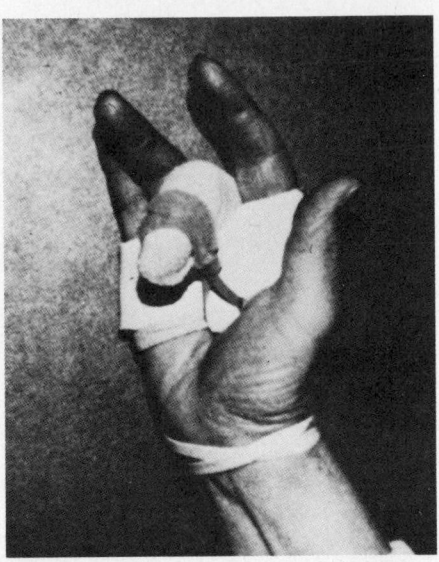

Fig. 18-41. Dynamic splint for maintaining PIP joint flexion; stockinette glove to reduce swelling.

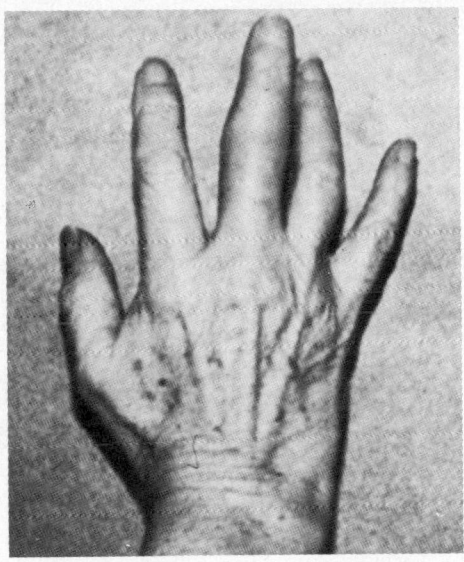

Fig. 18-40. Appearance of PIP joint at initiation of treatment.

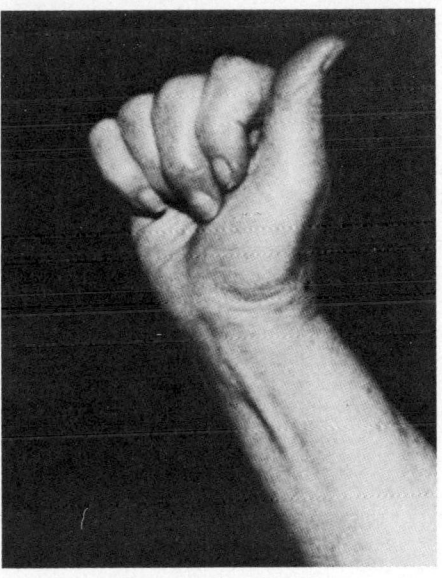

Fig. 18-42. Active range of motion at conclusion of treatment, 5 months following traumatic PIP joint injury, was 0 to 90 degrees flexion.

tion and pronation (Fig. 18-36). To increase metacarpal mobility and the palmar arch, dorsal/volar glide of the metacarpals is performed (Fig. 18-37). When joint mobilization is applied to the digits, a concave surface is moved on a convex one. After response to traction is ascertained, dorsal, volar, radial, and ulnar forces may be applied where appropriate (Fig. 18-38).

CASE STUDY

A case in which mobilization was used with a successful outcome involved a 64-year-old woman who was referred for severe restriction of PIP joint motion. Her history began with jamming her middle finger against the bathtub while housecleaning.

She had immediate sharp pain and slowly increasing pain and ecchymosis within the next 24 hours. However, she recalled that she was able to perform full range of motion after the incident. She did not seek medical attention but self-splinted the finger in extension for about 6 weeks until the pain subsided. At this time there was a marked loss of PIP joint flexion. She reported jamming the joint again and experiencing severe pain, which restricted function. She was seen by a physician, was diagnosed as having a "contusion of the right middle finger, possible sublimis rupture," and was referred for physical therapy to increase function. At the time of her referral, approximately 2 months after the initial injury, active flexion of the PIP joint was 0 to 5 degrees, passive flexion was 0 to 30 degrees, the sublimis was

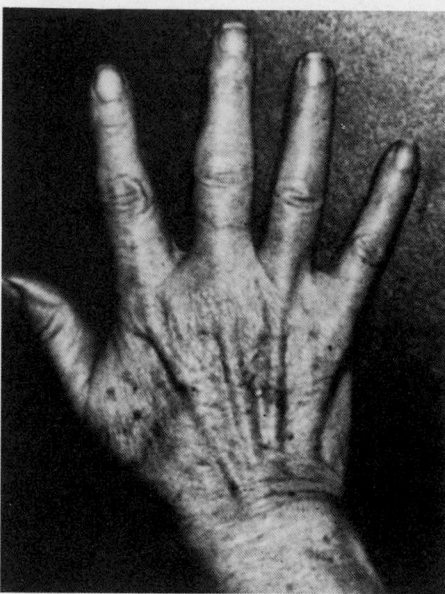

Fig. 18-43. Appearance of PIP joint at conclusion of treatment.

functional, and the rest of the hand was normal (Fig. 18-39). The joint was enlarged secondary to fibrotic edematous changes (Fig. 18-40). Pain was minimal with a capsular end-feel of movement being noted by the therapist well before the client's pain threshold was reached.

Joint mobilization treatment was initiated, and underwater ultrasound and massage were added the following week. The client was treated three times a week, and at the end of 1 month active range of motion was 0 to 50 degrees and passive range of motion was 0 to 70 degrees. A stockinette glove and dynamic flexion splint were constructed at this time to maintain the motion and reduced swelling that were achieved during treatment (Fig. 18-41). The client was instructed in a home program of active, passive, and resistive exercises, and physical therapy treatment was reduced to twice weekly. After 2 more months the client had achieved 90 degrees active range of motion and 100 degrees of passive range of motion (Fig. 18-42). Joint enlargement was markedly reduced (Fig. 18-43). The client and physician were satisfied with the results, and treatment was discontinued.

SUMMARY

The client with hand dysfunction desires the fullest recovery in the shortest time possible. This demands a fully coordinated team effort, with the client being prepared to take responsibility for lasting results. The therapist who rehabilitates such a client must have an in-depth understanding and working knowledge of the clinical anatomy, mechanics, and pathology of the hand, as well as be skilled in evaluation, interpretation, and treatment techniques. This chapter has attempted to correlate anatomical structure and function and pathological conditions that are commonly seen. Also a detailed format for evaluation and interpretation of results has been offered. Treatment considerations include the use of joint mobilization in selected cases.

REFERENCES

1. Beasley RW: Hand injuries, Philadelphia, 1981, WB Saunders Co.
2. Bell JA: Sensibility testing: state of the art. In Hunter JM et al, editors: Rehabilitation of the hand, ed 2, St Louis, 1984, The CV Mosby Co.
3. Bogumill GP: Anatomy of the wrist. In Lichtman DM: The wrist and its disorders, Philadelphia, 1988, WB Saunders Co.
4. Boswick JA: Rehabilitation of the burned hand, Clin Orthop 104:162, 1974.
5. Boyes JH: Bunnell's surgery of the hand, ed 5, Philadelphia, 1970, JB Lippincott Co.
6. Brown HC: Current concepts of burn pathology and mechanisms of deformity in the burned hand, Orthop Clin North Am 4(4):987, 1973.
7. Cailliet R: Hand pain and impairment, ed 2, Philadelphia, 1975, FA Davis Co.
8. Cyriax J: Textbook of orthopaedic medicine, ed 6, vol 1, Baltimore, 1975, Williams & Wilkins.
9. Dellon AL: Evaluation of sensibility and reeducation of sensation in the hand, Baltimore, 1981, Williams & Wilkins.
10. Fess EE et al: Evaluation of the hand by objective measurement. In Hunter JM et al, editors: Rehabilitation of the hand, ed 2, St Louis, 1984, The CV Mosby Co.
11. Flatt AE: Care of the arthritic hand, ed 4, St Louis, 1983, The CV Mosby Co.
12. Harris C Jr and Rutledge GL Jr: The functional anatomy of the extensor mechanism of the finger, J Bone Joint Surg (Am) 54(4):713, 1972.
13. Hoppenfeld S: Physical examination of the spine and extremities, New York, 1976, Appleton-Century-Crofts.
14. Kapandji IA: The physiology of the joints, vol 1, Baltimore, 1970, Williams & Wilkins.
15. Kleinert HE and Meares A: In quest of the solution to severed flexor tendons, Clin Orthop 104:23, 1974.
16. Lampe EW: Surgical anatomy of the hand, CIBA Clin Symp 9(1), 1957.
17. Landsmeer JM: Power grip and precision handling, Ann Rheum Dis 22:164, 1962.
18. Matheson LN et al: Work hardening: occupational therapy in industrial rehabilitation, Amer J Occup Ther. 39(5):314-321, 1985.
19. McCue FC III et al: Hand and wrist injuries in the athlete, Am J Sports Med 7(5):275, 1979.
20. Moore KL: Clinically oriented anatomy, Baltimore, 1980, Williams & Wilkins.
21. Omer GE: Sensation and sensibility in the upper extremity, Clin Orthop 104:30, 1974.
22. Palmer AK and Werner FW: Biomechanics of the distal radioulnar joint, Clin Orthop 187:26-35, 1984.
23. Phalen GS: The carpal-tunnel syndrome, Clin Orthop 83:29, 1972.
24. Philips CA: Hand therapy in the early stages of rheumatoid arthritis. In Hunter JM et al, editors: Rehabilitation of the hand, ed 2, St Louis, 1984, The CV Mosby Co.
25. Salisbury RE, Reeves S, and Wright P: Acute care and rehabilitation of the burned hand. In Hunter JM et al, editors: Rehabilitation of the hand, ed 2, St Louis, 1984, The CV Mosby Co.
26. Smith RJ: Balance and kinetics of the fingers under normal and pathological conditions, Clin Orthop 104:92, 1974.
27. Souter WA: The problem of boutonniere deformity, Clin Orthop 104:116, 1974.
28. Spinner M: Injuries to the major branches of peripheral nerves of the forearm, ed 2, Philadelphia, 1978, WB Saunders Co.
29. Sprague BL: Proximal interphalangeal joint injuries and their initial treatment, J Trauma 15(5):380, 1975.

30. Swanson AB: Reconstructive surgery in the arthritic hand and foot, CIBA Clin Symp 31(6):1, 1979.

31. Swanson AB, Goran-Hagert C, and Swanson G: Evaluation of impairment of hand function. In Hunter JM et al, editors: Rehabilitation of the hand, ed 2, St Louis, 1984, The CV Mosby Co.

32. Swezey RL: Dynamic factors in deformity of the rheumatoid hand, Bull Rheum Dis (series) 22(1 and 2):649, 1971-72.

33. Warwick R and Williams PL, editors: Gray's anatomy, ed 35 (Br), Philadelphia, 1973, WB Saunders Co.

34. Weeks PM and Wray RC: Management of acute hand injuries, ed 2, St Louis, 1978, The CV Mosby Co.

35. Wynn Parry CB: Rehabilitation of the hand, ed 3, Sussex, 1973, Butterworth Publishers.

Chapter 19

THE ELBOW COMPLEX

Richard W. Bowling
Paul A. Rockar, Jr.

The cubital articulation is formed by the joints between the radius and humerus, the ulna and humerus, and the radius and ulna. All these joints share a common articular cavity. The first two are collectively known as the elbow and function as a hinge to allow flexion and extension of the forearm. The superior radioulnar joint belongs functionally to the joints of the forearm and participates in the movements of supination and pronation of the forearm along with the distal radioulnar joint.

The most common problem encountered by physical therapists in management of clients with dysfunction of the elbow complex is loss of motion as a result of trauma or immobilization. The goal of treatment in such cases is the restoration of a full and pain-free range of motion. The manner in which this should be accomplished, however, is controversial. Most textbooks of orthopaedic surgery advocate early active motion and state unequivocally that passive movement is contraindicated.[19,21] On the other hand, physical therapists who are experienced in the application of passive movement techniques are aware that properly selected and applied passive movement can supplement the effects of active exercise.[11,17]

The ability of the physical therapist to successfully manage the problems encountered at the cubital complex hinges on understanding functional anatomy, pathokinesiology, principles of examination, and the principles of treatment of the musculoskeletal system used in therapeutic exercise. Selection of the appropriate treatment modality is no different at the cubital complex than at any other region of the musculoskeletal system. It involves the ability to perform a clinical examination to determine the nature and state of the pathological condition present as well as the ability to select and apply therapeutic techniques that can influence the problem identified in a positive manner.

ANATOMY
Osteology

Distal humerus. The distal end of the humerus is flattened in the frontal plane and projects anteriorly from the shaft of the humerus at an angle of approximately 45 degrees.[13] It bears two articular condyles, a medial or trochlear surface, for articulation with the trochlear notch of the ulna and a lateral surface, or capitellum, for articulation with the proximal surface of the radial head.[22]

Three concavities, or fossae, are situated on the distal

humerus. Anteriorly, the coronoid fossa is located just superior to the trochlear surface. It receives the coronoid process of the ulna during flexion of the forearm. Similarly, the radial fossa lies on the anterior surface just proximal to the capitellum, and during flexion of the forearm it accommodates the radial head.[7] Both of these anterior fossae increase the potential for flexion of the forearm.[13]

On the posterior aspect of the humerus, the olecranon fossa is located just superior to the trochlea, and it receives the olecranon process of the ulna during extension of the forearm, thus augmenting the range of extension.[13]

The *trochlea* covers the anterior, inferior, and posterior aspects of the medial humeral condyle.[22] It is a sellar articular surface that is concave in the frontal plane and convex in the sagittal plane. The trochlea is marked centrally by a deep groove that dictates the path that the ulna must follow during flexion and extension of the forearm.[15] The axis of motion of the elbow joint lies perpendicular to this groove. Laterally, the trochlea is separated from the capitellum by the capitotrochlear groove.[22] Medially, the trochlea projects prominently downward below the rest of the bone.[22]

The *capitellum* is a roughly hemispherical body located on the anterior aspect of the distal humerus. Kapandji[13] has described this articular condyle as lying entirely in front of the distal end of the humerus. Thus the radial head does not fit congruently with the capitellum when the elbow is extended. The capitellum has an ovoid articular surface that is convex in all planes.

The *medial epicondyle* is a blunt projection on the medial side of the medial condyle of the humerus.[22] The flexor muscles of the forearm (flexor carpi radialis, flexor carpi ulnaris, flexor digitorum superficialis, palmaris longus, and part of the pronator teres) take their origin from the anterior aspect of the medial epicondyle.[22] This structure also serves as the proximal attachment of the medial collateral ligament of the elbow joint.[22] The ulnar nerve runs in a groove on the posterior aspect of the medial epicondyle and is easily palpable in this location. The nerve is susceptible to trauma at this site because of its superficial position.

The *lateral epicondyle* is the lateral portion of the nonarticular region of the lateral condyle of the humerus. It gives origin to the superficial extensor muscles of the forearm (extensor carpi ulnaris, extensor digiti minimi, and supinator) as well as the lateral collateral ligament of the elbow joint.[22]

Proximal radius. The proximal end of the radius includes the head, neck, and bicipital tuberosity. The radial head is shaped somewhat in the manner of a disk, and its superior surface bears a shallow, cuplike articular surface for articulation with the capitellum of the humerus.[13,22]

The circumference of the radial head also bears an articular surface. This convex surface articulates with the radial notch of the ulna.[13] Just distal to the head the shaft of the radius is constricted. This region is known as the neck of the radius, and it bears a roughened tuberosity on its medial aspect for attachment of the biceps brachii.

Proximal ulna. The upper end of the ulna bears two prominent processes, the olecranon and the coronoid. It also contains two articular surfaces. The articular surfaces are the trochlear notch and the radial notch, which articulate, respectively, with the trochlea of the humerus and the circumference of the radial head.

The *olecranon process* is the most proximal portion of the ulna. It projects upward and bends anteriorly to form a prominent beak that enters the olecranon fossa of the humerus when the elbow is extended.[22] The anterior aspect of the olecranon forms the upper part of the trochlear notch of the ulna.

The *coronoid process* is a small projection located on the anterior aspect of the bone. Its superior surface forms the lower part of the trochlear notch.[22]

The *trochlear notch*, like the trochlea of the humerus with which it articulates, is a sellar surface. It is concave in the sagittal plane and convex in the frontal plane. Centrally, it is marked by a prominent ridge that corresponds to the groove found on the trochlear surface of the humerus.[15]

The *radial notch* is a concave articular depression located on the upper portion of the lateral aspect of the coronoid process of the ulna. It articulates with the circumference of the radial head to form the proximal radioulnar joints.[13]

Arthrology

MacConaill and Basmajian[16] have classified the cubital complex as a paracondylar joint because one bone (the humerus) articulates with two others (the radius and ulna) by way of two facets. This enables one of the latter two bones to undergo a movement independent of the other (i.e., rotation of the radius during pronation and supination of the forearm). The complex has two degrees of freedom. Flexion and extension of the forearm occur in the sagittal plane, and supination and pronation of the forearm are permitted in the transverse plane.

Kinematic analysis of the cubital complex can be simplified if the joint is divided functionally into the following components: (1) the elbow, which permits the movements of flexion and extension, and (2) the joints of the forearm, which permit supination and pronation.

Elbow. The elbow is composed of the humeroulnar and the humeroradial joints. The former possesses sellar articular surfaces, whereas the latter is ovoid in configuration. For practical purposes these two joints can be considered to function as a uniaxial hinge joint.

Conflicting reports of elbow kinematics have been presented in the literature.[6,14,15,18] In a recent review London[15] has discussed some of the major contributions in this area and noted some deficiencies in analytical techniques that were employed. With what he considered an improved methodology, he determined that the instantaneous axes of rotation (IAR) for flexion and the IARs for extension of the humeroulnar joint were tightly clustered around the center of the arc formed by the trochlear sulcus of the humerus. Exceptions occurred during the last 10 degrees of flexion when the IAR moved proximally and anteriorly toward the coronoid fossa and during the last 10 degrees of extension when the IAR moved proximally and posteriorly toward the olecranon fossa.[15]

The IARs of the humeroradial joint demonstrated a similar distribution around the center of the arc formed by the capitellum.[15] During terminal flexion the IAR moved proximally and anteriorly toward the radial fossa, and on terminal extension the IAR moved toward the posterior aspect of the capitellum.

The axis of motion of the elbow can be approximated by a line that connects the center of the arc of the trochlear sulcus with the center of the arc of the capitellum. This axis makes an angle of 94 to 98 degrees with the humeral shaft that declines from lateral to medial.[15] The position of the axis is also internally rotated with respect to the plane of the humeral epicondyles by 3 to 8 degrees (Fig. 19-1).[15]

In the plane of flexion and extension of the elbow both of the moving surfaces (trochlear notch and radial head) are concave articular surfaces. Thus the swing of the two bones will be accompanied by gliding of the articular surfaces in the same direction.[16,22]

At the extremes of flexion and extension the gliding movement of the articular surfaces is augmented by rolling. The rolling movement also occurs in the same direction as the swing of the bones.[16,22] This rolling movement accounts for the displacements of the IARs that London[15] has reported.

The range of motion of elbow flexion and extension depends on whether the movement is produced actively or passively. From the anatomical position the elbow can flex through a range of 145 degrees actively and 160 degrees passively.[13] Movement from the position of full flexion back to the anatomical position is termed *extension*. In some individuals movement is permitted beyond the anatomical position. This motion is termed *hyperextension* and may reach a range of 5 to 10 degrees (Fig. 19-2).[13]

When the elbow is in the anatomical position (extended), a valgus angulation is evident between the arm and forearm. This angle is termed the *carrying angle* and usually ranges between 10 and 15 degrees.[13] The angle is generally larger in women than in men. There is some controversy over whether the valgus angulation remains constant or alters as the forearm is carried into flexion. Morrey and Chao[18] state that the carrying angle varies in a linear manner from a valgus angle in extension to a varus angle in flexion. On the other hand, Grant[7] and London[15] state that the carrying angle is relatively constant throughout the range of flexion and extension. On careful clinical observation the carrying angle does appear to remain constant if care is taken to prevent medial rotation of the humerus at the glenohumeral joint as the elbow is flexed.

Supporting structures of the elbow. The elbow is supported by static and dynamic structures. The static structures include the fibrous capsule, the collateral ligaments, and osseous structures, while the dynamic supporting structures include the muscles that cross the joint. The static supports of the elbow region will be described. The reader is referred to any standard anatomical text for a review of dynamic supporting structures.[22]

Static supporting structures

FIBROUS CAPSULE. The anterior portion of the fibrous capsule is thin and broad. It is attached to the anterior surface of the humerus just above the radial and coronoid fossae. Inferiorly, it attaches to the anterior surface of the coronoid process and to the annular ligament of the supe-

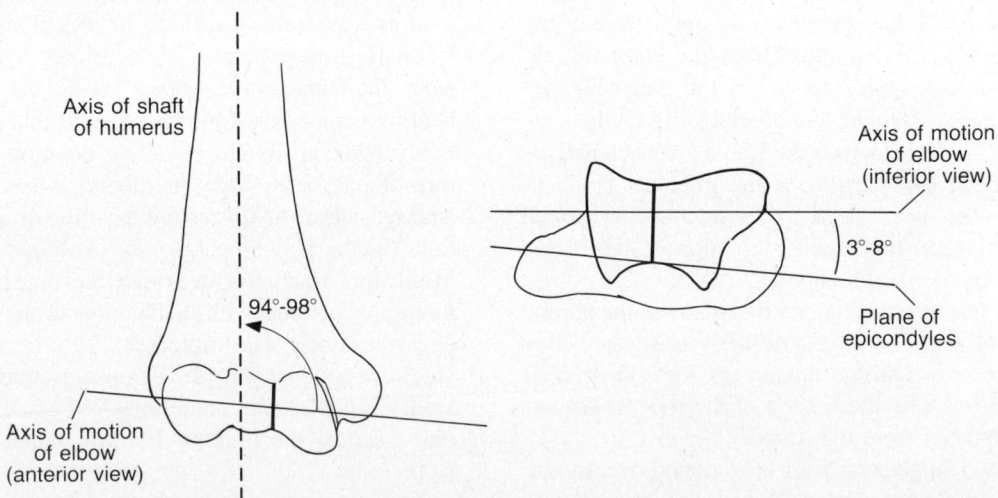

Fig. 19-1. Axis of motion of elbow joint.

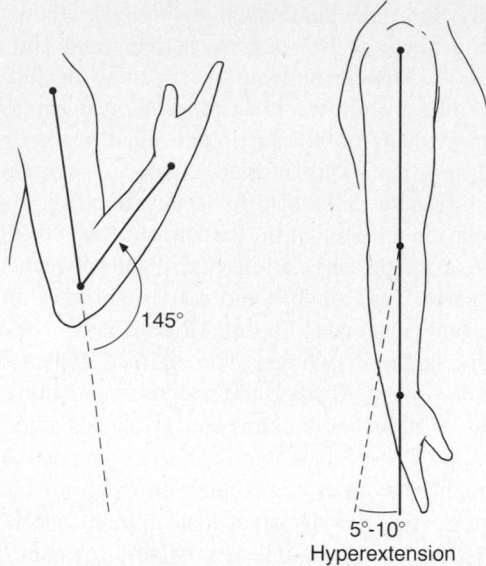

Fig. 19-2. Range of motion of elbow. From the anatomical position, the elbow can move through a range of 145 degrees of flexion actively. The joint is capable of 160 degrees of flexion passively. A range of 5 to 10 degrees of hyperextension is possible in some individuals. (Modified from Kapandji IA: The physiology of the joints, vol 1, The upper limb, London, 1970, E & S Livingstone, Inc.)

rior radioulnar joint. On either side it blends with the collateral ligaments.[22]

The posterior portion of the capsule is also thin and loose. Superiorly, it attaches to the humerus directly behind the capitellum and the lateral margin of the trochlea. It extends around the rim of the olecranon fossa and on to the posterior aspect of the medial epicondyle. Inferiorly, the posterior capsule is attached to the superior and lateral margins of the olecranon process. Laterally, it is continuous with the capsule of the superior radioulnar joint deep to the annular ligament.[22]

The *synovial membrane* extends from the margin of the articular surfaces of the humerus, lines the coronoid, radial, and olecranon fossae, and covers the flattened, medial, nonarticular surface of the trochlea. It is then reflected over the deep surface of the fibrous capsule and attaches inferiorly to the margins of the trochlear notch of the ulna and to the radial neck. It forms a saclike pouch below the radial head that permits rotation of the radius without tearing of the membrane.[22]

Between the fibrous capsule and the synovial membrane are three pads of fat. The largest of these is situated over the olecranon fossa. During flexion of the elbow it is pressed into the fossa by the tendon of the triceps. On extension it is displaced from the fossa.[22]

Anteriorly, two smaller fat pads are situated over the radial and coronoid fossae. These fat pads are pressed into their respective fossae during extension and are displaced during flexion.[22]

Normally the fat pads are not visible on a lateral radiograph of the elbow. If they are displaced from the fossae by an effusion or a hemarthrosis, they are visible as radiolucent zones. This *fat pad sign* may be the only radiographic evidence of an occult fracture of the elbow.[6]

ULNAR COLLATERAL LIGAMENT. The ulnar collateral ligament provides a major contribution to stability of the elbow.[20] It is composed of two functional bands, both of which emanate from the medial epicondyle. The most anterior portion, the anterior oblique ligament, passes downward and anteriorly to insert into the medial aspect of the coronoid process of the ulna. This band is further subdivided into two functional components, one of which is taut in all positions of flexion or extension of the joint.[20]

The posterior portion of the ulnar collateral ligament is weaker than the anterior oblique portion. It is shaped like a fan and attaches to the medial and posterior aspects of the olecranon process. This portion of the ligament is only taut when the joint is in full extension.[20]

RADIAL COLLATERAL LIGAMENT. The radial or lateral collateral ligament is not as strong as the ulnar collateral ligament. It passes from its origin on the lateral humeral epicondyle downward to insert into the annular ligament of the superior radioulnar joint.[20] A few fibers may pass over that ligament to insert into the superior portion of the supinator crest of the ulna.[22] The radial collateral ligament is not capable of providing much protection against varus stress to the elbow joint.[20]

Restraint to motion in the sagittal plane. The capsule of the elbow is designed to permit free movement in the sagittal plane and does not offer much resistance to movement under normal circumstances.

Extension is limited primarily by impact of the olecranon process with the olecranon fossa. In this position the humeroulnar joint is in its most stable state, the close-packed position.[11] Interestingly, while the humeroulnar joint is in its close-packed position, the humeroradial joint is in its least stable position, the maximal loose-packed position (resting position).[11] Therefore, when in full extension, the ulna would appear to be the primary weight-bearing bone of the forearm. A joint that is stressed abnormally while in its close-packed position is prone to fracture of one of its bony members, whereas a joint that is stressed while in its resting position is prone to dislocation.[16] This phenomenon may explain the mechanism of Monteggia fractures, in which the proximal ulna is fractured concomitant with dislocation of the radial head.

Extension is also limited, but to a lesser degree, by the anterior capsule and by the flexor musculature of the joint.[13] Under pathological conditions either of these structures may become the primary limiting factor to elbow extension.

Flexion of the elbow is limited primarily by contact and compression of the soft tissue masses of the anterior aspects of the arm and forearm.[2] When the movement is performed actively, the block to movement occurs at approximately 145 degrees because of the relative incompressibility of actively contracting muscle tissue.[13]

Passive flexion may also be limited by soft tissue compression in mesomorphic individuals (at 160 degrees) but is just as often brought to a halt by impact of the radial head and coronoid process into their respective fossae. As was the case with elbow extension, flexion may be limited by the posterior capsule and by the extensor musculature, although the role played by these structures under normal circumstances is insignificant.

It was noted that the humeroulnar joint reaches its close-packed position in full extension. The close-packed position of the humeroradial joint occurs at approximately 80 degrees of flexion with the forearm in the midposition between full pronation and full supination.[11] This position also corresponds to the resting position of the humeroulnar joint.[11] It might be expected that trauma in this position would produce a fracture of the humeroradial joint and dislocation of the humeroulnar joint.

Restraint to motion in the frontal plane. The collateral ligaments of hinge joints are typically designed to prevent motion outside of the normal plane of movement of the joint. The capsule of the elbow permits free movement in the sagittal plane, while the ulnar and radial collateral ligaments limit movement in the frontal plane. From a clinical standpoint the only restraint required is resistance to valgus stresses, since varus stresses at the elbow are rarely encountered in functional activities.

The principal restraint to valgus angulation is provided by the ulnar collateral ligament, a portion of which is taut in all positions of the joint.[20] Tearing of this ligament results in instability of the joint with a tendency to recurrent dislocation. A further buttress to valgus angulation is provided by the bony configuration of the humeroradial joint.[20] This joint is capable of resisting compressive stresses that occur on the lateral side of the joint with a valgus stress, particularly when the joint is in a semiflexed attitude.

Joints of the forearm. The joints of the forearm include the proximal radioulnar joint and the distal radioulnar joint, both of which are ovoid synovial joints. The middle radioulnar syndesmosis must also be included. Movement of the joints of the forearm depends on movement at the humeroradial joint, which permits the joints to function in any position of flexion or extension of the elbow.

The joints of the forearm permit rotation of the radius in a medial and lateral direction. Medial rotation of the radius is termed *pronation,* whereas lateral rotation is known as *supination.* Supination is usually permitted through a range of 90 degrees. Pronation is permitted through a somewhat smaller excursion of 85 degrees.[13]

On a cursory analysis supination and pronation appear to be simple rotations of the radius about a fixed or stationary ulna. However, closer observation reveals the move-

ments to be more complex. In fact, the axis of rotation of the radius appears to move in a manner that depends on the required functional activity.[13] That is to say, the axis of rotation appears to shift to the radial side of the forearm, the ulnar side of the forearm, or to any position between these two extremes.

An analysis of these movements must begin with the joints that participate. First, at the superior radioulnar joint the convex peripheral rim of the radial head articulates with a concave surface formed by the annular ligament and the radial notch of the ulna. The radial head is capable of rotating within this fibroosseous ring in a clockwise or a counterclockwise direction. The axis of rotation is at the center of curvature of the ring. Since the major portion of the ring is fibrous tissue, the axis may shift somewhat if the configuration of the ring is distorted. However, the axis does not displace to a significant degree because of this mechanism.

At the distal radioulnar joint the convex articular surface of the head of the ulna articulates with a concave facet on the medial aspect of the distal radius. The axis of rotation of this joint must lie at the center of curvature of the head of the ulna. This position is near the point of attachment of the articular disk to the base of the styloid process of the ulna.[13,14]

Since the shafts of the radius and the ulna are united at each end by a joint and are relatively inflexible, the radius must rotate in relation to the ulna about an axis that passes through the axes of both the proximal and distal radioulnar joints. If motion occurs about any other axis, it can only do so if one of the bones or one of the joints fails (Fig. 19-3).

The apparent shift in the axis of motion must occur through a concomitant movement of the ulna. The distal end of the ulna may be observed to move in a lateral direction (abduction) during pronation and in a medial direction (adduction) during supination. This movement of the ulna in the frontal plane carries the distal pole of the axis of rotation of the forearm with it.[13,22]

When the frontal plane movement of the ulna is minimal, the functional axis of motion is near the ulnar side of the forearm. When ulnar movement is maximal, the axis shifts to the radial side of the forearm.

Ulnar motion in the frontal plane may occur at the humeroulnar joint because of the sellar configuration of the joint.[22] Since this is the case, the humeroulnar joint should be included in the detailed examination of motion disturbances of the joints of the forearm.

Thus far the motion of the radius in space (osteokinematics) has been described. Also important are the articular movements (arthrokinematics) that occur when the radius moves in supination and pronation. Rotation of the radius depends on movement in the proximal radioulnar joint, the distal radioulnar joint, the middle radioulnar syndesmosis, and the humeroradial joint.

It is somewhat confusing to consider the long axis of

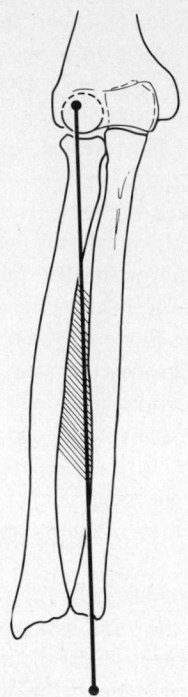

Fig. 19-3. Axis of joints of forearm.

the radius as the mechanical axis of the bone. For the sake of a better understanding of the arthrokinematics of these joints, it is helpful to construct a mechanical axis that is perpendicular to the plane of the concave joint surfaces.

The mechanical axis of the bone can be arbitrarily established as perpendicular to the plane of the distal articular surface of the radius. Supination, or lateral rotation, is a swing of the axis in a lateral direction, and pronation, or medial rotation, is a swing in a medial direction.

At the superior radioulnar joint the moving articular surface is the convex radial head. Thus the circumference of the radial head will roll in the same direction as the swing of the axis. It will glide in the opposite direction of the swing. Motion of the radial head at this articulation appears to be mostly gliding with little rolling.

The inferior radioulnar joint is formed by the articulation of the concave facet on the medial surface of the distal radius with the convex ulnar head. The concave radial surface is the moving surface. It rolls and glides in the same direction as the swing of the mechanical axis of the bone.

The shafts of the radius and ulna are connected by the oblique cord and by the interosseous membrane of the forearm. The latter is the most important structure functionally. Its fibers slant downward and medially from the interosseous border of the radius to that of the ulna. The fibers of the membrane are supposedly directed so as to transmit force from the radius to the ulna and hence to the humerus. However, the fibers of the membrane are only taut when the forearm is midway between full supination and full pronation and are relaxed at the extremes of these

positions.[22] Primarily, the membrane appears to increase the surface area for muscle attachment, but, as will be seen, it can limit the range of motion under certain pathological conditions.

Factors limiting supination. Supination is limited by the quadrate ligament at the proximal radioulnar joint and by the anterior ligament and capsule at the distal radioulnar joint. The pronating muscles, however, provide the greatest restraint to supination.[13,14]

Factors limiting pronation. Pronation is also limited by the quadrate ligament at the proximal joint. Movement is regulated by the posterior capsule and triangular ligament of the distal radioulnar joint. The primary restraint to pronation, however, is compression of the soft tissues covering the shafts of the radius and ulna as the two bones are crossed.[13,14]

As previously stated, the interosseous membrane is slack at the extremes of both supination and pronation. Thus it cannot be a factor in restricting either of these movements under normal circumstances. It becomes taut midway between full supination and full pronation and appears to play a role in providing stability to the joints in this close-packed position of the forearm. The joints of the forearm reach the close-packed position in approximately 5 degrees of supination.[11] The joints of the forearm cannot be placed in their resting positions simultaneously. The distal radioulnar joint reaches the resting position at 10 degrees of supination, whereas the proximal radioulnar joint is in the resting position at 35 degrees of supination, when the elbow is flexed to approximately 70 degrees.[11]

The complex bowing of the radius also appears to be an important factor that influences range of motion in pronation and supination. The radius is bowed in the opposite direction (laterally) in relation to the ulna when the forearm is in the close-packed position. This factor appears to produce tension in the interosseous membrane. Following fractures of the forearm, if the bones are allowed to unite with an angular malunion, a significant reduction in the range of motion of pronation and supination will occur.[1]

EXAMINATION OF THE ELBOW COMPLEX

The objective of the examination of any part of the musculoskeletal system is to provide data from which decisions regarding management can be made. All too often a diagnosis or naming of a disease process is over-emphasized. In many cases a traditional diagnosis is impossible to obtain. In other cases clients with the same diagnosis should be managed differently. This is one reason, in fact, for the disrepute of using passive movement exercises at the elbow joint.

The objectives of a physical therapist's examination may be different from those of the physician. The physician is concerned with identification of major disease processes that may produce disorders of the musculoskeletal system, whereas the primary concern of the physical therapist is the determination of the client's reaction to movement of the joint. Of course, the physical therapist must also be alert for signs of pathological conditions of a more serious nature.

Often, a diagnosis can only be stated in terms of altered motion. At other times, when a traditional diagnosis can be made, an understanding of the altered motion state that results from the pathological condition present is of more use. This can be stated in terms of an abnormal response to active motion, passive motion, or both.

Once the movement disorder has been identified through a thorough examination of the effects of movement on the symptoms, management is directed toward improving the dysfunction. The methods of management are derived from a continual, dynamic process that involves the selection and application of treatment technique, reevaluation of the dysfunction, and maintenance or alteration of the treatment program depending on the outcome. That is to say, if one movement in the examination scheme appears to have the most effect on the client's symptoms, that movement may be selected as a treatment technique. After the movement has been applied as a mode of therapeutic intervention, its effects on the symptoms are assessed during the reevaluation. If the dysfunction has improved, the treatment may be continued with no changes. If the dysfunction has not changed or become worse, a different treatment technique may be selected.

In this chapter only those portions of the subjective and objective examination that are most important to the physical therapist (see accompanying box) will be stressed. A thorough discussion of the numerous pathological conditions that affect the elbow has already been given in a number of standard orthopaedic texts, and the reader is referred to these for further information.* However, certain aspects related to pathological conditions at the elbow that are important to understanding the examination and treatment of movement disorders of this joint complex will be discussed.

Functional examination

The functional examination is that portion of the objective examination scheme (see accompanying box) from which the physical therapist derives the most useful information regarding movement dysfunction. The functional examination includes an assessment of (1) active movements, (2) passive movements, (3) accessory movements, and (4) resisted tests.[11]

Active movement. The examination of active movement serves the following purposes: (1) the willingness of the client to move the joint may be assessed, and (2) if the range of motion is abnormal or painful, a baseline may be established to measure the effects of treatment.[2]

Active movement, in and of itself, is not diagnostic be-

*See references 1, 2, 5, 8, 9, and 21.

Examination of the elbow complex

Subjective

What caused the client to consult a physician?
 If pain
  Where is the pain felt?
  Is it constant or intermittent?
 If constant
  Does it vary in intensity?
  What makes it worse?
  What eases it?
 If intermittent
  What brings it on?
  How long does it last?
 If loss of motion
  What are the functional limitations?
  How did this problem begin?
  Any history of the same, or a similar problem, in the past?
  Any related problems?

Objective*

 Inspection
  Functional movements
  Posture
  Shape
  Skin
  Aids
 Function
  Active movements
  Passive movements
  Accessory movements
  Resisted tests
 Palpation
  Skin and subcutaneous tissue
  Muscle and tendon
  Tendon sheaths and bursae
  Joints
  Nerves and blood vessels
 Neurological tests
  Nerve trunk
  Reflexes and key muscles
  Sensory examination
  Motor examination
  Coordination
 Additional examinations
  Radiography
  Laboratory tests
  Electrodiagnosis
  Punctures (e.g., biopsy, aspiration)
  Special examination (referral to other practitioner)

*Objective examination modified from Kaltenborn FM: Manual therapy for the extremity joints, specialized techniques: tests and joint mobilization, ed 2, Oslo, 1976, Olaf Norlis Bokhandel.

cause it stresses both contractile and noncontractile tissue.[2] The findings must be interpreted along with those of subsequent portions of the examination. The client's response to active movement may provide a valuable gauge in determining how to proceed with the remainder of the examination. For example, if a client complains of a considerable increase in pain while performing an active movement or if it takes a considerable length of time for the discomfort provoked by movement to subside, the examiner must be alerted to the fact that caution should be employed in the performance of passive and resisted tests. If, on the other hand, no pain is reported by the client and the range of motion is full, a more vigorous application of the remaining examination techniques may be indicated.

The client is instructed to perform the following active movements: flexion, extension, supination, and pronation. The last two movements should be performed with the elbow held in varying degrees of flexion. As stated previously, the examiner should note any abnormality, including pain, decreased range of motion, or increased range of motion, compared with the uninvolved limb.

Passive movement. Passive movements are intended to stress noncontractile tissues.[2] This portion of the examination may be the most valuable tool for the physical therapist. Much can be learned about the state of the tissues in and around the joint from a careful analysis of the passive range of motion permitted at the joint. While the movements are performed, the examiner must focus attention on three phenomena that follow: (1) the range of motion possible, (2) the nature of the motion barrier, and (3) the relationship of pain to the motion barrier.[2]

Range of motion. The passive movements included in the examination of the elbow joint are flexion, extension, pronation, and supination. On completion of these test movements, one of three possibilities will have been found. The range of motion will be normal, restricted, or excessive.

Excessive motion usually implies damage of the supporting connective tissues or muscles surrounding the joint. In an adolescent this finding may warrant the inclusion of stress radiographs to rule out the possibility of epiphyseal fracture near the joint.

If the range of motion is limited, it will be limited in one of two patterns. Cyriax[2] has termed these (1) the capsular pattern and (2) the noncapsular pattern.

The *capsular pattern* has been defined as a proportional limitation of the movements available at a particular joint. The capsular pattern of the elbow is usually such that a greater limitation of flexion will be found as opposed to extension. Generally, supination and pronation are not affected to a great extent. At times the restrictions of flexion and extension may be nearly equal, and in advanced cases of arthritis movement of the forearm may also be limited.[2] At the elbow, as at other joints of the musculoskeletal system, the finding of a capsular pattern signifies a total joint reaction; that is, an inflammation of the joint is present.[2]

The mechanism behind the proportional limitation of movement is not clearly understood. The joint may be splinted (by muscles surrounding the joint) in the position where the joint capsule can accommodate the greatest volume of fluid.[6] There is also some preliminary evidence that suggests an imbalance between the preaxial and postaxial musculature associated with a withdrawal reflex.[3,4] This area requires further investigation.

Although the finding of a capsular pattern does provide a diagnosis (a joint inflammation or arthritis), it does not provide enough information on which to base decisions regarding treatment. These data will be provided, as will be seen, in subsequent portions of the examination.

If the restriction of motion does not fit the proportional requirements of the capsular pattern, a noncapsular pattern of restricted motion is present. *Noncapsular patterns* may be caused by lesions that are capable of restricting range of motion but that do not involve the entire joint. The following categories of pathological conditions fit these requirements: (1) adhesions of ligaments (uncommon at the elbow), (2) internal derangements, and (3) extraarticular lesions.[2]

Noncapsular patterns of restriction at the elbow are usually caused by internal derangement, which results from a loose body of bone or cartilage within the joint.[2] Depending on which aspect of the joint is affected, movement will be limited in one direction and free in the other. For example, if a loose body lies in the anterior aspect of the joint cavity, flexion will be limited and extension unaffected. Conversely, if the loose body lies posteriorly, extension will be blocked and flexion will be free.

At times a confusing picture may appear with regard to the pattern of restriction. This occurs in the joint with a loose body that develops a simultaneous inflammation. The joint inflammation produces the characteristic proportional limitation of movement or capsular pattern. However, the loose body may block movement to a greater degree than expected in one direction. The identification of these cases is facilitated once the motion barrier is examined.[2]

Appraisal of the motion barrier. When a joint is moved passively, movement is brought to a halt when a barrier to motion is met. Under normal circumstances the motion barrier prevents excessive movement from occurring. This may be termed an *anatomical motion barrier* and may be provided by (1) apposition of bony surfaces, (2) the development of tension in the connective tissues, or (3) approximation and compression of the soft tissues.

In each of these situations, as the movement is brought to a halt at the anatomical motion barrier, a distinctly different sensation is imparted to the hands of the examiner. Cyriax[2] has termed this sensation *end-feel*.

When the barrier is provided by bony apposition of the members of the joint, the movement comes to an abrupt stop and no further movement is possible regardless of how hard the movement is forced.

If the motion is restrained by tension in the connective tissues, the movement will also come to an abrupt stop, but continued forcing of the joint will yield a small increase in the range of motion. Cyriax[2] has termed this sensation a *capsular end-feel*. The sensation is much the same as that obtained from stretching a piece of leather.

Contact and compression of the soft tissues overlying the moving members of a joint provides yet another sensation to the examiner. The movement is felt to slow down as contact occurs, but continued forcing yields considerably more motion as the soft tissues are compressed.

Before an account of pathological motion barriers can be given, the *normal barriers to movement* at the elbow and forearm need to be discussed. When the elbow is extended, movement is stopped as the olecranon process engages the olecranon fossa. In thin individuals flexion is stopped in a similar manner when the radial head and coronoid process are received, respectively, into the radial and coronoid fossae. The motion barrier in these situations is one of bony approximation.

In mesomorphic individuals, when the elbow is flexed, the anterior surface of the arm comes into contact with the anterior surface of the forearm before bony approximation can occur. The motion barrier to flexion in these individuals is soft tissue compression.

Supination of the forearm is limited by connective tissues and by the pronator muscles. It usually has a capsular end-feel. Pronation is limited by the soft tissues, which are interposed between the radius and ulna, thus producing a soft tissue approximation end-feel.

When motion of the joint is restricted, a *pathological motion barrier* impedes movement of the joint before the anatomical barrier is reached. The same factors that create an anatomical barrier may also constitute a pathological barrier; that is, movement can be limited by bony approximation, soft tissue compression, or tension in the connective tissues before the anatomical range of motion is attained. In order to make appropriate decisions regarding treatment, it is of the utmost importance to determine the quality of the motion barrier.

If the pathological motion barrier is one of bony approximation, no form of movement—active or passive—will increase motion in the direction of the barrier. If the motion barrier is soft tissue compression, which may occur prematurely if the arm or forearm is edematous, the initial objective may be to reduce the edema. On the other hand, if the movement is limited by contracture of connective tissues, a combination of active and passive movements may be used to improve the range of motion. The motion may be limited by a loss of flexibility in either the joint capsule or the accessory ligaments of the joint. Alternatively, the movement may be limited by shortening of the connective tissues of the antagonistic musculature, which will give rise to a similar motion barrier.

The length of these tissues can be modified with the application of appropriate stresses. The appropriate stress to induce lengthening of connective tissue is tension, which is produced by stretching. Although tension can also be induced with active movement, in many cases the optimal manner of providing the appropriate stress is with passive movement.

Two other types of motion barriers are encountered when passive movements are examined, and both are common at the elbow joint. These are (1) the *springy block* and (2) *muscle guarding*. If either type of barrier is encountered, forceful passive stretching in the direction of the barrier is clearly contraindicated. The failure of physical therapists to observe this contraindication is undoubtedly one of the reasons for the disrepute of passive movement treatment at this joint.

A springy motion barrier is usually found at the elbow when motion is limited by a loose body.[2] A loose body produces a noncapsular pattern of restriction, and either flexion or extension may be limited. As the joint is moved into the barrier, a sensation of resistance develops. The block to motion is not abrupt, and if the examiner persists in the movement, more range can be obtained. If the joint is moved toward the barrier to the position where resistance is first met and then suddenly moved into the barrier (through a small amplitude), the joint springs back in the opposite direction when the force is released.

Motion may also be limited by spasm of the antagonistic muscles to the movement. The muscles may arrest the movement by contracting involuntarily when passive movement is produced. The muscle guarding may be termed *slow guarding* or *fast guarding*. Both types of muscle guarding indicate an acute inflammation of the joint or the extraarticular tissues. Motion should never be forced in the presence of muscle guarding. If this rule is not observed, the good intentions of the physical therapist will have the opposite effect—the joint will lose even more motion.

The physical therapist must also keep in mind that the motion barrier may change. For example, if elbow extension is found to have a restriction of 30 degrees with a capsular barrier, appropriate treatment may include passive mobilization. If the restriction has been reduced to 20 degrees following the treatment, the motion barrier must be assessed at this point. If the barrier is still capsular, treatment may be continued with passive movement. However, if a bone-on-bone barrier occurs at the new position, this treatment is contraindicated.

Relationship of pain to the motion barrier. As the joint is moved passively, the client is instructed to inform the examiner when any sensation of pain is experienced. The pain may be related to the motion barrier in several ways. First, it may occur before the barrier is met, in which case it indicates an acute lesion. It may also occur simultaneously with engagement of the motion barrier. This, too, represents an acute lesion but differs from the former situation.[2] In both of these cases treatment must progress with caution, with the initial objective of treatment being relief of pain.

Finally, pain may be experienced after the barrier to motion is met.[2] In this case the pain is usually caused by stretching of contracted connective tissues (if the barrier has this quality), and the pain is typically not intense. The treatment goal in this instance should be directed toward improving the range of motion by increasing the flexibility of the connective tissues.

Accessory movement. Accessory movements or joint play movements are involuntary passive movements in a joint.[22] Two types of accessory movements are found at the elbow. The first type is characterized by abduction and adduction of the ulna at the humeroulnar joint. It is not possible to perform these motions voluntarily in isolated fashion, although they do occur when the forearm is supinated and pronated.[22]

The second type of accessory movement depends on the laxity of the supporting connective tissues. This type of accessory movement includes distraction of the articular surfaces and gliding movements of the surfaces. Through an examination of these accessory movements the examiner can determine whether isolated portions of the capsule and accessory ligaments are contracted or are excessively lax. Thus treatment decisions will be based on these findings. If, for example, an accessory movement reveals a limited range of motion and the corresponding passive movement is also limited, the treatment of choice is to restore the lost range of motion through passive stretching. Restoration of movement is best accomplished by using the accessory movement rather than the physiological movement. This eliminates problems associated with compression of the articular surfaces.

Alternatively, if the accessory movement is excessive in range and the corresponding passive movement is limited, passive stretching is not the treatment of choice. The limitation of passive motion is not caused by contracture of the capsule and accessory ligaments, since the accessory movement is excessive. The limitation of motion may be caused by an extraarticular lesion.

The accessory movements performed in the examination of the elbow complex are listed in Table 19-1.

Resisted tests. The primary objective of resisted testing is the identification of painful lesions on the contractile elements of the musculoskeletal system.[2] Examples of these types of lesions include tendonitis and tears of the elements of the contractile units. Disorders that result in weakness of the muscles tested may also be identified, although this may be better accomplished with a conventional manual muscle test.

The resisted tests are performed by placing the joint in its resting position. This step is included so that the tension on the noncontractile tissues is at a minimum.[2] The client is then asked to hold the joint in a static position while the examiner attempts to move the joint in a direc-

Table 19-1. Accessory movements at the elbow

Joint	Movement
Humeroulnar joint	Abduction of the ulna
	Adduction of the ulna
	Medial glide of the ulna
	Lateral glide of the ulna
	Distraction of the ulna
Humeroradial joint	Distraction of the radius
	Compression of the radius
	Ventral glide of the radius
	Dorsal glide of the radius
Proximal radioulnar joint	Ventromedial glide of the radius
	Dorsolateral glide of the radius

tion that will activate the muscle or muscle group being tested. In this manner as much movement as possible is prevented in the joint, while the stress or tension in the contractile unit is increased.

The theoretical basis of resisted testing rests on the following assumptions: (1) no movement occurs that will stress the noncontractile tissues, and (2) increasing the tension in the contractile unit will increase the client's complaint of pain by stressing a painful lesion.[2] In theory these assumptions may appear valid, but enough false positive and false negative results are found with this type of examination to warrant further discussion.

In general, the purpose of muscle force is to produce torque or moment across the joint. This force results in a torque that resists or does work against an external load. In addition, there are large compressive forces created at the joint between the two bones, and if the joint is not permitted to move, large shear stresses may also be created that tend to displace one bone with respect to the other. Therefore it may be concluded that it is impossible to eliminate stress on noncontractile tissue during a resisted test. When a muscle contracts, it has the capacity to compress a joint or to produce gliding movement in a joint without visible motion of the joint. If the joint is acutely painful, the resisted test may produce an increase in the client's pain that may be wrongly attributed to a lesion of contractile tissue.

In the above situation, although pain may have been elicited by a resisted test, the pain produced by examination of passive movement is usually worse. Correlation of the results of the entire functional examination is essential to eliminate this source of false positive resisted testing.

A similar situation may exist at locations where a contracting muscle can compress a painful, noncontractile structure. This may be observed in cases of acute bursitis, but, again, passive movements will generally elicit a more intense pain.[2]

Another type of problem may appear as a simple contractile lesion with pain on one or more resisted tests. Such pain may be caused by a fracture near the insertion of the muscle being tested (avulsion fracture). Contraction of the muscle produces pain that may be mistakenly diagnosed as tendonitis. If this is followed by treatment with deep friction massage, the therapist may exacerbate rather than alleviate the condition. Therefore, to prevent this possibility, an adequate radiographic examination must be carried out if there is any history of trauma.

False negative results of resisted tests are usually not a factor at the elbow, although they may be encountered in athletes. The lesion may be aggravated by stresses encountered in competition that are impossible to duplicate with clinical testing. In these situations it may be helpful to have the client engage in the activity that precipitates the symptoms before examination. This may produce sufficient irritation of the painful structure to permit localization of the lesion with resisted testing.

The resisted tests that are performed at the elbow complex usually include (1) elbow flexion, (2) elbow extension, (3) supination of the forearm, (4) pronation of the forearm, (5) extension of the wrist, and (6) flexion of the wrist.[2]

After completion of the examination procedures described above, the examiner must correlate the results. (Table 19-2 lists test movements and the muscles that may be involved with each test.) For example, a client may complain of an increase in pain with resisted flexion of the elbow. This may be caused by a contractile lesion located in the biceps brachii, the brachialis, or the brachioradialis. If the problem lies within the biceps, the client will also complain of increased pain with resisted supination. If the lesion is in the brachioradialis, pain may be exacerbated by resisted pronation in full supination and resisted supination in full pronation. If the lesion is in the brachialis, no pain will be elicited with resisted supination or pronation.

A similar process of elimination should be used for the remaining resisted tests. Once the lesioned muscle has been identified, the examiner may palpate the muscle to locate the lesion.

TREATMENT OF THE CUBITAL COMPLEX

After the examination of the cubital complex has been completed, the physical therapist should have sufficient data with which to formulate a plan of care. Client problems that require physical therapy will have been identified. At this point the therapist must establish a goal or objective of treatment for each problem and must design a plan of care that responds to each problem.

There are four primary goals that become evident through a detailed assessment of the elbow region. These include (1) reducing pain, (2) reducing mobility, (3) increasing mobility, and (4) preventing recurrence of the problem, if possible.[11]

Musculoskeletal dysfunction can be divided into the following broad categories: (1) lesions of the noncontractile tissues and (2) lesions of the contractile tissues.[2] The former is identified by an abnormal response to passive movement, whereas the latter is identified by an abnormal response to resisted testing.

Dysfunction of noncontractile tissues

The following noncontractile tissues may be involved in a pathological process at the cubital complex: (1) the bones or their articular surfaces; (2) the articular capsule, synovial membrane, synovial bursae, or the accessory ligaments of the joint; (3) the passive component of the muscles that cross the joint; and (4) nerves that are located in a position that subjects them to trauma near the joint.

Client problems that may result from lesions of the noncontractile structures include one or more of the following: (1) pain, (2) limited movement (hypomobility), (3) excessive movement (hypermobility), and (4) paresthesias.

Dysfunction of the capsule and accessory ligaments

The articular capsule and accessory ligaments of the elbow are connective tissues. Connective tissue dysfunction is characterized by an abnormal response to passive movement. The motion may be abnormal in that it may be restricted or excessive. Either type of dysfunction may be accompanied by pain. If pain is the predominant feature, it may in fact be difficult to determine the type of dysfunction that is present because of muscle guarding. Occasionally, the physician must examine the joint with the client under anesthesia to determine whether the joint is hypomobile or hypermobile.

Since pain and muscle guarding may obscure the nature of the problem, the initial objective in the acutely painful

Table 19-2. Interpretation of resisted tests at the elbow

Test	Affected muscle
Flexion	Biceps brachii
	Brachialis
	Brachioradialis
Extension	Triceps brachii
	Anconeus
Supination	Supinator
	Biceps brachii
	Brachioradialis (full pronation to neutral)
Pronation	Pronator teres
	Pronator quadratus
	Brachioradialis (full supination to neutral)
Wrist extension	Extensor carpi radialis longus
	Extensor carpi radialis brevis
	Extensor carpi ulnaris
	Extensor digitorum
Wrist flexion	Flexor carpi radialis
	Flexor carpi ulnaris
	Flexor digitorum superficialis
	Palmaris longus

joint is pain relief. Once this has been obtained, a more thorough examination of movement will be permitted and the type of dysfunction may be identified.

Regardless of the type of connective tissue dysfunction present—hypomobility or hypermobility—the goal of treatment is to return the joint to the best possible function in the shortest possible time. Obviously, the methods used to achieve this goal will vary, depending on the pathological condition identified in the examination and on the stage of the pathological process. The physical therapist should be aware that the client's primary problem may change during the course of treatment. When this occurs, the treatment plan should be modified accordingly.

When the connective tissues are traumatized (or affected by a systemic disease), an inflammatory reaction will occur. The inflammatory reaction will typically produce a capsular pattern of limitation at the joint. As noted previously, the presence of a capsular pattern of limitation of passive movement must be correlated with the results of other examination procedures in order to select the appropriate treatment modality. Treatment effectiveness will be enhanced if the stage of the inflammatory process is identified.

Early stage of inflammation. *Inflammation* is a term used in reference to a large group of normal processes provoked by injury or alien material. Acute inflammation as a response to trauma is caused by the function of collagen in the activation of molecular systems (chemical mediators) that set off the inflammatory process.[10,12]

When collagen is exposed by injury, the chemical mediators of inflammation produce vascular changes in the area of tissue injury that result in exudation.[10] Cells and solutes that are normally intravascular pour out into the injured area to neutralize the noxious stimuli (damaged tissue). Dead or dying tissue must be disposed of in preparation for the repair process.

The local vasodilation, leakage of fluid into the extravascular space, and interruption of lymphatic drainage produce the classic signs of inflammation (i.e., redness, swelling, and heat). Pressure and chemical stimulation of nocioceptors produce the fourth sign (i.e., pain).

In most noncontaminated injuries the early inflammatory period subsides in 3 to 5 days.[10] During this period an examination of the joint may reveal pain at rest or pain on movement that occurs before any barrier to movement is felt. If a motion barrier is reached, it is usually one of fast muscle guarding.

Although a capsular pattern of motion restriction is found during this period, restoration of motion is not the primary goal of treatment. The goal is the reduction of pain and limitation of the inflammatory process. Toward this end ice and other modalities, such as transcutaneous electrical nerve stimulation (TENS) or high-voltage galvanic stimulation, may be used.

The joint is usually immobilized with a sling or with a sling and splint to prevent further tissue damage. Immobi-lization should be maintained only long enough for adequate tissue healing to occur. Complications of management may arise if the joint must be immobilized for a prolonged period of time following an unstable fracture, dislocation, or a similar injury. A dense scar may form in the area of tissue injury, along with adhesions between adjacent tissue planes and generalized shortening of the connective tissue structures.

Intermediate stage of inflammation. As the damaged tissues are neutralized in the area of injury, the intermediate stage of inflammation—early repair—can begin. There is no sharp line of demarcation between the early and intermediate stages of inflammation. Both may exist simultaneously in different regions of the injured tissues.[10] For this reason it is sometimes difficult to distinguish between these two stages of inflammation on a clinical basis.

The intermediate stage is an early repair process that is characterized by an ingrowth of capillary buds into the injured region to reestablish circulation. As the circulation is being reestablished, fibroblasts appear in the injured region and begin to manufacture collagen and ground substance. Collagen may be found in the healing region as early as the first day after injury, but peak production occurs 5 to 7 days after injury.[10]

The early collagen is a gel-like substance that serves as a support for the new, fragile capillary system.[10] The tissue formed during this stage is termed *granulation tissue*. It is a highly vascularized connective tissue that is very fragile and easily torn by the application of tensile stress.

During the intermediate stage of inflammation the motion barrier to passive movement is usually muscle guarding, and a capsular pattern of restriction will be found. The sequence of pain to the motion barrier is variable. Generally, the client will experience pain at the same time the examiner feels the motion barrier. However, the pain may be felt slightly before or slightly after the barrier to motion is felt.

Treatment during this phase of inflammation is important and has considerable bearing on the final outcome of the problem. It will require the coordinated efforts of the physician and the physical therapist.

Conceptually, one can think of treatment during this period as a balance between the immobilization that was required during the early stage of inflammation and the vigorous mobilization that will be required, in some cases, in the late stage of repair. In fact, the objective of treatment at this time is preventing the formation of dense, inflexible scar tissue that can create problems that require vigorous mobilization later.

The referring physician is responsible for determining when it is reasonable to begin movement of the joint. The physical therapist is responsible for supervision of the client during this period. He or she must ensure that movement is sufficient to produce desirable results without disruption of the healing tissues.

Movement during the intermediate stage is intended to

provide an adequate stimulus for the functional orientation of collagen fibers. If movement is not sufficient, the fiber orientation will be such that free movement of the joint will be impeded. If movement is excessive, the fragile connective tissues will be torn. When this occurs, the joint may develop a chronic inflammatory reaction with an even greater loss of motion. Alternatively, if the initial trauma involved a significant disruption of the capsule and ligaments, excessive movement may result in permanent lengthening of these tissues with resultant instability of the joint.

Active and passive movement of the joint may be used in the management of the joint during this stage. Both should be guided by the same treatment principle. Pain should not be experienced as the joint is moved, and no muscle spasm should be provoked. Between periods of exercise the joint should be protected with a sling.

Late stage of inflammation. The late stage of inflammation involves the maturation and remodeling of the young connective tissues that were formed during the intermediate stage. Again, there is no sharp line of demarcation between the intermediate and the late stages of inflammation.[10]

Maturation occurs through the formation of chemical cross-links between adjacent collagen fibers. If appropriate stresses are not provided during the repair process, excessive cross-linking may occur and the organization of the collagen fibers will be at random.[10] The tissues formed will be dense, inflexible, and ill suited to the needs of a freely movable joint, such as the elbow.

Examination of the joint during this stage reveals a problem that is primarily one of lost motion, not one of pain. Motion is restricted in a capsular pattern and limited by contracture of connective tissues. The motion barrier thus has a capsular end-feel. The accessory movements of the joint will also be limited.

If pain is produced on passive movement, it occurs only after the motion barrier is met and the pressure is maintained in a manner that forces movement into the barrier. The pain is usually not severe, and it generally abates once the force is released.

The goal of treatment at this stage is to increase the range of motion. This is accomplished by increasing the flexibility of the connective tissues. The most advantageous method of achieving this end is the application of tensile stress to the tissue.

Treatment of hypomobility associated with connective tissue dysfunction

Various forms of passive movement can be used in the treatment of hypomobility of the elbow complex that is caused by contracture of the connective tissues. These have been well described in the literature.[2,11,17] It is beyond the scope of this chapter to discuss, in detail, all passive movement techniques that can be used in the management of these problems. Furthermore, it is not the intention of this chapter to teach the reader how to perform passive movement techniques. This can be accomplished only through supervised practical experience. However, for the sake of illustrating the most important aspects of passive movement, selected techniques are described in some detail.

Passive movement can be divided into the following two groups: (1) accessory joint movement and (2) physiological joint movement.[17]

Accessory movements. The accessory movements used in the treatment of the elbow complex are identical to those used in the examination of the joints (see Table 19-1). During the examination the purpose of performing accessory movement is to assess the range of motion, which will be restricted in cases of hypomobility caused by connective tissue contracture. The purpose of using accessory movement in treatment is to restore the range of motion. When the range of motion of the accessory movement has been regained, that of the associated physiological movement will also be restored.[11]

Accessory movements are used in the treatment of joints during either the intermediate stage or the late stage of the inflammatory process. Since the demands of treatment in each of these stages vary, the application of the treatment movement must be modified accordingly. Modification of the accessory movement may be accomplished by (1) altering the position of the joint, (2) varying the amplitude of the movement, (3) varying the rate of movement, and (4) varying the number of movements performed.

First let us consider the position of the joint when the accessory movement is performed. Joint position has a definite effect on the accessory movement of distraction of the humeroulnar joint. During the intermediate stage of the inflammatory process (when pain is the predominant feature) the joint should be positioned in its resting position.[11,17] This position will minimize the tension on all portions of the fibrous capsule and on the ligaments of the joint. Theoretically, distraction performed in this position will increase the tensile stresses in all portions of the connective tissues, but the increase in stress will not be great in any area. Thus distraction of the humeroulnar joint in the resting position has the capacity to improve motion in flexion and extension and is relatively safe in that it does not produce significant increases in stress within the capsule (Fig. 19-4).

If distraction is used to treat the humeroulnar joint in the late stage of the inflammatory process (when loss of motion is the predominant feature), the joint is usually positioned at a motion barrier. When the joints move to the flexion motion barrier, the posterior aspect of the capsule will become taut, while the anterior portion of the capsule will be relaxed. A distraction movement applied to the joint in this position will produce a significant increase in the tension within the posterior capsule, while having little or no effect on the anterior capsule. Although treatment in this position is usually more effective because tensile stress can be increased more readily, it also carries more inherent danger. If the joint is not capable of tolerating the stress, the condition may be exacerbated.

Distraction can also be performed with the joint positioned at the extension barrier. In this situation the stress

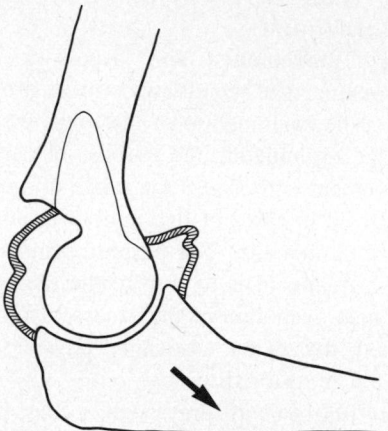

Fig. 19-4. Distraction of humeroulnar joint with joint in resting position. When the physical therapist performs distraction movement of humeroulnar joint in resting position, stress created in all portions of capsule is small. This is so because the capsule is relaxed in all regions. Note that direction of distraction force is perpendicular to the plane of concave joint surface (trochlear notch of ulna).

will be applied selectively to the anterior portion of the capsule (Fig. 19-5).

A second factor that can be used to modify the effects of accessory movement is the amplitude of the movement. Kaltenborn[11] and Maitland[17] have developed systems for describing the amplitude of passive movement. Maitland's grading system is used to describe both accessory and physiological movement, since he uses both of these in treatment. He has classified movement into four grades, which are based on how far the movement is carried into the available range of motion and also on the amplitude of the movement.

A *grade I movement* is a small amplitude movement performed at the beginning of the range. A *grade II movement* is a large amplitude movement performed within the range but not reaching the limit. A *grade III movement* is also a large amplitude movement performed up to the limit of the range. A *grade IV movement* is a small amplitude movement that is performed at the end of the range (Fig. 19-6).[17]

Kaltenborn describes three grades of movement. The first movement is always performed in the direction of distraction. In fact, this movement may not actually move the joint surfaces apart but neutralizes the compressive forces that tend to bind them together. Kaltenborn's remaining two types of movement are based on the feel of the connective tissues rather than on the range of motion. The first of these is performed in the selected direction of motion

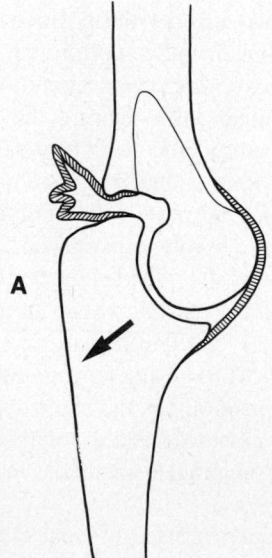

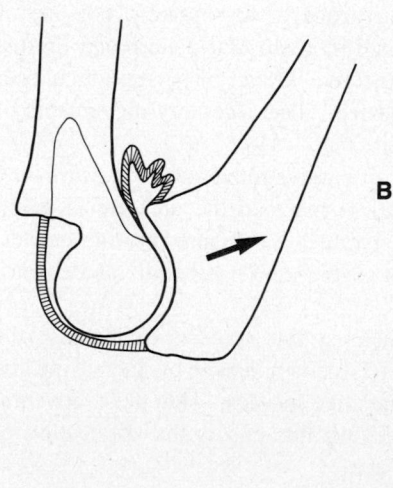

Fig. 19-5. **A,** Distraction of humeroulnar joint with joint positioned at motion barrier. When the joint is moved to motion barrier before application of distraction force, a portion of the capsule becomes taut while another portion becomes relaxed. Extension relaxes posterior capsule and tightens anterior capsule. **B,** The converse is true on flexion. Posterior portion of capsule becomes taut while anterior aspect is relaxed. When distraction force is applied in either of these positions, it will have greater influence on the area of capsule that is prestressed. Thus, when movement is performed at flexion barrier, flexion will be improved. When movement is performed at extension barrier, extension will be improved.

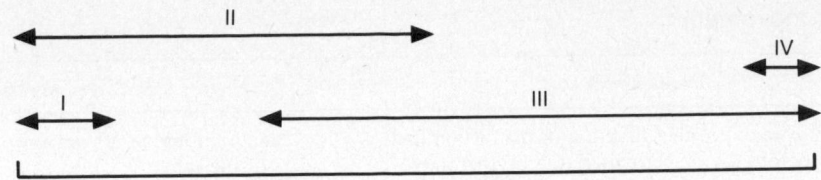

Fig. 19-6. Maitland's grades of movement.

but only until the *slack* is taken out of the connective tissues. The final grade is performed in such a manner that movement is carried beyond the slack in an attempt to stretch the connective tissues that restrain the joint movement. (Fig. 19-7).

In treating a joint in which pain is the predominant feature, the physical therapist can perform accessory movements starting with Maitland's grade I and progressing to grade II as the inflammatory process subsides. Similarly, if the therapist uses Kaltenborn's system of grading accessory movement, the treatment may begin with a grade I, or small distraction movement, and progress to taking up the slack in the direction of the movement selected.

When the predominant feature of the dysfunction is loss of motion, as occurs in the late stage of repair, the therapist may select Maitland's grade III and progress to grade IV. If Kaltenborn's system is used, the accessory motion will be taken to stretch.

The rate of movement can also be varied in treatment with accessory movements. Maitland[17] performs these movements as a series of oscillations, whereas Kaltenborn[11] performs the movement in a slower, rhythmical manner, with the joint held at the terminal point in the movement for several (5 to 8) seconds. Table 19-3 gives a comparison of Maitland's and Kaltenborn's grades of movement.

Of course, the intensity of treatment will also be affected by the number of treatment movements that are performed. Generally, acutely painful joints are treated with a much smaller number of movements before the joint is reexamined, whereas the stiff joint can tolerate more treatment movements before reexamination.

Physiological movement. Physiological movements can also be used in the treatment of dysfunction at the elbow complex. Maitland[17] has provided a detailed description of the use of these movements in the treatment of the elbow. He also has provided a description of the use of physiological movements in combination with accessory movements.

When physiological movements are used in the treatment of hypomobility, they can also be graded. Maitland's grading system is well suited for describing physiological movement. In general, grade I and grade II movements are used in the treatment of painful conditions, whereas grade III and grade IV movements are used in the treatment of stiff joints.

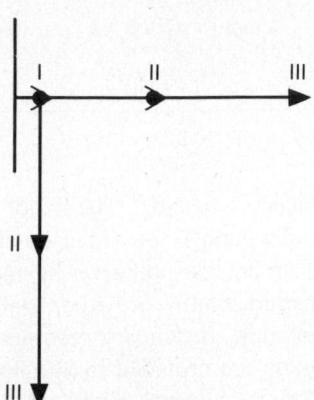

Fig. 19-7. Kaltenborn's grades of movement.

Although passive movement is useful in the management of dysfunction caused by connective tissue contracture, the ultimate success of the treatment program hinges on the physical therapist's ability to instruct the client in the performance of active exercises. Often, considerable time and effort are spent in the performance of passive movement and little attention is paid to instruction in a home exercise program.

Active exercises should be governed by the same factors that guide the use of passive movement. In the intermediate stage of the inflammatory process the client must be instructed to perform active range of motion within the pain-free range. During this stage of the inflammatory process the fragile granulation tissue may just as easily be damaged by improper application of active movement as by excessive passive motion. The client must be carefully instructed as to which motions can be performed and the frequency with which the movement should be done. It is very important for the client to realize that pain and muscle guarding should not be provoked by the exercises.

With a dysfunction in the late stage of repair, the exercises are further modified by increasing the frequency of the movement rather than the intensity of active effort. Again, the exercises should not provoke pain.

Accompanying dysfunction of the capsule and accessory ligaments (hypermobility)

The most common form of instability seen at the elbow complex is medial laxity.[20] This is evidenced by excessive

Table 19-3. Grades of movement

	Kaltenborn	Maitland
Grade I	A small movement in the direction of distraction that is done before the performance of a gliding movement (only enough movement to neutralize the joint compression forces)	Small-amplitude movement performed at the beginning of the range
Grade II	A movement that takes up the slack in the soft tissues	Large-amplitude movement performed within the range but not reaching the limit of the range
Grade III	A movement that is taken beyond the slack (an attempt to stretch the soft tissues)	Large-amplitude movement performed up to the limit of the range
Grade IV		Small-amplitude movement performed at the limit of the range

motion on valgus stress testing. The major contribution to stability in this direction is provided by the anterior oblique portion of the medial collateral ligament.[20] This ligament is also instrumental in providing stability in the anteroposterior direction. Secondary restraints to motion in the valgus direction are provided by the flexor muscles of the forearm and by the humeroradial joint, which is able to resist compressive forces that occur on the lateral side of the joint complex with this motion.[20]

Although it is important for the physical therapist to recognize the existence of instability, treatment of this problem is within the realm of the orthopaedic surgeon. If the surgeon does not feel that the client is a candidate for surgical stabilization, the client may be referred to physical therapy for strengthening of the flexor muscles. The exercises performed should not cause engagement of the motion barrier, since this may result in further stretching of the already compromised connective tissues.

Hypomobility as a result of dysfunction of the noncontractile component of the muscle

If the joints of the elbow complex demonstrate a limited range of motion of physiological movement but a normal or slightly hypermobile range of accessory movements, the limitation of motion may be caused by insufficient length of the antagonistic muscles to the movement being tested. The pattern of motion restriction may be noncapsular, since the problem is extraarticular.

When this situation exists, the muscles may be lengthened with a contract-relax procedure. The joint is positioned at the motion barrier, which is provided by the shortened muscle, and the client is instructed to contract the muscle to be treated against the unyielding force of the therapist. This contraction is maintained for 5 to 10 seconds; then the client is instructed to relax. Once relaxation has been obtained, the joint is moved into the motion barrier again. At this point the client performs another isometric contraction, then relaxes, and the joint is again moved into the motion barrier. A series of 5 to 10 procedures is generally required.

When contract-relax techniques are used, the therapist must follow the same guidelines for repositioning the joint at the motion barrier as those described for the use of any passive movement. Pain and protective muscle guarding should not be provoked.

These techniques must be used with particular caution when elbow extension is limited. Extension may be limited by myositis ossificans. If this is the case, the use of contract-relax procedures or any form of passive stretching is contraindicated.

Hypomobility as a result of articular surface dysfunction (springy motion barrier)

If a springy motion barrier is present on either flexion or extension of the elbow, a loose body of cartilage or bone may be lodged between the articular surfaces. Cyriax[2] has described the passive techniques that may be used to reduce the displacement (move the loose body from its position between the articular surfaces). However, he stresses that recurrence of the block is common and advocates surgical removal of the fragment.

Hypomobility as a result of articular surface dysfunction (bone-on-bone motion barrier and capsular barriers resistant to treatment)

Perhaps the most important consideration in the treatment of limited passive movement that results from trauma at the elbow joint is the establishment of realistic goals of treatment.

Following a fracture in the elbow region, it is not likely that a full range of motion will be obtained if the fracture fragments cannot be anatomically reduced. This is also true if the fracture is complicated by a significant soft tissue injury.

During the course of treatment the physical therapist must constantly reassess the nature of the motion barrier. When a barrier to motion changes, the goals of treatment will often need to be changed accordingly.

If, at any time, a bone-on-bone barrier is encountered, continued efforts to regain motion in the direction of the barrier are futile and contraindicated. Several situations in the management of fractures of the bones around the elbow require special consideration.

If a compression screw has been used to stabilize the fragments of a fracture of the distal humerus, and the screw passes through or projects into the olecranon fossa, motion in extension will be blocked.[5] The motion barrier will most likely be one of bone-on-bone—a hard, abrupt end-feel. Obviously, efforts to regain extension in this situation will exacerbate the condition (Fig. 19-8).

If an intercondylar fracture of the humerus is reduced

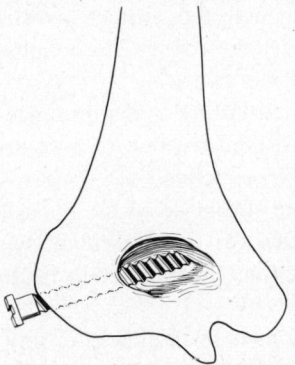

Fig. 19-8. Compression screw used to stabilize humerus, causing motion barrier.

with a residual rotary deformity or malalignment of one of the humeral condyles, the biomechanics of the joint will be disturbed.[5] Motion of the elbow in the sagittal plane will be limited as a result of malalignment of the axes of the humeroulnar and the humeroradial joints. If, for example, the lateral condyle (capitellum) is tilted ventrally with respect to the humeral shaft, bone-on-bone contact may occur prematurely as the forearm is flexed at the elbow. During extension the humeroradial portion of the joint will reach the limit of its excursion prematurely. In this situation a bone-on-bone end-feel will be present in flexion and a capsular end-feel will be present in extension. Neither barrier will respond to treatment with active or passive movement (Fig. 19-9).

Fractures of the forearm that are permitted to unite with malalignment will also permanently limit the range of motion of pronation and supination of the forearm. If the radius is fractured and unites with the proximal fragment in supination and the distal fragment in pronation, forearm rotation will be restricted. The loss of motion will be in a one-to-one proportion to the rotational malalignment.[1] During supination the proximal rdioulnar joint will reach its anatomical motion barrier prematurely, and on pronation the same will occur at the distal radioulnar joint. Limitation of the range of motion may be present with no pathological condition at either the proximal or distal radioulnar joints. This condition may be suspected when the

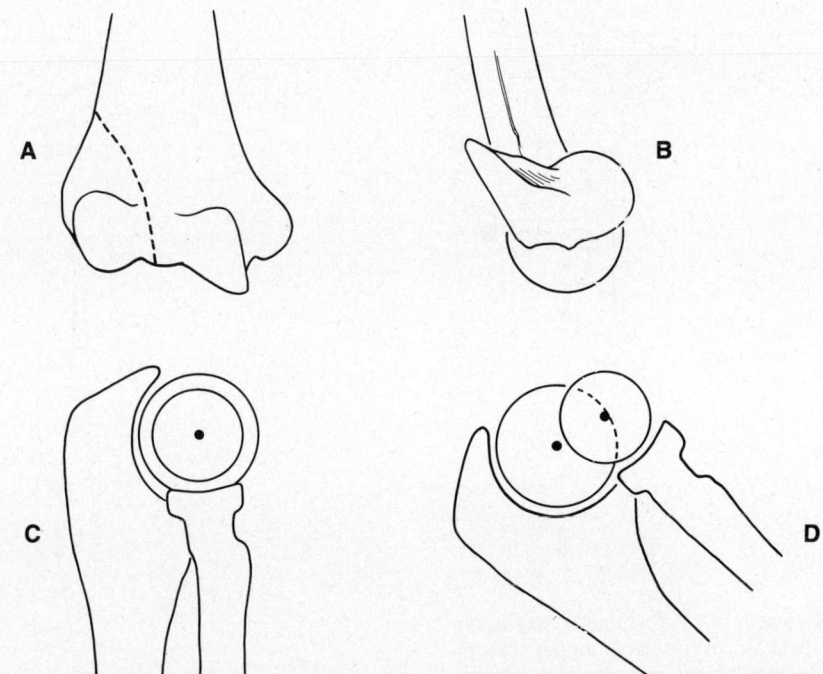

Fig. 19-9. Effects of condylar malalignment. Centers of articular arc of separate condyles are located on same horizontal line through distal humerus **(A,C).** When there is malalignment of one condyle with another **(B,D),** flexion and extension of elbow are blocked. (Redrawn from Magnuson PB and Stack JK: Fractures, ed 5, Philadelphia, 1949, JB Lippincott Co.)

physiological range of motion is limited and the range of motion of the accessory movements is normal.

Treatment of a problem of this nature with active or passive movement may convert a painless limitation of motion into a painful condition. (Fig. 19-10).

The complications of angular malunion of the forearm have already been mentioned. When normal curvature of the radius is disturbed, the range of motion in pronation and supination will be limited (Fig. 19-11).[1] This probably occurs because of the development of abnormal or premature tension within the interosseous membrane.

When the joint in question presents a bone-on-bone motion barrier or fails to respond to an adequate program of treatment, one of the above problems may be the cause. If the range of motion present is sufficient to allow reasonable function, further attempts to regain motion should be terminated. If the range of motion is nonfunctional, the client should be sent back to the physician for further care.

Noncontractile lesions (nerves and bursae)

Lesions of the nerves that traverse the cubital region are discussed in Chapter 18.

The most common type of bursitis seen at the elbow is

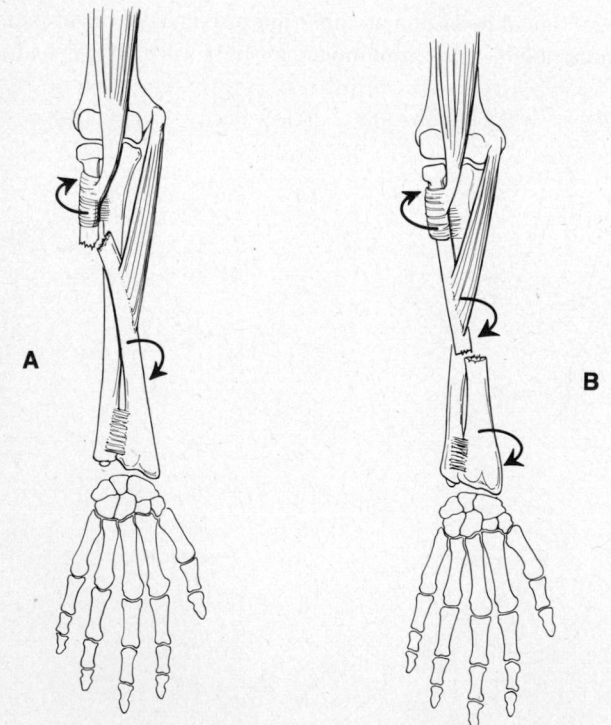

Fig. 19-10. Rotational malalignment of shaft of radius may occur following fracture of radial shaft. **A,** In fracture of upper shaft of radius between insertion of supinator and pronator teres, proximal fragment is supinated and lower fragment pronated. **B,** In fracture of middle or lower shaft between insertions of pronator teres and pronator quadratus, proximal fragment is in midposition.

olecranon bursitis. Pain at the elbow exists and is usually not aggravated by motion or by resisted testing.[2] The diagnosis is usually based on palpable thickening or tenderness over the olecranon bursa.

Dysfunction of contractile tissues

Dysfunction of contractile tissues is identified by an abnormal response to resisted testing.[2] An abnormal response may include weakness of the muscle or muscles being tested, pain that occurs as the muscle contracts isometrically, or a combination of the two. Pain combined with weakness is often associated with serious pathological conditions in the region and requires further investigation.[2]

If weakness is detected, further investigation is also indicated to uncover the cause. The treatment for weakness is described in Chapter 18.

Pain on resisted testing in the presence of a strong contraction indicates the presence of a contractile lesion.[2] A *contractile lesion* is defined as a macroscopic or microscopic tear of the substance of the musculotendinous unit. This unit includes (1) the muscle belly, (2) the musculotendinous junction, (3) the tendon, and (4) the tenoperiosteal junction.

The unit may have been injured or torn by a single violent contraction of the muscle or, as is more often the case, by repeated overuse. Regardless of the mechanism of injury, an inflammatory reaction identical to that previously described will occur. Inflammatory reactions that in-

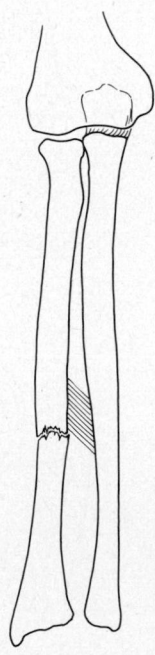

Fig. 19-11. Angular malalignment of radial shaft. When normal lateral bow of radius is lost, length of interosseous membrane will not be maintained. Shortening of membrane will impede rotation of forearm.

volve the contractile units can be divided into two broad categories—acute and chronic. These categories are based more on the irritability of the tissues (severity of pain) than on the longevity of the symptoms. For example, a client with a long history of a contractile lesion may have an acute problem because of a recent exacerbation of the condition.

Treatment of contractile lesions. The objectives of treatment for contractile lesions will vary depending on the phase of the inflammatory process and on the severity of the tear. In the acute phase the goals of treatment are to reduce pain and to prevent the formation of adhesions between tissue planes. While this is being done, care must be taken to ensure that no further tissue damage occurs. In chronic cases with existing adhesions the objectives of treatment include improvement of the gliding function between tissue planes by stretching of adhesions with transverse friction massage.[2]

Ultimately, the client should be provided with a treatment program designed to prevent recurrence of the problem. This may include an exercise program designed to develop strength, power, and endurance in the musculotendinous unit if deficiencies are identified and a stretching program to promote flexibility. The total program should include instruction in activities of daily living, which will prevent overload of the structures involved. In the athlete this may require instruction in technique or alterations in equipment.

Contractile lesions in the elbow region may involve the flexors and extensors of the elbow joint as well as the pronators and supinators of the forearm.[2] These lesions are not encountered frequently. The precise identification of these lesions and their treatment has been described by Cyriax.[2]

By far the most common contractile lesions found in the elbow region involve the proximal attachments of the wrist extensors and wrist flexors. If the wrist extensors are involved, the condition is known as lateral epicondylitis, or *tennis elbow*. This syndrome is identified by pain produced by isometric contraction of the wrist extensors with the elbow in the extended position. The lesion is usually caused by overload of these muscles by repetitive use. It is common in tennis players but also occurs frequently in persons whose occupation demands repeated use of the muscles in question.

When the wrist flexors are involved, the condition is termed medial epicondylitis or *golfer's elbow*. Medial epicondylitis is not seen as commonly as lateral epicondylitis. It, too, results from repeated overuse of the musculotendinous units and is often found in athletes who engage in the action of throwing.

A treatment program for contractile lesions has been outlined below. The plan can be modified for any contractile lesion found in this region.

I. Acute stage
   A. Ice
   B. Aspirin
   C. Oral or injected antiinflammatory agents
   D. Electrical stimulation (muscle placed in shortened position to prevent excessive tension)
   E. Gentle transverse friction massage (to prevent formation of adhesions)
II. Chronic stage
   A. Heat applications before periods of activity
   B. Ice following periods of activity
   C. Deep transverse friction massage to mobilize adhesions
   D. Ultrasound (may be used before transverse friction massage)
   E. Orthosis (tennis elbow splint)
III. Prevention of recurrence
   A. Exercise for strength, power, and endurance of involved muscle
   B. Exercise to promote flexibility
   C. Activities of daily living to improve technique, avoid stressful situations, modify equipment

SUMMARY

This chapter provides a description of the functional anatomy of the elbow complex, which is essential for understanding the examination and treatment of this region of the musculoskeletal system.

An outline of the examination protocol has been provided with an emphasis on the functional examination and its interpretation. Attention to the details of this examination should enable the physical therapist to identify movement dysfunctions of the elbow. These can be divided into (1) dysfunctions of the noncontractile tissues and (2) dysfunctions of the contractile tissues.

Interpretation of the results of the examination is most important. The physical therapist must determine which tissues are involved and the state of the pathological process. From this information goals or objectives of treatment can be set on a rational basis.

If the physical therapist follows the examination and treatment principles that have been described, the client may benefit from a more rapid return to optimal function. This is not to say that all clients will attain a full and pain-free range of motion. In many situations this is not possible. However, the client should not be made worse as the result of treatment. When treatment is directed toward unattainable goals, the final outcome of the process is usually unfavorable. Improper goal setting and failure to heed the principles of treatment of the musculoskeletal system have both contributed to the disrepute of physical therapy in the management of movement dysfunction of the elbow complex.

Before attempting to treat movement dysfunctions of

the elbow complex the physical therapist should receive supervised instruction in the examination and treatment of the musculoskeletal system. This is particularly true if passive movement is used in the management of problems found at this joint.

REFERENCES

1. Anderson LD: Fractures of the shafts of the radius and ulna. In Rockwood CA and Green DP, editors: Fractures, vol 2, Philadelphia, 1975, JB Lippincott Co.
2. Cyriax J: Textbook of orthopaedic medicine, vol 1, Diagnosis of soft tissue lesions, ed 5, Baltimore, 1969, Williams & Wilkins.
3. deAndrade JR et al: Joint distension and reflex muscle inhibition in the knee, J Bone Joint Surg (Am) 47(2):313, 1965.
4. Dunn JS: Personal communication, 1981.
5. Eppright RH and Wilkins KE: Fractures and dislocations of the elbow. In Rockwood CA and Green DP, editors: Fractures, vol 2, Philadelphia, 1975, JB Lippincott Co.
6. Eyring EJ and Murray WR: The effect of joint position on the pressure of intra-articular effusion, J Bone Joint Surg (Am) 46(6):1235, 1964.
7. Grant JCB: A method of anatomy, Baltimore, 1937, William Wood & Co.
8. Heppenstall RB: Fractures of the forearm. In Heppenstall, RB, editor: Fracture treatment and healing, Philadelphia, 1980, WB Saunders Co.
9. Heppenstall RB: Injuries of the elbow. In Heppenstall RB, editor: Fracture treatment and healing, Philadelphia, 1980, WB Saunders Co.
10. Hunt TK and VanWinkle W: Wound healing. In Heppenstall RB, editor: Fracture treatment and healing, Philadelphia, 1980, WB Saunders Co.
11. Kaltenborn FM: Manual therapy for the extremity joints, specialized techniques: tests and joint mobilization, ed 2, Oslo, 1976, Olaf Norlis Bokhandel.
12. Kang AH: Connective tissue: collagen and elastin. In Kelly WN et al, editors: Textbook of rheumatology, vol 1, Philadelphia, 1981, WB Saunders Co.
13. Kapandji IA: The physiology of the joints, vol 1, The upper limb, London, 1970, E & S Livingstone Inc.
14. Kapandji IA: The inferior radioulnar joint and pronosupination. In Tubiana R, editor: The hand, vol 1, Philadelphia, 1981, WB Saunders Co.
15. London JT: Kinematics of the elbow, J Bone Joint Surg (Am) 63(4):529, 1981.
16. MacConaill MA and Basmajian JJ: Muscles and movements: a basis for human kinesiology, Baltimore, 1969, Williams & Wilkins.
17. Maitland GD: Peripheral manipulation, New York, 1970, Appleton-Century-Crofts.
18. Morrey BF and Chao YS: Passive motion of the elbow joint: a biomechanical analysis, J Bone Joint Surg (Am) 58(4):501, 1976.
19. Muller ME et al: Manual of internal fixation: techniques recommended by the AO-Group, ed 2, New York, 1979, Springer-Verlag New York, Inc.
20. Schwab GH et al: Biomechanics of elbow instability: the role of the medial collateral ligament, Clin Orthop 146:42, 1980.
21. Sisk TD: Fractures. In Edmonson AS and Crenshaw AH, editors: Campbell's operative orthopaedics, ed 6, vol 1, St Louis, 1980, The CV Mosby Co.
22. Williams PL and Warwick R, editors: Gray's anatomy, ed. 36 (Br), Philadelphia, 1980, WB Saunders Co.

Chapter 20

THE SHOULDER

John W. Halbach
Robert T. Tank

This chapter presents a systematic approach to the evaluation, prevention, and rehabilitation of shoulder injuries. Although the concepts discussed apply to the general orthopaedic population, emphasis will be placed on injuries to the athlete.

An understanding of the pathomechanical demands placed on the shoulder complex in sports is based on understanding specific anatomical and biomechanical considerations. Once these are defined and an appropriate evaluation is performed, the subsequent rehabilitation techniques can be systematically applied. The rehabilitation program should be firmly based on the physiological principles of active and passive exercise in an attempt to address the specific problems identified in the client evaluation.

ANATOMY

A study of shoulder injuries must take into account the anatomical relationships of the entire upper quadrant. This becomes even more essential when the biomechanics of any one of the many associated joints is being analyzed.[76] The shoulder complex can be divided into five articulations: glenohumeral, humerocoracoacromial (suprahumeral or subdeltoid), acromioclavicular, sternoclavicular, and scapulothoracic.[14]

Joint articulation

Glenohumeral joint. The glenohumeral joint is more mobile and less stable than the acetabular-femoral joint. This mobility and lack of stability can be attributed to the shallow glenoid fossa, the large and round humeral head, and capsular laxity. The glenoid fossa is shaped like an inverted comma (i.e., broad below and narrow above[8]). Some stability is provided by a fibrocartilaginous rim (glenoid labrum) that surrounds the fossa. This labrum, along with its bony attachments, may be disrupted through traumatic dislocations of the humeral head and has been implicated as a possible cause of chronic instability of the shoulder.[52]

The capsule surrounding the glenohumeral joint has a volume that is twice as large as the humeral head.[8] The

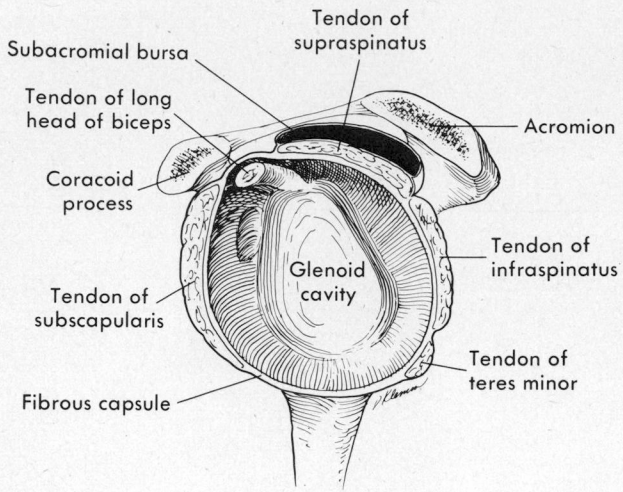

Fig. 20-1. Orientation of the tendinous insertions of the rotator cuff on the capsule. (From Pettrone FA, editor: AAOS symposium on upper extremity injuries in athletes, St Louis, 1986, The CV Mosby Co.)

capsule originates from the glenoid labrum and its surrounding bone and attaches to the periosteum of the humeral shaft and the upper portions of the anatomical shaft. Posteriorly and superiorly, it is reinforced by the tendinous insertions of the rotator cuff (Fig. 20-1). Bland, Merrit, and Boushey[8] describe these tendons as being broad, flat, only an inch in length, and so intricately attached to the capsule that they cannot be dissected apart. The supraspinatus, which is the most superior of these tendons, inserts into the greater tuberosity after crossing the superior capsule (Fig. 20-2). The infraspinatus and teres minor tendons also insert on this tuberosity, but more inferiorly and posteriorly.

Kummel[52] reports that the anterior capsular mechanism is comprised of four interrelated structures: the subscapularis tendon (attaching to the lesser tuberosity of the humerus after spanning the anterior aspect of the humeral head), the labrum, the anterior capsule (consisting of the coracohumeral and the glenohumeral ligaments), and three

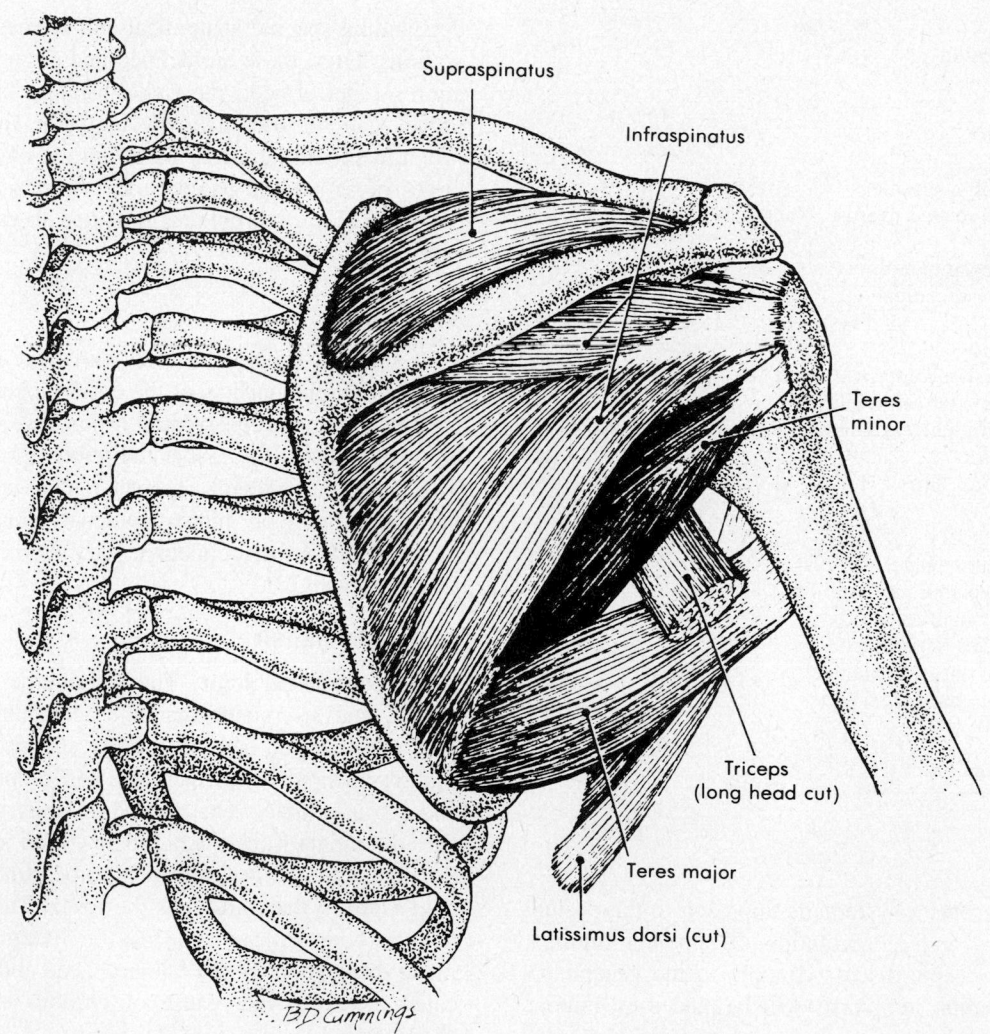

Fig. 20-2. Anatomical relations of the posterior shoulder musculature. (From Travall J and Simons D: Myofascial pain and dysfunction, the trigger point manual, Baltimore, 1983, Williams & Wilkins.

anterior synovial pouches of the shoulder. The most superior recess is the subscapular bursa, which normally communicates with the glenohumeral joint. The axillary pouch lies inferiorly and is separated from the superior bursa by the width of the subscapularis tendon. The middle, or anterior glenoidal, bursae may become contiguous as a result of recurrent dislocation, but normally they are distinct entities.

The superior, inferior, and middle glenohumeral ligaments have been described as being "pleated horizontal folds of the anterior capsule in a fan-shaped appearance."[13] These ligaments are considered to be thickenings of the anterior capsule. An opening may exist between the superior and middle ligaments, which may be covered by a thin capsular layer or which may communicate with the subscapular recess. This opening, referred to as "the foramen of Weitbrecht," may have some predisposing significance in anterior glenohumeral dislocations.

The fourth anterior capsular ligament is the coracohumeral ligament, which arises from the lateral edge of the coracoid process of the scapula and inserts on the greater tuberosity of the humerus. Engin[24] describes this structure as limiting external rotation of the humerus as well as providing a *suspension service* to the humerus as it hangs along the torso, unsupported from above.

The glenohumeral capsule is lined with synovial tissue

that is closely associated with the hyaline cartilage of the humeral head but does not blend with the cartilage of the glenoid fossa. The capsule folds and incorporates the bicipital tendon down into the intertubercular sulcus of the humerus.[13] As a result, the long head of the biceps invaginates the capsule but does not enter the synovial cavity.

Because of the winding attachment of the glenohumeral capsule, the amount of rotation available in this joint depends on the amount of abduction. One hundred and eighty degrees of rotation is possible with the arm adducted to the side. This is diminished to 90 degrees of rotation with the arm at 90 degrees of abduction, and only a trace of rotation is available in the position of full abduction.[5]

Humerocoracoacromial joint. The humerocoracoacromial joint can be thought of as providing protection against direct trauma to the subacromial structures. It is bound superiorly by a ligamentous coracoacromial arch that connects the two processes for which it is named. It is a strong, triangular ligament that serves as a roof over the greater tuberosity of the humerus, the rotator cuff tendons, portions of the biceps tendon, and the subdeltoid bursa. However, if these tissues become inflamed and swollen from overuse or biomechanical trauma, they may become pinched between the humerus and the anterior acromion or the coracoacromial arch (see the section on biomechanics of impingement).

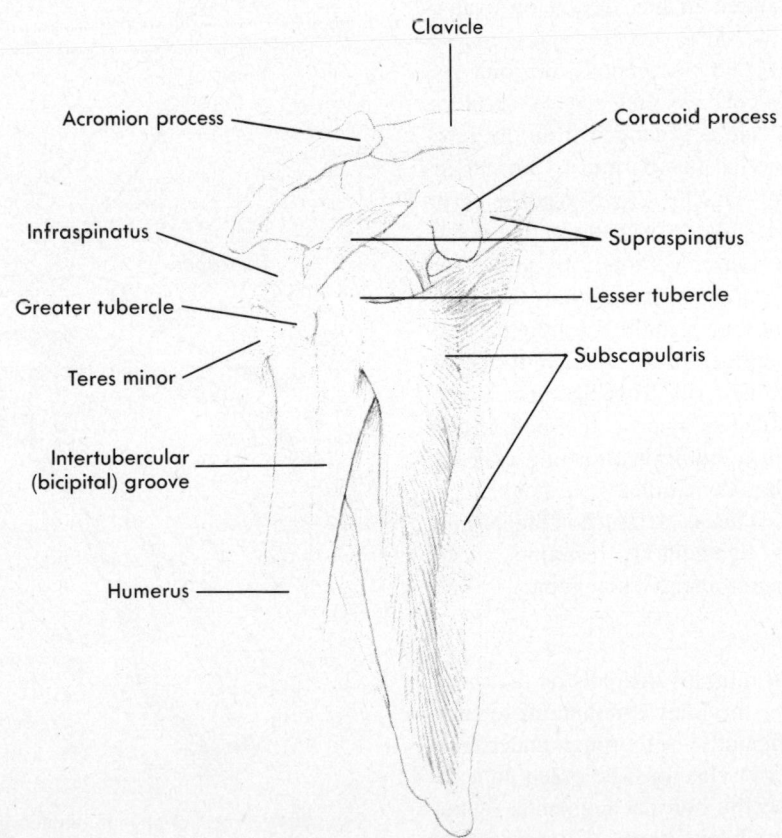

Fig. 20-3. Lateral view of the shoulder complex revealing the subacromial bursa. (From Seeley RR, Stephens TD, and Tate P: Anatomy and physiology, St Louis, 1989, The CV Mosby Co.)

Lying above the greater tuberosity and supraspinatus tendon and below the deltoid muscle and acromial process is the subacromial bursa (Fig. 20-3). Codman[18] describes this as the only significant bursa in the shoulder and reports that the terms *subdeltoid, subcoracoid,* and *subscapularis* are used for extensions of the subacromial bursa. The bursa is attached at its base to the greater tuberosity, the distal portion of the conjoined rotator cuff tendon, and the bicipital groove. The superior aspect is attached to the underside of the acromion and to the coracoacromial ligament. These two layers, which are in intimate contact, are lined with a synovial membrane that can increase or decrease the amount of synovial fluid available on minimal stimulation.[8]

Acromioclavicular joint. The acromioclavicular articulation is located between the convex lateral facet of the clavicle and the concave anteromedial portion of the acromial process. An intraarticular disk is present for several years after birth but undergoes thinning and fibrillation as early as the first or second decade.[13] The actual joint integrity relies on the bridging and surrounding ligaments rather than the shape of the joint surfaces. The joint is supported both superiorly and inferiorly by acromioclavicular ligaments. The clavicle is also held firmly to the scapula by the clavicular ligament. This ligament has two separate fascicles: a medial band (conoid) and a lateral portion (trapezoid). The pathological significance of injury to these ligaments is discussed in the section on evaluation.

Sternoclavicular joint. The sternoclavicular joint is a saddle joint that has both concave and convex surfaces. The medial end of the clavicle is separated from the superior lateral aspect of the sternal manubrium by an intraarticular meniscus. The two clavicles are connected by an interclavicular ligament that crosses over the sternal notch. The actual joint capsule is reinforced anteriorly and posteriorly by sternoclavicular ligaments. In addition, the costoclavicular ligament adds further stability by obliquely securing the inferior medial surface of the clavicle to the superior medial aspect of the first rib. This ligament is necessary to stabilize the clavicle against the pull of the sternocleidomastoid muscle in addition to acting as a fulcrum for motions of the shoulder girdle.[13]

Scapulothoracic joint. This is a free-floating physiological joint without any ligamentous restraints except where it pivots about the acromioclavicular joint.

Muscles

The complex network of muscles that acts on the shoulder complex is essential for the joint articulations to function synchronously and efficiently. A thorough understanding of the actions of these muscles must be based on accurate knowledge of their specific bony attachments. Fundamental muscular actions will be discussed further in the section on biomechanics.

The individual muscles acting on the shoulder complex can be grouped according to their origins and insertions:

1. Scapulohumeral-subscapularis, teres major, teres minor, infraspinatus, supraspinatus, coracobrachialis, and deltoid.
2. Scapuloradial and scapuloulnar biceps and triceps.
3. Axioscapular-trapezius, latissimus dorsi, serratus anterior, rhomboids, pectoralis minor, and levator scapulae.
4. Axiohumeral-latissimus dorsi and pectoralis.

BIOMECHANICS
Force couples

A *force couple* is the application of combined forces to produce a specific type of rotation.[5] The combined actions of the deltoid and rotator cuff muscles result in elevation of the humerus. The deltoid muscle is hinged at its origin and therefore forces the humerus upward on the glenoid labrum at 0 degrees of abduction.[5] As abduction progresses, the pull of the deltoid forces the humerus more directly into the glenoid cavity. Similarly, at the end range of abduction the deltoid exerts a force that is directed toward translating the head of the humerus downward out of the glenoid cavity. For normal mechanics it is necessary that

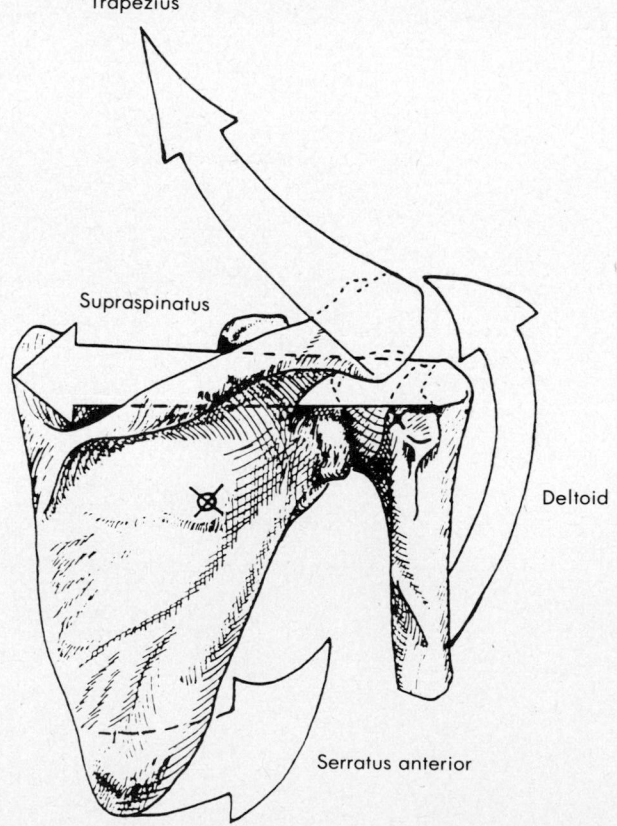

Fig. 20-4. Force coupe of abduction. (From Kapandji IA: The physiology of the joints, vol 1, New York, 1970, Churchill Livingstone, Inc.)

this potentially abnormal force be counteracted by the pull of the fan-shaped rotator cuff muscles that work to fix the humerus within the glenoid (Fig. 20-4). Staples and Watkins[79] have shown that, in the absence of the deltoid muscle, the rotator cuff is able to fully abduct the glenohumeral joint at about 50% of normal power.

Full active range of abduction can also be accomplished, even if the supraspinatus muscle is paralyzed. In this case abduction can be initiated at about 80% of normal force. This power, however, is rapidly lost as abduction increases, and, at approximately 90 degrees of combined scapular and humeral motion, the arm can barely resist the pull of gravity. Abduction in the absence of the supraspinatus muscle is therefore possible, but the deltoid must rely on the three remaining rotator cuff muscles to help stabilize the head of the humerus in the glenoid cavity (Fig. 20-5). In a classic study Inman, Abbott, and Saunders[36] were able to show that all four of the rotator cuff muscles were active throughout active abduction, although their relative contributions depend on the range of abduction.

In the absence of strength, or as a result of weakness, of the deltoid muscle, the long head of the biceps may assume the deltoid's role if the humerus is externally rotated to 90 degrees. This compensation will allow for full abduction, although strength is greatly decreased.[79]

Another example of a force couple is the combined action of the three parts of the trapezius muscle. The upper segment elevates the acromion, the lower segment downwardly rotates the base of the scapular spine, while the middle fibers act to maintain contralateral alignment. Unassisted, however, the trapezius is not properly aligned to prevent the weight of the arm from tilting the inferior angle of the scapula posteriorly, resulting in *winging*. In flexion, therefore, the serratus anterior muscle must function to prevent this instability in the scapula. The serratus anterior also acts as a force couple in conjunction with the trapezius muscle during upward rotation of the glenoid fossa, an action that is necessary for full abduction. It does so by tracking the scapula anteriorly, laterally, and superiorly.[18]

Scapulohumeral rhythm

The importance of upward scapular rotation to the glenoid fossa becomes obvious when the scapulohumeral rhythm is investigated. In 1934 Codman[18] first reported that abduction of the humerus to 180 degrees overhead requires the clavicle, scapula, and humerus to move through essentially their full range of motion in a very specific pattern of interaction. He described the following rhythm that exists throughout active abduction: for every 15 degrees of arm abduction, 10 degrees of abduction occur at the glenohumeral joint and 5 degrees of abduction occur as a result of scapular movement, laterally, anteriorly, and superiorly.

In a slightly different investigation Bland, Merrit, and

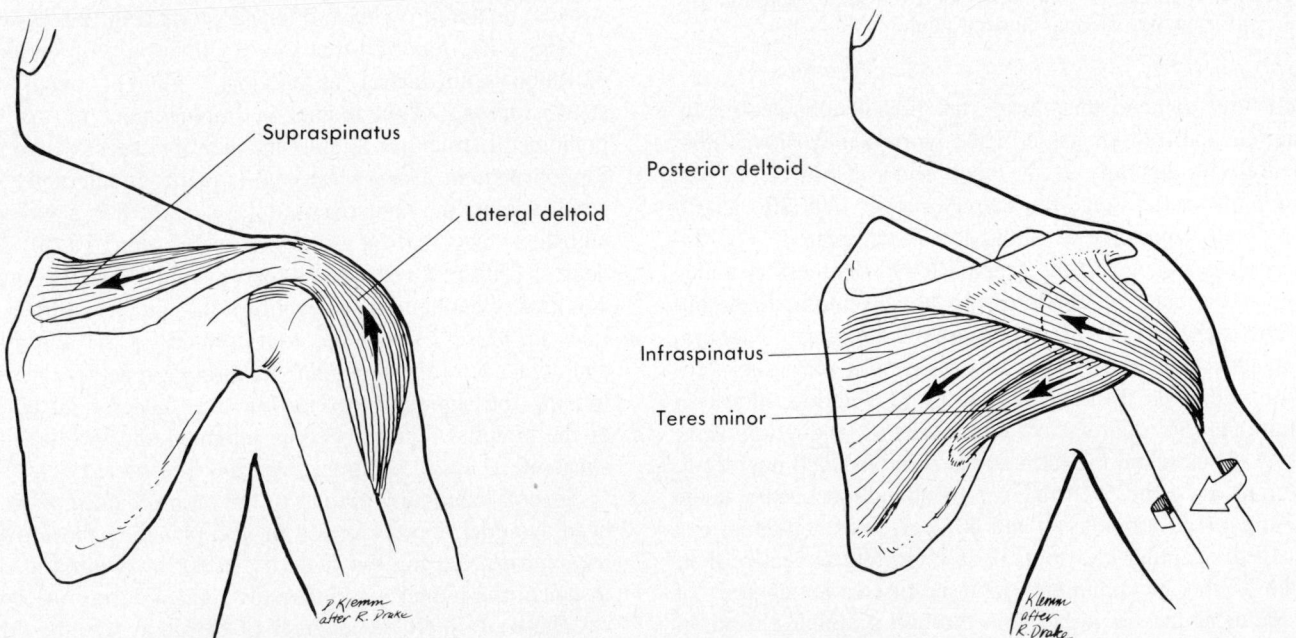

Fig. 20-5. The rotator cuff and deltoid muscle forces at the onset of abduction (zero degrees) and with the arm elevated 90 degrees. The deltoid force changed from a shear to a compressive force. Thus, a damaged or weakened supraspinatus muscle causes loss of counterbalance and allows the vertical force of the deltoid muscle to compress the tissue more. (From Bogamil GIN: AAOS Symposium on upper extremity injuries in athletes, Pettrone FA, editor, St. Louis, 1986, The CV Mosby Co.)

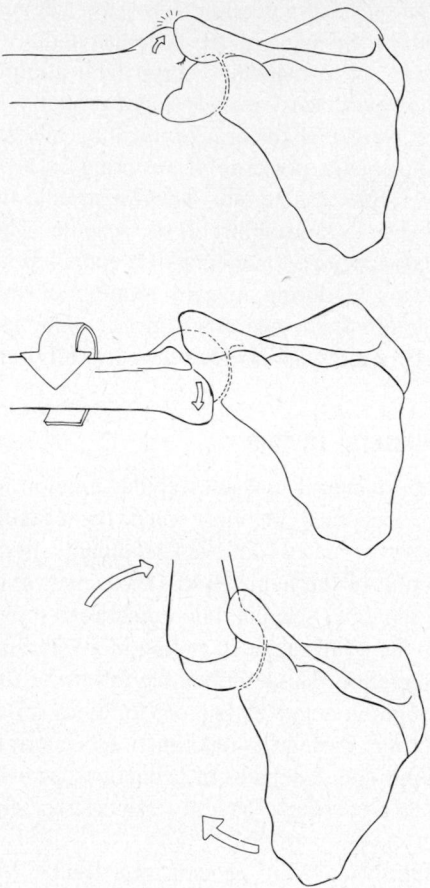

Fig. 20-6. Clearing greater tuberosity from under acromium to gain full abduction at glenohumeral joint.

Boushey[8] contend that during the first 45 degrees of abduction, the inferior angle of the scapula may move either medially or laterally as the bone seeks stability, but past this point in the range the scapula moves laterally, anteriorly, and superiorly as abduction is completed. The humerus can abduct on the scapula to 90 degrees, at which point the greater tuberosity abuts the acromium. If the humerus is externally rotated before 90 degrees of glenohumeral abduction, the greater tuberosity will clear the acromion and avoid locking against it. This action allows an additional 30 degrees of glenohumeral abduction (Fig. 20-6). Thus when the humerus is abducted 180 degrees to straight overhead, 120 degrees of abduction occurs at the glenohumeral articulation and 60 degrees of abduction is a result of scapular elevation. It is important to realize that, even if the glenohumeral joint is fused, 60 degrees of scapular abduction is possible through scapular elevation. This scapular rotation is important not only for attainment of full abduction, but also because (1) it improves the deltoid length-tension relationship throughout the full range of abduction, and (2) as the scapula rotates upward, the glenoid labrum remains almost perpendicular to the head of the humerus. Therefore there is a decreased caudal

shear force, which might otherwise sublux the humerus inferiorly.

Full clavicular motion at both the acromioclavicular and sternoclavicular joints is essential for full scapulothoracic motion to occur. Inman and Saunders[37] have shown that, for full abduction of the arm to occur, the clavicle must rotate 50 degrees posteriorly. This movement becomes important in clients who have had complete acromioclavicular tears treated by pinning the clavicle to the coracoid. Perry[72] reports that this may limit abduction to only 100 degrees.

There is some disagreement in the literature concerning the available range of clavicular motion. Those interested should consult the following sources: Kapandji,[47] Cailliet,[13] Lunggren,[59] and Engin.[24]

Impingement syndrome

The impingement syndrome results from repetitive microtrauma to the tissues that are enclosed in the humerocoracoacromial space. Any or all of the following tissues can be affected: the supraspinatus tendon, the long head of the biceps, the subacromial bursa, or the acromioclavicular joint. These tissues may be subjected to repetitive impingement between the greater tuberosity and either the acromion, if the humerus is in neutral or external rotation, or the thick and sharp coracoclavicular ligament, if the humerus is internally rotated when the arm is elevated above 80 degrees. The impingement can occur during an overhand tennis stroke, the butterfly or front crawl swimming strokes, or the throwing motion in sports (Fig. 20-7).

Neer[62] has reported that the functional arc of shoulder elevation is not lateral, as previously thought, but is, instead, forward. This results in impingement of the suprahumeral structures against the anterior aspect of the acromion and, in cases where the humerus is internally rotated, against the coracoacromial ligament. It is a well-established fact that at somewhere between 70 to 120 degrees (different researchers report slightly different numbers) of glenohumeral elevation, the greater tuberosity rides up closely under the roof formed by the acromion and coracoacromial ligament. If, through repetitive microtrauma, the supraspinatus tendon, the subacromial bursa, or the bicipital tendon become inflamed and swollen, the subacromial space becomes even more restricted.

Several examples relating to the biomechanics of overhead shoulder sports can aid in understanding these overuse injuries. During the butterfly stroke in swimming, for instance, the humerus is internally rotated during the critical phase of 70 to 120 degrees of elevation. On the other hand, the humerus is externally rotated from the windup in pitching. This external rotation helps to clear the greater tuberosity by pulling it down and allowing it to ride under the coracoacromial structures. Internal rotation may account for the greater percentage of impingement syndromes in butterfly swimmers compared to baseball pitch-

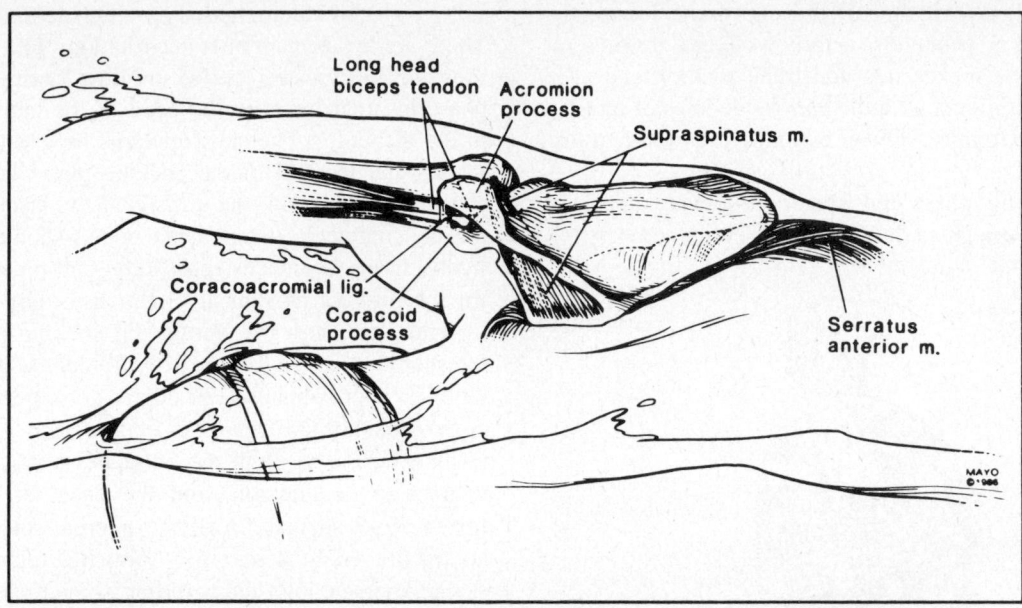

Fig. 20-7. Impingement of supraspinatus and biceps tendons between humeral head and coracoacromial arch can occur with abduction and internal rotation of humerus, as in recovery phase of freestyle stroke. Note how serratus anterior muscle rotates scapula into abduction as humerus is abducted to allow a greater range of shoulder motion. Scapular rotation also delays impingement of greater tuberosity under coracoacromial arch until humerus is maximally abducted to near 180 degrees. With fatigue or underdevelopment of serratus, humeral impingement may occur at an earlier point in recovery stroke at a lower angle of shoulder abduction. (From Johnson JE, Sim FH, and Scott SG: Mayo Clin Proc 62:289-304, 1987.)

ers. It is interesting to note that studies by Atwater[3] have shown that pitchers hold their arms at nearly 95 degrees of abduction in relation to their trunk, regardless of whether they are throwing overhand, three-quarter, or sidearm.

Other sports-related overuse syndromes

The biomechanical actions in overhead sports require extremely coordinated movements in order for the athlete to function maximally and without injury. The ballistic and repetitive nature of these sports can lead to overuse microtrauma if the musculature is too tight or underconditioned or if the overhand stroke or delivery is the result of faulty technique. It is important for the clinician to appreciate proper techniques in order to prevent future injury. Proper techniques and pitching mechanics will be discussed.

The pitching sequence can be broken down into four phases: The *windup phase* begins when motion first occurs and ends when the ball is taken out of the glove; the *cocking phase* then begins and lasts until the shoulder is in the apprehensive position; the *acceleration phase* starts from the apprehensive position until the ball is released; and the *follow-through phase* starts from the point from where the ball is released until motion is stopped.[41]

Approximately 60% of the speed comes from the legs, 25% from the trunk, and about 15% from the shoulder.[81,87] The arm is essentially used as a guidance system

during acceleration and ball release, which may result in a ball speed of anywhere from 70 to 100 miles per hour.[12] The vast majority of the speed comes from the trunk and legs because of the rotary movements and the larger linear forces of the lower extremity as compared to the upper extremity. A pendulum swing in the opposite direction of the arm and leg occurs during the windup and cocking phase. Movement of the ball is determined by the pressure points and grasp of the wrist and fingers on the ball. During pitching, most of the muscles usually begin their concentric contractions in the stretched position, which results in the greatest electromyographic (EMG) activity and allows for a greater arc of force to develop from acceleration and speed of movement.[41,42]

The windup phase begins with a rocker step. A pitcher will rock step backwards, which begins the momentum change of the lower extremity transferred through the trunk to the upper extremity. This results in the pendulum movement of the arms and legs in the opposite directions and also the movement of weight transfer through rotation. During the windup phase balance is important because of the inverted pyramid that occurs with pitching. Correct balance of the foot that is on the rubber is extremely important. Proper and smooth transmission of movement requires at least 90 degrees of hip rotation, 20 degrees of dorsiflexion, and 15 degrees of knee flexion. The hip will be in about 20 degrees of flexion. In summary, the windup phase establishes rhythm of the upper and lower extremity through a pendulum action with the shifting of weight during the rocker step and trunk rotation and also serves to distract hitters with the various degrees of motion in the upper extremity, lower extremity, and the trunk (Fig. 20-8).[87]

In the cocking phase the shoulders elevate approximately 80 to 110 degrees throughout the entire activity, resulting in continuous activity of the deltoid (Fig. 20-9). There are 90 degrees of trunk rotation. The supraspinatus fires for the greatest period of time during the cocking phase in order to retain the head of the humerus centered in the glenoid.[42] The subscapularus fires with the greatest intensity at the end of the cocking phase because it fires eccentrically to slow the arm down.[42] Also, at this point the noncontractile components of the shoulder are coiled tightly in the apprehensive position and provide a fulcrum for the forward movement of the arm. The external rotators fire concentrically during the cocking phase because the shoulder moves from exactly 90 degrees of internal rotation to approximately 130 degrees of external rotation.[42] Approximately 60 degrees of abduction is required in the pushoff leg, along with the 90 degrees of rotation and 20 degrees in dorsiflexion, and the knee, at this point, is flexed at 45 degrees. With the internal rotators and noncontractile components in a stretched position and the scapulothoracic joint ready to fire isometrically, the kinetic chain is prepared to transfer all the energy from the legs and trunk to the arm, which will result in forward acceleration of the upper extremity.

The acceleration phase, the shortest of the four phases, begins in the apprehensive position and lasts less than one tenth of a second (Fig. 20-10). There is very little EMG activity of the rotator cuff muscles. The vast majority of the EMG activity during this phase is produced from an isometric contraction of the serratus anterior and rhomboids (for stability of the scapulothoracic joint) and the acceleration firing of the pectoralis major, latissimus dorsi, and subscapularus.[41] The rotator cuff muscles are surprisingly quiescent. The triceps fire concentrically and the biceps fire eccentrically during the last 20 degrees of elbow

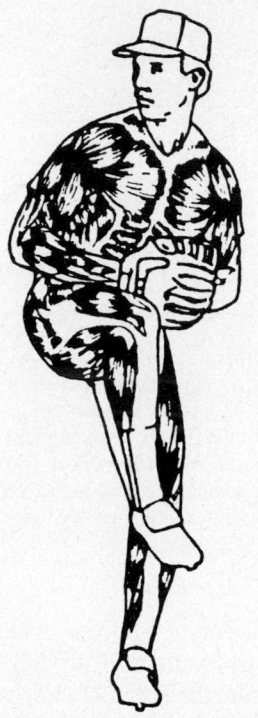

Fig. 20-8. Windup phase.

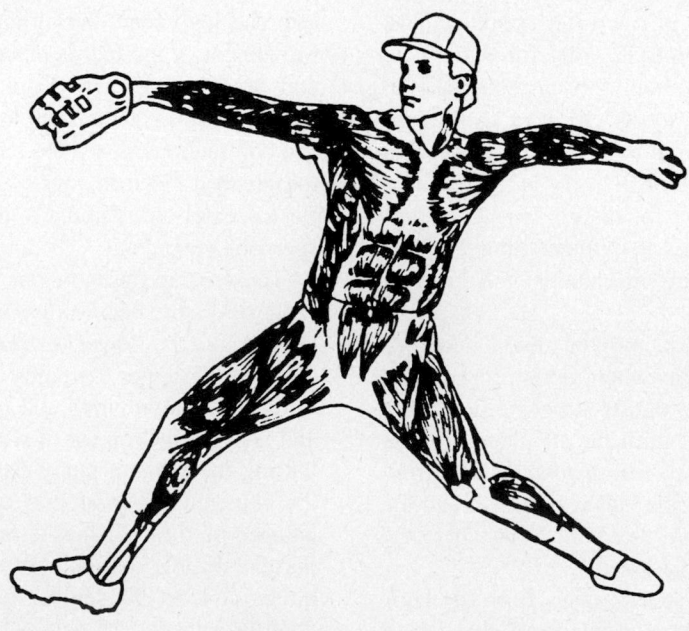

Fig. 20-9. Cocking phase.

extension.[42] The ball is released at approximately 20 degrees of elbow flexion, with the forearm in pronation.[69,70] There is a concentric contraction of the wrist flexors and pronators until the ball is released. The range of motion at this time is directed toward internal rotation and horizontal flexion. The arm is accelerated at 500,000 degrees per second, with the average velocity of the shoulder being 6,200 degrees per second, and the elbow moves at 4,600 degrees per second.[70] At 90 degrees of abduction, the rotator cuff is only 59% efficient because of the length to tension ratio. Since the cuff is in the shortened position, the stress-strain curve for soft tissue efficiency is at 85%, which will result in soft tissue microtrauma that occurs with every pitch.[83] It is interesting to note that with underhand pitching the stress-strain curve is at 79%, and fastball underhand pitchers usually can pitch for a much longer time and with fewer arm problems than someone who throws overhand. [38,87] During the acceleration phase the ankle plantar flexes to 40 degrees and the hip extends 30 degrees. In addition, a very long stride length places stretch demands of greater than 90 degrees on the hamstring musculature.

The final phase of throwing is the follow-through phase (Fig. 20-11), which results in the greatest EMG activity. It includes eccentric contractions of the rotator cuff, deltoid, and biceps (during the last 20 degrees of elbow extension) to decelerate the arm. There is also a continuing isometric firing of the scapulothoracic muscles.[38,39,41,42]

At this point maximal traction stresses are applied to the medial aspect of the elbow, and maximal compressive force results on the lateral aspect of the elbow because of linear compressive forces.[67,70]

In summary, pitching is a very complicated coordina-tion activity that requires finite synchrony of force transmission between the lower extremity, trunk, and upper extremity. Proximal stability must be matched with glenohumeral static flexibility and dynamic stability in order to minimize the stress to surrounding soft tissue.

EVALUATION

A systematic approach to the shoulder examination is needed to suit the needs of the physical therapist working with orthopaedic and sports injuries. A thorough review of both subjective and objective data will allow the therapist to refer the athlete to proper medical personnel, if a physician is not present during the initial injury, and to initiate a comprehensive rehabilitation program directed toward symptomatic relief and prevention of reinjury.

The preventive phase of rehabilitation is often overlooked. Many injuries of the shoulder in athletes can be classified as overuse problems that result from repetitive stresses on what may only be minimal structural abnormalities; overuse injuries of swimmers and pitchers may fall into this category. These abnormalities, whether they represent deficits in strength, flexibility, or technique, are often easily remedied through appropriate intervention by a skilled therapist trained in anatomy, biomechanics, physiology, and therapeutic exercise. The key to rehabilitation lies in effectively evaluating the injury, the person, and the sport. This evaluation should be an ongoing process. The initial examination is important, not only in identifying the structures involved but also in providing a set of baseline data that can be referred to in subsequent evaluations. Without such information the therapist will lack any objective measure of the efficacy of the prescribed treatments. The collection of an initial data base can be most helpful in providing positive reinforcement to the client regarding his/her progress during therapy.

The format of the evaluation can be modified easily to

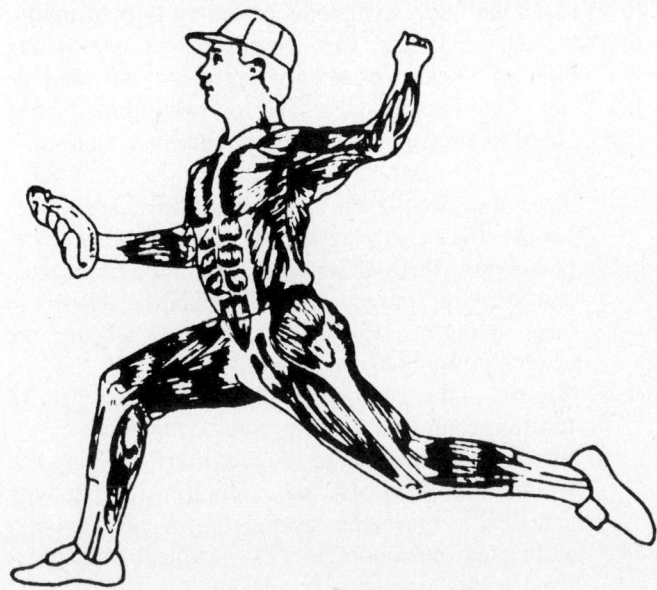

Fig. 20-10. Acceleration phase.

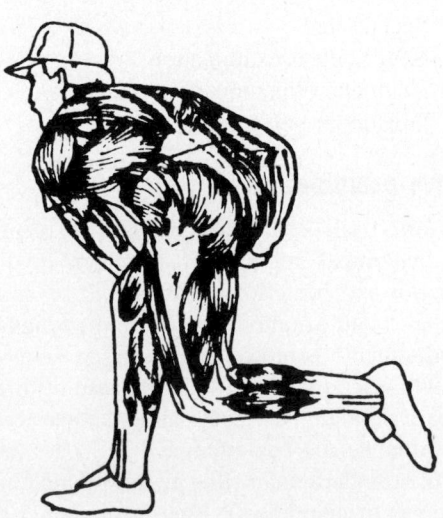

Fig. 20-11. Follow-through phase.

suit the needs of the therapist, whether the evaluation is performed on the field, in the clinic, in the classroom, or within the structure of a preseason examination. The two major subdivisions of the evaluation are the subjective and objective examinations. The subjective portion of the evaluation is often overlooked and not given the attention it merits. It not only enhances communication between client and therapist but also serves to help identify the mechanism, irritability, severity, stage of progression, functional loss, and client's perception of the injury. The objective examination is necessary to further identify the structures involved and to supplement the baseline information. Cyriax[20] stressed that "though many different lesions exist, they can all be distinguished: identification is merely an exercise in applied anatomy." However, this statement appears to be rather idealistic. Clancy[17] believes that "the shoulder is perhaps the most difficult of all joints to evaluate because of the number of important structures located in such a small area, the poorly understood biomechanical demands placed on these structures during the different phases of the act of overhead acceleration and deceleration, and the inability to predict excessive wear and tear on these structures."

An outline of a shoulder evaluation follows:

1. Subjective examination
   a. Location
   b. Present history
      (1) Onset
      (2) Symptoms
   c. Past history
2. Objective examination
   a. Gait
   b. Posture
   c. Referral joints
   d. Active movements
   e. Passive movements
   f. Palpations
   g. Special tests
   h. Neurological examination
   i. Isokinetic dynamometer testing
   j. Functional performance

Subjective examination

Location. Body charts can be used in identifying the general anatomical regions of shoulder involvement.[31] Both anterior and posterior charts should be used and can easily be included in one form. These drawings should include prominent contours representing major muscle groups and skeletal structures. In the case of diffuse or radiating pain dermatome charts can be shown to the client, but only after he/she has attempted to locate these symptoms on the standard chart (this avoids prejudicing the subjective report of symptoms). The client should be encouraged to fill out the chart according to the examiner's in-

structions, which should include locating the central site of greatest sensory change (x), the boundaries of altered sensation (. . .), the directional spread of symptoms ($\rightarrow$), and any other pertinent information (e.g., symptoms at proximal or distal regions). During subsequent evaluations this information will be a valuable reference for mapping the progression of symptoms. It should be emphasized that body charts are, at best, a gross tool used to locate symptoms and that further identification of the actual structures involved depends on the remainder of the subjective and objective findings.

Present history. This section of the evaluation is important in establishing the onset and sequential behavior of the symptoms. It provides information that may assist the clinician in directing the client's rehabilitation (what treatment modalities have been used in previous disorders and with what success), evaluating the tissues involved (Was a snap heard?), assessing the severity of the injury (Did immediate swelling and discoloration occur?), and instituting preventive measures (understanding the mechanism of injury).

The history of the injury indicates whether or not the onset was sudden (usually associated with a specific incident) or gradual (suggesting an overuse syndrome or systematic involvement). In the case of sudden onset the mechanism of injury should be identified (i.e., Was it a direct and localized external force or an excessive resistance to motion?). If the onset was gradual, the client should be questioned as to any changes made (before the initial symptoms) in the following: activity (type, technique, frequency, duration, or intensity), environmental conditions, equipment, medication, body weight, or symptoms elsewhere in the body (indicating related disease requiring compensatory biomechanical changes).

While discussing the onset of the injury, it is important to focus on the initial symptoms regarding type of injury, severity, and irritability. Through appropriate questioning the subsequent behavior of the symptoms can then be traced up to the current stage. The following three factors can be used in assessing the initial or current symptoms:

1. Type of injury—esthesia (hyperesthesia, hypoesthesia, anesthesia, or paresthesia), hypermobility or hypomobility, thermal sensation, coloration, crepitus, and strength (fatigue and/or weakness). These, in turn, should be evaluated according to whether the symptoms are constant or variable.
2. Severity—the amount of initial pain and loss of function compared to the present symptoms.
3. Irritability—in response to (1) activity (walking and specific use of the affected extremity), (2) inactivity (standing, ipsilateral side-lying, and gravity-eliminated positioning), (3) treatment modalities (heat, cold, compression, elevation, massage, traction, splinting or slinging, and medication), (4) cir-

cadian behavior, and (5) any additional means of increasing or decreasing the symptoms.

Past history. An appropriate review of the client's medical history can provide information that may demonstrate the integrity of the musculoskeletal system (possibly revealing weak linkages in the kinetic chain) or that may serve to uncover underlying visceral, systemic, or psychological disorders that have contributed to the injury indicated by shoulder pain. The client's past athletic history should also be obtained and may be an important factor to consider when setting up a treatment regime appropriate to the individual's goals.

The past history should focus on previous injuries to the shoulder complex. When identified, these disorders should be reviewed in terms of onset, treatment, duration, and anatomical or functional loss. It is also important to review any previous musculoskeletal disorders elsewhere in the body that may influence the transfer of forces through the upper extremities. A weakness or hypomobility in an associated joint (cervical, thoracic, lumbar) may influence the biomechanics and resultant forces of the shoulder complex.

This history should also touch on disorders of the cardiac and visceral organs that may be found to refer pain to the shoulder region (e.g., cardiac ischemia; gallbladder, hepatic, gastric, and pancreatic disease; and diaphragmatic irritation).[10]

Objective examination

Gait. The client should be observed during ambulation. This will assist the examiner in gauging the severity of the disorder in terms of functional loss of motion in the shoulder complex. Asymmetry of motion may lead to additional compensatory dysfunction within, or distant to, the original site of the injury. The following patterns may indicate that a significant loss of function is present:

(1) upper body or cervical listing to the affected side and
(2) loss of rhythmical tandem arm motion during gait.

Posture. A standing examination should be carried out for the anterior, lateral, and posterior aspects of the upper body. This will indicate any gross joint abnormalities. A glenohumeral dislocation is indicated by a prominent acromion laterally, a depressed scapula, and a slightly abducted humerus, while a separation of the acromioclavicular, coracoacromial, and coracoclavicular ligaments is obvious because of an abrupt stairstep positioning of the distal clavicle above the acromion.[1] The examination will also reveal any significant muscle atrophy that results from neurological or disuse problem. Loss of proper muscle contour may also be the result of ruptures in the musculotendinous unit, such as a *Popeye* biceps following a complete rupture of the bicipital tendon, although this is rare in the case of younger athletes. An abnormal concavity in the supraspinatus and/or infraspinatus fossa is some-

times observed. Usually these fossae should be convex in nature, but occasionally, with either an underdeveloped muscle or a problem with the suprascapular nerve, they will be concave. Another postural abnormality is a hollowness where the teres minor and teres major attach to the lateral border of the scapula (Fig. 20-12). This is hard to see in the presence of a well-developed latissimus dorsi. Again, this can be caused by disuse, misuse, or neurological injury to the axillary nerve.

Other postural variations may include spinal kyphosis or scoliosis (acquired or congenital), protracted shoulders because of tight pectoralis major and minor muscles (often seen in weight lifters), and a distracted or winged scapula, resulting from an injury to the long thoracic nerve or a general weakness of the serratus anterior muscle.

Referral joints. Several neurologically related joints may refer symptoms to the shoulder region. These include the cervical spine, temporomandibular joint, cardiovascular system, and the elbow. Careful consideration of the mechanism of injury may help determine the number of additional joints that need evaluation. Joint clearing tests need only be performed if symptoms or questions from the subjective examination reveal possible involvement of particular joints. Clearing examinations are carried out by having the client perform each available active motion with the examiner applying a steady overpressure at the end of the range. The therapist should be careful not to involve the shoulder.[31] Any symptoms or signs should be checked bilaterally for a determination of their significance.

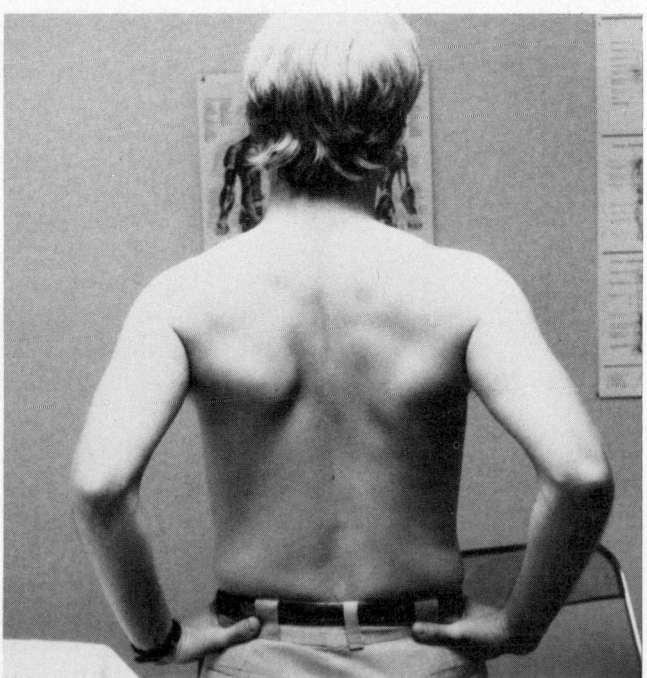

Fig. 20-12. Observation for atrophy.

With joint clearing tests the examiner must consider the cervical spine, especially C-4–C-5 and C-5–C-6 that have contributory branches to the axillary nerve, dorsal scapular nerve, long thoracic nerve, and subscapular nerve.[48] A client with any type of trauma to the C-4–C-5 area or any of the muscles that are attached to it, such as the levator scapula, splenius capitus, cervicus, or trapezius, could experience referred pain to the shoulder. Therefore it is very important that the examiner also do accessory movements to the levels of C-4, C-5, and C-6.

Active movements. Active movements provide useful information when assessing the severity of a shoulder lesion in addition to providing a means of stressing the contractile and noncontractile tissues.

Goniometric measurements should be recorded, including body position for the 3 degrees of freedom of the shoulder to establish a data base for rehabilitation as well as provide information concerning the specific disorder.

During active abduction, the examiner should observe component motions at both the scapulothoracic and glenohumeral joints. This movement can be tested by marking the resting position of the inferior angle with the examiner's thumb and then having the client actively abduct. The relative movement at these joints should be similar to that discussed in the biomechanics section of this chapter. Baseball pitchers should be observed from behind as they raise their arms into a simulated cocking position of combined abduction, horizontal extension, and external rotation. Any loss of smooth synchrony or range of motion or occurence of fasciculations indicating fatique should be noted (Fig. 20-13).

The sternoclavicular and acromioclavicular joints should also be palpated for range of motion. Hypomobility of these joints will decrease the measured values obtained for abduction, flexion, and extension of the shoulder (see biomechanics section for discussion of normal value). Hypomobility can be grossly tested by placing a finger in the supraclavicular groove and asking the client to elevate his/her arm. The component motions of the clavicle should cause the finger to be pushed out of the groove.

During active abduction the client may experience acute pain between 60 and 120 degrees and then report relief at a point beyond this range. Kessel and Watson[50] reported that this behavior suggests the presence of a subacromial disorder (bursa and rotator cuff insertions). This range of motion anatomically represents the sequence in which the greater tuberosity and its overlying bursae and tendons are closely articulating beneath the acromium and the coracoacromial ligament. It is important to realize that this painful arc may be overlooked if clients are reluctant to abduct through pain. If the concept of the test is explained to them, they will often report that they notice a cessation of pain once they have passed the critical range of 120 degrees. Then the examiner should systematically test the acromioclavicular joint.

Passive movements. Passive movements can assist in

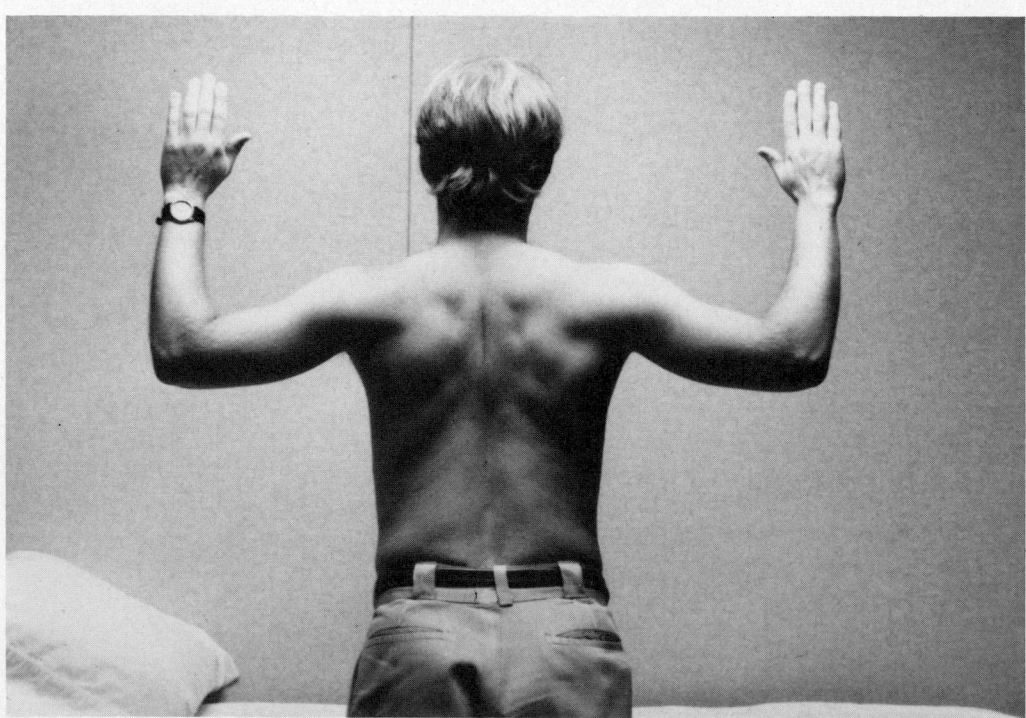

Fig. 20-13. Observing for synchrony of movement in pitchers: combined abduction, horizontal extension and external rotation.

the differentiation between contractile tissue (muscle, tendon, muscle-tendon junction, and tendoperiosteal complex) and noncontractile tissue (bursa, bone, ligaments, joint capsules, and neurovascular structures) problems. In order to rule out the involvement of contractile tissue during passive movements, it is essential that the muscles acting on the joint not be in a state of spasm. In addition, if these same muscles exhibit decreased flexibility, they will undergo a passive stretch at the extreme range—which is opposite to their function. Flexibility can be assessed during range of motion in order to further differentiate between capsule and muscle. The contractile tissues that oppose the passive motion, causing pain or discomfort, should always be tested isometrically. These tests should be performed at midjoint position, where the noncontractile tissues are relaxed, and should be very specific in isolating the muscles (see Daniels and Worthingham[22] or Kendall, Kendall, and Wadsworth[48] for further discussion of these tests). With the above qualifications in mind, pain at the extreme range of pure passive motion would implicate involvement of the noncontractile tissues. In other words, if active and passive movements are painful in the same direction, noncontractile structures are involved. If active movements are painful in one direction and passive movements painful in the opposite direction, involvement of a contractile unit is indicated.[45]

Passive movements can be divided into two basic types: physiological and accessory. Physiological movements can be defined as those movements directly under control of the client, such as flexion, extension, rotation, abduction, and adduction. Accessory movements are those movements not under control of the client but necessary for normal movements to occur at a joint.[60] Table 20-1 gives a description of the accessory movements that can be tested, along with the pathological implications of any restriction in movement. As is the case with all measures of range of motion, accessory movements should be compared bilaterally because there is variability within the normal population. As these unconscious movements account for the intrinsic hypermobility of the shoulder joint, even minor decreases in any of these component motions will result in rather drastic limitations in active physiological movements. Once these limitations are identified, appropriate mobilization to improve the accessory movements can be instituted to restore normal joint play.

End-feel. Cyriax[21] has emphasized the importance of the end-feel imparted to the examiner's hands during passive motion. The end-feel can not only serve as a valuable means of assessing the type of disorder present, but it can also indicate the severity or stage of the problem, help in prognosticating the percentage of possible recovery, and, therefore, assist the therapist in selecting treatment modalities and rehabilitation goals. The following is a list of six end-feel findings possible at the extreme range of passive motion.

Capsular end-feel. This represents a distinct end-feel

Table 20-1. Assessment of accessory movements of the shoulder joint and their pathological implications

Accessory movement	Implication
Glenohumeral joint	
Lateral traction (movement of the head of the humerus away from the glenoid cavity)	Hypomobility of the shoulder joint
Posterior glide (posterior movement of the head of the humerus within the glenoid cavity)	Restricted flexion
Anterior glide (anterior movement of the head of the humerus within the glenoid cavity)	Restricted abduction and external rotation
Posterior shear (posterior movement of the head of the humerus with the arm in 90° of shoulder flexion)	Restricted flexion
Caudal glide (inferior movement of the head of the humerus within the glenoid cavity)	Hypomobility of the shoulder joint (results in a compromised subacromial space)
Sternoclavicular joint	
Cranial glide	Restricted depression
Caudal glide	Restricted elevation
Ventral glide	Restricted protraction
Dorsal glide	Restricted retraction
Acromioclavicular joint	
Cranial glide	Restricted abduction
Caudal glide	Restricted adduction
Ventral glide	Restricted flexion/abduction
Dorsal glide	Restricted extension/abduction
Combined cranioventral glide	Restricted external rotation
Combined caudodorsal glide	Restricted internal rotation

that has some give to it and can be compared to the stretching of leather. It is easily found in a normal shoulder at the extreme of passive external rotation. Cyriax[21] claims that each joint has a general capsular pattern that occurs when there is a lesion to the joint capsule or synovial tissue. This pattern for the shoulder is a greater limitation in external rotation than abduction and creates less restriction in internal rotation than in abduction. Mobilization is the indicated treatment. A procedure with this type of end-feel will be discussed in the rehabilitation section of this chapter.

Bone-on-bone end-feel. This is an abrupt, nonyielding end-feel in the range where two bony surfaces approximate each other. It is normally found in the shoulder at 90 degrees of passive abduction, when the humerus comes in contact with the acromion. With this type of end-feel, the prognosis for increasing range of motion with physical therapy is very poor.

Spasm end-feel. This sensation is one in which a vibrant twang comes into play and leads to the end-feel imparted from a normal maximal muscle test. It indicates a protective muscle spasm in the case of an acute lesion. Palpation will readily reveal the muscle in spasm. For further information refer to Travell and Rinzler's book on myofascial pain and dysfunction.[82]

Specifically, one should look for trigger points in the trapezius, levator scapula, rhomboids, and the remainder of the shoulder complex.

Springy block end-feel. This is identified by a rebound sensation present in the joint that results in a decrease in the normal range of motion. It represents the presence of a loose body within the joint and indicates internal derangement. This is encountered in the glenohumeral joint with a positive Clunk test, which will be discussed under special tests. You may also have a springy block end-feel

in the sternoclavicular joint if the meniscus becomes displaced.

Tissue approximation end-feel. This results when range of motion is not limited by the joint structures themselves but rather is limited because of the engagement of extraarticular body tissue. It is present in the shoulder complex during horizontal adduction.

Empty end-feel. This occurs when a client stops any further movement of the joint before the examiner is able to sense any organic resistance to the movement. An empty end-feel may be indicative of an acute bursitis, extraarticular abscess, neoplasm, or hysteria.[21]

The scapulohumeral motion should be observed during passive abduction by placing the web space of the examiner's hand at the inferior angle of the scapula and the thumb along the lateral edge. The examiner should passively abduct the arm and observe the component glenohumeral and scapular motion (Fig. 20-14).

It should be emphasized that passive movements the examiner thinks will be most painful should be tested last. This will avoid a tendency to come to a premature conclusion without carefully ruling out other tissues that may be involved. It will also avoid client apprehension, enhance client cooperation, and prevent excessive symptomatic reaction from clouding the issue. This same principle also applies to palpation.

Palpation. Six different findings as a result of palpation will be described. They are crepitus, change in temperature, swelling, point tenderness, cutaneous sensation, and vascular pulses. The unaffected side should serve as a control.

Crepitus. The presence of crepitus suggests irregular joint articular surfaces, tenosynovitis of the biceps tendon, or an inflamed subacromial bursa.[16]

Temperature. This is best sensed on the dorsum of the

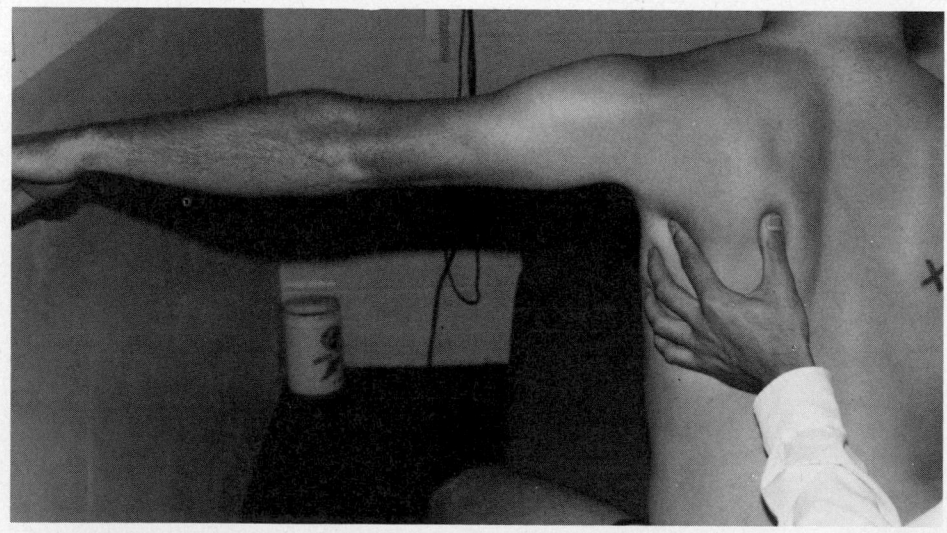

Fig. 20-14. Hand placement to allow pure glenohumeral motion by restricting scapular motion.

examiner's hand and may indicate an increase in vascular activity, indicative of an inflammatory process, or a decrease in temperature, indicative of compromised circulation.

Swelling. A check for localized swelling as well as diffuse intraarticular effusion should be carried out. With effusion, the client may be unable to fully adduct the shoulder toward the trunk.

Point tenderness. A test for point tenderness should be done with as little pressure as needed and will be valuable in localizing the source of pain and trigger points.

Cutaneous sensation. A test for cutaneous sensation is necessary to determine if the neural tissues are functioning properly. The various dermatome levels can be tested for pain and light pressure. Any change in sensation should lead to further neurological testing, which is described in the section dealing with special tests.

Vascular pulses. The brachial artery may be palpated just medial to the biceps tendon, and the axillary artery can be found with firm pressure to the axilla. The radial pulse should be checked for quick assessment of overall circulation.

Hoppenfeld[35] has presented an excellent review of the anatomical structures that can be palpated when examining the shoulder complex. In this chapter the systematic mechanisms of point-by-point palpation will not be presented (since these have been adequately covered by Hoppenfeld), but rather, some of the aspects of clinical importance in examining components of the shoulder complex will be discussed.

Sternoclavicular joint. The available range of motion in this joint has been discussed earlier. Crepitation may be felt and should be related to the presence of any pain or change in range of motion. The clavicle will normally protrude superiorly above the manubrium of the sternum. The sternoclavicular joint usually subluxes in an anterior or posterior direction. The anterior displacement is reportedly three times as frequent and appears as an obvious deformity, whereas a posterior displacement may be more damaging because of potential injury to the structures in the superior mediastinum.[63]

Clavicle. Inspection should reveal any localized swelling or superficial inflammation in this area. Firm tapping along the clavicle may result in localized sharp pain that can be reproduced even with distant percussion. This may reveal the presence of a fracture, and appropriate measures should be instituted to stabilize the shoulder until a physician can diagnose the pathology.

Acromioclavicular joint. Because of its mobility, this articulation, if injured, can result in a significant loss of total shoulder motion. A painful arc can result with degenerative disease injury to this joint. Horizontal adduction, forward flexion, and abduction above 90 degrees are usually all symptomatic. Hawkins and Kennedy[33] report that, in the case of acromioclavicular injury, pain is reproduced by "forcibly adducting and internally rotating the humerus across the chest to jam the acromioclavicular joint together." As with all suspected sprains, the joint should be carefully mobilized during assessment in order to check for excessive motion that would indicate a second-degree or third-degree sprain. As mentioned earlier, a third-degree sprain may be indicated by a stairstep posture at the point of articulation, depending on the integrity of the coracoclavicular and coracoacromial ligaments. If, in fact, these ligaments have also been injured, a total separation may occur, resulting in excessive acromioclavicular motion and associated soft tissue swelling. The mechanism of injury to this joint most commonly results from a direct caudal force exerted on the acromion (e.g., a fall on the shoulder—as in football), although a cephalad force directed up through the humerus may also disrupt the acromioclavicular and coracroclavicular ligaments.

Greater tuberosity of the humerus. The insertion of the supraspinatus, infraspinatus, and teres minor tendons can best be palpated with the arm **passively** placed behind the client's back, which will result in internal rotation, extension, and horizontal adduction. This brings the insertion out from under the acromion. Neer and Welsh[63] have shown that the insertion of the supraspinatus and anterior portion of the infraspinatus tendons all lie anterior to the acromion when the humerus is in the anatomical position of slight external rotation. These tendons move anteriorly with internal rotation of the humerus. They insert just lateral to the superior bicipital groove and wrap around the superior portion of the greater tuberosity as they intermesh with the shoulder capsule posteriorly. From an anterior to posterior direction, they are aligned in the order described above. It should be noted that the subdeltoid bursa overlies this area of palpation and therefore should be considered when pain on palpation needs to be differentiated. The superior portion of the greater tuberosity may be painful to deep palpation on otherwise asymptomatic individuals. Therefore care should be taken not to apply excessive pressure and to palpate bilaterally if any positive signs are elicited.

Lesser tuberosity of the humerus. The superior medial surface of the lesser tuberosity is clinically important in that this is where the subscapularis tendon attaches. This region can best be palpated with the humerus in extension and external rotation. It should be noted that some researchers believe that this region lies too far anterior to be palpated.

Bicipital groove. This area can be palpated with the humerus in external rotation, since the groove lies between the greater and lesser tuberosities. It should be palpated with minimal pressure because the tendon of the biceps and its surrounding sheath are sensitive. If these structures have been irritated, a thickened sheath may be apparent. In some people it is impossible to discern this tendon because the mass of the deltoid intervenes.[17]

Coracoid process. It is important to realize that this structure is angulated in an anterolateral direction and therefore should be palpated from an anteromedial approach. The pectoralis minor muscle attaches on the medial edge, while the short head of the biceps and the coracobrachialis originate from the anterior aspect, which faces laterally. Also present is the attachment of coracoacromial ligament.

Medial and lateral scapular borders. From a superior to inferior direction the following muscles originate from the lateral margin of the scapular border: long head of the triceps, teres minor, and teres major. From the same approach the following muscles insert into the medial aspect: levator scapulae, rhomboideus minor, and rhomboideus major. The supraspinatus and infraspinatus muscles also originate from the medial border. If the scapula is passively raised or winged from the thorax by a gentle posteromedial force applied to the anterolateral shoulder complex, the insertion of the serratus anterior muscle can be palpated as it arises from the entire ventral surface of the medial scapula.

Muscle palpations. Hoppenfeld[35] or a good anatomy text can be consulted for the specific anatomical position of the musculature surrounding the shoulder. The muscles should be palpated from one attachment to the other, and, optimally, they should be checked in both a tightened and a relaxed state. Palpation will reveal any abnormalities in gross structure, such as hematomas, other masses, major tears, tenderness to pressure (indicating possible mi-

crotears and inflammatory reaction), and trigger points that refer pain to the shoulder region. Travell and Rinzler[83] have identified the following muscles as potential sites for trigger points that refer pain to the shoulder complex in a fairly predictable pattern: levator scapulae, rhomboideus minor, supraspinatus and infraspinatus, scaleni, deltoid, subscapularis, teres major, trapezius, serratus anterior, and the pectorals.

Subacromial bursa. With the humerus in passive extension, this bursa may be palpated as inferior to the acromion, lateral to the bicipital groove, and beneath the deltoid. Crepitation may result if the bursa becomes thickened and the thickening can be felt with passive abduction.

Special tests. The following tests are usually supplementary to a standard examination and are selected in accordance with the preceding findings.

Test for bicipital tendonitis. Yergason[86] developed the most commonly used test (Figure 20-15). This test is positive if pain in the anterior inner aspect of the shoulder results from the client's active attempt to supinate against resistance while the elbow is kept at 90 degrees of flexion. If it is possible to palpate the tendon through the overlying muscle, Lippman's test[55] may produce sharp pain when the tendon is displaced from side to side with a probing finger and then released. This is done about 3 inches from the shoulder joint with the elbow flexed at 90 degrees. In Ludington's test[58] sharp pain is elicited when the biceps are contracted while the client clasps his/her head. Hawk-

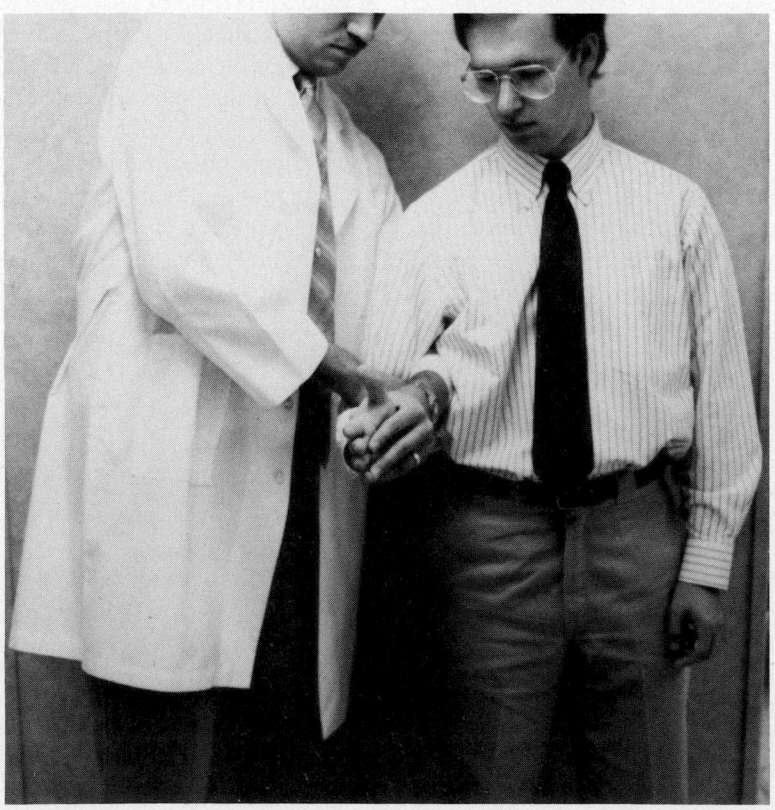

Fig. 20-15. Yergason test for bicipital tendonitis.

ins and Kennedy[33] also have reported on a straight-arm-raising test that produces pain in the area of the bicipital groove during resisted forward flexion of the humerus with the elbow extended.

Test for a ruptured transverse humeral ligament. Booth and Marvel[10] have described a maneuver that tests the integrity of this ligament. The client's arm is abducted and externally rotated with the examiner's fingers placed along the bicipital groove. The arm is then internally rotated while the examiner feels for the tendon snapping in and out of its groove. The mechanism of injury to this ligament occurs as a result of an excessive overload to the arm, which is in a position of abduction and external rotation. Such an injury often results in an audible or palpable snap. Neer and Welsh[63] claim that this disorder is rarely found in younger athletes.

Test for a complete tear of the supraspinatus tendon. The *drop arm test* is positive in evaluating for a tear in the supraspinatus tendon if the client is unable to slowly and smoothly lower his/her arm from a position of 90 degrees abduction.

Test for the impingement syndrome. This syndrome has been best described by Neer.[62] He reports that the most common structures involved are the supraspinatus tendon (with overhead activity), the anterior aspect of the infraspinatus tendon, and the bicipital tendon (with butterfly movements in swimming). He emphasizes that the possible involvement of adjacent soft tissues (subacromial bursa, coracoacromial ligament, and the acromioclavicular joint) may render a specific assessment of single anatomical structures inappropriate. He further characterizes the impingement to be more intimately related to shoulder flexion than to abduction. This flexion will cause the rotator cuff tissues to abut against the **anterior** third of the acromion, if the arm is in an anatomical position, and against the coracoacromial ligament, if the humerus is internally rotated. Based on this finding, Neer and Welsh[63] described an impingement test (Fig. 20-16) that "consists

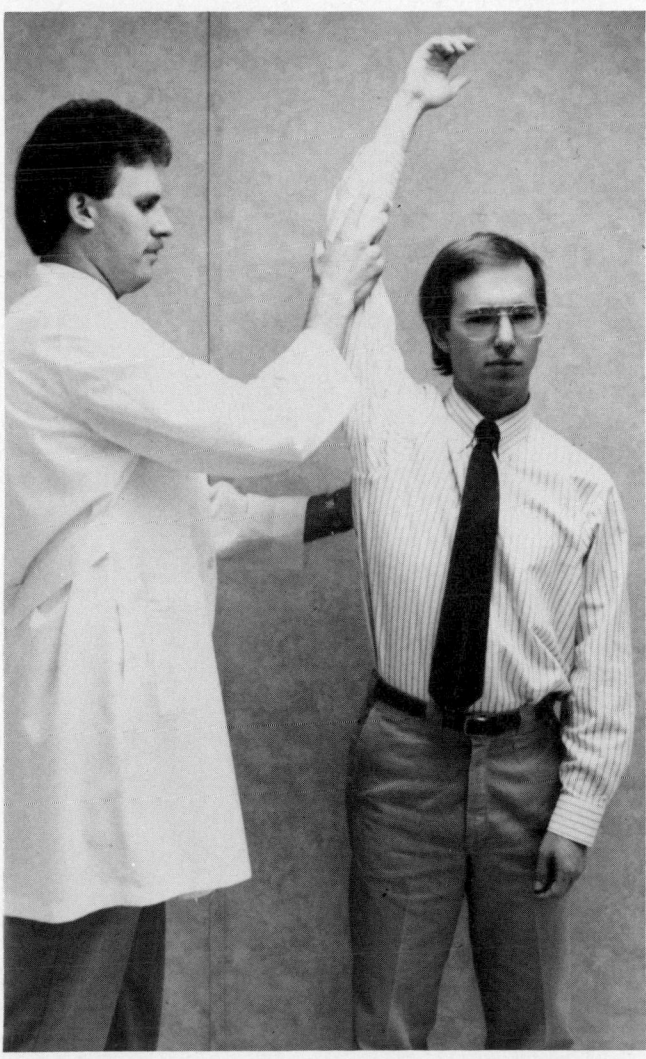

Fig. 20-16. Testing for impingement of the rotator cuff against the anterior, inferior acromial surface.

of forced elevation of the humerus against the anterior acromion, which causes pain that can be relieved by injecting 10 ml of 1% Xylocaine beneath the acromion." Hawkins and Kennedy[33] have described a similar maneuver in which the humerus is flexed to 90 degrees and then forcefully and internally rotated in order to drive the greater tuberosity further under the coracoaromial ligament. Clancy[16] reports that the test for impingement should be done by initially abducting the humerus to 90 degrees and then adducting the arm across the chest, while internally rotating the arm and maintaining 90 degrees flexion (Fig. 20-17).

The Clunk test, performed with the athlete supine, is the most common test for a torn labrum. The examiner's left hand is placed posteriorly on the humeral head while the right hand is secured on the distal humerus (Fig. 20-18). The patient's arm is taken into full abduction, with the humerus forced anteriorly, while the left and right hands assist in externally rotating the shoulder. This may result in an anterior subluxation or dislocation. The examiner then repositions the humeral head by lifting the arm into horizontal adduction. A clunk sensation during this relocation my be suggestive of the humerus snapping or rolling over a tear in the labrum.[87]

Test for anterior glenohumeral dislocation. The apprehension test for glenohumeral dislocation is performed by slowly abducting and externally rotating the humerus while the client is in a relaxed supine position (Fig. 20-19). If the client will not allow the examiner to carry this motion to its extreme or is very apprehensive about the

motion, as reflected by facial reaction, it is considered a positive sign. This motion should never be forced because it may result in a subsequent dislocation. Cailliet[13] reports that the most common cause for this injury is falling on an outstretched arm. Whenever a dislocation is suspected, thorough neurological and vascular examinations should be performed.

Test for posterior glenohumeral dislocation. Neer and Welsh[63] recommend that the apprehension test for posterior instability be carried out by transmitting a posterior force with the humerus held in various angles of flexion and internal rotation (Fig. 20-20). They report that this type of dislocation can be caused by impact with the shoulder flexed, as occurs when a person falls on a ball or pushes forward. A chronic posterior subluxation will often result in involvement of the teres minor and infraspinatus muscle because of the location of their insertion into the humerus. As a result, a posterior subluxation can be misdiagnosed as tendonitis.

Test for the thoracic outlet syndrome. This syndrome,

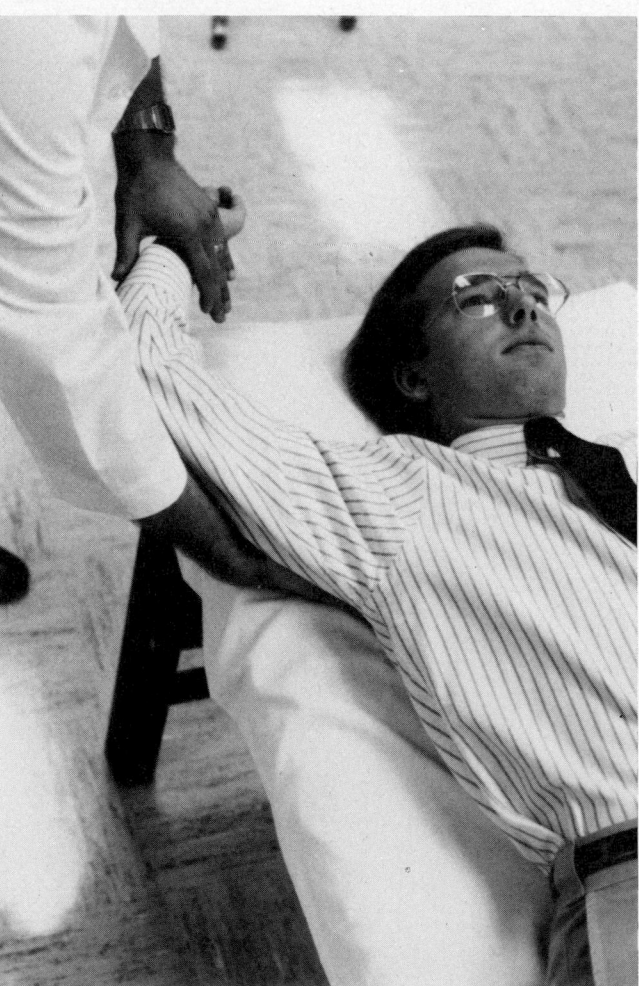

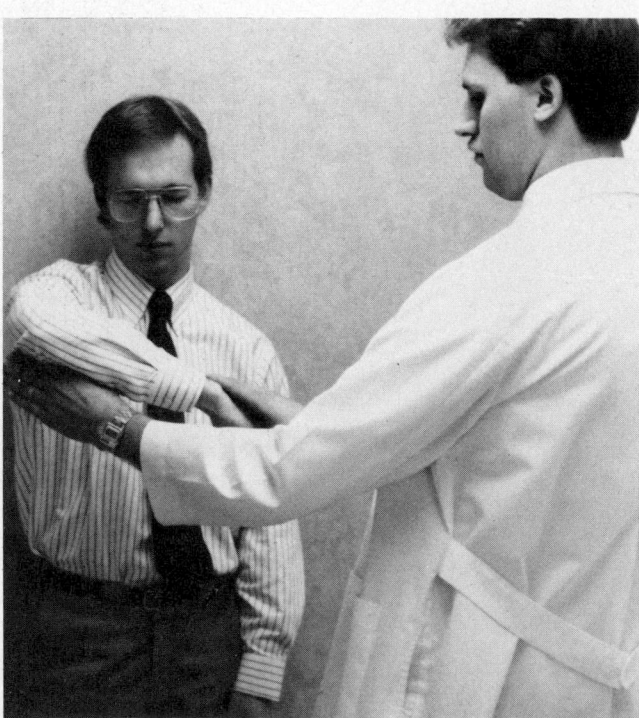

Fig. 20-17. Testing for impingement of the rotator cuff against the anterior surface of the coracoacromial ligament.

Fig. 20-18. The clunk test for a tear to the anterior glenoidal labrum.

which may result from several different causes, should be referred to appropriate medical personnel for a thorough investigation. The Adson maneuver may be used to confirm the presence of this syndrome. The client is asked to hold his/her breath in deep inspiration while fully extending the neck and turning the chin toward the side being examined. The examiner palpates the radial pulse, checking for any obliteration or dampening. Lord and Rosati[57] discuss further discriminating tests for this type of disorder.

Neurological tests. There are several injuries that necessitate a specific neurological evaluation—for instance, any suspicion of a fracture or dislocation. Both of these also require a vascular assessment.

A common injury encountered in football is a traction stretch to the brachial plexus, often referred to as a *stinger*. It results when forced rotation of a flexed or extended cervical spine occurs along with traction in the arm. It can occur if a player is tackled or held by the arm while at the same time being struck on the helmet in a direction away from the arm. It also can occur if a tackler's neck and shoulder are forced apart through contact with the ball carrier.

Wallace[85] has reported on several cases of injury, occurring during sports activities, to the long thoracic nerve. The resulting winging of the scapula may not be easily detected. Nevertheless, it should be evaluated any time that an athlete suffers a stinger or a blow to the shoulder complex. For a specific discussion of the test see Daniels and Worthingham[22] or Kendall, Kendall, and Wadsworth.[48]

The spinal accessory nerve, because of its superficial location along the vertical aspect of the trapezius, may be injured by a direct blow. O'Donaghue[66] reports that there

may be serious paralysis for a few days, but in most cases recovery of motor function is rapid.

The following three areas should also be evaluated during the neurological examination: sensation, reflexes, and results of resisted tests.

Sensation. The cervical region and entire upper extremity should be tested for sharp and dull touch as well as for temperature sensitivity. Each dermatome (C-5 to T-2) should be tested. If an axillary nerve has been damaged from a fracture or a dislocation, there may be an anaesthetic patch over the lateral deltoid region.

Reflexes. Three different muscle reflexes should be tested: biceps (C-5), brachioradialis (C-6), and triceps (C-7). These tests should be performed bilaterally by an experienced examiner. The client should be relaxed, and the elbow should be positioned so as to place the tendon on a slight stretch.

Resisted test. Manual muscle testing can be done on the following muscles: deltoid (C-5), biceps (C-6), triceps (C-7), long-finger flexors (C-8), and the interossei (T-1). Further manual testing will assist in evaluating any weak-

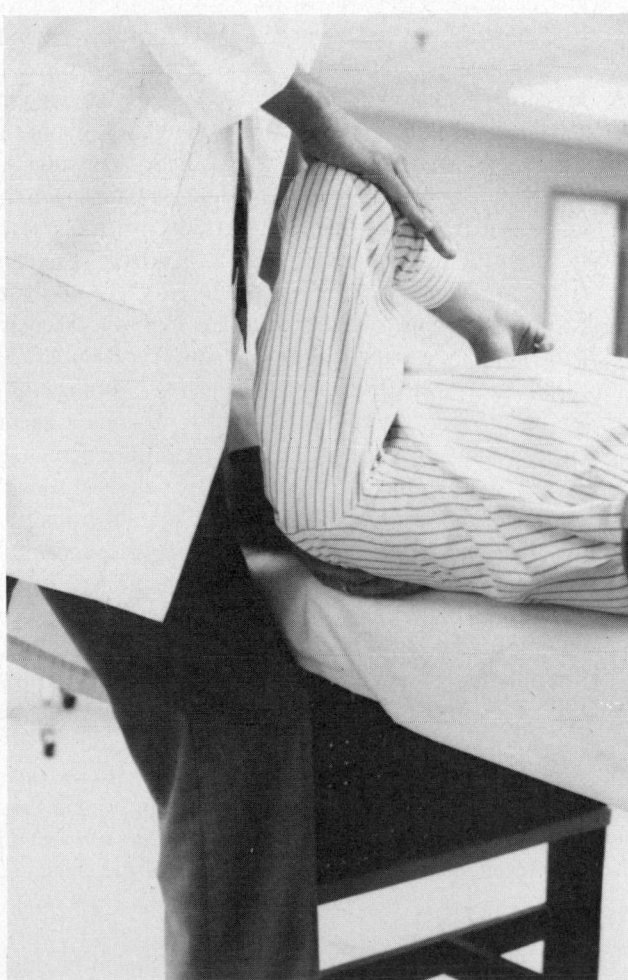

Fig. 20-20. Testing for posterior glenohumeral instability.

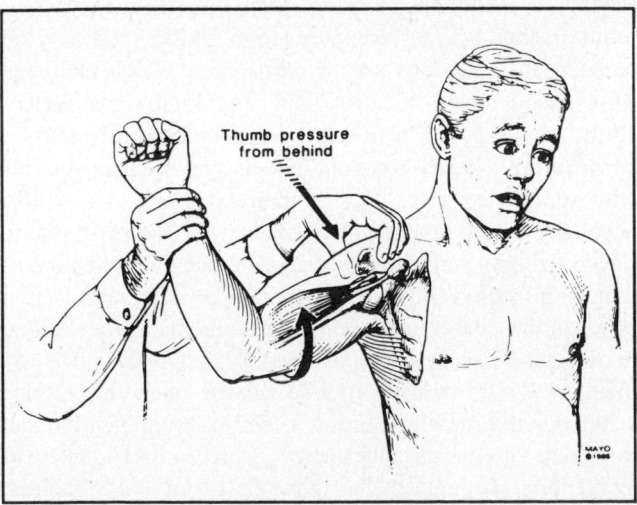

Fig. 20-19. Shoulder apprehension test. Shoulder is placed in 90° of abduction and stressed in maximal external rotation, while the humeral head is pushed anteriorly with the examiner's thumb from behind. A positive test result reproduces pain or sensation of impending subluxation. (From Johnson JE, Sim FH, and Scott SG: Mayo Clin Proc 62:289-304, 1987.)

ness discovered in the above tests. The following nerves can be injured through a direct blow or through a stretching activity: the axillary nerve for the deltoid muscle, the suprascapular nerve (as it goes through its fossa along the lateral aspect of the scapula and provides the motor function for the infraspinatus and supraspinatus muscles), the dorsal scapular nerve to the rhomboids and levator scapula, long thoracic nerve (which results in the winging of the shoulder because of a weakness in the serratus anterior), and the subscapularis nerve (which results in weakness in the subscapularis muscle and also the teres minor). Most of this nerve damage can be treated with some type of electrical stimulation and rested from further trauma.[44] The damaged nerves usually return to normal.

Objective strength testing. Isokinetic machines, such as Cybex, Kincom, Lido, Biodex, Merak, and Humac, hand-held dynamometers, cable tensiometers, or maximal isotonic weight lifting can be used to test objective muscle strength if such testing is not contraindicated. The following are some general guidelines for data analysis from concentric isokinetic testing. The torque and total work will decrease as the speed increases with isokinetic testing. Power will increase as speed of testing is increased. Slow-speed Cybex testing has revealed the following general trends in agonist and antagonist relationships: internal rotators are stronger than external rotators by approximately a 2 to 1 ratio, shoulder extension is stronger than shoulder flexion by approximately 2 to 1, shoulder adduction is stronger than shoulder abduction by approximately 3 to 1, and horizontal shoulder adduction is stronger than horizontal abduction by approximately 4 to 3. Also noted is that the dominant side is usually anywhere from 5% to 10% weaker than the uninvolved side. Care must be taken in applying normative data to clinical situations. Published values are specific to the speeds of testing, stabilization, subject positioning, age, sex, activity level, and type of isokinetic machine used. Testing may need to be modified in the case of a hypermobile shoulder (i.e., the test should be performed in a shortened arc to avoid apprehension positions), an impingement lesion (i.e., avoid the painful range rotations by testing in a modified neutral position) (see Fig. 20-30), and acute injuries or early postoperative rehabilitation.

Functional performance. If a shoulder injury occurs because of overuse, a biomechanical assessment can be made by observing the athlete in motion. The use of videotapes can be very helpful in this regard. See Richardson, Jobe, and Collins,[75] Jobe,[38] Fowler,[26] Larson,[53] and Pappas, Zawacki, and Sullivan[70] for information relevant to the pathomechanics of overuse syndromes of the shoulder.

REHABILITATION

Rehabilitation of the shoulder complex should be done in the context of a problem-oriented approach based on the results of a comprehensive evaluation. Some of the problems common to many different injuries will be discussed. Specific treatment techniques, which are aimed at correcting these problems, will be outlined. Finally, guidelines specific to some of the most common injuries will be presented.

Pain

Transcutaneous electrical nerve stimulation (TENS) or microelectric nerve stimulation (MENS) can be used throughout the course of rehabilitation in order to decrease muscle spasms and promote use of the extremity. MENS provides the normal electrical field for normal cellular activity to occur, which results in decreased pain and promotes cellular healing.[6,44] The application of hyperstimulation of the sensory nerve afferents using high-intensity electrotherapy is also effective in reducing pain because it stimulates the thalamus to increase the production of serotonin and endorphins.[15,61] In acute conditions cryotherapy is effective not only as an anesthetic but in decreasing the permeability of the capillaries and slowing down the effects of histamines in the bloodstream.[4] Immobilization also can be used to reduce pain, since it reduces the mechanical source of pain. It is important that the healing tissues be rested from function (load bearing) but not necessarily from motion altogether. Massage and mobilization are also effective in stimulating the sensory nerve afferents, which can trigger the gating mechanism of pain at the spinal cord level.[21,31] Iontophoresis also can be used to decrease pain using an antiinflammatory or anesthetic agent for pain reduction.[23]

Hypomobile noncontractile tissue

Mobilization should be the modality of choice for restoring or maintaining normal joint play of the synovial joints in the shoulder complex (Fig. 20-21).[47] It may be preceded by judicious use of ultrasound, which has been shown to decrease viscosity and alter membrane permeability in the collagen fibers.[29] Early emphasis should be on restoring external rotation. This is important in patients who splint their arms against their abdomen and is also necessary to the attainment of abduction free of impingement. Anterior and inferior (caudal) accessory glenohumeral mobilization will allow for an increased subacromial space in the case of impingement lesions that have resulted in decreased accessory movement.[46] Transverse friction massage should be used after soft tissue injury to produce a functionally mobile scar and to aid in the prevention and treatment of fibrous adhesions.[21] Care must be taken to avoid this technique in the presence of an acute bursitis. Table 20-1 lists some of the specific techniques for shoulder mobilization.

Hypomobile contractile units

Static stretching of the musculotendinous tissue has proved to be very effective in increasing the flexibility of

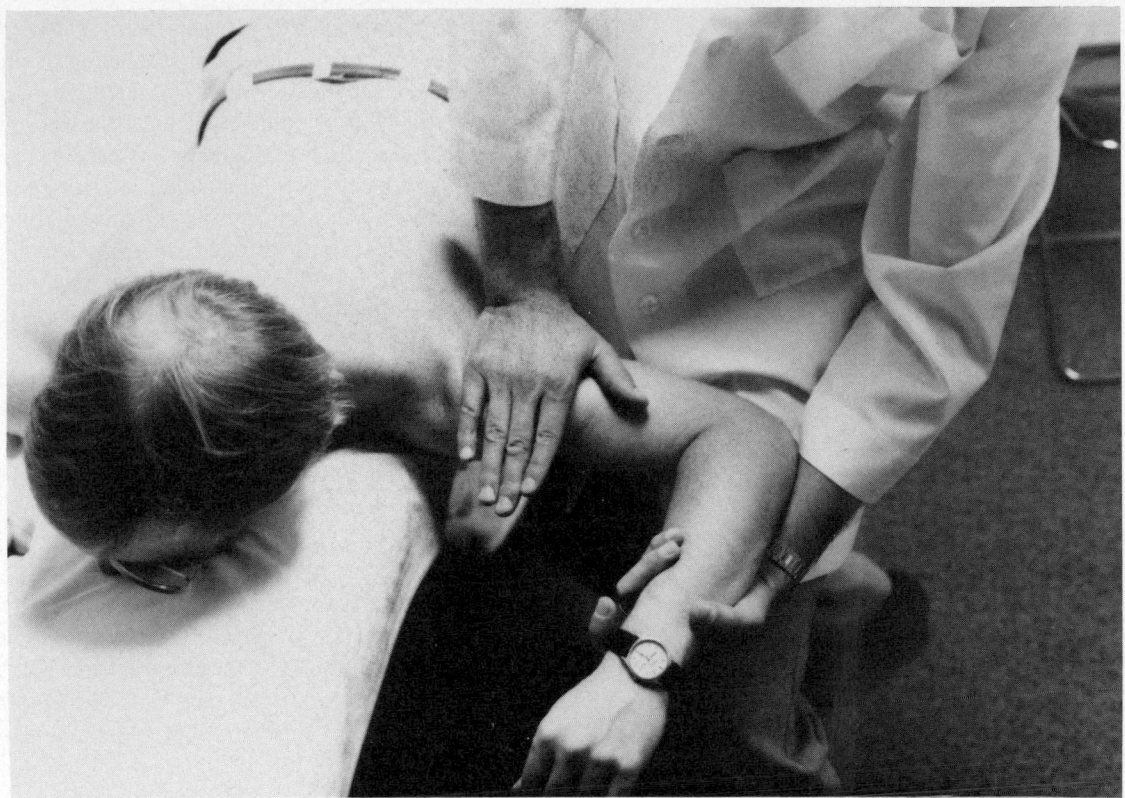

Fig. 20-21. Mobilization of anterior capsule with the humerus externally rotated.

the shoulder complex. As previously discussed, this can effectively alter the mechanics of overhead throwing and racquet sports and is mandatory in athletes involved in heavy resistive weight lifting. Static stretching is very important in the presence of a tight pectoralis major muscle. The stretch should be preceded with mild muscle contractions in order to warm the tissues through increased circulation and metabolism. The static position should be held for 90 seconds or longer in order to maximize the effects. The following positions are recommended (Fig. 20-22):

1. Leaning into a corner with each forearm on a different wall. This position stretches the internal rotators. This should be performed in several different positions of shoulder abduction.
2. Straight-arm hangs from a chinning bar, with palms supinated will clear the greater tuberosity from the coracoacromial constriction.
3. Glenohumeral hyperextension (biceps, anterior deltoid) with slight positional alterations will allow these exercises to be very specific to the biomechanical demands of the sport.

Proprioceptive neuromuscular facilitation (PNF) techniques are also very effective in increasing flexibility through biasing the muscle spindle. For the exercises to be

safe and effective, however, careful instruction and demonstration are essential.

The combined use of vapocoolant sprays, MENS, and static stretching can result in muscle relaxation and elongation, especially if the muscle is in spasm or exhibits specific trigger points.[23,64] This technique is indicated in the presence of a spasm end-feel.

Deep heating modalities may be helpful adjuncts in the treatment of chronic strains to the contractile units. They act by increasing the fluid dynamics in the involved area, thereby facilitating the rate of healing,[29] in addition to preparing the muscle for static stretching.

Decreased muscular strength, power, and endurance

Isometric, isokinetic, isotonic, or elastic tubing exercises can be used to improve strength, power, and endurance. There are five principles of exercise that apply when dealing with these problems: readiness, specificity, overload, progression, and trainability.

The principle of *readiness* is concerned with whether the client is at the level of rehabilitation where muscle development training can begin. The therapist should determine if the client has any pain with resisted motion that could irritate the problem. There may be pain when the muscle is in a lengthened position because of increased

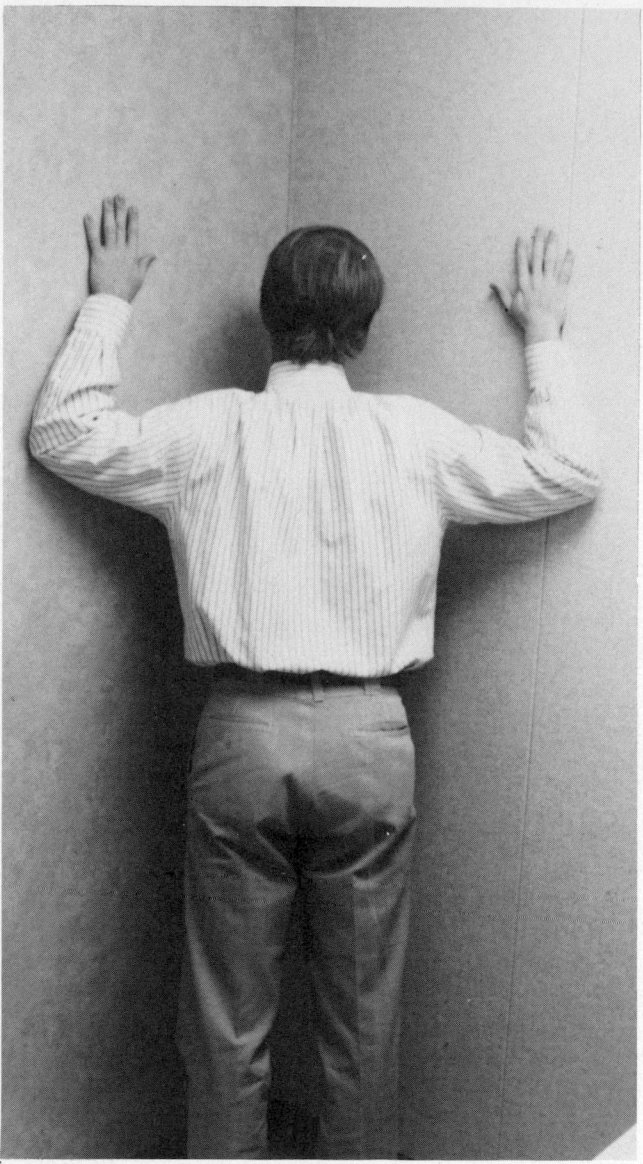

Fig. 20-22. Stretching internal rotators and anterior capsule.

traction on the muscle fibers and connective tissue. In this case, if contraction is pain free in the shortened position, the client may begin training within this pain-free range.[20] In the case of dynamic reconstructions for capsular instability, it is important to allow for primary revascularization of the transplanted tendon. This generally requires 6 to 20 weeks.[31]

The second principle, *specificity,* deals with whether the client should concentrate on strength, power, endurance, or a combination of these. This can be determined by isokinetic dynamometer testing and careful consideration of the type of activity to which the client will be returning (i.e., aerobic or anaerobic).

The third principle is *overload.* In order to functionally improve a muscle, the structure must be sufficiently stressed in a position of function.

The fourth principle of exercise is that of *progression* (i.e., to avoid a leveling off or plateauing of physiological responses, an overload of either intensity, duration, frequency, or type of contraction must be maintained). This is brought about by a systematic increase in these parameters. The concept of periodization addresses this need to constantly vary the demands on the muscular system in order to provide continual overload. This technique is used during off-season conditioning or in exercise programs lasting more than 6 weeks. It involves a cycling of the intensity of the workout.[80]

The fifth principle, *trainability,* determines the rate of progression. For example, the intensity, duration, and frequency of exercise for an individual at a low level of training should increase at a faster rate than for an Olympic athlete, who would require more time for a given increase in strength.

Recent studies by East Germans, Russians, and Americans have suggested that various forms of electrical stimulation can maintain or possibly increase muscle strength, power, and endurance. The proposed mechanism is used to increase the recruitment and rate coding of the motor units for a specific muscle group.[32,34] More research is indicated in this area.

It is important for an athlete involved in a particular sport, such as swimming, to develop strength, power, and endurance in specific muscle groups for preventive reasons. For instance, a swimmer's supraspinatus muscle should be as strong and powerful as possible. As discussed earlier, in the butterfly or freestyle stroke there is repetitive trauma to the muscle tendon unit, which can cause inflammatory reactions or microtears.[26] Animal studies have shown that repetitive stress to a ligament or tendon can increase the capabilities of these tissues to withstand stress and deformation. Pool therapy is a very effective and functional modality for power and endurance training. With the use of hand paddles and a modified D2 reversal proprioceptive neuromuscular facilitation (PNF) pattern, the butterfly stroke can be replicated using the "pseudo" isokinetic resistance of water. Similarly, a D2 pattern can be used for the backstroke and, for the freestyle, a D1 pattern. Care should be taken to avoid any overuse injuries from excessive or improper use of this technique.

With any type of hypermobile shoulder, it is very important to make sure that the rotator cuff is strengthened, especially with chronic subluxations of the shoulder. The subscapularis muscle should be strengthened because it is a dynamic anterior stabilizer of the glenohumeral joint. The cuff external rotators also are very important in patients with anterior instability. Cain et al[13a] have shown the role they play in helping to position the humeral head posteriorly in the glenoid.

Specific exercises for building strength in the serratus anterior muscle include doing wall pushups and progressing to floor pushups and bench presses. Care must be taken when performing bench presses because hyperextension of the glenohumeral joint can result in anterior laxity in the capsule.[7]

For throwing and racquet sports the primary accelerators (latissimus dorsi, teres major, pectoralis major, and triceps) can be strengthened by performing dips on the parallel bars or wheelchair pushups in a chair or, with blocks under the hands, on the floor. In the case of an unstable shoulder capsule these should not be done past 50 or 60 degrees of shoulder abduction. The use of an isokinetic pulley can allow for even more specific strengthening of shoulder movements, especially at high speeds of contraction.

Just as important in preventing ballistic injury to the shoulder in sports is the need to strengthen the decelerators. In throwing sports the decelerators include the teres minor, rhomboids, and the posterior deltoid. These can be strengthened through prone airplane exercises, consisting of horizontal extension and some external rotation (see Fig. 20-26). Surgical tubing can also be used with emphasis on the eccentric contraction. Eccentric modes on isokinetic machines can also be used to specifically load the decelerators, but care must also be used so as to not create too much microtrauma to the muscle tendon complex. Ideal muscle training programs should specifically address the needs of the sport or activity and incorporate all types of muscle contractions (isometric for stabilizers, eccentric for decelerators, concentric for accelerators), all types of resistance (isotonic, isokinetic and plyometric), different velocities of training through all planes of movement, high loads alternated with low loads, multiple repetitions, and isolated as well as integrated patterning of muscle groups.

Training errors

Training errors usually have a gradual onset, resulting from faults in either frequency or duration. Errors in frequency, for example, occur when a pitcher throws after only 3 days' rest instead of the usual 4, or a tennis player plays 5 times a week instead of the usual 3, or a nonathletic individual shovels the walk 5 times in a week instead of the usual once or twice.

Duration, the second type of training error, occurs when an inappropriate amount of time per session is spent on an activity. For example a swimmer may swim 7,000 yards per workout instead of 5,000 without a gradual progression in the distance. If a pitcher throws 150 pitches instead of 100, he would also be committing an overuse error.

A third training error is related to the type of workout or its intensity. Errors in this area can be seen in a weight lifter, for instance, changing directly from a DeLorme to a pyramid protocol during the season. It is also seen in a baseball player working on a new pitch, such as a slider or a screwball, or an individual raking the lawn for the first time in the fall. In order to prevent training errors, frequency, duration, or intensity should be increased by a maximum of 5% per week.

Biomechanical flaws

If an abnormal shoulder use problem results from biomechanical flaws, it is very important to get a knowledgeable coach's opinion and information because this problem often recurs from season to season. One biomechanical flaw found in swimmers occurs when the opposite shoulder is dipped during the stroke and an impingement syndrome results. Temporary relief can be obtained by having the swimmer use a higher power arm entry into the water (see section on impingement syndrome, page 488).[26] Another swimmer's problem is the hypermobile shoulder on the flip turn of the backstroke, which puts the shoulder in the apprehensive position (Fig. 20-23). With this problem either a change in the swimmer's event or a change in the style of flip turn is indicated.[16,38]

Another common biomechanical flaw is frequently found in baseball players who face the direction of throwing with the arm lagging behind—that is, opening up too

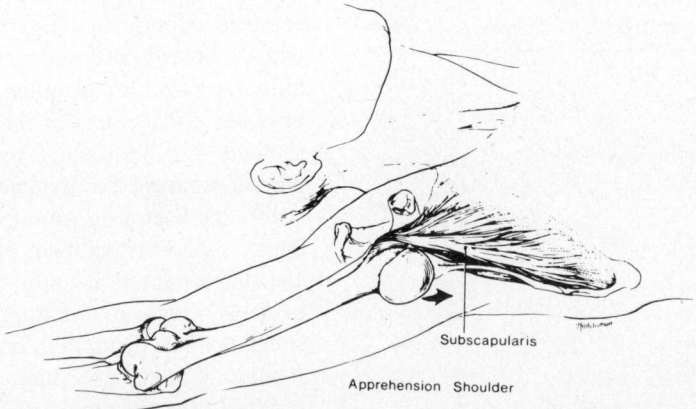

Fig. 20-23. Apprehension shoulder with vulnerable position of full abduction and external rotation as found in the backstroke turn. (From Kennedy JC, Hawkins R, and Krissoff WB: Am J Sports Med 6:309, 1978.)

soon.[38] As a result, the elbow is dropped, which allows the shoulder to catch up and puts additional stress on the anterior aspect of the shoulder. It is very important for baseball players to have at least 120 degrees of external rotation at the beginning of the acceleration phase to at least 90 degrees of internal rotation during the deceleration phase. If this motion is not present, the player will compensate, which may result in a problem in another part of the arm (see rehabilitation of pitching injuries).

Swelling

In acute conditions ice can be used to decrease inflammatory effects. This is especially important to reduce swelling in the impingement zone. Elevation also works since the effect of gravity pulls the fluid proximally. Electrotherapy has been used effectively as a means of decreasing swelling, since the mechanism increases the hemostasis of arteries and veins in addition to having the electrostatic effect of pulling the fluids proximally.[51] Pneumatic pumps can also be used externally to alter the pressure gradient, which will serve to move the fluids proximally.

Return to activity

It is important that the client not progress to the next level of activity until he/she is asymptomatic at the previous level. Only one parameter should be varied at any given time in order to assess its effect on irritability and function. For example, a therapist could vary three individual parameters in pitching: number of throws, distance of throws, and percentage of effort given. Table 20-2 outlines a throwing progression for baseball fielders. They should progress in accordance with individual signs and symptoms. Maximal progression without symptoms would be one new level per day. The same program could be modified for tennis, with the protocols changed to number of hits, number of strokes, and percentage of effort. For

Table 20-2. A fielder's progressive throwing program

Number of throws	Distance (in feet)	Percentage of effort
20	30	50
25	30	50
25	45	50
25	45	60
30	45	60
30	60	60
30	60	70
35	60	70
35	75	70
35	90	70
35	90	80
35	105	80
40	105	80
40	120	80
40	120	90
40	120	100

swimming the parameters could be changed to types of strokes, distance, and effort given. In a similar manner, a worker could go back to work gradually for half days before going full days or to light duty before heavy duty.

Neurological damage

The mechanisms that cause these injuries have been briefly outlined in the section on evaluation.

Specific shoulder-strengthening exercises are indicated in the case of a brachial plexus stinger injury if neurological damage results in any weakness to the muscles. Prevention should be aimed toward increasing the strength and power of the neck musculature. In football neck rolls can be fitted to the shoulder pads to prevent excessive lateral cervical motion.

With early detection of injury to the long thoracic nerve, O'Donaghue[66] recommends immobilization of the shoulder in abduction and external rotation. Wallace[85] describes a pad that can be used to dynamically stabilize the scapula against the thorax. Specific exercises for the serratus anterior muscle have been discussed earlier in this section.

Conservative treatment of the thoracic outlet syndrome is specifically directed toward its cause and may involve posture alterations; mobilization of the scapulothoracic, acromioclavicular, or sternoclavicular joints; or flexibility stretching to the scalene and pectoral musculature.[77]

Acromioclavicular (AC) injuries

Injuries to the AC joint typically result from a downward directed force to the lateral edge of the scapula subsequent to falling with the arm adducted to the side. Tension is initially directed to the acromioclavicular ligaments and, in more severe cases, the coracoclavicular ligaments (Fig. 20-24). A first-degree sprain does not involve any laxity or loss in continuity of the ligamentous restraints and is treated with ice and progressive range of motion and strength exercises as pain allows. No immobilization is usually necessary. A second-degree sprain results in a complete rupture of the acromioclavicular ligament without any loss of coracoclavicular stability. Horizontal instability (A-P) is present in the absence of significant superior instability. Placement of the involved hand to the opposite shoulder is painful, and abduction and flexion to 90 degrees is weakened to manual testing. Treatment usually involves the use of an immobilizer designed to hold the humerus superiorly and the clavicle inferiorly. Ice is used, and the patient is usually started on gentle, early glenohumeral range of motion exercises for tolerance and strengthening, depending on the length of immobilization. A third-degree tear results in a complete separation of the acromioclavicular and coracoclavicular ligaments and partial tears of the deltoid and trapezius insertions with resulting A-P and superior instability. A visible stairstep drop off is seen between the lateral clavicle and the acromion.

Treatment of this injury is somewhat controversial and can be classified in three ways: (1) nontreatment (pain relief and early movement), (2) conservative management (4-to-6 weeks in AC splint, ice, isometrics to tolerance, range of motion exercises after 4-6 weeks, and progressive strengthening when mobilization is allowed), and (3) surgical treatment, to reduce the joint with internal fixation. If reduction is through screw fixation, the arm is usually immobilized in a sling, with early gentle active range of motion exercises and isometrics followed by active range of motion exercises to 90 degrees, usually after 7 to 10 days. Progressive strengthening and range of motion exercising begins at 4 to 6 weeks with gradual progression to activity-specific strengthening. With wire fixation isometrics are performed as pain allows, and active motion usually begins at 2 to 4 weeks postoperatively, progressing to active strengthening at 4 to 6 weeks. A custom made donut-relief pad can be constructed from pastizote or other padding material and worn under the shoulder pads of football or hockey players for contact-related pain relief in first-degree, second-degree, or third-degree sprains.[11]

Rotator cuff injuries

Rotator cuff tendonitis is a common overuse injury that occurs predominantly from activities involving repetitive overhead use of the arm. It frequently occurs in swimmers and baseball pitchers and occurs less frequently in tennis players. Neer and Welsh[63] have reported that the lesion involves an impingement phenomenon occurring in the suprahumeral space. They cited the anatomical involvement of, primarily, the supraspinatus tendon and, at times, the anterior part of the infraspinatus tendon and the long head of the biceps. They also identified the source of the impingement as being the anterior one third of the acromion and the coracoacromial ligament and, in some cases, hypertrophic spurring at the acromioclavicular joint. Removal of these offending structures allows a decompression of the suprahumeral space and has been

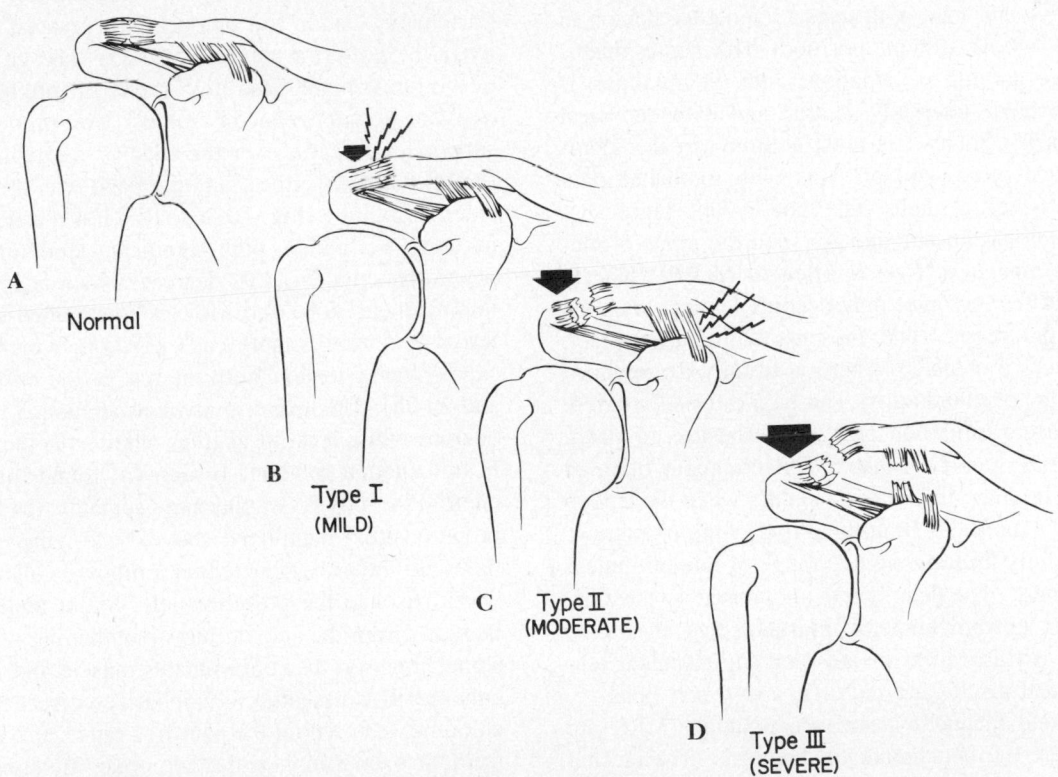

Fig. 20-24. These schematic drawings illustrate the ligamentous injuries that occur to the acromioclavicular joint. **A,** Normal anatomic relationships. **B,** In type I injury, a mild force is applied to the point of the shoulder, which stretches only the acromioclavicular joints but does not disrupt the fibers of the joint. **C,** In type II injury, a moderate force applied to the point of the shoulder displaces the acromion process ditally, disrupts the acromioclavicular ligaments, and may partially stretch the coracoclavicular ligaments. **D,** In type III injury, the severe force applied to the point of the shoulder drives the acromion and accompanying coacoid process downward, disrupting both the acromioclavicular ligaments. (From Pettrone FA, editor: AAOS symposium on upper extremity injuries in athletes, St. Louis, 1986, The CV Mosby Co. Modified from Allman FL: J Bone Joint Surg 49A:774, 1967. In Rockwood CA and Green OP, editors: Fractures in adults, ed 2, Philadelphia, 1984, JB Lippincott Co.)

practiced for years for resistant cases of rotator cuff pathology.

Rotator cuff tendonitis has been pathologically identified by Nirschl and Pettrone[64a] as being characterized by angiofibroblastic hyperplasia and viewed as an infarct of the tendon. Repeated microtrauma sets off a vicious debilitating cycle of inflammation-edema–increased-tendon volume and subsequent decreased suprahumeral space, which results in further impingement and microtrauma.[74]

Over a period of years the pathology progresses through four stages: (1) edema and hemorrhage, (2) fibrosis and tendonitis, (3) tendon degeneration, and, ultimately, (4) complete tendon rupture. Stage I is reversible and presents with a toothache discomfort felt after activity. General avoidance of the precipitating movements provides relief. A painful arc, which is most painful at 90 degrees, is often present and the standard impingement tests of forced flexion at the end range (see Fig. 20-16), as well as forced internal rotation while the arm is horizontally adducted with the shoulder at 90 degrees (see Fig. 20-17), will be painful. If the biceps are involved, there will be pain over the bicipital groove and pain with resisted shoulder flexion in the palm up, elbow straight position. The supraspinatus tendon will be painful to palpation, with the shoulder, if primarily involved, internally rotated and extended (arm behind the back). Stage II is most common in the 25-to-40-year-old age group and presents with toothache pain most frequently felt at night. The tendons and bursae become thickened and fibrotic and the shoulder range of motion begins to decrease. Rest is often of limited value in this stage, and the AC joint may become tender. Stage III is a further progression and presents with partial tears, which may buckle or catch. There is usually a prolonged history of refractory tendonitis. The pain is usually severe enough to cause a limitation of activity and loss of sleep. The patient may report weakness and complain of more stiffness than in Stage II. Stage IV occurs when the tendon has completely ruptured, limiting active range of motion, while not severely limiting passive range of motion, unless chronic or painful. The deltoid acts unopposed by the cuff, resulting in an upward humeral migration and an altered glenohumeral rhythm. Infraspinatus and supraspinatus tendon wasting will result, and the drop arm test is positive. Arthrograms and magnetic resonance imaging (MRI) are positive and are the benchmark of diagnosis. The mechanism of rupture commonly involves a fall on an outstretched or adducted arm. Rupture is also associated with dislocation or greater tuberosity fractures. In the elderly patient, a rupture may occur with minimal trauma.

Treatment of Stage I lesions usually involves decreasing the inflammation with aspirin, NSAID, ice, heat, ultrasound, and, occasionally, injections into the subacromial bursa. The shoulder is rested from function but not motion. Pain-limited stretching into external rotation in several positions of abduction is initiated in the subacute stage. This is important because external rotation allows the greater tuberosity to swing back from under the anterior acromion during active abduction of the shoulder. If the requisite amount of external rotation is not available, the greater tuberosity is forced against the acromion during elevation and the tendonitis will worsen. As the inflammation subsides, specific rotator cuff strengthening exercises are begun in order to help centralize the humeral head in the glenoid during elevation. If the deltoid overpowers a weak rotator cuff, the humeral head will migrate superiorly during abduction, further compromising the suprahumeral space. A strong rotator cuff can counteract this by maintaining the humeral head in the center of the glenoid. This is especially important in athletes who traditionally overdevelop their deltoids while neglecting the cuff musculature. EMG studies by Jobe and Moynes[39] and Blackburn[7] have helped to clarify the correct mechanics of isolating the supraspinatus, infraspinatus and teres minor muscles. Blackburn found that horizontal abduction to eye level in the prone position, with the arm in full external rotation, was found to elicit the greatest activity in the supraspinatus tendon and produced the greatest overall activity in the posterior cuff (Fig. 20-25). The greatest activity in the teres minor (also high levels of infraspinatus activity) was found when the subject was prone, upper arm supported, forearm over the edge of the table, elbow and shoulder at 90 degrees, and the hand was brought up into external rotation (Fig. 20-26). This last position should not be used in a patient with significant tendonitis because it places the shoulder at 90 degrees, which is associated with impingement. Jobe and Moynes[39] described a position referred to as the "empty can" position, which isolates the supraspinatus tendon from the rest of the cuff (Fig. 20-27 and 20-28). This exercise involves abducting the arm to 90 degrees while it is 30 degrees anterior to the midline and in full internal rotation. Blackburn[7] found this position to elicit less activity in the supraspinatus tendon than the prone position mentioned above. Side-lying external rotation with the arm abducted on a pillow is also an effective way to isolate the posterior cuff. Slight abduction of the humerus from the side during strengthening will avoid tensional stress on the supraspinatus muscle and its microvasculature. It is essential to emphasize correct form and positioning, stay within the pain-free range, use light weights (seldom over 5 lbs), and incorporate stretching exercises, with emphasis on external rotation.

Stage I tendonitis in athletes will recur unless the pathomechanics of their movements are corrected. Tennis players can irritate their cuff during the follow-through of an overhead shot, when they allow the racquet to twist their shoulder into internal rotation and extension lateral to their hip. This is corrected by letting the racquet finish the overhead stroke across the front of the body. A proper toss during the serve can also greatly decrease the faulty mechanics associated with rotator cuff tendonitis. Generally,

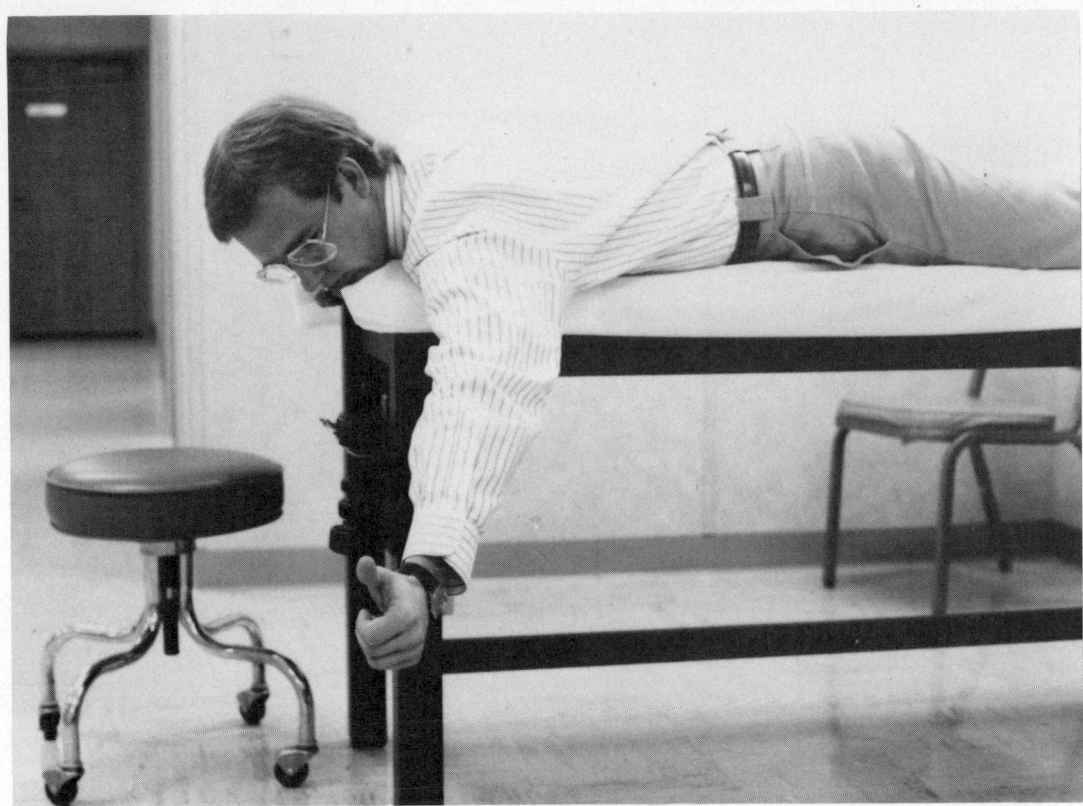

Fig. 20-25. Position for maximizing supraspinatus activity (also results in greatest overall activity in the posterior cuff.)

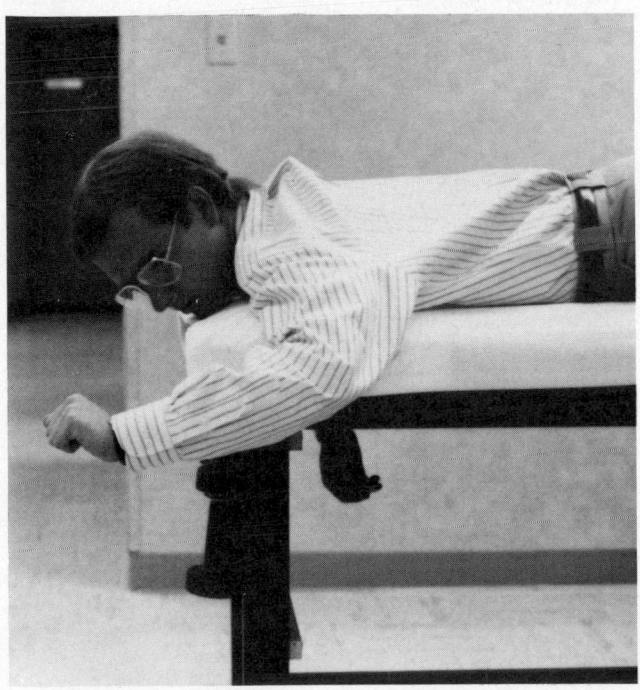

Fig. 20-26. Position for maximizing teres minor activity (also results in high activity levels of the infraspinatus.)

tennis players can work on ground strokes (minus the overspin) and volleys as long as they keep the racquet low during the healing phase of shoulder tendonitis. Swimmers are prone to overuse tendonitis of the supraspinatus and biceps tendons. Johnson[43] reported that average competitive swimmers subject their shoulders to up to 16,000 revolutions per week as compared to the 1,000 per week of a professional tennis player or baseball pitcher. The mechanics of the freestyle, backstroke, and butterfly strokes are similar in that they result in repeated combined abduction and internal rotation during the recovery phase, which can result in an impingement syndrome (see Fig. 20-7). It has also been speculated by Penny and Welsh[71] that when the arm is adducted to the side during the late pull-through phase, the microvascularity is wrung out in the distal 1 cm of the biceps and supraspinatus tendons, which could lead to degenerative changes. Treatment of the impingement syndrome should include decreasing the internal rotator of the arm as it enters the water (thumb should not touch first), increasing the body roll during the freestyle and backstroke, and increasing the body lift in the butterfly. Richardson, Jobe, and Collins[75] recommended that hand paddles be avoided because they are associated with increased incidence of shoulder pain. Blatz[9] has reported a 90% success rate in treating painful shoulders of swimmers by the use of a neoprene upper arm counterforce

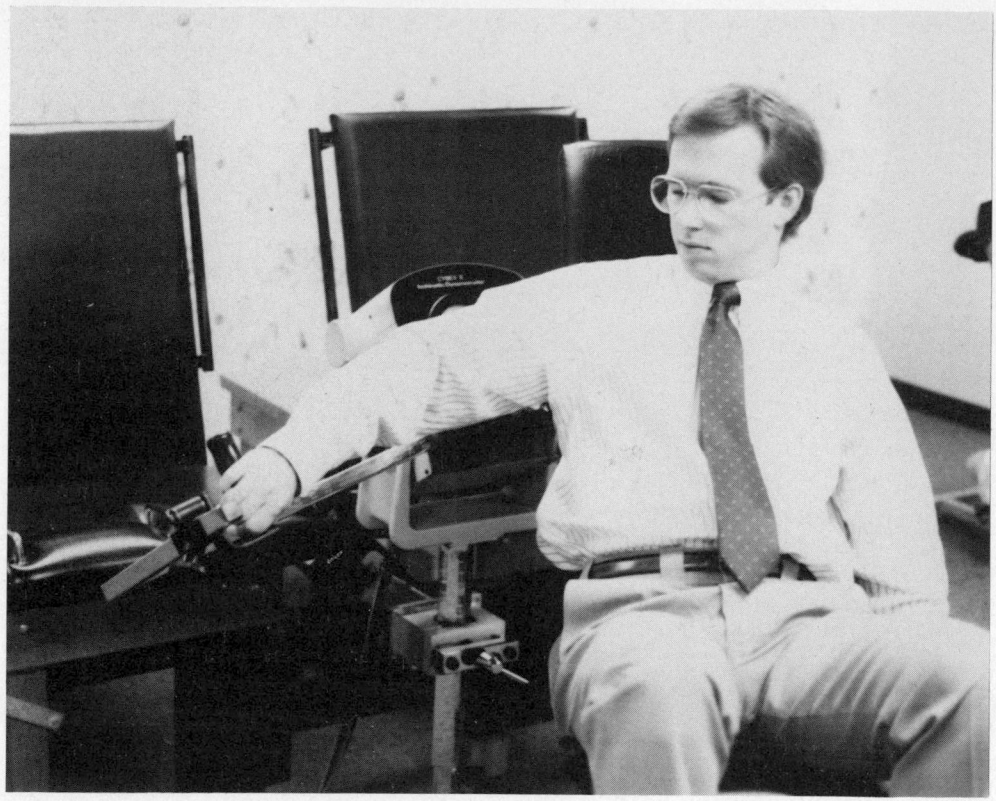

Fig. 20-27. Isokinetic strengthening of supraspinatus.

brace. It is thought to have a tenodesis effect on the biceps tendon, which makes it a more efficient humeral head depressor, and thereby increases the space beneath the coracoacromial arch. Nuber et al[65] studied the function of eight shoulder muscles with fine wire electromyography during both aquatic and dry land performance of the freestyle, breaststroke, and butterfly strokes. They state:

"the supraspinatus, infraspinatus, and middle deltoid were predominately recovery phase muscles. Their function is important to fully abduct the arm and externally rotate the extremity to prepare it for a new pull-through phase. The serratus anterior appears to have an important function during recovery: preparing the shoulder for the transition to pull-through. This allows the scapula to rotate clear of the abducted humerus and also to supply a stable glenoid on which the arm may rotate. Although we were unable to quantify our data while in the water, the dry land data indicate that the serratus anterior works at a nearly maximal level to accomplish this. If over the course of a number of cycles this muscle fatigues, scapular rotation may not coincide with humeral abduction and impingement may precipitate. Thus a vigorous program to strengthen the serratus anterior and other scapular rotators may be an important prophylactic measure to alleviate impingement."

Finally, if a kick board is used to rest the shoulder, the elbow on the involved side should be held slightly flexed so as to keep the shoulder out of the impinge-

ment test position of forced flexion with the forearm pronated.

Weight lifters are also prone to rotator cuff tendonitis if they emphasize the pectoralis muscles and deltoids and neglect the smaller external rotators. Overdevelopment of the anterior chest can result in protracted scapulae, which may result in *stretch weakness* in the rhomboids and other scapular retractors. The anteriorly protracted shoulders will alter the mechanics of glenohumeral elevation by requiring greater external rotation of the humerus to position the hand overhead at any given point of abduction. This situation of the arm, resting in an internally rotated position due to tightness of the pectoralis, can also cause the bicipital tendon to track excessively against the medial side of the intertubercular groove. Weight lifters must be advised in the importance of balancing their shoulder muscles through strengthening the external rotators and scapular retractors in addition to stretching the tight internal rotators. The pectoralis muscles should be stretched in several positions of abduction, which can be accomplished while supine with weights, with therapist-assisted contract/relax techniques, or by doing a corner lean. The corner lean is performed with both forearms resting on the walls that form a corner (see Fig. 20-22). The patient leans in toward the corner being careful to avoid compensatory lumbar and hip extension. This stretch is performed in two or three positions of shoulder abduction.

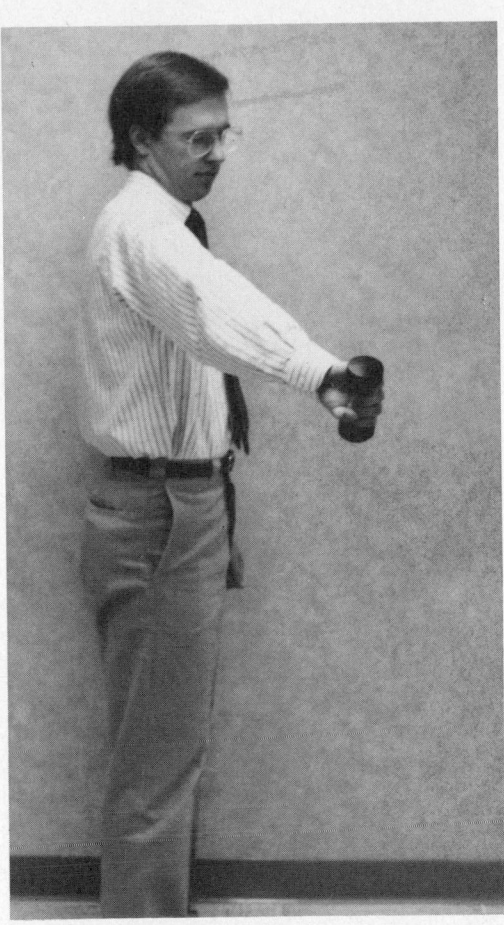

Fig. 20-28. Position for emphasizing supraspinatus activity (also results in high activity levels of the deltoid.)

The function of the rotator cuff during golf has also been analyzed and can be found in the article by Jobe et al.[41]

Common to all cuff overuse syndromes, regardless of sport, are several very basic rules for rehabilitation. Warm-up should never be overlooked. Intensity, duration, and frequency should be carefully controlled, and any increases should be gradual. Flexibility should be an integral part of both the warm-up and cool-down with emphasis on external rotation and the sport-specific positions. The cuff muscles should be strengthened in isolated positions, both concentrically and eccentrically, depending on the demands of the sport.

Surgical treatment of resistant rotator cuff tendonitis in the absence of significant disruption of the tendon is sometimes necessary in the case of Stage III lesions. The operation of choice is generally an anterior acromioplasty to decompress the anatomic region of impingement.[71] This is seldom performed on patients under 30 years old and is usually preceded by a lengthy period of conservative treatment, involving judicious rest, injections, oral antiinflammatory agents, and varying use of heat, ice, and exercise. Surgery involves excision of the anterior one third of the

acromion, release of the coracoacromial ligament, tendon debridement as needed, distal clavicle excision (in the instance of AC arthritis), and related spurring. Rehabilitation usually begins within the first postoperative week with the institution of passive range of motion movements below 80 degrees of flexion or abduction. Elevation above 80 degrees is initiated usually after 2 weeks, depending on the degree of inflammation present within the shoulder. Active range of motion movement is delayed for at least 2 weeks because the surgery involves limited detachment of the deltoid muscle. Progressive strengthening involves minimal resistance at first, and attention should be directed toward isolating the rotator cuff and avoiding positions that might cause impingement (i.e., 80 to 120 degrees of elevation). It is essential that external rotation range of motion is fully returned prior to overhead activity in order to allow the greater tuberosity to rotate out from under the remaining suprahumeral structures. Attention should also be paid to ensuring that the scapular stabilizers, including the serratus anterior, rhomboid, and levator scapula, are strong and contributing to a normal scapulohumeral rhythm.

Treatment of Stage IV lesions of the cuff is generally directed at the surgical reattachment and advancement of the torn tendon complex into a bony trough created on the greater tuberosity. Also, an anterior acromioplasty usually is performed at the time of surgery, while care is taken to disrupt as little of the deltoid attachment as possible. Postoperative care depends on the surgeon's assessment of the viability of the repaired structures. Longitudinal repairs can be mobilized earlier than repairs of transverse tears. If an abduction splint or pillow is used for 4 to 6 weeks, passive range of motion movement above the splint is usually initiated at 1 to 2 weeks after the repair. Passive motion is best performed while the splint is in place and the patient is relaxed in a supine position. If the patient is sitting, there is a greater risk that he/she will assist in the antigravity movement. Passive movements involve elbow extension and flexion, shoulder external rotation, shoulder flexion, and shoulder abduction while in a position of external rotation. Horizontal adduction, internal rotation, and adduction are avoided during the initial 4 to 6 weeks after surgery. Active range of motion movement generally is allowed at 6 weeks and should progress from gravity-eliminated to gravity-resisted positions. Active assistive exercise with wands and pulleys on the uninvolved extremity may be necessary during the initial active rehabilitation stages in order to ensure the return of full range of motion. Passive external rotation is emphasized early on, as in the case of postoperative acromioplasties. Abduction and flexion should be strengthened both in a standing and a lying position. Standing emphasizes the midrange of strengthening, while supine flexion and sidelying abduction challenge the muscles' ability to initiate the movement. During the early stages of the active exercises it may be necessary to bend the elbow past 90 degrees in order to shorten the lever arm. It may also be necessary to work on gravity-resisted eccentrics prior to full range of motion concentrics if the patient is unable to actively overcome the pull of gravity. These are easily performed with the assistance of a wand or pulley, but the patient should be encouraged to assist only in the range that they are limited. Resistance training is generally begun at 7 to 8 weeks following the operation and is initiated with 1 lb weights, which are slowly increased in 1 lb increments. Specific cuff isolating exercises, as discussed previously, are emphasized prior to the initiation of multiple plane movements in order to ensure the cuff's ability to centralize the humeral head in the glenoid. Rhythmic stabilization and PNF patterns are effective at this stage (Fig. 20-29). As the cuff function improves, weight-bearing exercises, such as rocking on all fours and chair push-ups, may be initiated. Scapular stabilizers can be further trained with push-ups, progressing from a wall to a table and from a table to a chair. Finally, in advanced cases, pushups may be performed on the floor.

Isokinetics are usually initiated at 3 to 8 weeks. These exercises should be limited-range concentric submaximal efforts at intermediate velocities that allow the patient to

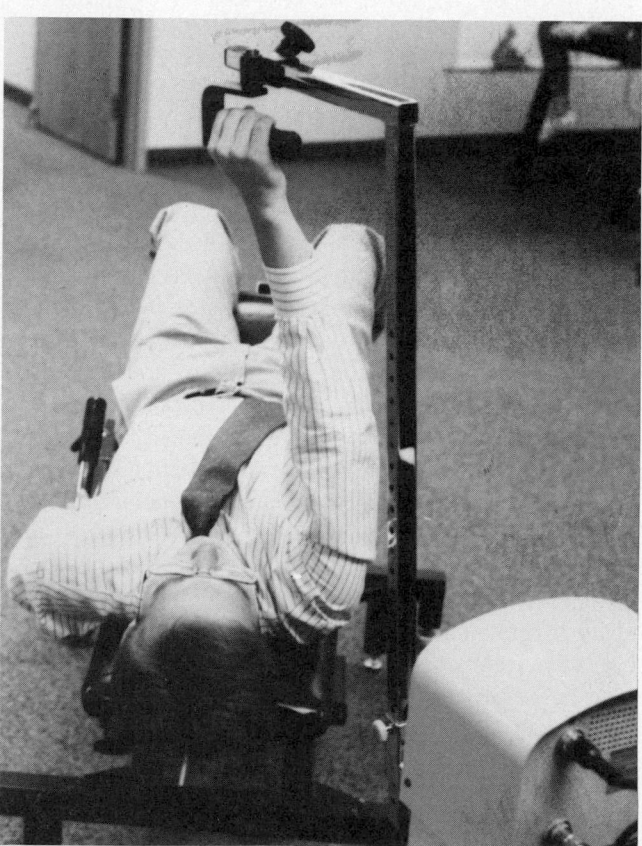

Fig. 20-29. Positioning for PNF D-1 diagonal strengthening on an isokinetic dynomometer.

catch the machines at low torque outputs while carefully avoiding positions of impingement. A modified neutral position for strengthening the rotators is used (Fig. 20-30). As symptoms allow, the isokinetics are progressed to maximal efforts at faster velocities and then finally progressed to slower velocities. The slower velocities result in increased tension placed on the contractile structures. The faster velocities should not cause discomfort and should not be so fast that the patient cannot exert force throughout the range.

Rubber tubing or bands are often used for home exercises at 4 to 6 weeks and allow for a great variety of strengthening patterns. General guidelines are to start with the most flexible grade of rubber, avoid excessive impingement positions, progress from isolating to general patterns and submaximal to near maximal efforts, and emphasize controlled concentric and eccentric contractions. Pool exercises are very helpful in rehabilitation of rotator cuff injuries. Gravity is greatly reduced, and the patient often can relax better in the water. Movements are somewhat isokinetic in that attempts to accelerate the limb are met with increased resistance. Fanning the fingers apart will increase the drag and result in more resistance. Rotations, flexion, extension, abduction, and PNF patterns all can be performed in chest-high water. Overhead strokes should be discouraged.

Pitching injuries. Pitching is a very complicated coordination activity that requires extreme synchrony of force transmission between the lower extremity, trunk, and upper extremity. Proximal stability must be matched with glenohumeral static flexibility and dynamic stability in order to minimize the stresses to the surrounding soft tissue (see the section on biomechanics).

Injury prevention to the throwing arm should emphasize accuracy and moderation of intensity. The number of pitches should reflect the growth plate and collagen maturation.[56,87] The following are recommendations: Children under the age of 10 should not pitch competitively; children between the ages of 11 and 12 should be limited to approximately 40 to 50 pitches every 4 days; children between the ages of 13 and 14 should be limited to approximately 60 pitches; children ages 15 to 17 should be limited to approximately 70 pitches; and children ages 18 to 19 should be allowed approximately 85 to 95 pitches. It is also important for pitchers to throw long distance at least two times per week to maintain dynamic flexibility.[83,87]

A classic example of a pitching overuse syndrome occurs when a pitcher opens up too soon. The arm and trunk should come out of the windup phase (which involves backward trunk rotation and abduction and external rotation of the humerus) at approximately the same time. If not properly synchronized, the arm may lag behind the trunk during the delivery phase, in which case the muscles that initiate the forward acceleration of the arm are

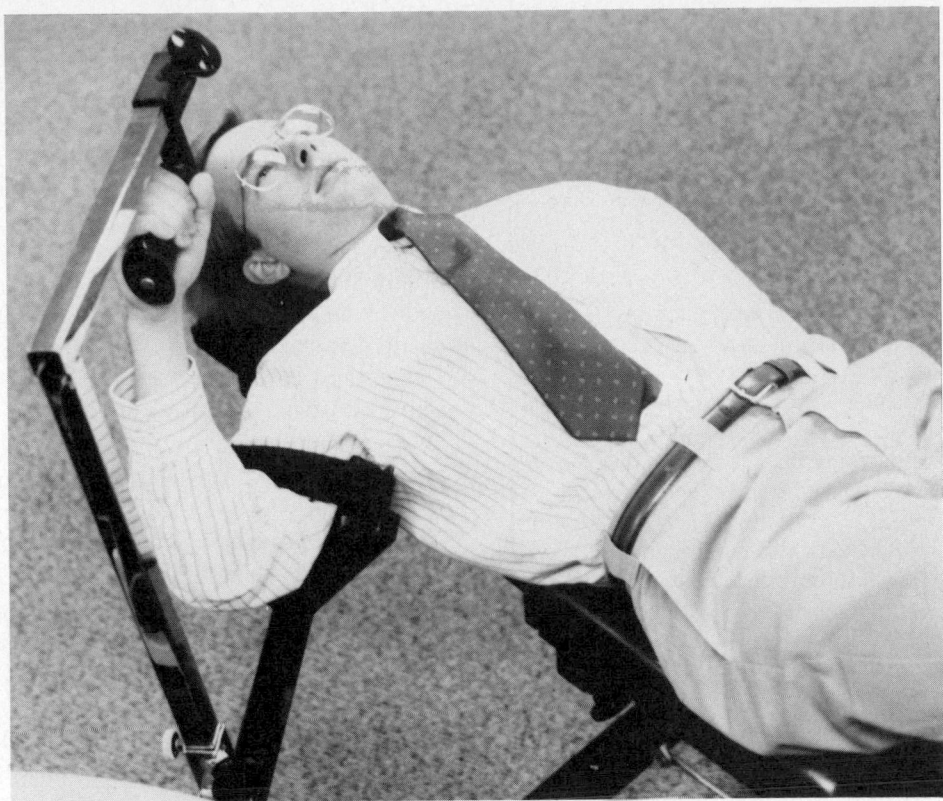

Fig. 20-30. Isokinetic strengthening of rotators with shoulder at 60 degrees to avoid impingement.

stretched at the same time that they are powerfully contracted. This could result in greater microtears to the biceps and internal rotators than what normally occurs with pitching. Larson[53] has pointed out that in the transition between windup and delivery the internal and external rotators of the shoulder must quickly change roles of relaxation and contraction. If the external rotators are not properly warmed up or are fatigued, they may not undergo normal relaxation as the internal rotators take over. This could result in muscle strain or minute tearing. In much the same way, during the postdelivery follow-through, the accelerators must relax while the decelerators slow the forward motion of the arm. This could result in repetitive injury to the posterior deltoid, long head of the triceps, rhomboids, posterior capsule, or external rotators.

The following is an 8-day rotation over a 12-week period of time for starting pitchers with a goal of being able to complete an entire game by the end of spring training or after recovery from an injury.

The first day begins with the normal warm-up protocols (see accompanying box). After warming up the pitcher then works off the mound. The number of pitches that he throws begins at approximately 33% of what is required to pitch a complete game. For example, a high school pitcher's goal is to throw 90 pitches in a complete game, so in the first practice session he begins with 30 pitches

Table 20-3. Spring training pitching program

	High School (17 to 18)		Babe Ruth (14 to 15)	
Day	**# of pitches**	**% of effort**	**No. of pitches**	**% of effort**
1	30	75	20	75
5	30	75	20	75
9	35	75	25	75
13	35	75	25	75
17	40	80	30	80
21	40	80	30	80
25	45	80	35	80
29	45	80	35	80
33	50	85	40	85
37	50	85	40	85
41	55	85	45	85
45	55	85	45	85
49	60	90	50	90
53	60	90	50	90
57	65	90	55	90
61	65	90	55	90
65	70	95	60	95
69	75	95	60	95
73	80	95	65	95
77	85	95	65	95
81	90	100	70	100

Warm-up protocol for baseball pitchers

1. Manual warm-up

   a. Mobilization of the ST, AC, GH, and T-spine
   b. Massage of entire upper quarter
   c. Physical agent as necessary (e.g., ultrasound, MENS, and hot packs)

2. Static stretching

   a. Codman's exercise with 5 lb weight for 30 seconds in each direction
   b. Horizontal hang bar for 60 seconds
   c. Pectoralis stretch for 60 seconds; push-up against wall
   d. Proprioceptive neuromuscular facilitation, D2 and reversal pattern (10 times contract and relax both ways)
   e. Lower extremity stretch for calf, hamstring, hip, and trunk (1-2 minutes for each muscle group)

3. Ballistic stretching

   a. Trunk twister, with arms horizontal, 10 times
   b. Jumping jacks 15 times
   c. Sprints of 20 to 30 yards, 10 to 15 times (70% effort)

4. Basic rules

   a. Begin throwing easily (a 90-degree recommended arc) at a distance greater than 60 feet 6 inches and work up to the distance at the pitcher's mound, decreasing the arc as you approach 60 feet.
   b. Do not throw curve balls until your arm is warm.
   c. On windy days warm up with the wind behind your back.
   d. Work up a sweat before forceful throwing.
   e. Put on your jacket immediately after the warm-up.

5. Throwing

   a. 15 to 25 pitches, slowly increase to medium velocity
   b. 6 curve balls, sliders, screwballs, etc.
   c. 6 changeups
   d. 8 fast balls; increase velocity to maximum
   e. 10 pitches of varying types

(Table 20-3). A professional pitcher whose goal is to throw 110 to 120 pitches begins with 40 pitches at the first workout. A Babe Ruth league pitcher begins with approximately 20 pitches. During the first day the intensity of effort should be at approximately 75%. Over the 12-week period the pitcher progresses by increasing the number of pitches by five every other cycle and increasing the intensity by 5% every 2 weeks (see Table 20-3). Immediately (within 5 minutes) after throwing the entire upper extremity and shoulder complex needs to be iced for 15 to 20 minutes. Salicylite loading then begins with the postgame meal. The amount depends on the prescription from the team physician.

The second day begins with gentle mobilization, soft tissue treatment modalities, and physical agents, as indicated, for the entire upper quarter. Stretching of the entire trunk and lower extremity follows gentle active and passive movements. The pitcher then jogs approximately 2 to 3 miles, followed by 20 repetitions of 30 yard sprints at approximately 80% of intensity. This day of rest is then finished with 15 to 20 minutes of cryotherapy for the entire upper quarter and the continuation of salicylate medication.

The third day begins, again, with gentle mobilization, active and passive movements for the entire upper and lower quadrants, and use of massage and physical agents as indicated. Salicylite loading is discontinued. After the warm-up the pitcher plays catch for approximately 15 to 20 minutes, throwing approximately 60 to 75 feet. Following catch, the pitcher continues a stretching program for the lower extremity and trunk. Next, the pitcher begins the isotonic strengthening program, emphasizing an isometric workout for the following stabilizing muscle groups: serratus anterior, rhomboids, levator scapula, and upper trapezius. The isotonic program is performed with light weights (5 to 8 pounds) and incorporates concentric and eccentric exercises at 90 degrees of abduction for the internal and external rotators. The pitcher should perform three sets of 20 repetitions, concentrating on the eccentric phase (with the muscles in the mid to shortened position) and the concentric phase (with the muscles in the stretched position). The type of muscle contraction and position of the joint (and subsequent length/tension relationship) should approximate the demands placed on each particular muscle throughout the pitching sequence. The pitcher does isotonic triceps work, with the shoulder in 90 degrees of elevation. The biceps are strengthened concentrically from 90 to 20 degrees and eccentrically from 20 to 0 degrees. Isolation of the supraspinatus follows in either the *empty can* position or in the prone position, as previously described in this article. The program finishes with wrist rolls in the pronated position, using approximately 5 pound weights for about three sets of five repetitions. Again, the pitcher should concentrate on slow rhythmic contraction of both the eccentric and concentric phase. Immediately after the isotonic program the entire upper quarter should be iced for 15 to 20 minutes, and the pitcher should finish the day with a 2-mile jog.

The fourth day begins with mobilization and flexibility exercises for the upper quarter, trunk, and lower extremity. The pitcher then plays catch for a period of approximately 5 minutes, throwing from 60 to 75 feet, and progresses to a long toss period of 15 to 20 minutes, throwing from 120 to 150 feet to stretch out the entire throwing linkage in a more functional position. After the long toss session the pitcher does 20 repetitions of 30-yard sprints followed by cryotherapy.

The fifth day is a day of throwing, and it is identical to day one, following the recommendations under Table 20-3.

The sixth day is the same as day two, a day of rest with an emphasis on salicylite loading, cryotherapy, and soft tissue treatments.

The seventh day is identical to day three except that the isotonic program can be replaced with an isokinetic workout. It consists of a warm-up that begins with a 3-minute bout on the upper body ergometer at approximately 120 RPMs, with 30-second increments of increased intensity in RPMs starting at 600, 900, 1200, 1500, and 1800 RPMs, and finishes with a 30 second maximal bout. Internal and external rotation is strengthened in a modified neutral position (see Fig. 20-30), using 10 repetitions from 120 degrees per second to as fast as the dynamometer will go, increasing every 30 degrees per second. A linear stress pattern, using D2 PNF in the prone position to replicate the cocking phase of pitching, can be performed using 10 repetitions every 30 degrees per second from 90 degrees per second to 210 degrees per second. The third isokinetic sequence is a supine D2 pattern that replicates the acceleration and follow-through phase using 10 repetitions from 180 degrees per second and going to the highest speed that the dynamometer can go. Another isokinetic exercise would be scapulothoracic elevation/depression (Fig. 20-31) and protraction/retraction (Fig. 20-32), with the pitcher doing 10 repetitions from 15 to 75 degrees per second. The final isokinetic exercise works the internal and external rotators in the 90-degree apprehensive position using 10 repetitions from 180 to 300 degrees per second, with 30 degrees per second increments. This can then be followed by using the Impulse inertial eccentric deceleration machine* for three sets of 10 repetitions. Cryotherapy should be applied to the entire upper quarter for approximately 15 to 20 minutes immediately following the workout.

The eighth day is identical to day four. The cycle then repeats itself for approximately 12 weeks.

Once the season begins, this 8-day rotation remains the same except that the isotonic and isokinetic workouts are decreased by approximately one third in both intensity and duration. The weight-training aspect of the rotation becomes a maintenance program. In a 5-day rotation an extra day of rest follows the pitching day of the sequence.

Total shoulder replacement

Total shoulder replacement (TSR) is considered an option in arthritic conditions when conservative treatment (i.e., physical therapy, medications, rest) fails, moderate to severe pain is present, active and passive range of motion is 50% or less (particularly abduction and external rotation), the medical history permits the procedure, and the

*EMA, PO Box 2312, Newnan, Ga, 30264.

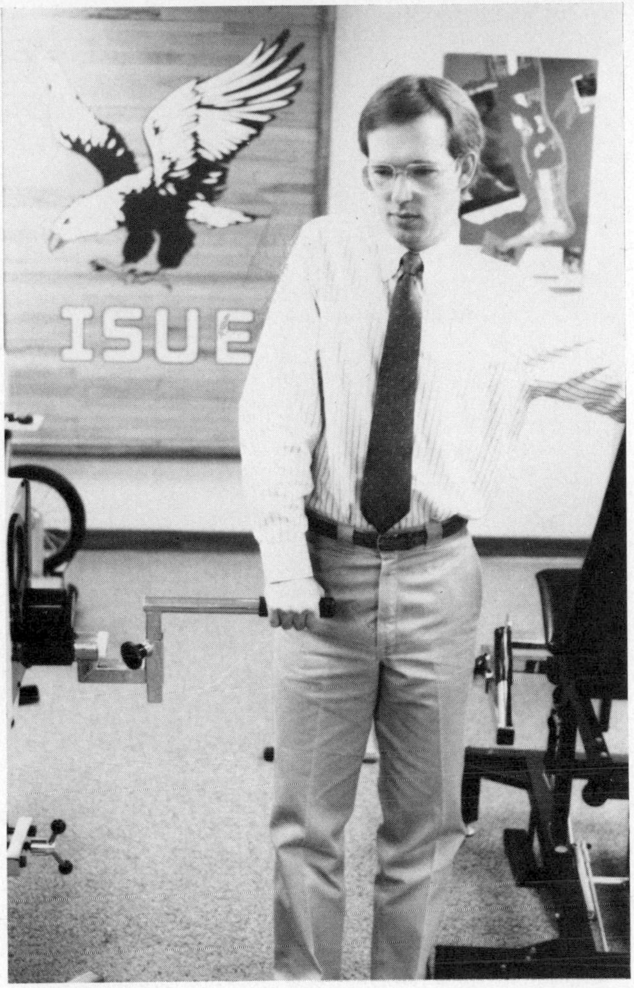

Fig. 20-31. Isokinetic strengthening of scapular elevators and depressors while keeping the elbow extended.

patient is motivated to work through extensive postoperative rehabilitation.

In the operation the head of the humerus is excised[1] above the tuberosities, if possible, in order to maintain anatomical attachment of the rotator cuff musculature. The prosthesis is inserted in 30 to 40 degrees of retroversion and fixed with methylmethacrylate, if needed.[19]

Postoperatively, the arm is placed in an elastic binder, with the forearm resting at 90 degrees over the abdomen. The rehabilitation program has been reported by Viadero, Harrison, and Farbent.[84] Immediately after surgery the binder should be secure when the patient is transferred from the bed. Patient education should include emphasis on avoiding rolling onto the TSR or using the involved arm to assist in repositioning in bed. On the second postoperative day the therapist can replace the binder with a Velpeau's sling. The patient is permitted to remove the sling 3 to 4 times daily for hygiene and exercise. Initial exercise involves gentle active assistive range of motion movements to the elbow and forearm. Pendulum exercises

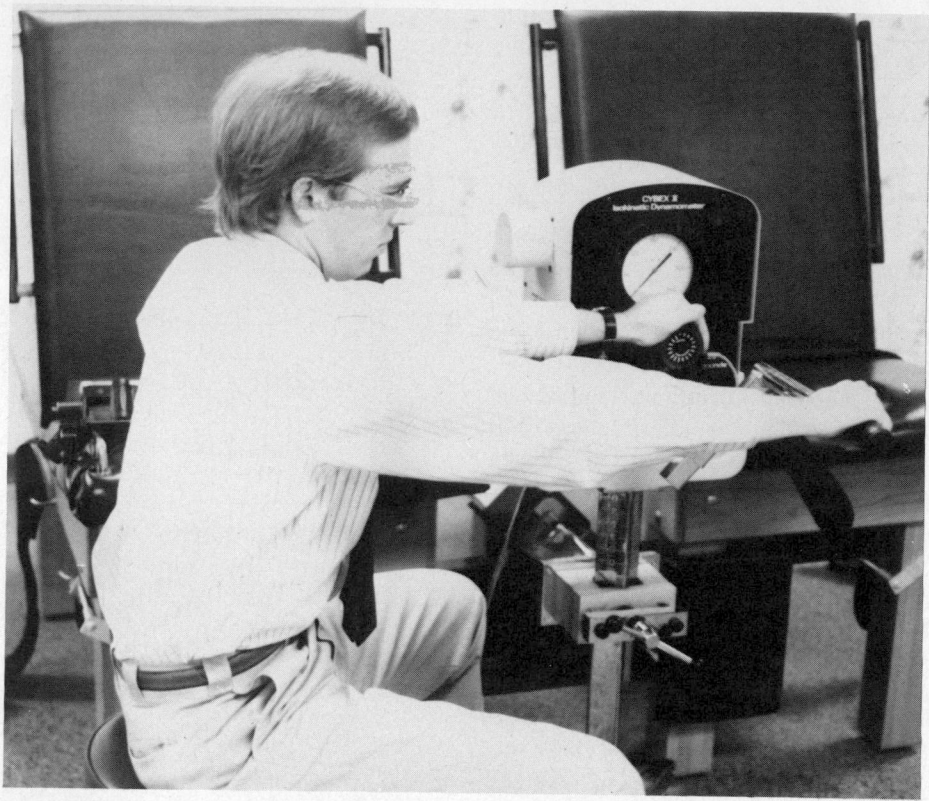

Fig. 20-32. Isokinetic strengthening of scapular retractors and protractors while keeping the elbow extended.

are followed by supine flexion and rotations. Hyperextension is done while the patient is seated on the the bed, and the patient is encouraged to work on assisted range of motion movement throughout the day. The patient can be progressed to gentle pulley exercises for flexion and extension with external rotation. Routine cane exercises are performed for assisted rotations while the patient is supine or seated. Isometrics are initiated (in the absence of a cuff repair) toward the middle or end of the hospital stay and are performed for all the associated muscle groups. These are progressed to low resistance rubber tubing exercises and gravity resisted exercises at discharge. Home programs should be designed for low repetition (10 to 20 repetitions for each exercise) and high frequency (at least 4 times a day) rather than 1 or 2 exhaustive workouts. The sling is worn only in crowds or prolonged outings. After 6 to 8 weeks postoperatively the patient is permitted to wash and brush his/her hair and to lift light items above shoulder level. Lifting or pulling heavy items is not allowed. Periodical visits to the therapist are necessary to progress the patient further and to reinforce the importance of the exercises. Minor changes in technique and resistance may help keep the patient motivated. Full function of the arm should be accomplished by 6 months. The above exercise program will have to be modified if a significant tear of the rotator cuff is present at the time of surgery. Those with a repaired cuff will necessarily be immobilized longer (sometimes in an abduction splint for 6 to 8 weeks) and have more pain and less motion postoperatively.

Cofield[19] reported on the range of motion attained following TSR in a follow-up study. Those with predisposing osteoarthritis could actively abduct to an average of 141 degrees and externally rotate to an average of 49 degrees. The rheumatoid arthritis group abducted to 103 degrees and externally rotated to 35 degrees, while those with traumatic arthritis attained an average of 109 degrees of abduction and 45 degrees of external rotation. The amount of abduction achieved was clearly related to the condition of the rotator cuff at surgery. If the cuff was normal or nearly so, the postoperative active abduction averaged 143 degrees. This value dropped to 102 degrees in patients with a thin and scarred cuff, 93 degrees in patients needing osteotomies of the tuberosity, and 63 degrees in the patients who underwent a repair of a major cuff tear at the time of surgery. Cofield[19] also reported that the ultimate range of motion is dependent on the patient's performance in the rehabilitation program.

Postsurgical unstable shoulder

Rehabilitation following surgery to repair a hypermobile glenohumeral joint is tailored to the specific type of reconstruction. If the contractile structures (e.g., deltoid and subscapularis tendon) have been violated during surgery, the postoperative program will be less stressful during the initial month, whereas, if firm fixation via bone-to-bone healing and screw fixation has been achieved, the exercise program can be progressed faster.[30]

Direct repairs attempt to restore the normal anatomy, as opposed to indirect repairs, such as some muscle transfers, which are designed to alter the biomechanics extrinsic to the glenohumeral joint. The Bankart repair is a direct procedure that involves suturing the capsule and labrum back down to the anterior glenoidal rim. It requires a healthy capsule and results in probably the best postoperative range of motion, but it is technically more difficult to perform. The patients generally wear an internal rotation sling for 2 to 3 weeks after surgery and may begin submaximal isometrics during the first several weeks because the contractile tissues were not cut during the operation. From weeks 3 to 6 after the operation the sling is worn only at night, and active abduction is allowed to 90 degrees, while external rotation is limited to neutral. After 6 weeks external rotation and abduction are slowly increased as pain and active motion allows. Progressive isometrics, isotonics, concentric isokinetics, and, finally, eccentric isokinetics are introduced, using range-limiting devices as needed. Rubber tubing and hand weights are used at home for isolated cuff, deltoid, and pectoralis strengthening, and later multiple plane strengthening (such as PNF patterns) is incorporated into a well balanced program. Attention is focused on the internal and external rotators and adductors but not to the exclusion of the prime movers. More aggressive range of motion is initiated at 7 to 8 weeks if motion is slow in returning. Functional activities can be performed from 8 to 12 weeks postoperatively.

Staple capsulorrhaphy is another surgical procedure designed to reattach the anterior capsule and labrum to the glenoid and can be performed as an open repair or through the arthroscope. The advantage of this procedure is that range of motion (Codman's pendulum) can begin within the first week following the operator. A sling is usually worn for 1 week. From 1 to 2 weeks active assistive range of motion is allowed within pain tolerance. This is progressed to active range of motion at 2 weeks, and then a functional strengthening program can be instituted from 3 to 6 weeks using light resistance.[28]

Putti Platt repairs limit external rotation by overlapping, and therefore shortening, the subscapularis tendon and anterior capsule. The patient is usually kept in an internal rotation sling for 2 to 4 weeks. Active range of motion to tolerance is generally encouraged from 3 to 6 weeks, at which time strengthening and passive range of motion are initiated. Maximal internal rotation efforts are usually delayed until 8 weeks, but 10 to 15 repetitions (RM) can begin at 6 weeks.

Magnuson-Stack repairs transfer the subscapularis tendon and capsule to a point lateral to the biceps groove and inferior to the greater tuberosity. This effectively reduces external rotation by about 50% and serves as a dynamic active anterior sling to the head of the humerus as the arm is abducted and externally rotated. Freeman[27] reports that the success of this procedure relies on limitation of external rotation by 50%. Therefore aggressive range of motion beyond this range would not be appropriate. The time frame for rehabilitation is similar to that for Putti Platt repair.

The Bristow and modified Bristow procedures use screw fixation to transfer the lateral coracoid process and its attached biceps tendon to the anterior aspect of the scapular neck through a slit in the subscapularis tendon. This then serves as a dynamic buttress when the arm abducts and externally rotates and generally results in only a 10- to- 15-degree loss of external rotation. The patient generally spends 3 to 4 weeks in an internal rotation sling. Circumduction exercises usually begin at 3 weeks. Active elbow flexion and active or passive elbow extension are avoided for 6 weeks. Progressive strengthening and range of motion begin within pain limits between 3 and 6 weeks, as dictated by the referring physician.

The Eden-Hybbinette reconstruction involves the placement of a bone graft against the anterior aspect of the neck of the scapula and rim of the glenoid in order to mechanically block the anterior excursion of the humeral head. It is used in cases where the anterior glenoidal rim is eroded. After surgery the shoulder is kept in an internal rotation sling for 2 weeks. At 2 weeks active range of motion is allowed, avoiding external rotation. Isometrics and gentle strengthening are allowed and slowly progressed.

Posterior reconstructions for posterior dislocations are directed at decreasing posterior capsule laxity. The reverse Putti Platt uses the infraspinatus joint instead of the subscapularis joint. The patient is usually positioned in neutral or external rotation after surgery. Abduction and internal rotation movements are avoided early on, and emphasis is placed on strengthening the posterior deltoid and rotator cuff. Push-ups and bench presses should be avoided in the locked-out position.

Glenoid labrum tears. Vertical, circumferential, and longitudinal tears of the glenoid labrum can result from shearing forces that occur as the head of the humerus is forced through the extremes of motion or from traction stresses of the biceps tendon onto its attachment to the superior labrum. The latter forces are common during the acceleration phase of throwing,[68] while the shear forces are usually produced in cases of capsular hypermobility. Anterior shoulder subluxation or dislocation can result in anterior labral tears, while posterior shoulder instability can result in posterior labral injuries. The most common sites of injury are the anterosuperior and/or anterior third quadrants.

Symptomatic to tears of the labrum are sensations of popping or catching during quick movements, pain with forced end range positioning, capsular hypermobility, and a positive clunk test. Surgical treatment usually involves resection, suturing, or stapling of the offended structure and is often accompanied by reconstruction or repair of an associated torn or stretched glenohumeral capsule.

Rehabilitation of the postoperative shoulder that involves repair or resection of a portion of the labrum has been described.[25] Several key concepts are important to keep in mind. Therapeutic exercises should not be very aggressive during the first 3 to 4 weeks in order to minimize traumatic synovitis and pain. Ice should be used after exercise in order to further control inflammation. Submaximal isometrics are important for reestablishing neuromuscular control and should be performed in midrange positions. Early forceful stretching should be avoided. Early use of the biceps is avoided in cases where the lesion involved the superior aspect of the labrum, and the apprehension position of combined abduction and external rotation should be avoided in the presence of an anterior injury. Strengthening progresses from submaximal midrange isometrics to short arc isotonics and isokinetics. Isolated rotator cuff strengthening is performed in positions that avoid subacromial impingement and movements associated with subluxation or instability. Forced flexion is contraindicated during the early stages of rehabilitating patients with tears in the posterior labrum because this is the position that often causes the tear. Rehabilitation of injuries to the glenoid labrum is presently in its infancy and will no doubt evolve, along with the advances in the diagnosis and surgical treatment of the injury.

Nonsurgical unstable shoulder

Hypermobility of the glenohumeral joint can symptomatically result in recurrent subluxations or dislocations. The head of the humerus actually passes through the capsular mechanism and remains alongside of the glenoid during a dislocation. A subluxation occurs when the humerus slips over the rim but spontaneously relocates without any external force other than instantaneous muscle contraction.[73] These subluxations result in a sudden pain that is followed by a sense that the arm goes dead and usually result during rapid overhead activities, such as throwing a ball, swimming (especially during the backstroke or flip turns), or serving a tennis ball. Dislocations are anterior in 95% of the cases, with the majority of these resting in the subcoracoid position. The patient generally is positioned with the arm in slight abduction, the elbow flexed, and the acromion prominent, and the shoulder has a flattened appearance. Reduction is best accomplished early on, before muscle spasms occur, and may involve traction in the plane of the humerus with adduction and gentle internal and external rotation. The mechanism of anterior dislocations is usually forced external rotation that occurs while the humerus is abducted. Associated injuries can include the Bankart lesion (avulsion of the anterior capsule

and labrum from the glenoid), fracture of the anterior glenoid rim, Hill-Sachs compression fracture of the posterior humeral head, fracture of the greater tuberosity (seen in 10% of the cases), and injuries to the brachial plexus (25% of these are to the axillary nerve) and vascular structures (this is rarely seen but necessary to evaluate because of its potential seriousness). Fifty to sixty percent of acute dislocations will recur. Age of the patients is a major factor in incidence of recurrence, as 80% to 85% of those younger than 20 years old will suffer repeated dislocations and only 15% of those older than 50 will have recurrences. Those with associated fractures of the greater tuberosity have only a 5% to 7% chance of a repeated dislocation, while those with a fracture of the anterior glenoid rim have a 60% reinjury rate. Aronen and Regan[2] have reported a 75% success rate (average of 36 month followup) in the conservative treatment of first time dislocations in members of the naval academy. They followed a well-supervised program of isometrics, isotonics, isokinetics, and rubber tubing exercises. Other reports have not been as successful.

Conservative care of anterior dislocations usually involves wearing an internal rotation sling for 2 to 4 weeks, unless the patient is elderly and at a risk of developing excessive contractures. Pain-free isometrics are begun early on to prevent atrophy while range of motion is avoided in the combined planes of external rotation and abduction. These are often progressed at 2 to 4 weeks to isotonics, isokinetics, and rubber tubing exercises, as pain allows, taking care to avoid positioning the shoulder simultaneously in both external rotation and abduction. Traditionally, strengthening has been directed toward the internal rotators and adductors in order to dynamically control or limit external rotation and abduction. The subscapularis muscle and its broad tendon also play a significant role in the anterior stability of the glenohumeral joint. It is important to incorporate eccentric strengthening because this matches the functional demands on these muscles when they are recruited to resist forced abduction and external rotation. At 4 to 6 weeks the dynamic strengthening programs are progressed, as pain allows, to include strengthening with the arm no longer adducted to the side. External rotation strengthening is added to help centralize the humerus in the glenoid. Cain et al[13a] have reported that activation of the infraspinatus tendon and teres minor draws the humeral head posteriorly and helps to unload the stress on the anterior capsule. This is analogous to the effect that the hamstrings have on the anterior cruciate ligament of the knee. Adduction and abduction can now be strengthened up to 90 degrees of elevation while the arm is kept in internal rotation. Flexion and extension strengthening is allowed overhead. Internal and external rotation strengthening are now performed in three different positions: 0 degrees of abduction, 45 degrees of abduction, and 90 degrees of forward flexion. Isokinetics are performed, both eccentricly and concentricly, at a variety of speeds and using appropriate range of motion limiting stops. Higher velocities (> than 210 degrees per second) are avoided initially until the patient is able to catch resistance throughout the limited range. Slow velocities (< than 90 degrees per second) are avoided early due to soft tissue healing. Ramping can be used to educate the patient in catching faster velocity (> than 210 degrees per second). Exercise tubing and hand weights are used at home, incorporating high repetition with low weight as well as low repetition with high weight, in order to increase endurance and strength, respectively. Pool exercises with hand paddles can be performed within the above mentioned limitations. Upper body ergometers, which exercise the shoulder in flexion and extension, are also quite helpful at this stage of rehabilitation. The exercises are progressed to include multiple planes of movement in accordance with the functional demands of each individual patient. The patients are advised to avoid the following: routine stretching into external rotation, standard Nautilus arm cross exercises on the double chest machine (these can be done sitting 90 degrees to the seat or side-saddle), behind the head military presses or latissimus pull-downs, wide grip presses (narrow gripping positions the bar more in the forward flexed plane), and lowering the bench press too far into horizontal extension. Sometimes it is necessary to try to limit external rotation and abduction with special braces and/or taping.

Smith and Brunolli[78] have shown that shoulder kinesthesia is significantly reduced in patients who have had a history of glenohumeral joint dislocations. This suggests the need to incorporate kinesthetic challenges, such as PNF routines, balancing on all fours, and repeated attempts to match the positioning of the shoulder in the total rehabilitation of the upper extremity.

Kennedy, Hawkins, and Krissoff[49] have reported an overuse injury found in swimmers, which they call the *apprehension shoulder*. It occurs most frequently during the backstroke, when the athlete enters the flip turn. At this instant the shoulder is in full abduction and external rotation, while the hand pushes forcefully from the wall. While investigating this movement with cineradiography, the researchers found that the humeral head can actually luxate anteriorly onto the rim of the glenoid fossa.

Posterior dislocations are infrequent and differ from anterior instability in that the shoulder is more susceptible to dislocating if the arm is internally rotated. External rotation and posterior deltoid strengthening are usually emphasized during rehabilitation, while push-ups and bench presses are avoided.

Prevention

Preseason screening and conditioning in athletics are of infinite importance to orthopaedic and sports physical therapy. Areas of vulnerability to injury can be detected and corrected before the season starts.[7] A preseason evaluation for the shoulder should include the following parameters: flexibility, posture, joint clearing tests, isokinetic dynamometer evaluation, a neurological evaluation, and videotape analysis of pitchers.

An example of preventive conditioning, a warm-up protocol for baseball pitchers that can minimize shoulder injuries, is outlined in the boxed material, in Table 20-3, and in the text. The procedure has three basic parts: static stretching, ballistic stretching, and a gradually increased throwing period. The total time expended for the program is approximately 25 minutes.

SUMMARY

The scheme that has been presented in this chapter outlines a comprehensive approach to the evaluation and rehabilitation of shoulder injuries. The program is based on a detailed and comprehensive knowledge of anatomy and biomechanics. It is hoped that, by applying these concepts, physical therapists will be better equipped to treat shoulder disorders and direct treatment toward prevention of reinjury, in contrast to simply alleviating symptoms without regard for the underlying pathological condition or the predisposing weakness.

REFERENCES

1. Allman FL: Fractures and ligamentous injuries of the clavicle and its articulations, J Bone Joint Surg (Am) 49:774, 1967.
2. Aronen JG and Regan K: Decreasing the incidence of recurrence of first time anterior shoulder dislocations with rehabilitation, Am J Sports Med 12(4):283-291, 1984.
3. Atwater AE: Biomechanics of overarm throwing movements and of throwing injuries, Exerc Sport Sci Rev 7:43, 1979.
4. Barnes L: Cryotherapy in sports injuries, Phys Sport Med 7(6):130, 1979.
5. Bechtol CO: Biomechanics of the shoulder, Clin Orthop 146:37, 1980.
6. Becker RO and Selden G: The body electric, New York, 1985, William Morrow & Co, Inc, pp. 275-325.
7. Blackburn TA: Shoulder injuries in sports, Ohio State APTA annual meeting, Columbus, 1981.
8. Bland JD, Merrit JA, and Boushey DR: The painful shoulder, Semin Arthritis Rheum 7(1):21, 1977.
9. Blatz D: Upper arm strap, Swimming World, February, pp. 43-44, 1985.
10. Booth RE and Marvel JP: Differential diagnosis of shoulder pain, Orthop Clin North Am 6(2):353, 1975.
11. Bowers KD: Treatment of acromioclavicular sprains in athletes, Physician and Sports Medicine 11(1): 79-89. 1983.
12. Braatz JH and Gogia PP: The mechanics of pitching, J Orth Sports Phys Ther 9(2):56-69, 1987.
13. Cailliet R: Shoulder pain, Philadelphia, 1966, FA Davis Co.
13a. Cain PR et al: Anterior stability of the glenohumeral joint — a dynamic model, Am J Sports Med 15(2): 144-148, 1987.
14. Carmichael SW and Hart DL: Anatomy of the shoulder joint, J Orth Sports Phys Ther 6(4):225-228, 1985.
15. Cheng RSS: The mechanism of electrode acupuncture and TENS, Ontario J Med Assoc 18:372, 1980.
16. Clancy WG: Shoulder problems in overhead-overuse sports: introduction, Am J Sports Med 7(2):138, 1979.
17. Clancy WG: Personal communication, November 1981.

18. Codman EA: The shoulder, Boston, 1934, Thomas Todd Co.
19. Cofield RH: Total shoulder arthroplasty with the Neer Prosthesis, J Bone Joint Surg (Am) 66A(6):899-906, 1984.
20. Cyriax J: Textbook of orthopaedic medicine, vol 1, ed 6, Baltimore, 1975, Williams & Wilkins.
21. Cyriax J: Textbook of orthopaedic medicine, vol 2, ed 10, London, 1975, Bailliere Tindall.
22. Daniels L and Worthingham C: Muscle testing, ed 4, Philadelphia, 1980, WB Saunders Co.
23. Delacerda FG: A comparative study of three methods of treatment for shoulder girdle myofascial syndrome, J Orth Sports Phys Ther 4(1):51-54, 1982.
24. Engin AE: On the biomechanics of the shoulder complex, J Biomech 13:575, 1980.
25. Engle RP and Canner GC: Shoulders and glenoid labrum tears, Clin Management, 8(5):14-17, 1988.
26. Fowler P: Shoulder problems in overhead-overuse sports: swimmer problems, Am J Sports Med 7(2):141, 1979.
27. Freeman BL: Recurrent dislocations. In Edmonson AS and Crenshaw AH, editors: Campbell's operative orthopaedics, ed 7, vol 3, St. Louis, 1987, The CV Mosby Co.
28. Grana WA, Holder S, and Schelberg-Karnes E: How I manage acute anterior shoulder dislocations, Phys Sports Med 15(4):88-93, 1987.
29. Griffin JO: Physical agents for physical therapists, ed 2, Springfield, Ill, 1975, Charles C Thomas, Publisher.
30. Grinsburg JH, Whiteside LA, and Piper TL: Nutrient pathways in transferred patellar tendon used for anterior cruciate ligament reconstruction, Am J Sports Med 8(1):15, 1980.
31. Gould JA: Lecture notes, University of Wisconsin—La Crosse, Fall 1978.
32. Halbach JW and Straus P: A comparison of electromyo-stimulation to isokinetics in increasing power of the knee extensor mechanism, J Orthop Sports Phys Ther 2(1):20, 1980.
33. Hawkins RJ and Kennedy JC: Impingement syndrome in athletes, Am J Sports Med 8(3):151, 1980.
34. Hollman MW and Hettinger TH: Sports medicine and training, Stuttgart, 1976, FK Schattauer Verlag.
35. Hoppenfeld S: Physical examination of the spine and extremities, New York, 1976, Appleton-Century-Crofts.
36. Inman VT, Abbott L, and Saunders JB: Observations on the functions of the shoulder, J Bone Joint Surg (Am) 26:1, 1944.
37. Inman VT, and Saunders M: Observations on function of clavicle, Cal Med 65:158, 1946.
38. Jobe FW: Shoulder problems in overhead-overuse sports: thrower problems, Am J Sports Med 7(2):139, 1979.
39. Jobe FW and Moynes DR: Delineation of diagnostic criteria and a rehabilitation program for rotator cuff injuries, Am J Sports Med 10(6):336-339, 1982.
40. Jobe RW et al: An EMG analysis of the shoulder in throwing and pitching: A preliminary report, Am J Sports Med 11:3, 1983.
41. Jobe FW et al: An EMG analysis of the shoulder in pitching—a second report, Am J Sports Med 12:32, 1984.
42. Jobe FW, Moynes DR, and Antonelli DJ: Rotator cuff function during a golf swing, Am J Sports Med 14(5):388-392, 1986.
43. Johnson D: In swimming, shoulder the burden, Sports Care and Fitness 1(2):24-30, 1988.
44. Kahn J: Low voltage technique, New York, 1978, Syosset.
45. Kaltenborn FM: Mobilization of the extremity joints, Oslo, 1980, Olaf Norlis Bokhandel, pp. 92-113.
46. Kaltenborn FM: Personal communication, March 1981.
47. Kapandji IA: The physiology of the joints, vol 1, New York, 1970, Churchill Livingstone, Inc.
48. Kendall HO, Kendall FP, and Wadsworth GE: Muscle testing and function, ed 2, Baltimore, 1971, Williams & Williams Co.
49. Kennedy JC, Hawkins R, and Krissoff WB: Orthopaedic manifestations of swimming, Am J Sports Med 6:309, 1978.
50. Kessel L and Watson M: The painful arc syndrome, J Bone Joint Surg (Br) 59:2, 1977.
51. Kingsman AJ: Clinical effects and uses of interferential TENS. Paper presented at Australian Physiotherapy Association Congress, Sidney, Australia, 1975.
52. Kummel BM: Spectrum of lesions of the anterior capsular mechanism of the shoulder, Am J Sports Med 7(2):111, 1979.
53. Larson RL: Throwing injuries to the upper extremity. Paper presented at the Nineteenth Conference on the Medical Aspects of Sports, Monroe, Wis, 1978, American Medical Association.
54. Larsen E, Bjerg-Nielsen A, and Christensen P: Conservative or surgical treatment of acromioclavicular dislocation, J Bone Joint Surg (Am) 68:552-555, 1986.
55. Lippman RK: Frozed shoulder: periarthritis, bicipital tenosynovitis, Arch Surg 47:283, 1943.
56. Little league baseball: official regulation and playing rules, Section 6, pp. 12-13, 1984.
57. Lord JW and Rosati LM: Thoracic outlet syndromes, Clin Symp 23(2):1, 1971.
58. Ludington NA: Rupture of the long head of biceps flexor cubiti muscle, Ann Surg 77:358, 1923.
59. Lunggren AE: Clavicular function, Acta Orthop Scand 50:261, 1979.
60. Maitland GD: Peripheral manipulation, Boston, 1977, Butterworth Publishers.
61. Melzac R and Wall P: Pain mechanism: a new theory, Science 150:971, 1965.
62. Neer CS II: Anterior acromioplasty for the chronic impingement syndrome in the shoulder, J Bone Joint Surg (Am) 54:41, 1972.
63. Neer CS II and Welsh RP: The shoulder in sports, Orthop Clin North Am 8(3):583, 1977.
64. Niclsen JA: Myofascial pain of the posterior shoulder relieved by spray and stretch, J Orthop Sports Phys Ther 3(1):21, 1981.
64a. Nirschl RP and Pettrone F: Tennis elbow: the surgical treatment of lateral epicondylitis, J Bone Joint Surg 61A:832, 1979.
65. Nuber GW et al: Fine wire electromyography analysis of muscles of the shoulder during swimming, Am J Sports Med 14(1):7-11, 1986.
66. O'Donaghue DH: Treatment of injuries to athletics, Philadelphia, 1976, WB Saunders Co, pp. 439-444.
67. Pappas AM: Elbow problem associated with baseball during childhood and adolescence, Clin Orthop 164:30, 1982.
68. Pappas AM, Goss TP, and Kleinman PK: Symptomatic shoulder instability due to lesions of the glenoid labrum, Am J Sports Med 11(5):279-288, 1983.
69. Pappas AM, Zawacki RM, and McCarthy CF: Rehabilitation of the pitching shoulder, Am J Sports Med 13(4):223-235, 1985.
70. Pappas AM, Zawacki RM, and Sullivan TJ: Biomechanicis of pitching, Am J Sports Med 13(4):216-222, 1985.
71. Penny JN and Welsh RP: Shoulder impingement syndromes in athletes and their surgical management, Am J Sports Med 9:11-15, 1981.
72. Perry J: Anatomy and biomechanics of the shoulder, Clin Sports Med 2:10-83, 1983.
73. Perry J: Normal upper extremity kinesiology, Phys Ther 58(3):265, 1978.
74. Rathbun JB and Macnab I: The microvascular pattern of the rotator cuff, J Bone Joint Surg [Br] 52:540-553, 1970.
75. Richardson AB, Jobe FW, and Collins HR: The shoulder in competitive swimming, Am J Sports Med 8(3):159, 1980.
76. Schenkman M and DeCartaya VR: Kinesiology of the shoulder complex, J Orth Sports Phys Ther 8(9):438-450, 1987.
77. Smith KF: The thoracic outlet syndrome, a protocol of treatment, J Orthop Sports Phys Ther 1(2):89, 1979.

78. 78. Smith RL and Brunolli J: Shoulder kinesthesia after glenohumeral joint dislocation, Phys Ther 69(2): 106-112,1989.

79. Staples OS and Watkins: Full active abduction in traumatic paralysis of the deltoid, J Bone Joint Surg (Am) 25:85, 1934.

80. Stone MH et al: A theoretical model of strength training, Natl Strength and Condition Assoc J 4(4):36-39, 1982.

81. Toyoshima S, Hoshkawa T, Miyashita M: Contribution of body parts to throwing performance, Biomechanic IV, Baltimore University, 1974, Park Press.

82. Travell J and Rinzler SH: The myofasical genesis of pain, Postgrad Med 2(5):425, 1952.

83. Tullos HS and King S: Throwing mechanism in sports, Clin Orthop North Am 4:709-711, 1973.

84. Viadero A, Harrison B, and Farbent J: Postoperative care of the TSR patient, Clin Management 7(4)14-15, 1987.

85. Wallace LA: Injuries to the serratus anterior in athletics, Paper presented at the Annual PPTA meeting, Washington, DC, 1981.

86. Yergason RM: Supination sign, J Bone Joint Surg (Am) 13:160, 1931.

87. Zarin A, Andrew J, Carson M: USOC Injuries to the throwing arm, Philadelphia, 1985, WB Saunders Co, pp. 10-106.

Chapter 21

THE SPINE

James A. Gould III

The omnipresence of spinal disorders in various populations has been well documented.* The spine, because of its multiple segments and numerous articulations, has a high potential for disorders to become manifest. Andersson[1] indicates that 50% to 80% of all adults will suffer from back pain during their lifetime. Industrial back injury accounts for 25% of all compensation claims,[1,42] and work loss in England alone has been estimated at 18 million days per year.[63,64] Treatment programs vary from rest and physical exercise to surgery. Recently the emphasis has been on client education with the formation of the back school, which has produced a better response to treatment in clients than other conservative measures.[2,38,76] Forms of prevention range from doing radiographic studies for job determination[18,54,66,68] to employing exercise tests, which have proved less than conclusive.

Unfortunately, medical management frequently recommends single-treatment programs as the therapy for all back problems no matter what the cause. In the past, rest and Williams' exercise[71] have been the prevalent conservative treatment. At present we have the potential of substituting and applying exclusively extension exercises for flexion exercises as the conservative mode of care. However, while both Williams' flexion[71] and McKenzie's extension[47] programs are excellent for some cases, it is the intent of this chapter to provide a clinical foundation in anatomy, biomechanics, and examination so that the clinician can then select a treatment technique based more on understanding spinal disorders and their signs and symptoms than on employing standard treatment for all cases of spinal pain.

ANATOMY

Understanding the anatomy of the spine forms the essential basis for any examination and subsequent treatment. This discussion is divided into segments to allow discussion of each component of the spine.

Osteology

The 33 bones of the full spinal column are divided into five areas. The cervical area is composed of the uppermost seven vertebrae, the thoracic area is comprised of the next twelve vertebrae, the lumbar spine consists of the five lowest mobile vertebrae, the sacrum is composed of the five fused vertebrae, and the coccyx has four to five vertebrae, which are usually fused. This chapter focuses on the 24 mobile vertebrae found in the cervical, thoracic, and lumbar regions.

Lumbar osteology. Lumbar vertebrae are characterized by large ovoid-to-kidney shaped bodies, short, broad pedicles, stout articular pillars, relatively small transverse processes, and quadrangular spinous processes. The pedicles are primarily responsible for the trefoil or triangular vertebral canal. The acute lateral angles of the canal are narrow, forming a potential stenosis problem for the nerve

*See references 1, 21, 63, 66, 67, and 72.

roots that traverse the pedicle to exit through the intervertebral foramen.

Each vertebral body has its primary nutrient foramen located in the center posterior aspect and in situ is covered by the posterior longitudinal ligament.[58] The vertebral bodies alter in shape, from the first lumbar vertebra (which is more squared) to the fifth lumbar vertebra (which is more rectangular), giving the articular endplate a broader surface area.[48] The fifth lumbar vertebral body is also deeper anteriorly than posteriorly (this may also occur to a lesser degree at L-4).

The articular pillars also vary in shape and direction for facet alignment. In the upper four lumbar vertebrae, the articular pillars are longer, thinner, and closer together than in the fifth vertebra.[48] The facets face in an almost lateromedial direction and are therefore aligned in the sagittal plane.[57] This alignment limits the total rotation available in the lumbar spine to 13 degrees of rotation. The articular pillars of the fifth lumbar vertebra are shorter and more wide set, and the facets face obliquely forward and laterally toward the frontal plane. The alignment allows for the most rotation in the lumbar area to occur at this articulation level. All the articular pillars of the lumbar vertebrae have convex surfaces on the inferior articular pillar and concave surfaces on the superior.

Unique to the articular pillars of the lumbar vertebrae are roughened, raised areas at the superior border of each superior articular pillar that serve for muscle attachment for the multifidus. These areas are called the *mammulary processes*.[70] Also unique to the lumbar area are the accessory processes, found on the articular pillars, and the adjoining transverse processes, both of which serve as attachment sites for the psoas and quadratus lumborum muscles.[27]

Thoracic osteology. The thoracic vertebrae are characterized primarily by two features: the presence of articular facets on the bodies (for articulation with the ribs) and the long and thin spinous processes that angle downward. Unlike the spinous processes in the cervical and lumbar areas, where the tip of the spinous process is found directly posterior to the body of the vertebra, the tip of the spinous process in the thoracic area lies posteriorly and inferiorly to the body of that vertebra.[70]

The bodies of the thoracic vertebrae are taller and more squared in the transverse plane. The bodies of the middle thoracic vertebrae often appear almost heart shaped because of the pressure of the descending aorta. The first, tenth, eleventh, and twelfth vertebral bodies have full facets on the lateral aspects of the body for articulation with the ribs at these levels. Thoracic levels T-2 to T-9 have demifacets at the superior and inferior border of the body posterolaterally for articulation of the ribs to adjacent vertebral bodies.[27] The articulation of the ribs to adjacent vertebral bodies limits lateral flexion at these levels. The nutrient foramen is located in a posterocentral location and is

covered in situ by the posterior longitudinal ligament. The pedicles are longer than in the cervical or lumbar area, thus giving the vertebral canal an oval or circular appearance and diminishing the possibility of stenosis of the canal.

The transverse processes are characterized by being angled backwards, so that the tips of the transverse processes lie posteriorly to the articular facets, encouraging rotation movements by attached muscles. Each thoracic transverse process also articulates with the tubercle of the appropriate rib. These costovertebral and costotransverse articulations add stability to the thoracic area.

The articular pillars of the thoracic vertebrae are short and have broad facets that lie nearly on the frontal plane. The superior facet faces posteriorly and slightly laterally, and the inferior faces anteriorly and slightly medially.[35] The superior facet is slightly convex and the inferior facet is slightly concave, which is opposite to the facets in the lumbar spine. Because of the facet alignment and stabilization of the vertebral bodies laterally, rotation is the most accessible movement.

Cervical osteology. The cervical vertebrae can be divided into two categories: typical (C-2 to C-7) and atypical (C-1 and C-2). The typical vertebrae are characterized by transverse processes with foramina (foramen transversarii) through which the vertebral artery passes. Also unique to the typical cervical vertebra are lateral prominences, called uncinate processes, on the superior surface of each vertebral body, which articulate with the beveled edge of the inferior surface of the vertebral body. At this junction there is usually a synovial joint called the *joint of Lushka*.[26,70] The uncinate processes add lateral bony support to the intervening disks. The transverse processes of the typical vertebrae are formed by a true transverse process and the costal process, which together form the anterior and posterior borders of the bone surrounding the vertebral artery.[70] The tips of the transverse and costal processes are called the anterior (costal) and posterior (transverse) tubercles and serve as attachment sites for muscles. The scalenus anterior muscle attaches to the anterior tubercle, and the scalenus posterior and medius and the multifidus muscles attach to the posterior tubercle.[27]

The spinous processes, C-3 to C-6, which are usually bifid, become progressively longer in descending order. The seventh cervical vertebra, which has the longest spinous process in the cervical area and is not bifid, is called the vertebra prominens but is often times not the most prominent spinous process.[48]

The cervical facets are located on short, stout, articular pillars and are angled about 45 degrees obliquely backward and downward. The angle increases at descending levels, and it approaches vertical at C-7. The superior facet surface is convex, and the inferior facet surface is concave, similar to the facet surfaces in the thoracic area. The angulation of the facet joints allow for movement in flexion, extension, lateral flexion, and rotation.

The atypical cervical vertebrae (C-1 to C-2) are characterized by the absence of a body in C-1 (atlas) and by the embryological fusion of the C-1 body with C-2 (axis), forming a prominent pillar on the superior surface of C-2 called the *odontoid process* or dens.[70] The atlas is also characterized by large dishlike articular surfaces for articulation with the occiput superiorly and the atlas inferiorly. These specialized articulations allow flexion and extension at the atlantoccipital joint, with slight lateral flexion and rotation, and predominantly rotation at the atlantoaxial articulation.[31] The component movements allowed at the atlanto occiput and atlanto axial joints comprise approximately 50% of the movement of the cervical spine. The inferior articular pillar of C-2 forms a relatively normal articulation with the superior facet of the third cervical vertebra. The spinous processes of the upper cervical vertebrae are unusual in that the atlas has a tubercle that is not really palpable, whereas the axis has a very prominent bifid spine.

The transverse processes of the atlas and axis are also unique in that the atlas has proportionately very large transverse areas called lateral masses, which have foramen transversarii and serve as attachments for the inferior and superior oblique, splenius cervicis, rectus capitus lateralis, and levator scapulae muscles. The axis has very small transverse processes containing foramen transversarii. The atlas projects further laterally than the subjacent axis, which facilitates rotation between the atlas and the axis.

Intervertebral foramen. The intervertebral foramen is a canal rather than a hole. The canal is primarily osseous, being formed by the dorsal vertebral bodies, pedicles, and articular pillars of adjacent vertebrae, with some soft tissue areas in the form of a disk anteriorly and the capsule of the facet and ligamentum flavum posteriorly. Spur formation within the foramen can decrease the available space and create compression forces on the spinal nerves exiting through the foramen. The foramen has structures that pass through it while both entering and exiting the spinal canal. The nerves as they exit use between a fourth and a third of the available space usually in the upper half of the foramen.[24] Accompanying the nerves are sections of the dorsal branch from the segmental arteries that come directly from the aorta.[53] These arteries, as well as corresponding veins, traverse the foramen to provide nutrients to and remove wastes from the dura, ligaments, and vertebral bodies. There is also a small nerve, called the *sinuvertebral nerve,* which reenters the foramen and innervates the posterior longitudinal ligament. The rest of the space is filled with adipose tissue that supports these structures.

Noncontractile soft tissues of the spine

In discussing the noncontractile soft tissue structures of the spine, those structures common to all areas will be discussed first, followed by a description of the structures unique to each area.

Ligaments. Ligaments are fibrous noncontractile structures that are present throughout the spine. Some are also located in specific areas of the spine. All ligaments have a poor blood supply but a good nerve supply.

General ligaments. Ligaments common to all areas of the spine are the anterior longitudinal ligament, posterior longitudinal ligament, ligamenteum flavum, interspinous ligament, and supraspinous ligament. These ligaments are found in all areas of the spine, whereas the ligaments described in the sections on different areas of the spine are found primarily or uniquely in those areas.

Anterior longitudinal ligament. The anterior longitudinal ligament (ALL) extends the full length of the spine from occiput to sacrum. It begins as a rather narrow band at the occiput through C-2 and broadens as it descends from C-3 to the sacrum. The ALL is adherent to the anterior vertebral bodies and the intervening disks, creating an extended support for both structures. It has a tensile strength of nearly 3,000 psi.[12] The ALL, in concert with the musculature about the spine, keeps a preloaded beam condition in the spine, which helps to strengthen the spine during lifting. Because of the ALL's breadth and tensile strength, it provides strong support and reinforcement to the anterior disks during the lifting of heavy loads.

Posterior longitudinal ligament. The posterior longitudinal ligament (PLL) begins at C-3 and extends to the sacrum. The PLL begins as a relatively broad band in the cervical area, gradually narrowing as it descends, becoming so narrow in the low lumbar area that during lifting, it is of little protective value for the lumbar disks.

The tensile strength of the PLL approximates that of the ALL. The difficulty in the lumbar area is one of quantity rather than quality.[12] The PLL is adherent to the disks at each level, with both vertical and transverse fibers that spread across the posterior annulus.[57,58] The PLL is not attached to the dorsal surface of the vertebral bodies. Branches of segmental arteries run under the PLL to arrive at the central posterior nutrient foramen of the vertebral body. In flexion the PLL becomes taut and acts to compress the vessels running anterior to it against the dorsal vertebral body. This ligamentous value holds fluids within the vertebral body during forward bending and increases the vertebral bodies ability to withstand compressive forces.

Ligamentum flavum. The ligamentum flavum spans adjacent vertebrae and is an elastic ligament. It serves to protect the spinal canal from encroachment by soft tissue on flexion movements. It has a tensile strength of 113N compared with the anterior longitudinal ligament strength of 676N.[50]

Interspinous ligament. The interspinous ligament is not considered an elastic ligament but, unless diseased, it is loose enough to allow full flexion. The interspinous ligament is located between adjacent spinous processes.

Supraspinous ligament. The supraspinous ligament is an extension of the nuchal ligament of the cervical area. It is a loose, but not elastic, ligament that serves to limit segmental flexion. Located between or on top of adjacent spinous processes, the supraspinous ligament is the most superficial of the spinal ligaments and the farthest from the axis of flexion; therefore it has a greater potential for sprain.[35] It is assisted in its ability to resist spinal flexion by the spinalis portion of the erector spinae muscle.

Lumbar area. The lumbar area is affected by two main ligaments: the iliolumbar ligament and the thoracolumbar fascia.

Iliolumbar ligament. The iliolumbar ligaments are located at L-5, and sometimes at L-4, with attachment from the transverse process to the inner iliac crest just above the posterior superior iliac spine (PSIS). The iliolumbar ligaments that are located posteriorly, inferiorly, and laterally serve to stabilize the L-4 and L-5 segments during flexion and rotation. In flexion both sets of ligaments become taut as full range is approached; on rotation the opposite side becomes taut. The iliolumbar ligaments have been identified as adaptations of the quadratus lumborun muscle which resists shear forces at the L-4–5 and L-5–5, levels.[40]

Thoracolumbar fascia. Although not technically a ligament, the thoracolumbar fascia has a tensile strength of nearly 2,000 psi and serves as one of the most important noncontractile structures in the lumbar area.[12] It spans the area from the iliac crest and sacrum up to the thoracic cage and envelops the paravertebral musculature. On full flexion, as the muscles become electrically silent, the thoracolumbar fascia becomes the major resisting factor against further flexion.[41] On extension from a fully flexed position, the gluteus maximus and hamstrings act in concert with the thoracolumbar fascia to initiate the extension movement. As the muscles become active, the tense fascia serve to increase the efficiency of the muscle contraction.

Bogduk and Macintosh[4] and Bogduk and Twomey[5] have identified three layers of the thoracolumbar fasica with fibers aligned vertically, horizontally and obliquely. The vertical fibers are tensed by the gluteus maximus in the act of lifting. The horizontal fibers are tensed through forces applied by the transversus abdominus and internal obliques, which exert an extension force on the spinous processes.[22,65] The latissimus dorsi muscle is in direct line with the oblique fibers, translating forces coming into the back by the lifting of an object with the arms. Through these layers and the attachment of muscles to the fascia the thoracolumbar fasia has gained new prominence in its function as a vital component of a healthy back.

The thoraco lumbar fascia and the intervening fascia coverings of the deep back muscles have been identified as forming a series of compartments in the back that run its

length.[55] These compartments can fill with fluid on injury and create some of the findings of acute back strain. The fluid in a compartment can create a *Bourdon tube effect*, which acts to straighten the tube therefore acting to flatten the lumbar lordosis as seen in back injury. The increased pressure caused by fluid accumulation will create an ischemic condition in the area, which promotes necrosis of tissue and destruction of the receptor input essential for proper spinal feedback.[8] In addition the accumulation of fluid in the compartment may give the appearance of what was previously identified as muscle spasm or tight muscles in the spine. Treatment of fluid accumulation in these compartments would be indicated in acute and sometimes chronic back problems. The movement of this accumulated fluid may also be a basis for the response to treatment using the McKenzie extension exercises and some of the deep connective tissue techniques.

Thoracic area. The ligaments unique to the thoracic area are those that serve to attach the ribs to the vertebral bodies and transverse processes. The ligaments can be discussed as a group. The ligaments are the radiate, superior costotransverse, inferior costotransverse, and lateral costotransverse. The radiate ligament is merely a thickening of the anterior capsule of the costovertebral joint, whereas the other ligaments are separate anatomical entities.[27] All the ligaments act to provide protection and to guide movement of the costovertebral and costotransverse synovial joints during respiration and exertion. Because of the nature of synovial joints, capsules can become impinged by the edges of the joint through unguarded movements, and the resultant irritation can effect the intercostal nerve (as well as the sympathetic chain ganglia) that traverses the anterior capsule of the costovertebral joint.

Cervical area. The upper cervical area has a number of special ligaments that assist in the movement of the head on the neck.

Suspensory or apical ligaments. The apical ligament is a thin ligament that extends from the tip of the dens to the anterior border of the foramen magnum. It acts to hold the dens in position and serve as an axis for rotation.

Alar ligaments. The alar ligaments extend from the lateral aspects of the dens cranially and laterally to the anteromedial border of the foramen magnum. These ligaments, along with the apical ligament, serve to stabilize the dens and to keep proper alignment with the foramen magnum medially and laterally.[70] The alar ligaments also act to limit rotation of the atlas on the axis through their lateral attachments.

Cruciform ligament. The cruciform ligament has three bands of fibers; the transverse band is the thickest and is often identified in anatomical texts as a separate ligament, yet it remains part of the total cruciform.[53] In some texts the vertical portions are termed the *transverse occipital* and the *transversoaxial ligaments*.[53,70] The function of the cruciate is to maintain the odontoid bone snugly against the posterior aspect of the anterior arch of the atlas. This avoids compression of the spinal cord, which runs immediately posterior to it. Laxity of the cruciform ligament and other ligaments in clients with rheumatoid arthritis preclude strong traction or strong mobilization movements to the upper cervical spine in these clients.

Tectorial membrane. The tectorial membrane, which originates at the foramen magnum, inserts into the second and third cervical vertebrae, becoming continuous with the posterior longitudinal ligament. The tectorial membrane is located in the vertebral canal, just posterior to the cruciform ligament, and serves to hold the odontoid process against the anterior arch.

Ligamentum nuchae. The ligamentum nuchae is one of two elastic ligaments in the body, the other being the ligamentum flavum. The ligamentum nuchae is an anteroposteriorly thick band that extends from the inion or external occipital protuberance to the spinous process of C-7, where it becomes continuous with the supraspinous ligament. In addition to serving as an attachment site for muscles of the neck, it guides and limits flexion of the head on the neck.

Capsules. Capsules encompass all zygapophysial joints and the articulation of the head with the atlas.[49] They function with ligaments to guide and to limit joint movements. The capsule serves as support and protection for the synovial membrane and is one of the primary limiters of movement. In full flexion of the lumbar spine, capsules support approximately 40% of the body weight using their tensile strength of 319N.[50]

Capsules are also integral in forming the close-packed and loose-packed positions of facet joints of the spine. In the spine, the close-packed position of the facets from the third cervical level to the fifth lumbar level is when the joint is in full extension, whereas the close-packed position for the atlas and axis is when the joint is in full flexion. The *military salute* position is the maximum close-packed position for the entire spine; in this position, the spine is most rigid. The close-packed position, although rarely held for any period of time, is needed for full movement and is used when creating a rigid spinal lever for lifting. Following trauma or long periods of poor posture, the ability to attain a full close-packed position is often lost. The close-packed position is also the hardest position to reattain. A person who cannot assume a full-range close-packed position will be, as a consequence, positioned in a more unstable loose-packed position, where the potential for dysfunction is increased.

Synovial lining. Within the joint capsule of the diarthroidal facet is a synovial lining supported and protected by the capsules discussed previously. (The composition and function of the synovial lining are best described in Chapter 4). The synovial lining is mentioned here since it has been demonstrated that there are intraarticular synovial protrusions, sometimes called *meniscoid inclusions,* which

can, on aberrant movement, become trapped between the hyaline articular cartilages.[20,37] These can, in essence, block the joint surfaces from gliding, create pain from compression of the subsynovial layer, and produce a splinting response from the spinal musculature (perceived clinically as spasm). The synovial lining, when traumatized, will create effusion into the joint and position the joint into flexion creating a loose packed position that is less stable.

Disk. The disk consists of two portions: the annulus fibrosis and the nucleus pulposus.

Anulus fibrosus. The anulus fibrosus consists of 12 to 20 fibrous layers that insert and originate on adjacent vertebral bodies and end plates.[35] The layers of the anulus contain collagen fibers aligned at acute angles with alternate layers of fibers running in opposite directions.[28]

The anular layers act together much the same as a radial ply on a tire. Working together, the layers have half the fibers on stretch in each direction of rotation. The anulus acts to absorb forces that arrive at the joint, and it contains the nucleus pulposus, which acts as the fulcrum of movement for the three degrees of freedom available at each vertebral level.[35] When sprained or overstretched, the outer fibers of the anulus that attach to the vertebral body periosteum can result in pain of sclerotomal distribution.[24] If a third-degree sprain results from trauma, there can be ingrowth of new innervated tissue from the periosteum of the adjacent vertebral bodies. The ingrowth of new tissue can lead to an increased sensitivity of the area to pain during movement.

Nucleus pulposus. The nucleus pulposus is a mucopolysaccharide gel that changes in its biochemical characteristics with age and damage.[28] The biochemical change decreases the strength of the water-binding capability of the nucleus. Hendry[29] demonstrated that a disk will give up water more readily if it is degenerated because of age or damage. When the water-binding capability is at normal functional levels, the nucleus contains approximately 88% water, which makes it nearly incompressible. Therefore it acts as a distributor of force that arrives at that vertebral level. The nucleus also serves as a major contributor to the mechanism of disk nutrition through release of bound water during weight-bearing activities and imbibition of fluids when a person is recumbent. A more detailed description of the disk can be found in other sources and will not be covered here.*

Peripheral nerves. Peripheral nerves are noncontractile structures that originate from the spinal cord within the vertebral canal and exit through the intervertebral foramen. The roots exit laterally from the cord and aggregate to form the peripheral nerve as it exits the vertebral canal. The nerves of the cervical spine leave the cord and exit through the intervertebral foramen at a 90-degree angle to

*See references 28, 32, 57-59, 69, and 70.

the cord. The nerves angulate more at descending levels to the conus medularis, where the nerves leave the cord almost vertically and exit the intervertebral foramen by making a near 90 degree angle turn around the pedicle. The angulation of exit from both the cord and the intervertebral foramen is a factor in the effect of space-occupying lesions on the compression of the nerve.[6] Lumbar nerves have more potential to be compressed as they exit the vertebral canal than cervical nerves.

Peripheral nerves and their roots are sensitive to pain, and irritation or compression results in signs and symptoms that are most dominant distally.

Contractile soft tissues of the spine

Contractile tissues of the spine consist of muscle, the musculotendinous junction, the tendon (when present), and the insertion of the tendon to the bone through the periosteum via Sharpey's fibers.[70] Discussion of the contractile elements will be divided into two groups: those common to most areas of the spine and those more specific to each of the three major areas.

Contractile tissues common to most areas of the spine

Trapezius and latissimus dorsi. Combined, the origins of the trapezius and the latissimus dorsi span the entire spine from occiput to sacrum. The trapezius spans the occiput to T-12, and the latissimus overlaps six segments, spanning T-6 to the sacrum. The trapezius then inserts on the stable portion of the shoulder complex—the scapula—whereas the latissimus dorsi inserts onto the mobile humerus. Together they act to position the shoulder and retract it during lifting. In essence, the two muscles spread the load of the upper extremity across the entire span rather than concentrating the force in the upper thoracic area.

Erector spinae (sacrospinalis). The sacrospinalis is another combination of muscles that has a common origin in the sacrum and extends to the occiput. As the muscle group ascends, three divisions are delineated: the iliocostalis, longissimus, and spinalis.[27]

Iliocostalis. The most lateral portion of the sacrospinalis, called the *iliocostalis,* inserts into the ribs near the rib angle. Therefore, if the iliocostalis portion is restricted in function, it can have an effect on ribcage elevation. Clients with back pain often have a shallow breathing pattern because of the pain, which in turn causes improper ventilation of the lungs, increasing the carbon dioxide concentration of the blood that in turn increases the perception of pain.[73]

Longissimus. The longissimus is the longest portion of the sacrospinalis. Located just medial to the iliocostalis, it attaches to the rib and transverse processes. If tight, it can affect breathing and go into spasm or splint the area if mechanical impingement of the costotransverse joint occurs. The longissimus creates the major cross-sectional area of the erector spinae and is most involved in the action of extension of the spine.

Spinalis. The spinalis is the most medial of the sacrospinalis group. On dissection, the spinalis is seen to be composed mostly of tendon with only small muscle bellies. The spinalis muscle tendons attach from spine to spine and probably serve as a sensory feedback mechanism for spinal flexion and extension. Additionally the spinalis acts as a check reign to limit flexion of the spine in concert with the posteriorly located ligaments of the spine.

As a total group, the sacrospinalis acts to extend the spine and head and functions to create a solid lever of the trunk for lifting.[15]

Interspinalis. This muscle series spans from spine to spine, functioning in spinal extension. Because of its size, the interspinalis probably serves more of a sensory function than that of a prime mover of extension.

Intertransversarii. The intertransversarii, which are located between adjacent transverse processes, function in a manner similar to the interspinalis, but they monitor lateral flexion. An interesting fact regarding the intertransversarii is that the posterior primary ramus of the segmental peripheral nerves exits through the medial and lateral portions of this muscle. Spasm or tightness of the muscle can compress the nerve.[6]

Multifidus. The multifidus is most prominent in the lumbar area and to some extent in the cervical area. The multifidus originates on the transverse processes or mammalary processes and inserts into the spinal processes of vertebrae one to four segments above. Rotation, as well as sensory monitoring of the position of rotation, is its primary function when acting singly. When the multifidus acts bilaterally, it functions to create extension of the spine toward a more close-packed position for stability. It also counteracts the shear forces that act on the lumbar spine.

Contractile tissues by specific area. In addition to the muscles already described, some muscles are found only in certain areas or are most prominent in a particular area of the spine. These muscles will be described by area.

Lumbar area. The lumbar area contains three groups of contractile tissues: the quadratus lumborum, the abdominal muscles, and the psoas muscle.

Quadratus lumborum. The quadratus lumborum is a flat muscle forming the posterior abdominal wall and spanning the iliac crest to the last rib. It is described as a *hip hiker,* which is active in gait on the swing side to hold the pelvis in a neutral position.[30] If painful or restricted, it will also restrict chest or rib cage expansion. Additionally the muscle attaches to the transverse processes of the lumbar vertebra and acts as a medial-lateral support and guidance system for the lumbar area. The position of the lower fibers of the quadratus also provide resistance to shear forces acting at the lumbo sacral junction. The iliolumbar ligaments are considered to be adaptations of some of the fibers of the quadratus lumborum.

Abdominal muscles. Forming the lateral and anterior walls of the abdominal cavity, the abdominal muscles are intricately involved in creating a semirigid column in combination with the chest cavity by compressing the abdominal contents. This acts as a temporary force attenuation for the spine during lifting. The function of increasing intraabdominal pressure is primarily used in heavy lifting for extra support and cannot be held for very long because it compresses the vena cava and reduces the return of blood to the heart from the lower extremities.

RECTUS ABDOMINIS. The rectus abdominis has always been the primary focus of exercise routines, but its origin on the pubis and insertion on the xiphoid process and costochondral junction places it in a poor position to add support. Interestingly, the longest muscle fibers are located in the lower rectus. There are tendinous intersections at regular intervals from the umbilicus to the sternum but none from the umbilicus to the pelvis.

OBLIQUUS INTERNUS AND EXTERNUS ABDOMINIS. The oblique muscles run in opposite directions and act to create tension when the trunk is rotated in either direction. The internus fibers attach to the thoracolumbar fascia and are thought to actively bring about spinal extension via tension on that fascia.

TRANSVERSUS ABDOMINIS. The transversus abdominis runs from the spine to the linea semilunaris at the lateral edge of the rectus abdominis. It is an important tie between the muscle-fascia column formed anteriorly by the rectus abdominis and the column formed posteriorly by the sacrospinalis muscle and thoracolumbar fascia.[27] Transverse force applied by the transversus abdominus has been implicated in a mechanism to extend the spine through tension on this throacolumbar fascia.

Psoas. The psoas is a muscle that is associated with the hip but acts directly on the lumbar vertebrae.[39] The psoas originates on the anterolateral aspects of the vertebrae and disks L-2 to L-5 and inserts on the femur. The psoas is described as a hip flexor, but it can act on the lumbar area when contracted, causing a lordosis or a scoliosis if acting singly. Cocontraction of the psoas with the quadratus lumborum acts to stabilize the lumbar spine with in anteroposterior direction.

Thoracic area. The thoracic area is affected by the rotatory muscles and those that position the scapula and humerus.

Rotatories. Although the rotatories are frequently present at other levels, they are most prominent in the thoracic spine.[27] The rotatories belong to the transversospinalis group, having their origin on the transverse process and traversing upwardly and medially to the spinous process of a vertebra one to four levels above. These muscles bring about rotation of the vertebrae in the direction opposite the side of the muscle and probably have a sensory role in monitoring rotation.

Muscles positioning the scapula and humerus. Also worthy of note in the thoracic region are the thoracic muscles, which alter the position of the scapula and humerus. These are the serratus anterior, rhomboids, pectoralis minor, and pectoralis major, in addition to the trapezius and latissimus dorsi that have already been discussed. (The levator scapulae will be discussed in the cervical area.) It is important for the clinician to be aware of the proper length, muscle tone, and strength of these muscles with regard to both the movement of the arm and the thorax. For proper arm flexion and abduction, the thoracic spine must allow rotation, extension, and lateral flexion for full range of limb movement. Therefore full limb movement depends on proper flexibility of the noncontractile and contractile tissues of the spine that affect the area.

Cervical area. In the cervical area, special attention must be paid to a balance of the length and strength of posterior, anterior, and lateral musculature that controls head-on-neck and neck-on-thorax movements.[35]

Clinicians are aware of the bulk of posterior musculature that serves as an antigravity muscle as well as a primary mover of the head.[35] Little attention is given, however, to the anterior musculature, which is associated with ventilation, phonation, and mastication. These muscles, although not primary movers of gross head and neck movement, are nonetheless important in consideration of neck symptoms and must be addressed regarding proper length and function for full rehabilitation.

Posterior neck muscles. Posteriorly located are the cervicis and capitis portions of the sacrospinalis group, which includes the iliocostalis, longissimus, and spinalis. Along with these muscles, the semispinalis capitis, cervicis, and splenius capitis assist in general head and neck positioning and movement.[70] These muscles bring the cervical spine into extension to create a rigid stability to the area during lifting.

In addition to these muscles that have their origin and insertion on the spine or occiput, there is a clinically important muscle, which originates on the first four cervical transverse processes and inserts on the superior angle of the scapula, called the *levator scapulae*. It is clinically important in two ways. First, its origin allows the muscle to move the C-1 to C-2 area, especially when the shoulder is fixed. Second, it has a propensity for transferring symptoms from the upper cervical area to the superior angle of the scapula.[23] Pain in the upper cervical area creates an increased tension in the levator, which acts to elevate, downwardly rotate, and forwardly migrate the scapula, resulting in rounded shoulders.

In addition to the muscles that act on the neck, there is a group of four muscles that function to move the head on the neck. These four muscles, which comprise the suboccipitales, are the rectus major and minor and the obliquus superior and inferior.[48]

The rectus minor and the obliquus superior originate on the atlas and insert on the occiput. This places them in good position to monitor and move the head into extension. The rectus major and the obliquus inferior originate on C-2, the rectus traverses upward and laterally to the nuchal line of the occiput, and the obliquus inferior traverses upward and laterally to the transverse process of C-1 (atlas). These two muscles act to move the head and C-1 in rotation and are important in small neck movements necessary for reading.

The suboccipital group of muscles becomes tender and go into spasm when the muscles are asked to function in a shortened range of motion. This more often occurs when the head and neck are in a forward position relative to the trunk. This position is common in persons with occupations that use computer work stations.

Lateral neck muscles. Two muscles in the lateral neck are especially important: the sternocleidomastoid (SCM) and the scalenus (taken as a group). Tightness in these two muscles limits lateral flexion of the head and neck to the opposite side. SCM tightness creates or facilitates a forward head position and limits rotation toward the side of the tight muscle. The scalene muscles, if unable to maintain the proper length, have a constrictive effect on the subclavian artery and vein as well as on the brachial plexus, all of which exit from the thoracic cavity and neck to the upper extremity.[27]

Anterior neck muscles. Anteriorly, there are two deep muscles that assist in flexion of the spine and are in good position to monitor movements. The longus capitis and the longus coli lie deep to the esophagus and are positioned in such a way that head and neck flexion and extension, rotation, and lateral flexion are resisted or assisted by the oblique or vertical fibers that make up these muscles.[35]

The muscles that serve the functions of ventilation, phonation, vocalization, and mastication are collectively known as the suprahyoid and the infrahyoid muscles. The infrahyoid muscles consist of the sternohyoid, sternothyroid, cricothyroid, and omohyoid. These muscles span the sternum and the hyoid and generally act to depress the larynx or raise the larynx in response to desired speech and breathing patterns.[70] Stretching of these muscles in a forward head posture can create difficulty with speech and swallowing.

The suprahyoid muscles are the geniohyoid, mylohyoid, digastric, tongue, stylohyoid, and palatopharyngeus. These muscles, in addition to positioning for speech, are active in the acts of chewing and swallowing. Improper positioning of these muscles can cause stress on the temperomandibular joint and lead to symptoms from that area.

BIOMECHANICS

During development, the spine is in a position of total flexion. At birth the baby is described as having a C-shaped spine. The C curve means that the facets and the posterior elements have developed with the articular surfaces distant from each other or in the loose-packed position as described by MacConiall.[41]

Reversed or lordotic curves appear in the cervical spine as the baby bears the weight of the head on lifting it and in the lumbar spine as the child assumes the upright posture for gait. The lordotic curve places the facets in a more close-packed position, which adds stability to the spine and guides movements in weight bearing. The thoracic area maintains a kyphotic curve on bearing weight because of the lateral stabilization supplied by the ribs and their articulation to two adjacent vertebrae via demifacets.

The head, thoracic area, and pelvic area form the rigid portions of the total span of the trunk, with the lordotic, cervical, and lumbar areas acting as springs. Dynamic stabilization depends on muscular, capsular, and ligamentous systems and their interplay with the facets to allow movement, yet they remain stable during weight bearing.

The cervical, thoracic, and lumbar curves have been described as functioning to increase the ability of the spine to withstand axial compression.[13,35] Calculations have determined that a three-curve system can withstand more compressive forces than a straight system.[35,61]

Within each area there are areas of most and least biomechanical movement. In the cervical spine there are two such areas. The upper two cervical vertebrae are reported to accomplish approximately 50% of the movements of flexion and extension and rotation of the head and neck.[31] The greatest movement in the lower cervical spine occurs at C-5 to C-6, with C-6 to C-7 being the second most active.[31] Restriction of movement in these two areas by either pain or spasm results in significant decrease in the total movement available.

Descending from the occiput to the sacrum, the vertebrae change in their characteristics as discussed in the osteology section of this chapter. The facets or zygapophysial joints are formed by the articulation of the inferior articular pillar of the vertebra above with the superior articular pillar of the vertebra below. As indicated earlier in the chapter, the facets in the cervical spine are angled at approximately 45 degrees in the anteroposterior direction at C-3, with a transition to near vertical by C-7. The 45 degree angulation allows the greatest freedom of movement with the least resistance of any area in the spine. The large amount of cervical movement is accompanied by protective elements consisting of a trough-like arrangement in the cervical transverse process. The laterally positioned uncinate processes add external support to the disks. In addition to bony protective elements, the ligaments are also broad and strong.

In the thoracic area the facets are aligned nearly vertically, allowing predominantly lateral flexion and rotation, while limiting flexion and extension. Since the ribs attach between vertebral bodies, they limit lateral flexion, leaving rotation as the dominant movement allowed in the thoracic area.

In the lumbar spine the facets lie in the sagittal plane and limit rotation to the greatest extent, lateral flexion to a lesser extent, and flexion/extension least. The facets are most sagittal near L-1 to L-2 and move toward the frontal plane at the L-4 to L-5 and L-5 to S-1 levels.[69] Therefore the least rotation is allowed in the upper lumbar area and the most rotation allowed in the lower lumbar region.

Spinal mechanics are unique compared to any other mechanics of the body in that the 24 mobile bony vertebrae are connected by disks that serve as semielastic axes for spinal movements as well as force transmitters and absorbers.[19] The disks located between each vertebra from the second cervical vertebra to the sacrum consist of two portions: the nucleus pulposus and the anulus fibrosus, which together act as a force couple to transmit, disperse, and absorb axial forces entering the spine. Intradiskal pressures on the lumbar spine are greatest in sitting position and least in the supine position.[51] The anulus fibrosus consists of rings of fibrous tissue composed of collagen, ground substances and cells.[17] The collagen fibers are arranged at an oblique angle and therefore are most taut on rotation in one direction. Each layer of the anulus has fibers on stretch when rotated in either direction. The anulus is least protected when in a transition stage from one direction of rotation to the other. This occurs in the lumbar spine when the individual flexes and side-bends, picks up a load, or tries to come to the upright position while maintaining a side-bent position.

In the lumbar spine, when the trunk is flexed and undergoes side-bending, the vertebra undergoes a component motion of rotation. In the flexed position, because of ligamentous and facet factors, the vertebra will rotate to the same side as the side-bending. Inherent in the rotation of one vertebra on another is a tautening of one half the anular fibers. For instance, if an individual picks up a load in the flexed side-bent position and maintains that side-bent position while trying to assume the upright position, the mechanics acting on the vertebrae change so that, as the upright position is assumed, the rotation of the vertebrae shifts to that opposite of the side-bending. Therefore, at an intermediate point between full flexion and full upright position, the anular fibers move from having one half the fibers on stretch to having no fibers on stretch and then again to having the other half of the fibers on stretch. At the extremes of the movement described, the anulus has good protective qualities; at the midpoint the situation is precarious. Should there be any weakness in the anular wall, the contents of the nucleus may protrude, causing herniation or extrusion of the nuclear contents.

The phenomenon of component rotations with side-bending (and vice versa) occurs in all regions of the spine, but the shift in the direction of rotation in flexion and in the upright position is unique to the lumbar area. In the cervical spine side-bending and rotation occur to the same side no matter what the position of the neck, while in the thoracic area the rotation and side-bending occur in opposite directions.

The anular layers take origin and insert in three areas on the vertebral body. The outermost fibers attach a few millimeters up onto the vertebral body itself, being anchored by Sharpey's fibers through the periosteum. The middle layers of the anulus attach to the growth ring of the body, and the inner layers attach to the cartilaginous end plates of adjacent vertebral bodies. Although controversy has existed as to whether the disk, especially the anulus, is innervated, it is now generally accepted that at least the outer fibers of the anulus are innervated. Although an excellent point for researchers to investigate, it is clinically insignificant since it is accepted that the outer fibers of the anulus originate and insert on the vertebral periosteum. The periosteum is innervated, and therefore strain of the outer fibers will be painful. It is also logical that the body's attempt at healing such sprains could entail the ingrowth of vascularized—therefore innervated—tissue into the outer annular layers.[24] Clinically, a client with a sprain has symptoms of scleratomal pain, locally dominant, with the possibility of some referred pain.

The nucleus pulposus is composed of chondroitin-6-sulfate and keratin-4-sulfate, both of which have hydrophilic characteristics. The nucleus, encased in the anulus, acts as a ball-bearing type fulcrum, which allows the movements of flexion, extension, lateral flexion, and rotation. The amount of each movement is dependent on the facets and external muscles and ligaments.[35] The nucleus, being primarily water, is nearly incompressible and therefore acts in force distribution more than absorption.

The nucleus, during aging or when damaged, undergoes biochemical changes that decrease its ability to form strong bonds with water.[29,52] The nucleus then gives up the imbibed fluids more rapidly than the fluid can be reabsorbed, increasing pressure laterally. The fluid can work its way between the adherent layers of the anulus. As the fluid progressively separates them, the fibers of the anulus begin working as individual units rather than as a cohesive whole. The nucleus can continue to progress through the concentric layers of the anulus until a bulge appears on the outer fibers and pain is generated.

EXAMINATION

A thorough knowledge of the tissues of the spine is meaningless without an adequate vehicle to affect the status of these tissues in a client with symptomatic pain. An examination of the client is the essential process by which a clinician obtains this information. Questions and tests should focus on determining which tissues are symptomatic and obtaining a baseline to assess future progress. The client's complaints (symptoms), as well as objective restrictions or excesses of movement (signs), serve as the basis for treatment selection and progression throughout the rehabilitation process.

The examination entails two modes of information acquisition. The first is the subjective questioning of a client regarding the onset of symptoms and their present status. The second mode consists of actual tests and measures of the symptomatic area, whereby a data base is obtained. Various examination formats are available* that demonstrate subtle nuances, but the examination format presented here will allow a clinician to obtain adequate baseline information.

Subjective examination

The subjective examination should begin by determining the location of the symptoms described by the client. Use of a body chart is encouraged for rapid visualization and accuracy when the clinician reviews the chart for treatment progression. When ascertaining the location of symptoms, the clinician is advised to concentrate not only on the most symptomatic area but to inquire also about the areas above and below (Fig. 21-1).

Pain, anesthesia, and paresthesia are recorded, as well as structural deviations, scars, or other pertinent information that is quickly observable. The clinician should use the body chart throughout the examination to relate symptoms to signs and to add measurements to the body chart.

The next area of interest is determining the onset of the symptoms. The mode of onset may be insidious or sudden. Whatever the client describes as the original cause should be recorded. If an incident was involved, the mechanism of injury should be determined, if possible. The clinician should be persistent in the attempt to obtain information regarding onset. In case of an accident, the following questions can be asked: From which direction was the object of destruction coming? In what position was the client at onset? What was the initial response if disability was immediate? Muscle injury is a likely cause for immediately present symptoms, but, if the disability was progressively apparent (that is, over a period of hours), the relatively nonvascular, noncontractile structures should be the focus of examination.

After establishing onset and mechanism, the clinician should inquire as to any previous occurrences of the same or similar symptoms. The number of previous occurrences, treatment, and recovery time are important.

The behavior of the symptoms over the course of a day and night are important to establish as part of the baseline for future comparison. Are the symptoms constant? If constant, do they vary? This is important since, if a musculoskeletal problem is present, movement of the system during a day should exacerbate or alleviate the symptoms to some extent.[44,45]

The clinician should always question constant, unchanging symptoms, inquire specifically as to activities of daily living and their effect on the client's symptoms, and

*See references 9, 11, 14, 33, 36, 42, 43, 45, 46, 59, 63, and 75.

establish the effect of rest and movement. What induces the pain or increases the symptoms? The symptomatic responses help the clinician establish the irritability of the joint, which in turn determines the vigor possible in physical tests and the intensity that can be used in treatment techniques.

Other questions that should be asked are: Is there any night pain associated with the condition? If so, is it associated with rolling, or is it a spontaneous exacerbation (commonly associated with nonmusculoskeletal problems)? Also, when symptoms arise, what can the client do to relieve them? Usually a client with a musculoskeletal problem will mention any positions that afford some, if not complete, relief. The clinician should note the positions(s) described and assess the mechanics of the action as a possible treatment technique.[45]

The client should relate to the clinician the intensity and effect of symptoms from first rising to the end of the day, as well as whether they affect the quality of sleep. Careful notation and listening skills will allow the clinician to correlate events described in the history with the behavior of the symptoms described.

Special questions can be asked for each area of the spine, based on recognized anatomical and physiological properties as well as known pathological syndromes. Examples of special questions and the reason for asking them are presented by area in Table 21-1 (these questions are not intended to be all-inclusive).

The last area of the subjective questioning is directed at determining any contraindications to treatment or suggesting further medical tests. In this section the client's general health should be assessed. Are there other associated or nonassociated problems or conditions that may bear on the symptoms? Is there any family history of arthritis, back problems, spinal disease, heart disease, or diabetes? Is the client experiencing unexplained weight loss (which may indicate carcinoma if other factors accompany this symptom)? Have radiographic films been taken that demonstrate any fractures? Is the client taking any medications, and, if so, what and how much? These factors are important in assessing the client's present condition as well as establishing goals for a rehabilitation program.

Once the subjective questions have been asked and answered, the clinician should take a moment to assess the information obtained. Do the client's statements correlate with the location, onset, past history, and behavior of the symptoms? Is there concern that the complaint is not of musculoskeletal origin? Should further medical tests be considered at this point? To what degree must the clinician protect the client from increases in symptoms when completing the tests for movement restrictions?

The clinician's next step is to initiate objective physical tests. Prejudgment should be avoided, and facts should be recorded.

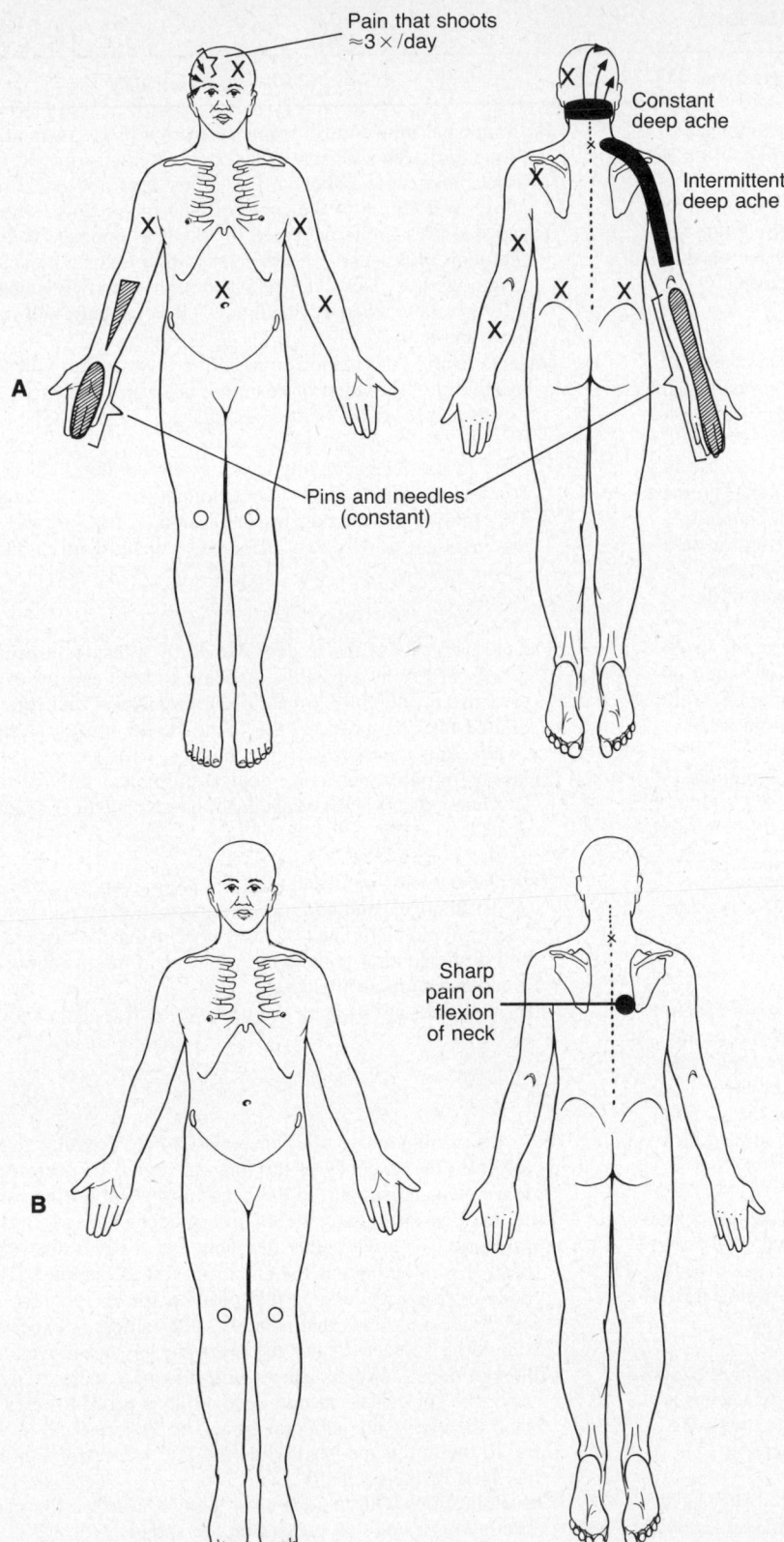

Fig. 21-1. Body charts, showing **(A)** C-7– and C-2–level symptoms and **(B)** possible C-7 distribution of referred pain.

Table 21-1. Special questions

Area	Question	Rationale
Lumbar	What position does the client sleep in?	Before spinal injury most people sleep in a prone or modified prone position. Prone-lying for a person with restricted extension will compress the posterior tissues and cause ischemia. Often this does not give rise to pain until movement allows restoration of the compromised blood flow (similar to "theater" sign).
	What effect does sitting have on the symptoms?	Intradiskal pressure is increased in sitting as opposed to lying or standing. Disk problems will cause exacerbated symptoms for a person who sits for an extended length of time. However, a person with spondylolisthesis will find that sitting affords relief, whereas standing or slow walking will increase the aching into the back and legs.
	Is there a change in symptoms in rising from a sitting position?	Pain on change of position from sitting to standing indicates possible ligamentous instability. The action of changing position is painful; yet, when an upright position is acquired, the pain is diminished.
	Does an increase in abdominal pressure (as in coughing, sneezing, or defecating) create changes in the symptoms?	If there is a space-occupying lesion in the vertebral canal, the increase in intraabdominal pressure creates a concomitant increase in cerebral spinal fluid pressure. This presses the dura against the lesion, increasing the symptoms. These pressure increases are usually very painful for clients with disk extrusion.
	Are there any problems urinating or any numbness in the groin area?	Flaccid paralysis of the bladder caused by a disk protrusion affecting the sacral nerves will bring a positive response to both aspects of this question. Pain can give rise to difficulty urinating, but numbness indicates a compressive lesion. Should these be positive, the client should consult a physician immediately as cauda equina compression is a medical emergency.
(for women)	Do the symptoms have any alteration related to menstruation?	Menstrual problems or gynecological problems can give rise to back symptoms. If any relationship is established, the proper medical examination should be conducted.
Thoracic	Are the symptoms changed by deep respiration?	Articular pinching or irritation of the pleura can give rise to symptoms that change as the lungs expand and the chest rises in deep inhalation. To differentiate, the client should slump and then breathe, using the diaphragm. The costovertebral and costochondral joints will not move in this position, so increased pain implies a nonmusculoskeletal cause.
	Does the pain seem to go up and down between the spine and the medial border of the scapula?	If there is pain in this area, the neck, as well as the area of symptoms, should be assessed.
Cervical	What kind of pillow is used?	Cervical symptoms are often increased when a regular foam pillow is used, resulting from the tendency of the foam to regain its normal shape. In addition, the foam gives no support to the head in rotation during rolling.
	Is any dizziness experienced on rotation or extension of the head from a flexed position?	Inner ear disorders and vertebral artery occlusion can cause dizziness and should be ruled out. To test whether the inner ear needs further examination, the client's head should be held as the client faces the examiner. The client then rotates the body to one side, holding that position for 10 seconds, and then rotates to the other side and holds that position. If dizziness is experienced, the vertebral artery should be suspected since the inner ear has not moved.
	Does the client experience headaches associated with the problem?	Although there are many causes of headaches, there are characteristic referral areas from the spine. The second cervical level tends to refer to an ipsilateral pain behind the eye in the temporal area. The first cervical level has a tendency to referral to the top of the head while the lower cervical area has a tendency to refer to the base of the occiput.
	Does the client have any bilateral numbness or tingling of the hands or feet? Any disturbance of gait?	These questions will be positive if there is a protrusion of the disk or other space-occupying lesion that presses on the spinal cord.
	Is there any difficulty swallowing?	An anterior protrusion of the nucleus pulposus will infringe on normal esophageal flow and make swallowing difficult.

Objective examination

The objective portion of the spinal examination will be discussed in two parts: those tests that are done for all areas and those tests unique to one particular area. Tests required in every orthopaedic examination are observation, attempts to clear joints or areas above and below the symptomatic area, evaluation of movement restrictions, a neurological survey, palpation, and mobility assessment.

Observation. As noted in other chapters, the static and dynamic posture of the client can add insight to musculoskeletal problem-solving. The clinician should attempt to gain awareness not only of gross alterations (such as shoulder height or iliac crest height) but also of subtle changes in muscle tone or subtle disruptions of rhythm.

Referral joint clearing. The clinician should be aware that the site of the symptoms is not necessarily the site of the cause and that the tissue that is creating the symptoms may be affected tissue rather than tissue that is causing the problem.[9] This necessitates examination not only of the area of symptoms but of all sites that could refer to this area. If spinal symptoms are present, the extremity joints are tested to see if they contribute to the described complaint. In addition, it is suggested that at least two levels above and below the symptomatic area be tested for symptom reproduction.[45] The specific tests for the peripheral joints will be discussed in detail later.

Movement tests. Movement tests have two forms: active and passive.

Active movement tests. Active movement tests of the spine evaluate all movements in the three degrees of freedom: flexion/extension, lateral flexion, and rotation. While observing these movements, the examiner should record the quanity of movement as well as the quality. Is the movement smooth? Are there deviations within the arc of movement or at the end? The clinician should look not only at the quanity and quality of the movement but also at where in the spine the movement occurs. Are there observable areas that do not respond to the movement attempted? Is there a correlation between these areas and the area of symptoms? Often hypomobile segments will have symptomatic hypermobile segments above or below. Scoliosis or a short leg, for instance, can be determined in the position of full flexion (Fig. 21-2).

When a client is able to attain his or her full range, no matter how restricted, the clinician should apply an additional passive overpressure if the movement is asymptomatic. This tests the noncontractile tissues as well as osseous junction of the tendon.

Although active movements can give the clinician an indication of the client's willingness to move, they are not diagnostic as to the tissue involved.[9]

Passive movement tests. Passive movement tests in the spine play a very important role, once active movements have been assessed, in focusing on the tissue involved. With the contractile tissue at rest, passive movement

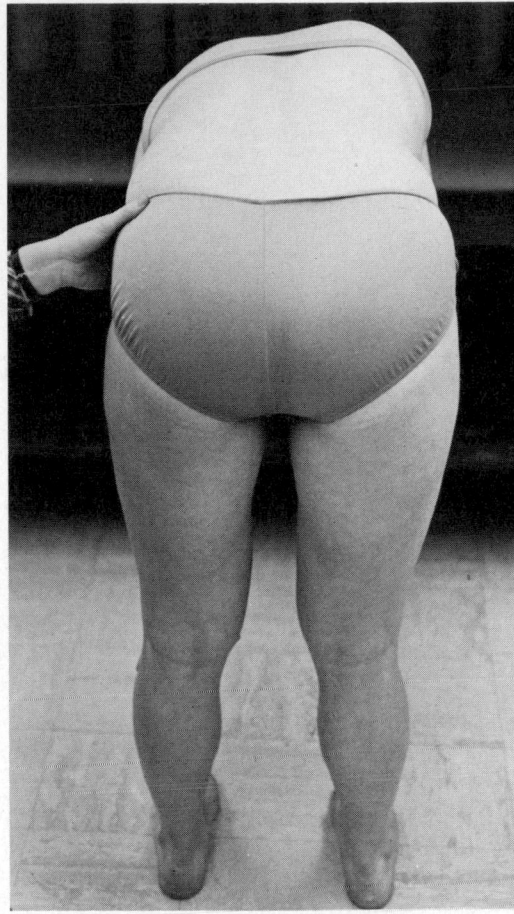

Fig. 21-2. Position of full flexion demonstrating rib hump of scoliosis.

places stretch on the noncontractile tissue. The clinician should look for a correlation between passive movement and symptoms, according to Cyriax's view of contractile versus noncontractile tissue examination.[9]

Physiological passive movements. Evaluation of passive movement should be conducted in two ways. First, the client should be assessed for the amount of movement available and the intensity of response to the passive movement using the same movements that were previously accomplished actively. The examination of passive movements of flexion/extension, lateral flexion, and rotation allows the examiner to check for hypermobility or hypomobility of each segment. There are different ways of testing these passive physiological movement. Some clinicians advocate testing in a weight-bearing position[34], others prefer the non–weight-bearing position for adequate feedback and client comfort.[45] The clinician is advised to try both methods and to use the method that affords maximal information with minimal energy expenditure. It is many times preferred to assess movement restrictions of cervical and thoracic complaints with the client sitting and lumbar complaints with the client side-lying.

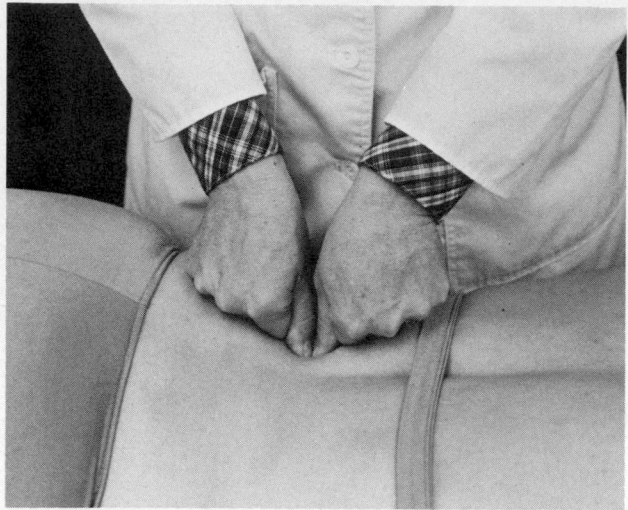

Fig. 21-3. Accessory movement testing using thumbs.

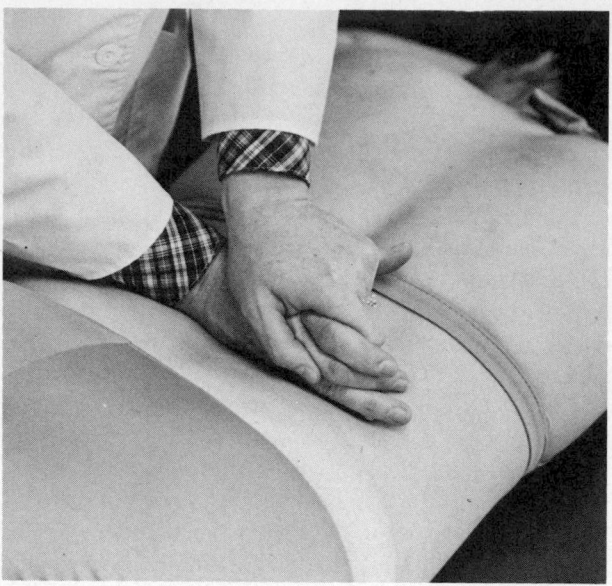

Fig. 21-4. Accessory movement testing using a point just distal to pisiform.

Table 21-2. Classification of resisted movements

Response	Problem
Strong and painless	Normal
Strong and painful	Minor tear
Weak and painful	Major problem
Weak and painless	Complete rupture or neurological problem

Modified from Cyriax J: Textbook of orthopaedic medicine, vol 1, Baltimore, 1969, Williams & Wilkins.

Accessory passive movements. The other movement assessment that should be made passively is the testing of accessory movements. The three accessory movements in the spine are (1) anteroposterior (AP) glide, in which the spinous process is used to spring the vertebrae one on the other to assess relative movement and tissue response; (2) rotation (segmental), in which the transverse process or articular pillar is used to apply an AP pressure, causing rotation of an individual segment on the two adjacent vertebrae, and (3) traction, in which a distractive force is applied manually during examination. The first two accessory movements in the spine are performed with the client prone. The clinician uses the thumbs (Fig. 21-3) or a point just distal to the pisiform on the ulnar side of the hand to apply the force (Fig. 21-4).

Information from the passive physiological and accessory tests should be correlated with the active tests to focus on the involved spinal levels as well as to determine the irritability of the tissue involved.

Neurological survey. The neurological survey examination—a quick testing of sensation, muscle strength, and reflexes—is performed if a possible nerve impingement is suspected. Two indications that a neurological examination is needed as part of the musculoskeletal examination are complaints of numbness into the extremities or pain symptoms radiating below the buttocks in back problems and below the tip of the acromion in cervical cases.

Testing for sensation. Testing for sensation should involve both light touch and pinprick and can be conducted rapidly unless an area of actual numbness is found, in which case that area of actual numbness should be well delineated. All dermatome areas should be covered in the examination. Both Maitland[45] and Grieve[24] provide excellent clinical dermatome charts, or other anatomical texts can be consulted.[27,70]

Testing for reflexes. Testing for reflexes should be done when numbness is demonstrated. The integrity of the reflex is an important baseline determination and an easily checked reference for the integrity of the peripheral nerves. The reflexes usually tested in the lower extremity include the infrapatellar tendon (knee-jerk) reflex and the Achilles tendon (ankle-jerk) reflex. In the upper extremity the reflexes usually tested are the biceps reflex, triceps reflex, and the brachioradial is reflex.

Resisted muscle testing. A muscle test, performed to check both the integrity of innervation to the musculature and the general state of strength, is an integral part of the neurological survey. If a neurological problem is present, the client's response should be one of nonpainful weakness.

Pain associated with the muscle test would suggest a muscle strain more than a decreased nervous innervation. The Cyriax responses to muscle testing can be used (Table 21-2).

The quick tests used in screening of a spinal problem can be supplemented by further manual muscle tests found

Table 21-3. Quick test of muscle strength for nerve involvement

Area	Muscle	Innervation tested
Lumbar	Psoas and iliacus	L1-2
	Rectus femoris	L3-4
	Vastus intermedius, media-lis, lateralis	L3-4
	Anterior tibialis	L4
	Extensor hallucis longus	L5
	Extensor digitorum commu-nis	L5 (S1)
		S1 (L5)
	Peroneal	S1-2
	Gastrocnemius—soleus	
Cervical	Trapezius	C2-4 and spinal accessory
	Deltoid	C5
	Supraspinatus	C5
	Biceps—brachioradialis	C5-6
	Triceps—wrist extensors	C7
	Extensor pollicis longus	C8
	Flexor digitorum sublimis	C8
	Flexor digitorum profundus	C8
	Interosseous and lumbricalis	T1

Modified from Maitland GD: Vertebral manipulation, ed 4, Woburn, Mass, 1977, Butterworth Publishers.

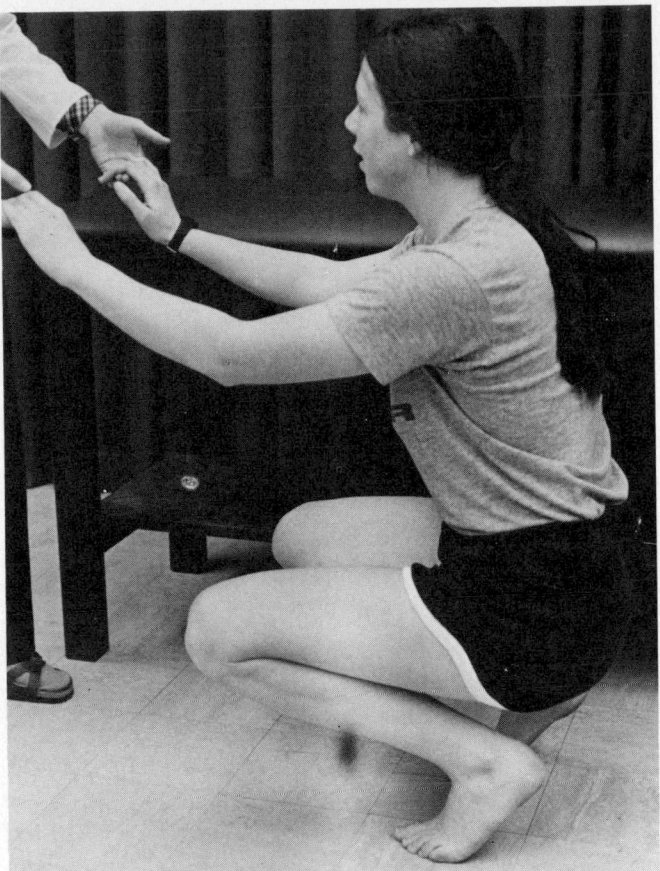

Fig. 21-5. Squat test for peripheral joint involvement.

in appropriate texts. Table 21-3 lists quick muscle tests and the innervation that is predominately checked.

Palpation. Palpation is the point in the examination where the clinician's perceptive skills are maximally tested. An understanding of anatomy is essential for adequate palpation to be a decisive examination tool. The area of symptoms should be approached slowly from a distance so as to palpate the client's more normal skin and underlying tissue and to gain an appreciation for that which will be felt as the clinician approaches the symptomatic area. Subtle changes in tissue texture and muscle tone should be appreciated. Side-to-side comparisons should be conducted. The client should be instructed to indicate any painful sensations.

The palpation should begin very lightly and progress deeper into the tissue; notation of tissue tension and pain response should be recorded. The clinician should be aware at all times of what tissue is beneath his or her fingertips and should correlate it with the subjective and objective information already obtained. Muscle spasms should be noted, and referred pain, if any, should be investigated. Palpation should act as the point where the data collected during previous general tests are used to focus on a particular level and particular side.

Tests by specific area. Specific tests conducted for each area are discussed here, with rationale for their application. These tests are useful for data collection in one area and can further incriminate or clear specific tissues.

Lumbar objective tests. The tests presented here may

be beneficial for testing symptoms in the lumbar area. They are not all-inclusive but can be supplemented by other tests known to the clinician.

Balance testing. Based on the information provided by Wyke,[74] balance testing is conducted to appraise the receptor integrity in the joints of the lower extremities and lumbar area. The test is not specific but can be indicative of balance problems that may initiate pain. A simple Stork standing test can be conducted, or a sophisticated digital balance board can be used to assess balance. Treatment using balance boards, rocker boards, or other balance activities should be instituted if deficits are found.

Active peripheral joint test. Squatting on the heels from standing and returning to upright position puts and peripheral joints through a full active range of motion (Fig. 21-5). The hip, knee, and ankle are involved, with minimal back movement. Changes in symptoms should be noted, as well as where in the range they occurred.

Passive peripheral joint tests. The sacroiliac joint tests consist of compression and distraction of the sacroiliac joint. The procedure uses the anterior superior iliac spine (ASIS) and iliac crests as levers to compress and distract the sacroiliac joint (Fig. 21-6 and 21-7). A positive test produces pain over the area of the sacroiliac joint.

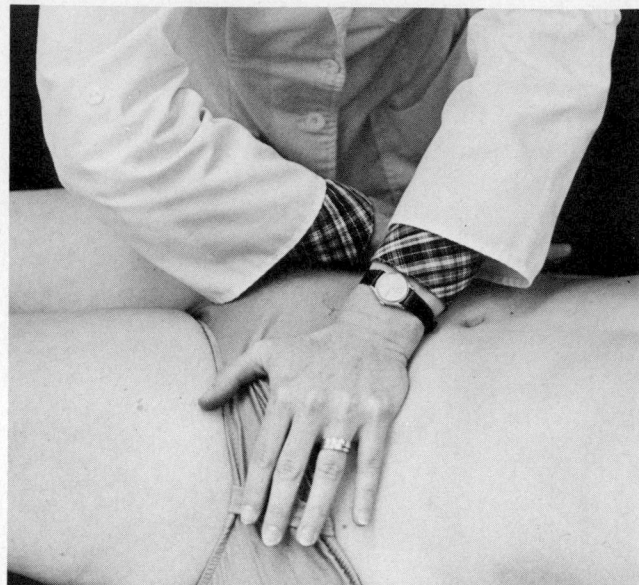

Fig. 21-6. Sacroiliac clearing tests: compression.

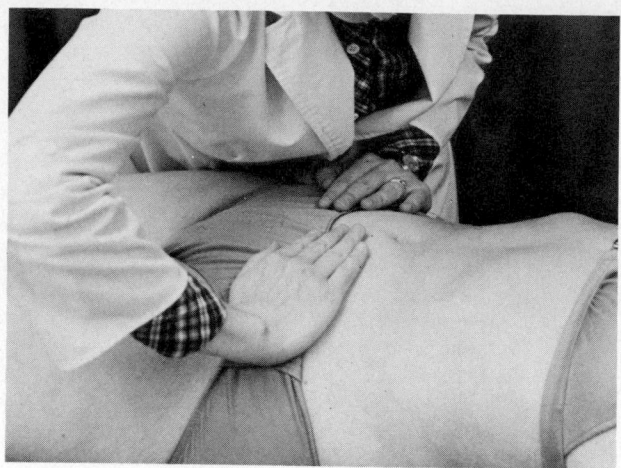

Fig. 21-7. Sacroiliac clearing tests: distraction.

Other tests that assess the sacroiliac while also testing the hip and clearing it are the hip flexion-adduction-internal rotation test (FADIR) (Fig. 21-8) and the flexion-abduction-external rotation test (FABER or Patrick's test) (Fig. 21-9).

The FADIR test uses the femur as a lever and stretches the posterolateral and inferior portions of the hip capsule and compresses the superior and medial portions of the capsule. The opposite is true of the FABER test. Symptoms should be posterior and lateral if there is sacroiliac and low lumbar involvement and anterior if the hip is irritable.

To clear the knee from possible involvement, two tests are conducted. One is to place the knee into full extension and apply a varus and valgus stress. This tests the collateral joints and the posterior cruciate as well as the posterior capsule. The other is to glide the tibia forward on the femur when the knee is flexed, testing the anterior cruciate ligament.

To clear the ankle, the talus is glided in the mortise anteriorly and posteriorly. Then inversion and eversion are tested by applying an overpressure to the end of the range.

Nerve sensitivity tests. A series of tests are performed to place stress on the dural and peripheral nerves, from both above and below, to determine if there is a space-occupying lesion or extreme irritability of the nerve roots.

The first of these tests involves passively lifting the head toward the chest while the client is recumbent. This increases the length of the vertebral column and stretches the dura. Symptoms in the area of the original complaint should be elicited before 50% of the movement is completed.

The second test is the straight-leg raise, which stretches

the dura after about 30 degrees of hip flexion. Positive symptoms should be located in the buttocks and back area (Fig. 21-10).[7]

The third test is the prone knee-bend test, in which the clinician flexes the knee to 90 degrees while the client is prone. This applies stretch to the femoral nerve to test its sensitivity. The test movement can be carried further into the range to test the length of the vastus and rectus femoris muscles. If the hip flexes (i.e., the pelvis rises from the table), the response is noted; a shortening should be suspected and tested. Palpation of the bony and soft tissue structures complete the specific examination of the lumbar spine.

Cervicothoracic examination. Observation in clients with cervicothoracic symptoms is critically important. The position of the head on the neck, the neck on the thoracic cage, and the shoulders should be noted for asymmetries. A forward head posture and rounded shoulders are common, and postural realignment should be stressed as part of rehabilitation.[59]

Active peripheral joint-clearing tests. In addition to the general tests, the clinician should perform an active clearing test of the shoulder, elbow, and wrist. This can be easily accomplished by having the client actively complete a full range of motion at the wrist (flexion and extension and ulnar and radial deviation in full supination, then in full pronation). The elbow should undergo full flexion and extension with the forearm supinated and then fully pronated.[34] The shoulder should undergo full flexion, extension, abduction, adduction, internal rotation, and external rotation. To test both the muscular units and the capsule, mild pressure should be applied at the end of the active ranges that are not symptomatic. While the client is performing the movements, deviations in normal biomechanical rhythm should be observed and noted.[31]

Passive peripheral joint-clearing tests. Testing of the temporomandibular joint to determine its contribution to

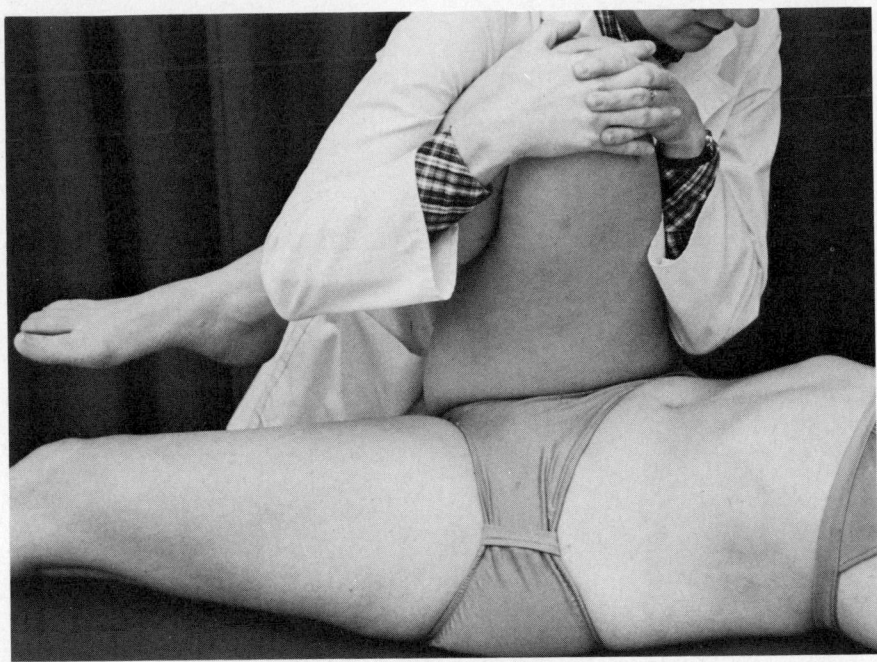

Fig. 21-8. Flexion-adduction-internal rotation test of hip.

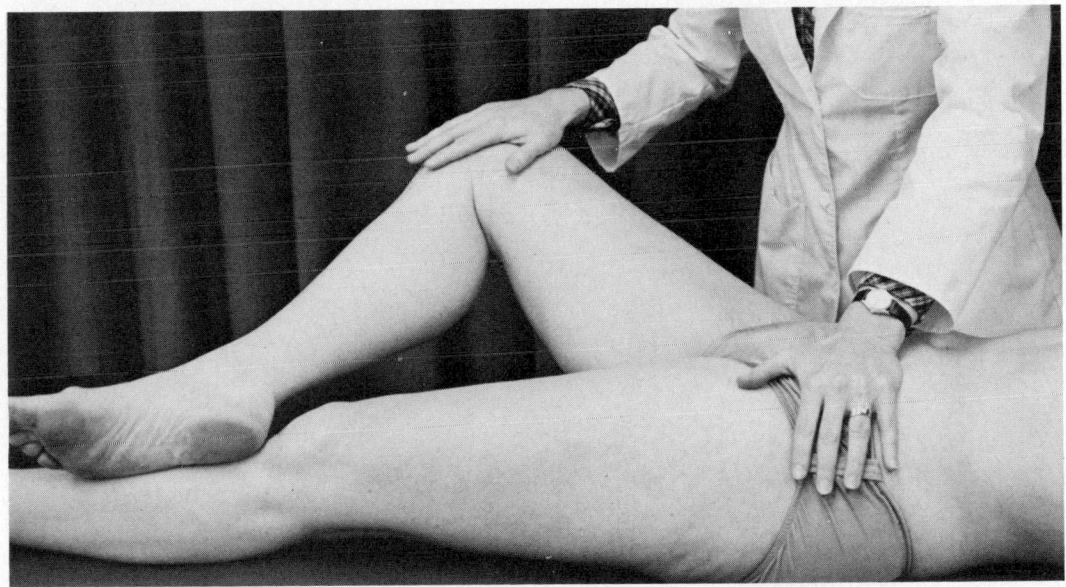

Fig. 21-9. Flexion-abduction-external rotation test of hip.

cervical symptomatology is an important aspect of the cervical spine examination and one that is easily overlooked.[23] (See Chapter 24 for the specific procedures.)

The shoulder should be cleared of possible symptoms by using overpressure at the ends of range and placing the shoulder into a combined movement of extension and abduction and then externally rotating it. When the shoulder is extended and abducted, external rotation should be restricted. This positioning places the humerus up against the acromion and stretches the anterior capsule while compressing the posterior capsule (Fig. 21-11). The attempted external rotation is stopped by the approximation of the greater tuberosity against the acromion. If symptoms are produced, the shoulder should be examined in more detail. To stress the inferior capsule and compress the superior capsule, the arm should be abducted as far as possible and then glided laterally over the acromion with mild pressure (Fig. 21-12).[45] Again, symptoms that appear should be further investigated (see Chapter 20).

The elbow is cleared passively by a varus and valgus

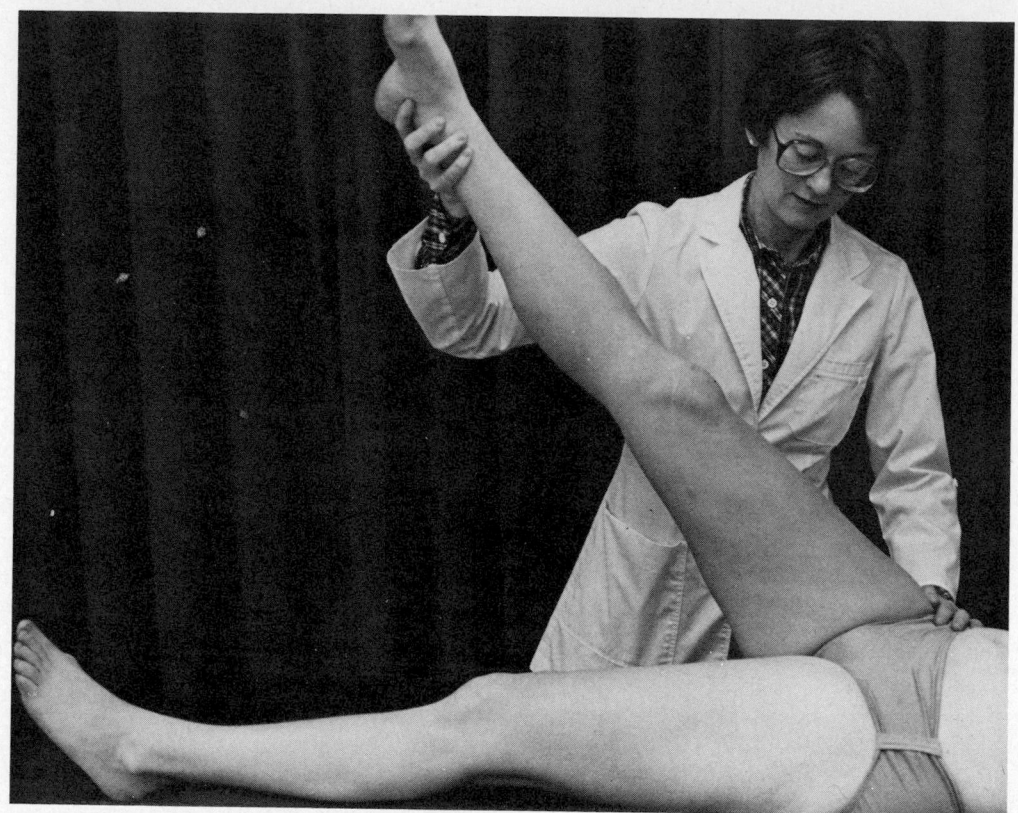

Fig. 21-10. Straight-leg raise.

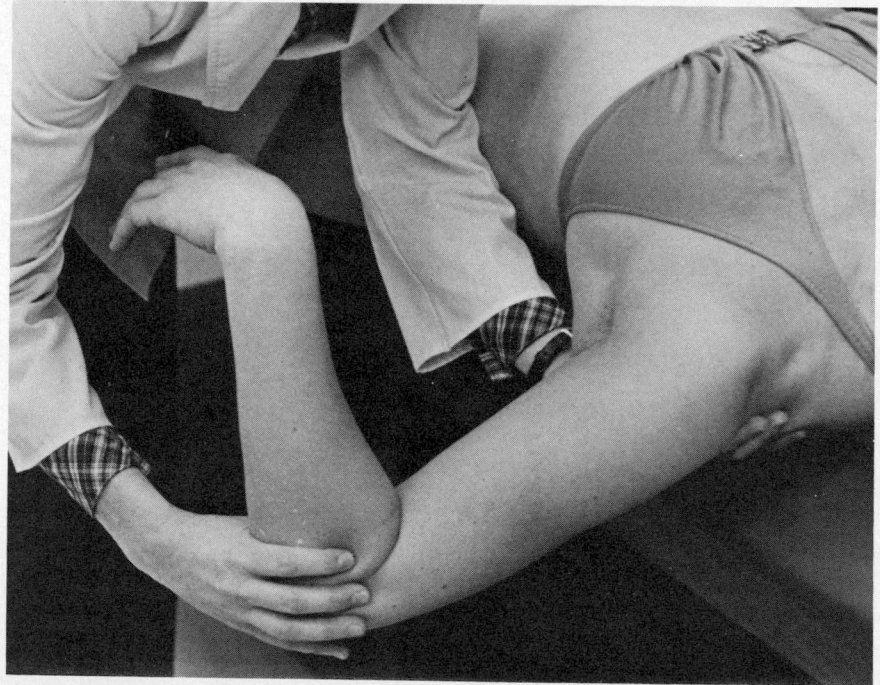

Fig. 21-11. Clearing test of shoulder for anterior and superior capsule.

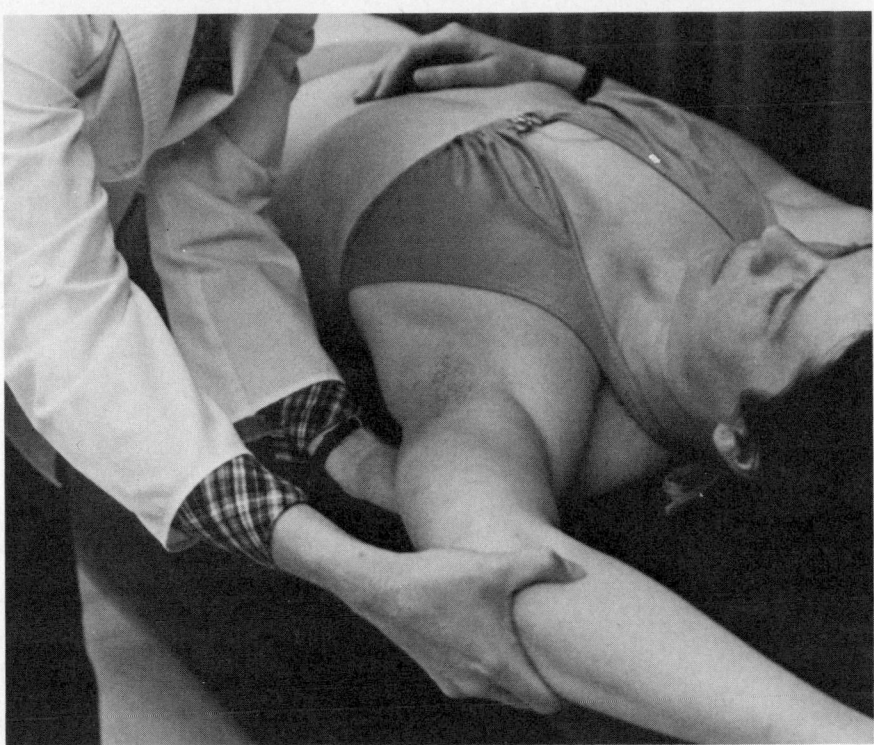

Fig. 21-12. Clearing test of shoulder for inferior and posterior capsule.

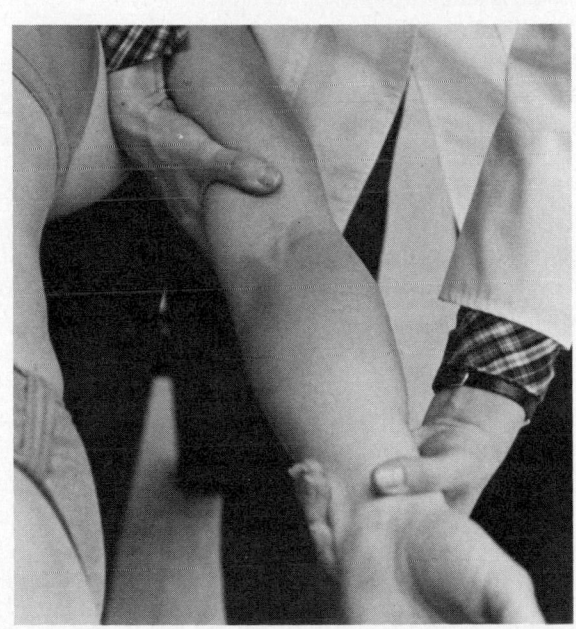

Fig. 21-13. Elbow clearing.

stress applied at full extension, 10 degrees from full extension, and at full flexion. This stresses the collateral ligaments and the anterior and posterior capsule (Fig. 21-13).[45]

The wrist can be cleared by applying overpressure at the end of the range in flexion and extension and ulnar and radial deviation.

Movement testing

Active movements of the neck. The movements of the neck should include flexion/extension, lateral flexion, and rotation. Both quantity and quality of movement, as well as the area of the symptom occurrence, should be observed and recorded.[9] For all movements that are completed without increase in symptoms, an overpressure should be applied.

On completion of the objective tests, the clinician must correlate the subjective examination with the objective tests. Do they correlate, and, if so, to what degree? Were the symptoms the client described reproduced? If not, was there a sign of tenderness or increased tension at a level that could refer to the area of complaint? Should further tests be done? If the tests indicate that a musculoskeletal problem truly exists, then an appropriate rehabilitation program for the involved tissues should be planned.

TREATMENT

Many treatment programs are available for the various areas of the spine.*

To adequately plan a treatment program, determination of the tissue type involved is critical.[60] If the symptoms arise from the noncontractile tissue, determination of hypomobility or hypermobility should be derived from mobility testing of physiological and accessory movement. Classifications of movement range from ankylosed to un-

*See references 9, 17, 47, 56, and 62.

stable, all of which guide the clinician to assess the hypomobility or hypermobility of the joint and treat it accordingly. Maitland[45] has developed guidelines ranking the status of the mobility, which allow the clinician to treat the signs according to the symptomatic response of the tissue in question. Maitland's scheme is predicated on determining not only whether resistance or lack of it is the major factor but also on allowing for the influence of pain as an inhibiting factor.

Schools of thought seem to be polarized and favor either treating biomechanical resistances or laxity without regard to pain or treating the pain in light of resistance encountered. I find that, since most clients seek assistance with their problems because of pain, incorporation of both ends of the spectrum is the safest and most clinically valuable approach to client treatment, especially for the inexperienced therapist. When pain is the dominant factor inhibiting full range of motion, the logical approach is to select techniques to treat the pain first and then to proceed to the abolition of the mechanical hypomobility. To treat only pain, without removing the cause of the biomechanical restriction, leaves the client half treated and will most likely result in recidivism. To treat only the biomechanical fault without regard to the pain factor can result in increased pain and a distrustful client.

If pain is the dominant factor, treatment should be initiated to ameliorate the symptoms and gain client cooperation. Therefore the noncontractile structures should be initially treated with techniques that accomplish a goal with a minimum of exacerbation. This usually entails positioning of the joint in a neutral or nonpainful range and selecting techniques that reduce inflammatory response and gait the pain. Accessory movement techniques are usually best for this approach. If the structure treated gives signs and symptoms of being irritable or severe, or the nature of the response leaves questions in the clinician's mind, modalities and rest may be initially indicated.

When movement is indicated, the clinician should begin with a small amplitude movement near the beginning of the pain-free range and progress in amplitude as the response indicates. An intermediate amount of treatment should be given in the painless range of the first visit. To determine if alteration of the symptoms has occurred, the client should be assessed after 24 hours in light of the behavior of the symptoms described in the initial examination. If the response has been positive, both subjectively and objectively, the clinician can continue with the same treatment intensity or can increase the intensity a moderate amount to assess further progress. In using mobilization movements in treatment, the technique is usually oscillatory at approximately 2 amplitudes per second for 30 seconds to 1 minute. Although this seems a minor treatment, the clinician should be cognizant that 60 to 120 repetitions of the selected technique have been performed. If the therapist were prescribing active push-ups rather than passive

movement, the client would be required to perform 60 to 120 push-ups. A workout of this intensity should rarely be increased without assessing the soreness or progress that results from the initial treatment.

If the symptoms and signs have improved, more of the same or additional passive movement can be added with assessment at each visit for progress. If there is an increase in symptoms or reduction of the range available on the second visit, the intensity of the treatment or the applicability of the technique should be reassessed and modifications should be made. In mobilization techniques the number of 60-second applications should rarely exceed four to five or 480 to 600 repetitions in one session.

If they are accomplishing an increase in range, the techniques can be increased in amplitude and/or applied further into the range in order to adequately treat the symptoms and restore movement. The rest position (position of maximum laxity) of the joint, aptly described in Kaltenborn,[34] can be used if such a position is obtainable. Otherwise a neutral position between the beginning and limit of range should be selected. If 50% to 60% of the normal available range is obtainable, the clinician can use physiological movements as treatment techniques instead of accessory movements. Treatment away from—or close to—the limit or range is predicated on the initial examination and subsequent client response.

Once pain is diminished and movement restriction becomes stiffness, Cyriax's guidelines can be incorporated.[9] If pain occurs synchronously with resistance, large-amplitude movements up to the limit are viable as a treatment. If pain occurs before the limit, neutral painless techniques are advised. If pain occurs only after engaging the resistance, then a stretching technique at the limit is indicated. If pain is elicited during the treatment session (as it will be when stretching), a large-amplitude movement in the pain-free range should be used at the end of the treatment session to gate the symptoms produced from the desired technique. This approach allows the clinician to stretch the range of motion restricted by stiffness and give the greatest change of client comfort following treatment—a factor that definitely enhances client enthusiasm for further treatment. In all protocols, the ultimate goal is a full, pain-free range of motion—a goal that should not be compromised unless surgical or other intervention prohibits it. This method of incorporating the philosophies of Maitland,[44,45] Kaltenborn,[33,34] and Cyriax[9] is a logical, rewarding treatment approach.

If the contractile elements are determined to be the problem tissue, the protocol of PRICE is advocated initially to resolve the inflammatory response. PRICE stands for:

1. Protection from further injury
2. Rest from function
3. Ice or cryotherapy

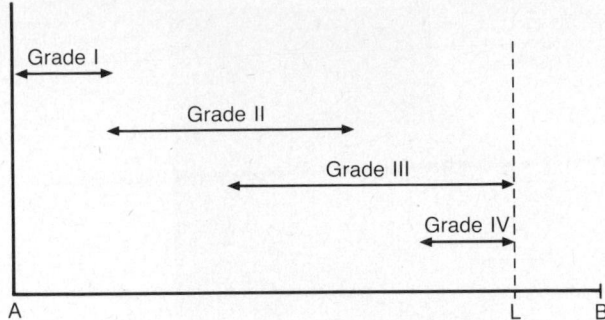

Fig. 21-14. Maitland's grades of movement.

4. Compression of the inflamed area
5. Elevation to facilitate removal of excess fluid

As the inflammatory response is controlled, the initial focus should be directed at exercise, beginning with isometrics (no joint movement). The progression is to submaximal exercise (isotonic or isokinetic); if minimal or no exacerbation of symptoms occurs, maximal exercises follow. The arc of movement should be limited initially in both submaximal and maximal exercise with progression of both to full range.

Treatment techniques

Treatment techniques are presented in two categories: passive and active resistive. Although these techniques are not all-inclusive, they should be useful in treating properly selected cases when they are applied in terms of the guidelines already presented.

Passive movement techniques*. Before applying passive techniques, the therapist should review from the examination findings the amount of movement available. In light of the guidelines on pain and resistance, the clinician should decide if pain inhibition or stretching is the intent. From the amount of movement available and the intention of treatment, the clinician can determine the amplitude of passive movement to use in treatment. Maitland[44] has delineated four grades of movement (Fig. 21-14), which are based on amplitude and the portion of the available range of motion. (See the chapters on mobility and examination for a full discussion of these four grades of movements.)

There are two kinds of passive movement techniques, physiological and accessory, which can be described by area and by kind of treatment applied.

Spinal mobilizations: lumbar and lower thoracic area.

A. *Movement:* Posteroanterior central pressure (Fig. 21-15).
   Position: Client lies prone with arms at sides. Therapist stands at client's side, placing pisiform of one hand just lateral to the spinous process of the lum-

*For more details on passive techniques, the reader is directed to Maitland.[45]

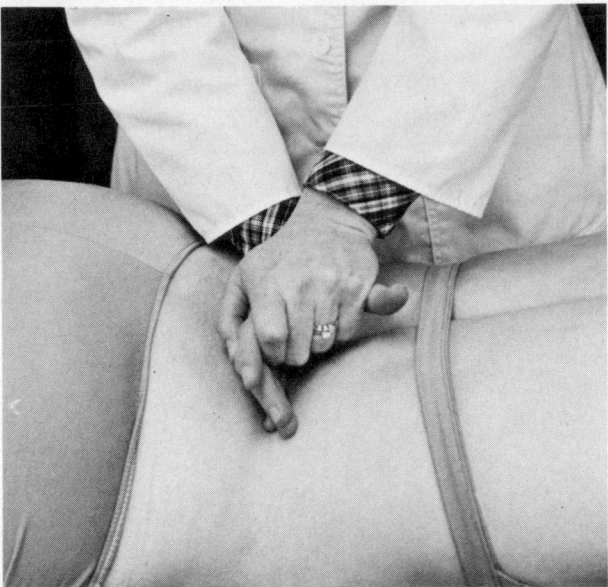

Fig. 21-15. Lumbar posteroanterior central pressure.

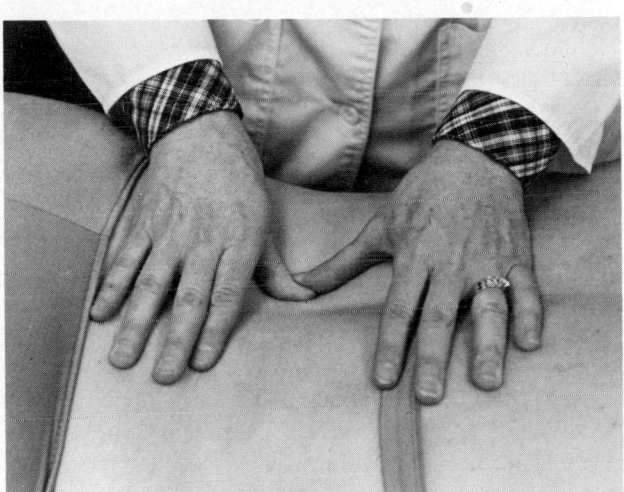

Fig. 21-16. Horizontal vertebral pressure.

bar vertebra. The wrist is extended and reinforced by the other hand. Pressure is applied directly over the spinous process.
   Procedure: The various grades of movement are applied by gradual movement of the therapist's body weight over the client's vertebral column, using oscillating movements at a rate of two per second.
   Indications: Pain that is evenly distributed.

B. *Movement:* Posteroanterior unilateral pressure (see Fig. 21-3).
   Position: Client lies prone with arms at sides. Therapists places both thumbs (back to back) over the transverse processes of the lumbar vertebra. (Because of the muscle bulk, it is difficult to feel the transverse processes in the lumbar spine.)

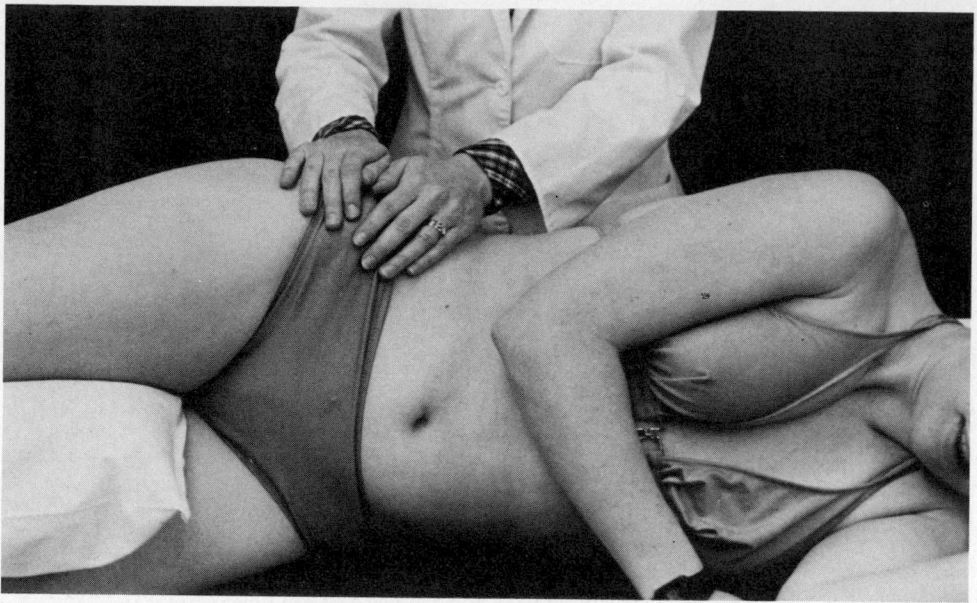

Fig. 21-17. Rotation (grades I and II).

Procedure: A posteroanterior force is applied on the transverse process by moving the therapist's body weight directly over client's vertebral column in oscillatory movements.
Indications: For use on the side of muscle spasm and pain.

C. *Movement:* Horizontal vertebral pressure (Fig. 21-16).
   Position: Client lies prone with arms at sides. Therapist faces client's side. Therapist places thumbs on the side of the spinous process.
   Procedure: A horizontal force is applied to the spinous process, using oscillatory movements. Therapist applies transverse pressure, pushing the spinous process toward the painful side, thus opening the facet on he painful side.
   Indications: Unilateral symptoms.

D. *Movement:* Rotation: grades I and II (Fig. 21-17).
   Position: Client lies on side, with painful side up, facing away from therapist. Therapist flexes client's knees and hips to place desired vertebral level in midposition. Client's trunk is in a neutral position. Client's upper arm, in grade I position, is flexed to 90 degrees at elbow and placed along the chest, with the hand on the plinth. In grade II movement, the therapist's arm is comfortably extended with the forearm resting on the client's side. Therapist grips the anterior superior iliac spine (ASIS) and the buttocks to apply movement.
   Procedure: A rotation force is applied through the pelvis by a posteroanterior movement.
   Indications: Unilateral symptoms.

E. *Movement:* Rotation: grades III and IV (Fig. 21-18).
   Position: Client lies on pain-free side, bottom leg extended, foot off the edge of the plinth. The upper leg is flexed and extended to position the desired vertebral level in midposition. The trunk is rotated to the desired level, and client's upper arm is extended. The elbow is flexed, and the forearm rests comfortably on the client's side.
   Procedure: The rotational force is applied by a posteroanterior pressure to the client's pelvis, with a counterforce applied to the client's shoulder.
   Indications: Same as rotation grades I and II.

F. *Movement:* Unilateral manual traction (Fig. 21-19).
   Position: Client lies supine. Therapist stands at client's side, facing his/her feet. Grasping the ankle, therapist raises it off the plinth, flexing and extending the hip to the neutral position for the pelvis.
   Procedure: Therapist applies a graded force in the caudal direction.
   Indications: Unilateral symptoms with origin below L-4. (For more detail, the reader is directed to Maitland.[45]

Spinal mobilizations: Cervical spine and upper thoracic area.

A. *Movement:* Manual traction (Fig. 21-20).
   Position: client lies supine, neck level with the plinth. Therapist supports client's occiput with right hand, then comfortably grasps client's chin with the left hand, laying the forearm long the side of client's face.
   Procedure: A traction force is applied through ther-

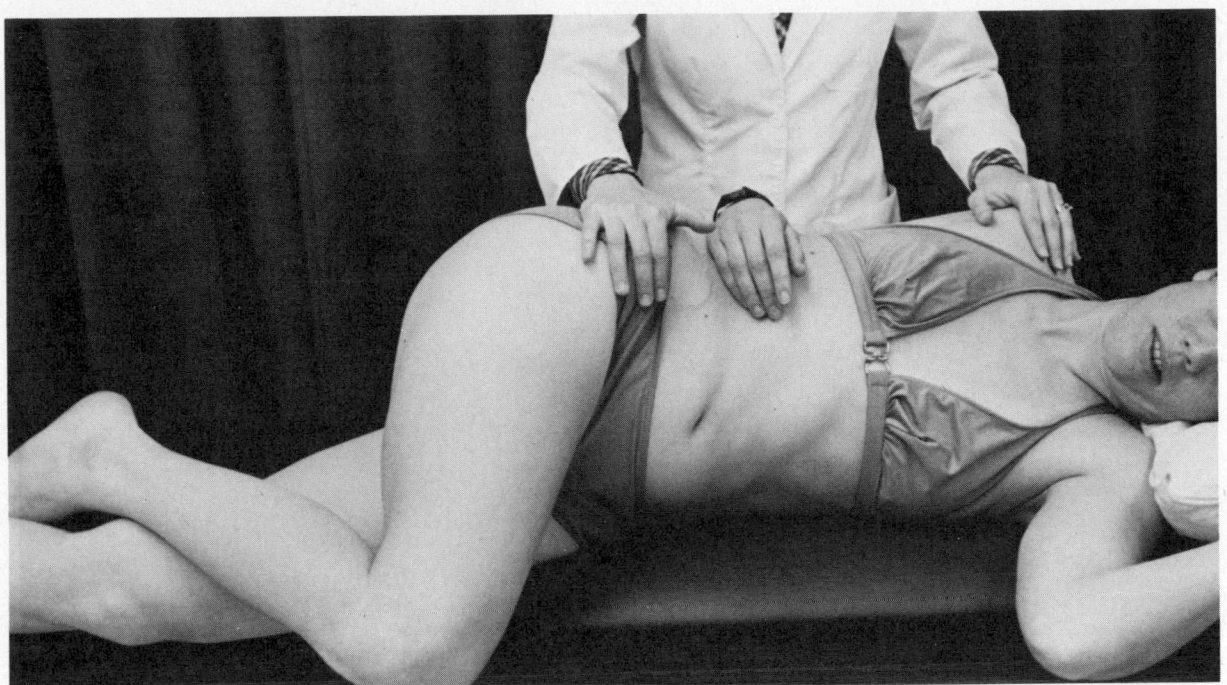

Fig. 21-18. Rotation (grades III and IV).

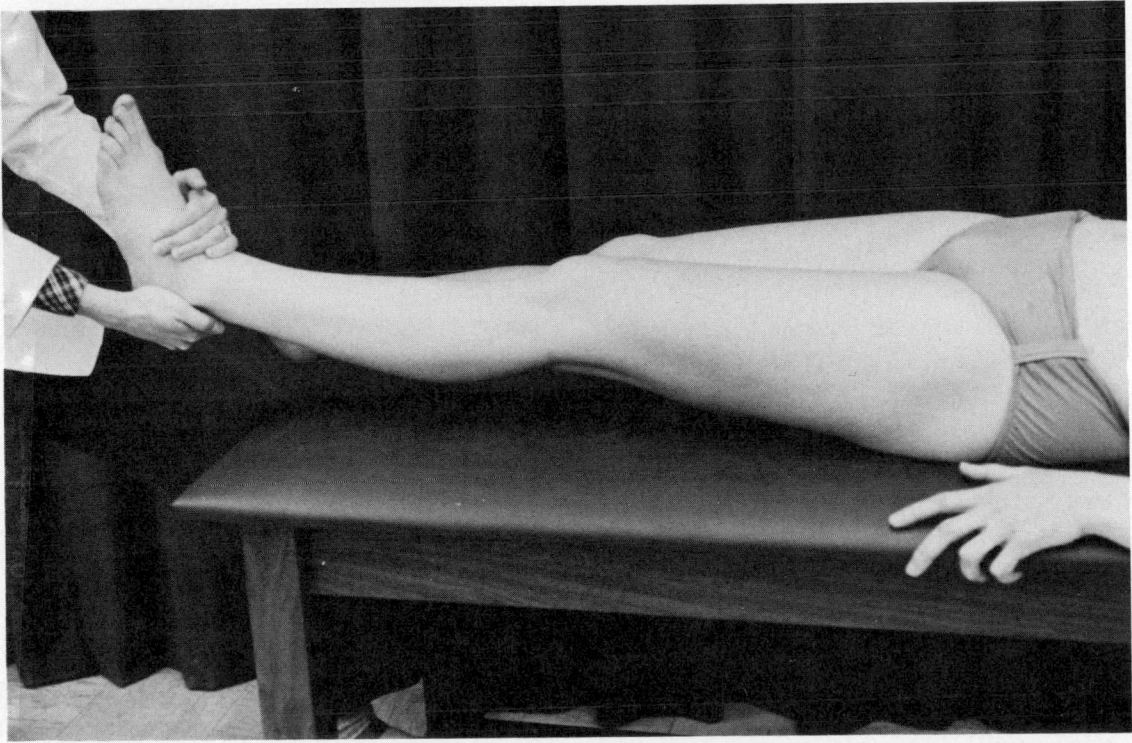

Fig. 21-19. Unilateral manual traction.

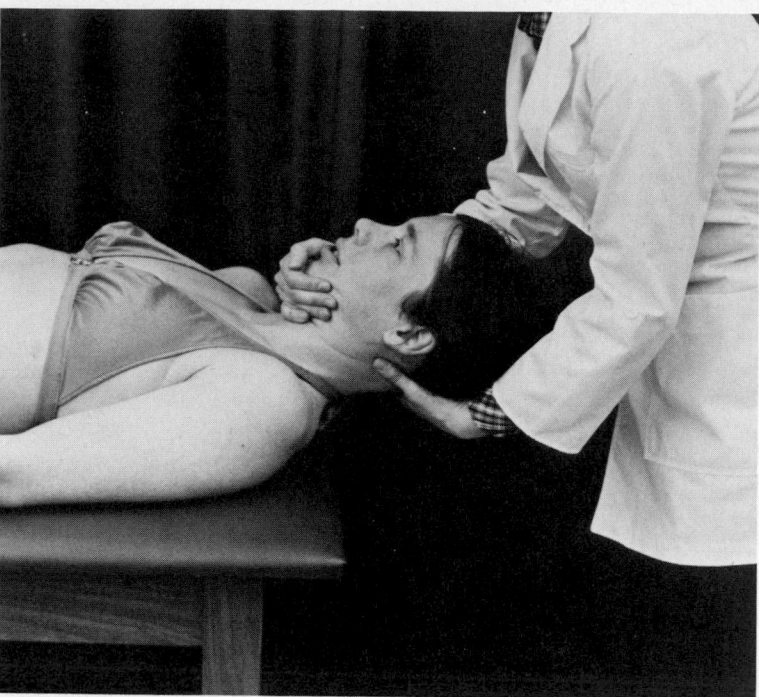

Fig. 21-20. Manual cervical traction.

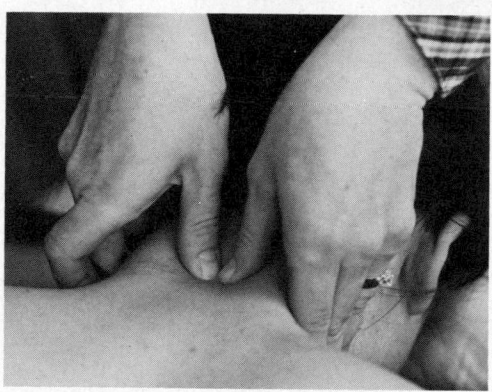

Fig. 21-21. Posteroanterior cervical central pressure.

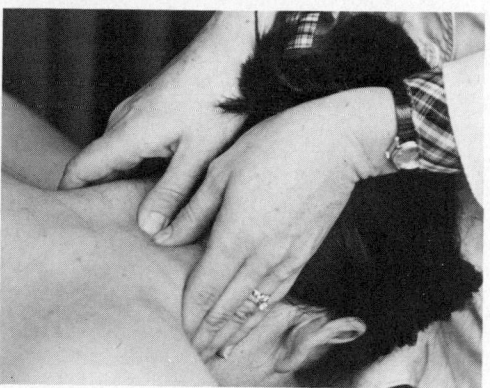

Fig. 21-22. Posteroanterior unilateral cervical pressure.

apist's hands with slight backward movement of therapist's body followed by an equal relaxation.
Indications: This is a good initial treatment to test and treat a client with an acute cervical complaint. It is also very useful in treatment of torticollis.

B. *Movement:* Posteroanterior central pressure (Fig. 21-21).
Position: Client lies prone, forehead cradled in hands. Therapist stands at client's head, placing both thumbs on spinous process of desired cervical vertebra. Therapist's fingers are spread along sides of client's neck to stabilize thumb positions.
Procedure: Therapist applies a graded pressure through the thumbs in an anterior direction. NOTE: Use gentle pressures in the neck as therapist-felt

sensation is different from client-felt sensation. The tendency is for the therapist to apply too much pressure.
Indications: Central pain.

C. *Movement:* Posteroanterior unilateral pressure (Fig. 21-22).
Position: Same as preceding except on the articular pillars.
Procedures: Same as preceding, applying unilateral pressure on he side of the pain.
Indications: Unilateral symptoms.

D. *Movement:* Transverse pressure to the atlas (Fig. 21-23).
Position: Client lies prone with head turned to side. Therapist's thumbs are placed on tip of the lateral

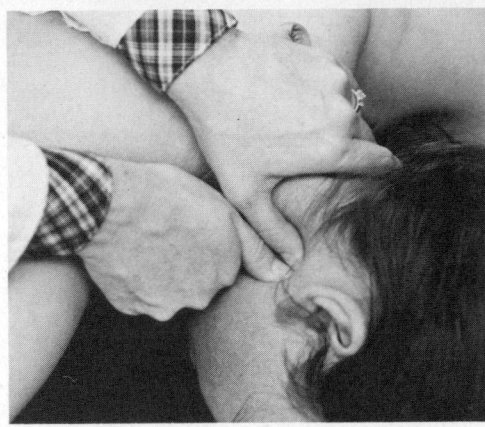

Fig. 21-23. Transverse pressure to atlas.

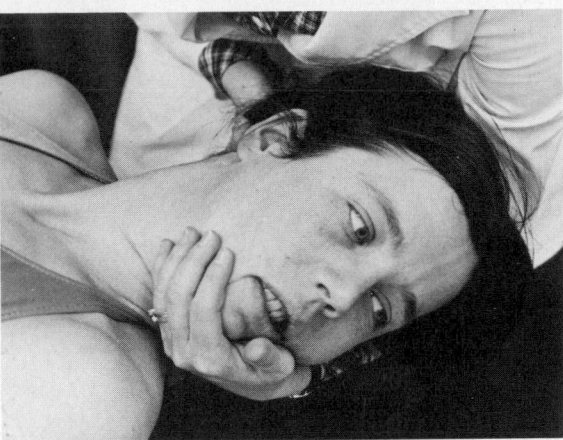

Fig. 21-25. Cervical rotation (grades III and IV).

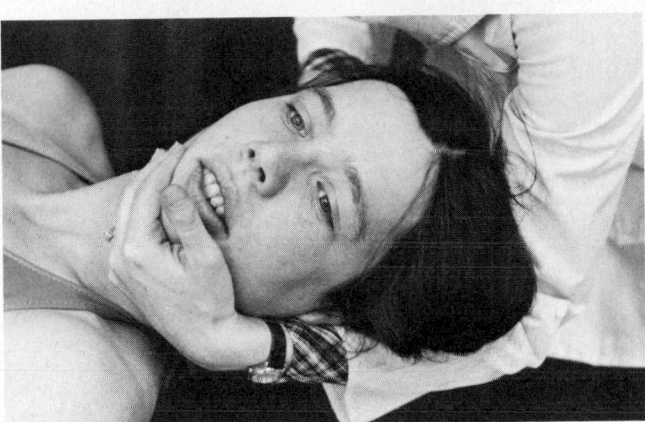

Fig. 21-24. Cervical rotation (grades I and II).

mass. (This is found just below the mastoid process and near the angle of the jaw.) Therapist's fingers are spread to stabilize.

Procedure: Gentle oscillatory pressure is applied through the thumbs.

Indications: Upper cervical pain: pain-free side if unilateral; both sides if bilateral.

E. *Movement:* Cervical rotation: grades I and II (Fig. 21-24).

Position: Client lies supine, head and neck extended beyond edge of plinth. Standing at client's head, therapist cradles the neck and occiput. Therapist then comfortably grasps client's chin with one hand, forearm lying alongside face.

Procedure: Therapist stands at client's head, facing the feet, and rotates head in direction toward the hand holding the chin. Therapist moves both hands equally, creating a rotation force of the head on the neck. NOTE: Always rotate away from painful side.

Indications: Unilateral neck symptoms.

F. *Movement:* Cervical rotation: grade III (Fig. 21-25).

Position: Same as preceding, except that the hand holding the occiput is moved laterally toward the hand holding the chin. The tip of the middle finger is placed in the client's are for better hold. Therapist stands at almost a 90-degree angle to the neck, forearm cradling the head.

Procedure: Same as preceding.

Indications: Same as preceding.

Traction. Traction is a technique that is used in many treatment programs. The forces applied vary from a few pounds to 400 to 700 pounds as advocated by Frazier.[16] Grieve[24] presents the following guidelines for using traction as a treatment technique.

Initial traction for the cervical spine should be 8 to 15 lbs, based on palpation of the desired vertebral level for movement. The length of sustained traction application should be 5 minutes, followed by 15 minutes of rest. (If mechanical traction of the head is being used, the head halter should not be removed since lifting of the head will compress the vertebral interspace.) Intermittent traction can be applied for 10 minutes, but, at the start, long holds and short relax periods are recommended. As symptoms and signs improve, both the hold and the relax time can be decreased.

The first application of lumbar traction should be a trial procedure using 30 pounds. This trial traction can sense whether a phenomenon known as the *imbibition phenomenon* is present. Clients exhibiting this phenomenon have a nucleus pulposus gel composition that imbibes (takes on) water from the vertebral body very quickly and will do this during the short traction period. Then when the client rises and weight is applied to the disk, this fluid is released, putting great pressure on the annulus and increasing the client's symptoms. Therefore 30 lbs of traction will create a small amount of imbibition and increased symptoms, although not enough to debilitate the client. If the phenomenon is present, traction should not be applied. The 30-lb trial should be applied for 5 minutes, but no rest following

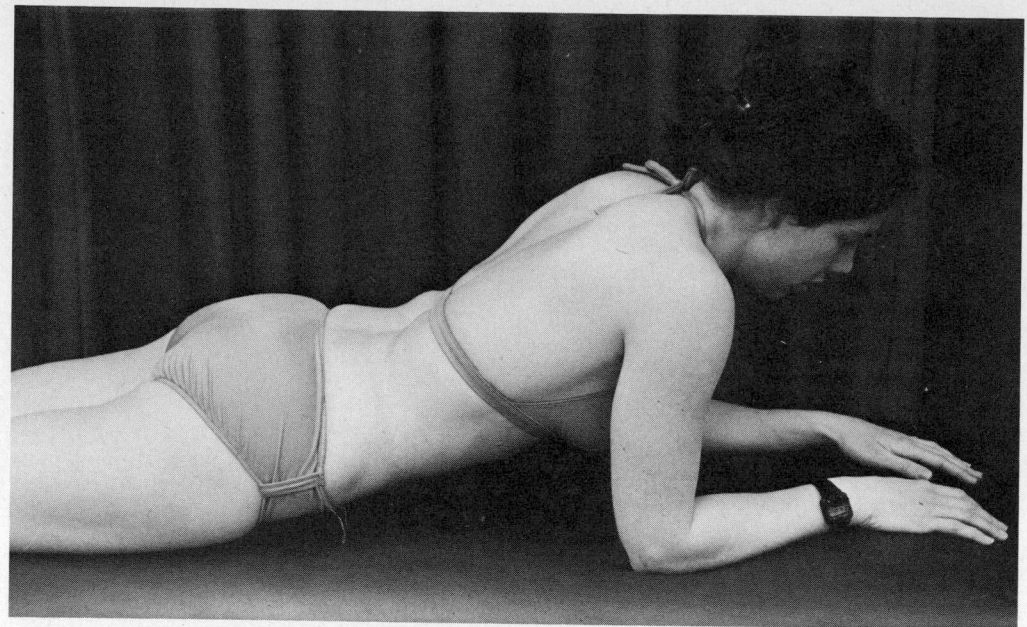

Fig. 21-26. Prone on elbows.

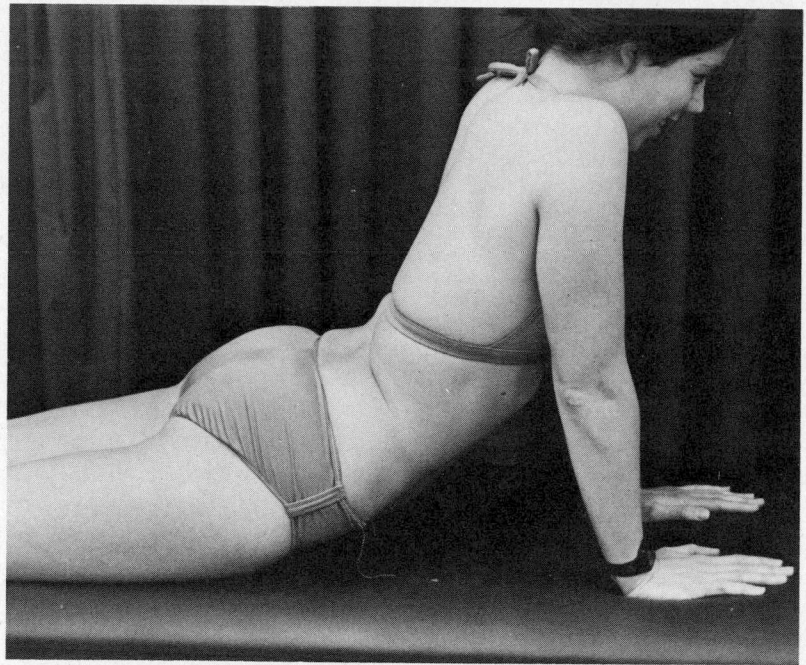

Fig. 21-27. Prone press-up.

Table 21-4. Guidelines for the application of traction

Symptoms	Signs	Duration	Weight
Improved	Improved	Same as initial traction	Keep the same as previous treatment
Unchanged	Unchanged	Increase by 5 minutes	Increase by 5 pounds
Improved	Unchanged	Increase by 5 minutes	Keep the same as previous treatment
Same	Improved	Increase by 5 minutes	Keep the same as previous treatment
Worse	Same	Keep the same as previous treatment	Decrease weight by half
Same	Worse	Keep the same as previous treatment	Decrease weight by half
Worse	Worse	Decrease time by half	Decrease weight by half

Modified from Grieve G: Common vertebral joint problems, London, 1981, Churchill Livingstone, Inc.

CONCAVE MOVING ON CONVEX

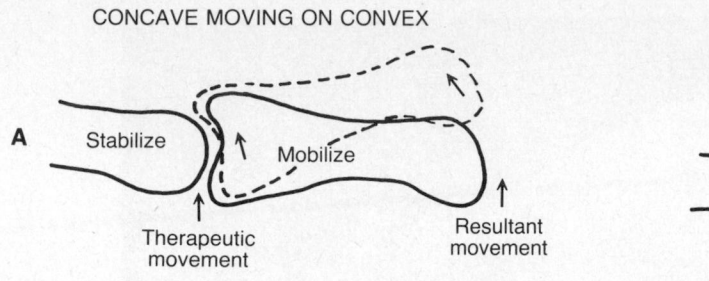

CONVEX MOVING ON CONCAVE

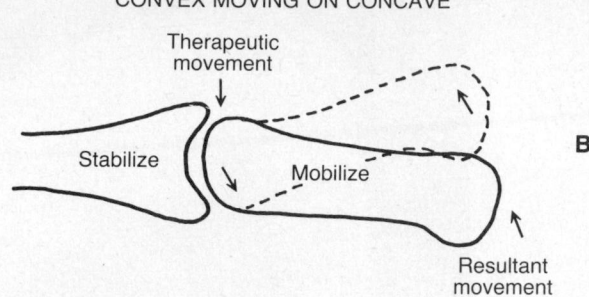

Fig. 21-28. Joint relationships. **A,** Concave on convex. **B,** Convex on concave.

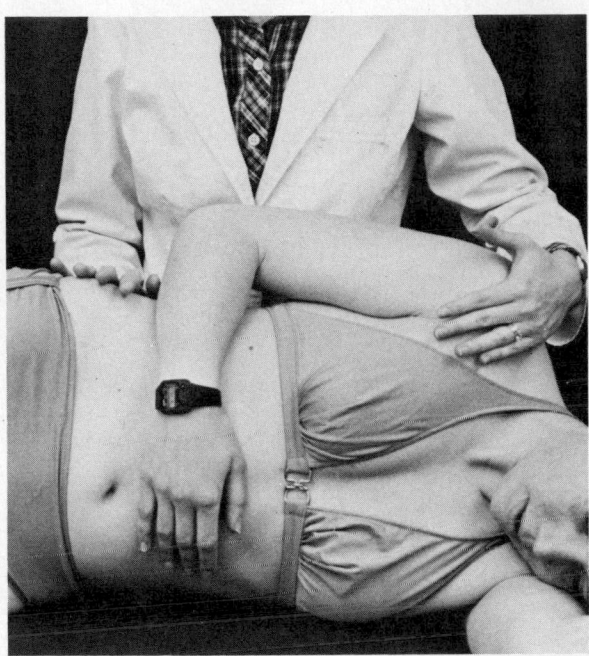

Fig. 21-29. Rhythmical stabilization for muscle strengthening of back with acute pain.

treatment is necessary. On the second visit the traction on a client not exhibiting the imbibition phenomenon can be increased to 45 to 80 lbs, depending on the client's actual body weight. I find that poundage equal to half or more of the client's body weight is often necessary. All weights indicated are for friction-free table application; if not friction free, then one eighth of the body weight must be added to overcome friction.

On subsequent visits for treatment of the cervical area, the poundage can be increased by 3- to 5-lb increments and the time increased in 5-minute increments if indicated. In the lumbar spine increases in weight are accomplished in 5- to 10-lb increments, and the time is increased in 5-minute blocks.

When a client returns after the first treatment, the decision to increase, decrease, or leave the traction constant is based on he client's response to previous treatment (Table 21-4).

Spinal exercises: lumbar. When applying exercises to the spine, the clinician should take into consideration both the examination findings and treatment goals. If the client has a restriction of extension with stiffness being the dominant limiting factor, the following progression of exercises can be considered.

Physiological movements. The client is positioned prone on elbows, progressing to a prone press-up.[46,47] These two activities work to increase extension, but the pelvis should be kept on the mat surface and relaxed. This adds a traction aspect to the extension movement, which to some extent reduces intradiskal pressure and bulging of the posterior annular fibers into the vertebral foramen (Figs. 21-26 and 21-27).

Accessory movements. Grade IV central pressure on spinous process and unilateral pressure on the transverse process can be used (see Figs. 21-3 and 21-15). The pressures should be applied to the superior vertebra of the involved vertebral segment because of the convex-on-concave relationships of the facet surfaces (Figs. 21-28 and 21-29).

Active movement techniques. Once passive movement has been instituted to increase the range of motion, active exercises should be added, as signs and symptoms allow, to facilitate smooth, reliable control of the increased movement. A decision should be made as to whether mobility or stability is desired. If stability is desired, then isometrics should be instituted, progressing to isotonics and isokinetics as mobility is added. If mobility is desired, then isokinetics and isotonics should be started, with isometrics at various points in the range of motion to increase strength (multiple-angle isometrics).

Stability exercises. There are three main stability exercises that can be performed by the client.

Isometric abdominal stabilization. The client can contract the trunk musculature isometrically, being sure to breathe to decrease the influence of intraabdominal pressure. This can be done by the client throughout the day.

Rhythmic stabilization. The *hold and hold* proprioceptive neuromuscular facilitation (PNF) command should be used while the clinician applies equal but opposite force on the pelvis and shoulder. The client's trunk should not

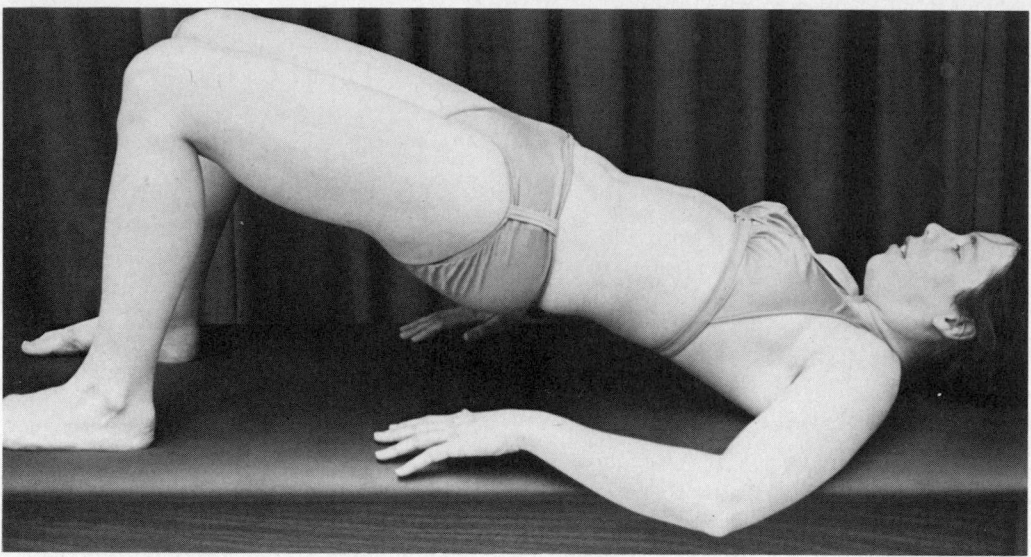

Fig. 21-30. Bridging.

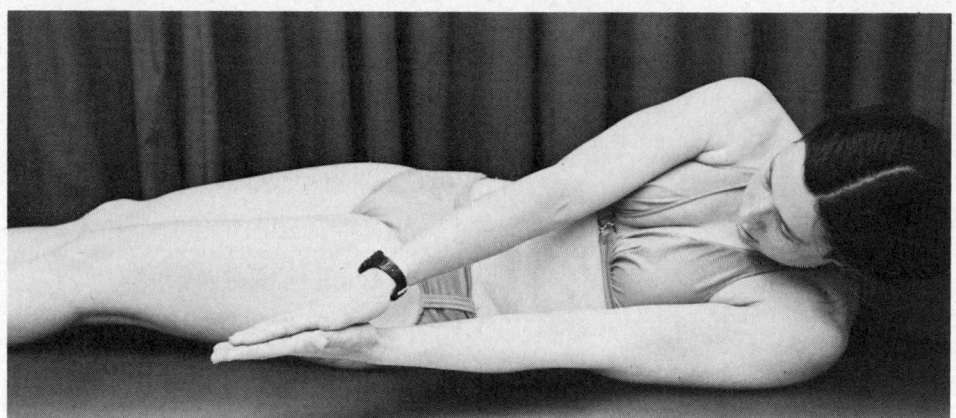

Fig. 21-31. Trunk twist.

move; if it does, the clinician is overpowering the client (see Fig. 21-29).

Bridging. The client should flex the hips and knees to a comfortable footflat position and lift the buttocks up from the surface as far as in pain-free. This activates the extensor muscles of the back and legs, with the client controlling the movement (Fig. 21-30).

Mobility exercises: trunk strengthening. Trunk strengthening can be accomplished by exercises involving the trunk or the legs.

Trunk twist. Active abdominal strengthening is best accomplished via an exercise called a *trunk twist.* This activity is used to actively involve all components of the abdominal group. The client places the palms together with elbows straight. The upper body and arms are rotated and flexed overhead. The upper extremities are brought down through a diagonal to the opposite hip. The client's shoulder and head should rise only to the point where the infe-

rior angle of the scapular comes off the mat surface (Fig. 21-31).

Prone leg lifts. Initial extensor strengthening is started in the prone position with one or two pillows under the pelvis. To avoid active lumbar hyperextension, straight-leg extension is performed, one leg at a time, only to the horizontal position. This exercise can progress to the client positioned prone over a table with the trunk supported and legs over the edge. The legs are lifted bilaterally to horizontal and then returned to the flexed position (Fig. 21-32).

With increased tolerance and decreased irritability, the client can progress to strength, power, and endurance extensor training. At that point, occupational or athletic requirements must be taken into consideration so that rehabilitation can be directed toward the demands of the client's life-style. In the near future, use of velocity specific isokinetic equipment will enable health professionals to

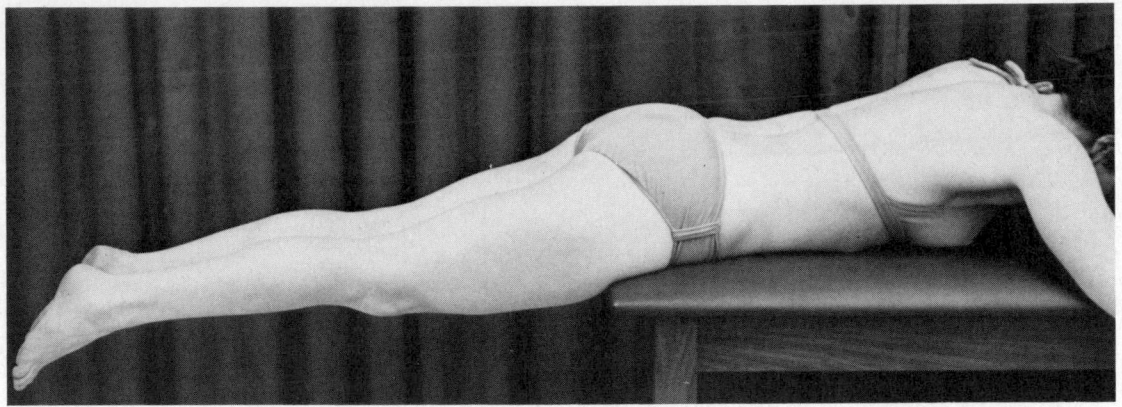

Fig. 21-32. Bilateral leg lifts.

test and rehabilitate the trunk for the demands placed on it by the individual.

Trunk muscle strengthing can continue using resistive exercises with PNF or Isokinetic exercise equipment to assess the strength and to increase it. A review of the literature on isokinetic testing is found in an article by Beimborn and Morrissey.[3]

Spinal exercises: cervical. The application of exercise to the cervical spine tends to be more difficult because of the different characteristics of the typical vertebrae C-3 to C-7 versus the atypical upper cervical group (occiput to C-2). Gross applications of stability and mobility activities can follow the guidelines described for the lumbar area.

Stability exercises. Isometrics performed supine, standing, or sitting can begin by manually applied resistance while the head and neck are in a neutral position. Rhythmical stabilization exercises can also be persued.

Mobility exercises. Routines can follow planar range of motion with resistance applied manually or by simply designing concentric or eccentric gravity-resisted movements. PNF diagonals encourage mobility and strengthening through functional patterns.

Isometric endurance exercises to the anterior, posterior, and lateral cervical muscle groups can be reinforced by horizontal positioning, eliminating head support as a concomitant activity, or by having the client lean against a wall in the appropriate positions for extended periods of time.

SUMMARY

The spine consists of 24 mobile segments with 23 disks and 48 facet joints along with numerous muscle attachment sites. Each area of movement has the potential for dysfunction, so it is essential that clinicians working with spinal problems have a firm anatomical background and the ability to examine each aspect and to treat each component with techniques based on sound physiological principles. This chapter cannot encompass the total of all areas but attempts to give a basis for clinical understanding and informed treatment of spinal conditions.

REFERENCES

1. Andersson G: Epidemiologic aspects on low-back pain in industry, Spine 6:60, 1981.
2. Attix EA and Tate MA: Low back school: a conservative method for treatment of low back pain, J Orthop Sports Phys Ther 1:4, 1979.
3. Beimborn DS and Morrissey MC: A Review of the Literature Related to Trunk Muscle Performance, Spine 13(6):655, 1988.
4. Bogduk N and Macintosh JE: The applied anatomy of the thoracolumbar fascia, Spine 9:164-170, 1984.
5. Bogduk N and Twomey LT: Clinical Anatomy of the Lumbar Spine, New York, 1987, Churchill-Livingstone, Inc.
6. Bradley KC: The posterior primary rami of segmental nerves. In Idczak RM, editor: Aspects of manipulative therapy, Carlton, Victoria, Austria, 1980, Lincoln Institute of Health Sciences.
7. Breig A and Troup JDG: Biomechanical considerations in the straight-leg-raising test, Spine 4(3):242, 1979.
8. Carr D et al: Lumbar Paraspinal Compartment Syndrome, Spine 10(9):816, 1985.
9. Cyriax J: Textbook of orthopaedic medicine, vol 1, Baltimore, 1969, Williams & Wilkins.
10. Dixon ASJ: Diagnosis of low back pain. In Jayson M, editor: The lumbar spine and back pain, New York, 1976, Grune & Stratton, Inc.
11. England R: The cervical spine: some clinical and practical considerations, JAOA 71:129, 1971.
12. Farfan HG: Mechanical disorders of the low back, Philadelphia, 1973, Lea & Febiger.
13. Farfan HF: The biomechanical advantage of lordosis and hip extension for upright activity, Spine 3(4):336, 1978.
14. Finneson BE: Low back pain, ed 2, Philadelphia, 1980, JB Lippincott Co.
15. Floyd WF and Silver PAS: The function of the erector spinae muscle in certain movements and postures in man, Physiology 129:184, 1955.
16. Frazier EH: The use of traction in backache, Med J Aust 2:694, 1954.
17. Friberg, S and Hirsch C: Anatomical and clinical studies on lumbar disc degeneration, Acta Orthop Scand 19:222, 1949.
18. Fullenlove TM and Williams AJ: Comparative roentgen findings in symptomatic and asymptomatic backs, Radiology 68:572, 1957.
19. Geden LC: A comparison of biomechanical factors in weight bearing in the lumbar and cervical spine. In Idczak RM, editor: Aspects of

manipulative therapy, Carlton, Victoria, Austria, 1980, Lincoln Institute of Health Sciences.

20. Giles LGF and Taylor JR: Intra-articular synovial protrusions in the lower lumbar apophyseal joints, Bull Hosp Joint Dis 42(2):248, 1982.

21. Gilula L: Degenerative disease and injury of the back, Occup Health Saf 50(1):14, 1981.

22. Gracovetsky S, Farfan HF, and Helleur C: The abdominal mechanism, Spine 10:317-324, 1985.

23. Grieve GP: Manipulation therapy for neck pain, Physiotherapy 65:136, 1979.

24. Grieve GP: Common vertebral joint problems, London, 1981, Churchill Livingstone, Inc.

25. Grieve G: Modern manual therapy of the vertebral column, Edinburgh, 1986, Churchill Livingstone, Inc.

26. Hall MC: Lushkna's joint, Springfield, Ill, 1965, Charles C Thomas, Publisher.

27. Hamilton WJ, editor: Textbook of human anatomy, ed 2, St Louis, 1976, The CV Mosby Co.

28. Happy F: A biophysical study of the human intervertebral disc. In Jayson M, editor: The lumbar spine and back pain, New York, 1976, Grune & Stratton, Inc.

29. Hendry NGC: The hydration of the nucleus pulposus and its relation to intervertebral disc derangement, J Bone Joint Surg (Br) 40:132, 1958.

30. Inman VT et al: Human walking, Baltimore, 1981, Williams & Wilkins.

31. Jackson R: The cervical syndrome, ed 4, Springfield, Ill, 1977, Charles C Thomas, Publisher.

32. Jayson M, editor: The lumbar spine and back pain, New York, 1976, Grune & Stratton, Inc.

33. Katlenborn FM: Manual therapy for the extremity joints, Oslo, Norway, 1976, Olaf Norlis Bokhandel.

34. Kaltenborn F: Test segmenti mobilis columna vertebris, Oslo, Norway, 1975, Freddy Kaltenborn, Publisher.

35. Kapandji IA: The physiology of the joints, vol 3, ed 2, London, 1974, Churchill Livingstone, Inc.

36. Kessler RM and Hertling D: Management of common musculoskeletal disorders, Philadelphia, 1983, Harper & Row, Publishers Inc.

37. Kos J and Wolff J: Intervertebral menisci and their possible role in intervertebral blockage, Bull Orthop Section APTA, 1(3):8, Winter 1976.

38. Kvien TK et al: Education and self care of patients with low back pain, Scand J Rheumatol 4(10):318, 1981.

39. LaBan MM et al: Electromyographic study of function of iliopsoas muscle, Arch Phys Med Rehabil 46:676, 1965.

40. Luk L: The iliolumbar ligament: A study of its anatomy, development, and clinical significance, JBJS, 68.

41. MacConaill MA and Basmajian JV: Muscles and movement, Baltimore, 1969, Williams & Wilkins.

42. MacNab I: Backache, Baltimore, 1977, Williams & Wilkins.

43. Maigne R: Orthopedic medicine, Springfield, Ill, 1972, Charles C Thomas, Publisher.

44. Maitland GD: Peripheral manipulation, ed 2, Woburn, Mass, 1977, Butterworth Publishers.

45. Maitland GD: Vertebral manipulation, ed 4, Woburn, Mass, 1977, Butterworth Publishers.

46. McKenzie RA: The lumbar spine: mechanical diagnosis and therapy, Waikanae, New Zealand, 1981, Spinal Publications.

47. McKenzie R: Treat your own back, Waikanae, New Zealand, 1980, Spinal Publications.

48. McMinn RMH and Hutchings RT: Color atlas of human anatomy, Chicago, 1977, Year Book Medical Publishers, Inc.

49. Mooney V and Robertson J: The facet syndrome, Clin Orthop 115:149, 1976.

50. Mykelbust JB et al: Tensile strength of spinal ligaments, Spine 13(5):526, 1988.

51. Nachemson A: Lumbar intradiscal pressure, Acta Orthop Scand Suppl 43:122-147, 1960.

52. Naylor A: Intervertebral disc prolapse and degeneration, Spine, 1:108, 1976.

53. Netter FH: The CIBA collection of medical illustrations, vol 1, Nervous system, Summit, NJ, 1972, CIBA Medical Education Division.

54. Park WM: Radiological investigation of the intervertebral disc. In Jayson M, editor: The lumbar spine and back pain, New York, 1976, Grune & Stratton, Inc.

55. Peck D, Nicholls PJ, and Beard C: Are there compartment syndromes in some patients with idiopathic back pain? Spine, 11:468-475, 1986.

56. Rogoff JB: Manipulation, traction, and massage, ed 2, Baltimore, 1980, Williams & Wilkins.

57. Rothman RH and Simeone FA: The spine, vol 1, Philadelphia, 1975, WB Saunders Co.

58. Rothman RH and Simone FA: The spine, vol 2, Philadelphia, 1975, WB Saunders Co.

59. Rubin D: Cervical radiculitis: diagnosis and treatment, Arch Phys Med Rehabil 41:580, 1960.

60. Saunders HD: Classification of musculoskeletal spinal conditions, J Orthop Sports Phys Ther 1:3, 1979.

61. Schultz AB and Andersson GB: Analysis of loads on the lumbar spine, Spine 6(1):76, 1981.

62. Simon G: Drug therapy in the management of back pain, Occup Health Saf 1:10, 1981.

63. Stoddard A: Manual of osteopathic practice, New York, 1969, Harper & Row Publishers, Inc.

64. Strachan A: Back care in industry, Physiotherapy 65(8):249, 1979.

65. Tesh D, Dunn L, and Evans J: The abdominal muscles and vertebral stability, Spine, 12:501–508, 1987.

66. Torgerson WR and Dotler WE: Comparative roentgenographic study of the asymptomatic and symptomatic lumbar spine, J Bone Joint Surg (Am) 58(6):850, 1976.

67. Troup JDC et al: Back pain in industry, Spine 6(1):61, 1981.

68. Valtonen EJ et al: Comparative radiographic study of the effect of intermittent and continuous traction on elongation of the cervical spine, Ann Med Interne 57:143, 1968.

69. Vernon-Roberts B: Pathology of degenerative spondylosis. In Jayson M, editor: The lumbar spine and back pain, New York, 1976, Grune & Stratton, Inc.

70. Warwick R and Williams P: Gray's anatomy, ed 35, (Br), Philadelphia, 1973, WB Saunders Co.

71. Williams PC: Low back and neck pain, Springfield, Ill, 1974, Charles C Thomas, Publisher.

72. Wolf S et al: Normative data on low back mobility and activity levels, Am J Phys Med 58(5):217, 1979.

73. Wyke B: Neurological aspects of low back pain. In Jayson M, editor: The lumbar spine and back pain, New York, 1976, Grune & Stratton, Inc.

74. Wyke B: Articular neurology and manipulative therapy. In Idczak RM, editor: Aspects of manipulative therapy, Carlton, Victoria, Austria, 1980, Lincoln Institute of Health Sciences.

75. Yates A: Treatment of back pain. In Jayson M, editor: The lumbar spine and back pain, New York, 1976, Grune & Stratton, Inc.

76. Zachrisson-Forssell M: The back school, Spine 6(1):104, 1981.

Chapter 22

THE SACROILIAC JOINT

James Allen Porterfield
Carl DeRosa

The hub of weight bearing in the human body for both static and dynamic activities is the lumbopelvic region. It is a key region of extraordinary stability, since the trunk and ground forces converge in this region. The two sacroiliac joints form an integral part of this lumbopelvic unit.

The lumbopelvic region consists of seven bones (the fourth and fifth lumbar vertebrae, the right and left innominate, the sacrum, and two femurs), six synovial joints (the related four apophyseal joints of the last two lumbar vertebrae and the sacrum and the two hip joints), two joints of synovial and fibrous makeup (sacroiliac joints), and one amphiarthrodial joint (the pubic symphysis).

The pelvis is a stable system of joints maintained by extremely strong ligaments.[16] The normal physiological movements of this region are influenced by lumbar and hip joint mechanics. Abnormal or asymmetrical forces reaching the hip or lumbar area are ultimately translated to the pelvis and render the weight-bearing joints vulnerable to injury.[9] Until the progression of forces to the pelvis from-

above and below are evaluated, a client may not respond favorably to treatment.

Considerable effort has been expended to study and quantify the normal range of movement of the sacroiliac joints* Mitchell[29] suggests that the ilium rotates in a posterior direction at heel strike and progresses in an anterior direction as the individual passes through the stance phase. He describes the movement of the sacrum on the ilium as occurring around three horizontal axes. Weisl[45] has a different view. He identifies different axes around which the sacrum and ilium move and estimates approximately 6 degrees of movement at the sacroiliac joint. Colachis et al[5] have suggested a 5 mm translation between the ilium and the sacrum. Most recently, Sturesson et al [40] have suggested that these estimates of normal sacroiliac joint mobility are most likely overestimated.

Forces reaching the sacrum are governed by movements and forces directed from the so called *trunk forces* (Fig. 22-1). The innominate bones are also governed by forces reaching them via the lower extremities, the *ground forces* (Fig. 22-2). These forces are attenuated through the nine joints, bones, and soft tissue of the lumbopelvic region. When the forces that reach the pelvis are normal and symmetrical, the lumbopelvic region becomes stressed within the limits of physiological tolerances. However, when these forces exceed the normal physiological adaptive capacity of its tissues, a chronic, painful condition can re-

We wish to acknowledge the assistance of Valory Murray, Ph.D., and Diane Winters, P.T., in the editing of this chapter; the staff of the Library and Media Center of Akron City Hospital, Steve King for modeling for the pictures, and Rajena Quinn for manuscript preparation.

*See references 4, 5, 7, 8, 12, 16, 23, 25, 26, 28, 29, 34, 38, 37, 40, and 45.

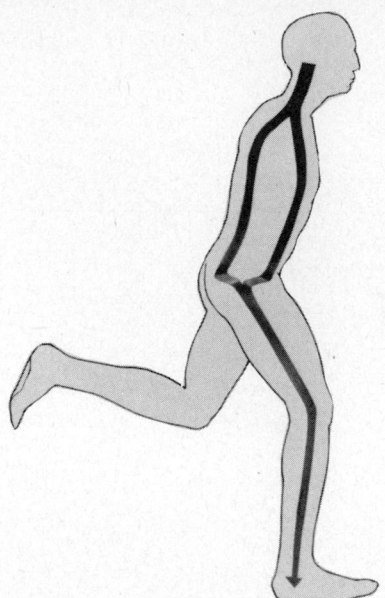

Fig. 22-1. Inferior progression of the superior trunk forces.

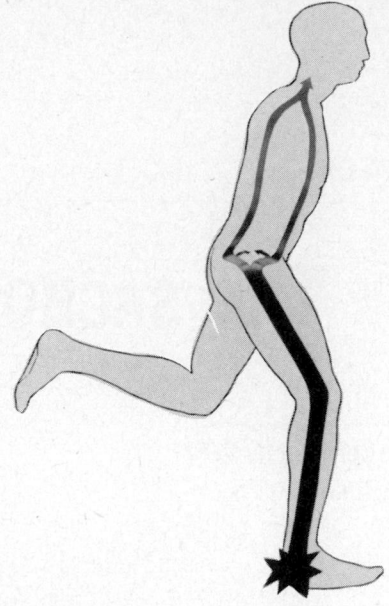

Fig. 22-2. Superior progression of the ground forces in the closed kinetic chair.

sult.[6,27] The exact mechanism of this lesion has been quite controversial.

The theories include everything from iliac rotation lesions and hip rotational imbalances to pelvic subluxations. To date, the technology necessary to measure the exact mechanism has not been refined enough to differentiate these lesions. It is also unlikely that only one tissue is involved in the painful syndrome. Therefore identification of the exact lesion is not pertinent to the proper management of continued pain in this region. The overall key appears to lie in (1) determining the weight-bearing pattern of the sacroiliac (lumbopelvic) region from above and below that results in the familiar pain of sacroiliac dysfunction, (2) assessing the status of the injured tissues, and (3) intervening with the proper treatment protocols that maximize the body's healing processes.

The purpose of this chapter is to provide a comprehensive overview of the sacroiliac joint's tissues and biomechanics, as well as concepts of evaluation and treatment. This overview is aimed at assisting the clinician in identifying the forces that are potentially destructive to the lumbopelvic tissues.

LUMBOPELVIC ANATOMY
Lumbar vertebrae and pelvis

Study of the osteology of the lumbopelvic region begins with attention to the vertebrae. The body of the vertebrae is composed of cancellous bone perfused with blood and surrounded by a cortical shell. The body of the L-5 vertebrae is the largest in the spine; it is here that weight from the trunk is transmitted to the pelvic via the sacrum.

Normal transference of trunk force from the standing

position creates a flexion force on the sacrum around a horizontal axis. The location of this axis has been described by many,[5,12,29,45] although most agree the axis occurs at the intersection of the cranial and caudal portions of the sacroiliac articular surface.

The left and right innominate bones are composed of the fusion of three segments: ilium, ischium, and pubis. These bones provide four surface projections that can serve as landmarks for palpation. These projections are the anterior superior iliac spine, the iliac crest, the posterior superior iliac spine, and the pubic tubercle.

The sacrum is a mass of irregularly shaped bone formed by the fusion of five sacral vertebrae and perforated by four pairs of neuroforamina. Solonen[38] has found that approximately 87% of the articular surface of the sacroiliac joint is formed by the S-1, S-2, and S-3 segments. The sacrum is wider superiorly than inferiorly and broader anteriorly than posteriorly. Its overall shape roughly resembles a truncated pyramid, with the base located superiorly and anteriorly.

The sacrum articulates at its apex with three coccyx bones that result in the terminal portion of the spine. The posterior aspect of the sacrum includes bony landmarks that can also be used for palpation. These include the sacral hiatus, the sacral cornu, and the spinous processes of the sacral vertebrae (Fig. 22-3).

The body of S-1 articulates with the body of L-5 via the lumbar intervertebral disk, facilitating the transmission of weight from the trunk to the pelvis. Posteriorly, the apophyseal joints link the two segments. The plane of the apophyseal joints between L-5 and S-1 varies between individuals and can also be asymmetrical when comparing

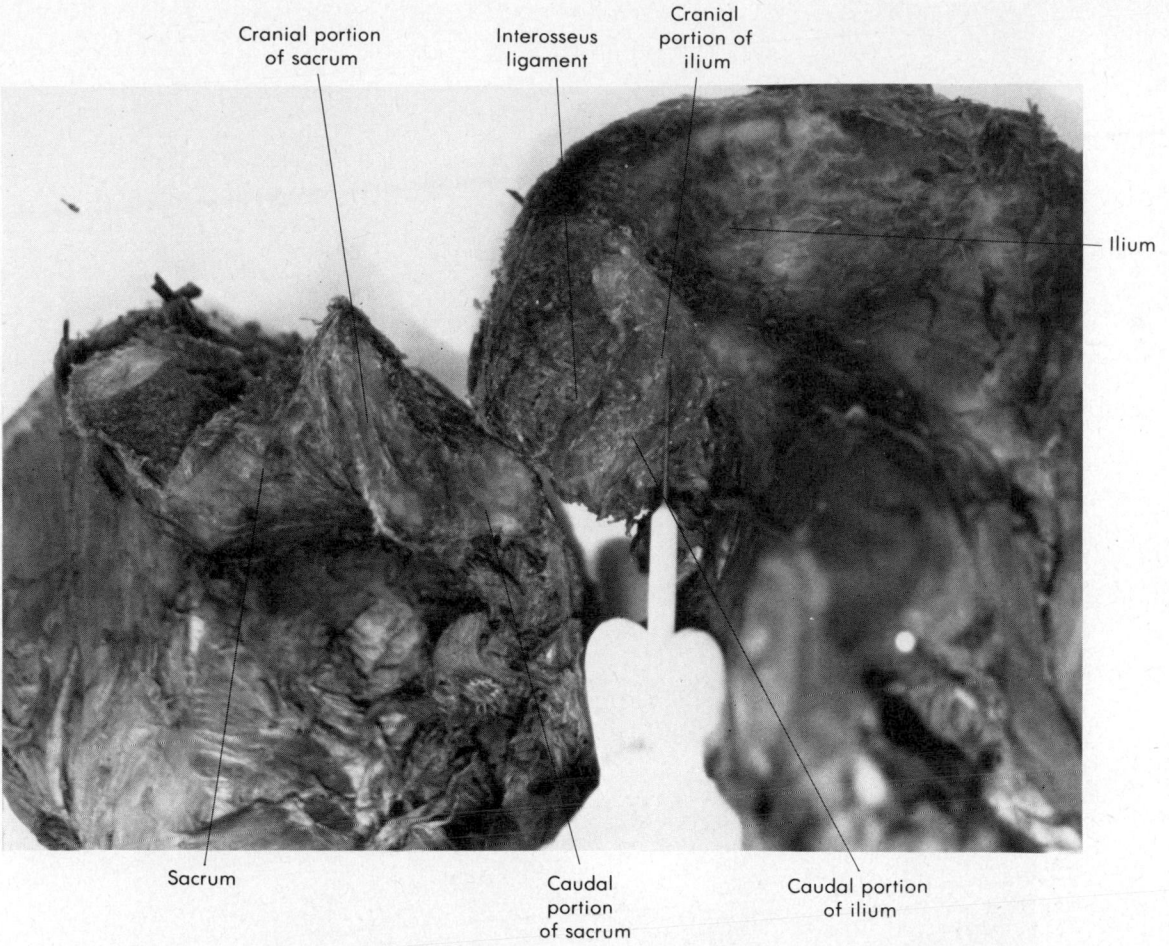

Cranial portion
of sacrum   Interosseus   Cranial
                              ligament   portion of
                                                      ilium

                                                                                    Ilium

Sacrum   Caudal   Caudal portion
                            portion   of ilium
                            of sacrum

Fig. 22-3. A disarticulated pelvis showing the cranial and caudal portions of the left sacroiliac joint. The probe is pointing to the cranial portion of the sacral component of the SI joint. (From Porterfield JA and DeRosa C: Lumbopelvic function and dysfunction, Philadelphia, 1990, WB Saunders Co.)

right side to left. The orientation is usually a combination of frontal and sagittal plane positions.[41]

The two sacroiliac joints are L or auricular shaped when viewed from the side. Their surfaces are divided into cranial and caudal segments (Fig. 22-4), the caudal usually being larger.[31,45] Weisl's extensive studies[45] of these joints have shown that a central depression can often be found at the junction of the cranial and caudal segments.

The sacral component of the joint is concave and lined with hyaline cartilage that is 1.7 to 5 times greater than the iliac component.[1,3] The iliac component is generally convex and lined with a thin fibrocartilage. As these two joints articulate and become compressed, cartilage deformation results. This accommodation by the cartilage is one method of force acceptance as trunk and ground forces converge into the region.

Fig. 22-4 reveals a transverse section of the sacrum at three descending levels. The reader should recognize the differences in the cartilaginous surfaces of the sacral and iliac components of this joint. Also, the configuration of

the interosseous ligament should be noted. This thick, fibrous band fills the gap between the ilium and the sacrum as the sacrum angles posterior and medially. The membrane apparently acts to provide stability to the sacroiliac joints and simultaneously permits small deforming translational movements proportional to the way in which the trunk and ground forces react during function.

The sacroiliac joint changes as we go through the aging process.[3,32,36,43] Osteophytes become more abundant, and a decrease in mobility with physiological joint fusion generally becomes evident in the third and fourth decade.[3,31,36]

The public symphysis is an amphiarthrodial joint that permits limited mobility. Borell[2] and Laban et al[22] have observed that the symphysis undergoes significant articular changes in multiparous women. This joint also appears to be affected by excess mobility in the sacroiliac joints and can be a source of anterior pelvic symptoms.

The hip joints are also an integral part of the pelvic unit because it is through the hips that ground forces reach the

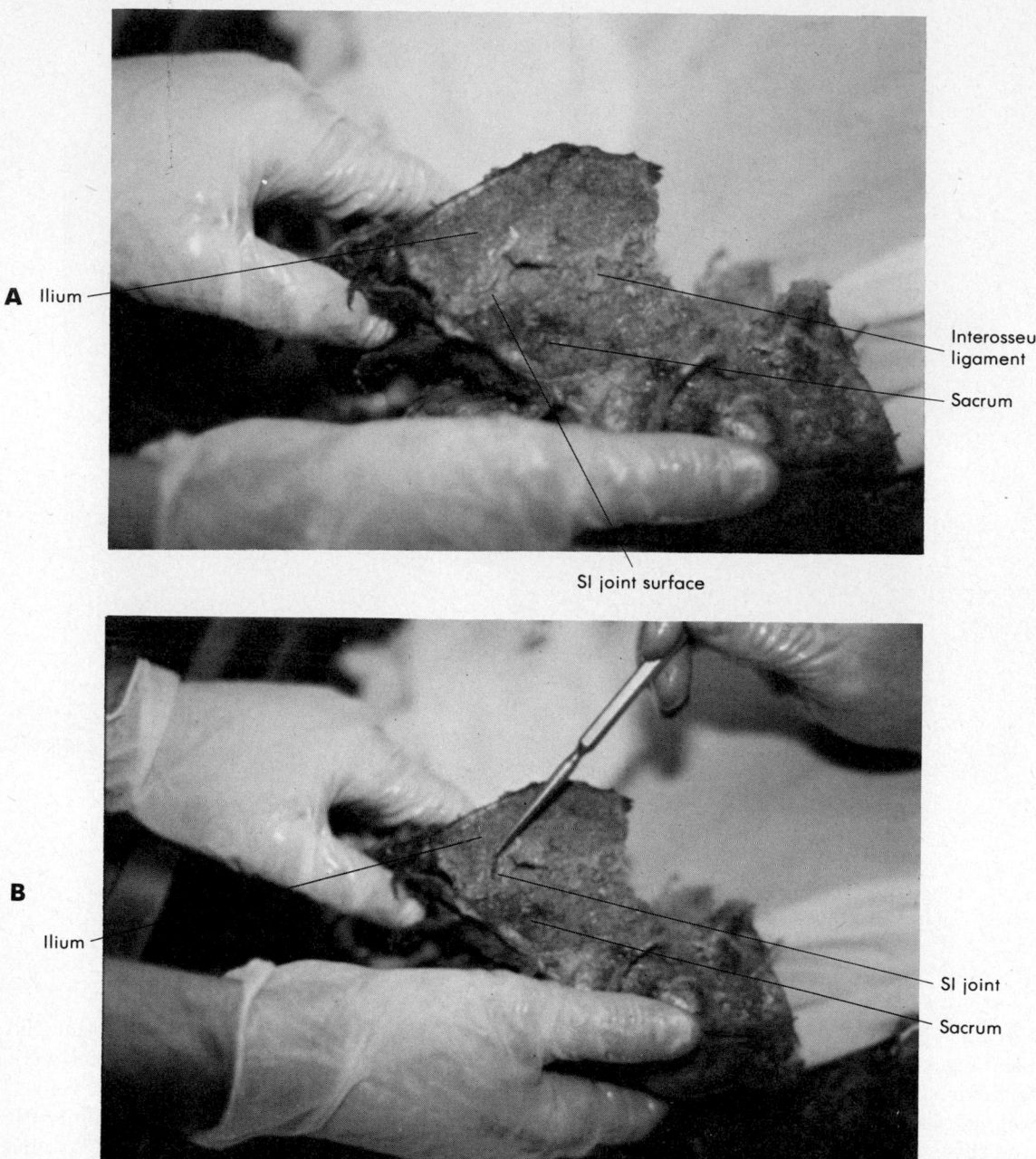

A Ilium

Interosseus
ligament

Sacrum

SI joint surface

B

Ilium

SI joint

Sacrum

Fig. 22-4. A, Transverse section of the right sacroiliac joint at the second sacral level. **B,** The probe is pointing to the joint surface. **C,** The probe is pointing to the interosseus ligament, and **D,** reveals a separated ilium and sacrum showing the angle of the sacroiliac articulation and the probe is pointing to the joint surface. Note: the thicker hyaline cartilage on the sacral portion and the thinner cartilaginous covering of the ilial portion of the SI joint. (From Porterfield JA and DeRosa C: Lumbopelvic function and dysfunction, Philadelphia, 1990, WB Saunders Co.)

pelvis. A loss of hip range of motion potentially impacts on the type and degree of forces that reach the sacroiliac and lumbar joints. Based on clinical experience, adaptive changes in the hip joint are a major contributor to lumbar and sacroiliac pain. This area should not be overlooked when the clinician is attempting to assist the patient in the management of problems in this region.

LIGAMENTS

The pelvis is an extremely stable area, largely because of its strong ligaments. While muscles offer a degree of dynamic stabilization, the ligamentous complex offers static stabilization. Forces from above and below are thus accepted and transferred because of the interplay between the musculature and ligaments.

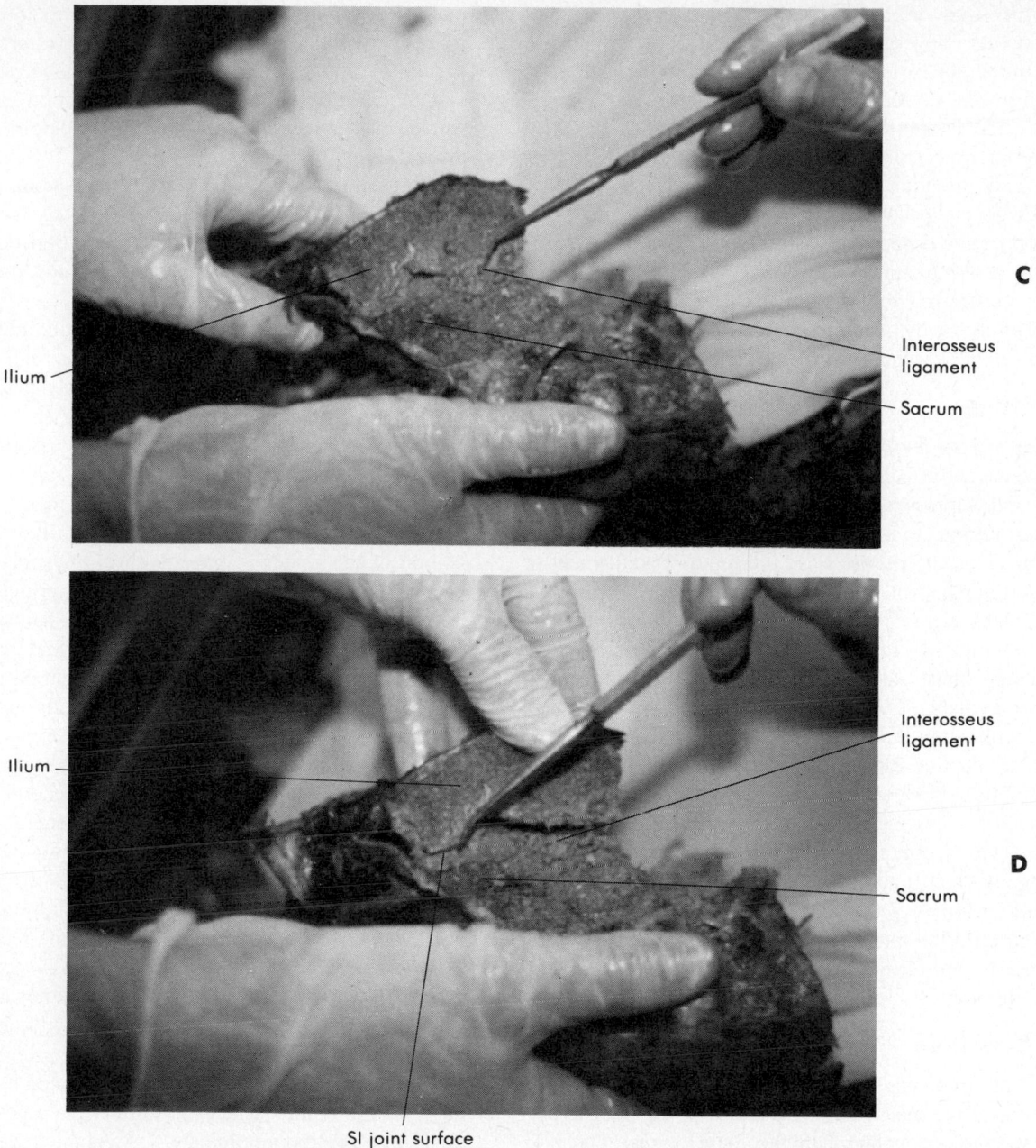

Ilium

Interosseus
ligament

Sacrum

C

Ilium

Interosseus
ligament

Sacrum

D

SI joint surface

Fig. 22-4. For legend see opposite page

The iliolumbar ligament is an excellent example. Its major insertion is to the transverse process of the fifth lumbar vertebrae, although it can reach as far superiorly as the fourth lumbar vertebrae. Luk et al[24] have suggested that formation of the iliolumbar ligament occurs because of metaplasia of the quadratus lumborum muscle as we age. The iliolumbar ligament is divided into multiple component bands, which are named for both their attachments and direction. The multidirectional aspect of these bands allow the ligament to check various motions of the L-5 vertebrae on the sacrum, such as shear motion and torsion, as well as forward, backward, and lateral bending. The ligament is extremely important in squaring the L-5 vertebrae on the sacrum.

The sacroiliac joints are reinforced by the anterior and posterior sacroiliac ligaments. The posterior ligaments are extremely thick and strong and significantly contribute to the stability of the sacroiliac joint directly.

The sacrotuberous and sacrospinous ligaments are attached to the sacrum and ischium. Their function becomes evident in weight-bearing positions because they act to check the forward flexion moment of the sacrum on the innominate as trunk forces converge on the sacrum. The interplay of these ligaments and the sacroiliac ligaments is discussed in the section on biomechanics.

The intrinsic capsular ligaments of the hip are the iliofemoral, ischiofemoral, and pubofemoral. These ligaments are named for the aspect of the innominate bone from which they originate. The iliofemoral and pubofemoral ligaments converge and attach to the intertrochanteric line of the femur, whereas the ischiofemoral ligament originates from the posterior acetabulum and travels superior, anterior, and lateral around the femoral neck to attach to the anterior aspect of the femur. As the hip becomes extended and the joint reaches the close-packed position, these ligaments become tight. As these ligaments reach their connective tissue limits and the lower extremity continues to move toward hyperextension, forces are subsequently transferred to the sacroiliac joints and then the lumbar joints. A dysfunction of the hip can thus alter pelvic and lumbar mechanics.

Musculature

Twenty-eight muscles originate or insert on the pelvis and subsequently exert a variety of forces on the bones, joints, and supporting structures of the sacroiliac (lumbopelvic) region. In a closed kinetic chain the hip muscles exert forces on the pelvis, since the femoral attachment of these muscles becomes the fixed point of origin while the pelvic bones become the moveable insertion. When the lower extremity is in the swing phase, the lumbopelvic musculature must contract isometrically to control and maintain a balance of the weight-bearing properties in this area. Decreases in the length or strength of these muscles, caused by adaptive shortening and/or afferent/efferent neuromusculature imbalances, can thus alter normal pelvic mechanics.

The external oblique, internal oblique, transversus abdominis, and rectus abdominis are also important in the attenuation of forces as they reach the pelvis. These muscles help to control the manner in which trunk forces reach the lumbopelvic unit,[42] as will be further discussed in the section on mechanics.

BIOMECHANICS

The biomechanics of the female pelvis are different than those of the male pelvis. Structurally, the female pelvis is shorter and wider than the male pelvis. The hormonal changes of menses and pregnancy render the female pelvis slightly more mobile, suggesting an increased vulnerability to sprain and strain.[2,10,13] Hisaw[17] was the first to describe the release of the hormone relaxin during pregnancy. Weiss[46] later added to this information. This hormone appears to decrease the integrity of the supporting structures of the pelvis so that excess motion is available to expand the pelvis and open the pelvic outlet to facilitate childbirth. The ischial tuberosities are closer together before the fetus has moved into the pelvic canal. However, as the fetus migrates down the pelvic canal, the ischial tuberosities spread, causing an inward motion of the ilia.

While the biochemical changes may facilitate childbirth, they may potentially render the weight-bearing joints of the pelvis vulnerable to sprain caused by excessive mo-

tion for up to four months after childbirth, depending on whether the infant is breast-fed. The longer breast-feeding occurs, the longer the titers of this hormone remain in the system. Specific sacroiliac joint dysfunction can occur in women who have suffered trauma just before or just following childbirth.

The subject of movement of the sacroiliac joint is controversial.* The concept of normal physiological movement of the female pelvis during parturition is generally well accepted, but physiological movements of the male and female sacroiliac joints during other functional activities has led to lively debate in the literature.

Because of the attachments of the sacrum to the fifth lumbar vertebra that have been previously described, forward and backward motions of the lumbar column influence the way in which forces reach the sacrum. For example, while bending forward from the standing position, there is an extension moment on the sacrum. This extension moment is crucial to counterbalance the forward migration of the center of gravity during the forward movement. This counterbalance is provided primarily by the contraction of the gluteus maximus and hamstrings muscles. In returning to the erect position and restoring the original lordosis, there is a flexion moment on the sacrum.

These applied moments on the sacrum influence the sacroiliac joints. While appreciable or excessive movement may be possible in some individuals, especially multiparous women and individuals with general connective tissue laxity, this is not the rule for the general population. Small accommodating movements are most justifiable because of cartilage deformation that occurs as the sacroiliac joint surfaces engage and compress together during weight bearing. Perhaps it is better to consider the resultant force as a *moment* rather than a *movement*. The cartilaginous surfaces compress and seat into one another as the trunk and forces are accepted and transferred by the lumbopelvic region during weight bearing.

The innominate bone is mainly influenced by the movement of the femur. At heel strike there is a posterior rotational force on the innominate.[29,39] As the lower extremity proceeds through the stance phase and approaches push off, there is a resultant anterior rotational force.

When there is a leg length discrepancy or any other frontal plane asymmetry, the pelvis must drop a distance equal to the amount of the discrepancy with every step. This transference of ground force reaches the lumbopelvic tissues in an abnormal, asymmetric manner.[11] For example, with a short right leg or sacral tilting to the right side, the right sacroiliac joint is in a more horizontal position, while the left sacroiliac joint is more vertical. This results in comparatively more compressive force applied to the right sacroiliac joint and more shear stress to the left. The

---

*See references 4, 5, 7, 8, 12, 16, 20, 23, 25, 26, 28, 29, 34, 36, 37, and 45.

tilted position of the sacrum also results in sidebending motion at the lumbosacral joint complex away from the short side. Consequently, compressive forces are placed on tissues on the concave side of the curve and tensile forces on the convex side. If these forces exceed the supporting capabilities of the tissue, microtearing occurs and symptoms of overuse appear.

The abdominal wall is also important in controlling how

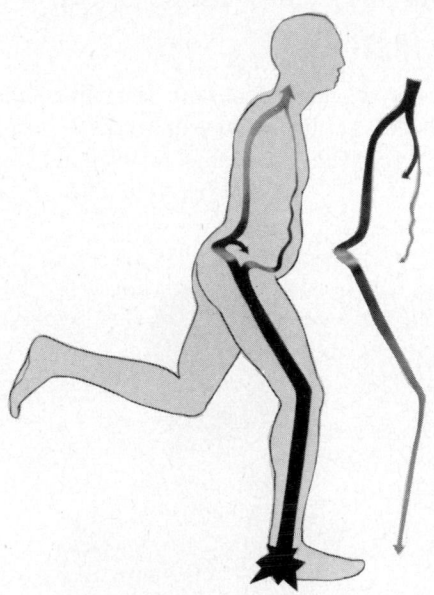

Fig. 22-5. Ground and trunk force changes with weak abdominal musculature, resulting in an anterior tilting of the pelvis and an increase in wcight bearing to the apophyseal joint.

forces reach this region. The abdominal wall contributes to the attenuation of trunk and ground forces as they converge into the lumbopelvic area.[43] A weak abdominal wall permits the anterior aspect of the pelvis to drop, thus creating an anterior migration of the individual's center of gravity (Fig. 22-5). In order to counter the anterior migration and maintain postural equilibrium, the individual must increase the extension of the lumbar spine with a posterior movement of the weight line. This will result in an increased load to the posterior structures, primarily the articular surfaces and capsule of the apophyseal joints. These synovial joints now take on the task of added weight bearing. Many authors[18,25,30,33] have suggested that the apophyseal joints are important sources of low back pain. Maintaining the integrity of the abdominal wall and the mobility of the spinal segments can normalize the amount of stress transmitted to the lumbopelvic region.

As can be seen in Fig. 22-6, the ground force, R, causes a posterior rotary force on the ilia, $N2$. The trunk forces, P, produce the exact opposite motion in the sacrum, $N1$, which is an anterior rotary force or flexion of the sacrum, $N1$. These forces ligamentously lock the sacroiliac joints and in essence create a *screw home mechanism* in the pelvis because of their fiber direction and attachments, the tension of the sacrotuberous, and sacrospinous and posterior sacroiliac ligaments increases. Thus stability is enhanced.

CAUSES OF DYSFUNCTION

Symptoms emanating from the sacroiliac joint are primarily caused by three types of events. The first of these is

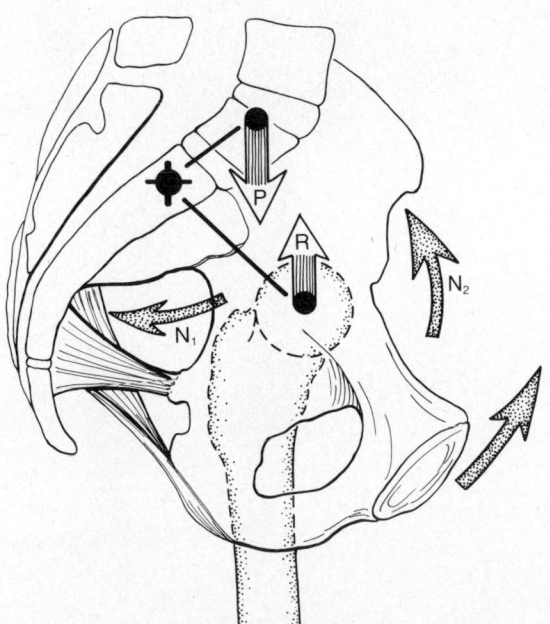

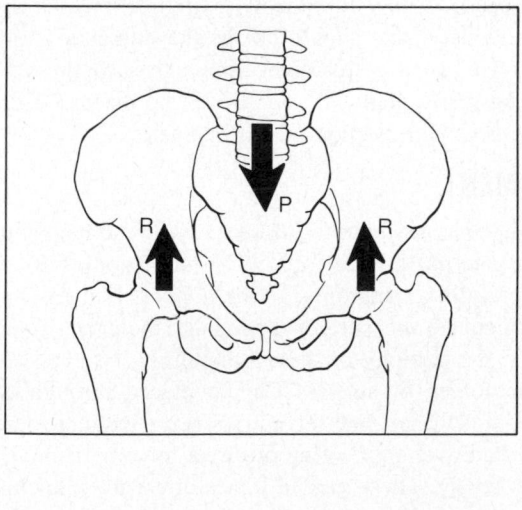

Fig. 22-6. Convergence of trunk forces, P, and ground forces, R. (Modified from Kapandji IA: The physiology of the joints, vol 3, Edinburgh, 1974, Churchill Livingstone Inc).

direct trauma, as when someone slips on ice or falls down stairs. This force to the ischial tuberosity moves the innominate in a posterior direction and causes an anterior stress on the sacrum. The resultant force thus has rotary and shear components.

The second kind of event that generates symptoms in this region is *indirect trauma.* This commonly results from one of two physiological or kinesiological problems: skeletal asymmetry or stress to the joint when it is in an extreme range.

Skeletal asymmetry can render the joint vulnerable to abnormal wear patterns.[11] These patterns increase the duties on supporting structures, thus altering the normal function and predisposing the musculoskeletal system to injury.

Any position that takes the pelvic joints to their end range, such as combined forward and side bending or backward and side bending, renders the area vulnerable to injury. If the limits of sacroiliac joint motion are reached and a force is then imparted through the lower extremities toward this region, there is a potential to sprain or strain the various lumbopelvic supporting tissues.

The third common source of symptoms in the lumbopelvic region is *pregnancy.* Stress on the joints results from the altered placement of the weight line as it reaches the lumbopelvic tissues and the increased elasticity of the supporting structures because of release of the hormone relaxin. It is quite common for the therapist to see low-back pain originating from the apophyseal joints or sacroiliac joints in the pregnant female. Pregnant women who have asymmetrical skeletons often run a higher risk of musculoskeletal symptoms.

However, it is often difficult to accurately differentiate the exact cause of any lumbopelvic dysfunction. As discussed previously, this should not be the clinician's foremost concern because treatment approaches to these lesions are basically identical. These will be discussed further in the treatment portion of this chapter.

ASSESSMENT

The goal of assessment of the sacroiliac/lumbopelvic region is to determine what force or combination of forces reproduce familiar symptoms. In the lumbopelvic region it is very difficult to measure or distinguish the exact tissues involved in the etiology of these symptoms.

Specific forces or stresses can be placed through the sacroiliac joint via manual techniques (i.e., indirect forces created through weight bearing or direct force by using the femur as a lever). These graded forces often give the clinician valuable information as to the inflammatory or irritability status of the tissues in the sacroiliac joint region.

This assessment approach is used to regionalize the site of symptoms by directing the various combinations of mechanical forces and determining which make the symptoms worse. This approach follows the same rules of evaluation

as any other weight-bearing region. The overall goal is to reproduce the symptom (i.e., recreate the symptom that is familiar to the patient in the weight-bearing posture and then substantiate it by reproducing the force and position that increases pain in the prone, supine, sitting, or sidelying positions). It is important to note that the clinician should examine each sacroiliac joint and lumbopelvic region in the same manner. Repetition of the evaluation in this way allows for comparison and some degree of quantification of each low back that is evaluated.

CLIENT HISTORY

The history of the patient with sacroiliac joint pain typically includes: (1) unilateral pain over the sacroiliac joint and/or buttock with occasional referral into the hip and

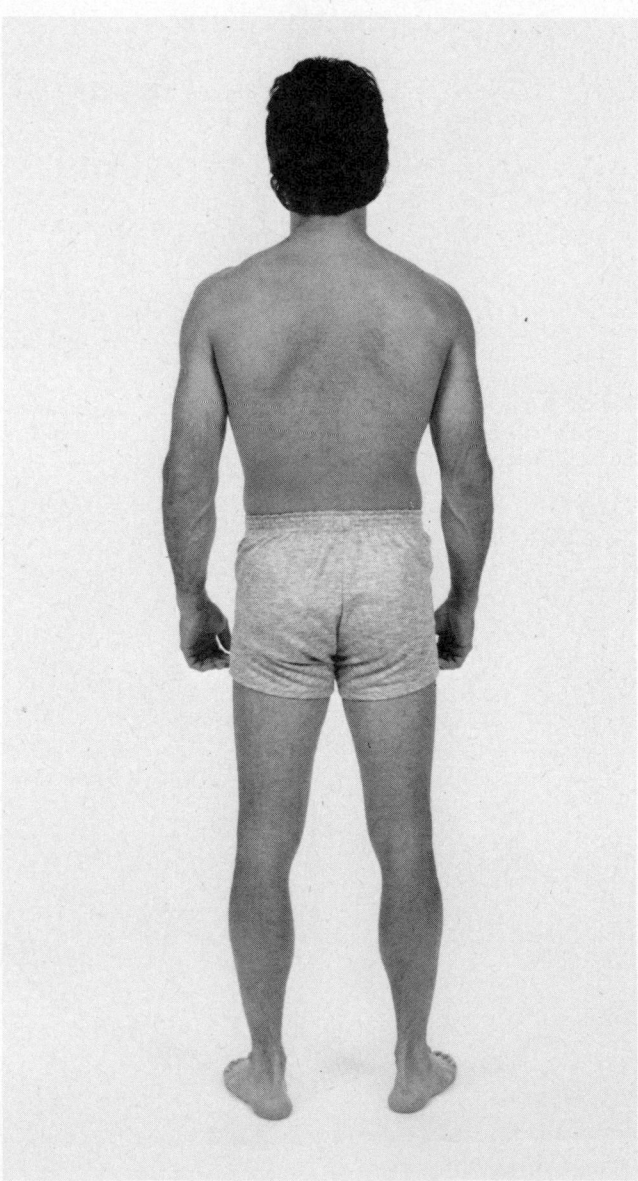

Fig. 22-7. Posterior view for initial stages of skeletal inspection.

groin, (2) increased pain with standing or sitting on the affected side, (3) increased pain with prolonged postures, (4) difficulty raising from a seated position accompanied by pain, (5) difficulty in climbing stairs, especially when leading with the affected leg, (6) relief of symptoms through pressure of the hand over the sacrum, and (7) morning stiffness that eases after a short period of weight bearing.

An understanding of the normal mechanics of this region amplifies the fact that it is very difficult to distinguish an isolated sacroiliac joint problem, since many lumbopelvic tissues are ultimately affected with an insulting force.

Standing examination

The observant clinician begins collecting pertinent information by watching the client rise from the sitting position and walk into the examining room. The extremes of movement in the sacroiliac joint appear to occur at end ranges of stance and long sitting,[40] and from rising from a seated to a standing position.[5] During this activity the pel-

vis is vulnerable to stress and can thus potentially elicit symptoms. Consider the opposing forces that are generated at the sacroiliac joint during this motion. Initially, the gluteal musculature produces a posterior force on the pelvis, while the sacrum is stressed in an anterior direction. This region is designed to accommodate these types of forces, however, this position places the supporting structures at an end range of stress and therefore increases their vulnerability for injury or reinjury.

For the formal examination the client should be attired so as to expose as much of the spine and buttock area as circumstances and discretion permit. The clinician is initially observing for atrophy or asymmetry as well as general postural position (Fig. 22-7).

A frontal plane inspection of the spine should be substantiated by palpating the iliac crest, posterior iliac spines, anterior superior iliac spines, and greater trochanters. Figs. 22-8 through 22-11 show these palpations. Palpation of these bony landmarks, combined with visual inspection, give the clinician an adequate impression as to

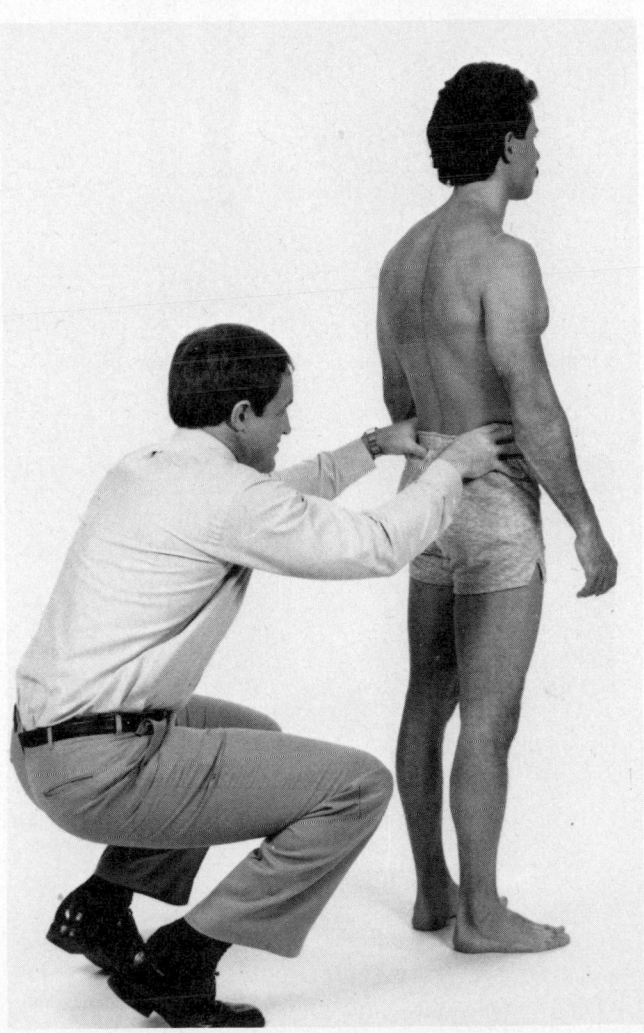

Fig. 22-8. Palpation of the iliac crests.

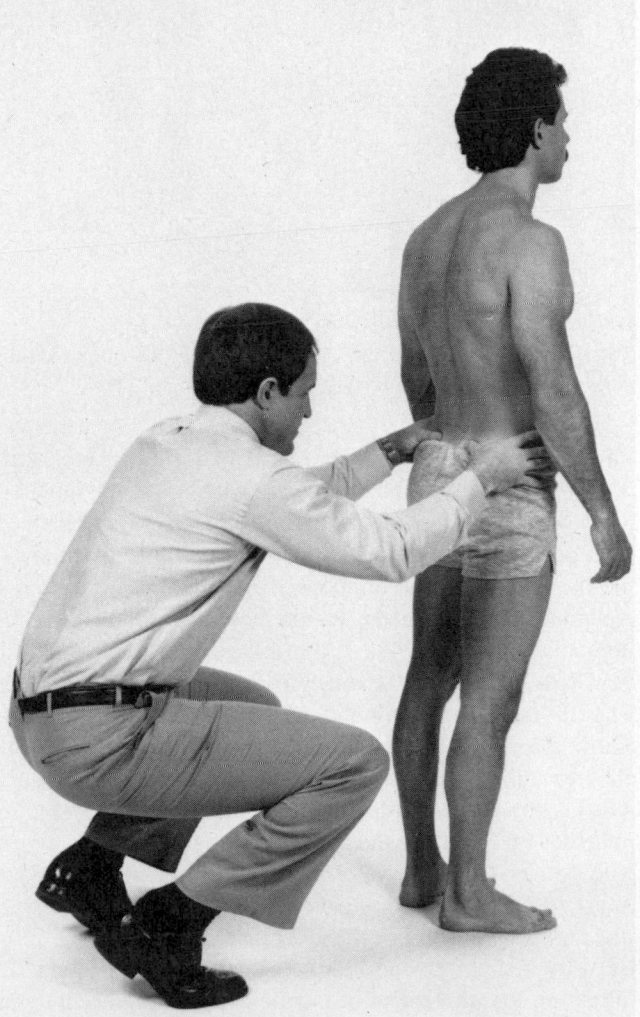

Fig. 22-9. Palpation of the posterior superior iliac spines (PSIS).

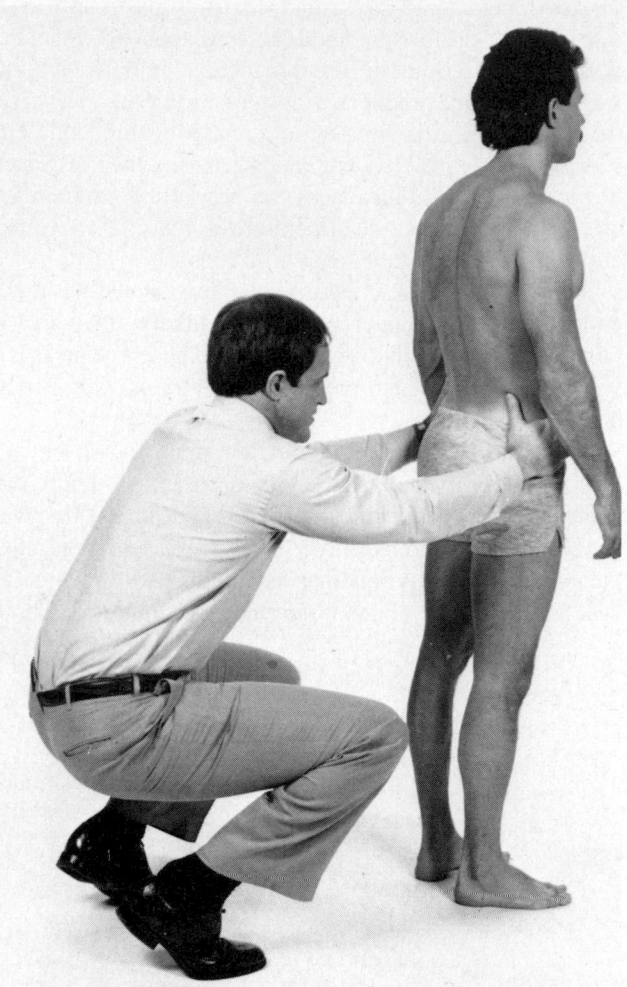

Fig. 22-10. Palpation of the anterior superior iliac spines (ASIS) with the middle fingers from behind.

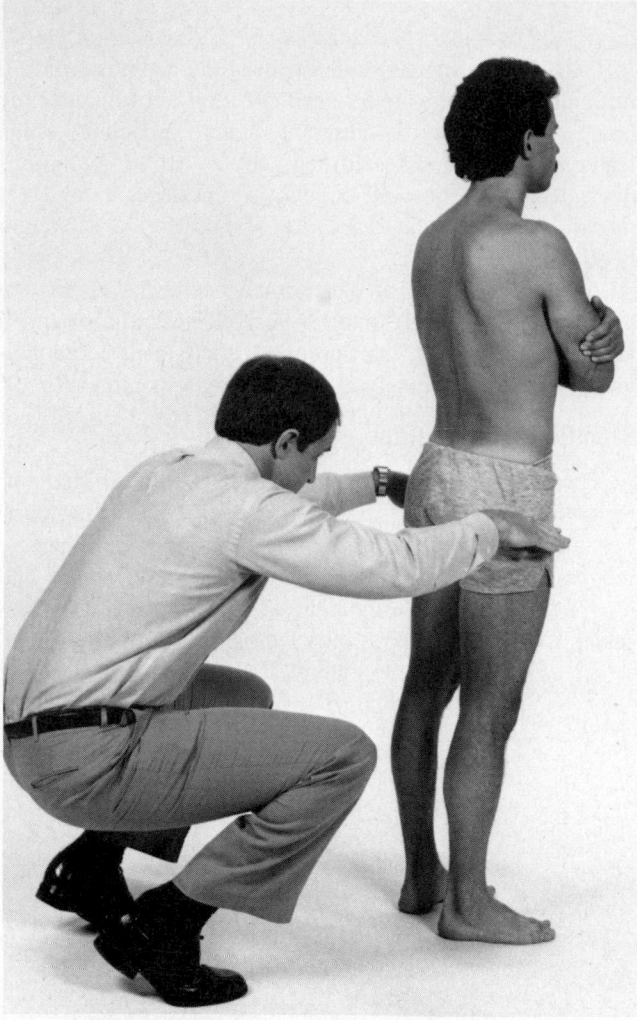

Fig. 22-11. Palpation of the greater trochanters bilateral.

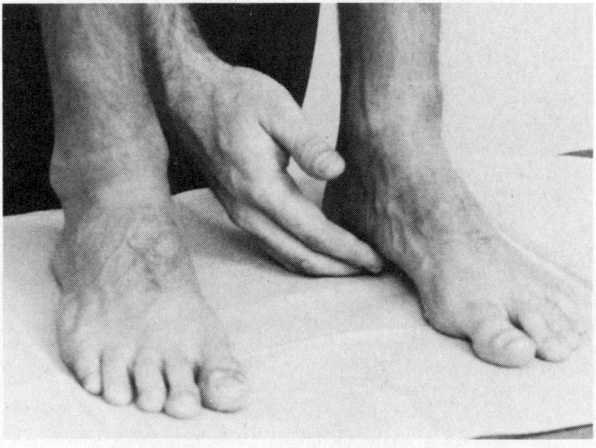

Fig. 22-12. Palpation of longitudinal arch.

the presence or absence of a relative frontal plane asymmetry that involves the lumbopelvic unit. The alignment of the knees and position of the foot (Fig. 22-12) supplement this postural information. It is important that the foot not be overlooked in the lumbopelvic evaluation because it is an important link in the transference of ground forces to the pelvis.[40]

Gross movement testing from the standing position should then be performed. Figs. 22-13 through 22-15 show the important single plane and multi-plane motions. The examiner should also attempt to apply overpressure, when possible, while being extremely cognizant of whether this overpressure is increasing compressive or tensile forces to the area. The forces of these movements must reach the lumbopelvic tissues. Often, it is necessary for the examiner to direct the weight line through these tissues by manually controlling the requested movement. By directing the movement in this manner a more accurate interpretation of the movement and loading pattern that gives rise to familiar pain can be recognized.

For example, the extension-sidebending test (Fig. 22-15), if performed correctly and with adequate overpressure, can significantly load the sacroiliac region (L-5-S-1

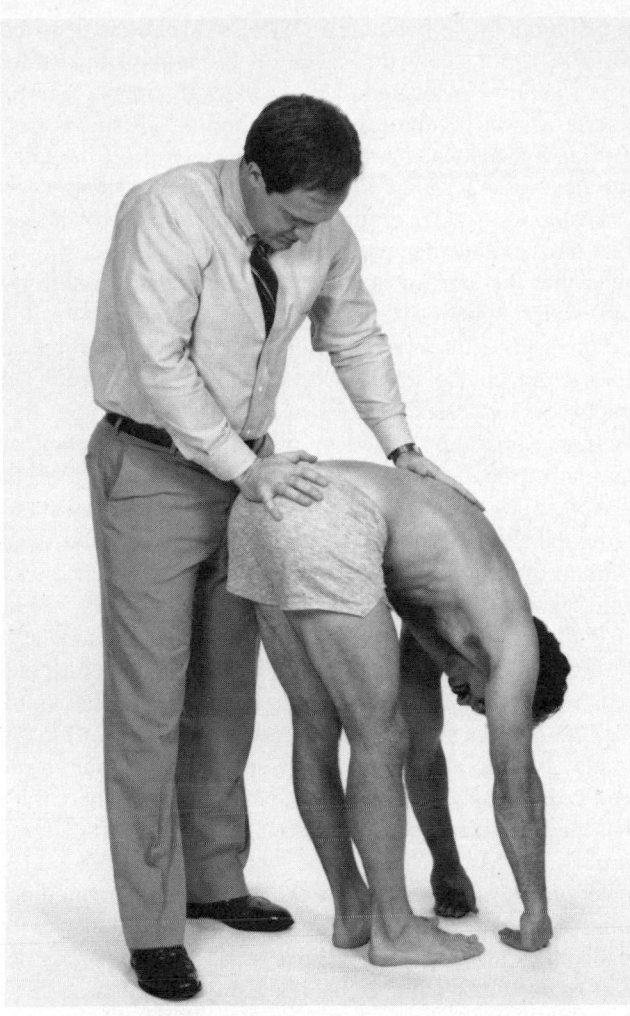

Fig. 22-13. Gross movement testing—forward bending.

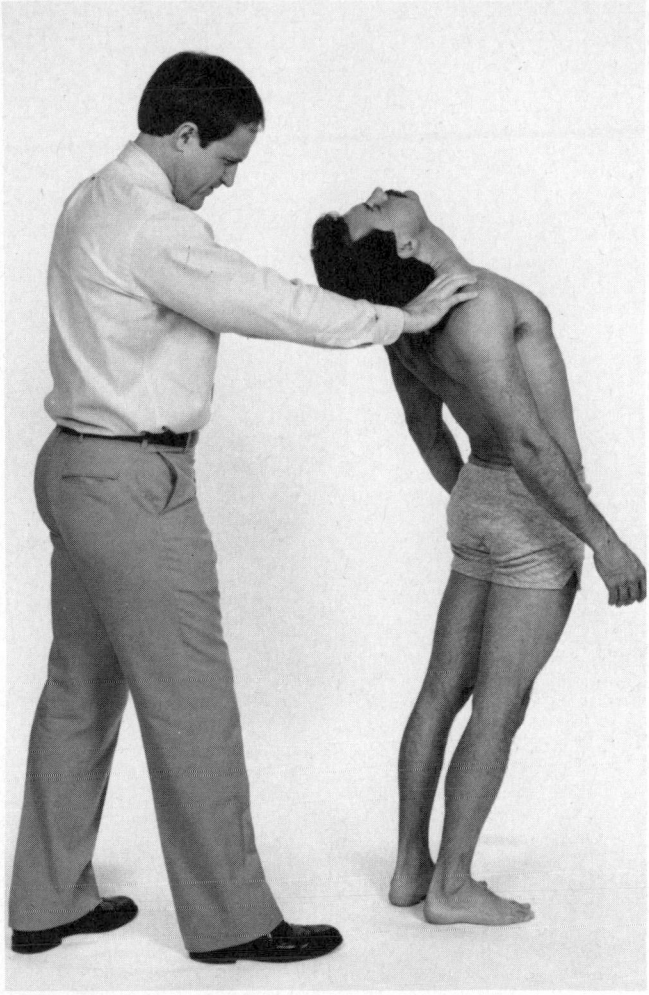

Fig. 22-14. Gross movement testing—backward bending.

apophyseal joint, iliolumbar ligament, and sacroiliac joint structures) and reveal whether forces to this region may be the source of symptoms. The examiner must control the motion to direct the weight line through these tissues for the test to be effective. More important, the examiner should be able to visualize the various compressive, tensile, shear, and torsional forces that are being imparted into the region when any test is performed.

Supine and prone examination

Examination of the standing, antigravity posture should reveal various positions and forces that increase the patient's symptoms. The supine and prone exams substantiate these findings. This section will focus on specific stresses that can be placed through the sacroiliac region during a low-back evaluation in non–weight-bearing positions.

In the supine position the hip is taken through full passive flexion. This flexion motion creates a loose-pack position of the hip joint until the femoral extensors (buttocks muscles) become tight. At this point the force is trans-

ferred through the hip to the pelvis. A posterior rotary force acts on the innominate, and a small amount of rotary accommodation results at the sacroiliac joint. Continuation of this movement causes the force to transfer through the sacrum and ultimately produces flexion of the lumbar spine. The clinician must be cognizant of the specific point in the range of motion and the amount of force used to reproduce the symptoms in order to establish whether the hip, pelvis, or lumbar spine created the symptoms.

The Figure 4 test position (Fig. 22-16) assesses flexibility of the hip joint. Asymmetrical Figure 4 tests are often encountered with chronic low-back problems. Tightness in this position usually indicates that passive hip hyperextension from the prone position will also be limited.

As previously mentioned, tight hip structures can cause increased forces on the sacroiliac joint and lumbar spine during activities of daily living.

The sacroiliac joint can also be stressed directly by using the femur as a lever. The examiner should place the femur in a slightly flexed, abducted, and externally rotated

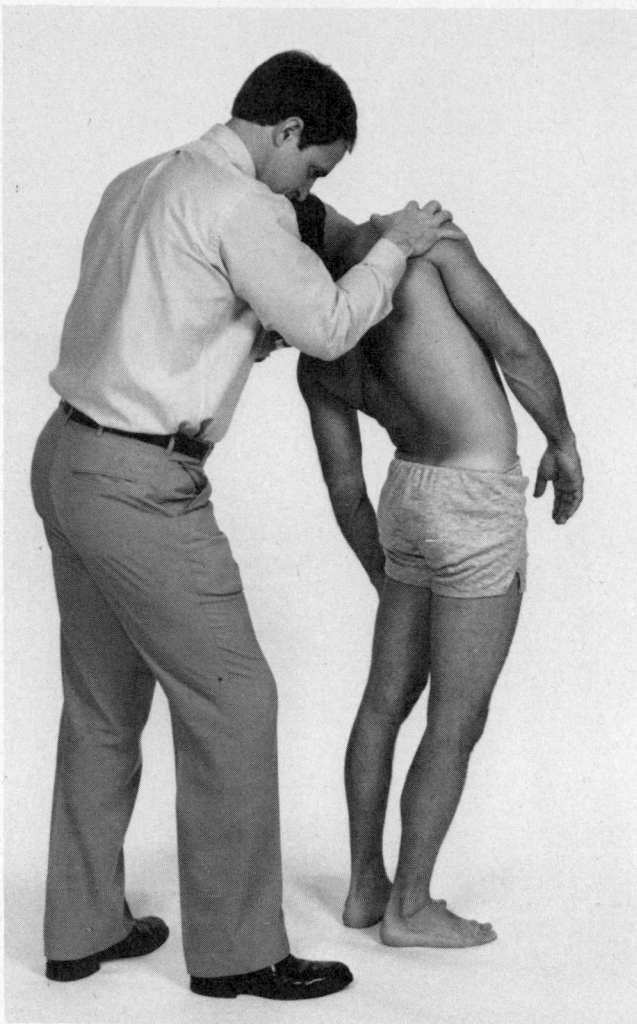

Fig. 22-15. Gross movement testing—combined backward bending and sidebending to the right, creating overpressure into the right lumbosacral triangle (L-5–S-1 apophyseal joint, iliolumbar ligament, and sacroiliac joint).

position, approximately 45 degrees from the midline (Fig. 22-17). From this position a graded force can be placed through the long axis of the femur and subsequently cause an anterior to posterior shear force to the sacroiliac joint.

A different force on the sacroiliac joint results when the hip is placed in flexion with a slight degree of adduction (Fig. 22-18). A graded force is generated along the femur until the slack[19] is taken up in the hip joint and the external rotators, and then a small adduction force is added to the distal femur resulting in a gapping or distraction force on the posterior aspect of the sacroiliac joint.

There are many specific tests designed to stress the tissues of the sacroiliac joint. However, it is more important that the clinician be able to evaluate the direction and intensity of the applied forces with a three dimensional appreciation of the anatomy. With this understanding any variation of these tests can be logically interpreted.

From the prone position a variety of sacroiliac tests are possible. Once again the status of the anterior hip structures should be evaluated. This includes the rectus femoris muscle as well as the hip flexors. Fig. 22-19 shows passive hip hyperextension that will ultimately direct the force into the hips, sacroiliac joints, and the lumbar spine.

Posterior to anterior pressures can be placed directly over the sacrum, diagonally in the joint plane, keeping in mind that the sacrum is wider anteriorly than posteriorly and wider superiorly than inferiorly. Pressure on the sacrum will result in a posterior to anterior shear force of the sacrum on the ilium. Although there is a significant amount of soft tissue directly over the sacroiliac joint line itself, the pressure is used in an attempt to elicit familiar pain rather than attempting to quantify the small degrees of motion. The sacroiliac joint can also be stressed by stabilizing the sacrum and applying a posteriorly directed shear force to the ilium. This will also provoke an irritated sacroiliac joint.

If further evaluation of the sacroiliac joint is necessary, the side-lying position can be used. Manually, forces can be applied to the innominate bone in the manner shown by Fig. 22-20. The femur can be used as a lever, in this example, to place an anterior rotary and posterior shear force into and through the sacroiliac joint. It is only necessary that the clinician be able to follow the application of force through the tissue to determine what type of stress is ultimately being placed on the hip, sacroiliac, or lumbar joints. The ability to progressively direct these forces with graded intensity to the exact area is the most important aspect of sacroiliac joint evaluation. Any forces directed to the sacroiliac joint region have the potential to be an excellent test, if one adheres to this concept.

Since this chapter emphasizes the sacroiliac joint, description of a complete lumbopelvic evaluation is beyond its scope. However, it should be recognized that the complete lumbar spine and hip regions should be carefully screened, since sacroiliac joint lesions occur in combination with tissue injury to other lumbopelvic tissues.

TREATMENT OF THE SACROILIAC (LUMBOPELVIC) REGION

Treatment of the lumbopelvic region is designed around the science of soft tissue healing and recognition of the mechanisms by which forces converge in this area. While some syndromes have a straightforward history with a logical sequence of signs and symptoms, many lumbopelvic problems take years to become symptomatic enough to cause the person to seek professional help. Consequently, the treatment program requires active involvement by the patient in order to address both short and long term goals.

It is important to educate patients to the fact that management of their lumbopelvic problem is ultimately their responsibility. The therapist's role is to guide the patient through a program that facilitates independent manage-

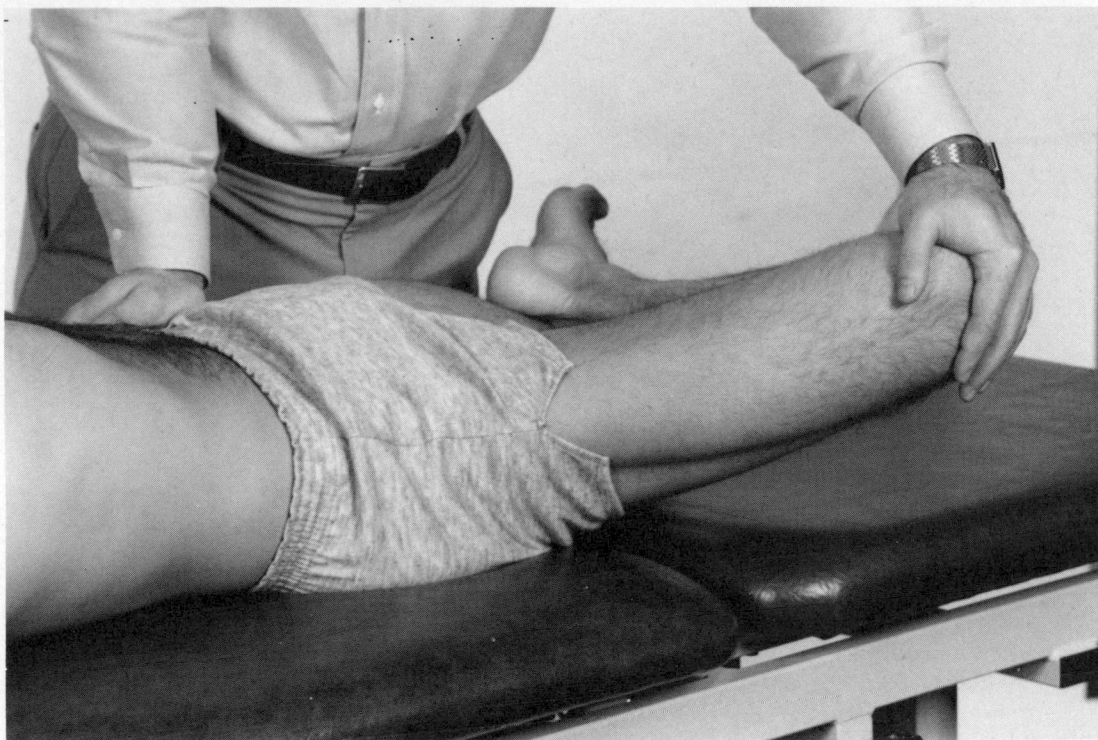

Fig. 22-16. Fabere's or figure 4 test (testing the integrity of the right hip in flexion, abduction, and external rotation).

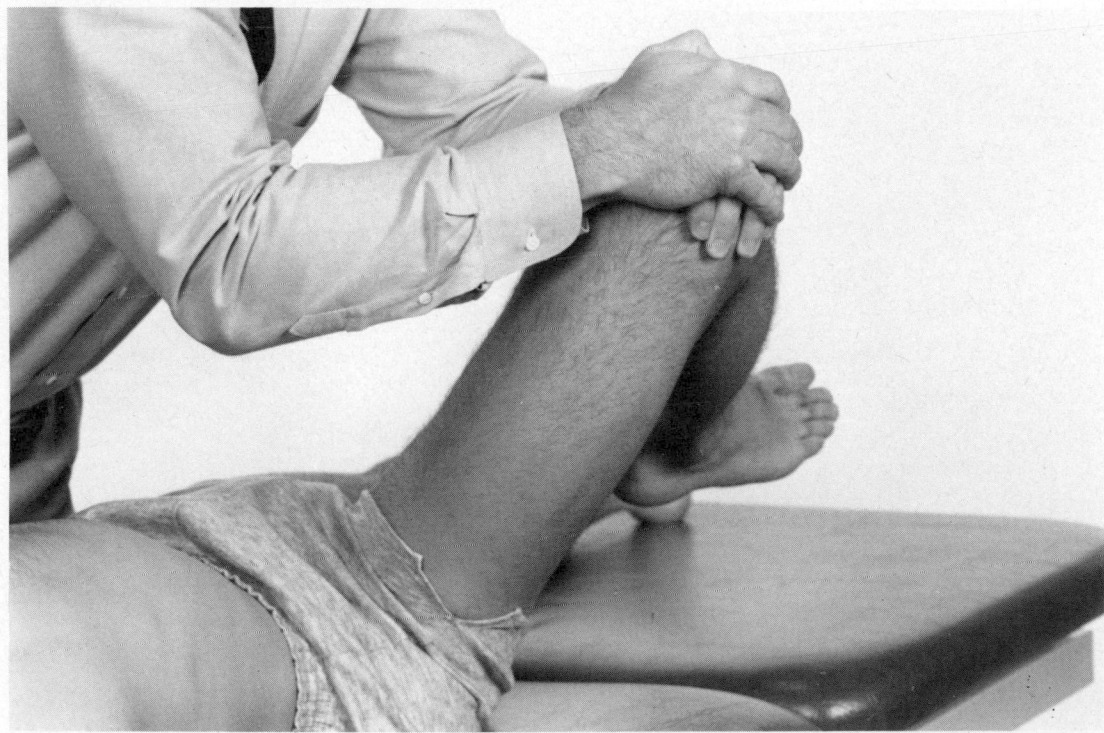

Fig. 22-17. Using the femur as a lever—femoral flexion, abduction, and external rotation, resulting in anterior to posterior shear of the ilium on the sacrum.

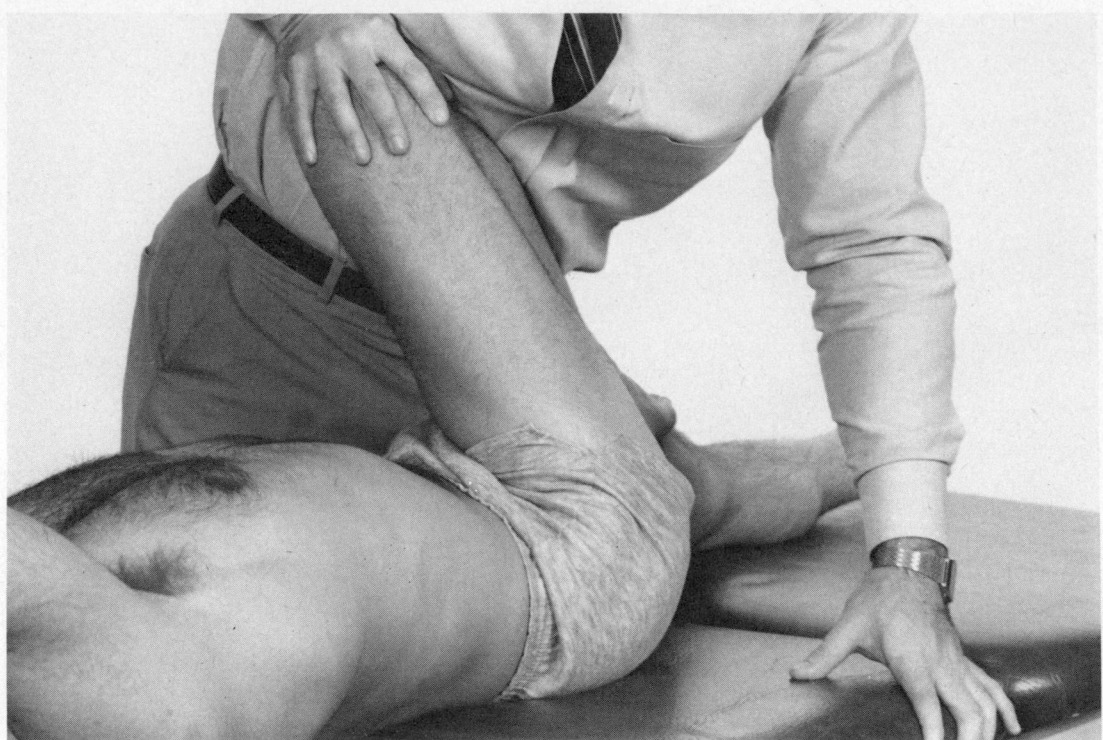

Fig. 22-18. Using the femur as a lever—femoral flexion and adduction, resulting in compression of the anterior aspect of the sacroiliac joint and a gapping or tensile stress to the posterior aspect of the sacroiliac joint.

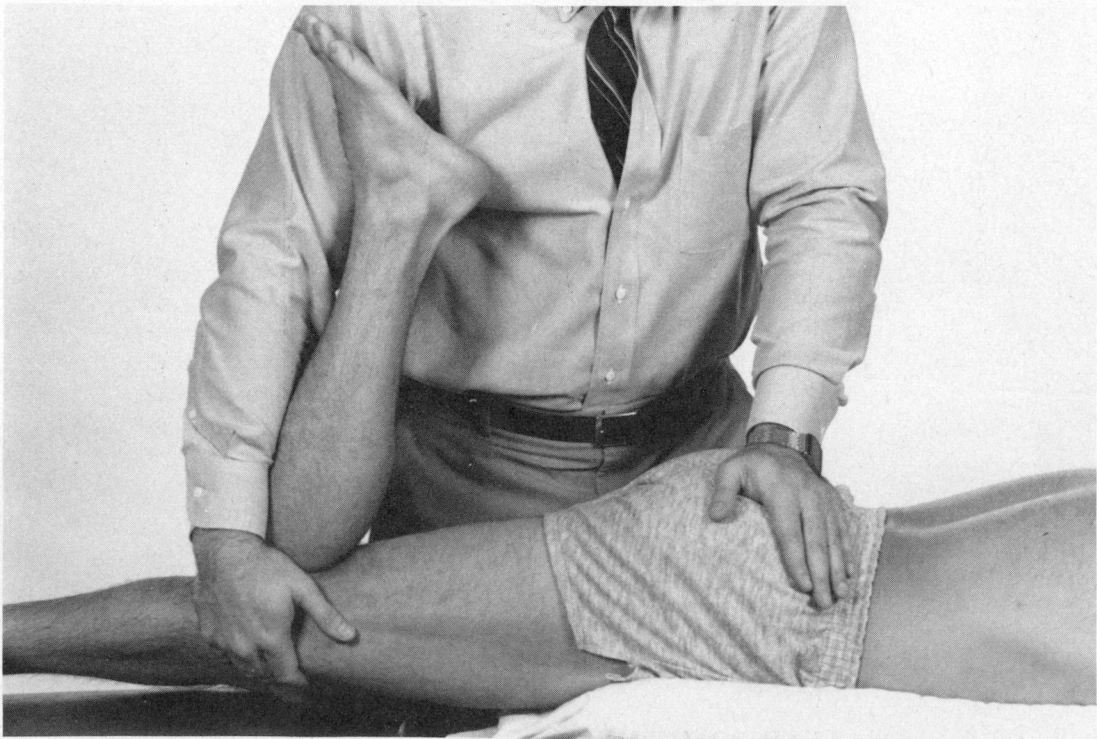

Fig. 22-19. Prone positioned passive mobility testing of the length of the rectus femoris and the anterior hip musculature, mainly the iliopsoas.

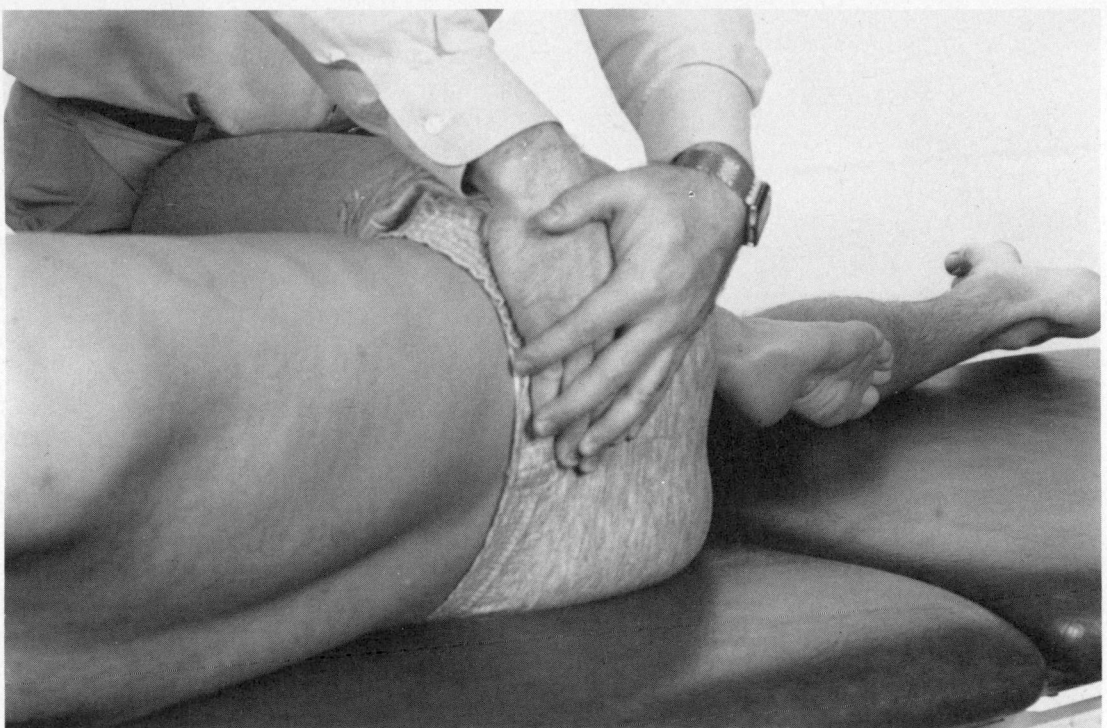

Fig. 22-20. Using the femur as a lever—sidelying manual stresses to the pelvis. The clinician pushes horizontally along the femur and pulls up and forward on the right ilium, resulting in an anterior rotary force on the sacroiliac joint.

ment. Education in the form of biomechanical counselling becomes one of the most important aspects of treatment. The purpose of the evaluation is to enable the therapist to recognize the destructive stimuli that creates the perception of pain. Biomechanical counselling is the teaching process that informs the patient about how his/her daily activities involve these same potentially destructive mechanics.

In all but a few instances a quick cure is not available for a sacroiliac (lumbopelvic) problem for two main reasons. First, it is unreasonable to think that one isolated structure is injured in this area. The joints, disks, muscles, and connective tissue structures do not act in isolation but rather work in concert with each other. Injury to any component of this region alters the function of the remaining structures.

Secondly, scar tissue is not an exact match of the tissue that was injured. The healing process in the lumbopelvic region is similar to that of the rest of the body. A common misconception is that the tissues of this region are governed by different rules, when in fact the physiological principles of connective tissues and bone appear to be constant throughout the body. Injured tissue is repaired by the formation of granulation and scar tissue.[21] As this process progresses, physical function and neuromuscular communication can be expected to undergo alterations. It is this phenomenon that motivates the individual to seek professional assistance.

One clear example of this is the anterior cruciate ligament disorder of the knee. Once this ligament is torn or sprained to a degree that its viscoelastic properties have changed, function of the knee is permanently altered. The therapist's role in this case is to rehabilitate the knee in order to allow the patient to optimally perform normal activities, while recognizing the fact that this joint will never be normal again.

The same is true for the sacroiliac (lumbopelvic) region. Once a major connective tissue structure is torn by injury, its function is permanently altered. As with the cruciate ligament, the goal of rehabilitation is to teach the patient how to manage his/her problem with an understanding that torn, and subsequently repaired tissue, is unlike noninjured, healthy tissue.

There are certainly variations to the above discussion. For example, sacroiliac pain is quite common in multiparous women and young females with a highly elastic connective tissue makeup. Subluxation of the joint appears reasonable if forces exceed the capacity of the stabilizing tissues. If this is the case, mobilization or manipulation of the joint, followed by external support of the region, may offer dramatic relief.

In addition, the pregnant female may place excessive strain on otherwise normal tissue because of the change in the location of the weight line as it traverses the lumbopelvic tissues. To accommodate this altered weight line, a

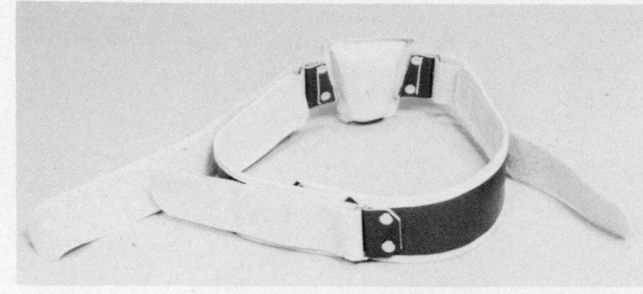

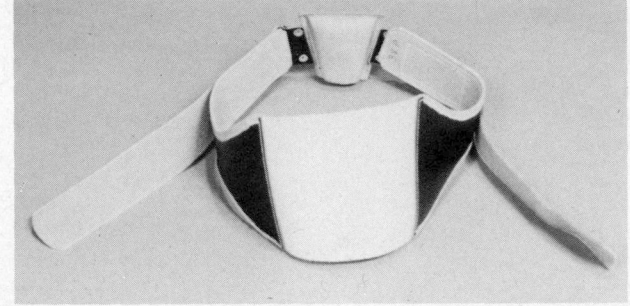

Fig. 22-21. A, Regular sacroiliac support. **B,** Pregnancy sacroiliac support.

sacral support can be used to help provide a counter force that redirects the weight line and marginally unload the soft tissues so that the painful stimulus can be diminished.

These examples are certainly the exception rather than the rule with the most common sacroiliac (lumbopelvic) disorders. In the more common clinical syndromes the history is extended over a greater period of time, and the patient presents with a chronic problem featuring acute episodes of symptoms.

The intent of treatment of the lumbopelvic region follows the same guidelines as other areas of the body. The first objective is to heal the wound.[48] While the term *wound* may conjure thoughts of skin lacerations, we need to extend this concept to include any tissue, superficial or deep, that has a ruptured cell membrane or fibers. The initial phases of rehabilitation should be designed to maximize the healing process. This process includes sequential phases that start with the inflammation and culminate in a functional repair that can allow nondestructive movement patterns to the injured region. Many patients with lumbopelvic disorders continually reinjure themselves and, consequently, never effectively complete the task of functional healing.

The second intent of treatment is to maintain normal relations between injured and noninjured tissue. At some point controlled nondestructive motions must be properly introduced into the area so that the injured tissues will heal according to appropriate stress lines.

The third intent is to maintain normal function of noninjured tissue. Regard must be given to maintaining the health and strength of the various tissues, with specific attention given to preventing the effects of disuse. Maintain-

ing neuromuscular balance between the afferent and efferent receptors is critical to the control needed for smooth, noninjurious movement (see Chapter 2).

The fourth intent is to prevent putting excessive strain on the affected tissue. This requires knowledge of the basic science of tissue healing[21] and subsequent initiation of an appropriate rehabilitation (training) program that does not continually disrupt the healing process. Since the lumbopelvic tissues are the hub of weight bearing, musculoskeletal and neuromuscular training is important to facilitate normal, nondestructive acceptance and transference of continual loads during weight-bearing activities. However, the training program must be performed in a manner that does not cause or prolong injury. The results of mismanagement are compromised function, frequent reinjury, and persistent chronic symptoms.

For purposes of description the treatment protocol is divided into four phases. *Phase I* is the period when pain is treated and rest becomes an important consideration. The physical therapist has multiple modalities available in order to deal effectively with the patient's pain. Modalities and medications are very often used in combination during this initial phase.

The patient needs to understand the importance of recognizing changes in pain frequency, duration, and intensity. The clinician should make every attempt to increase the client's sensitivity to any of these changes. The clinician must also take time to educate the client, for the more the client understands, the quicker and more attainable will be the long-term rehabilitation goal.

Unless the patient is appropriately counselled, he/she will be unable to keep the area at rest. This is one of the most important aspects of the first phase of treatment. Keeping the area at rest refers to the ability to keep destructive forces away from the injured tissue. This is why the evaluation system previously discussed is so important. As mentioned earlier, it is often not important to identify the tissues at fault, but rather those combinations of abnormal or excessive forces that stimulate the nociceptive or pain carrying system.

The evaluation attempts to determine these potentially destructive forces, and biomechanical counselling educates the patient as to how these same forces reach the affected region from above and below during his/her daily activities. For example, the patient must understand that a standing back extension maneuver places a similar force on the sacroiliac and lumbar tissues as the pushoff phase of gait. The hip is now in maximal hyperextension, and the lumbopelvic region has the same extension force applied to it. Successful treatment thus requires that the patient understand which forces minimize their chance to "heal the wound."

During this initial phase a support is used in an attempt to help stabilize the area in order to enhance soft tissue healing and minimize reinjury. The support cannot be expected to completely immobilize the area, however, the proprioceptive stimulus, in combination with the external support, helps to increase awareness of lumbopelvic position and motion. Fig. 22-21, *A* and *B,* shows two types of sacroiliac supports (pregnant and nonpregnant styles) for the pelvic and lower lumbar region. The most significant aspect of these supports is that they tighten from the back. This directs an extension force to the sacrum and a posterior-to-anterior force on the sacroiliac or lumbar tissues. These supports are angled inferiorly to superiorly as they track anteriorly to posteriorly creating a lifting force to the anterior aspect of the pelvis.* These temporary supports are used mainly in the first two phases of rehabilitation to help create optimal conditions for soft tissue healing.

Resting the region may also require altering the way in which forces reach this area. A common clinical example is the use of a heel lift. A heel lift can redirect the convergence of ground and trunk forces in a frontal plane, which in turn may lessen the destructive stimulus to the lumbopelvic region. For example, when the standing evaluation demonstrates that all palpated boney landmarks are lower on the right, it can be deduced that the right sacroiliac joint has more compressive forces applied to it, while the left has more of a shear force, as compared to the normal, symmetrical anatomical position. This is primarily because of the horizontal and vertical positions, respectively, that result with the change in the weight-bearing pattern. Likewise, because of the sidebending motion of the lumbar spine away from the sacral tilt, the right intervertebral foramen at the lumbosacral junction has a tensile or opening force applied to it, while the left has an increased compressive or closing force. This frontal plane asymmetry may be caused by an actual short leg, an asymmetrical muscular imbalance, or a combination of all of the above. The significance to this shift of forces is that the tissues on both sides are stressed at their upper limits. At the sacroiliac joint it appears that shear forces are potentially more destructive than compressive forces, therefore rendering the side of the body that is positioned more vertically or the sacroiliac joint opposite of the sacral tilt (the long leg side) vulnerable to injury and symptoms.[11]

Thus heel lifts may be a valuable adjunct during the tissue healing phases of rehabilitation. Heel lifts can be easily fabricated by using commercially available cork with soft foam rubber material glued to it. Heel lifts are also commercially available. The rule of thumb is to place one-half of the measured pelvic difference into the shoe.

Only up to ⅜ inch can be comfortably placed into the shoe without altering the affectiveness of the rearfoot counter. The clinician should recognize that the frontal plane should be assessed for at least the first four visits to assure that the frontal plane difference is skeletal and not neuromuscular. If the difference is caused by a neuromuscular imbalance, then the heel lift will generally provide temporary relief, but it will ultimately create an imbalance to the other side and should be removed. The proper use of heel lifts can be quite effective in the successful management of problems in this region.

Phase II represents a significant crossroads with respect to the progression of the treatment process. During this phase the therapist works carefully to avoid a setback that could revert the patient back to Phase I. At the same time this second phase cannot be the final stage. Very often physical therapy and medical treatment throughout this phase is prolonged or stops after successful completion. This, in turn, contributes to the chronicity of lumbopelvic problems.

Use of supports is continued during Phase II. The patient must recognize that supports cannot offer complete immobility of the region, and it is a significant mistake to design a rehabilitation program without a goal to discontinue its use. In order to ensure a successful rehabilitation process, the patient must be cognizant of his/her activities to avoid reinjury.

During this phase nondestructive movements should be started. These movements have a twofold effect. First, the tissue is stimulated to adapt along appropriate lines of stress (i.e., forces are directed to the injured tissues in a nondestructive manner so as to stimulate fibroblasts to lay down collagen in a functional pattern). Second, the important afferent neurological system is activated (see Chapter 2), which has the potential to modulate pain as well as provide proprioceptive input to the central nervous system (CNS).[46]

The physical therapist has a variety of ways in which to introduce active or passive nondestructive forces into the tissues. Unfortunately, these techniques have a variety of different names. Joint mobilization, soft tissue mobilization, traction, muscle energy procedures, prolonged stretching, transverse friction, and contract-relax exercises are but a few in a family of nondestructive movement techniques. Whether the therapist is actually repositioning such an inherently stable complex as the sacroiliac joint, or reducing a subluxation of apophyseal joints, is certainly open for question and at this point is highly suspect. However, the unifying element to nearly all of these and other manual techniques is that forces are placed on tissues and joints, and these forces result in an increase in afferent input to the CNS.

With this in mind, it is easy to understand why such a variety of techniques can all be successful in this phase. Figs. 22-22 and 22-23 are examples of such techniques. Fig. 22-22 exemplifies a muscle energy technique that places an anterior rotary moment on the right innominate bone. In this example the iliopsoas muscle creates the desired force because the therapist is stabilizing the femur

*Further information regarding supports can be obtained from I.E.M. Orthopaedics, 7108 State Route 14, Ravenna, Ohio 44266.

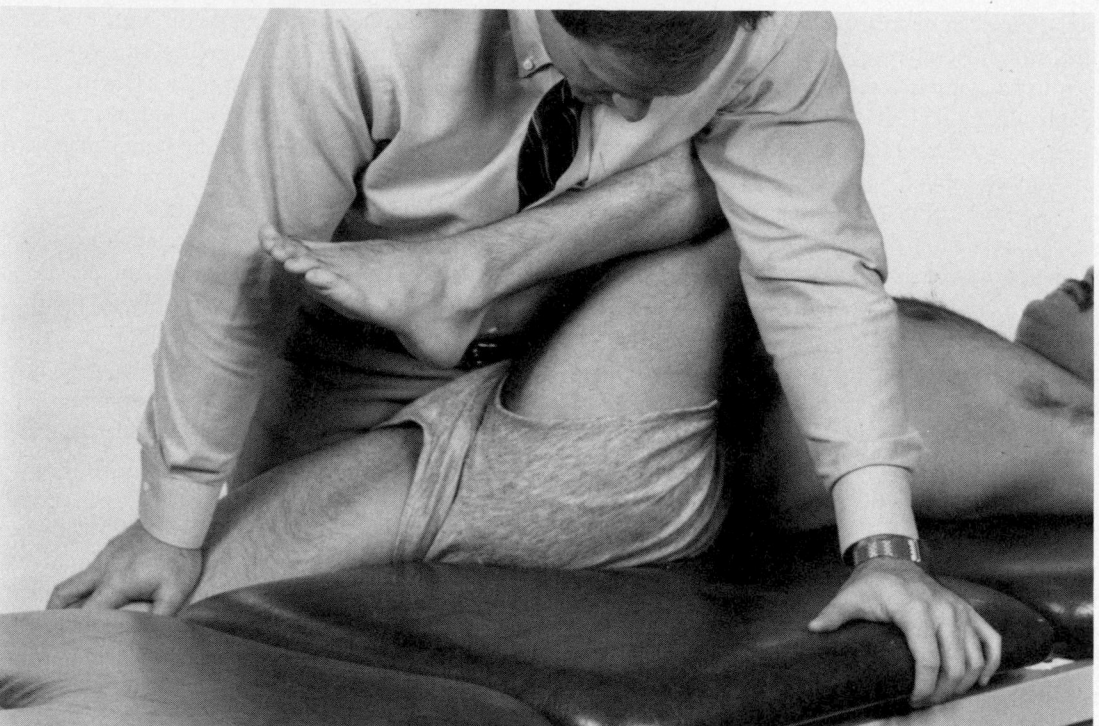

Fig. 22-22. Use of the right iliopsoas to create an anterior rotary force to the right ilium and a slight extension force to the lumbar spine.

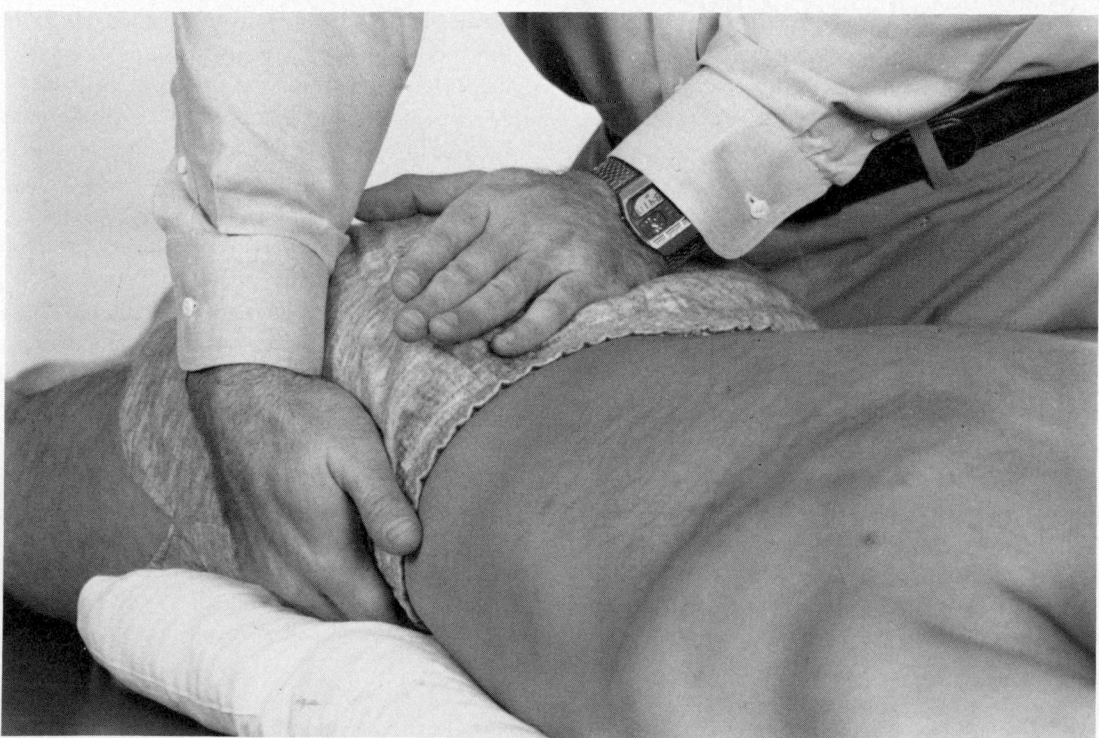

Fig. 22-23. Manual technique to create a posterior rotary and posterior shear force to the tissues of the right sacroiliac joint.

while asking for an isometric contraction of the muscle. The isometric contraction results in the anterior rotary moment on the pelvis.

The clinician is not necessarily repositioning a bone, but rather is generating a nondestructive stimulus into the region and increasing CNS afferent activity. The result is a positive step in developing or regaining a balance in information to the musculature of this region.

The second example, Fig. 22-23, represents a manually directed force to the tissues. In this example, the resultant force is a posterior rotary and posterior-to-anterior shear force to the right ilium and an anterior rotary and a posterior-to-anterior shear force to the sacrum. The patient is positioned prone, with the pelvis stabilized on a pillow. Consideration must be given to placing the lumbar spine in a neutral position. The clinician's right hand grasps the patient's right anterior superior iliac spine (ASIS) and anterior ilium, and the clinician's left hand is comfortably placed on the midsacrum. Graded, equal, and opposite forces are directed to the patient's ilium and sacrum to create the desired mechanical stimulus.

What is more important is that these techniques are all based on the skill of the clinician to successfully apply controlled forces into the area. With an understanding of the biomechanical and neuromuscular implications of controlled movement and an in-depth knowledge of the functional anatomy of this region, the reader can easily add to this list of manual techniques.

A common finding in the examination of sacroiliac dysfunction is decreased passive range of motion on the side of the lesion. Hip capsular and/or muscular tightness creates a biomechanical alteration, which makes the sacroiliac joint vulnerable to overuse and sprain from what would otherwise be activities within normal tolerance. Stretching adaptively shortened tissues or directing elongating forces to a muscle that has an increased efferent output are effective techniques to normalize forces in this phase of treatment. In the management of pelvic dysfunction, stretching techniques for the hip are extremely important in that if the hip does not have normal mobility, adaptations in the form of excessive forces will result proximally. For example, during the evaluation the clinicians will often find a tightness in the figure 4 position or a tightness in hyperextension and internal rotation of the hip on the side of sacroiliac (lumbopelvic) pain. It is important to recognize that tight anterior hip structures have the potential to cause anterior torsional forces of the ilium on the sacrum, and extension forces on the lumbar spine, when the individual is in an upright posture.

The client should be taught stretching techniques for lengthening the musculature and capsular ligaments of the hip.

Lastly, the patient must be continually counseled as to the movement patterns or static postures that have the potential to replicate the offending forces, or conversely, they must recognize their optimal resting postures. For example, an extended hip posture in a prone or standing position is an ideal posture to remove tensile force on all tissues posterior to the axis of rotation in order to counteract flexion of the lumbar spine. Flexion patterns, on the other hand, put a tensile force on these same tissues and are a potentially destructive stimulus. The evaluation process should help guide the thought process of optimal rest positions.

Phase II is the phase in which the various patient educational programs are most effective because the patient starts to develop an understanding of the functional anatomy of the region. For example, a one-legged standing posture has the potential to increase the rotary and upward shear force of the ilium on the sacrum of the stance leg because of the convergence of forces as they reach this area. If the evaluation has determined that these same forces reproduce this pain, then it is important for the patient to realize that it is not only one-legged standing that has the potential to be a painful stimulus but any posterior rotary or upward shear force of ilium on sacrum. The therapist must then review the client's daily activities and create a recognition within the client as to when these destructive forces might occur. We recommend four rules for the successful management of sacroiliac lesions.

Rule 1: Stair climbing two at a time is strictly prohibited, and if the patient is carrying anything up the steps, like a basket of clothes or a bag of groceries, then the patient should climb one step at a time leading with the unaffected limb. Consider the forces generated in this region when the foot is fixed on a step and the hip and thigh musculature is asked to generate the forces required to lift the body weight up the step. There is a tremendous accumulation of stresses in the sacroiliac (lumbopelvic) region; usually enough to continue the inflammatory process of an injured pelvic tissue.

Rule 2: When getting up from a seated position, unload the affected limb and transfer the weight to the unaffected leg. Once upright, lean over the unaffected leg. This decreases the accumulation of unwanted forces to the area.

Rule 3: Avoid squatting down on the affected leg or full hip flexion while weight bearing. As mentioned earlier, the greatest force appears to be generated in this region during a return from the seated or squatting position.[25]

Rule 4: Femoral flexion, abduction, and external rotation in the nondominant sexual position should be avoided. The hip joint, in this position, transfers the forces applied to the femur proximally to the pelvis and sacroiliac joints.

The avoidance of these forces allows the patient and the therapist to succeed at the goal of resting the area, while continuing to perform nondestructive activities. Each patient with the syndrome that has been described in this chapter should be educated with these four rules.

After the patient has been gradually and successfully assisted through the first two phases of the rehabilitation process, therapy proceeds to Phase III. During this phase supports are discontinued, except for periods when the individual is involved in strenuous physical activity. Training of the neuromuscular system with resistive exercises is initiated but directed away from the extremes of range.

The patient must learn to recognize the difference between the highly vulnerable and less vulnerable position of his/her lumbopelvic tissues. This position is unique to the individual and is dependent on the injury. For example, if someone has a great deal of pain with the extended posture, and the pain increases with overpressure, then any exercise that subjects the lumbopelvic region to an increased extension and compression force leaves this area vulnerable to reinjury.

In an individual whose pain is reproduced with flexion movements, exercises that have a minimal chance to introduce a flexion force are preferable. A position of spinal extension or normal lumbar lordosis is desired for this individual. For example, a curl up that creates trunk flexion is an inappropriate exercise for this individual. The same thought processes need to occur with torsional, compressive, shear, or multi-plane forces.

In both of the above examples the goal was to initiate resistance exercises by teaching the patient to maintain a less vulnerable position of the spine and pelvis. This phase is extremely important because it is the first attempt to train the lumbopelvic muscles as stabilizers, rather than prime movers. We prefer to call this type of activity proprioceptive training of the trunk, since the muscles are asked to control spinal position based on proprioceptive awareness. The exercises used in this phase of treatment should be single plane movements to avoid undesired component movement.

Phase IV consists of advanced proprioceptive training of the spine, with an emphasis on multi-plane motions. This phase requires that resistance exercises for the upper and lower extremities be initiated. It is critical that the less vulnerable spinal position be maintained throughout the exercise. For example, a pulley exercise that uses a pulling motion requires a coordinated effort of the shoulder extensors, scapula retractors, and spine extensors. If the therapist superimposes this activity on a less vulnerable position of the spine, significant involvement of the muscles controlling the pelvis and lumbar spine are added. Muscles that are recruited for this activity are the deep erector spinae, multifidus, abdominals, hip extensors, adductors, and abductors. This activity occurs by virtue of the muscle's attachments to the pelvis and lumbar spine.

The therapist must remember that to make gains in muscle strength or endurance, the point of momentary failure must be approached in order to provide the stimulus for the necessary biochemical and anatomical changes in the muscle. The muscle must be given the opportunity to respond to these new stresses. In the above example it may not be the shoulder extensors that fail as endurance repetitions are accomplished, but an inability of the musculature to stabilize the trunk. Proper affective stabilization of the spine during weight bearing, especially in the lumbopelvic region of a back injured individual, is critical in successful rehabilitation and spine management programs. The physical therapist must analyze the complete movement pattern with cognizance of all the functioning muscle groups, while critiquing the exercise. The point of failure for the activity is when any one of the components of this activity no longer occurs correctly. Many times this failure occurs in the trunk, and excessive torsional, flexion, or extension motions result. Obviously with this type of training program, the concept of three sets of 10 repetitions is no longer appropriate. While the individual may still be able to do the shoulder extension component of the exercise, the clinician may immediately recognize the inappropriate activity of the lumbopelvic segments. At this point the clinician needs to alert the patient as to the importance of all the components working synchronously and avoid overload of one area.

For many individuals with long-standing sacroiliac (lumbopelvic) problems, moving the lower or upper extremities independent of the spine is extremely difficult. The patient has difficulty stabilizing the lumbopelvic area because his/her internal information system in the form of afferent/efferent pathways has lost its acuity.

Excessive torsional, shear tensile, and compressive forces are thus imparted to the sacroiliac and lumbar joints when the upper and lower extremities move through their range of motion. The muscles of the trunk must therefore be trained to dynamically stabilize this region.

It is important to recognize the carryover of this type of training to activities of daily living and the industrial work environment, thus the fourth phase of rehabilitation must be instituted. There are certainly many names for the various efforts to return the worker to industry in optimal physical condition and with an awareness of his/her spinal posture. From the scientific perspective the common link between many of these programs is that they teach proprioceptive awareness of spinal motion, and they attempt to increase the fitness level of the participant.

The added benefit of training the upper and lower extremity with the trunk muscles in this manner is the effect this has on the muscles attached to or indirectly affecting the many fascial planes in the lumbosacral region. There appears to be a positive relationship between muscle and thoracolumbar fascia in providing dynamic stability of the trunk.[14,35]

Prompt identification of the injury and a goal oriented rehabilitation program designed to optimize the patient's ability to functionally heal should be the aim of physical therapy. The treatment goal in all cases is to normalize stresses in the lumbopelvic region by balancing specific systems, including anatomical structure, ground and trunk forces, muscular length and strength, and afferent/efferent neuropathways. This treatment protocol takes time and patience, but without normalization of these systems the therapist has no hope of producing lasting results in the treatment of lumbopelvic disorders. If this approach is not taken, the client develops a lifestyle that inherently weakens the various tissues and leaves them prone to continued injury.

SUMMARY

This sacroiliac (lumbopelvic) region is a fascinating area of biomechanics, and it can potentially play a significant role in many low-back pain syndromes. The continued study of the manner in which the musculoskeletal system destructively and/or nondestructively absorbs and transfers loads (forces) in normal and abnormal conditions has heightened our understanding of the lumbopelvic region. This improved knowledge of the design and function of this region has formed the basis for the successful management of painful conditions affecting this area.

REFERENCES

1. Beal MC: The sacroiliac problem: review of anatomy, mechanisms and diagnosis, Jr. of AOA, 81 (10):667-679, 1982.
2. Borell U: The movements of the sacroiliac joints and their importance to changes in pelvic dimensions during parturition, Acta Gynecol 36:1, 1957.
3. Bowan V and Cassidy JD: Macroscopic and microscopic anatomy of the sacroiliac joint from embryonic life until the eighth decade, Spine 6:620-628, 1981.
4. Chamberlin WE: The symphysis pubis in the roentgen examination of the sacroiliac joint, J Bone Joint Surg (Am) 24(6):621, 1930.
5. Colachis SD et al: Movement of the sacroiliac joint in the adult male: a preliminary report, Arch Phys Med Rehabil 44:490, 1963.
6. Coventry MB and Tapper EM: Pelvic instability, J Bone Joint Surg (Am) 54:83-101, 1972.
7. Drerup B and Hierholzer E: Movement of the human pelvis and displacement of related anatomical landmarks on the body surface, J Biomechanics 20(10):971-977, 1987.
8. Egund N et al: Movement in the sacroiliac joints demonstrated with roentgen stereophotogrammetry, Acta Radiol (Stockh) 19:833, 1978.
9. Erhard R et al: The recognition and management of the pelvic components of low back sciatic pain, J of Orthop Section APTA, Fall 1967.
10. Fraser DM: Postpartum backache: a preventable condition? Orthop Section APTA 3(1):14-16, 1978.
11. Friberg O: Clinical symptoms and biomechanics of lumbar spine and hip joint in leg length inequality, Spine 8(6):643-650, 1983.
12. Frigerio NA et al: Movement of the sacroiliac joint, Clin Orthop 100:370, 1974.
13. Golighty R: Pelvic arthropathy in pregnancy and the puerperium, Physiotherapy 68:216-220, 1982.
14. Gracovetsky S and Farfan H: The optimal spine, 11(6):543-572, 1986.
15. Gray H: Anatomy of the human body, Philadelphia, 1973, Lea & Febiger.
16. Grieve E: Lumbo-pelvic rhythm and mechanical dysfunction of the sacroiliac joint, Physiotherapy 67:171-173, 1981.
17. Hisaw TL: Corpus luteum hormone: experimental relaxation of pelvic ligaments of guinea pigs, Physiol Zool 2:59, 1929.
18. Hoppenfeld S: Physical examination of the spine and extremities, New York, 1976, Appleton-Century-Crofts.
19. Kaltenborn F: Personal communication regarding the sacroiliac joint, Akron, Ohio, 1981.
20. Kapandji IA: The physiology of the joints, vol 3, Edinburgh, 1974, Churchill Livingstone, Inc.
21. Kellet J: Acute soft tissue injuries—A review of the literature, Med Sci Sports Exerc 18(5):489-500, 1986.
22. Laban MM et al: Lumbosacral-anterior pelvic pain associated with pubic symphysis instability, Arch Phys Med Rehabil 56:548, 1975.
23. Lavignolle B et al: An approach to the functional anatomy of the sacroiliac joints in vivo, Anat Clin 5:169-176, 1983.
24. Luk KDK et al: The iliolumbar ligament, a study of its anatomy, development and clinical significance, J Bone Joint Surg (Br) 68(2):197-200, 1986.
25. Lumsden RM et al: An in vivo study of axial rotation and immobilization at the lumbosacral joint, J Bone Joint Surg (Am) 50(8):1591, 1968.
26. Maitland GD: Vertebral map, ed 3, London, 1973, Butterworth Publishers.
27. McKenzie RA: Mechanical diagnosis and therapy of the lumbar spine, Waikanae, New Zealand, 1981, Spinal Publications.
28. Mennell JM: Diagnosis and treatment using manipulative techniques: joint pain, Boston, 1964, Little, Brown & Co.
29. Mitchell FL: An evaluation and treatment manual of osteopathic muscle energy procedures, ed 1, Valley Park, Mo, 1979, Mitchell, Moran & Pruzzo.
30. Money V et al: The facet syndrome, Clin Orthop 115:149-156, 1976.
31. Oakland O et al: The "axial sacroiliac joint," Anat Clin 6:29-36, 1984.
32. Paquin JD et al: Biochemical and morphologic studies of cartilage from the adult human sacroiliac joint, Arthritis Rheum 26(7):887-895, 1983.
33. Paris S: Introduction to joint mobilization, continuing education course, Atlanta, Ga, 1975.
34. Pitkin IID et al: Sacrathrogenetic telalgia, J Bone Joint Surg (Am) 18(2):365, 1936.
35. Porterfield JA: Dynamic stabilization of the trunk, J Orth Sports Phys Ther 6(2):271-277, 1985.
36. Sashin O: A critical analysis of the anatomy and the pathological changes of the SI joints, J Bone Joint Surg (Am) 12:891, 1930.
37. Schunke GB: The anatomy and the development of the sacroiliac joint and their relation to the movements of the sacrum, Acta Anat 23:80-91, 1955.
38. Solonen KA: The sacroiliac joint in light of anatomical, roentgenological, and clinical studies, Acta Orthop Scand (Suppl) 27:1, 1957.
39. Stoddard A: Manual of osteopathic technique, London, 1959, Hutchinson & Co.
40. Sturesson B, Selvik CT, and Uden A: Movement of the sacroiliac joints: A Roentgen stereophotogrammetric analysis, Spine 162-165, 1989.
41. Subotnick S: Podiatric sports medicine, Mount Kisco, NY, 1975, Futura Publishing Co.
42. Taylor JR and Twomey LT: Age related charges in the lumbar zygaphophyseal joints, Spine 11(7): 1986.
43. Tesh KM et al: The abdominal muscles and vertebral stability, Spine 12(5): 1987.
44. Walker JM: Age-related differences in the human sacroiliac joint: A histological study; implications for therapy, J Orth Sports Phys Ther 7(6):325-334, 1986.
45. Weisl H: The movements of the sacroiliac joint, Acta Anat 23(1):80, 1955.
46. Weiss M, Nagelschmidt L, and Struck H: Relaxin and collagen metabolism, Horm Metab Res 11:408-414, 1979.
47. Wyke B: The lumbar spine and back pain, Marshfield, Mass, 1980, Pitman Publishing, Inc.
48. Zarins B: Soft tissue injury and repair—biomechanical aspects, Int J Sports Med 3:9-11, 1982.

Chapter 23

THE TEMPOROMANDIBULAR JOINT

Mark H. Friedman
Joseph Weisberg

The temporomandibular joint (TMJ) is one of a very few synovial joints in the body that physical therapists do not usually evaluate or treat. The fact that TMJ dysfunction is widespread and is often the cause of varied symptoms throughout the head and neck is becoming recognized among health professionals. Currently, dentists are the primary professionals involved in treatment to enhance physical therapists' knowledge about the TMJ so that their expertise in joint and soft tissue management can improve treatment of this joint. Evaluative and treatment techniques for synovial joint management, such as range-of-motion measurements, muscle function, and joint-play tests, and mobilization techniques, can be adapted by physical therapists to TMJ management.[14] This will improve treatment and enlarge the scope of the physical therapy practice.

Furthermore, since the TMJ is a link in the chain of synovial joints connecting the human body, it interrelates anatomically and kinesiologically with adjacent joints in this chain and those of the cervical spine.[34] Because of this relationship, a greater understanding of the TMJ will aid physical therapists in treating the cervical spine.

FUNCTIONAL ANATOMY AND KINESIOLOGY
Bony structures

The TMJ, located just anterior to the external ear, is the articulation between the condylar process of the mandible and the mandibular fossa and articular eminence of the cranium (Fig. 23-1). These articulating surfaces are covered by fibrocartilage rather than hyaline cartilage. The condylar head of the mandible resembles a football, with blunted ends pointing mediolaterally. When the mouth is closed, the condyle fits into the mandibular fossa of the temporal bone. The anterior boundary of this fossa is

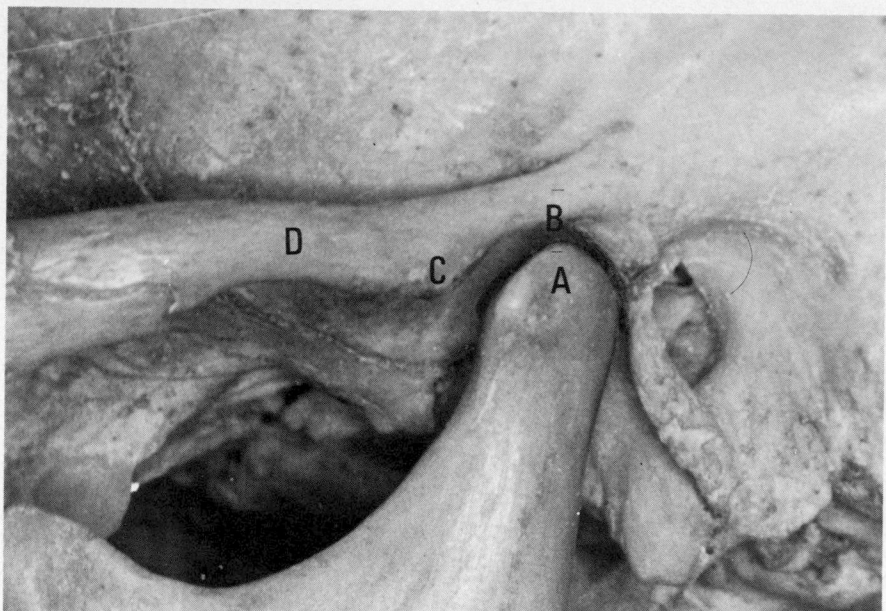

Fig. 23-1. *A*, Mandibular condyle; *B*, mandibular fossa; *C*, articular eminence; *D*, zygomatic arch.

formed by a transverse bony ridge, the articular eminence.[8]

Soft tissues

Soft tissues such as joint capsules, masticatory muscles, and ligaments articulate the mandible to the skull. The articulating components of the TMJ are separated and cushioned by an articular disk, which divides the joint space into an upper and a lower compartment. The disk is composed of fibrocartilage, is thinner at the center than anteriorly or posteriorly (Fig. 23-2), and is attached to the condyle only at the medial and lateral poles.[35] The anterior portion of the disk is joined to the superior head of the lateral pterygoid muscle. Posteriorly, the disk is attached to a thick layer of loose vascularized elastic connective tissue (Fig. 23-2).

The TMJ is surrounded by a loose, relatively thin fibrous joint capsule. Superiorly, the capsule encircles the mandibular fossa. Inferiorly, it is attached to the condylar neck, below the attachment of the disk. Posteriorly, the capsule fuses with the posterior attachment of the disk. Anteriorly, disc and capsule are fused, allowing the attachment of some lateral pterygoid fibers (upper head) directly to the disk. Thus the capsule is attached to the disk around its entire circumference. The lateral surface of the capsule is reinforced by a triangular thickening, the temporomandibular ligament.[23]

The inner surface of the TMJ capsule is lined by a single layer of cells known as the synovial membrane. This thin membrane reflects onto the superior and inferior surfaces of the disk. The highly specialized cells that form this membrane perform various functions, such as (1) pro-

ducing hyaluronic acid (the main component of joint lubrication), (2) cleansing the joint of debris (phagocytosis), and (3) participating in immune reactions.

The temporomandibular ligament, the most important ligament of the TMJ, originates at the inferior aspect of the zygomatic arch and runs obliquely and inferoposteri-

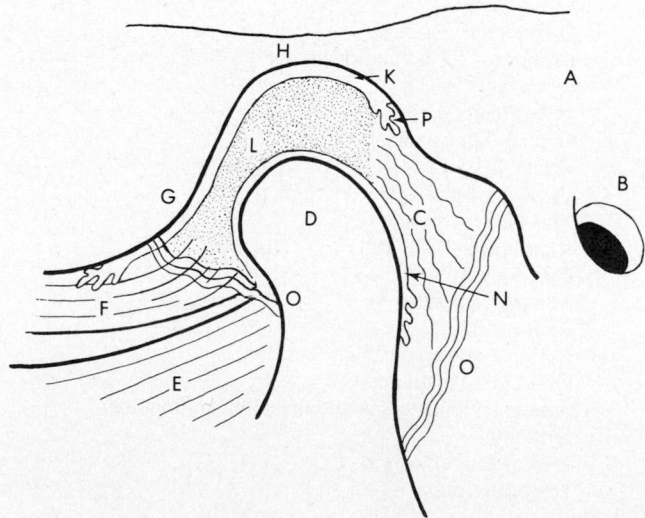

Fig. 23-2. Anatomy of TMJ. *A*, Temporal bone; *B*, external auditory meatus; *C*, loose areolar connective tissue; *D*, mandibular condyle; *E*, inferior belly of lateral pterygoid muscle; *F*, superior belly of lateral pterygoid muscle; *G*, articular eminence of temporal bone; *H*, mandibular fossa; *K*, superior joint cavity; *L*, articular disk; *N*, inferior joint cavity; *O*, posterior aspect of joint capsule; *P*, synovial reflection. (Reprinted from Physical Ther 62:597, 1982, with permission of American Physical Therapy Association.)

orly. This ligament limits excessive lateral or posterior movement of the condyle. Two accessory ligaments, the sphenomandibular and stylomandibular ligaments, have little influence on mandibular function.

The muscles of mastication are primarily responsible for mandibular movements and include the lateral pterygoid, medial pterygoid, masseter, and temporalis muscles. They originate on the skull and insert on the mandible (Fig. 23-3). Their neural innervation is from the mandibular division of the trigeminal nerve; blood is supplied by the muscular branches of the maxillary artery.

The lateral (external) pterygoid muscle consists of a large lower and a small upper head; the two heads function separately. The muscle generally lies in a horizontal plane running backward and laterally. The lower head arises from the lateral surface of the lateral pterygoid plate and extends to the anterior surface of the condylar neck. The upper head arises from the infratemporal surface of the greater wing of the sphenoid bone and extends to the articular disk.

The medial (internal) pterygoid muscle is almost perpendicular to the lateral pterygoid muscle, originating on the medial surface of the lateral pterygoid plate. It inserts on the inner mandibular surface, forming the inner portion of the mandibular sling. Its shape and anteroposterior direction are similar to those of the masseter muscle. However, its fibers are directed medially.

The masseter muscle is the most superficial and the strongest of the masticatory muscles. This muscle arises from the zygomatic arch and passes inferiorly and posteri-

orly to insert on the outer surface of the mandibular ramus; its inferior extent is close to the angle of the jaw. This muscle is divided into a superficial and a deep portion; the deeper fibers are directed vertically. The parotid gland overlies this muscle posterolaterally.

The fan-shaped temporalis muscle arises from the temporal fossa and inserts by a strong tendon into the coronoid process of the mandible. Because of its broad origin and narrow insertion, this muscle is well suited for delicate positional changes of the mandible.

The masseter and medial pterygoid muscles are powerful mandibular elevators and aid in mandibular protrusion. The lateral pterygoid muscle is the main mandibular depressor and is also responsible for anterior and lateral mandibular movements. The temporalis muscle assists the medial pterygoid and masseter muscles in elevating the mandible; its posterior fibers retract the mandible.[8] The temporalis muscle is responsible for maintaining the postural position of the mandible.

The four suprahyoid muscles—digastric, mylohyoid, geniohyoid, and stylohyoid—are considered accessory muscles of mastication. They aid in mandibular depression when the hyoid bone is fixed by contraction of the infrahyoid muscles—thyrohyoid, sternothyroid, sternohyoid, and omohyoid. When the mandible is fixed, as in swallowing, the suprahyoid muscles raise the hyoid bone. The digastric muscles are the most important of the suprahyoid muscles in mandibular function. They are responsible for the complete opening of the jaw and also aid in retraction of the mandible.

Associated structures

The equilibrium of forces around the teeth in the oral cavity is maintained intraorally by the tongue and extraorally by the orbicularis oris and buccinator muscles. At rest, the anterior third of the tongue should be located on the incisive papilla, just behind the upper incisors. The middle third of the tongue should rest on the roof of the mouth, and the posterior third should form a 45-degree angle between the hard palate and the pharynx. During normal swallowing the tongue moves smoothly up and back, with the lips closed and immobile.

The average adult mouth contains 32 teeth, 16 in the maxilla and 16 in the mandible. They are fixed in the maxillary and mandibular alveolar processes. The mucous membrane covering the dental arches near the teeth is called *gingiva,* or *gum.* Normal gingiva is pink and firm and is called *attached gingiva.* Between adjacent teeth the gingiva is extended in a V shape, called the *interdental papilla.* The gingiva is continuous with the mucous membrane of the oral cavity. These two tissues join at a distinct line, the mucogingival junction. The dark-pink or reddish mucous membrane just beyond this line covers the alveolar processes and is called *alveolar mucosa.* It is absent in the palate[3] (Fig. 23-4).

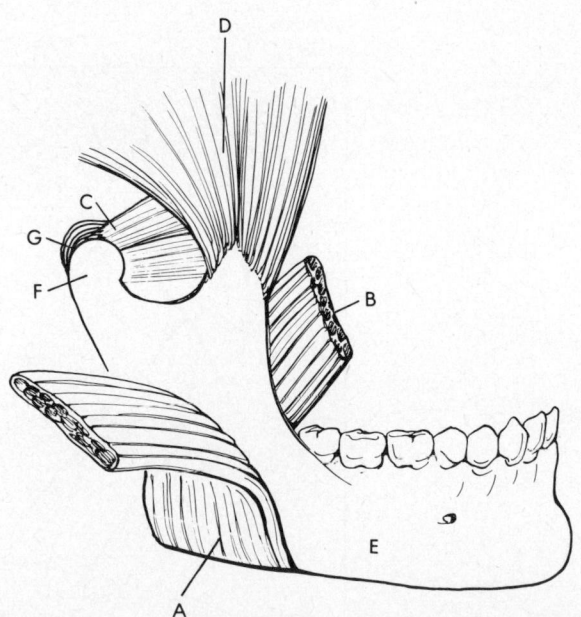

Fig. 23-3. Muscles of mastication. *A,* Masseter muscle; *B,* medial pterygoid muscle; *C,* lateral pterygoid muscle; *D,* temporalis muscle; *E,* lateral surface of body of mandible; *F,* mandibular condyle; *G,* articular disk.

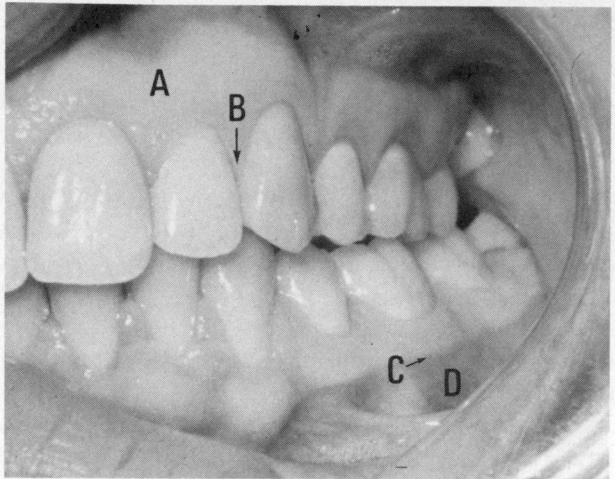

Fig. 23-4. *A,* Attached gingiva; *B,* interdental papilla; *C,* mucogingival junction; *D,* alveolar mucosa.

Certain characteristics common to the normal adult dentition are illustrated in Fig. 23-5. When the mouth is closed and the teeth contact maximally (centric occlusion), the mandibular teeth occlude anteriorly to the corresponding maxillary teeth by a distance of one half the width of a bicuspid. This anterior mandibular position is extremely stable, because it allows each tooth (except for the lower central incisors and the upper third molars) to interdigitate with two opposing teeth. Posterior teeth have cone-shaped projections (cusps) and depressions (fossae). When the teeth occlude, cusps fit into fossae.

The teeth of each dental arch normally have a close proximal contact; dental floss passes between adjacent teeth with difficulty. The maxillary teeth overlap the mandibular teeth in a vertical and horizontal direction[3] (Fig. 23-6). The overbite covers about one third of the labial surface of the lower anterior teeth. This vertical and horizontal relationship exists to a lesser degree in the posterior region of the mouth.

Basic mandibular movements

The TMJ is a hinge joint, which, with its disk, acts as a movable socket.[8] This movable socket permits condylar translation, which prevents mandibular encroachment of the anterior structures of the neck during jaw opening. A simple hinge joint permits adequate opening for four-footed animals, whose necks lie behind, rather than below, their mandibles.

Initially the jaw opens when the closing masticatory muscles—the masseter, temporalis, and medial pterygoid—relax. Condylar rotation then depresses the mandible by gravitational pull. When the jaw has opened approximately 1 cm, the lateral pterygoid muscles contract, causing condylar translation to maximal jaw opening. The relatively large synovial reflections (Fig. 23-2) unfold, allowing translation to occur without tearing the synovial lining.[23] Bilateral contraction of the digastric muscles occurs toward the end of the opening range. In normal jaw opening the condyles move forward about 15 mm, often extending beyond the articular eminence. As the condyles translate from the mandibular fossa to the convex articular eminence, the pliable disks change their position and shape to fill the space between the two bones.[35] The artic-

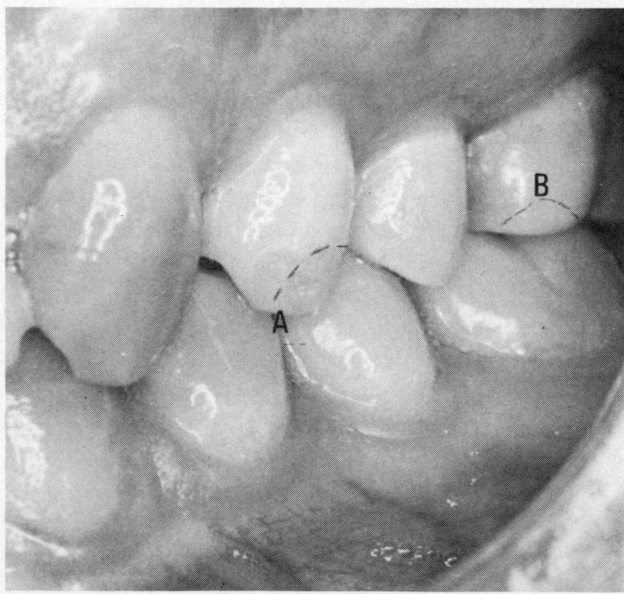

Fig. 23-5. *A,* Upper bicuspid occluding with two lower bicuspids; *B,* distobuccal cusp of lower molar occluding with fossa of upper molar.

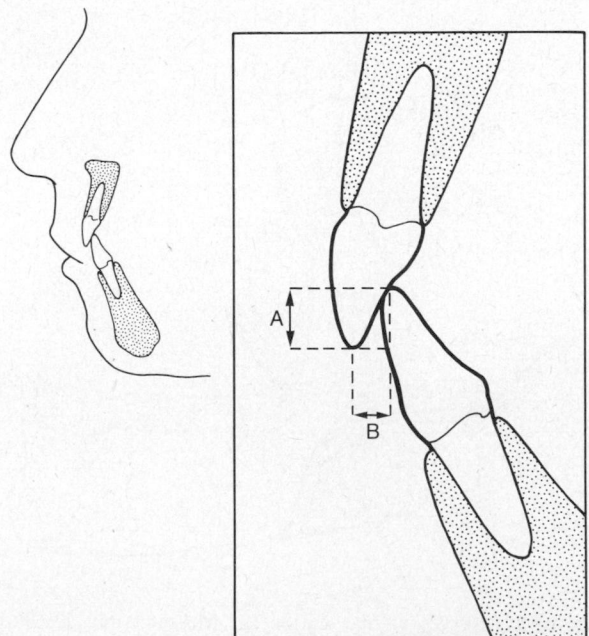

Fig. 23-6. Overlap of maxillary anterior teeth. *A,* Vertical overlap (overbite); *B,* horizontal overlap (overjet).

ular disk can move somewhat independently of the condyle, because it is attached only to the medial and lateral poles of the condyle. As the jaw opens the disk moves forward about 7 mm, half as far as the condyle (Fig. 23-7).[30]

Mandibular closure occurs as the temporalis, masseter, and medial pterygoid muscles contract. The disk is retracted by the elastic fibers in its posterior attachment. The superior heads of the lateral pterygoid muscles contract at the beginning of closure, preventing excessive posterior movement of the disk.[23]

Lateral movements are asymmetrical, whereas opening and closing movements are symmetrical. As the mandible moves laterally, one condyle and its disk slide downward, medially, and forward, as the other rotates laterally, around a vertical axis.[8] These movements are caused by contraction of the ipsilateral temporalis and masseter muscles and the contralateral medial and lateral pterygoid muscles.

Protrusion of the mandible is accomplished by the simultaneous contraction of the inferior heads of the lateral pterygoid muscles, assisted by the masseter and medial pterygoid muscles. The lateral pterygoid muscles pull the condyles forward; the masseter and medial pterygoid muscles pull the body of the mandible forward. The medial pterygoid muscles exert the stronger force. Mandibular retrusion occurs as the digastric and posterior fibers of the temporalis muscles contract.

Basic mandibular positions

A basic position of the mandible can be defined as a position assumed frequently during function. The most important basic mandibular positions are the intercuspal position (centric occlusion) and the postural (rest) position.

The intercuspal position occurs when the cusps and fossae of the maxillary and mandibular teeth mesh tightly (maximal contact between opposing teeth), with the mandible in its most cranial position. Proprioceptive impulses from the periodontium cause a reflex mechanism that guides jaw closure directly into the intercuspal position. This closing mechanism must be reinforced repeatedly, which normally happens when opposing teeth occlude maximally during swallowing.[31]

When the head is held erect in a relaxed state, opposing teeth do not contact. This relationship of the mandible to the skull is called the *rest* or *postural position* and represents a balance of various soft tissues—muscles of the head and neck, joint capsules, ligaments, and articular disks. This position changes with various body and head positions; it is influenced by the occlusion as well as by physiological and pathological conditions. The masticatory muscles are relaxed in the postural position. The gap between opposing occlusal surfaces that occurs in the postural position is called the *interocclusal distance* or *freeway space*. It normally varies between 2 and 4 mm.[8,31]

TEMPOROMANDIBULAR JOINT DYSFUNCTION
Causes of dysfunction

A faulty occlusion may be the most common cause of TMJ dysfunction. One of the unique features of the TMJ and its associated structures is the influence exerted on them by the teeth. Complete mandibular closure is dictated by tooth position. If a malocclusion exists, the mandible will still close to maximal tooth contact, often creating muscle imbalance and faulty condylar position, a common cause of disk derangements. The relationship of the first molars (upper and lower) to each other forms the basis for classification of malocclusions:

Class I: Mesiodistal first molar relationship normal, tooth irregularities elsewhere.
Class II, Division 1: Lower first molar posterior to upper first molar, mandibular retrusion usually reflected in client profile, upper anterior teeth flared.
Class II, Division 2: Lower first molar posterior to upper first molar, deep overbite often reflected in client profile.
Class III: Lower first molar anterior to upper first molar, mandibular prognathism usually reflected in client profile (i.e., prominent chin).

A bimaxillary protrusion exists when the occlusion is normal but the entire dentition is forward with respect to the facial profile. The condition in which a vertical space exists between the upper and lower anterior teeth in centric occlusion is called an *open bite*. Both the bimaxillary pro-

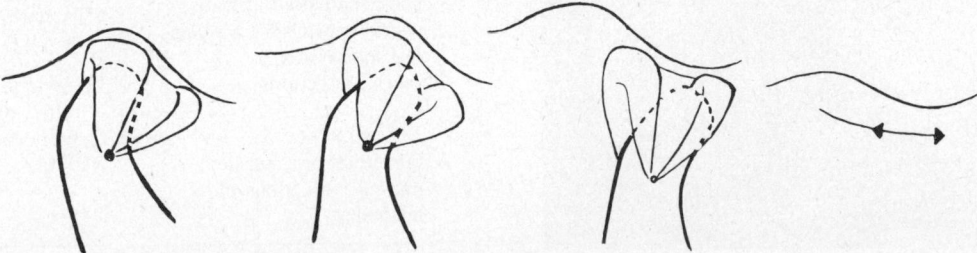

Fig. 23-7. Normal opening movements of condyle and disk. (From Weisberg J and Friedman MH: J Orthop Sports Phys Ther 3:62, 1981.)

trusion and the anterior open bite encourage soft-tissue disorders of the tongue and lip.

Severe malocclusions often result when posterior teeth (excluding third molars) are removed and not replaced. Tipping of teeth and a loss of vertical dimension usually result from this condition (Fig. 23-8).

The most difficult malocclusion to recognize is traumatic occlusion in a normal-appearing dentition. In this condition opposing teeth are related to each other in such a manner that cuspal interferences occur on closure or during gliding movements of the jaw. The consequences of traumatic occlusion may be TMJ dysfunction, bone loss on radiographs, excessive tooth mobility, and muscle disorders.

Developmental abnormalities and disease (e.g., rheumatoid arthritis, juvenile rheumatoid arthritis) can exert a strong influence on the TMJ by disruption of the occlusion.[28]

Systemic factors can also cause or aggravate TMJ dysfunction. If TMJ synovitis cannot be attributed to local factors or trauma, systemic disease must be considered as a possible cause.[17] Systemic inflammatory disease, infections, or viruses can cause TMJ synovitis (Table 23-1), but osteoarthritis is the most common cause. The hallmark of osteoarthritis is degeneration of the cartilage and, ultimately, the subchondral bone in the articulating components of the TMJ. TMJ synovitis occurs as a secondary phenomenon of osteoarthritis. Recent evidence points to the systemic nature of osteoarthritis as opposed to strictly "wear and tear"; it is caused by a disturbance in mucopolysaccharide metabolism.[25] Disk dysfunction is common in osteoarthritis of the TMJ. Complete disintegration of the disk is often seen in advanced osteoarthritis.

Predisposition is a major factor in most disorders, and

TMJ dysfunctions are no exception.[7] Gross malocclusions with healthy joints and adjacent musculature are commonly seen, as are slight occlusal deformities that produce acute dysfunctions. Poor condylar position, as determined by joint palpation and radiography, often exists with no joint problems. Constitutional factors are significant causes of arthritis,[25] the most common disease affecting the TMJ. Because clients without a predisposition for TMJ dysfunction can remain problem free in this area in spite of structural abnormalities, prophylactic treatment is not performed in the absence of signs and symptoms.

Psychological factors and tension can induce or aggravate TMJ symptoms.[22] Nevertheless, concentrating on this aspect instead of on the basic cause will not resolve the problem. When a pathological condition produces pain, management of the pain (or other symptoms) should be only one aspect of total client management. The correction of structural problems that cause TMJ dysfunction will enable the client to better resist harmful effects caused by psychological factors. Tension might be a significant factor in those cases where clenching or bruxism is the main cause of the dysfunction. Many clinicians believe that psychological factors are the main cause of TMJ dysfunction and that the most important aspect of treatment should be counseling. This course of treatment is recommended even when objective signs of joint dysfunction—limitation of motion, clicking, and inflammation—are present.[22] They cite the fact that many more women than men suffer from this disorder. However, the most widespread joint disease (rheumatoid arthritis and osteoarthritis) afflicts women more often than men. Rheumatoid arthritis is three times more common in women than men, and osteoarthritis oc-

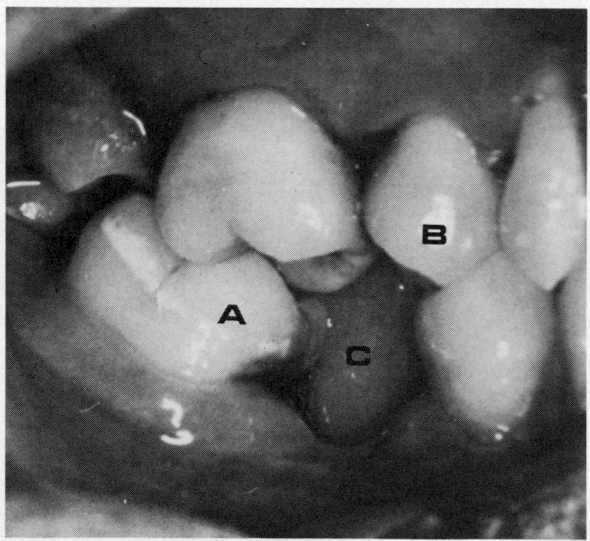

Fig. 23-8. *A,* Mesially tipped lower molar; *B,* rotated upper bicuspid; *C,* space formerly occupied by lower bicuspid.

Table 23-1. Causes of TMJ synovitis

Disease	Mechanism
Degenerative joint disease	Microtrauma, malocclusion, disk dysfunction, retrodiscitis, constitutional factors
Retrodiscitis	Posteriorly placed condyle, prolonged openings, disk dysfunction, trauma
Inflammatory joint disease: rheumatoid arthritis, juvenile rheumatoid arthritis, psoriatic arthritis, ankylosing spondylitis	Systemic inflammation or autoimmunity
Bacterial infections	Local extension from chronic otitis, direct penetration, or septicemia
Viral infections: measles, mumps, infectious mononucleosis	Viremia

Modified and condensed from Friedman MH, Weisberg J, and Agus B: Diagnosis and treatment of inflammation of the temporomandibular joint, Semin Arthritis Rheum 12:44, 1982.

curs twice as often in women than men.[2] With experience, the practitioner will be able to determine which persons will benefit from counseling.

Functionally, the cervical spine, the TMJ, and the articulations between the teeth are intimately related. Abnormal function or malposition of one of these can affect the function or position of the others. For example, a change in head position changes mandibular position, thus affecting occlusion. The balance between the flexors and extensors of the head and neck is affected by the muscles of mastication and the syprahyoid and infrahyoid muscles (Fig. 23-9). Dysfunction in either the muscles of mastication or the cervical muscles can easily disturb this balance.[34]

This balance between opposing muscle groups is seen in the relaxed posture. A common postural defect is the forward placement of the head (Fig. 23-10). This position leads to hyperextension of the head on the neck as the client corrects for visual needs, flexion of the neck over the thorax, and posterior migration of the mandible.[34] These factors often lead to pain and dysfunction in the head and neck.

The TMJ is vulnerable to trauma occurring anywhere in the head or neck. Whiplash in particular can cause a TMJ synovitis. Prolonged opening of the mouth is a common cause of TMJ synovitis or an anteriorly displaced disk.[17] Frequent or prolonged dental appointments and general-anesthetic procedures that require maximal opening of the mouth can stretch or tear the posterior attachment of the disk.

Poor habits can also affect the TMJ. The most obvious are clenching and bruxism. Mouth breathing and poor posture are often classified as habits, and they can affect the TMJ. The clinician must question the client carefully concerning habits. Excessive use of the telephone, for example, may be a factor in certain cases. It has recently been reported that violin and viola players have a high incidence of TMJ dysfunction. In a TMJ with an inherent structural weakness, certain habits such as singing and gum chewing, that require excessive use of the joint may be responsible for causing symptoms of TMJ dysfunction.

Symptoms

The client may complain of jaw pain and tenderness that relates to function or of limitation of opening. Many times, however, symptoms are not related to function. Instead, head or neck symptoms resembling a myriad of other disorders may occur.[18]

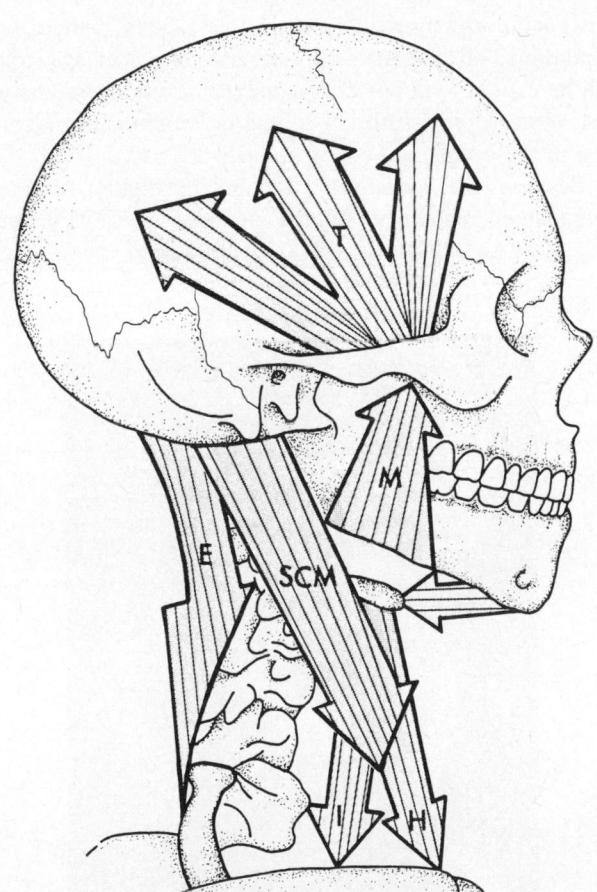

Fig. 23-9. Muscular balance of the head and neck. *M*, Masseter muscle; *E*, neck extensors; *SCM*, sternocleidomastoid; *T*, temporalis; *IH*, infrahyoid muscle. (From Friedman MH and Weisberg J: Temporomandibular joint disorders: Diagnosis and treatment, Chicago, 1985, Quintessence Publishing Co, Inc.)

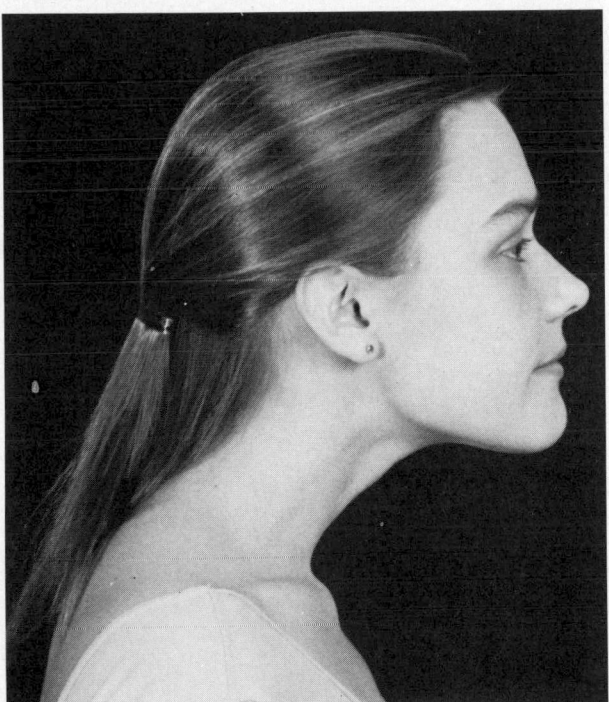

Fig. 23-10. Anterior head position. (Modified from Friedman MH, Weisberg J, and Agus B: Semin Arthritis Rheum 12:44, 1982.)

Clicking of the joint on movement and restricted opening of the jaw are the symptoms most commonly seen in clients suffering from TMJ dysfunction.[32] Pain related to jaw function is also a common finding.

Generalized headache, occurring as referred pain from masticatory muscles or the joint itself, is an important symptom of a TMJ disorder; clients with this symptom may initially seek medical aid.[17] Pain or tenderness or both are often seen in specific areas of the head, such as the temples, occiput, or muscles of mastication. Related pain may be felt in the dorsum of the neck, sternocleidomastoid region, or trapezius muscle.[18]

In addition to clicking and limitation of movement, symptoms specific to the joint itself include pain in the joint, tenderness to lateral or posterior joint palpation, and crepitus.[32]

Ear symptoms such as tinnitus, vertigo, hearing loss, ear pain, and stuffiness in the ear are sometimes seen.[21] Nasopharyngeal symptoms such as swallowing difficulties or numbness or burning sensations in the tongue, palate, or throat are occasionally seen.[32]

Classification

The TMJ develops problems similar to those of other synovial joints. The various dysfunctions will be discussed separately for clarity. A clinical presentation, however, often includes more than one of the following disorders.

Synovitis. Inflammation of the joint lining can occur in the TMJ, as it does in any synovial joint in the body. The acutely inflamed joint usually shows symptoms similar to those of a typical "hot joint," with the client complaining of pain and soreness, particularly relating to function. Palpation of the affected area elicits pain, and increased temperature and, occasionally, swelling may be noted.[17] If significant effusion is present in the posterior aspect of the joint, mandibular deviation toward the affected side on full opening and deviation away from the affected side at the mandibular rest position can occur.[9] The client's ability to open the mouth may be impaired. Protective spasm of adjacent musculature may confuse the examiner as to the true nature of the complaint. More often, the synovitis is less acute. The hallmark of chronic TMJ synovitis is tenderness to either lateral or posterior joint palpation or to both. Pain may be unrelated to function and can occur anywhere in the head or neck.[17]

Localized synovitis. Synovitis of the TMJ can occur from systemic causes, as described earlier. More commonly, a localized synovitis of the posterior aspect of the TMJ occurs, with a buildup of edema in the posterior joint space. This condition is referred to in dental literature as *posterior capsulitis*[9] or *retrodiscitis*. Since symptoms of this condition may overlap or simulate other pathological conditions, misdiagnosis can occur.[17] Posterior capsulitis can be caused by a posterior condylar position, trauma, or disk dysfunction (Table 23-1) and can often cause disruption of the occlusion.

Because the retrodiscal tissues are highly vascular, condylar encroachment of this area can cause inflamma-

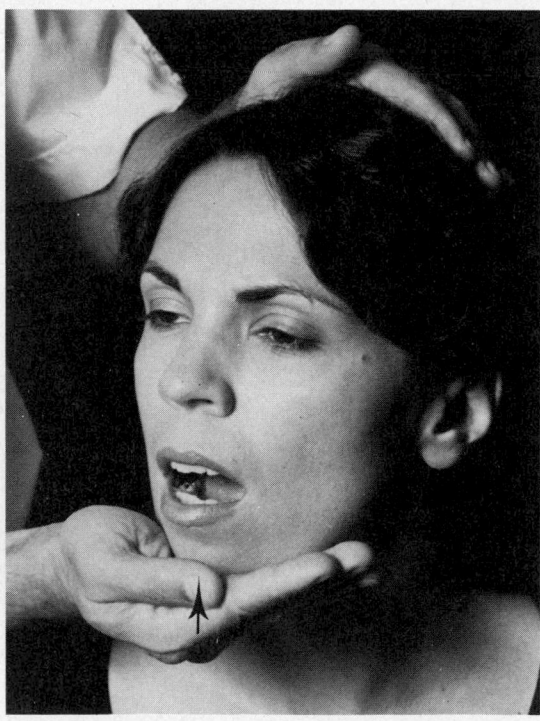

Fig. 23-11. Resistive opening. Client's occiput is supported to prevent backward head movement during testing.

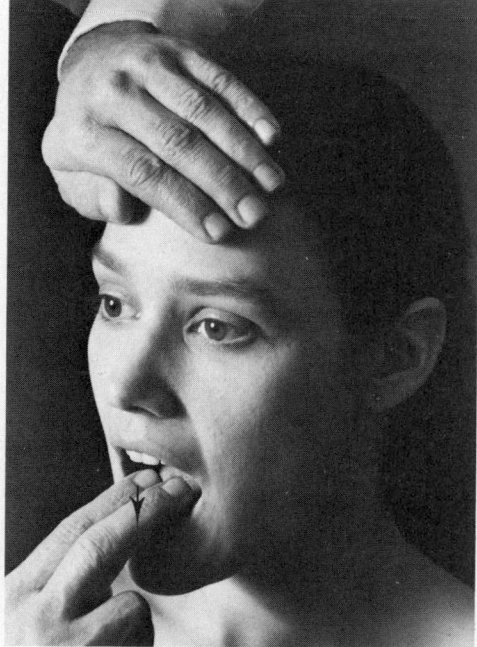

Fig. 23-12. Resistive closing. Client's forehead is supported to prevent forward head movement during testing.

tion. Because of the TMJ's loose joint capsule and nonlimiting bony configuration, muscular, postural, or occlusal factors can force the mandible posteriorly. Occlusal conditions that cause a loss of vertical dimension (mandibular overclosure), such as loss of posterior teeth or excessive tooth wear, encourage this type of condylar position.

Systemic synovitis. Degenerative joint disease (osteoarthritis) is the most common primary joint disease of the TMJ and predisposes the client to TMJ synovitis. Degenerative joint disease is frequently unilateral and usually occurs in people over the age of 40 years; it is twice as common in women as in men.[17] The cause of inflammation in this disease is not clear. Evidence suggests that crystals of hydroxyapatite, which were formerly thought to be inert, participate in the inflammatory process in acute osteoarthritis. A similar process is seen in gout or pseudogout.

Signs of TMJ synovitis occur in the systemic inflammatory arthritides, such as rheumatoid arthritis and its variants, particularly juvenile rheumatoid arthritis and psoriatic arthritis (Table 23-1). In these conditions evidence of arthritis in other joints is usually seen, although TMJ synovitis is occasionally seen as an initial presentation.[5,28]

Infections, although rare, can occur in the TMJ.[19] Usually, adjacent infection is also present in the inner ear. Direct joint penetration of blood-borne infection can be the cause of TMJ synovitis in the diabetic client, the immunologically compromised client, or the chronic drug abuser.[27] We have noted TMJ synovitis in a variety of viral infections. The most notable is mumps, which causes synovitis directly or by referring pain from an adjacent parotitis. Other viruses capable of causing synovitis in the TMJ are influenza and rubella.

Disk derangements. In centric occlusion the correctly positioned disk sits atop the condyle, separating it from the mandibular fossa. An anteriorly displaced disk is probably the most common TMJ dysfunction. In this condition, when the mandible is in centric occlusion or in the postural position, the disk is anterior to its normal position and the condyle rests beneath the stretched posterior attachment of the disk.[10]

Reciprocal clicking. The client demonstrates a click on opening and a click on closing (often less noticeable). The clicks may or may not be audible; they can easily be felt during opening and closing jaw movements while the posterior aspect of the TMJ is palpated[15] (Fig. 23-14). After the opening click the disk is in normal position over the superior aspect of the condyle until some point in the closing cycle when the condyle glides past the posterior edge of the disk (Fig. 23-15). The closing click occurs as the closing condyle slips off the posterior edge of the disk while the disk remains anteriorly displaced. Usually this condition worsens with time as the stretched posterior portion of the posterior ligament further deteriorates. This allows the disk to advance still further forward. The opening click occurs later, since the condyle must translate further forward to reach the disk. The posterior ligament is less able to retract the disk during jaw closure; therefore the closing click occurs sooner. A complete anterior dislocation of the disk can eventually occur. The client has a full range of motion, with no clicking. In a susceptible individual severe osteoarthritic changes may be seen as the protection of the disk is lost.[11]

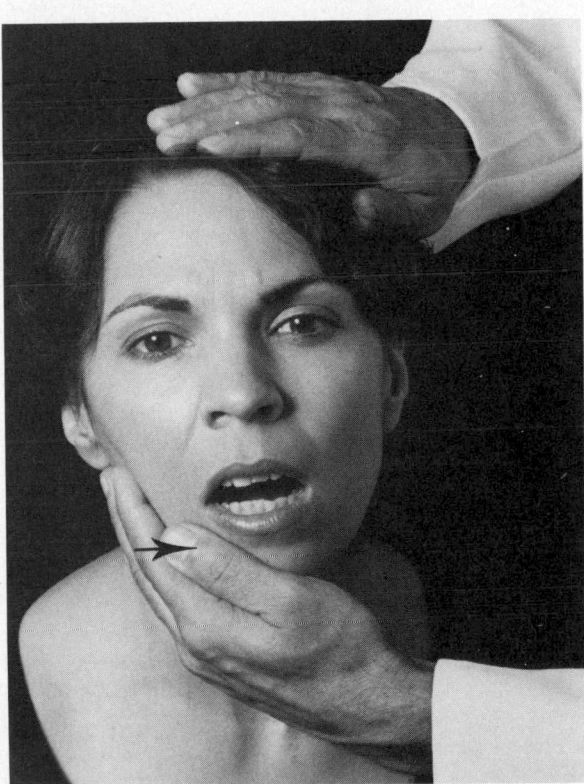

Fig. 23-13. Resistive lateral excursions. Opposite side of head is supported to prevent tilting of head during testing.

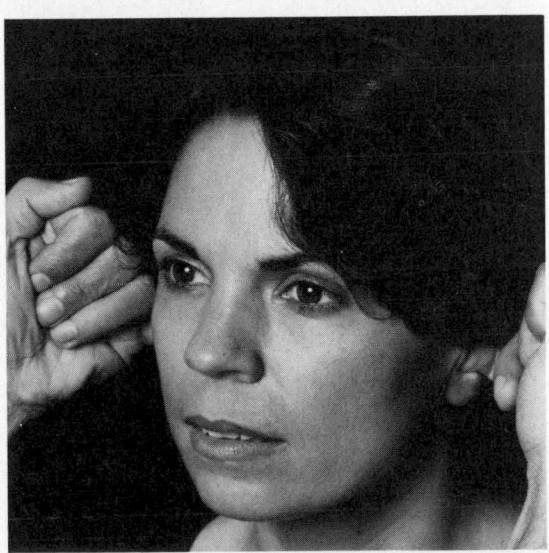

Fig. 23-14. Posterior joint palpation.

Locking. Another common type of disk derangement is an anteriorly displaced disk that limits condylar translation. This is referred to as *locking*. In this situation the client will have a sudden limitation of opening. Deviation toward the affected side will be seen on active opening, and lateral movement to the opposite side is limited. This condition is closely related to reciprocal clicking; clients with locking invariably report a history of clicking. Clients with an anteriorly displaced disk often shuttle between clicking (with full mandibular opening) and sudden episodes of locking. If locking persists, it can become chronic. In chronic locking the mandibular opening will increase slightly. The disk is still lodged anteriorly, but range of motion is increased as the posterior ligament is further stretched.[13]

Occlusomuscular dysfunction. Occlusomuscular dysfunction occurs when a malocclusion causes an incorrect mandibular position, ultimately causing masticatory muscle dysfunction in the susceptible client.[4,14] The symptoms are similar to those of TMJ synovitis. The client may complain of pain and soreness relating to function. However, a wide range of seemingly unrelated symptoms—headache and pain anywhere in the head or neck—is commonly seen.[18]

Differential diagnosis of this condition is accomplished by masticatory muscle tests (Figs. 23-11 to 23-13) to identify pathological conditions that may exist in the muscles. Muscle palpation is used in accessible areas to corroborate results of muscle function tests.[16] A critical occlusal evaluation is often necessary.

Hypermobile joint. In this condition the TMJ capsule

is abnormally stretched. The client's active jaw opening is wider than normal. Opening deviations may be inconsistent if the muscles of mastication cannot efficiently handle this excessive range of motion. Jaw dislocation is more likely to occur when this condition is present.

Hypomobile joint. The client's active jaw opening is less than normal. If only one joint is restricted, deviation toward that side will be seen.[34] Hypomobility of the TMJ can result from a restricted joint capsule that is caused by immobilization, localized inflammation, trauma, or systemic disease. A displaced disk will also cause TMJ hypomobility.

Dislocated joint. Dislocation of the TMJ occurs when one or both condyles are locked forward of the eminence(s), preventing jaw closure. This is the only joint in the body that can dislocate spontaneously (without an external force).

Differential diagnosis

The physical therapist is often confronted with clients who suffer from TMJ dysfunctions. A functional evaluation will enable the practitioner to distinguish between the various components of the syndrome—synovitis, muscle dysfunction, range-of-motion abnormalities, disk dysfunction, or cervical dysfunction.[14]

Differential diagnosis is complicated by the fact that symptoms can occur anywhere in the head or neck and may be caused by many other problems. Headache, for example, can be caused by over 100 different disorders.[12] The practitioner must also be alert to the possibility of systemic disease being superimposed on TMJ dysfunction.

A complete history must be obtained. This will help the practitioner to determine which additional health professionals, if any, the client should consult.

A dentist is best able to treat such signs of TMJ dysfunction as masticatory muscle dysfunction, malocclusion, posteriorly placed condyle, clenching or grinding, disk derangements, or synovitis from local causes.[14] If the occlusion is suspected as a causative factor but clear-cut signs are lacking, a diagnostic appliance can be inserted to separate the posterior teeth.

The physical therapist can aid treatment when a client has postural abnormalities (including an anteriorly displaced head), various muscle imbalances, history of trauma, breathing dysfunction, or cervical dysfunction. The use of various modalities to treat muscle disorders and inflammation can be helpful.

Many situations can be treated by either a dentist or a physical therapist, depending on background, training, and interest. These include TMJ hypermobility or hypomobility, dislocated joint, trigger point therapy, and various oral habits such as faulty tongue position and lip habits.

The client should be questioned as to history and famil-

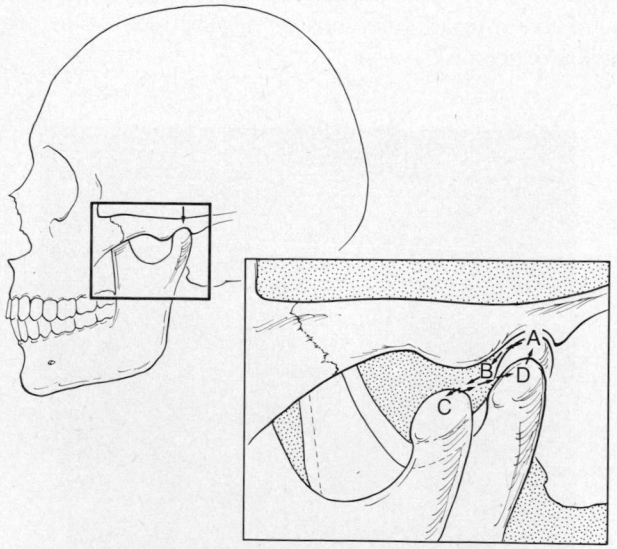

Fig. 23-15. Condylar path during reciprocal clicking. *A*, Position of condyle when mouth is closed (maximal intercuspation of teeth); *B*, point at which opening click occurs; *C*, maximal opening; *D*, point at which closing click occurs.

ial history of arthritis and previous problems with other joints. Many clients with a history of various joint problems may never have been evaluated for arthritis. We often refer clients to a rheumatologist if arthritis is suspected. A careful case history and examination of the hands for deformities will aid in making this determination.[2] Since psoriasis afflicts up to 2% of the population and the potential effect of psoriatic arthritis on the TMJ is so severe, the possible presence of this genetic disease is investigated with every client. A rheumatological consultation is indicated when unexplained TMJ synovitis exists or when the client cannot tolerate antiinflammatory medication. Other rheumatological diseases may affect the TMJ. These include scleroderma with restricted jaw opening and Sjögren's syndrome with parotid gland enlargement, dryness of the mouth, and red tongue.

Head pain is one of the most aggravating symptoms of TMJ dysfunction. If the headache does not appear to be related to the TMJ (e.g., pain at night, constant head pain, headaches of a cyclical nature [every 10 days, for example], headache accompanied by a visual aura or nausea, or pain set off by a trigger area), we refer the client to a physician. A medical consultation is also indicated in cases of suspected tumors or possible nerve involvement or where assistance in the management of pain is needed. Many situations indicate a referral to a primary physician or experienced internist. These include the medically compromised client with TMJ problems, a client who is suspected of having a systemically induced TMJ synovitis, and a client who shows evidence of infection, such as fever, glandular swelling, or lymphadenopathy. Any elderly client who has pain in the upper quarter of the body or in the head should be referred for diagnosis of possible polymyalgia rheumatica or temporal arteritis. These situations, which are easily detectable by a greatly elevated sedimentation rate, are correctable by administration of steroids. Untreated temporal arteritis can lead to sudden irreversible blindness by rupture of the ophthalmic arterial system.

Since symptoms of ear disease and TMJ dysfunction (earache, tinnitus, vertigo, hearing loss[21]) overlap, many situations require a consultation with an otolaryngologist. An ear inflammation may be suspected when the external auditory meatus is palpated (see Fig. 23-11) and pain not related to closing is elicited.

If signs of depression, anxiety, or extreme tension are detected at the initial interview, psychological counseling should be considered.

If the client has a history of trauma, a radiologist, oral surgeon, or both should be consulted. When the client exhibits a severe malocclusion or gross discrepancy in jaw size and these conditions seem to be related to TMJ symptoms, an orthodontist knowledgeable in joint dysfunction should be consulted.

EVALUATION OF THE TEMPOROMANDIBULAR JOINT AND ASSOCIATED STRUCTURES
Client history

The information that the physical therapist initially obtains from the client includes the following: (1) general history of the complaint, (2) dental history, (3) medical history, (4) previous medical consultations or treatment, (5) medications being taken, (6) history of trauma, (7) symptoms (ear, head, or neck), (8) pain or sensory deprivation to other areas, (9) previous TMJ treatment, and (10) habits.[14]

General appearance

The client is physically evaluated. Posture and abnormalities in standing or walking are observed. Asymmetry of the face and neck is noted, as are signs of soft tissue stress, such as hypertrophied masseter, mentalis, or sternocleidomastoid muscles. Postural abnormalities such as scoliosis or an anteriorly displaced head are identified.[14]

Dynamic evaluation of jaw movement

The amount and direction of active jaw opening are recorded—range-of-motion abnormalities are common in TMJ disease. Because clients vary greatly in size, we determine their normal TMJ range of motion in a functional way, which allows for this size variation. The client's knuckles are used to measure the widest opening between the upper and lower anterior teeth. The width of two to two and a half knuckles is a normal amount of jaw opening to expect (Fig. 23-16). If the TMJ is hypermobile, the client may be able to insert three knuckles or more between the teeth. If the joints are restricted, the client will

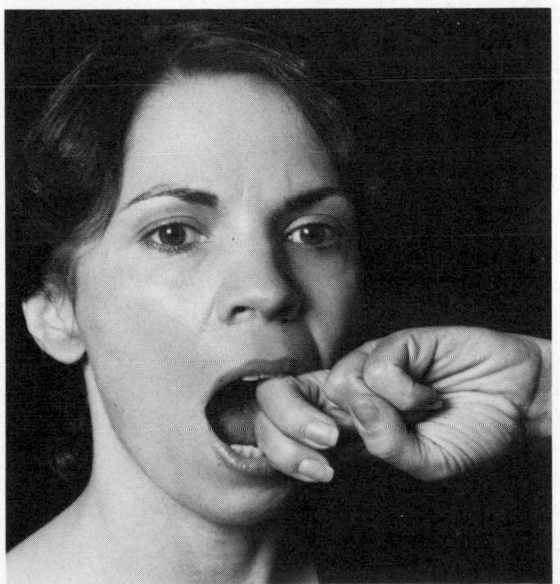

Fig. 23-16. Technique for measuring TMJ range of motion.

not be able to insert two knuckles.[34] Additionally, a linear measurement is taken.

If a reference point on the lower central incisors is selected and visualized on a frontal plane, side-to-side deviations of the mandible on active opening can be studied and recorded (Fig. 23-17). The same reference point can be used to examine lateral jaw excursions. The client is asked to open the jaw slightly (just enough to eliminate tooth contact) and move the jaw as far as possible to the left and right. A transparent ruler is used to record the movement of the reference point (Fig. 23-18). Pain, restriction, or significant differences in the amount of movement to either side are noted. The client is also asked to separate the teeth slightly and protrude the jaw as far as possible. Direction of protrusion can be observed by checking the movement of the same reference point previously used. The amount of jaw protrusion is measured in the following way. The client's overjet (Fig. 23-6) is measured with the teeth together and again measured at the end of the protrusive range. The difference is the amount of protrusion.[34]

All of this information is recorded in the client's chart. The causes of mandibular deviations are numerous; this information will aid in establishing a correct diagnosis.

Passive range of motion

Passive range of motion can be used in a TMJ evaluation to assess ligamentous damage in trauma cases. A disorder is determined by the presence of pain or excessive range on the side toward the direction of movement when the mandible is extended passively and laterally as far as possible. Passive range of motion may also be used to check the state of the opening muscles.

In the TMJ, joint play is in a downward and a lateral direction (Fig. 23-19). To determine the state of the joint play, downward and lateral mobilization of the condyle is performed gently.[14] This portion of the evaluation should be terminated if pain is produced; it should not be performed in the presence of inflammation or obvious disease. Mobilization is extremely valuable in treatment of the hypomobile joint. A complete discussion of joint play techniques and indications will be found in the treatment section.[14,26,34]

Masticatory muscle tests

Masticatory muscle testing is essential in diagnosis of TMJ malfunction. If a pathological condition exists in a muscle, pain will be elicited on application of maximum resistance.[6] To effectively test the muscles of mastication, the following rules should be observed: (1) The head must be supported to eliminate head movement or rotation, (2) the mouth should be partially opened (about 1 cm), (3) the application of force must be gradual enough to enable the client to build maximal resistance,[13] and (4) hand contact with the TMJ should be avoided; pain elicited in the presence of acute joint disease might be confused with the results of muscle testing.[14]

To test the main opening muscles of the jaw (inferior head of the lateral pterygoid), the client opens his/her jaw slightly and resists the therapist's strong closing force applied to the client's chin. Muscle testing of the closing masticatory muscles consists of the reverse of this test. The client opens slightly. The therapist applies a strong downward force to the incisal edges of the client's lower anterior teeth and attempts to further open the client's mouth against strong resistance.[14] In these tests (see Figs. 23-13 and 23-14) the client does not attempt to open or close the jaw but resists the therapist's attempt to do so. If these tests were done in the reverse manner (the client attempting to move the jaw against the resistance of the therapist), the therapist would not be able to judge or control the amount of applied force.

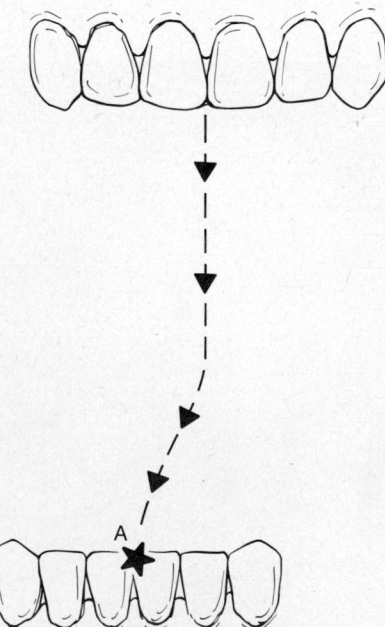

Fig. 23-17. Recording of active opening path. *A,* Reference point between incisal edges of lower central incisors.

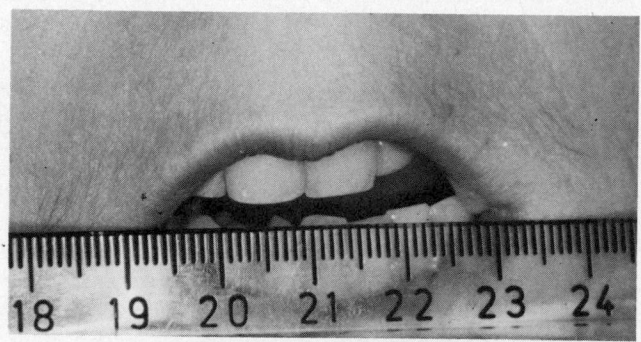

Fig. 23-18. Recording of lateral jaw excursions.

Resisted lateral excursions test the medial and lateral pterygoid muscles simultaneously (Fig. 23-15). A weak lateral pterygoid muscle might not be obvious on resistive opening muscle tests but would be evident by comparison with the opposite side. Because of the decided medial direction of the medial pterygoid muscles, they are also stressed during this test.

A muscle test of resisted protrusion is useful to test all four pterygoid muscles simultaneously. The client opens and protrudes the jaw slightly. The therapist supports the client's occiput and attempts to force the jaw posteriorly as the client resists.

Resisted retrusion can be used to test the digastric and posterior fibers of the temporalis muscles. The therapist places the fingers on the lingual surfaces of the client's lower anterior teeth and attempts to advance the mandible as the client resists.

Joint noises

Among the signs of TMJ dysfunction, joint noises occurring during mandibular movement are the most common; they can be heard unaided or with a stethoscope. The presence or absence of noise in each joint and its character (clicking, popping, or crepitus) should be noted. If clicking is present during functional movements, an abrupt mandibular shift can be seen or felt as the click occurs.[11] The exact point in the opening and closing cycles when the click occurs can be determined by the examiner during posterior palpation of the condyles, as the client opens and closes. Crepitation, if present, can be felt during the later stages of opening and indicates a roughening of the surfaces of the condyle and articular eminence and possible destruction or displacement of the disk, which normally separates the articulating surfaces. The presence of crepitus raises the possibility of osteoarthritis, which should be investigated.[17]

Joint palpation

Palpation of the lateral and posterior aspects of the TMJ is important in determining the existence of capsular inflammation. The tip of the forefinger is placed just anterior to the tragus of the ear; the client is asked to repeatedly open and close the mouth. At maximum opening the examiner's finger will identify a depression overlying the joint. Tenderness may be elicited. If the inflammation is severe, swelling and elevated skin temperature may be noted.[29] The joint capsule cannot be palpated except in the presence of severe inflammation.

The posterior aspect of the TMJ must be correctly palpated, because synovitis of the posterior aspect of the TMJ will not be appreciated on lateral palpation.[17] The therapist places the tips of the little fingers in the client's external auditory canals bilaterally, with the fingernails pointed posteriorly (see Fig. 23-11). Pressure is exerted anteriorly as the client opens and closes the mouth several times.[18] If inflammation is present, pain will be elicited as tissue is compressed between the examiner's finger and the client's condyle. As the examiner gains experience, he/she will be able to identify a posteriorly positioned condyle as it exerts pressure on the examiner's finger when the client closes.[1] Abnormal condylar movement caused by disk dysfunction can be appreciated during this phase of the evaluation.[14]

Muscle palpation

Palpation of the muscles of the head and neck cannot be used to distinguish between local pathological conditions in the muscle and referred pain.[6] Accessible muscles (portions of the closing muscles of mastication, for example) should be palpated to corroborate results of muscle tests and to determine the exact site of the dysfunction.[14] Through palpation the following information can be gained: skin temperature, tenderness, muscle tone, swell-

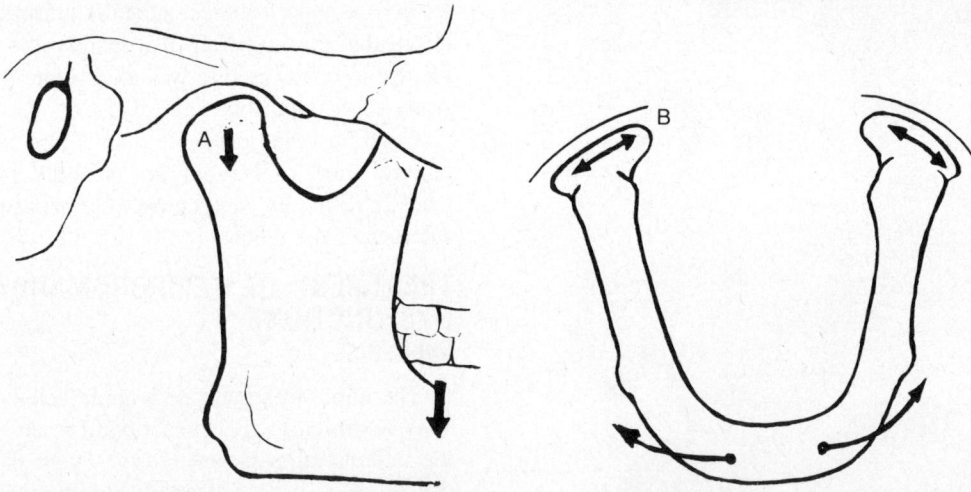

Fig. 23-19. TMJ joint play. *A*, Downward joint play; *B*, lateral joint play. (Reprinted from Physical Ther 62:597, 1982, with permission of American Physical Therapy Association.)

ing, skin moisture, and location of trigger points and their reference zones.[16]

The belly of the masseter muscle can be palpated more easily if the client clenches the teeth during palpation. This procedure will help to identify the actual muscle fibers from surrounding soft tissue. The muscle should be palpated from the angle of the jaw to the inferior surface of the zygomatic arch. The temporal muscle should be palpated through its full extent, from above the eye to the posterior auricular areas. The medial pterygoid muscle is palpated externally on the inner aspect of the angle of the jaw and intraorally in the area of the mandibular ramus.[14] The lateral pterygoid muscle cannot be palpated.[20] Attempts to palpate this muscle often elicit pain as soft tissue is compressed against the sharp edge of the lateral pterygoid plate.[16] The suprahyoid and infrahyoid muscles as well as the extensor and flexor muscles of the head and neck should be palpated. To palpate the pervertebral neck flexor muscles, the examiner should stand behind the client and retract the trachea and esophagus with the left hand while palpating the muscles with the right hand (Fig. 23-20).[14]

Radiography

We have found radiographs to be of limited use in evaluation of the TMJ; they can be correlated with the client's symptoms, or they can help in determining the course of treatment. Radiographic examination is particularly necessary in cases of suspected fractures, systemic diseases capable of affecting the TMJ, or suspected tumors.

Generally TMJ dysfunction involves disorders of radiotranslucent movable tissues—ligaments, muscles, and disks. These structures are not visible on conventional ra-

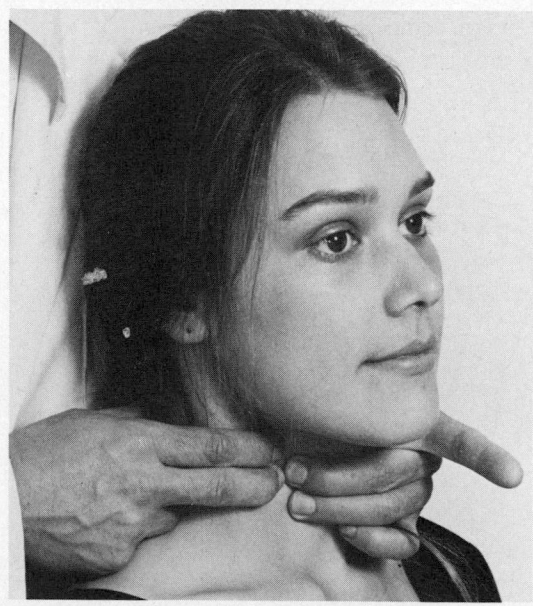

Fig. 23-20. Palpation of neck flexor muscles.

diographs. TMJ radiographs can be misleading even where hard tissues are involved. Since cartilage is radiolucent, osteoarthritis of the TMJ can exist for many years before bony changes are evident; by this time extensive damage to the cartilage may have occurred. Alteration of joint dynamics (orthodontia, mandibular repositioning) should be done before radiographic changes are seen.

Cervical spine screening

Active range-of-motion tests should be performed. Any of these tests that elicit a response indicate the need for further investigation by passive range-of-motion and appropriate muscle tests. If cranial symptoms are induced or exaggerated, the neck should be fully evaluated.

Oral cavity evaluation

The tongue should be evaluated with regard to its size, its position at rest, its function, the length of the frenulum, and oral habits. Tongue size is an important factor. A small tongue (microglossia) will not exert enough pressure against the teeth, whereas a large tongue (macroglossia) will exert too much pressure. In addition, an excessively large tongue may interfere with occlusion. Surgery is indicated in extreme cases. The mucous membrane under the tongue is reflected in the midline to the floor of the mouth; this reflection is called the *lingual frenulum*. A short frenulum will interfere with normal tongue position and function. A normal frenulum permits an opening of 2 cm or more between the incisors when the tongue is against the palate.

Lip size and strength should be assessed. The upper lip should cover at least two thirds of the upper incisors. Excess mentalis muscle activity should not be evident when the lips meet. A short upper lip accompanied by a large everted lower lip is a common dysfunction. This overdeveloped lower lip results from the client's attempts to meet the upper lips for esthetic needs. This condition usually leads to a hypertrophied mentalis muscle. It should be realized that the insertion of a mandibular repositioning appliance to open the bite will exaggerate the effect of an already short upper lip.

Good buccinator muscle tone is also important in maintaining good oral function. A weak buccinator muscle leads to difficulty in keeping food between the articulating surfaces of the teeth.

TREATMENT OF TEMPOROMANDIBULAR JOINT DYSFUNCTIONS
Synovitis

The initial treatment of a noninfected, acutely inflamed TMJ is similar to that prescribed for any inflamed joint. If the inflammation is severe, the client is told to limit the degree of opening and to rest the joint. This includes eating a liquid or soft diet, limiting movement, and refraining from talking and singing. Application of heat or cold is effective in reducing symptoms of acute inflammation and associated muscle spasm. If the inflammation is less acute, the preceding procedures are not necessary. Aspirin or one of the newer nonsteroidal antiinflammatory drugs is indicated, in either case.[17]

Aspirin, because of its long record of use (more than 100 years), potency, and cost, may still be the drug of choice. Aspirin and the nonsteroidal drugs work by inhibiting prostaglandin formation. Prostaglandins are short-lived hormones formed at the site of injury. In addition, aspirin acetylizes the platelets, thereby reducing their stickiness. This action prolongs bleeding time by inhibiting platelet aggregation. Therefore aspirin and ibuprofen should not be prescribed for anyone undergoing anticoagulant therapy. The effect on bleeding time of even one aspirin can last for several days.

If aspirin therapy is indicated, regular dosage schedules must be adhered to in order to achieve satisfactory blood levels (18 to 25 mg/100 ml).[17] The client can be sent to a medical laboratory for a determination of salicylate level if a question arises or if long periods of aspirin therapy are required. For most people a starting dose of 10 grains four times a day is satisfactory. People with high gastric acidity require a lower dosage; those taking barbiturates will require more aspirin. Since dosage can vary widely, clients should be cautioned for signs of aspirin toxicity, which include tinnitus, hearing loss, and headache.

The most common problem is gastrointestinal intolerance. This can be circumvented by taking aspirin on a full stomach or together with an antacid such as milk or by taking any of the commercial buffered preparations. These preparations delay the absorption of aspirin until it reaches the small intestine. In some individuals, however, aspirin can affect the gastric mucosa systemically and may have to be discontinued.

For clients who cannot tolerate or are allergic to aspirin, several excellent nonsteroidal drugs are available. These include ibuprofen (Motrin), indomethacin (Indocin), tolmetin (Tolectin), naproxen (Naprosyn), sulindac (Clinoril), and meclofenamic acid (Meclomen). The main advantages of these compounds are convenience (since fewer pills are needed to achieve the same effect), a higher compliance rate, and selectivity for the client who responds to only one of the drugs.[17] These drugs are much more expensive than aspirin.

Further treatment decisions depend on whether the TMJ synovitis is caused by systemic or local factors. In the case of an excessively posteriorly placed condyle, dental treatment would be indicated. Synovitis caused by systemic inflammatory disease, osteoarthritis, or an infection would require medical treatment. In the case of a severe infection, the client would require hospitalization for intravenous administration of antibiotics and surgical drainage.[33]

Since an anteriorly positioned head (Fig. 23-10) forces the mandible posteriorly, postural improvement may be required if an anterior mandibular shift is needed. Axial extension must be done by the client for 30 seconds, five to eight times daily. Correct posture should be demonstrated to the client, and it must be practiced constantly. Many times, muscle length has shortened and mobility has been lost as a result of years of incorrect posture. In these cases the therapist will have to stretch soft tissues in the neck to enable the client to assume correct posture.

Modalities can aid in the treatment of the inflamed joint, as they are used in treating other inflamed joints. Heat and cold are often used. Electrical stimulation and ultrasound are particularly effective when they are used with medication.

Mobilization of the TMJ is also indicated in treatment of TMJ synovitis.[26] Mobilization should not be used while the inflammation is acute. A complete discussion of this technique will be found in the section on treatment of the hypomobile joint.

Disk derangements

Reciprocal clicking. If the disk is not positioned too far anteriorly and if deterioration of the posterior ligament is not too far advanced, reciprocal clicking can be successfully treated. Fig. 23-21 represents the anteriorly displaced disk in centric occlusion. The clicks occur as the condyle crosses line *AB* in either direction (opening or closing). The disk-condyle relationship is normal to the left of line *AB;* the disk is anteriorly displaced if the condyle is located to the right of line *AB*. If condylar position in centric occlusion were changed (moved to the left along line *CD*), the client could go through a complete cycle with the disk in position and no clicking. If the client's occlusion were satisfactory in regard to condylar position and vertical dimension of the jaw, a permanent occlusal change would probably not be necessary.

If a small shift in condylar position is adequate to correct the malocclusion, a good response to treatment can be anticipated. A later opening click usually indicates an extremely anteriorly positioned disk, with advanced deterioration of the posterior ligament; the disk cannot be repositioned.[11]

At the client's initial visit the amount of condylar shift necessary to recapture the disk is determined. Centric occlusion is changed by having the client close in a more protrusive (tip-to-tip) position or by inserting a tongue depressor between the posterior teeth. If this is not sufficient to eliminate the click, two or three tongue depressors are used. These procedures are done after the opening click. For example, the client opens, a click is heard or felt, and a tongue depressor is placed between the posterior teeth. The client closes into this new centric occlusion. If the disk has been repositioned, the click will disappear as the client continues to open and close with the tongue depressor still in position. When the tongue depressor is re-

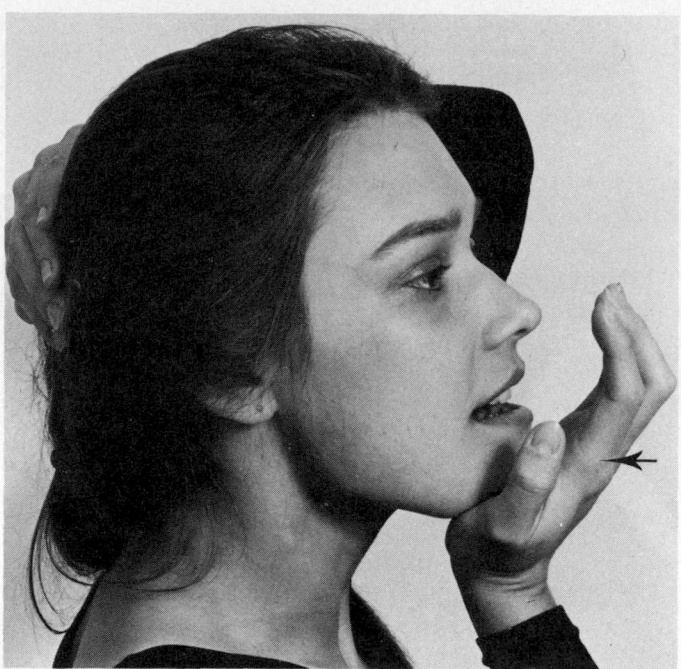

Fig. 23-21. Resistive-protrusive exercise. Client supports occiput with opposite hand.

moved, the click recurs. Various combinations of opening the bite or moving it anteriorly are tried.

If treatment is indicated, the condyles are moved anteriorly in centric occlusion by means of a removable mandibular orthopaedic repositioning appliance. If treatment requires a large change in centric occlusion, complex long-term procedures, such as orthodontics or permanent dental restorations at a new intercuspal position, would be necessary to effect a permanent condylar shift.

In addition to mandibular repositioning, a resisted-protrusion exercise may be prescribed in the treatment of reciprocal clicking. Resistive exercises are similar to the masticatory muscle tests, except that the client applies resistance. Resisted-protrusion exercises aid in repositioning the mandible forward by strengthening the muscles most responsible for mandibular protrusion—the lateral and medial pterygoids. The client is instructed to advance the mandible slightly (about ½ inch) and perform a resisted-protrusion exercise (Fig. 23-22) for 1 to 2 seconds. The exercise is prescribed six to ten times, and the entire sequence is performed five to eight times daily. The client should be instructed to perform the exercise with the tongue in normal resting position on the palate. If pain or other symptoms are produced, the exercise program should be discontinued. Resisted protrusion and the other resistive exercises, such as resisted opening and resisted lateral movement, can be used isometrically when the muscle is weak. In this case the force is applied for 6 seconds.

Locking. When the anteriorly positioned disk blocks condylar translation, mobilization techniques are required to permit the disk to reposition itself. A strong distraction

is applied to the client's mandible to drop the condyle. If the locking occurs closer to the end of the opening range, a more forward position of the lodged disk is indicated. In this situation a downward-forward movement is added to the mobilization technique (see treatment of the hypomobile joint).[35]

To prevent newly repositioned disks from dislocating again, dental intervention is usually necessary. Intervention consists of immediate insertion of an acrylic occlusal splint to move the condyle downward and forward. This will allow the posterior ligament to retract, which will take at least 2 weeks. The client is instructed to wear the appliance constantly, removing it only for oral hygiene (with the mouth kept open).[35] Once the lock is successfully reduced, treatment is similar to that for reciprocal clicking: insertion of a mandibular orthopaedic repositioning appliance to move the condyles downward and forward and prescription of resisted protrusion exercises. In treatment of reciprocal clicking or locking, the client's mandible is occasionally positioned too far anteriorly, which causes headaches. Adjustment of the appliance to move the mandible slightly posteriorly usually affords the client prompt relief.

Occlusomuscular dysfunction. This pathological condition results from an incorrect relation of the mandible to the maxilla in and near centric occlusion that is usually caused by a malocclusion. One of the unique features of the TMJ and associated muscle is the influence exerted on them by the teeth. Complete mandibular closure is dictated by tooth position. If a malocclusion exists, the mandible will still close to maximum tooth contact, often creating

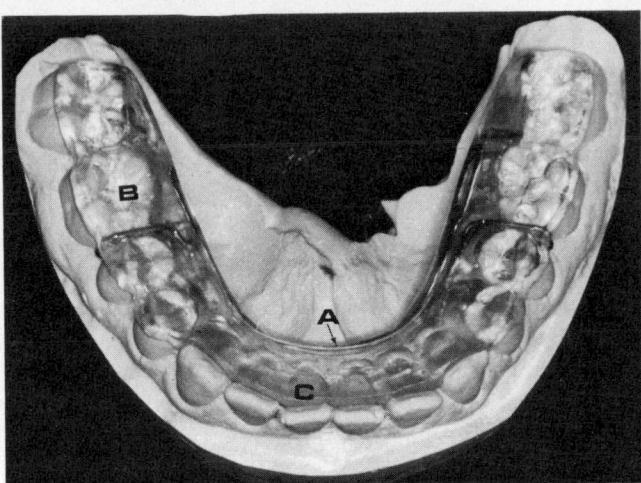

Fig. 23-22. *A,* Stainless steel lingual bar; *B,* plastic covering posterior teeth; *C,* plastic covering lingual surfaces of lower anterior teeth.

muscle imbalances and faulty condylar position. Head and body position and various conditions such as TMJ synovitis or disk disorders, degenerative joint disease, muscle disorders, and growth and developmental abnormalities can also affect jaw relationships. Pernicious habits such as bruxism and clenching can also cause occlusomuscular dysfunction, even if jaw relationships and occlusion are satisfactory.

The malrelationship of the mandible to the maxilla occurs in three planes. It can involve various combinations—lateral mandibular shifts to either side, protrusion or retrusion, or rotations around a vertical or horizontal axis. An upward mandibular shift that reduces the vertical dimension is most often seen. This can occur bilaterally, unilaterally, or anteroposteriorly.

This faulty jaw relationship may be extreme. In the susceptible client, however, even a slight discrepancy in tooth position, which is often difficult to diagnose, can initiate a wide range of symptoms. In some individuals the reflex avoidance of a single interfering cusp can cause occlusomuscular dysfunction.

Mandibular repositioning is usually needed to correct a faulty jaw relationship. This is done either by removing tooth structure through grinding or reshaping or by adding tooth structure through appliance therapy. If the teeth are ground, the modification is permanent; vertical dimension may be reduced by excessive grinding. Appliance therapy, however, increases the vertical dimension and is temporary; therefore removable appliances are used.

These procedures are dental in nature. Nevertheless, familiarity with mandibular repositioning will enable the physical therapist to better understand overall treatment and to enhance his/her relationship with the dentist.

If mandibular repositioning is indicated by TMJ symptoms and positive response to masticatory muscle tests, but

the client's vertical dimension is correct, the vertical dimension should be maintained. Mandibular repositioning should be accomplished by occlusal adjustment. (Such occlusal adjustment procedures are beyond the scope of this chapter.) Nevertheless, the following principles are used in selectively grinding the teeth: (1) elimination of premature contacts in centric occlusion, (2) elimination of bicuspid and molar contacts when the mandible assumes a protrusive position (anterior tip-to-tip tooth contact), and (3) elimination of balancing cusp contacts on posterior teeth. These contacts, which occur on the opposite side when the mandible moves laterally with maximal tooth contact, are damaging to the natural dentition.

If the client's vertical dimension is deficient, selective grinding may temporarily provide relief. Ultimately, however, the client's condition will worsen. These procedures should not be performed in the absence of signs and symptoms. Asymptomatic clients treated by extensive occlusal procedures often develop a positive occlusal sense. They become conscious of their occlusion, which indicates that it never feels quite right. When this situation exists, the closing reflex cannot function correctly.

If appliance therapy is indicated, plaster models of the teeth and gums are required. An appropriate appliance can be constructed from these models by an orthodontic laboratory.

A mandibular appliance is the best, where possible, because it is well tolerated by the client since the palate and the lingual surfaces of the upper anterior teeth are not involved (Fig. 23-22). A stainless steel lingual bar is embedded in plastic, which covers the posterior teeth and the lingual surfaces of the lower anterior teeth. Missing teeth are replaced by extending the plastic in these areas. To obtain the most effective occlusion, an appliance should be constructed for the jaw with the most missing teeth. For this reason a full maxillary appliance is sometimes indicated.

A maxillary appliance affords slightly more control than the mandibular appliance, because all of the opposing teeth occlude with the plastic, whereas there is usually no anterior occlusal contact with the mandibular appliance. Where minimal bite raising is indicated, the occlusal plastic will be quite thin. Breakage of the plastic occurs less often in the maxillary appliance because of the additional palatal support.

The anterior bite planc is a variation of the full maxillary appliance. Occlusal contact is limited to the six anterior teeth. This appliance is indicated in younger clients, because it does not limit posterior tooth eruption. It can alter the client's vertical dimension but cannot reposition the mandible anteroposteriorly because of its lack of posterior occlusion.

The functional portion of this appliance is the occlusal aspect. The plastic overlying the teeth functions as new tooth structure. Opposing tooth cusps fit into indentations in the plastic. Jaw closure is controlled by changing the position of these indentations.

When an ideal neuromuscular mandibular position is required, the Myomonitor* or the Neuropac IV Dental Unit† is helpful in establishing proper jaw relations. These electrical modalities deliver transcutaneous electrical neural stimulation (TENS) to the preauricular areas of the face at the appropriate frequency to override proprioceptive impulses from the periodontium. Muscle memory created by tooth-oriented closure is overpowered; the client's mandible shifts to the position of greatest neuromuscular relaxation regardless of tooth position (Fig. 23-23).[36] The discrepancy between maxillary and mandibular teeth that may become evident is then filled in with the occlusal plastic of the appliance.

These modalities are not used when a major change in condylar position is required, as in treatment of disk dysfunction or localized synovitis caused by an excessively posterior condylar position. In these cases soft acrylic is added to the occlusal portion of the appliance and the clinician guides the client into the desired anterior position.

Long-term response to appliance therapy in treatment of occlusomuscular dysfunction cannot be related to the severity of symptoms. After several months of treatment most clients can gradually discontinue wearing the appliance or use it at night only. Some clients will require a permanent change to the new jaw position. This is accomplished by extensive restorative procedures involving crowns and bridges, orthodontics, or the insertion of a

*Myotronics Research, Inc., Seattle, Wash.
†Ruderman Health Products, Inc., Forest Hills, N.Y.

metal removable appliance similar to the initial plastic appliance.

The use of physical agents in the treatment of occlusomuscular dysfunction is similar to that with other muscles. However, equipment has been modified or developed specifically for this joint. The high-voltage galvanic stimulator is equipped with an electrode for intraoral use. The medial pterygoid muscle can be stimulated with this electrode. The Myomonitor and Neuropac can also be used as electrical stimulators to the superficial muscles of mastication. The type of current in these units enables them to be used for extended periods of an hour or more, because they do not fatigue the muscle. Ultrasound is delivered with a small head attachment because of the size and location of the TMJ. However, only small doses should be used (0.3 to 1 W/cm).[2]

Muscle spasm is often seen in the initial phases of treatment. When relaxation of the muscle is desired, exercise based on the principle of reciprocal inhibition is prescribed. Spasm of the left lateral pterygoid muscle, for example, can be recognized by a positive response to resisted opening and resisted left lateral movement (Figs. 23-13 and 23-15) as well as by an early opening jaw deviation to the right side. In this case the closing muscles would be exercised. The procedure is identical to the resisted-closing muscle test (Fig. 23-14) except that the client applies the opening force and prevents head flexion with the opposite hand. As in resisted protrusion, a force is applied for 1 to 2 seconds for six to ten repetitions, and this is done five to eight times a day.

Neuromuscular reeducation is often used to correct de-

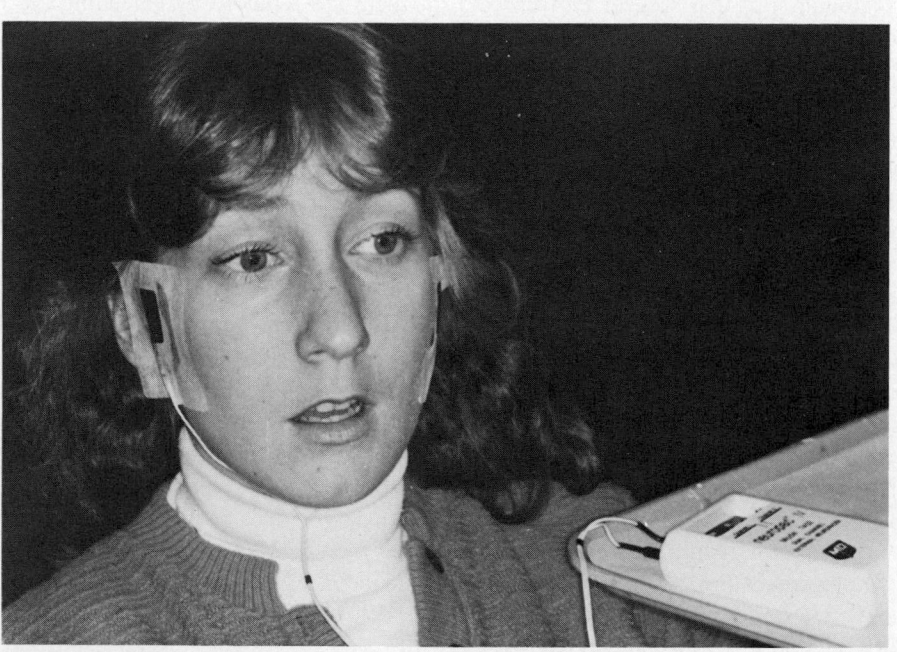

Fig. 23-23. Neuropac delivering TENS to preauricular areas of face. (Courtesy Ruderman Health Products, Forest Hills, NY.)

viations during the opening cycle. The client is asked to open as wide as possible without deviation and then to close, using a mirror at first. The tongue should be in its normal resting position. This is done several times in the course of a minute, five to eight times daily. The goal is to increase the opening but without deviation. The client is taught to palpate the condyles laterally during the opening cycle and to recognize and control premature anterior condylar movement. The goal is to increase the rotational opening of the mandible, where necessary. The client is instructed to feel deviations by opening to the right or left so he/she can learn to control them. Resisted–lateral movement exercises, where indicated, are done with the mouth opened to the position where the deviation occurs.[13] An opening deviation caused by muscle imbalance usually occurs toward the middle of the cycle. The weak muscle is strengthened by resisted–lateral movement exercises. In the case of muscle weakness the resistance is applied for 6 seconds, as opposed to 1 to 2 seconds for muscle reeducation.

Hypomobility. Joint mobilization is the technique of choice to increase range of motion of the TMJ.[26] Clients often notice an immediate result as adhesions are stretched or torn. The cumulative effect of mobilization on the TMJ capsule will lead to realignment of collagen fibers in such a way as to permit more movement. Fig. 23-19 illustrates the direction of joint play in the TMJ.[14]

The condyle must drop as it moves forward (translates) in order to clear the eminence. In the hypomobile joint this downward movement is restricted; the joint capsule must first be stretched before a full opening can be obtained.

Fig. 23-24 illustrates a strong downward force applied to the client's posterior molar with the thumb and a simultaneous upward pressure applied to the front of the mandible with the therapist's other fingers. After initial downward stretching is obtained, either at the first visit or later, a forward-downward movement is added. When this additional movement is performed, the therapist's index finger is hooked around the angle of the mandible. Immediately after the condyle is distracted and held briefly, the entire mandible is moved anteriorly at approximately a 40-degree angle, which coincides with the angle of the eminence. The therapist's forearm extends outward in the same direction as the thumb. If the forearm is not held in the sagittal plane, however, an undesirable element of rotation may be introduced to the mobilization.[35]

Sometimes a much more delicate lateral movement is also incorporated. When either downward or lateral mobilization is performed, the therapist usually stands on the side opposite that being treated. The basic body position of the therapist during lateral mobilization is similar to that in the previous procedure, except that the therapist's elbow is brought toward the body to permit the rotation (Fig. 23-25). The therapist's thumb applies a gentle force to the lingual surface of the posterior molar or to the lingual gum tissue on the side to be treated. Just before each downward or lateral mobilization, the client is instructed to relax the jaw. Pressure is applied laterally to move the condyle in the desired direction. At the same time, force is applied in the opposite direction to the anterior part of the mandible. Slight pressure is all that is required to gain the desired lateral condylar movement.[34] The client is cautioned to im-

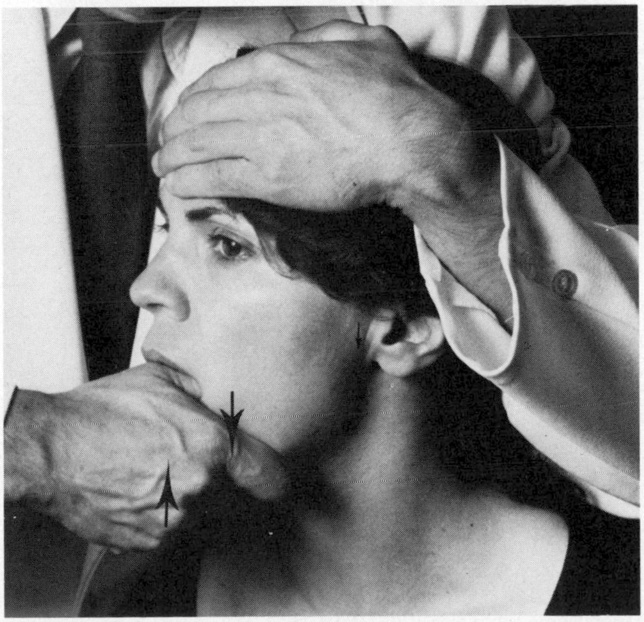

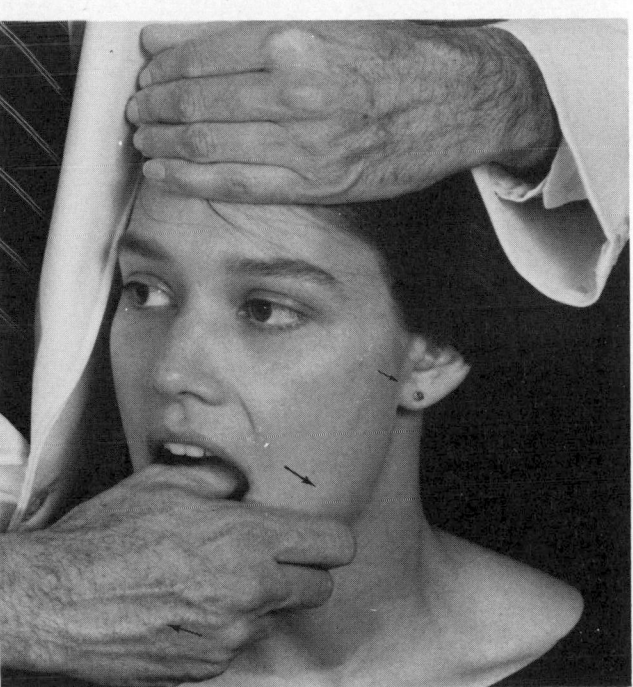

Fig. 23-24. Downward mobilization of TMJ. Note firm head stabilization by therapist's hand, forearm, and chest.

Fig. 23-25. Lateral mobilization of TMJ.

mediately report pain on the opposite side, which is indicative of use of excessive force.

If treatment of the hypomobile joint is anticipated, the initial opening is measured in standard units, as opposed to a functional measurement (see Fig. 23-16), so that improvement from treatment can be noted. The greatest increase in opening is often seen after the initial mobilization.

A minimum restriction may require downward stretching of 3 seconds' duration for each joint if hypomobility is bilateral. This is repeated five times, with a few minutes between each application so as not to tire the client. The gentle lateral mobilization is performed between each downward mobilization. Each treatment session is always finished with a bilateral joint mobilization, even if only one joint is involved, in order to leave the client with a good sense of balance. When the downward and downward-forward mobilization is performed bilaterally, the client's head must be stabilized (Fig. 23-26) to prevent forward movement. If this procedure is performed in a dental chair without an assistant, the client's head can be tied to the headrest with a strap.[34]

A few treatments will suffice in most cases. A severe case may require six or more visits. In these cases follow-up exercises by the client to maintain the increased opening should be prescribed (Fig. 23-27). Extraoral mobilization of the TMJ may be necessary in cases where the opening is extremely limited. These techniques are well described in the literature.[24]

Joint mobilization is useful in various other situations.

For example, a client may complain of a tight or restricted feeling caused by the intrusion of a newly inserted orthopaedic appliance into the freeway space. Joint mobilization will make the client more comfortable. Clients who experience tightness when yawning or opening widely often notice an immediate result, since adhesions are stretched or torn when mobilization is performed. Balancing the amount of joint play bilaterally often has a beneficial effect on small opening deviations. After much experience the therapist will be able to check the amount of vertical and lateral "give" in the condyles by applying minimal forces, as described in the evaluation section.[34] When downward mobilization is used to unlock the mandible because of an anteriorly positioned disk, lateral and bilateral mobilization are not used.

Hypermobility. Neuromuscular reeducation is used to limit the excessive opening in this condition. The client is taught to open with the tongue against the palate to control the amount of opening. Resisted-opening exercises are performed at midrange. The principle is to increase sensitivity to the stretch reflex. In addition to this exercise, a 1- to 2-second mild resistive force is applied five to ten times in all directions (posterior, left, right, superior, inferior) with the mouth slightly opened (1 cm).

Dislocated joint

Bilateral manipulation (see Fig. 23-27) is the treatment of choice to reduce the dislocation. If this is not done immediately, severe muscle spasm may necessitate use of strong medication or general anesthesia.[33] Immediately af-

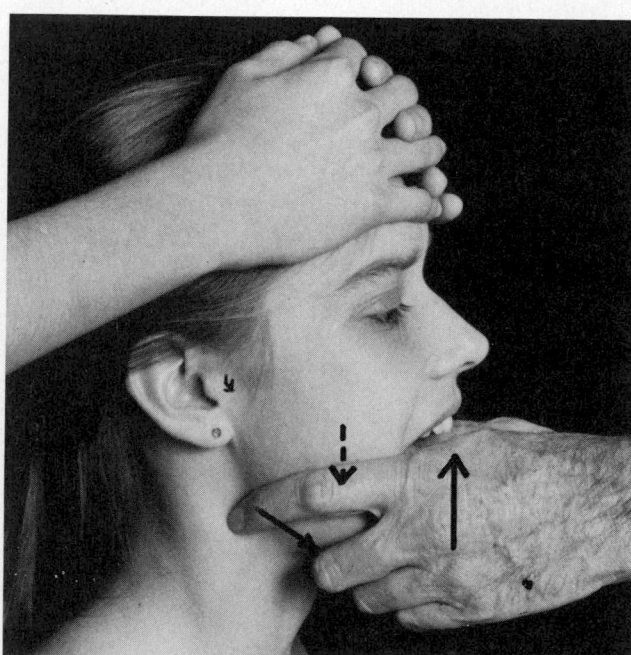

Fig. 23-26. Bilateral mobilization of TMJ. Note therapist's index finger around angle of mandible to assist downward-forward mobilization.

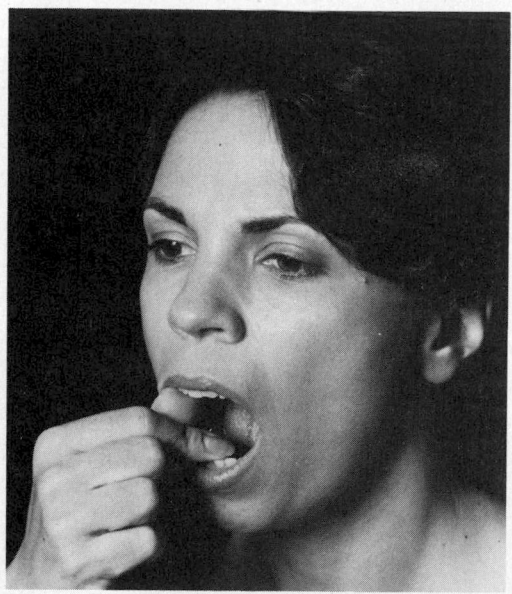

Fig. 23-27. Maintenance exercise. Client's thumb and forefinger are placed as far posteriorly as possible. Fingers are spread as wide as possible to aid in stretching jaw. Duration and frequency are similar to resistive exercises and may be prescribed bilaterally.

ter the dislocation is reduced, continued downward pressure should be maintained to prevent injury to the clinician as a result of reflex closure. The client should be put on a restricted diet and told to limit jaw opening.

SUMMARY

A dislocated TMJ is a relatively uncommon dysfunction. Nevertheless, the practitioner should have the knowledge to treat this acute condition if required.

REFERENCES

1. Arlen H: The otomandibular syndrome: Diagnosis, Ear Nose Throat J 57:553, 1978.
2. Arthritis teaching slide collection—Instructional guide, Atlanta, 1980, Arthritis Foundation.
3. Ashley R and Kirby T: Dental anatomy and terminology, New York, 1977, John Wiley & Sons, Inc.
4. Basmajian JV: Muscles alive, Baltimore, 1978, Williams & Wilkins, p 380.
5. Blair GS: Psoriatic arthritis and the TMJ, J Dent 4:123, 1976.
6. Cyriax J: The diagnosis of soft tissue lesion. In Cyriax J, editor: Textbook of orthopaedic medicine, vol 1, ed 7, London, 1978, Bailliere Tindall.
7. De Steno CV: The pathophysiology of TMJ dysfunction and related pain. In Gelb H, editor: Clinical management of head, neck, and TMJ pain and dysfunction, Philadelphia, 1977, WB Saunders Co.
8. Dubrul EL: Sicher's oral anatomy, ed 7, St Louis, 1980, The CV Mosby Co.
9. Farrar WB: Diagnosis and treatment of painful temporomandibular joints, J Prosthet Dent 20:345, 1968.
10. Farrar WB: Differentiation of temporomandibular joint pain to simplify treatment, J Prosthet Dent 28:630, 1972.
11. Farrar WB: Characteristics of the condylar path in internal derangements of the TMJ, J Prosthet Dent 39:319, 1978.
12. Friedman AP, editor: Symposium on headache and related pain syndromes, Philadelphia, 1978, WB Saunders Co.
13. Friedman MH, Anstendig HS, and Weisberg J: Case report: Treatment of a disc dysfunction, J Clin Orthodont 16:408, 1982.
14. Friedman MH and Weisberg J: Application of orthopedic principles in evaluation of the temporomandibular joint, Phys Ther 62:597, 1982.
15. Friedman MH and Weisberg J: Screening procedures for temporomandibular joint dysfunction, Am Fam Physician 25:157, 1982.
16. Friedman MH and Weisberg J: Pitfalls of muscle palpation in TMJ diagnosis, J Prosthet Dent 48:331, 1982.
17. Friedman MH, Weisberg J, and Agus B: Diagnosis and treatment of inflammation of the temporomandibular joint, Semin Arthritis Rheum 12:44, 1982.
18. Gelb H: Patient evaluation. In Gelb H, editor: Clinical management of head, neck, and TMJ pain and dysfunction, Philadelphia, 1977, WB Saunders Co.
19. Goodman WS, et al: Infections of the temporomandibular joint, J Otolaryngol 8:250, 1979.
20. Johnstone DR and Templeton M: The feasibility of palpating the lateral pterygoid muscle, J Prosthet Dent 44:318, 1980.
21. Jonck LM: Ear symptoms in temporomandibular joint disturbances, S Afr Med J 54:782, 1978.
22. Laskin DM: Etiology of the pain-dysfunction syndrome, J Am Dent Assoc 79:147, 1969.
23. Mahan PE: The temporomandibular joint in function and pathofunction. In Soldberg WK and Clark GT, editors: Temporomandibular joint problems, Chicago, 1980, Quintessence Publishing Co, Inc.
24. Maitland GD: Peripheral manipulation, ed 2, London, 1977, Butterworth Publishers.
25. Mankin HJ and Lippiello L: The glycosaminoglycans of normal and arthritic cartilage, J Clin Invest 50:1712, 1971.
26. Mennell J: Joint pain, Boston, 1964, Little, Brown & Co.
27. Nies KM: The infective arthropathies. In Bluestone R, editor: Rheumatology, Boston, 1980, Houghton-Mifflin Co, pp 332-339.
28. Oshrain HI and Sackler A: Involvement of the temporomandibular joint in a case of rheumatoid arthritis, Oral Surg Oral Med Oral Pathol 8:1039, 1955.
29. Polley HF and Hunder GG: Rheumatologic interviewing and physical examination of the joints, ed 2, Philadelphia, 1978, WB Saunders Co.
30. Possult U: Components. In Possult U, editor: Physiology of occlusion and rehabilitation, ed 2, Oxford, 1969, Blackwell Scientific Publications.
31. Possult U: Positions and movements. In Possult U, editor: Physiology of occlusion and rehabilitation, ed 2, Oxford, 1969, Blackwell Scientific Publications.
32. Possult U: Dysfunctions. In Possult U, editor: Physiology of occlusion and rehabilitation, ed 2, Oxford, 1969, Blackwell Scientific Publications.
33. Poswillo D: Surgery of the temporomandibular joint, Oral Sci Rev 6:87, 1974.
34. Rocabado M: Head, neck, and TMJ dysfunction, Read before Institute for Graduate Dentists, New York, April 1979.
35. Weisberg J and Friedman MH: Displaced disc preventing mandibular condyle translation: Mobilization technique, J Orthop Sports Phys Ther 3:62, 1981.
36. Wessberg G, et al: Transcutaneous electrical stimulation as an adjunct in the management of myofascial pain-dysfunction syndrome, J Prosthet Dent 45:307, 1981.

Sports physical therapy

Chapter 24

PRESEASON ATHLETIC PHYSICAL EXAMINATION

John S. Eggart
David Leigh
Greg Vergamini

Purpose of screening
Responsibilities
Frequency and timing
Utilization/dissemination
Scope of screening and program planning
The examination
    Medical history examination station
    Physical screening stations
Summary

The preseason athletic physical screening is beneficial for the physical therapist, and for the trainer, coach, athlete, and physician. In order to outline a comprehensive preseason screening program, we will first present the background philosophy. This includes the purpose for performing the screening, the responsibilities of various personnel, the timing and frequency of the screening, the uses and dissemination of the data obtained, and the scope of the screening.

PURPOSE OF SCREENING

The reason for performing a detailed preseason screening is twofold. The primary purpose is prevention of injury. This is accomplished by evaluating body structures to identify areas that have an increased susceptibility to injury during sports-related activities. With this structural identification and a knowledge of normal kinesiology and biomechanics as a base, a program to rectify or minimize the effect of abnormalities or weaknesses may be initiated to decrease the risk of injury. If modification of risk factors cannot significantly decrease the likelihood of injury, a conference should be arranged with the athlete, coach, parents, physician, and examiner to discuss the options available to the athlete. This entire process of prevention follows the recommendation of the American Medical Association's Committee on the Medical Aspects of Sport to recognize the athlete's rights; the rights include adequate health supervision, good coaching, capable officiating, and proper equipment and facilities[10] (see boxed material).

A second use of the preseason screening is to collect data that can be used for comparison during rehabilitation should an injury occur during the season. These baseline data give the health care team an idea of "normal" for the specific athlete. This "normal" can be used as a goal that must be reached before an athlete can be considered for return to preinjury status and activity without having an increased probability of reinjury.

RESPONSIBILITIES

The responsibilities of the physical therapist or athletic trainer are to (1) initiate the process of the preseason athletic physical screening, (2) organize and perform the screening, and (3) make recommendations to appropriate personnel based on the results of the screening. The coach and administrative personnel are primarily responsible for the enforcement of the recommendations made at the completion of the screening process.[15] The ultimate responsibility for the preseason screening rests with the physician.

American Medical Association recommendations on the medical aspects of sport

Rights of the athlete

Participation in athletics is a privilege involving both responsibilities and rights. The athlete has the responsibility to play fair, to give his best, to keep in training, and to conduct himself with credit to his sport and his school. In turn, he has the right to optimal protection against injury. This protection can be assured through the following:

Proper conditioning.

By strengthening the body and increasing resistance to fatigue, proper conditioning of the athlete is a significant factor in lowering the incidence and decreasing the severity of injuries.

Good coaching.

The importance of careful technical instruction in protecting the health and safety of athletes cannot be minimized. Good coaching not only leads to skillful performance, but discourages tactics—outside either the rules or the spirit of the rules—that may increase the hazard and thus the incidence of injuries.

Capable officiating.

Rules and regulations governing athletic competition are made to protect players as well as to promote enjoyment of the game. To serve these ends effectively, the rules of the game must be thoroughly understood by players as well as coaches and be properly interpreted and enforced by impartial and technically qualified officials.

Proper equipment and facilities.

There can be no question about the protection afforded by proper equipment and facilities. Good equipment is now available and is being improved continually; the problem lies in the false economy of using inexpensive, outmoded, worn-out, or ill-fitting gear and in the improper use of equipment. Provision of proper play areas and their careful maintenance are equally important.

Adequate health supervision.

(1) A thorough preseason history and medical examination must be performed. Many of the sports tragedies that occur each year result from unrecognized health problems. Medical contraindications to participation in contact sports must be respected. (2) A physician must be present or readily available during practice sessions and contests. Leaving to a trainer or coach decisions such as whether an athlete should return to play or be removed from a game after injury is unfair. In serious injuries the availability of a physician can make the difference in preventing disability or even death. (3) Medical control of the health aspects of athletics must be exerted. In medical matters the physician's authority should be absolute and unquestioned. Coaches and athletic trainers assist the physician.

Safeguarding the health of the athlete

Periodic evaluation of each factor involved in protecting the athlete against injury will help to assure a safe and healthful sports experience. The following are examples of questions to be answered in such an appraisal:

Proper conditioning

- Are prospective players given directions and activities for preseason conditioning?
- Is there a minimum of 3 weeks of practice before the first game or contest?
- Are precautions taken to prevent heat exhaustion and heat stroke?
- Is each player required to warm up thoroughly before participating?
- Are substitutions made without hesitation when players evidence disability?

Good coaching

- Is emphasis given to safety in teaching techniques and elements of play, such as a progressive method of developing difficult skills?
- Are injuries analyzed to determine causes and to suggest preventive programs?
- Are tactics discouraged that may increase the hazards and thus the incidence of injuries?
- Are practice periods carefully planned and of reasonable duration?

Capable officiating

- Are players as well as coaches thoroughly schooled in the rules of the game?
- Are rules and regulations strictly enforced in practice periods as well as in games?
- Are officials qualified both emotionally and technically for their responsibilities?
- Do players and coaches respect the decisions of officials?

Proper equipment and facilities

- Is the best protective equipment provided for contact sports?
- Is careful attention given to proper fitting and adjustment of equipment?
- Is equipment properly maintained and are worn and outmoded items discarded?
- Are proper areas for play provided and carefully maintained?

Adequate health supervision

- Is there a thorough preseason health history and medical examination?
- Is a physician present for contests and practice sessions or can he be readily contacted?
- Does the physician make the decision as to whether an athlete should return to play after injury during games?
- Is authority from a physician obtained before an athlete can return to practice after being out of play because of a disabling injury?
- Is the care given athletes by coach or trainer limited to first aid and medically prescribed services?

Reprinted from Medical Evaluation of the Athlete, 1981, with permission of American Medical Association, 535 N. Dearborn St., Chicago Ill.

From a medical-legal viewpoint the physician is recognized as the head of the medical team and therefore assumes responsibility for recommendations of activity level and type for a particular athlete.[18,32]

FREQUENCY AND TIMING

A complete medical and musculoskeletal evaluation should be performed in the off-season, and a re-evaluation of noted deficiencies should be performed immediately before the start of practice or competition. An off-season examination allows the athlete and medical team to gain a base of knowledge as to the athlete's anatomical and physiological standing in relation to normal levels. This also allows adequate time to attain those normal levels before the athlete begins his/her specific activity. The specialized followup evaluation immediately preseason allows either final

---

UNIVERSITY OF WISCONSIN–LA CROSSE
Student Health Center

ATHLETIC EVALUATION

Sport(s)_____ Date_____

Name _____ SSN_____

==

MEDICAL EXAMINATION

PMD exam dated _____ Reviewed by _____ On_____

OK_____Should be seen by M.D._____Needs_____

R.N.: BP_____Vision (R) 20/_____ (L) 20/_____ Tetanus date _____

LAB: Hct_____UA_____ TB test_____

M.D.: Skin_____ Eyes—pupils (R)_____(L)_____

Dental _____ ENT _____

Lungs_____ Heart_____

Abdomen _____

MEDICATIONS:_____

RECOMMEND: NO PARTICIPATION_____ HOLD FOR _____ FULL ACTIVITY_____BY _____

==

ORTHOPAEDIC EXAMINATION

Height_____ Weight_____

Resting pulse_____After exercise_____ 1 min_____ 3 min_____

Neck_____

Upper extremities_____

Grip (R)_____lb (L)_____lb

Lower extremities_____

Quadriceps (R)_____/_____/_____/ (L)_____/_____/_____/

Hamstring (R)_____/_____/_____/ (L)_____/_____/_____/

Feet/ankles_____

Gait_____

Anterior torso_____ Sit-up_____

Back_____

Posture_____

Reflexes_____

Sensation_____ Balance (R)_____(L)_____

Referral_____ Reviewed by_____

==

Hold for_____ By_____

NO CLEARANCE card sent_____By_____ RECOMMENDATION GIVEN

Hold cleared_____By_____ _____

OK FOR UNRESTRICTED ACTIVITY_____By_____ _____

Card sent_____By_____ _____

Fig. 24-1. University of Wisconsin–La Crosse Student Health Center athletic evaluation.

clearance or imposition of limited activity until total rehabilitation is achieved (Fig. 24-1).

An alternative is to give the athlete a total physical evaluation initially, then follow up with repeat evaluations annually, spot-checking risk areas or a previously injured area (Fig. 24-2). This alternative examination procedure is not as desirable but is adequate when a great number of athletes need to be examined in a short period of time. The screening program will vary according to number of clinicians available, number of athletes to be tested, facilities, and funding.

UTILIZATION/DISSEMINATION

Use of information gathered is, as mentioned previously, principally aimed at prophylaxis. Recognizing the confidential nature of this information, consent of the athlete is needed to allow dissemination of the findings or to make recommendations to appropriate personnel (Fig. 24-

---

UNIVERSITY OF WISCONSIN-LA CROSSE
Student Health Center

ATHLETIC RE-EVALUATION

Sport(s)_____ Date _____

Name_____ SSN_____

===

Please circle correct answer:

1. Have you had any injury since your last athletic evaluation here?   Yes   No
   Explain.

2. Have you any symptoms or condition about which you should consult   Yes   No
   us before you participate in athletics?
   Explain.

3. Have you consulted an outside physician or dentist since your last   Yes   No
   athletic evaluation here?
   Explain.

4. Do you know of any reason you should NOT participate in any sport?   Yes   No
   Explain.

I certify the above information is accurate and correct and a true reflection of my present
physical condition.

                          Athlete's signature_____
===
Review of recent injury/illness_____

_____

_____

_____

_____

Weight_____ Blood pressure_____Tetanus date_____

Resting pulse_____ After exercise_____ 1 min_____ 3 min_____

                          Reviewed by_____
===
Referral _____ By _____

Hold for _____ By _____

NO CLEARANCE card sent_____ By_____ RECOMMENDATION GIVEN

Hold cleared _____ By_____ _____

OK FOR UNRESTRICTED ACTIVITY _____ By_____ _____

Card sent _____ By_____ _____

Fig. 24-2. University of Wisconsin–La Crosse Student Health Center athletic reevaluation.

3). Screening results may then be used to determine who is a high-risk individual and whether or not corrective measures are needed to prevent an injury.

Research is another use for the information accumulated in an athletic screening program. The vast amount of data gathered from screening large numbers of structures may be used to help establish norms for the various testing procedures used in the screening; they may also possibly open a myriad of opportunities for detailed research. One area of research is the relationship between body type and performance in individual sports.

SCOPE OF SCREENING AND PROGRAM PLANNING

The detail to which the screening is performed and the type of program planning will be dependent on many variables, including individual tester's skill levels, number of testers, number of athletes, location, space, equipment, level of competition, and the like. It should be emphasized that there is no correct procedure for the overall screening, although there may be more efficient or useful individual methods.[5]

Overall, a group physical screening seems more time-efficient when compared to individual screenings. In such a setup the athlete can move in assembly line fashion from one station to another, with individual systems or joints screened at each station (Fig. 24-4). A final review is con-

ducted so the findings from the individual stations can be collated and final recommendations made.

THE EXAMINATION
Medical history examination station

The initial portion of the examination involves taking the client's medical history, which can be done orally or by questionnaire (Fig. 24-5). This should include inoculation records, surgical history (including names of surgeons or physicians involved so that followup contact may be made for details), a record of injuries (including diagnosis and care/rehabilitation), family history (especially of cardiac, respiratory, neurological, joint, and hereditary diseases), childhood diseases, convulsions, and current medical problems or medications. Special emphasis is placed on a detailed history of cerebral concussions and any medical/dental visits or injuries since the last evaluation was performed.

The physical portion of the medical evaluation then involves height and weight measurements, visual acuity tests (including a record of use of glasses or hard or soft contact lenses), ear, nose, and throat examinations, dental evaluation, abdominal evaluation (including hernia check), auscultation, as well as other more specific examinations that are indicated. Laboratory tests routinely include urine and blood (hematocrit) analysis, with further tests based on findings that are ordered by the physician[4] (Fig. 24-6).

UNIVERSITY OF WISCONSIN-LA CROSSE
Student Health Center

RELEASE OF INFORMATION AUTHORIZATION FOR VARSITY ATHLETES

I,_____, DO / DO NOT (circle one) give my consent for the team physician, athletic trainers, or other medical personnel of the UNIVERSITY OF WISCONSIN-LA CROSSE to release information regarding my medical history, record of injury or surgery, record of serious illness, and rehabilitation results as may be requested by the scout or representative of any professional or amateur athletic organization seeking such information.

I understand that such scout or representative of the team has indicated to the team physician, athletic trainer, or other medical personnel of the UNIVERISTY OF WISCONSIN-LA CROSSE that the purpose of this request for medical information is to assist the organization in making a determination as to whether to offer me employment.

I understand that a record will be kept of all individuals requesting such information and the date of the request. This information is normally confidential and except as provided for in this form will not be otherwise released by the parties in charge of the information. This RELEASE remains in effect until revoked by me in writing.

Signed_____
Date_____

Fig. 24-3. University of Wisconsin–La Crosse Student Health Center release of information authorization for varsity athletes.

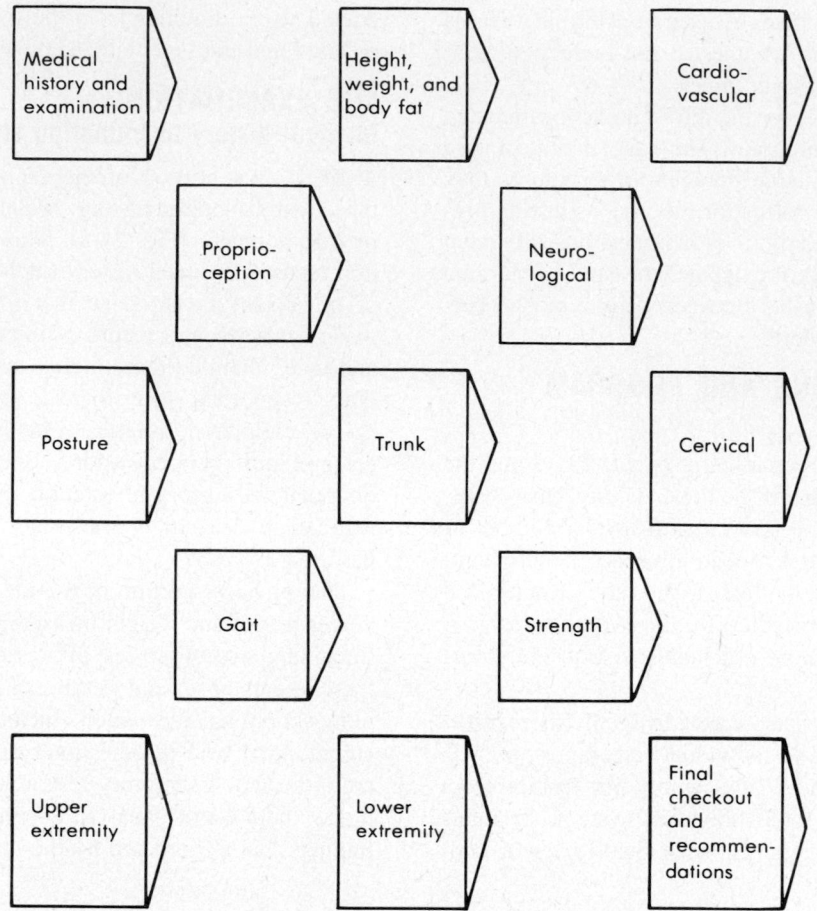

Fig. 24-4. Group physical screening assembly line stations.

Certain conditions are accepted as immediately disqualifying an athlete from participating in selected activities or levels of activities. The recommendations of the American Medical Association's Committee on the Medical Aspects of Sports regarding disqualification from participation are found in Table 24-1.[10]

Physical screening stations

A general physical fitness evaluation may involve analysis of cardiovascular endurance and recovery, body fat percentage, agility, muscle function, and lower extremity balance comparison. Any abnormalities are noted for further detailed examination at the final review station.

Cardiovascular recovery, cardiovascular endurance, and blood pressure. Cardiovascular recovery can be evaluated through the use of a bench-step maneuver, stationary cycle, or other standard stress tests. Resting heart rate and blood pressure are recorded and are followed by a standardized work performance activity (i.e., 50 bench steps or 3 minutes at a predetermined load on a cycle ergometer). Heart rate and blood pressure are then recorded immediately after exercise and at predetermined intervals (e.g., 1 minute, 3 minutes, 5 minutes) until the rates return to the preexercise level.

Cardiovascular endurance may be tested by using a timed run (i.e., 12 minutes) and measuring the distance covered. One can also use a preset distance (i.e., 880 yards or 1 mile) and record the time required to cover it.[16]

Body fat percentages. Body fat percentages are most accurately determined by underwater weighing techniques.[14] The technique involves submersion of the athlete and measurement of the water displaced. However, measurement of body skin fold can be used in lieu of underwater weighing. Skin fold measurement as a means of estimating percentage of body fat is both economical and expedient.[22,34] The Cramer Syndex caliper* (Fig. 24-7) has been shown to be a valid and reliable method of estimating percent of body fat.

Agility. Agility, the ability to change directions rapidly while moving at a high rate of speed, is dependent on elements such as strength, reaction time, speed of movement, and coordination. Whereas agility is difficult to assess,

---

*SYNDEX, Cramer Products, Gardner, Kan.

UNIVERSITY OF WISCONSIN-LA CROSSE
Student Health Center

ATHLETIC PARTICIPATION QUESTIONNAIRE

Name _____ Date _____

SSN _____ Insurance carrier and policy # _____

==

Please circle correct answer (Y = Yes, N = No) and indicate (R) Right or (L) Left.

1. Have you had a condition that required medical attention to:
   Muscle   Y N
   Joint   Y N
   Tendon   Y N
   Bone   Y N
   Explain _____
   _____

2. Do you get a rash from tape?   Y N
   Do you get a rash from linament? Y N

3. List date you had:
   Shoulder dislocation _____
   Knee trouble _____
   Knee cap dislocation _____ _____
   Ankle sprain _____
   Back pain _____
   Fracture _____

4. Have you ever had an injury pro-   Y N
   ducing weakness or numbness of
   arms or legs?
   Explain _____
   _____

5. Have you ever had a skull, neck,   Y N
   or spine fracture?
   X-ray of any of above?   Y N
   Explain _____
   _____

6. Have you ever been unconscious?   Y N
   Fainted?   Y N
   How many times? _____
   When? _____
   Hospitalized for this?   Y N
   Explain _____
   _____

7. Do you have frequent or severe   Y N
   headaches?

8. Have you ever had seizures or   Y N
   convulsions?

9. Have you ever had a brain wave   Y N
   test?
   When? _____
   Where? _____

10. Do you wear:
    Glasses _____ Contact lenses _____
    Bridgework _____ Dental braces _____
    Dentures _____
    Date of last visit to dentist? _____

11. Have you ever become weak or ill   Y N
    when exposed to high temperature?

12. Do you have loss or seriously im- Y N
    paired function of any paired
    organ?
    Eye _____ Lung _____
    Kidney _____ Testicle _____

13. Do you have or have you ever had:
    Asthma   Y N
    Hayfever   Y N
    Allergies   Y N
      To what? _____

14. List surgical operations you have had
    and approximate date(s). _____
    _____
    _____

15. Have you been seen by a physician Y N
    for any illness/condition lasting
    more than 1 week during the past
    year?
    Explain _____
    _____

16. Are you under a physician's care   Y N
    now?
    For? _____
    _____

17. Do you have or have you ever had:
    Diabetes   Y N
    Epilepsy   Y N
    Kidney disease   Y N
    Abnormal bleeding tendencies   Y N
    Tuberculosis   Y N
    Stomach/intestinal trouble   Y N
    Arthritis   Y N
    Heart disease   Y N
      (rheumatic fever, high blood
       pressure, heart murmur)
    Other problems? _____

Student signature _____

YOUR PERSONAL PHYSICIAN MUST COMPLETE THE REVERSE SIDE BEFORE YOU WILL BE EVALUATED IN THE STUDENT HEALTH CENTER FOR ATHLETIC PARTICIPATION.

Fig. 24-5. University of Wisconsin–La Crosse Student Health Center athletic participation questionnaire. (See Fig. 24-6 for reverse side.)

UNIVERSITY OF WISCONSIN-LA CROSSE
Student Health Center

MEDICAL EXAMINATION FORM

I have examined _____ on _____
                        (client's name)   (date)

Height _____ Weight _____ Blood pressure _____
Laboratory work _____
Findings _____
_____
_____

Has this client any of the following? (Please explain and give approximate dates.)
   Chronic health problem(s) _____
   _____
   _____

   Serious illnesses _____
   _____
   _____

   Injuries _____
   _____
   _____

   Surgeries _____
   _____
   _____

   On medication _____
   _____

Immunization dates:
   Dip-tet. _____ Tet. tox. _____
   Polio (oral) _____ Polio (injected) _____
   Rubella _____ Rubeola _____
   TB test _____ Chest x-ray _____

   _____ NO RESTRICTION FOR ATHLETIC PARTICIPATION
   _____ RESTRICTION   Participation limited to _____
Recommendation for continuing care of this student while at the University: _____
_____

                          Physician's signature _____
                          Printed name and address _____

Date _____

THIS FORM MUST BE RETURNED BY AUGUST 16 TO: Student Health Center
                                               University of Wisconsin-LaCrosse
                                               LaCrosse, WI 54601

Fig. 24-6. University of Wisconsin–La Crosse Student Health Center medical examination form. Reverse side of athletic participation questionnaire (see Fig. 24-5).

Table 24-1. Disqualifying conditions for sports participation

Conditions	Contact*	Noncontact endurance†	Other‡
General			
Acute infections; respiratory, genitourinary, infectious mononucleosis, hepatitis, active rheumatic fever, active tuberculosis	X	X	X
Obvious physical immaturity in comparison with other competitors	X	X	
Obvious growth retardation	X		
Hemorrhagic disease: hemophilia, purpura, other bleeding tendencies	X		
Diabetes, inadequately controlled	X	X	X
Jaundice, whatever cause	X	X	X
Eyes			
Absence or loss of function of one eye	X		
Severe myopia	X		
Ears			
Significant impairment	X		
Respiratory			
Tuberculosis (active or under treatment)	X	X	X
Severe pulmonary insufficiency	X	X	X
Cardiovascular			
Mitral stenosis, aortic stenosis, aortic insufficiency, coarctation of aorta, cyanotic heart disease, recent carditis of any cause	X	X	X
Hypertension of organic basis	X	X	X
Previous heart surgery for congenital or acquired heart disease	X	X	
Liver			
Enlarged liver	X		
Skin			
Boils, impetigo, herpes simplex gladiatorum	X		
Spleen			
Enlarged spleen	X		
Hernia			
Inguinal or femoral hernia	X	X	
Musculoskeletal			
Symptomatic abnormalities or inflammations	X	X	X
Functional inadequacy of musculoskeletal system, congenital or acquired, incompatible with contact or skill demands of sport	X	X	

Reprinted from Medical Evaluation of the Athlete, 1981, with permission of American Medical Association, 535 N. Dearborn St., Chicago, Ill.

*Lacrosse, baseball, soccer, basketball, football, wrestling, hockey, rugby, etc.

†Cross country, track, tennis, crew, swimming, etc.

‡Bowling, golf, archery, field events, etc.

§Each client should be judged on an individual basis. All things being equal, it is probably better to encourage a young boy or girl to participate in a noncontact sport rather than a contact sport. However, if a particular client has a great desire to play a contact sport, and this is deemed a major ameliorating factor in his/her adjustment to school, associates, and the seizure disorder, serious consideration should be given to letting him/her participate if the seizures are controlled.

‖The Committee approves the concept of contact sports participation for youths with only one testicle or with an undescended testicle(s), except in specific cases such as an inguinal canal undescended testicle(s), after appropriate medical evaluation to rule out unusual injury risk. However, the athlete, parents, and school authorities should be fully informed that participation in contact sports for such youths with only one testicle does carry a slight injury risk to the remaining healthy testicle. After such an injury fertility may be adversely affected. But the chances of an injury to a descended testicle are rare, and the injury risk can be further substantially minimized with an athletic supporter and protective device.

Table 24-1. Disqualifying conditions for sports participation—cont'd

Conditions	Contact*	Noncontact endurance†	Other‡
Neurological			
History or symptoms of previous serious head trauma or repeated concussions, controlled convulsive disorder§	x		
Convulsive disorder not completely controlled by medication	x	x	
Previous surgery on head or spine	x	x	
Renal			
Absence of one kidney	x		
Renal disease	x	x	x
Genitalia‖			
Absence of one testicle			
Undescended testicle			

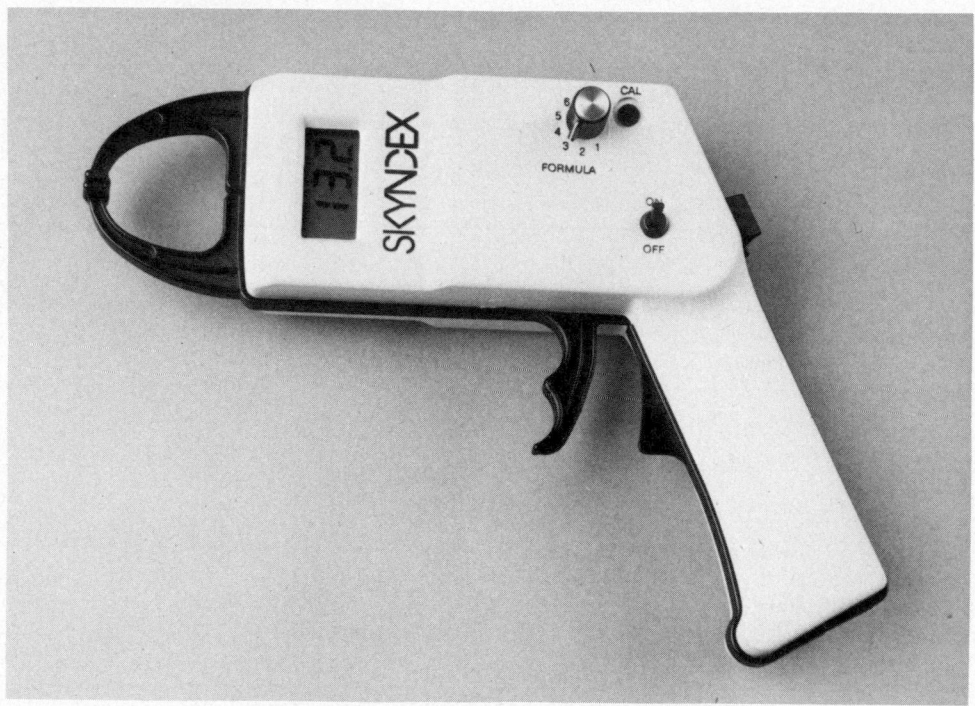

Fig. 24-7. The Cramer Skyndex caliper. (Photo courtesy of Cramer Products, Inc., Gardner, Kan.)

some specific tests can be incorporated in the preparticipation screening, depending on personnel and resources available. Tests should be as specific to the sport as possible.

Two tests that can be used to test agility of the lower extremity are the sidestep test and the shuttle run. The sidestep test is used primarily to test lateral movements (Fig. 24-8). An area 12 feet square is divided into 3-foot segments. A center line is marked at 6 feet and two other lines are marked at 3 feet to each side of center. Beginning at the center the athlete sidesteps to one side, then the other, changing direction as each line is touched. Ten seconds are allowed for the test, with 1 point scored with each line touched. A penalty of 1 point is subtracted for crossing of the feet or for not touching the line. Table 24-2 presents the raw score norms for the sidestep test.[22]

A second agility test that may be used is the shuttle run, which measures running agility.

Upper extremity agility is more difficult to assess, with reaction time being the most practical test. Several devices

Table 24-2. Raw score norms for side-step test

Performance level	College men	College women	High school girls	High school boys
Advanced	30-above	24-above	25-above	30-above
Advanced intermediate	26-29	20-23	21-24	26-29
Intermediate	16-25	14-19	14-20	15-25
Advanced beginner	12-15	10-13	10-13	11-14
Beginner	0-11	0-9	0-9	0-10

From Johnson BL and Nelson JK: Practical measurements for evaluation in physical education, Minneapolis, 1979, Burgess Publishing Co.

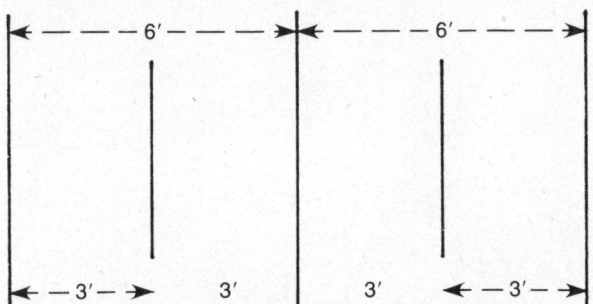

Fig. 24-8. Sidestep test diagram.

Manual muscle test grading system

Complete range of motion against resistance

6	AN	Above normal	With maximum resistance
5	N	Normal	With considerable resistance
4	G	Good	With some resistance

Completes range of motion

3	F	Fair	Against gravity
2	P	Poor	With gravity eliminated

No range of motion

1	T	Trace	Slight contraction
0	0	Zero	No contraction

Modified from Daniels L and Worthingham C: Therapeutic exercise, ed 2, Philadelphia, 1977, WB Saunders; and Kendall HO, Kendall FP, and Wadsworth GE: Muscles: Testing and function, ed 2, Baltimore, 1971, Williams & Wilkins.

can be used for testing reaction time to light stimuli. One such device is the AcuVision.* This device is designed (1) to improve an athlete's ability to concentrate on and track moving objects, (2) to enhance peripheral vision, (3) to increase speed and recognition, (4) to improve depth perception, and (5) to increase speed, time, and accuracy of response.

Muscle function. An assessment of strength, power, and endurance of major muscle groups is an important part of any preseason screening process for many reasons. Not only is there greater risk for injury if supportive muscular function is decreased, but there is also a decrease in athletic performance. Although often not practical, a precise muscular evaluation is ideal for all major muscle groups. In practice, however, it is usually necessary to concentrate on testing muscle groups most used for support in a given sport (for example, upper extremities in throwing or racquet sports and lower extremities in running or contact/collision sports).[31]

In assessing muscular strength, manual muscle testing (see accompanying box) will help show gross deficits but will be less than precise with a well-conditioned athlete.

With the healthy athlete it is difficult to apply enough resistance to measure weakness in many particular muscle groups (e.g., quadriceps). Use of a cable tensiometer[14] and isometric dynamometry will allow more accurate as-

sessment of strength. Tensiometers† can be used to measure up to 300 pounds, depending on the sensitivity needed for each test (Fig. 24-9). Dynamometers† can be used to determine grip strength (Fig. 24-10). A comparison between right and left grip should be made and any deficits noted. One must keep in mind that strength in the dominant hand may be 10% greater than that in the nondominant hand.

The most effective way to measure strength, power, and endurance is through isokinetic dynamometry. This is superior to these other methods, since it allows testing of strength and power at both slow and fast speeds and assessment of muscular endurance. Some examples of equipment available for this type of testing are MiniGym* (Fig. 24-11), Orthotron† (Fig. 24-12), Cybex† (Fig. 24-13), Biodex‡ (Fig. 24-14), KinCom§ (Fig. 24-15), and Portable Isokinetics‖ (Fig. 24-16). Reliability and accuracy of these isokinetic tests will depend on the quality of equipment used. Testing should be done at variable speeds to

*AcuVision Systems, Inc, New York, NY.

†J.A. Preston Corp., Clifton, NJ.
*MiniGym, Inc., Independence, Mo.
†Lumex, Inc., Cybex Division, Bay Shore, N.Y.
‡Biodex Corp., Center Moriches, N.Y.
§Chattecx Corp., KinCom, Chattanooga, Tenn.
‖Portable Isokinetics, Grand Rapids, Mich.

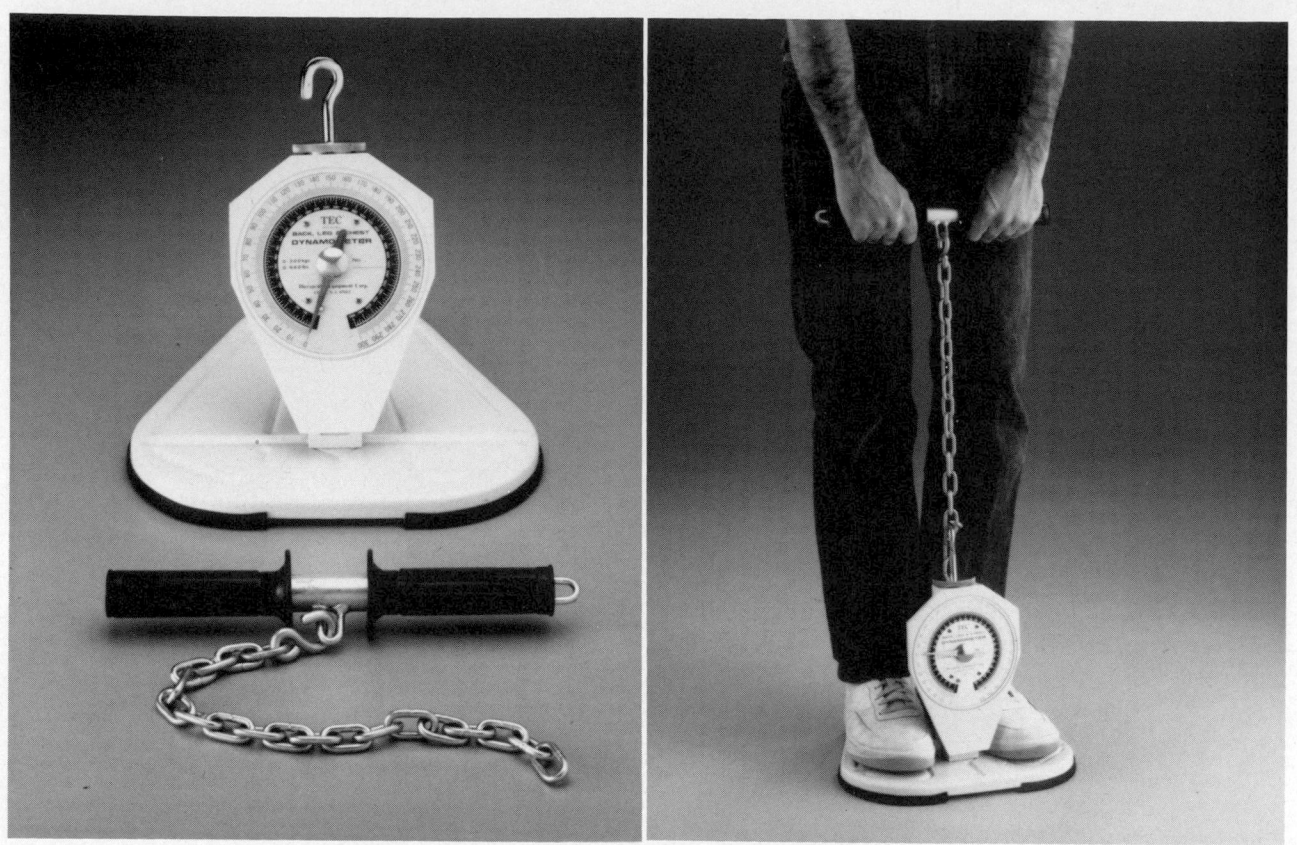

Fig. 24-9. The tensiometer. (Reprinted by permission of JA Preston Corporation, 1989.)

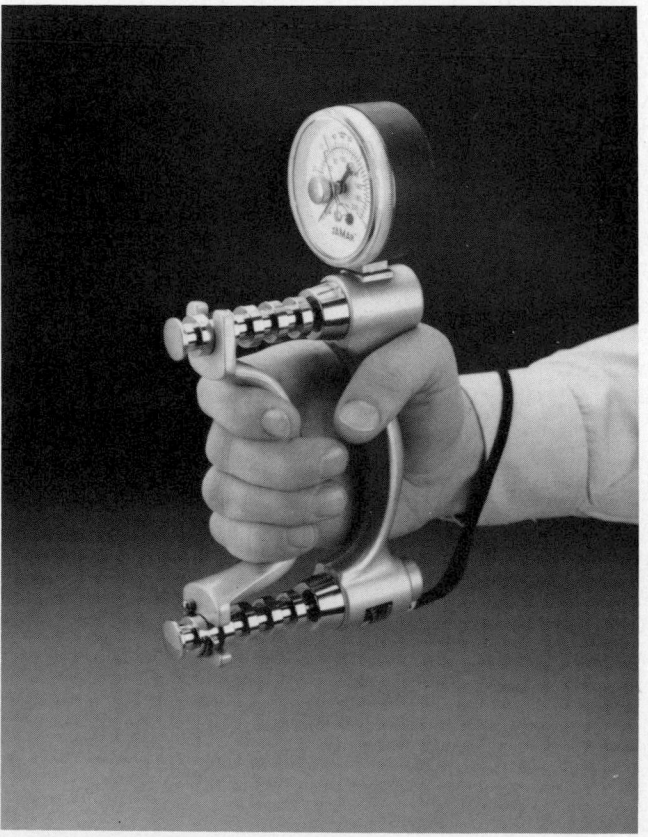

Fig. 24-10. The dynamometer. (Reprinted by permission of JA Preston Corporation, 1989.)

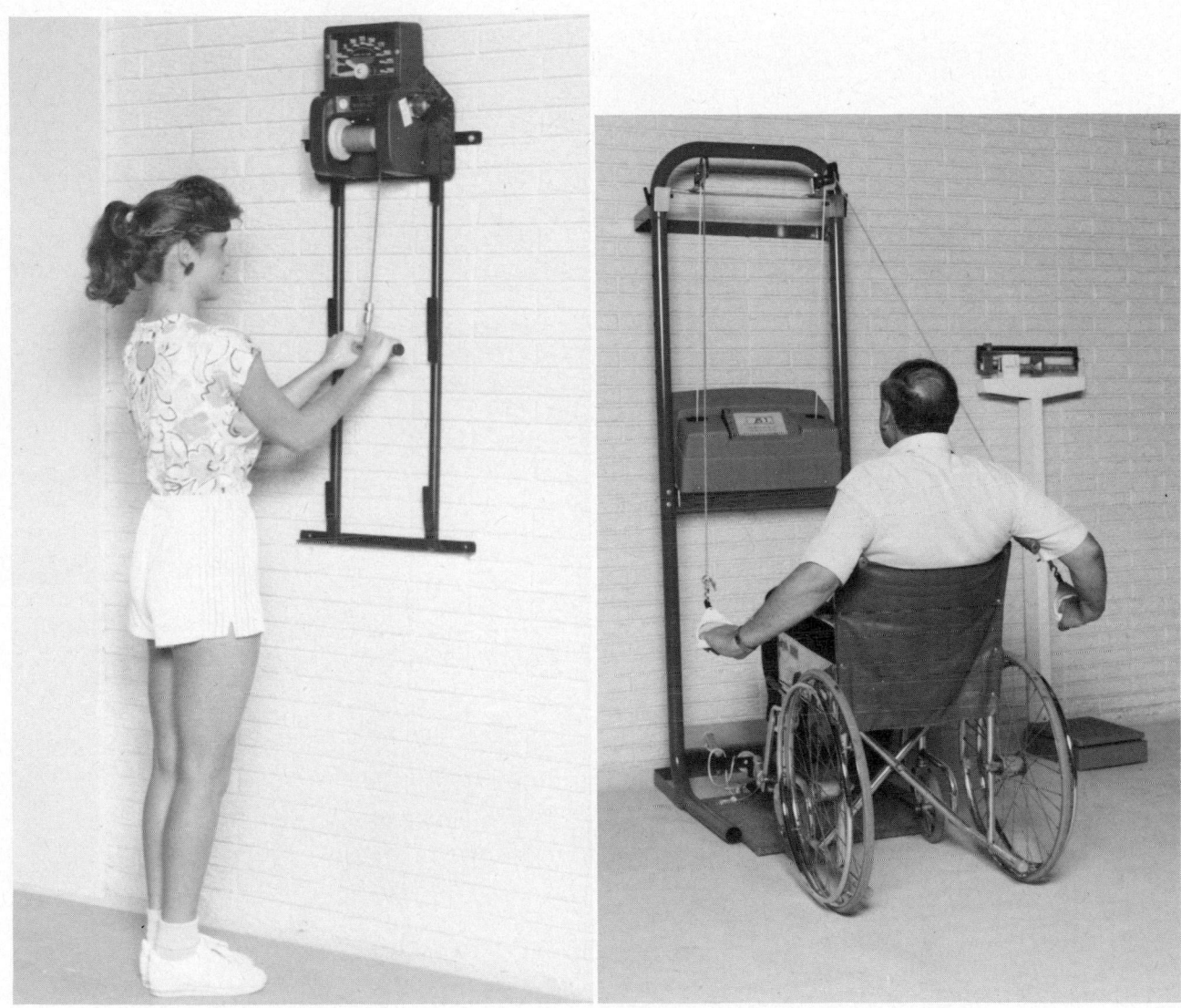

Fig. 24-11. MiniGym. (Photos courtesy of Fitness systems, Inc, Independence, Mo.)

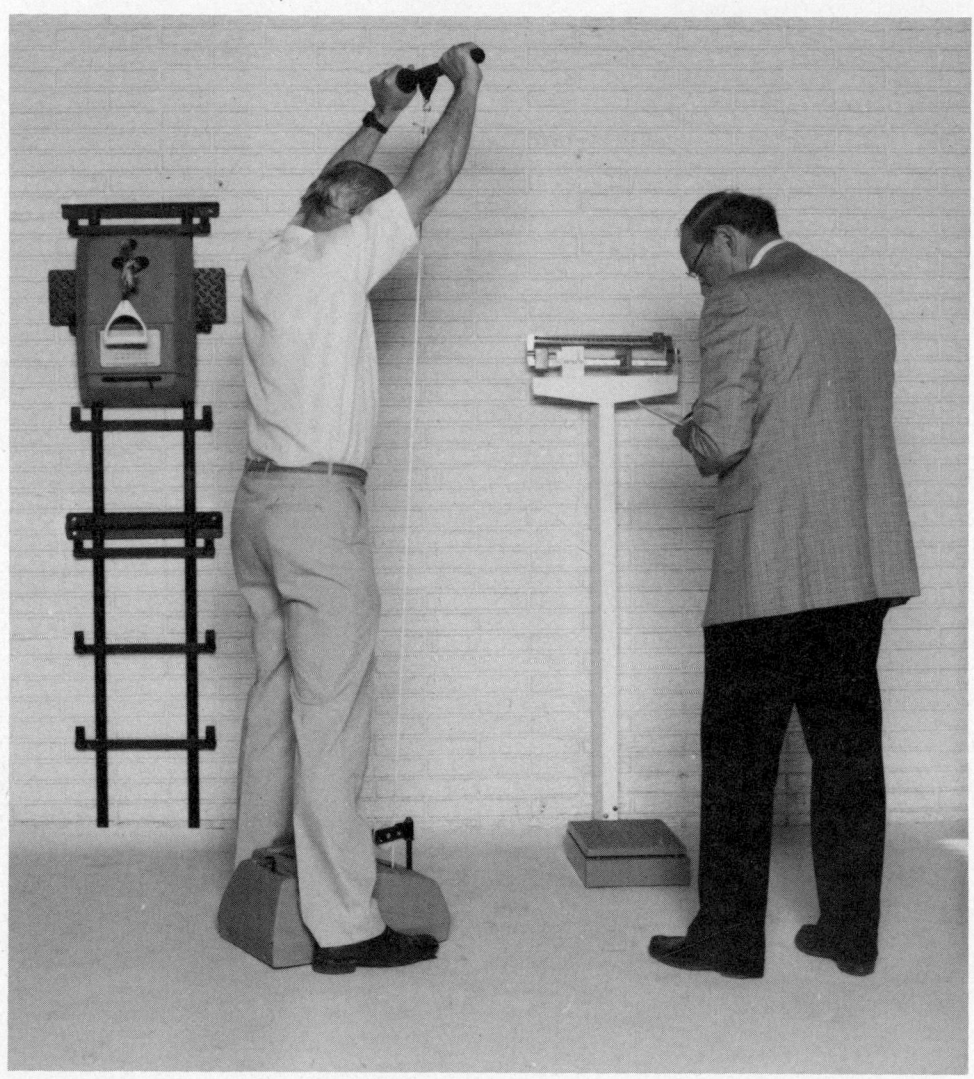

Fig. 24-11. cont'd.

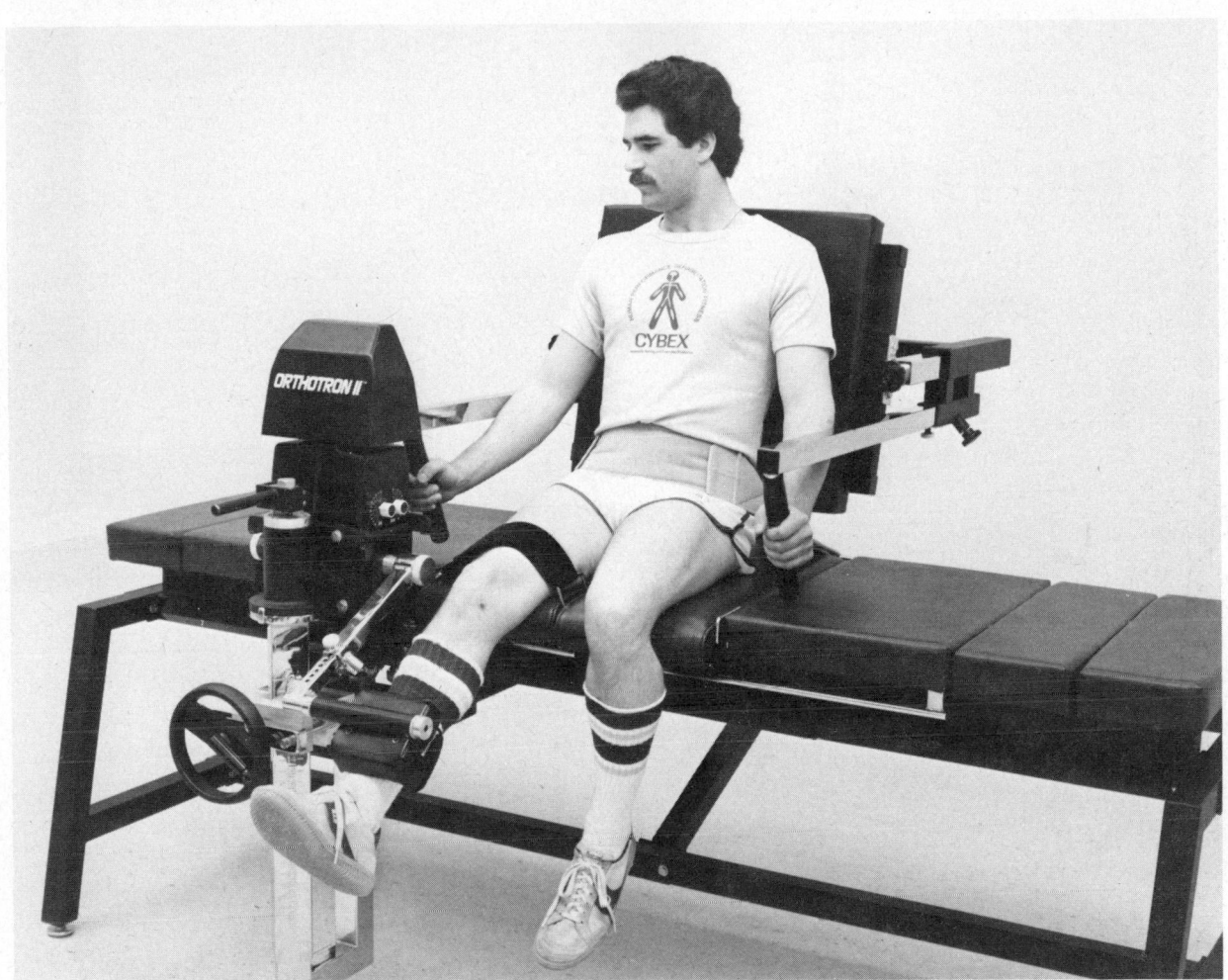

Fig. 24-12. Orthotron II strength testing for knee extensors. (Photo courtesy of Lumex, Inc., Cybex division, Ronkonkoma, NY.)

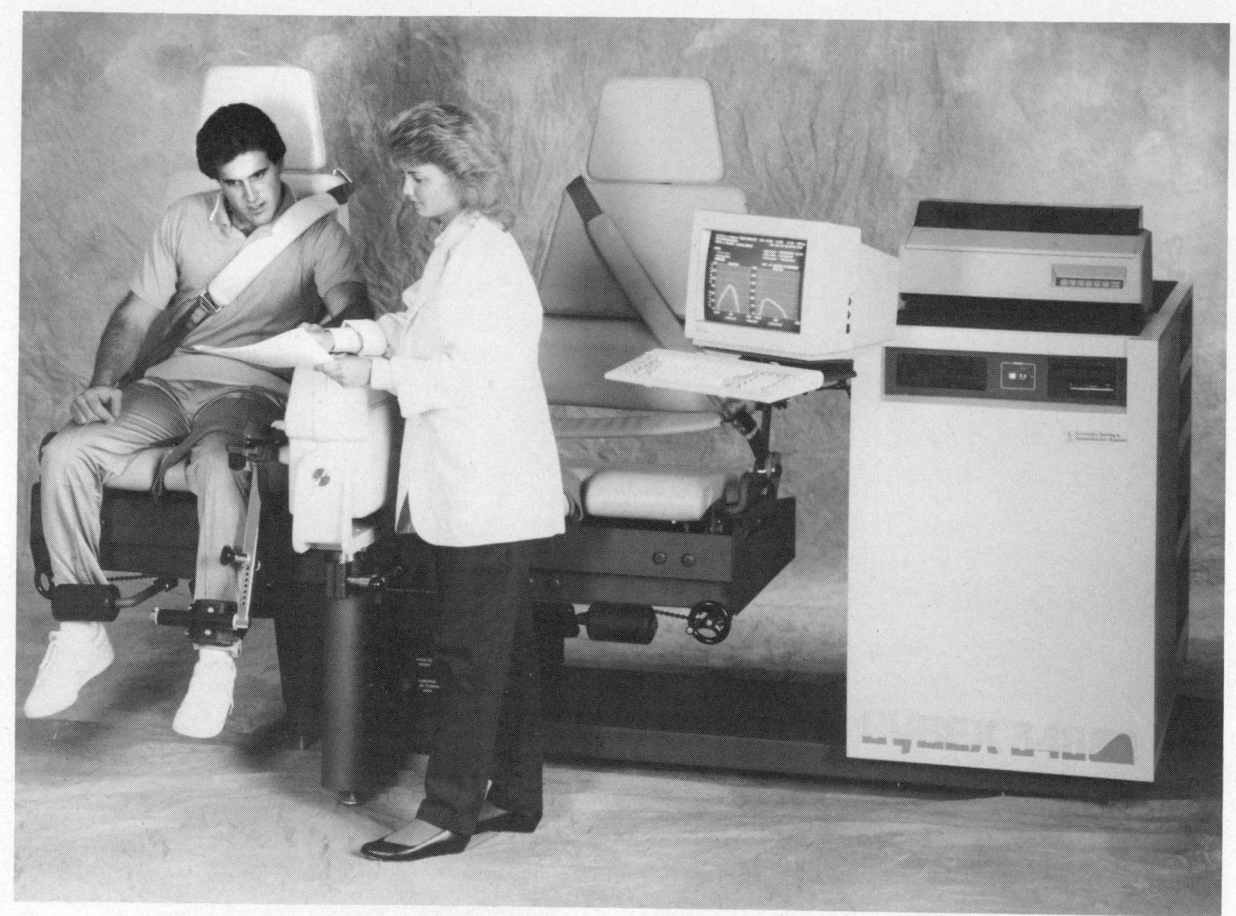

Fig. 24-13. Cybex 340. (Photo courtesy of Lumex, Inc., Cybix division, Ronkonkoma, NY.)

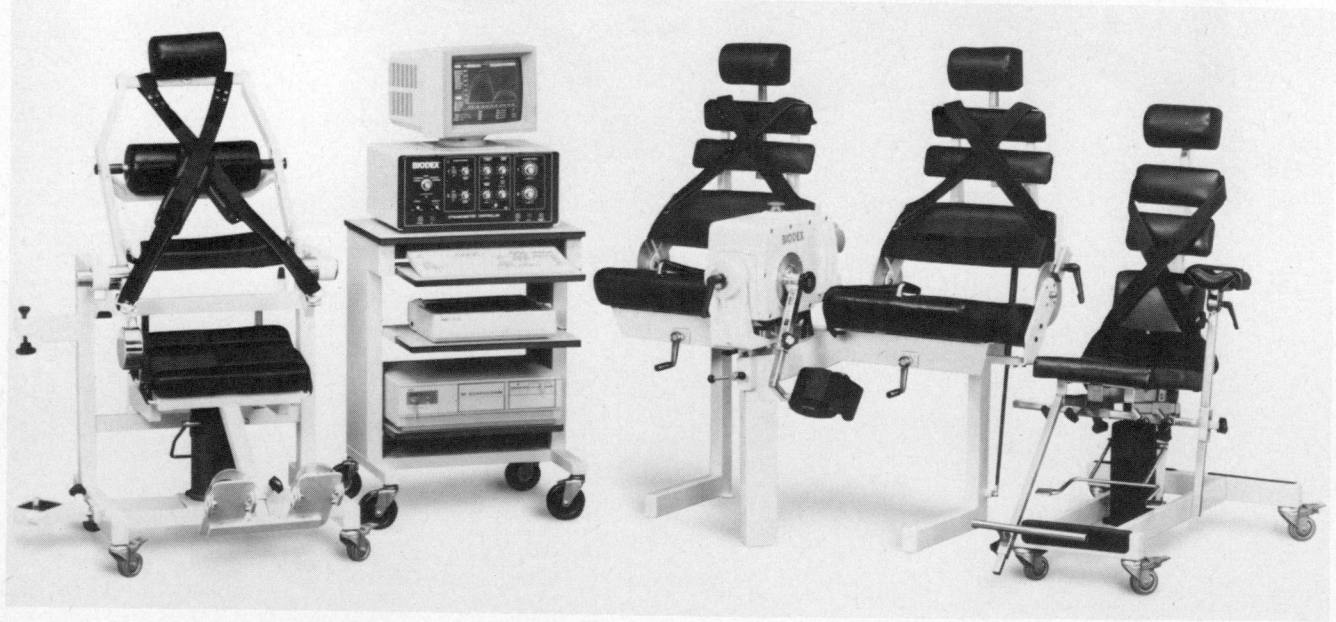

Fig. 24-14. Biodex. (Photo courtesy of Biodex Corporation, Shirley, NY.)

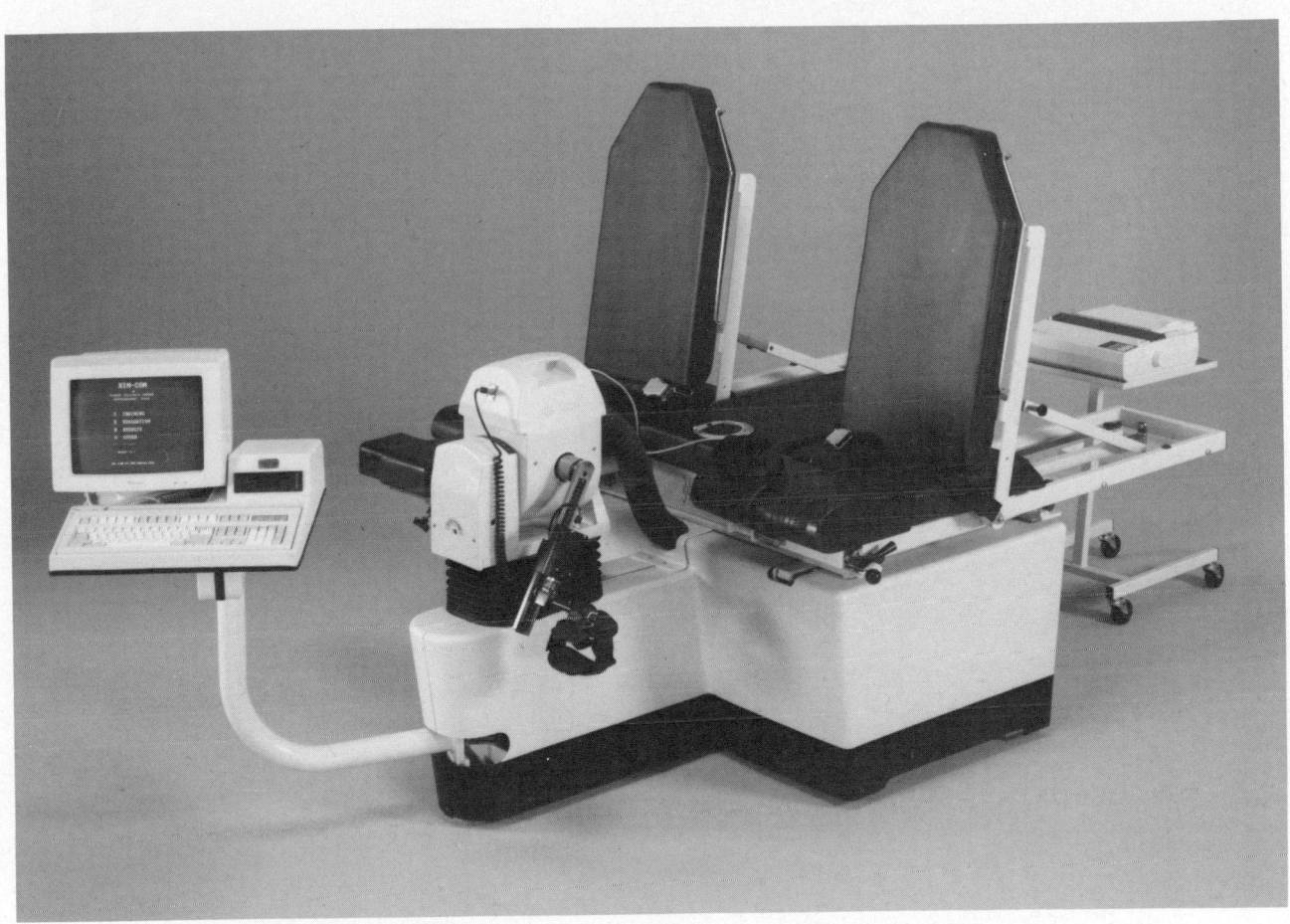

Fig. 24-15. KIN-COM500H. (Photo courtesy of Chattecx Corporation, Chattanooga, Tenn.)

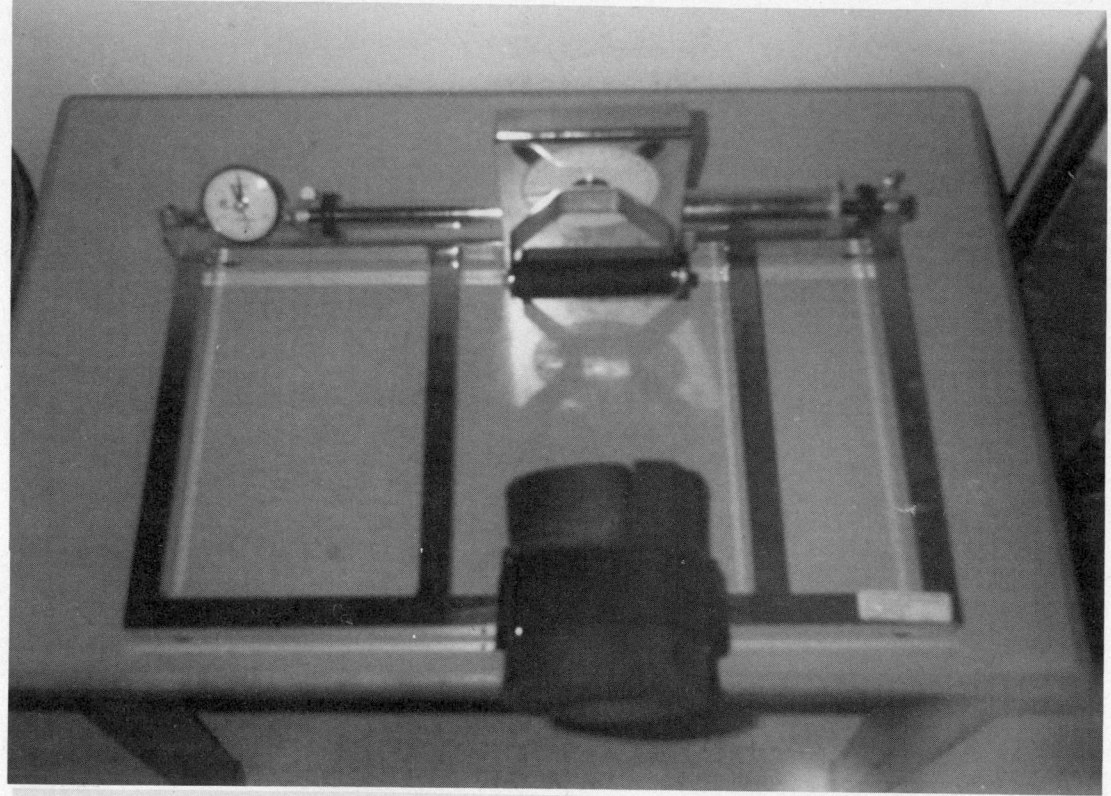

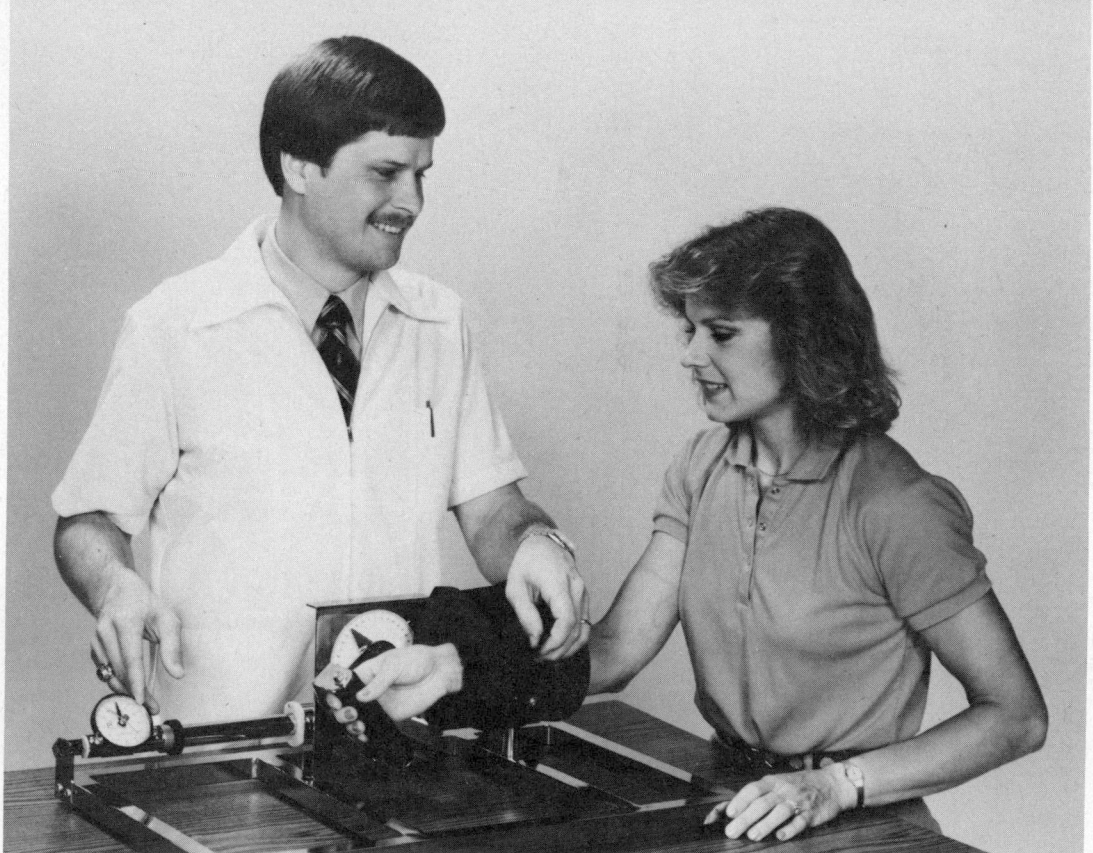

Fig. 24-16. Portable Isokinetics 3001 Wrist/Ankle Unit, which provides a full range of exercises for both the wrist and ankle. This is one of seven portable units that provide accommodating resistance exercise and isometric testing for the wrist, arm, shoulder, back/abdomen, hip, knee, and ankle. (Photo courtesy of Portable Isokinetics, Inc., Grand Rapids, Mich.)

allow for strength, power, and endurance testing. Protocols will vary according to the manufacturer's specifications.

Balance. Balance may be affected by injury as a result of deafferentation of proprioceptive joint receptors. This can enhance the possibility of reinjury even though muscle strength may be fully restored. A simple static test consists of having the athlete balance on one foot and then close the eyes (Fig. 24-17). The length of time before a lower extremity movement is required on the non-weight bearing side is recorded and compared bilaterally. Although no norms are yet described for such a static test, a discrepancy of more than 5 seconds should be further evaluated, with institution of balance training considered.

Dynamically, balance can be evaluated with a commercially available digital balance evaluator, which measures the number of seconds out of 30 seconds that an individual is out of balance. Norms are established for such data.

Neurological. The neurological evaluation is cursory in that only reflexes and dermatomal sensation are assessed. Other neurological tests, such as tests of specific muscles and specific functions (Table 24-3), are most efficiently performed at their respective stations.

Further neurological testing may be completed at the final station with the assistance of the attending physician.

Deep tendon reflexes, biceps brachii (C-5) (Fig. 24-18A), triceps brachii (C-7) (Fig. 24-18B), quadriceps femoris (L-4) (Fig. 24-18C), and triceps surac (S-1) are tested.[20] Discrepancies or absence of reaction is noted; such notes may be valuable as a data base in the event of later injury.

Clonus and Babinski reflexes are also checked in both

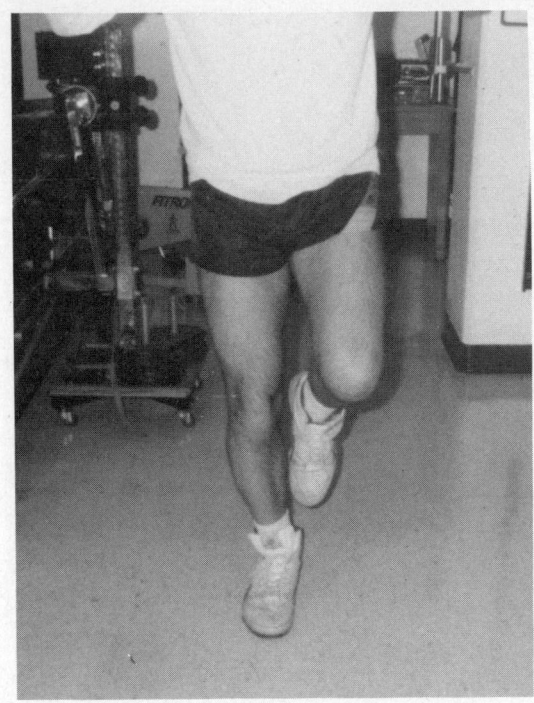

Fig. 24-17. Static test for balancing.

feet to note upper motor neuron involvement and as a data base. Once again, the athlete is specifically questioned about a history of convulsive disorders and cerebral concussion.

The neurological examination should also include a brief cranial nerve examination (Table 24-4).

Orthopaedic. Each of the orthopaedic stations is de-

Table 24-3.

Level	Motor	Reflex	Dermatome
C-1	Head/neck flexion	None	None
C-2	Head/neck flexion	None	Small area on upper mandible
C-3	Head/neck flexion	None	Ring around the collar
C-2–4	Shoulder shrug	None	
C-4	Breathing—diaphram	None	Top of shoulders
C-5	Shoulder abduction—arm and forearm	Biceps	Anterolateral
C-6	Wrist extension—forearm, thumb, index finger	Brachioradialis	Radial
C-7	Wrist flexion—finger to wrist	Triceps	Tip of middle
C-8	Finger flexion—hand and little finger	None	Ulnar border
T-1	Finger abduction and adduction—band and medial arm	None	Horizontal trunk
T-2–T-12	Breathing—bands	None	Horizontal trunk
T-5–T-12	Trunk flexion—bands	None	Horizontal trunk
L-1–L-3	Hip hiking	None	Groin
L-2–L-4	Knee extension		Groin
L-4	Diagonal front and inversion—diagonal front of thigh	Patellar	Anterior
L-5	Toe extension—2,3,4 dorsal	None	Lateral knee to toes
S-1	Foot eversion and plantar flexion—lateral thigh and leg[19,20]	Achilles	Posterior

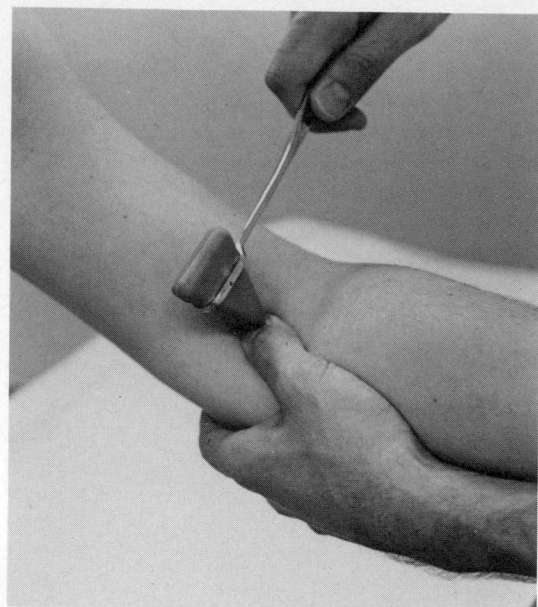

Fig. 24-18, A. Biceps reflex testing.

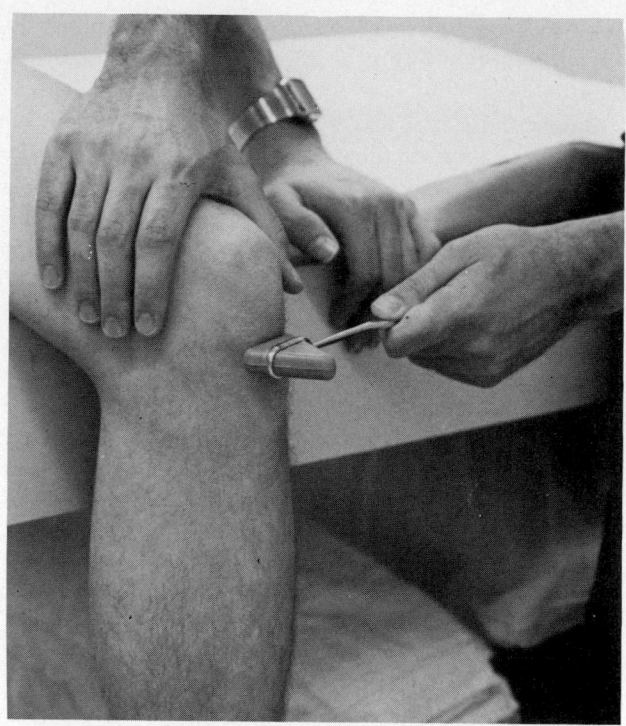

Fig. 24-18, C. Quadriceps reflex testing.

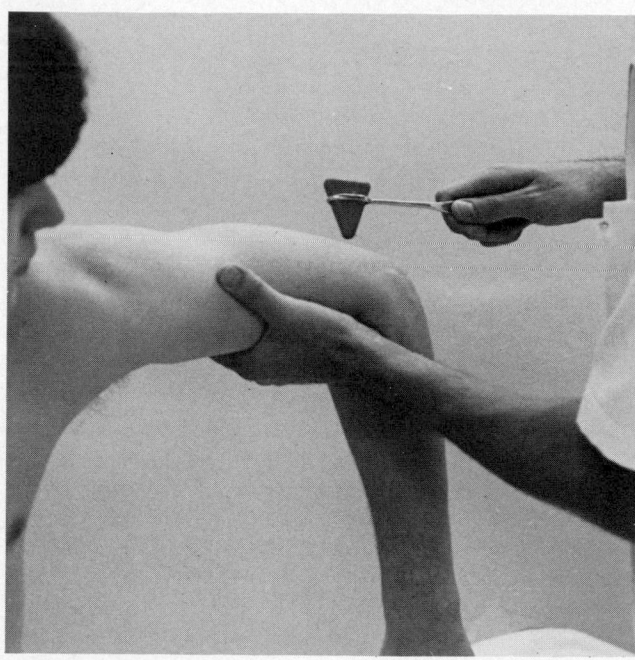

Fig. 24-18, B. Triceps reflex testing.

Table 24-4. Cranial nerves

No.	Name	Function
I	Olfactory	Can he smell?
II	Optic	Can he see (both eyes)?
III	Oculomotor	Droopy eyelids, diverted stabismus
IV	Trochlear	Move eyes up and in
V	Trigeminal	Pain on face and forehead
VI	Aducens	Internal stabismus—squinting
VII	Facial	Muscles of expression
VIII	Acoustic	Can he hear (both ears)?
IX	Glossopharyngeal	Difficulty swallowing, numb soft palate
X	Vagus	Deviated uvula, hoarseness
XI	Accessory	Torticollis (fixed twisting of the neck)
XII	Hypoglossal	Paralysis of tongue

signed to evaluate a specific body area. Evaluations will include range of motion, strength, and noncontractile structural stability, as well as any objective or subjective abnormalities or deformities noted. At each station the athlete is questioned about past injuries, present problems, and pain or discomfort with specific tests.

For each joint the evaluator first looks for scars or other visually noted deformities, such as swelling or discoloration. Range of motion is then evaluated actively (passively if motion is painful or limited) and with overpressure (Table 24-5).[1] A manual muscle test is performed for each major muscle group surrounding each joint to give a gross evaluation of contractile support (see the box on page 609). Stability of major ligaments or capsular structures is evaluated in detail to ensure noncontractile stability (see the box on p. 620). Anthropometric measurements are taken (e.g., circumference, leg length as measured from the anterior superior iliac spine to medial malleolus) when necessary. Each joint and the surrounding musculature should be palpated to determine if there are painful structures,

Table 24-5. Average ranges of joint motion

Joint	Sources 1	2	3	4	Averages	Joint	Sources 1	2	3	4	Averages
Elbow						**Hip—Cont'd**					
Flexion	150†	135	150	150	146	Rotation					
Hyperextension	0	0	0	0	0	In flexion					
						Internal rotation				45	45
Forearm						External rotation				45	45
Pronation	80	75	50	80	71	In extension					
Supination	80	85	90	80	84	Internal rotation	40	35	20	45	35
						External rotation	50	50	45	45	48
Wrist						Abduction					
Extension	60	65	90	70	71	In 90 degrees of flexion			45 to 60		
Flexion	70	70		80	73				(depending on age)		
Ulnar deviation	30	40	30	30	33						
Radial deviation	20	20	15	20	19	**Knee**					
						Flexion	120	135	145	135	134
Thumb						Hypertension			10	10	10
Abudction		55	50	70	58						
Flexion						**Ankle**					
Interphalangeal joint	80	75	90	80	81	Flexion	40	50	50	50	48
M—P	60	50	50	50	53	(plantar flexion)					
M—C				15	15						
Extension						Extension	20	15	15	20	18
Distal joint		20	10	20	17	(dorsiflexion)					
M—P		5	10	0	8						
M—C				20	20	**Hind foot (subtalar)**					
						Inversion				5	5
Fingers						Eversion				5	5
Flexion											
Distal joint	70	70	90	90	80	**Forefoot**					
Middle joint	100	100		100	100	Inversion	30	35		35	33
Proximal joint	90	90		90	90	Eversion	20	20		15	18
Extension											
Distal joint				0	0	**Toes**					
Middle joint				0	0	Great toe					
Proximal joint			45	45	45	Interphalangeal joint					
						Flexion	30			90	60
Shoulder						Extension	0			0	0
Forward flexion	150	170	130	180	158	Proximal joint					
Horizontal flexion				135	135	Flexion	30	35		45	37
Backward extension	40	30	80	60	53	Extension	50	70		70	63
Abduction	150	170	180	180	170						
Adduction	30		45	75	50	**2nd to 5th toes**					
Rotation						Flexion					
Arm at side						Distal joint	50			60	55
Internal rotation	40	60	90	80	68	Middle joint	40			35	38
External rotation	90	80	40	60	68	Proximal joint	30			40	35
Arm in abduction (90°)						Extension	40			40	40
Internal rotation				70	70						
External rotation				90	90	**Spine**					
						Cervical					
Hip						Flexion	30			45	38
Flexion	100	110	120	120	113	Extension	30			45	38
Extension	30	30	20	30	28	Lateral bending	40			45	43
Abduction	40	50	55	45	48	Rotation	30			60	45
Adduction	20	30	45	30	31	Thoracic and lumbar					
						Flexion	90			{ 80 / 4"	{ 85 / 4"
						Extension	30			20-30	30
						Lateral bending	20			35	28
						Rotation	30			45	38

Reproduced from Joint Motion, 1965, with permission of American Academy of Orthopaedic Surgeons, 430 North Michigan Avenue, Chicago, Ill.
*In degrees, unless otherwise specified.

Laxity grades	
0-5 mm	1+
5-10 mm	2+
Over 10 mm	3+

Table 24-6. Neck

Primary Tests	
Adson's	Thoracic outlet syndrome
Compression	Space-occupying lesion
Distraction	Facet joints
Quadrant (Spirlings)	Nerve or facet impingement
Spring test	Vertebral ligament lesion
Injury Tests	
Alar-odontoid test	Integrity of alar ligament
Hyperabduction	Thoracic outlet syndrome
Swallowing	Anterior cervical spine lesion
Valsalva	Cervical spine disorder
Vertebral artery test	Occlusion of vertebral artery
Wright's	Thoracic outlet syndrome

Table 24-7. Back

Primary tests	
Double leg lift	Lower abdominal strength
Long sit to supine	Innominate dysfunction
Patrick's (fabere)	Sacroiliac dysfunction
Situp (umbilical deviation)	Upper abdominal strength
Spring test	Ligament integrity
Straight leg raise	Space-occupying lesion
Chin to chest—supine	Space-occupying lesion
Injury tests	
Bowstring test	Sciatic nerve irritation
Heel slam	Irritated disk
Heel walk	Disk or L-4 nerve root lesion
Lesion	
Hoover's	Malingerer
Reverse SLR	Space-occupying lesion
Sacral push—caudal	Sacroiliac dysfunction
Sacral push—cranial	Sacroiliac dysfunction
Sciatic punch	Sciatic nerve irritation
Sacroiliac compression	Sacroiliac dysfunction
Sacroiliac distraction	Sacroiliac dysfunction
Siting flexion test	Innominate dysfunction
Sphinx	Sacral lesion
Standing flexion test	Innominate dysfunction
Toe flexion test	Malingerer
Toe walk	Disk or L-5 nerve root lesion
Well leg reverse straight-leg raise	Space-occupying lesion
Well leg straight-leg raise	Space-occupying lesion

Sources: references 8, 12, 19, and 21.

Table 24-8. TMJ

Primary tests	
Clicking	TMJ dysfunction
Deviation in range of motion	TMJ dysfunction[12,19,21]

Sources: references 12, 19, and 21.

calcium deposits, scar tissue, or other tissue abnormalities.[20,27]

The importance of bilateral comparison cannot be overemphasized. All findings are noted on the physical examination record and are in turn monitored and further evaluated at the final review station.

The following commonly used orthopaedic evaluation stations are discussed in detail: head, neck, and trunk; posture; upper extremity; lower extremity; foot and ankle; and gait.

Head, neck, and trunk. When observing the neck and trunk the examiner looks for scars, deformities, and any other abnormalities from all aspects. The athlete is then asked to perform active flexion, extension, lateral flexion to both sides, and rotation to both sides for the neck and trunk. Observation from the rear, front, and sides while these motions are performed is essential, since such observations may reveal hypomobile or hypermobile segments.[24] Palpation is performed over the spinous processes and the surrounding musculature. Any tenderness or palpable abnormalities are recorded.

Manual muscle tests for the trunk are done in flexion and extension. The extension muscle test is done with the subject lying in a prone position. The flexion tests are done in supine position with the legs extended.[23] Observation continues during these tests for muscle imbalance.

For special tests that can be used for assessing this area, refer to Tables 24-6 and 24-7.

The temporomandibular joint (TMJ) is also assessed at this station. While the TMJ is palpated bilaterally, the athlete is asked to open and close the jaw. The evaluator observes the mandible for deviation from the midline and palpates for clicking or popping. Deviation at the end of range is usually muscular in origin. Clicking or popping may be indicative of dental malocclusion or TMJ dysfunction. For TMJ special tests refer to Table 24-8.

Posture. The examination at the postural station should include both static and dynamic posture. Evaluation of dynamic posture would include a variety of movements, such as lifting, pushing or pulling an object, toe and heel walking, or backward walking. In both static and dynamic evaluations it is important to observe the overall bilateral comparison of body parts. Unilateral differences such as scars, prominences, and depressions should be noted.

Statically, the front view should afford a real or imaginary plumb line to bisect the nose, sternum, and umbilicus and to be equidistant from the knees and feet (Fig. 24-19). Rotation of the spine should be watched for, as should

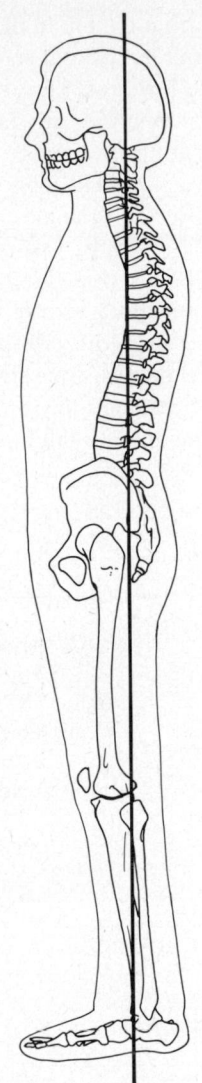

Fig. 24-19. The plumb line.

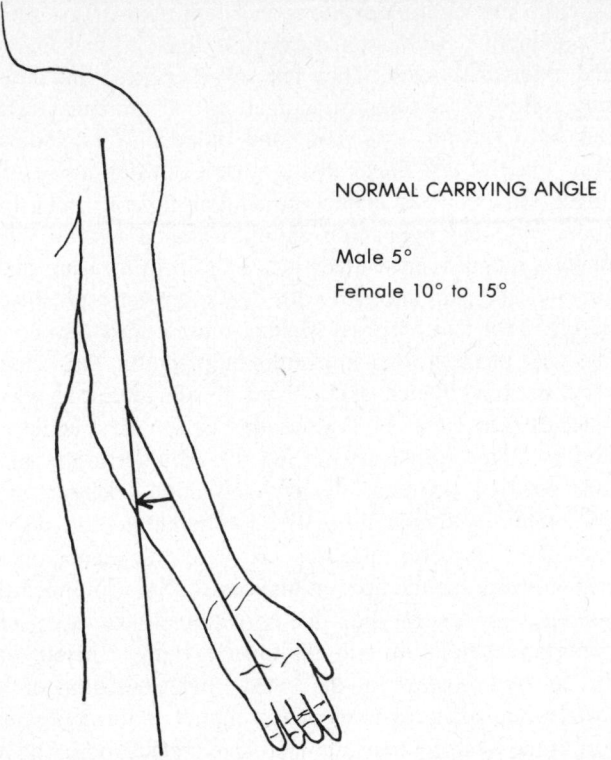

NORMAL CARRYING ANGLE

Male 5°
Female 10° to 15°

Fig. 24-20. Normal carrying angle: male, 5 degrees; female, 10 to 15 degrees.

symmetry of the shoulders, nipples, pelvis, hands, patellae, and malleoli.[3,8] The chest and rib cage are observed during a normal breathing pattern. Varus or valgus deformities in the knees, fore foot, and hindfoot; fore foot adduction or abduction; and tibial torsion should be noted if present. The back view affords easy viewing of the level of the earlobes, shoulders, iliac crests, greater trochanters, waist angles, gluteal folds, popliteal fossa and the malleoli. Scapular protrusion and any lateral spinal curves are also discernible in this position.

While viewing from the rear, the examiner should also have the athlete assume a flexed position (Adam's position). This position of flexing the trunk to a right angle allows the examiner to view the scapulae and rib cage tangenitally. Should scoliosis be present with a rib hump, the hump will appear in this position. If the deformity is functional, the hump will disappear in a non-weight-bearing position but will remain if the deformity is structural.[3,8,24]

Upper extremity. At this station the shoulders, elbows, wrists, and hands are evaluated. A bilateral examination is performed and any discrepancies are noted. Observation followed by palpation should be performed first.

At the shoulder observe the anatomical position, acromion heights, muscle mass, and inferior angles of the scapulae; palpate bone as well as soft-tissue structures including the clavicle, acromion, coracoid process, scapular spine, inferior angle of the scapulae, humeral head, and surrounding muscles and tendons; and note any trigger points or variance in muscle tone.

At the elbow observe the resting position and carrying angle (5 degrees in male subjects and 10 to 15 degrees in female subjects) (Fig. 24-20). Palpate the medial and lateral epicondyles, olecranon process, proximal radioulnar joint, common wrist extensor and flexor origins, and the ulnar nerve.

At the wrist and hand observe the resting position and palpate the radial sternoid and scaphoid (snuffbox) bones, as well as the rest of the bones in the hand.

Next, evaluate active range of motion with overpressure at the shoulder, elbow, wrist, and hand. While assessing the shoulder range, look for normal scapulohumeral rhythm. Note any crepitus, pain, or deviation from normal when assessing upper extremity ranges.

Now, perform a manual muscle test of the upper extremities. Beginning with the shoulder, test scapular protraction, retraction, elevation, and depression. Test shoulder abduction, adduction, flexion, extension, and internal and external rotation. Then test elbow flexion and extension followed by forearm supination and pronation. Then test wrist flexion, extension, and radial and ulnar deviation. Finally, test finger flexion and extension along with finger abduction and adduction. Thumb flexion, extension, abduction, and opposition should also be tested. When finger strength is measured, it is helpful to measure pinch strength and grip strength with dynamometers specifically designed for that purpose. Manual muscle tests also correlate with the neurological examination station. One should keep in mind which spinal cord levels innervate which muscles (see Table 24-3). Stability tests for the upper extremity include passively placing the shoulder in the quadrant position (extreme flexion–abduction–external rotation) while watching the axilla for humeral head protrusion. This not only assesses laxity of the glenohumeral joint toward subluxation or luxation but also mimics the apprehension test for the same conditions. Other especially important stability tests in the upper extremity include valgus and varus stress at the elbow and evaluation of the metacarpophalangeal joint of the thumb. Pain or discomfort in the stressed areas may indicate sprain, loose bodies, or other degenerative changes associated with overuse.

The ulnar collateral ligament of the metacarpophalangeal joint of the thumb is often mistreated. It is evaluated by applying an ulnar stress from the radial aspect of the joint while stabilizing the proximal phalanx.

Additional special tests for the upper extremity include those listed in Tables 24-9, 24-10, and 24-11.

Lower extremity. The lower extremity station actually covers only the area from the hip to the leg, with the ankle and foot as well as gait covered in separate stations.

Observation of the lower extremity may confirm abnormalities or reveal abnormalities missed at the posture station, such as genu varum or valgum, tibia vara, femoral anteversion or retroversion, and torsion of the tibia. Special attention is paid to the Q angle of the lower extremity[13] and to the definition of the vastus lateralis and vastus medialis obliquus muscles (Fig. 24-21). An abnormal Q angle may indicate propensity to patellofemoral problems, as may either an excessively hypertrophied vastus lateralis or an atrophied vastus medialis muscle.[13]

When the examiner palpates the lower extremity, he/she places emphasis on the anterior thigh, seeking nodules that

Table 24-10. Elbow

Primary tests	
Valgus stress	Medial collateral ligament
Varus stress	Lateral collateral ligament
Injury tests	
Compression ulna and radius	Fracture
Tennis elbow test— lateral	Lateral epicondylitis
Tennis elbow test— medial	Medial epicondylitis
Tinel's sign	Ulnar nerve tenderness

Sources: references 12, 19, 21, and 26.

Table 24-11. Wrist-hand

Primary tests	
Palpate snuffbox	Navicular fracture
Radial stress of thumb metacarpophalangeal joint	Radial collateral ligament
Ulnar stress of thumb metacarpophalangeal joint	Ulnar collateral ligament
Injury tests	
Allen's test	Radial and ulnar arterial blood supply
Axial compression	Fracture
Finkelstein's test	Stenosing tenosynovitis of abductor follicis longus and extensor follicus brevis
Flexor digitorum profundus (distal interphalangeal)	Integrity of flexor digitorum profundus
Flexor digitorum sublimus (proximal interphalangeal)	Integrity of flexor digitorum sublimus
Phalen's test	Carpal tunnel syndrome
Radial stress of joints	Radial collateral ligaments
Tinel's sign	Carpal tunnel syndrome
Ulnar stress of joints	Ulnar collateral ligaments

Sources: references 12, 19, 21, and 26.

Table 24-9. Shoulder

Primary tests	
Apley's scratch— adductor and internal rotator	Flexibility of shoulder
Apley's scratch— adductor and internal rotator	Flexibility of shoulder
Apprehension	Geniohyoid dislocation
Drop arm	Rotator cuff tear
Empty can	Supraspinatus tendon
Impingement	Impingement of supraspinatus
Yergason's	Biceps tendon dislocation
Injury tests	
Acromio-clavicular traction	Integrity of acromio-clavicular joint
Clavicular movement	Clavicular fracture or acromio-clavicular laxity
Locking	Capsule
Quadrant	Anterior capsule

Sources: references 12, 19, 21, and 26.

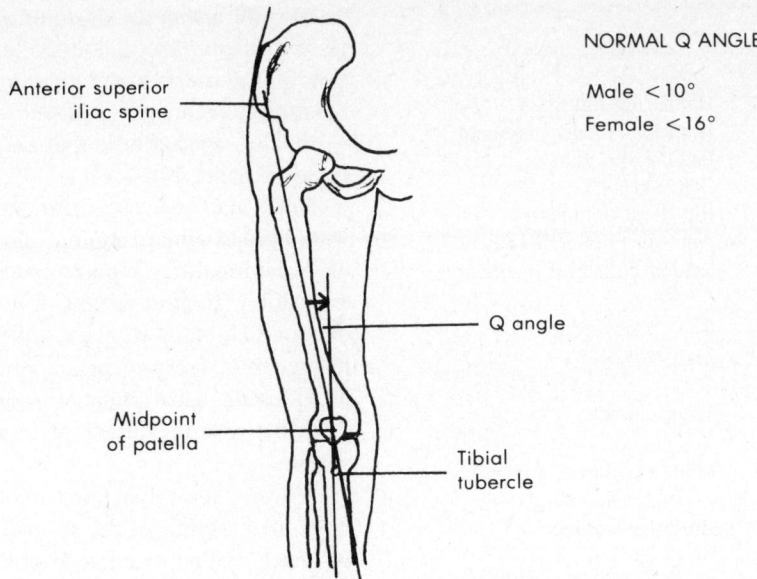

Anterior superior
iliac spine

NORMAL Q ANGLE

Male <10°

Female <16°

Q angle

Midpoint
of patella

Tibial
tubercle

Fig. 24-21. Normal Q angle: male, <10 degrees; female, <16 degrees.

may be manifestations of myositis ossificans. The medial patellar plica can be palpated along the superior medial patellar border.[2] The posteromedial tibial shaft and the anterior tibial compartment are also emphasized, since these are common sites of pain from overuse syndromes or faulty mechanics. Abnormalities found on palpation of the tibial shaft anteromedially are common; however, an isolated, painful area along the bone may be indicative of a stress fracture.

Active range of motion with overpressure should be evaluated for all motions of the hip and knee, and a special note should be made of any crepitus, pain, or abnormal movement.

Manual testing of muscles should then be done. Muscles tested at the hip include those that flex, extend, abduct, adduct, internally rotate, and externally rotate the hip. Knee motions that are evaluated for strength are flexion and extension.

Special tests that are used to assess hip and knee flexibility and stability include those listed in Tables 24-12 and 24-13.

Foot and ankle. At the foot and ankle station structures are observed in both weight-bearing and non–weight-bearing positions to check for abnormal differences in bony configuration, such as fore foot or hindfoot pronation or supination in each position, excessive splaying of the metatarsals, hypertrophy of the abductor hallucis (usually accompanying excessive hindfoot pronation), pes planus or cavus, and the like.

Emphasis is also placed on observation for fungal infections, verrucae or blisters, and callous formation, which may reveal abnormal biomechanics (i.e., at the second metatarsal head or along the medial or lateral calcaneus)

Table 24-12. Hip

Primary tests	
External rotator and abductor compression	Hip joint integrity—anterior capsule
Internal rotator and adductor compression	Hip joint integrity—posterior capsule
Leg length comparison	Real or apparent
Ober's test	Ilio-tibial band tightness
Straight leg raise	Hamstring tightness
Thomas' test	Hip flexor tightness
Trendelenburg's	Gluteus medius function
Injury tests	
Ely's test	Femoral nerve tension
Fabere	Joint capsule
Ilio-tibial friction test	Ilio-tibial friction syndrome

Sources: references 12, 19, 21, and 26.

and the position of the navicular tuberosity in relation to the Feiss line. The Feiss line is also observed in the weight-bearing and non–weight-bearing states (Fig. 24-22). This is discerned by drawing an imaginary line from the first metatarsal phalangeal joint to the medial malleolus. Ideally, the navicular tuberosity should be palpable along this line or very near by, both with and without weight bearing. Dropping of this bony landmark with weight bearing below the line leads to suspicion of flexible pes planus.

Stability of the major capsular ligaments is tested to assess their integrity. Palpable ligaments include the anterior inferior tibiofibular, deltoid, anterior talofibular, and calcaneofibular ligaments[29]; nonpalpable ligaments are the posterior tibiofibular and talofibular ligaments. In cases of re-

Table 24-13. Knee

Primary tests	
90-90 degree	Hamstring tightness
Anterior drawer	Anterior cruciate ligament
Apprehension	Patellar dislocation
Bounce home	Effusion
Ilio-tibial tightness	Ilio-tibial tightness
Lachman's	Anterior cruciate ligament
Lateral stress—20 degrees flexion	Lateral collateral ligament
Leg length comparison	Real or apparent
McMurray—valgus/external rotation	Meniscus tear
McMurray—varus/internal rotation	Meniscus tear
Medial stress—20 degrees flexion	Medial collateral ligament
Patellar grinding Roughness	Articular surface
Posterior sag	Posterior cruciate ligament
Screw-home motion	Intraarticular blockage
Squat	Meniscus injury

Injury tests

Apley—compression	Meniscus tear
Apley—distraction	Ligament integrity
Balance	Proprioception
Duck walk	Meniscus injury
Ilio-tibial friction	Ilio-tibial friction syndrome
Lateral stress—0 degrees flexion	Lateral stabilizers
Losse Instability	Anterolateral
Medial stress—0 degrees flexion	Medial stabilizers
Patella bollotment	Effusion
Pivot shift Instability	Anteromedial
Resisted quadriceps set	Patello-femoral pain syndrome
Slocum's rotary—external rotation	Anteromedial stability
Slocum's rotary—internal rotation	Anterolateral stability
Stutter	Plica[12,19,21,26]

Sources: references 12, 19, 21, and 26.

peated sprains calcifications of these structures may also be palpable.

Range of motion is evaluated, with care to evaluate active dorsiflexion of the ankles with both the knees flexed at 90 degrees and fully extended to eliminate the influence of the gastrocnemius muscle and to isolate the soleus, respectively. Range of motion once again should be measured both actively and passively with overpressure while carefully noting any complaints of pain or limitations during testing.

Manual testing of muscles is now performed. Whereas testing plantar flexion, dorsiflexion, inversion, and eversion is important, equal attention should be given to combination movements.

Finally, special tests that are done at the ankle are indicated in Table 24-14.

Gait. Gait is ideally evaluated both while the athlete is walking and while running, since the latter tends to magnify abnormalities (approximately three times). Although evaluation is most practical when the client runs on a treadmill, running in place will suffice if this equipment is unavailable. For any gait appraisal, however, a treadmill provides the ideal situation, since it allows constant distance between the athlete and examiner for close-up observation.

Whereas total dynamics are scanned in the gait station, from the carrying of the shoulders to pelvic flow, the area of concentration extends from the hips to the ground. The body's center of gravity lies approximately 2 inches anterior to the second sacral vertebra. In a normal gait pattern the center of gravity moves no more than 2 inches in a vertical direction. The pelvis and trunk will shift approximately 1 inch to the side bearing weight. The gait cycle should be analyzed in all phases: heel strike, footflat, midstance, push-off, acceleration, midswing, and deceleration. While observing these the examiner should especially notice rotational movements in the femurs, patellae, and tibiae. Normally, the extremities internally rotate from heel strike to midstance and externally rotate from midstance to push-off. Attention is also placed on the fore foot and hindfoot for abnormal pronation or supination. Whereas slight hindfoot pronation is normal and necessary between heel strike and midstance to absorb shock, this position should display supination from midstance to toe-off, affording a rigid lever for propulsion.

Abnormal wear of the shoes used in athletic activity can point out a gait abnormality. If possible, the shoes should be looked at during a gait evaluation. Since a runner's feet contact the ground 800 to 2,000 times per mile with a force three to eight times his/her body weight, a minor anatomical and biomechanical abnormality in walking may be very significant in running. It must also be remembered that since the foot and leg act in a closed kinetic chain, problems may be transmitted to the knee, hip, or lower back.*

Final review. This is the final stage of the preseason athletic screening. At this station all findings are reviewed and problem areas are identified. The final examiner then makes appropriate recommendations based on findings at the various stations. These recommendations also take into consideration the athlete's chosen sport and how any problems discovered in this evaluation relate to participation in

*See references 6, 7, 9, 11, 28, and 33.

NORMAL FEISS' LINE

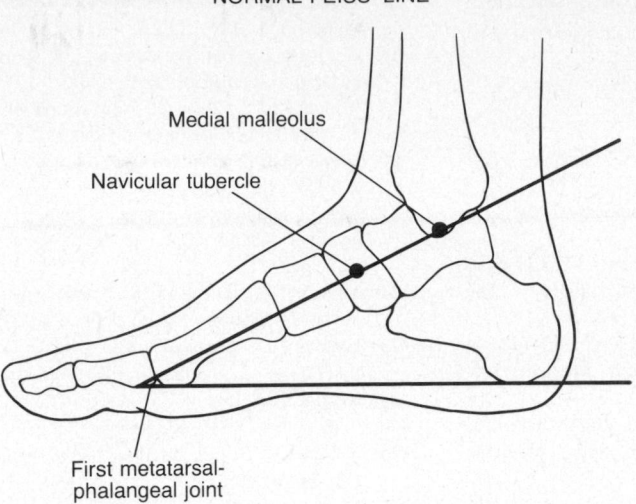

Medial malleolus

Navicular tubercle

First metatarsal-
phalangeal joint

A SECOND-DEGREE PRONATED FOOT

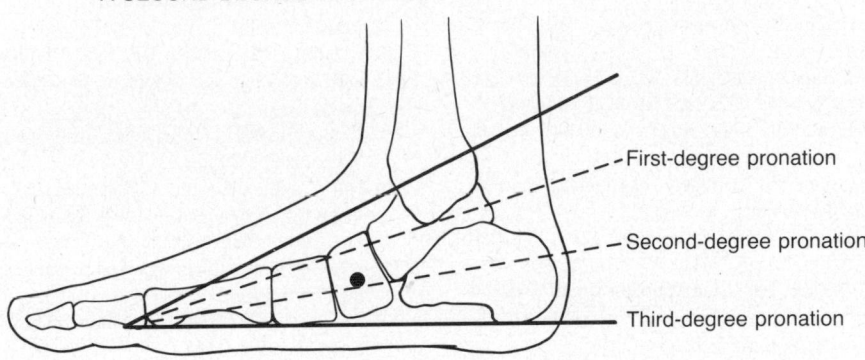

First-degree pronation

Second-degree pronation

Third-degree pronation

Fig. 24-22. Feiss' line.

Table 24-14. Ankle

Primary tests	
Anterior drawer	Anterior talofibular ligament
Balance	Proprioception
Lateral stability	Calcaneofibular ligament
Medial stability	Deltoid ligament
Injury tests	
Side to side	Anteroinferior tibiofibular
Thompson's test	Achilles continuity
Ankle dorsiflexion test—	Gastrocnemius tightness
knee 0 degree	
Ankle dorsiflexion test—	Soleus tightness[12,17,19,21,26]
knee 90 degrees	

Sources: references 12, 17, 19, 21, and 26.

the sport. Final recommendations and decisions are left up to the attending physician to determine.

Special equipment recommendations may also be made. These include protective harnessing, equipment modification, collision padding, specific shoe types, or special shoe inserts. External support such as taping, wrapping, or bracing of specific joints may also be recommended to fully clear an athlete for activity. In the event that restrictions are placed, it is essential to explain to all concerned (athlete, coaches, administrative personnel, parents) why these measures are taken as well as to emphasize options for the return to full activity.[30]

SUMMARY

A station-by-station method of preparticipation physical evaluation has been presented. The specifics of this particular format may or may not meet the needs or equipment allotments of all practitioners. Each individual involved in preseason screening will find it necessary to examine his/her own skills and expertise, take what is helpful, and leave the rest behind. However, the goal is to detect any problem that may threaten the life or quality of life of each athlete regardless of the level. Whereas an ideal format may be impossible at present, a more thorough musculoskeletal evaluation may complement any other current evaluation the athlete receives. As situations change and skills improve, every screening program should improve and thus the prophylactic quality increases. However, we can feel sure that if no thorough preparticipation screening is performed, an important chance to prevent injuries will have been neglected.[4,15]

REFERENCES

1. Joint motion—Method of measuring and recording, Chicago, 1965, American Academy of Orthopaedic Surgeons.
2. Anderson TL, et al: The year book of sports medicine 1981, Chicago, 1981, Year Book Medical Publishers, Inc.
3. Arnheim DD, Auxter D, and Crowe WC: Principles and methods of adapted physical education and recreation, ed 3, St Louis, 1977, The CV Mosby Co.
4. Beranek P and Eggart JS: Pre-participation physical evaluation at University of Wisconsin–La Crosse, APTA, Sports Medicine Section Newletter 2:1, 1976.
5. Blackburn TA, editor: Guidelines for pre-season athletic participation evaluation, Washington, DC, 1979, APTA, Sports Medicine Section.
6. Blake RL, Ross AS, and Volmassy RL: Biomechanic gait evaluation, Podiatric Sports Med 71:6, 1981.
7. Brody D: Running injuries, Clin Symp 32:4, 1980.
8. Cailliet R: Scoliosis: Diagnosis and management, Philadelphia, 1975, FA Davis Co.
9. Cailliet R: Foot and ankle pain, Philadelphia, 1976, FA Davis Co.
10. Committee on the Medical Aspects of Sports: Medical evaluation of the athlete: A guide, Monroe, Wis, 1979, American Medical Association.
11. D'Ambrosia RD: Prevention and treatment of running injuries, Thorofare, NJ, 1982, Charles B Slack, Inc.
12. Daniels L and Worthingham C: Therapeutic exercise, ed 2, Philadelphia, 1977, WB Saunders Co.
13. Davies GJ: Examining the knee, Physician Sportsmed 6:4, 1978.
14. DeVries HA: Physiology of exercise for physical education and athletics, Dubuque, Iowa, 1968, William C Brown Group.
15. Eggart JS: Causes of athletic injuries in the intercollegiate athletic program at the University of Wisconsin–La Crosse, unpublished graduate research paper, Winona, Minn, 1978, Winona State University.
16. Fox EL and Mathews DK: Interval training: Conditioning for sports and general fitness, London, 1974, WB Saunders Co.
17. Giannestras NJ: Foot disorders: Medical and surgical management, Philadelphia, 1973, Lea & Febiger.
18. Goldberg B, et al: Pre-participating sports assessment: An objective evaluation, Pediatrics 66:5, 1980.
19. Hoppenfeld S: Physical examination of the spine and extremities, New York, 1976, Appleton-Century-Crofts.
20. Hoppenfeld S: Orthopedic neurology, Philadelphia, 1977, JB Lippincott Co.
21. Irvin R and Roy S: Sports medicine: Prevention, evaluation, management and rehabilitation, Englewood Cliffs, NJ, 1983, Prentice-Hall Inc.
22. Johnson BL and Nelson JK: Practical measurements for evaluation in physical education, Minneapolis, 1979, Burgess Publishing Co.
23. Kendall HO, Kendall FP, and Wadsworth GE: Muscles: Testing and function, ed 2, Baltimore, 1971, Williams & Wilkins Co.
24. Kendall HO, Kendall FP, and Boynton DA: Posture and pain, Huntington, NY, 1977, RE Krieger Publishing Co, Inc.
25. Knight KL: Testing anterior cruciate ligaments, Physician Sportsmed 8:5, 1980.
26. Magee DJ: Orthopedic physical assessment, Philadelphia, 1987, WB Saunders Co.
27. Nicholas JA: Determining fitness for participation in sports, J Muscle Bone 1:2, 1981.
28. O'Sullivan SB, Cullen KE, and Schmitz TJ: Physical rehabilitation and evaluation and treatment procedures, Philadelphia, 1981, FA Davis Co.
29. Ramamutti CP: Orthopedics in primary care, Baltimore, 1981, Williams & Wilkins.
30. Ritter MA and Gosling C: The knee: A guide to the examination and diagnosis of ligament injuries, Springfield, Ill, 1979, Charles C Thomas, Publisher.
31. Ryan AJ and Allman FL: Sports medicine, New York, 1974, Academic Press, Inc.
32. Smilkstein G: Health evaluation of high school athletes, Physician Sportsmed 9:8, 1981.
33. Subotnick SI: Cures for common running injuries, Mountain View, Calif, 1979, World Publications, Inc.
34. Wilmore JH: Athletic training and physical fitness, Boston, 1978, Allyn & Bacon, Inc.

Chapter 25

MUSCULOSKELETAL INJURIES OF YOUNG ATHLETES: THE NEW TRENDS

Michael Zito

Athletes are participating in competitive sports at younger ages and in greater numbers than ever before.[19,44,80] Shaffer[80] has stated that today more than 20 million youngsters between the ages of 8 and 16 years are in nonschool, community-sponsored athletic programs and that more than 6 million are involved in a wide variety of high school sports. Whereas demands on maturing musculoskeletal tissues have caused concerns about subsequent tissue injury in the past, increased participation and heightened competitive spirits have now resulted in raising more than concerns. Musculoskeletal injuries to young athletes are now common and should be anticipated.

Over the last several decades the popularity of certain sports has affected the number and nature of the injuries sustained. This was most evident in little-league baseball during the 1960s when little-leaguer's elbow was prevalent and attention was focused on its management. Injury profiles changed in the 1970s as distribution of the participants was altered and the involvement of female athletes increased. Blum[13] reported, for example, that participation in high school sports rose 19% for boys and 700% for girls. Moreover, in gymnastics new standards of excellence attracted impressionable youngsters. Caine and Linder[19] reported a 461% increase in women's participation in gymnastics between 1974 and 1980, and it was significant that the gymnasts were younger and more susceptible to injury than were the postpubescent gymnasts of a decade earlier.

Later in the 1970s soccer rapidly increased in popularity and was considered by many experts to be safe, as well as health promoting and relatively free of the injuries associated with other more risky sports (Fig. 25-1). Soccer participation had increased by the 1980s, as had levels of competition, and any association with risk-free activity was quickly dispelled.

The 1980s have become an era of long-distance running. Training distances can vary, but running 60 to 70 miles a week in preparation for a marathon has become common, and a growing number of pubescent children are

My sincere appreciation to the following individuals for their assistance during this project: Joan Brady Levine and Donna Studdiford for drawing the figures; *Willimantic Chronical* photographer Harold Hanka, who contributed photographs; Pamela Roberts for her collegial support; and my wife Susan for her editorial suggestions. Thank you all.

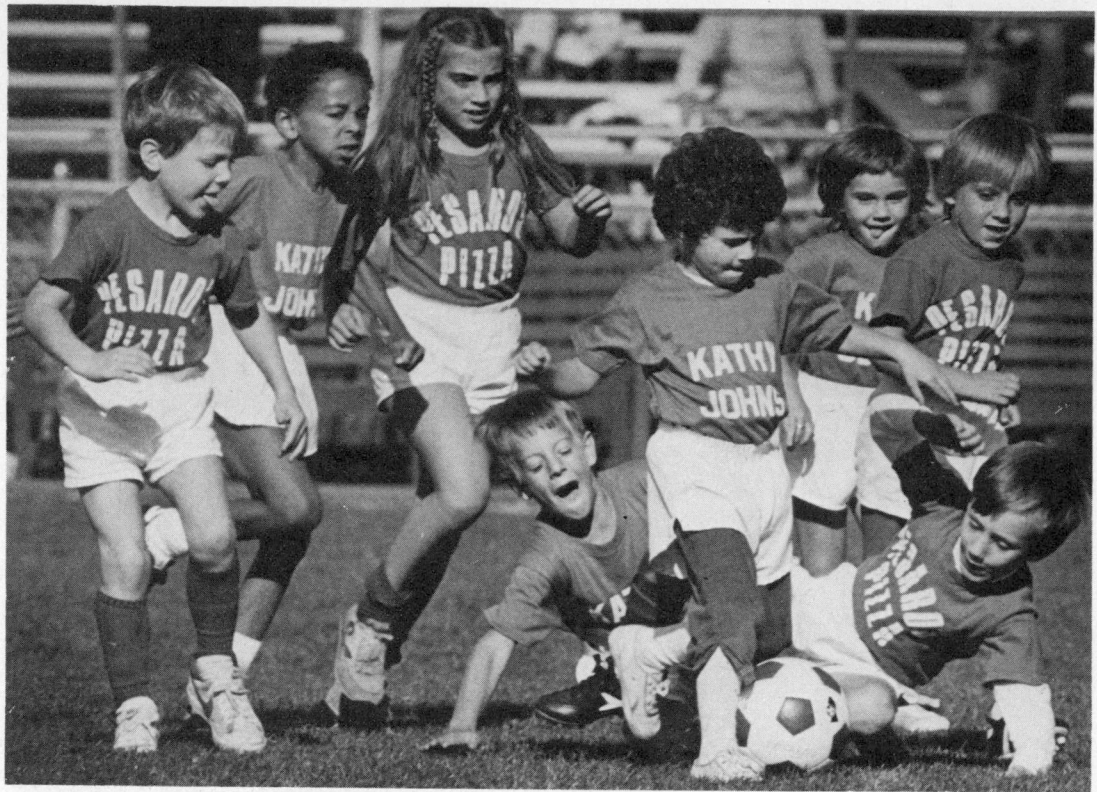

Fig. 25-1. Soccer is a sport gaining popularity with children and adolescents in the USA.

among those participants vying for the spoils.[2,19,48] Proliferation of youth sports over the last few decades has perpetuated a certainty of musculoskeletal injury, and the trend continues.[4,95]

This chapter provides an update of the status of the young athlete, with suggestions for the management of musculoskeletal injuries. Questions to be answered follow:

1. How are adolescent athletes unique, and what are their musculoskeletal risks of today?
2. What are the sports contributing to musculoskeletal injuries in the young athlete?
3. What factors contribute to increased injuries in this population?
4. What can be done to lessen the risks to musculoskeletal tissues and provide appropriate care?

STRUCTURAL CONDITIONS

The young athlete is musculoskeletally unique. Structural characteristics unique to young athletes predispose them to musculoskeletal injury, some of which have serious consequences.

Structurally the musculoskeletal system of the young athlete is not equivalent to its adult counterpart.[19,42] Differences range from structural anomalies (a more prevalent source of musculoskeletal injuries in younger athletes[22]) to a normal but susceptible immature structure. The differ-

ences greatly influence the likelihood, nature, and severity of musculoskeletal injuries unique to the young athlete. Important examples of those injuries for which the growing child has demonstrated a propensity are joint surface conditions, apophyseal disruptions, epiphyseal plate disturbances, and stress fractures.

Joint surface conditions

Articular cartilage is structured to resist repetitive loads and deformation[38]; these loads become excessive with athletic competition. When physical loading becomes prolonged or excessive, the normal growth is disturbed[19] and chondrocytes are destroyed.[38] Moreover, the joint surfaces in children are known to be less resistant to repetitive stress than those in adults.[19,22] Hettinga[38] has also suggested that fracture in adults is a shock-absorbing mechanism that spares the articular cartilage injury. Consequently, the bones of children are less brittle than bones in adults, and they transmit forces to articular surfaces.[38] Summarily, it follows that lesions of the joint surfaces in young athletes are common.

The joint surfaces of the little-leaguer's elbow clearly demonstrate the ill effects of excessive repeated compression. During the acceleration phase of pitching, compressive forces on the lateral aspect of the elbow occur between the capitulum and radial head.[36] Lack of rest, too many innings pitched, and accentuated stress from attempts to throw curveballs[22] contribute to the excessive compression and to destruction of the joint's articular surfaces. The condition, osteochondritis dissecans, was early evidence that in little-leaguer's elbow immature joint surfaces are susceptible to injury, and similar problems have since manifested in the more popular sports of today. For example, in female gymnasts the upper extremity is converted into a weight-bearing limb and osteochondritis has been found in the elbows of these athletes.[83] Excessive repetitions and technique advances have been cited as possible causative factors.[73]

Knees are another body area known to be susceptible to breakdown of articular cartilage. Chondromalacia, a softening of the patellar articular cartilage, is the most prevalent knee complaint seen in adolescents.[71] Thinner cortices and smaller, more delicate trabeculae in knees of females, as well as reduced muscle mass and increased mobility, differentiate the sexes.[65] Sports popular among young female athletes, such as soccer and running, are therefore likely to precipitate the condition (Fig. 25-2). Koenig's disease, a roughening of the articular surfaces of the femoral condyles, also exemplifies the susceptibility of joint surfaces to repetitive trauma.

Osteochondritic lesions of the foot have been reported in the talus, navicular, and cuneiform bones.[97] Long-distance running, with its increasing popularity among youth, is therefore a concern because of the severe strain placed on articular cartilage and the increased potential for injury and disturbed growth effects.[18]

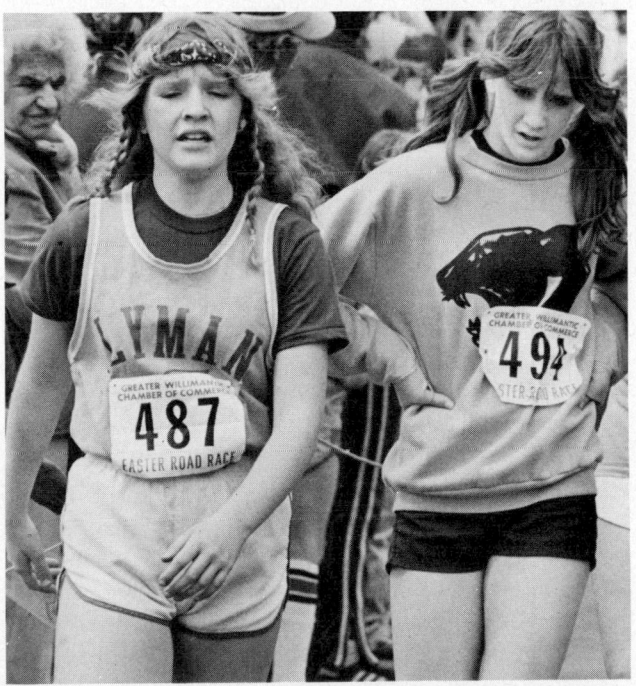

Fig. 25-2. The popularity of running is increasing in American women.

Apophyseal disruptions

The apophysis, or tendon insertion, is another important area predisposed to breakdown in young athletes. Apophyseal growth centers present as protuberances, such as tubercles and eminences, that are growth areas (although not considered to contribute much to bone length) and, as such, are considered as areas of weakness.[96] Skeletal growth at the apophysis occurs through the process of endochondral ossification in much the same manner as epiphyseal plates grow.[72,96] However, the apophysis receives its stimulus from muscular attachments that exert tensile forces and is therefore often referred to as *traction epiphysis*.[60,72,98]

Muscle forces imparted to immature apophyseal centers during athletic competition can result in tissue breakdown in two primary ways. First, the apophyses can partially or completely separate from the bone.[56,60,96] Separations or avulsions commonly occur at muscular attachments on the pelvis and femur.[88,96] Weight lifting and contact sports are most likely to produce injuries of this nature.[88] Wilkins[95] reported that hamstring tears occur in adults when the knee is extended while the hip is flexed; but in the skeletally immature ischial apophysis of the young athlete, an avulsion of the apophysis may result. Similarly, avulsions of the medial epicondyle occur with or without dislocation of the immature elbow. Here, a valgus strain or rotational injury that usually would sprain a matured elbow has a more severe consequence.[60]

The second way in which apophysis breakdown occurs is through overuse. Excessive physical loading applied over an extended period of time can result in a summation of acute structural changes from which the body is temporarily unable to recover.[18] The immature apophyseal attachment, instead of avulsing, develops microtears of the tendon and associated hemorrhage.[96] Some sites commonly having such injuries are at the tibial tubercle (Osgood-Schlatter disease),[6] the calcaneus (Sever's disease), and the inferior pole of the patella (Sinding-Larsen-Johansson disease).[96] Osgood-Schlatter disease, for example, is a tibial tubercle apophysitis, a condition that is unique to knees of adolescents.[6] Wong and Gregg[97] report that 10% of athletes between the ages of 10 and 15 years will have Osgood-Schlatter disease. In addition, Antich and Lombardo[9] report that males are affected more often than females and that unilateral involvement occurs more often than bilateral. Moreover, athletic activities seem to precipitate the condition, with basketball having the highest incidence (24%)[96] (Fig. 25-3). Information that describes the nature and trends of these injuries should be useful in determining preventive measures as well as offering management considerations after injury.

Epiphyseal plate disturbances

Perhaps more than any other site, the epiphyseal growth plate or physis has been implicated as an area of potential

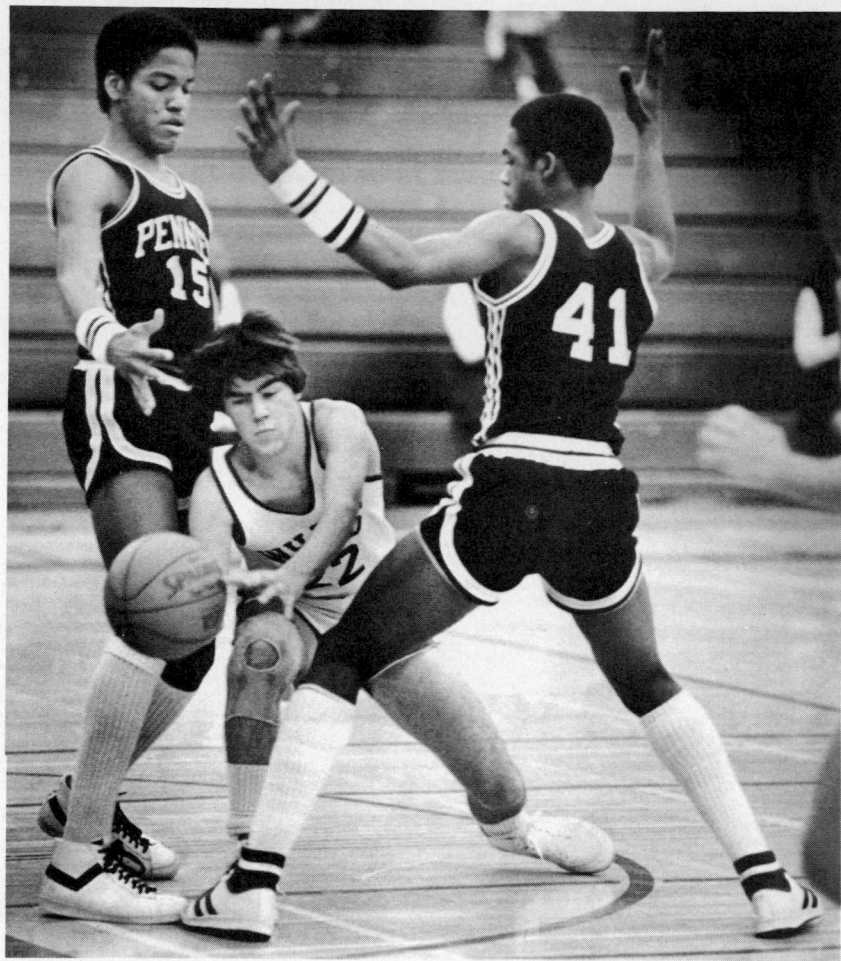

Fig. 25-3. Basketball is a contributing factor in some cases of Osgood-Schlatter disease.

injury in young athletes* (Fig. 25-4). Six to eighteen percent of sports-related injuries in children are reported to involve the physis area.[64,87] Consequently, epiphyseal fractures have been determined to be a direct consequence of sports-related activity, with the most frequent occurrences cited in football.[11]

Most linear bone growth occurs at the epiphyseal growth plate area, a movement permitting synchondrosis, which is usually depicted as a flat disk.[87] Speer and Braun,[87] however, have refuted this depiction and describe the growth plate as a complex system with contour as specific and unique as a fingerprint (Fig. 25-5). The contour serves an important biomechanical role in either resisting or augmenting forces imparted to the growth plate. For example, Speer and Braun suggest that with growth the epiphyseal plate in younger children unlocks the contours and provides an explanation for the predisposition in this age-group of the growth plate to disruption as a consequence of a sheer-type force. Further, injury to the physis region

could alter important architectural components of the physis region (such as its contours, height, and angles) as well as disrupt its collagen fiber systems (such as the perichondrium-periosteum, transphyseal-collagen fibers, and perichondrial rings), which provide major restraint to tensile and sheer forces.[87]

Physeal injuries of young athletes can occur from violent forces or chronic stresses. In skeletally immature children ligaments have been determined to be two to five times as strong as the epiphyseal plate.[19,22,60] It follows therefore that the physis has been identified as the weak link in the musculoskeletal system of adolescents.[11] For example, a violent force to the lateral aspect of a mature knee joint would likely result in a medial tibial collateral ligament sprain, but a similar force to an immature knee would likely result in an epiphyseal plate injury.

Likewise, when elbows of young athletes, usually those 6 to 10 years old, incur a varus stress with the elbow extended, fractures of epiphyseal growth plate of the lateral condyle may occur.[60] As described in these examples, violent mechanical forces that produce predictable injuries in

*See references 11, 15, 18, 19, 33, 60, 64, 76, 87, 88, 99.

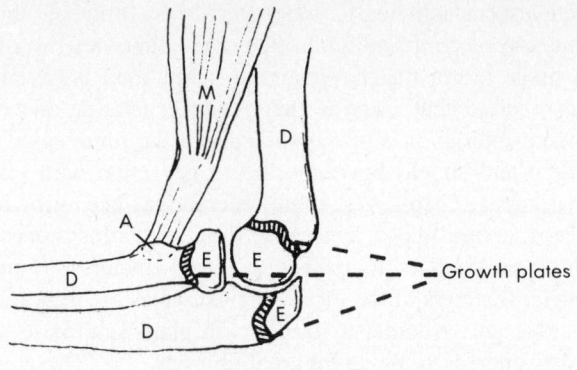

GROWTH STRUCTURES

Fig. 25-4. Growth structures. *A,* Apophysis; *D,* diaphysis; *E,* epiphysis; *M,* muscle.

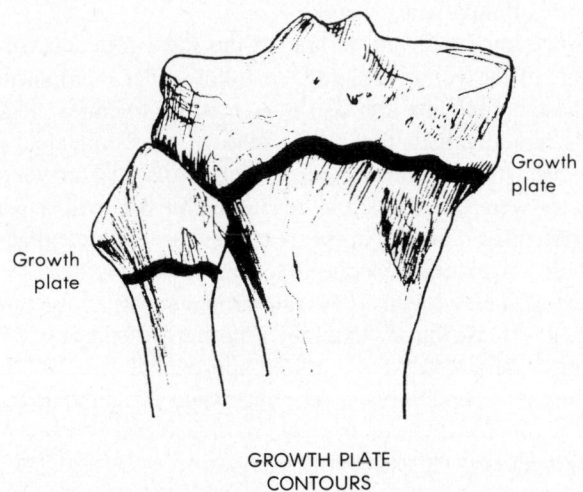

GROWTH PLATE
CONTOURS

Fig. 25-5. Growth plate contours

adults therefore have been shown to result in very different and unique musculoskeletal injury in the young athlete. Also, the very familiar rotator cuff lesions in the adult are rare in the adolescent, since the upper humeral physis when subjected to excessive loads sustains injury sooner than the more resilient musculoskeletal attachment.[22]

In addition, the type and nature of today's competitive sports have evoked changes in the locations of physeal fractures. For example, because of their combative nature, football and hockey continue to account for disproportionate numbers of physeal injuries in youth sports.[11] However, in the noncombative but highly skilled sports growing in popularity today, such as gymnastics, physeal injuries have also occurred as a result of unprecedented levels of musculoskeletal stress.[73] In one sports injuries clinic alone, stress changes related to the distal radial epiphysis were reported in 21 gymnasts.[73] Eleven of these had roentgenograms that showed changes indicative of possible stress fractures.[73] Caine and Linder[19] add that skeletal injuries to the upper extremity have recently been reported more frequently, and they explain that this is in part due to

the conversion of the upper extremity to a weight-bearing support.

However, as stated previously, it is not always a single violent force that overcomes the integrity of the physis; on the contrary, some experts believe that repetitive sports activity that causes overloading of immature tissue and results in inadequate rest is the primary cause of epiphyseal damage.[48,55,68] Micheli,[55] for example, attributes the current prevalence of back injuries in gymnasts to recurrent microtrauma, of which growth plate injuries have been included.[39] Speer and Braun[87] also explain the role of mechanical factors in predisposing the physis region to disruption through recurrent use; for example, they explain that the inclination of the plane of the proximal femoral physis departs from the more normal situation in which the physis is perpendicular to the axial loads placed on them. This biomechanical factor becomes a pathogenic mechanism in slipped capitofemoral epiphysis[87] (a displacement of the head of the femur on its neck); this should be carefully ruled out in any young athlete who complains of hip or medial knee pain and who participates in a repetitive sport activity, whether or not there is an identifiable mechanism of injury.

Goodshall et al[33] reported two cases of stress fracture through the distal femoral epiphysis in football players. In each case no mechanism of injury was reported; however, neither fracture occurred during football activity, but instead, both were precipitated by training periods that emphasized running. Perhaps more than any activity today, running exemplifies stressful, long-duration, repetitive activity. As more children and adolescents engage in competitive long-distance running, growth plate injuries have become an increasing concern.[4,18] Nevertheless, Caine and Lindner's[18] comprehensive review article examining the threat of growth plate injuries to young distance runners reported that evidence does not presently exist that unequivocally supports or condemns the effects of long-distance running on musculoskeletally immature children and adolescents.

The potential for growth plate injury in young athletes has therefore been well documented; however, it also has been reported that the incidence of physis injuries is not escalating and that most injuries are not severe.[64] Pappas[64] states that growth disturbances subsequent to epiphyseal fractures are estimated to occur in fewer than 5% of all epiphyseal injuries. However, it is precisely this potential for growth disturbances that has resulted in the attention to the physis in the literature and the continuing efforts to carefully scrutinize the frequency and severity of physeal injuries in rapidly growing sports. Complete or partial cessation of growth can ultimately result in limb-length inequality or angular deformity.[64] Moreover, the growth disturbance may be insidiously delayed, necessitating follow-up limb measurements and roentgenograms for several years after the injury.[64]

The prognosis of a growth plate injury is largely based on its potential for growth disturbances. Classification of epiphyseal injuries by Salter and Harris and by others assists in determining the likelihood of growth disturbance[77] (Fig. 25-6). In general, types I and II are less severe, are managed nonsurgically, and are less inclined toward growth disruption.

In summary, growth plate injuries remain a potential risk for young athletes participating in sport activity. In sports where velocity and contact are inherent in the activity, involvement of the "weak link" can present a significant risk. Major deformity, although rare, may result from physis disruption, and medical interventions with appropriate safeguards, including surgical correction, may be indicated.

Stress fractures

Fractures in young athletes are not limited to the growth plate region. Stress fractures of the tibia and fibula, for example, are common sports injuries and are typically seen in adolescent athletes[22]; moreover, this form of shin-splints can be confused with other shin-splint varieties of a soft tissue origin that have similar symptoms. It has also been reported that injuries that produce anterior cruciate ligament injuries in adults will fracture the tibial spine in children and should be suspected in any child with knee hemarthrosis.[97] However, there recently has been growing concern about upper extremity injuries*; this concern seems warranted with respect to stress fractures. Supracondylar fractures of the elbow are examples of stress fractures that are proximal to the growth plate, and these are not considered to be epiphyseal injuries.[60,66] These are among the most common elbow fractures in children and are often seen with ipsilateral forearm fractures.[60] In addition, stress fractures of the distal radius and scaphoid have been prevalent,[63,70] particularly in gymnastics, when the upper extremity bears weight.

Since low-back pain is among the most common complaints of the young athlete,[88] it follows that a proportion of these complaints are also due to stress fractures. Jackson[41] has identified that up to 40% of the complaints of low-back pain (persisting more than 3 months) in young athletes were due to "stress reactions" of the lumbar pars interarticularis area. Stress reactions are subroentgenographic, symptomatic conditions that often progress to a defect or spondylolysis (pars interarticularis stress fracture) (Fig. 25-7). Hoshina[37] examined the lumbar spines of 677 young male athletes and reported approximately a 20% incidence of spondylolysis. The incidence of spondylolysis

*See references 19, 20, 60, 66, 70.

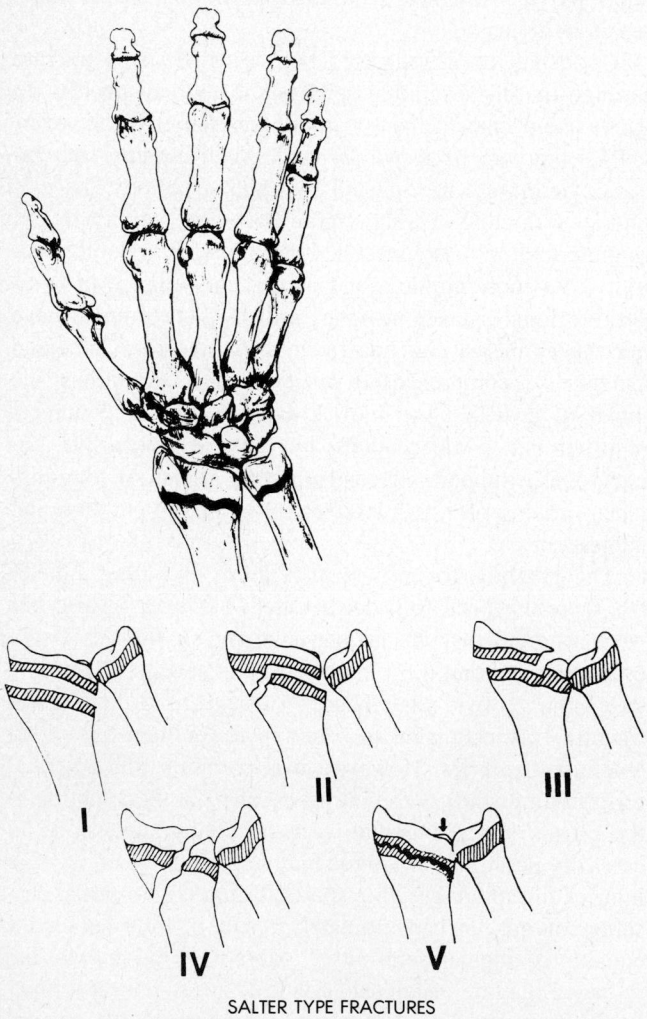

SALTER TYPE FRACTURES

Fig. 25-6. Salter type fractures I, II, III, IV, and V.

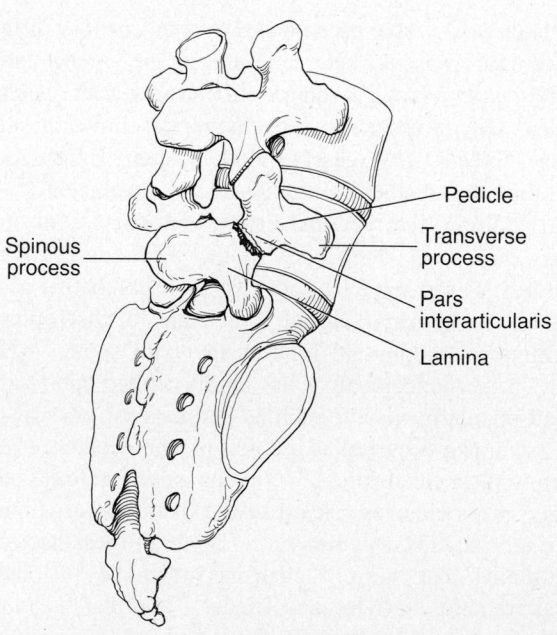

Spinous process — Pedicle — Transverse process — Pars interarticularis — Lamina

Fig. 25-7. Spondylolysis.

in a general, young, white female population has been reported to be 2.3%.[35]

Spondylolysis was initially explained as a genetic condition but is now considered an acquired defect as well.[19,39,55,88] Backaches occur for a variety of reasons, but when lumbar motions become repetitive, particularly in hyperextension, microtrauma presents as a stress reaction that can, without timely intervention, progress to a true pars stress fracture.[55,88] Hyperextension activities, such as blocking in football, the military press in weight training, pole vaulting, diving, pitching in baseball, training maneuvers in gymnastics, or serving in tennis, have all been cited as common aggravating activities that precipitate the condition.[39] Finally, it should be noted that although most pars interarticularis lesions involve the L-5 vertebra, they are not limited to L-5 and may be found at more than a single level.[88]

Summary

In review of the skeletal structure of children, it should be apparent that unmatured musculoskeletal tissue is unique and may therefore be predisposed to breakdown. Moreover, each of the tissues has properties of its own and its own manner of breakdown. The less resistant, maturing articular cartilage of an adolescent is likely to demonstrate degenerative changes when it is overloaded indiscriminately from repetitive compression; a traction apophysis can separate or become inflamed from overuse. However, the mechanisms of injury are usually tensile, with potentially greater consequences. The epiphyseal growth plate (the weak link) seems to be most vulnerable to torsional and linear shears, and since linear growth occurs here, injuries are considered severe.

The proliferation of new and different sport activities as well as "advancements" in technique should meet with a proportionate interest in the effects of these activities on maturing musculoskeletal tissue. Change in the nature and intensity of the sport or activity will alter the effects on the tissues. The increased incidence of upper extremity and low-back injuries in today's sports is important as an example of the redistribution of musculoskeletal injuries in young athletes subsequent to sports booms.

Finally, persistent low-back pain in young athletes has been discussed and attributed in part to growth disturbances (40%).[39] and pars interarticularis involvement (40%).[39] But the prevalence of disk lesions in this population and the relationship of these lesions to specific sports should also be considered. Disk-related lesions in children have been well document[39,42,55,88]; Jackson[39] has reported a 10% rate of discogenic disease in young athletes with pain present for longer than 3 months. Since low-back dysfunction is now the single most frequently encountered orthopaedic complaint of our adult population, continued vigilance of the effect of athletic participation on this particularly vulnerable area seems warranted.

EPIDEMIOLOGICAL REVIEW

Management and prevention of sports-related injuries in young athletes require more than an awareness of the athlete's unique structures and susceptibility to musculoskeletal injury. Attention should also be given the epidemiological trends, including the injuries sustained and the circumstances surrounding their occurrence.[31] Many of the causes of today's injuries to young athletes are not known. However, a review of recent studies that investigate particular sports, anatomical areas of injury, types of injury, the severity of injuries, and gender considerations will permit a more meaningful assessment of those factors that may be contributing to the injuries of young athletes.

Injuries in sports

Which sport activities result in the greatest number of injuries in young athletes? Dehaven and Lintner[26] reported 3,431 sports-related injuries over a 7-year period. More than 60% of the injuries reported were in young athletes in the 13 to 19 year age-group. Football was the most common sport causing injury and accounted for almost 64% of all the injuries. Males were injured 80% of the time; knees and ankles were the most commonly involved area, and sprains and strains were the most common type of injuries.

Through its national electronic information surveillance system (NEISS), the U.S. Consumer Product and Safety Commission estimated the frequency of medically attended sports injuries over a 1-year period.[92] Table 25-1 provides NEISS estimates for five highly visible sports, which, for a 1-year period, accounted for a total of 1,346,467 injuries. Although data were not available to calculate the injury rate for each sport (i.e., the number of injuries over the number of participants), the size and representativeness of the samples warrant proper consideration of the data. Basketball had the highest incidence of injury of the sports cited, with an estimated 457,746 injuries. Sprains and strains were again identified as the most common types of injury, accounting for 49% of the occurrences in basketball and nearly 37% of the occurrences in the five sports combined. Basketball alone caused 136,359 ankle injuries, accounting for one in every five injuries.

Other studies corroborate the high incidence of ankle injuries.[31,47] Investigating ankle and foot problems in the athlete, Garrick and Requa[31] reported sprains to be the most common ankle injury, occurring six times more than all other ankle injuries combined.[31] Wong and Gregg,[97] however, state that children with open growth plates rarely have ligamentous sprains but instead are susceptible to physeal or metaphyseal fractures. At about 13 years of age the lateral distal tibial physis remains open, and when an inversion force is sufficient to cause tissue damage, it usually results in a Salter-Harris type I or II fracture of the growth plate.[97] Diagnosis is confirmed on routine roentgenograms as well as by palpation of localized tenderness and swelling at the growth plate proximal to the ligamen-

Table 25-1. 1986 Injury profile by sport: Data adapted from the U.S. Consumer Product and Safety Commission through NEISS

Sport	Total no. of injuries	% of injuries by type			No. and % of injuries by area			No. and % of injuries by group			*% of injuries by gender		% of injuries considered severe
		Contusions/ abrasions	Strains/ sprains	Fractures	Area	No.	%	Age-group (yr)	No.	%	Male	Female	
Basketball	457,746	18	49	15	Ankle	136,359	30	5-14	104,678	23	68	32	3
					Finger	55,701	19	15-24	250,762	55	86	14	
Football	382,173	27	33	22	Finger	64,305	17	5-14	134,408	35	95	5	6
					Knee	41,249	11	15-24	216,675	57	94	6	
Baseball	361,552	30	28	19	Head/face	76,184	21	5-14	123,875	34	71	29	6
					Finger	55,701	15	15-24	114,133	32	71	29	
Soccer	103,735	30	37	19	Ankle	18,524	18	5-14	43,204	42	64	36	6
					Knee	15,262	15	15-24	45,742	44	74	26	
Gymnastic	41,261	22	47	18	Ankle	7,183	17	5-14	26,986	65	32	68	3
					Wrist	4,847	12	15-24	12,547	30	38	62	
Total	1,346,467												

*Percentage of injuries by gender is based on age.

tous injuries.[97] It would seem that prudent management of ankle injuries in younger athletes would strongly consider the likelihood of a growth plate fracture.

The NEISS number of medically attended football injuries was estimated at 382,173 (Table 25-1).[92] Football injuries were second only to basketball injuries in incidence, and they were most commonly reported to be contusions, sprains, and strains, which supported the observations of Dehaven and Lintner.[26]

Further, Table 25-1 shows that the 5 to 14 year age-group had fewer occurrences reported (35%) than had the 15 to 24 year age-group (57%), which suggests that football was safer when the participants were younger. When rates of injury have been available, youth football has shown a low rate of injury (<5%).[34,58]

The number of gymnastics injuries may not seem as significant as the other sports injuries listed in Table 25-1, but the proportion of injuries to the young female athlete, areas injured, and the types of injuries peculiar to this sport have been documented, and concern has grown.[19,41,55,73] The NEISS data reveal the ankle, the wrist, and knee areas accounted for 39% of all gymnastics injuries.[92] Additional sources provide strong evidence that each of these areas is at risk in this population. The prevalence of ankle injury warrants special attention because of the high incidence (17% of the reported injuries) and the identified risk of growth plate fracture to the immature ankles of younger athletes.[97] Gymnastics injuries at or about the wrist seem more prevalent than in other sports and account for 12% of the injuries.

In gymnastics, reported cases from numerous investigators corroborate the notion that the wrist of the young gymnast is particularly vulnerable to injury.* Chambers[20] may have been the first to suggest that reducing injuries in growing athletes could best be accomplished if attention were directed at reducing the risk of upper extremity injuries.

Nevertheless, an 8-year overview of NEISS data on sports-related injuries to persons 5 to 14 years of age lent strong support to the notion that younger children are in general more susceptible to upper extremity injuries. Across 15 selected sports, 5 to 15-year-old participants injured their arms more frequently than other regions, whereas persons under 5 years of age had more head injuries and older persons (>15 years old) injured their legs.[75] Moreover, Caine and Linder[19] reported that an increase in upper extremity injuries in female gymnasts is also apparent and that contributing factors include an increased and earlier involvement of participants as well as strenuous demands on the upper extremity that result from its conversion to a weight-bearing support.

In general, most injuries peculiar to gymnastics have been attributed to overuse.† Structurally immature tissues of very young athletes, such as the articular cartilage, apophyses, epiphyses, and bone, have been prime targets for the excessive load demands of this sport. Articular cartilage, with its limited capacity to withstand moderate repetitive loads, has been reported to yield under the excessive loading conditions of the sport.[35,83,93]

Singer and Roy,[83] for example, have cited several cases of osteochondrosis of the elbows of young gymnasts. The joint surface degeneration has been explained as a fatigue response of the tissues caused by overuse and as a sequela of an altered metabolism (hypovascularity).[43] Further, higher stress levels are necessary to cause similar responses in tissues such as tendon or bone.[43]

*See references 19, 52, 62, 70, 73, 83.

†See references 10, 19, 35, 60, 73, 83, 93.

Injury to the medial epicondyle of the elbow, Osgood-Schlatter disease, and Sinding-Larsen-Johannson disease are traction apophysis injuries attributed to overuse in gymnastics.[35,60,93] The more prevalently reported distal radial epiphysis injury to the gymnast's wrist has also been associated with repetitive torsional forces—or overuse. Including the lumbar spine in this scenario, Micheli[55] has remarked that it is the young female gymnast's back that is most susceptible to the overuse injury because of recurrent microtrauma. He adds that the "epidemic" of back injuries, in particular the stress fracture of the pars interarticularis, supports this contention. Overuse injuries in female gymnastics are prevalent and have prompted Caine and Lindner to conclude that the female gymnast is at considerable risk of incurring an overuse injury during her career.

Severity of injuries

Severe injuries should warrant our closest attention, because they are the athletic injuries that have the most serious consequences. Standardized methods for classifying an injury as "severe," however, do not exist, and comparisons of severe injuries across sports is usually unwieldy. Nevertheless, it is important to carefully examine each sport for those factors that needlessly contribute to the risk of serious injury.

Injuries in the NEISS data were classified on a 0 to 6 scale of severity. Severity percentages in Table 25-1 were calculated by collapsing all occurrences given severe ratings (5 or 6) in these data and dividing this number by the number of injuries (frequency). Six percent of the medically attended injuries in football, baseball, and soccer were then determined to be injuries of a severe nature. This should not suggest, however, that these sports are associated with an equal risk of serious injury. A particular sport's potential for causing severe injury will vary for each participant and is perhaps best determined without comparisons to other sports.

Because football involves collision, severe injuries have always been associated with this sport. Table 25-1 shows that in 1986, 6% of the football injuries reported, across all ages, were classified as severe and that 22% of all injuries were fractures. The NEISS has also revealed that more than 10,000 head and neck injuries from football alone are reported annually, the highest of any sport, and that concussions account for about 11% of the head injuries.[75]

In preadolescent football players severe injuries do not occur as often as in the young adult population, because younger children are smaller and yield less impact.[58] Nevertheless, catastrophic injuries such as paralysis, brain damage, and death occur.[75] NEISS data showed that over a period of 8 years 19 fatalities occurred in children 5 to 14 years old, and in two thirds of the fatalities the injury was to the victim's head or neck. Trends show that the incidence of severe injuries related to football has lessened, but despite closer scrutiny, improved equipment and facilities, and more responsible supervision, these tragic consequences remain a part of the sport.

In baseball severe cases are likely to involve fractures or lacerations of the fingers and hands. However, regarding catastrophic injuries, baseball has the highest number of fatalities involving children 5 to 14 years of age, and usually the child dies after being struck by a ball.[74] Although the problem has been identified and further analysis has been recommended, no current change in this trend is apparent. The severity of soccer injuries is also best understood when one considers that the rapid growth of soccer in recent years, its younger participants, the proportion of female athletes, and the emphasis on winning have contributed to a rapid change in the injury profile of this sport, including a rising number of injuries of a severe nature. The severity of sports injuries, as well as the factors that influence their trends, must continuously be explored if thoughtful interpretations and appropriate interventions are to be anticipated for young children.

Since most injuries in gymnastics involve young gymnasts, the severity of gymnastic injuries also warrants special consideration. Although studies exist that document the incidence of severe gymnastic injuries, the lack of controlled investigations has limited the extent to which meaningful comparisons of severe injuries with other sports injuries have been possible. The literature is replete with evidence that the physical loading during training and intense competition often results in demands on the growing bones of the gymnast that exceed the ability of musculoskeletal tissue to attenuate these loads.* An increasing number of investigators are concluding that the young gymnast is incurring a disproportionate number of severe injuries. Because no standardized criteria of what constitutes a severe injury have been reported for this sport, investigators have typically considered a gymnast's injury to be severe when (1) prolonged restrictions from the activity have been necessary, (2) surgery occurred, (3) the potential to impair musculoskeletal growth existed, or (4) there was a likelihood for a chronic problem in later life.

Reported severe wrist injuries commonly cited are stress fractures of the carpals and at the distal radius.[52,62,70,73] Of the distal radial fractures the epiphysis has most often been involved.[70,73] Consideration of these growth plate injuries as severe injuries seems well justified in that disruption of the physis can meet each or all of the criteria of a severe injury (listed previously). Roy et al.[73] investigated stress changes of the distal radial epiphysis in 21 young gymnasts; they reported that of the 11 athletes with roentgenographic changes, three required 3 months of inactivity before resuming gymnastic activity, five were inactive for at least 6 months, and one failed to return entirely after a year of recurring wrist symptoms. No evidence of growth disturbances was observed in this sample, but long-term medical supervision was suggested. It is also

---

*See references 19, 35, 52, 55, 62, 66, 70, 73, 83, 86, 93.

noteworthy that stress fractures of the distal radius were considered rare until recently, whereas involvement of the physis has been reported in young gymnasts exclusively.[73] Therefore the high incidence of wrist injuries in female gymnasts, the emergence of epiphyseal plate stress changes, and the tendency for these injuries to require unusually long periods to heal suggest the importance of determining the severity of these injuries, the factors that influence their incidence, and future trends.

The young gymnast's elbow is subject to excessive weight-bearing loads, as is the wrist. An exaggerated angle of the valgus in the female subject has been determined to predispose her to some serious injuries in this area.[35,66,83] Severe elbow injuries such as subluxations, dislocations, and fractures do not occur as frequently as the injuries associated with the wrist, knee, or ankle, but when the elbow is injured, the gymnast is more likely to be injured for a longer time or require surgery.

With weight borne by the upper extremity, the valgus alignment of the elbow contributes to a stretching of the medial structures, which can result in traction or apophyseal fractures of the medial epicondyle (the most commonly found elbow injury), subluxations, or dislocation.[35,66] The gymnast incurring these injuries is often left with a permanent elbow flexion deformity.[35] Priest and Weise[66] reported 32 elbow injuries in 30 female gymnasts. Thirty of the injuries were fractures or dislocations; the remaining two were osteochondrosis of the humeral capitulum (Panner's disease). Eleven of those injured required surgery, and the average time lost by those who returned to the sport was 4.1 months. Osteochondrosis of the capitulum is a manifestation of lateral compression forces that also occur when the upper extremity bears weight; these forces may become excessive with a pronounced valgus alignment. Singer and Roy[83] reported seven such patients, two of whom underwent surgery for removal of osteochondral fragments. In one of the remaining patients disease was too severe to permit a return to the sport. The investigators examined the capitullar blood supply and determined that vascular insufficiency and subsequent epiphyseal injury were induced by repetitive microtrauma at an early age. They expressed serious concerns about the long-term effects of this injury.[83]

The lumbar spine, as much as any area of the body, has been reported to incur injuries of a serious nature. Jackson et al.[39] stated that the demands placed on the back of the young female gymnast are unparalleled. Such demands test the structural limits of the lumbar musculoskeletal tissues and contribute to low-back conditions commonly seen in this population, some of which have been determined to be severe.

Spondylolysis is the most commonly occurring low-back condition seen in the gymnast[35,39,93] (see Fig. 25-7). Jackson et al.[41] reported an 11% incidence in 100 female gymnasts, an incidence almost five times the expected rate of a nonathletic but otherwise similarly matched group of young females. Jackson et al.[41] have also indicated that the disability period for the gymnast with a positive bone scan result is minimally 3 months, but they reported the average time off for a pars stress reaction to be 7.3 months. Typically, pars reactions, which are not managed with a commensurate restriction of activity, progress to a bilateral involvement and ultimately present as a defect (fracture) seen roentgenographically.[41] Complete bed rest until acute symptoms subside, brace or cast immobilization, and a progressive rehabilitation program are usually required for treatment of the patient with an acute symptomatic pars defect or reaction.[35] It is the severity of the symptoms then that often determines the duration of restriction from the sport. In some instances of persistent symptoms and evidence of a progressive defect, a surgical fusion is recommended.[93] However, returning an athlete to competition must not be the primary purpose for considering a fusion,[39] since a 1- to 2-year convalescence would preclude the athlete from returning to premorbid levels of competition in most instances.[39]

The long-term affects of pars defects have not been clearly determined. It has been reported that low-back pain in later life can frequently be traced to an unrecognized, untreated, vertebral fracture (i.e., pars defect) sustained earlier.[27] Jackson et al.[39] investigated adult patients with disk disease and found no evidence, however, of an increased incidence of pars defects.

The incidence of disk herniation in children is not what it is in adults.[42] Strenuous maneuvers such as in gymnastics do increase the likelihood that a child could sustain a disk injury,[35] and when this occurs the nature of the herniation is often severe.[39,42]

Disk herniations in children are associated with a high percentage of neurological signs,[42] and as such the most disk herniations in children are accompanied by a dermatomal sciatica.[39] Surgical removal of disk fragments, with or without partial laminectomy, is often recommended.[42] Jackson et al.[39] reported that surgery was necessary in about 30% of his patients with sciatica that persisted for more than 3 weeks. Treatment by fusion does not seem to affect outcomes in pediatric populations.[42] In addition, Jackson reported using epidural cortisone injection in 50% of young athletes with persistent symptoms.[39]

Anterior disk herniations through the growth plate, with a narrowing of the anterior disk space, has also been reported in skeletally immature athletes[39] and is most common in young gymnasts (and wrestlers) engaged in hyperextension maneuvers.[39] Recovery of children from disk herniations is much superior to that by adults.[42] Prolonged irritation of nerve elements can, however, result in persistent chronic effects, which in some instances have prevented a return to the inciting sport.[39]

Gender considerations

Gender differences can also assist in explaining the distributions of sports injuries in young athletes. The types of injuries to female athletes and the areas injured have been reported to be similar to those of their injured male counterparts.[26,31,82] As in males, sprains and strains have been identified as the most common type of athletic injury in females.[26,31] Knees and ankles seem to be the most commonly injured areas.[26] Garrick[31] investigated ankle and foot problems in a large sample of athletes and noted that ankle sprains were the most common of all injuries, that they were most often incurred in basketball, and that the injury was more prevalent in females. In a 7-year study of athletic injuries that considered age, sport, and sex, Dehaven and Lintner[26] reported that knees and ankles were most commonly injured areas, irrespective of age, and that these injuries accounted for 59.2% and 13.1%, respectively, of all injuries in females. The medial collateral and anterior cruciate ligaments were reported to be involved in 12.1% of all knee sprains.[26] In greater contrast to data reported for males, patellofemoral pain syndrome was diagnosed in nearly 20% of all the injuries involving the female athlete.[26] The increased genu varum of the female knee seems to predispose these athletes to overuse injuries such as chondromalacia and recurrent patella dislocation. The prevalence of knee injuries in female athletes has been well documented and warrants special attention.*

Gymnastics perhaps best exemplifies the importance of sex considerations in assessment of the risks of injury in particular sports (Fig. 25-8). In the large NEISS sample, females accounted for 66% of the gymnastic injuries reported (N = 41,261) for all ages.[92] Of note is that in this same sample, 65% of the gymnastic injuries were incurred by children 5 to 14 years of age. It is, then, the younger female gymnast who seems most susceptible to injury from participation in gymnastics. Moreover, Caine and Lindner's[19] comprehensive review of the young female gymnast concluded that these athletes have among the highest overall injury rates.

How much do sex differences contribute to the incidence, type, and nature of athletic injuries sustained? A decade ago Nilsson and Rohas[63] investigated soccer injuries and observed that the injury rates for girls doubled those of boys. The authors attributed their findings to a lesser skill level and lack of adequate training; conclusions that could be readily argued today. Michili[58] states that in similarly intensive athletic programs, given proper preparation, the risk of injury is similar in girls and boys. Only recently have studies been purposefully designed to permit comparisons of athletic injuries by gender. Garrick,[31] for example, recognized that gender comparisons of ankle injuries were misleading when football and wrestling, which have primarily male participants, were included in the analysis. When both sports were excluded from the sample of ankle injuries, the rates were then comparable for both sexes. Studies have not been found that compare the incidence of injuries in contact sports when male athletes compete against female athletes, but ongoing investigations of injuries by gender for each sport are necessary if meaningful conclusions for emerging sports with changing proportions of participants are to be reached.

Summary

Having culled from recent literature the incidence and severity of sports-related injuries, I have emphasized in this section the negative consequences of participation by children in sports. I therefore feel compelled to defend children's sports, since they provide young participants with untold benefits and essential opportunities for development. Although injuries do arise from athletic competition, they occur with some frequency and severity in a variety of nonathletic activities. Goldberg et al.[34] reported that sports-related injuries comprised only 1.7% of their total pediatric visits (N = 6,197). It would be no more appropriate to condemn or ban baseball than it would be to eliminate bicycle riding. The purpose then of epidemiological data such as these, despite their negative tenor, is to describe the extent of injuries and to provide a reasonable basis for ascribing contributing risk factors.

CONTRIBUTING RISK FACTORS
Intrinsic factors

Structural. Our knowledge of the factors contributing to musculoskeletal injuries in young athletes has not kept pace with the proliferation of new sports and their associated incidence of injury. Epidemiological techniques have been useful in detecting an increased frequency of sports-related injuries in young athletes[58,78]; however, many epi-

*See references 24-26, 30, 34, 65, 93.

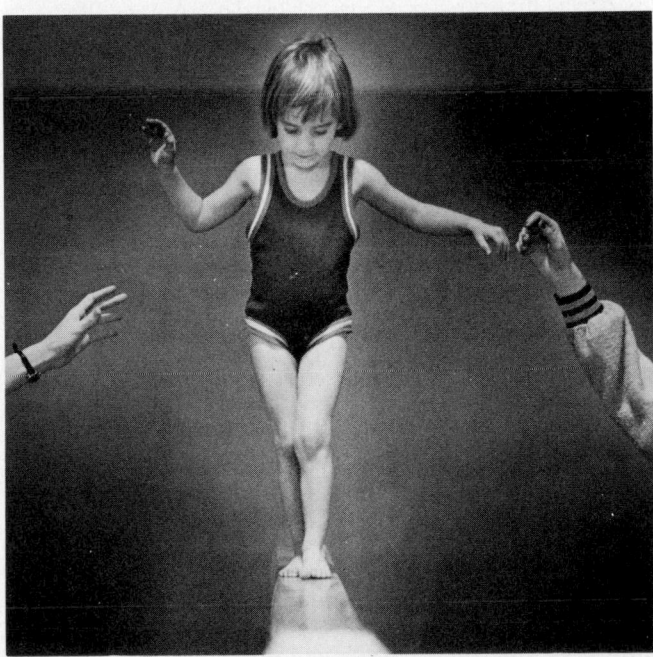

Fig. 25-8. Young females that participate in gymnastics are at risk for injury.

demiological studies, because of their ex post facto designs, do not provide explanations for these injuries and do not permit the findings to be generalized to athletes beyond the conditions observed.[16,58] Findings from surveillance systems (such as NEISS), for example, usually lack adequate controls and may be easily misinterpreted. Reported sports-related injuries must be well defined and the factors, which could explain the populations at risk, must be identified if valid explanations of the injury occurrences are to be expected.[78]

Intrinsic factors are those characteristics or attributes of the young athletes that predispose them to injury. Immature musculoskeletal structure described earlier, such as the less resistant articular cartilage and open epiphyses, exemplifies intrinsic or host factors warranting further consideration. These immature structures place the young athlete at greater risk than the adult athlete of sustaining either a macrotrauma (acute injury) or microtrauma (overuse injury) type of injury. Also, structurally related, unrecognized congenital defects are another contributing host factor that can increase the likelihood of a sports-related injury in young athletes.[2] An otherwise asymptomatic, congenital pars defect may become symptomatic in a young tennis player who hyperextends the arm while serving. Structural scoliotic or lordotic curves of the spine, true discrepancies in leg length, anterverted/retroverted hips, exaggerated genu recurvatum or valgum, and an abnormal foot type, to name a few, may all be factors that contribute to a sudden or eventual injury. The young athlete's structure with its unique conditions, potentially undetected congenital defects, and malalignments merits our attention as a risk factor.

Growth. Host contributing factors are not limited to the young athlete's structure. A child also has a special risk of incurring either macrotrauma or microtrauma musculoskeletal injuries because these tissues grow.[56] Moreover, growth itself has been identified as an important risk factor. It follows then that the potential for injury in the musculoskeletally immature athlete is increased.[19,46,58]

Growth involves an increase in the mass and size of the body's musculoskeletal tissues.[46] Within the normal growing process two growth spurts have been identified.[46] The "midgrowth spurt" occurs in children of both sexes between 5½ and 7 years of age. The second spurt or "adolescent growth spurt" begins in girls between 11 and 13 years of age but comes later in boys between 13 and 15 years. Females also grow faster and larger during their adolescent growth spurt, whereas males tend to have a more extended growth period[46] (Fig. 25-9).

Variations in growth have been a common concern in youth sports because of the associated risk of injury when athletes are unevenly matched.[3,44,46,58] Size and strength differences between male and female athletes, for example, should become a concern at the time of the adolescent growth spurt when growth differences may become appar-

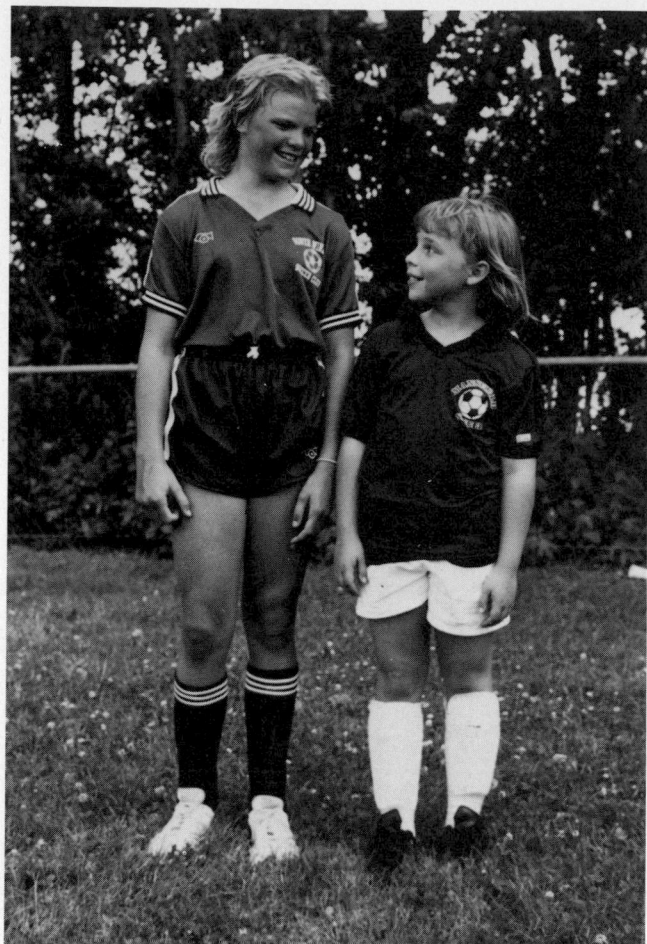

Fig. 25-9. Growth differences merit grouping according to physical maturation. The young female subject on the left, although taller and more physically mature, was not yet 11 years old (10 years and 8 months) when this photograph was taken. Her competitor, the smaller girl on the right, is already 12 years old.

ent. Before adolescence, however, separating children by sex may not be necessary.[3] Concerns regarding a size disparity related to age differences are also common because of wide variation in growth rates.[3,44] Grouping young athletes according to physical maturation rather than chronological age has been recommended so that variation in size and maturation may be reduced.[3,13,44,46]

Chronologically matched children at age 12 years may vary as much as 6 years in their maturity level.[44,68] Physical maturation, or "physiological age," is most often determined by breast development and pubic hair growth or age of menarch in females and pubic hair growth and genital development in males.[13,54,89] Tanner's[89] classification by sex characteristics is done by physical examination and affords a quick and inexpensive method of determining physiological age.[28] The skeletal age of a child can also be determined directly with roentgenograms, usually of the wrist, by comparison with standards for each growth period. Grouping of young athletes by means other than chronological age has therefore been widely recommended.[13,44,89] Strategies such as using physiological age, weight, skill, or the use of narrow chronological age ranges have merit and could reduce the risk of injury caused by variation in growth rate.

Growth spurts have also been reported to interact with a child's body type (somatotype) and augment the risk of an injury.[46] Although a child's somatotype does not change appreciably during the growth spurt,[51] the risks of injury for certain somatotypes are higher than for other types. During a growth spurt the more gangly, underdeveloped, uncoordinated adolescent athletes with poor muscle tone are more likely to sustain an injury than are their better developed counterparts.[46] The obese child with Frölich somatotype is at high risk of incurring a growth plate injury during a growth spurt and should be restricted from contact sports.[46] The physiques of young athletes then are more than just potential predictors of ability; during a growth spurt they require special attention as intrinsic risk factors.

Growth spurts have also been reported to result in a dramatic loss of flexibility by causing the contractile elements to tighten around the joints.[56] Micheli[56] states that this process of rapid growth with subsequent tightening of muscles and tendons predisposes young athletes' immature tissues to overuse. The traction epiphyses (apophyses) become stressed by additional tension forces; articular cartilage becomes more susceptible to sheer stresses[56,58]; and at the center of the growth spurt, epiphyseal plates are most susceptible to injury.[11,64,87] It is during the growth spurt that the interdigital contours of the growth plate are unlocked and the physis becomes most vulnerable to injury.[87] Therefore recommendations that 12- to 14-year-old children be restricted from collision sports such as football have been debated.[59] It is, however, also important to consider that predisposing risk factors that are restrictive for some sports may not rule out participation in another sport.

Physical activity. Any review of intrinsic risk factors in young athletes would be incomplete without some information regarding the effects of physical activity on the immature host. It is generally accepted that a well-balanced, progressive, physical activity initiated in early childhood promotes beneficial musculoskeletal growth and development.[50] However, any physical activity can be potentially injurious to a growing child.

How young is too young for a child to participate in a given sport?[10] The American Academy of Pediatrics, responding to its concern for the ill effects of long-distance running on children, issued this statement: "Long distance running events primarily designed for adults are not recommended for children prior to physical maturation." The International Athletics Association Federation suggested that up to age 12 years not more than 800 meters should be run in competition, with gradual progression up to 3,000

meters, for 14-year-old children.[79] Seefeldt et al.[79] expressed concern that this position may be too restrictive, since little scientific evidence exists to suggest that long-distance running is detrimental to a child's growth. In determining what age is too young to participate in a sport, consideration must be given to any evidence that suggests that the musculoskeletal risks to the child exceed the benefits of participation and, importantly, that the risks are attributable to the early exposure to the sport.

In collision sports, where risks to young athletes are usually due to an associated macrotrauma, restriction recommendations have been justifiably based on logic or reason. Unfortunately, many of today's sports produce a more insidious overuse injury, the microtrauma. Therefore carefully designed studies will be necessary so that the populations at risk can be validly identified. In the interim, erring on the side of conservatism remains in the best interests of the child.

If normal growth is to be expected, a certain minimum of physical activity is necessary.[50,72] Tensile and compressive forces from physical activity play a major role in the formation of new bone and growth[50]; moreover, athletics can provide strong mechanical stimuli to young athletes, and strong evidence attests to this phenomenon. For example, tennis players have been reported to have asymmetrically enlarged radius bones; femurs of soccer players demonstrate larger cross sections than those of nonathletes; and running causes the marrow cavity of the tibia to enlarge.[46] The intrinsic risk to the musculoskeletal structure occurs when the intensity and durations of the stimuli exceed the tissues' ability to attenuate the applied forces. The sport activity becomes excessive then when fatigue responses of tissues, such as inflammation, degeneration, or resorption, ensue. Morphological responses to exercise, however, do vary between children, so attention must be given to the individual's adverse reactions to excessive activity. It is recommended therefore that in planning appropriate physical activities for children engaged in athletic competition, consideration be given to the fatigability of the least physically developed child.[46]

Strength training. Strength training is at the cutting edge of physical activity in young athletes. There is general agreement that when modified appropriately to the young athlete, strength training can improve athletic performance and reduces the incidence of injuries.* This has resulted in the use of strength training in a growing number of sports such as football, gymnastics, and running to achieve these ends in younger athletes.[9] However, there remains considerable debate regarding (1) the attainability of strength gains in children, (2) the safety of the method of strength training, and (3) the benefits to the young athlete.[59]

Evidence supports the attainability of strength gains in

---

*See references 8, 17, 45, 51, 57, 68, 81.

adolescent males.[9,59] Adolescent females also demonstrate strength gains but less dramatically than do adolescent males.[8,9,23,59] Claims of similar gains in prepubescent athletes, that is, before the onset of any secondary sex characteristics, have been questioned because of the insufficient amounts of androgens (testosterone) in this population to permit strength gains.[81] Recent studies of the prepubescent weight trainee, however, reveal strength gains in this population of young athletes as well.[57,59] Yet age considerations do seem to bear on strength gains. Asmussen,[9] for example, has observed that at corresponding heights subgroups of younger children demonstrated less strength than their older counterparts. The American Academy of Pediatrics has also warned of the disproportionate strength in children.[3] Strength gains are attainable therefore in all subgroups of children, but variability in individuals as a result of genetic factors, such as body type and the growth variations, probably has more to do with the existing strength disproportions seen in children.

Is strength training a safe activity? Micheli[59] has stated that strength training in young athletes is safe if it is done under appropriate conditions and with proper techniques and equipment. Clearly not all "strength training" is appropriate in the young athlete. "Weight training" is a strength-training activity that uses submaximal, progressive, external resistance and has been generally accepted as a safe activity for children.[8,57,59,81] This is in contrast to a more rigorous strength-training activity, namely, "weight lifting," which is a training activity that demands a one-repetition maximum of an external weight such as in Olympic or power lifting. Because of its inherent risks on skeletally immature tissue, the American Academy of Pediatrics has condemned weight lifting in young athletes.[5] Moreover, since most strength gains in children are achieved at 70% to 80% of their projected best lift for a given exercise,[91] any additional gains from maximal lifting are not worth the added risks of injury.

Injuries are incurred during strength-training activities and have been reported.[11,14,59,81] The young athlete is at comparable risk to an adult-strength trainee of sustaining the typical joint dysfunctions of muscle sprains. More serious injuries that typically involve the growth plates are unique to the child and warrant special consideration. Growth plate injuries have occurred primarily in instances where poor training methods or maximal lifts were contributing factors.[58,76] In particular, military presses using excessive weight have been the mechanism of injury of fractures to the distal radial epiphysis.[59,76] These injuries to the growth plate tend to occur from a single macrotrauma incident. Available data do not suggest that young athletes involved in strength training are at much risk of sustaining the more insidious microtrauma injury usually associated with sports such as gymnastics or running. Also, pubescent (adolescent) children who lift weights seem at greater risk of incurring a growth plate injury than their prepubescent counterpart because of their increased susceptibility during the "adolescent growth spurt." No growth plate injuries to prepubescent children doing weight training have been reported.[59]

Back injuries have also been reported when poor training or maximal weight was used.[39,59] In adolescents with complaints of chronic low-back pain brought on or aggravated by lumbar extension maneuvers, as occur with squats or leg presses, medical attention is necessary to rule out a possible pars interarticularis injury. In summary, injuries in children do not appear prevalent when appropriate weight-training activities were used, but at this time epidemiological studies, which could determine their incidence, are lacking.

The benefits of strength training have been reported to include the enhancement of sport performance and the reduction of potential injuries.[9,45,57] Progressive resistive exercises designed to strengthen muscle groups, which are extensively relied on in given sports activities, have been shown to improve performance in that sport.[8] Moreover, the greater the similarity of the training activity with the sport activity, the greater the likelihood that the training gains will be transferred into athletic performance gains.[8,45] Enhanced sport performance has been well demonstrated for adolescents after weight training, whereas similar benefits have not yet been demonstrated in the prepubescent child.[59]

The risk of injury can be reduced in young athletes who effectively participate in weight training.[59] For example, Cahill and Griffith[17] investigated the effects of a preseason conditioning program, which included weight training, on knee injuries. Their findings showed a significant reduction in both the number and severity of knee injuries over a 4-year period.[17] Results of this kind are achieved through the stimulation and hypertrophy of collagen tissues, which increase the capacity of the musculoskeletal tissues to dissipate potentially harmful forces.[43] It should be noted that proportional increases in connective tissues have been shown to accompany training-induced muscle fiber hypertrophy.[49] Weight training then provides a means for strengthening in that an external force can provide a stimulus of sufficient magnitude to promote hypertrophy and can adequately simulate the extraordinary forces of athletic competition. Nonetheless, we must always be cognizant of the unique intrinsic risk factors of the skeletally immature child and temper our strength-training efforts and use of weight training accordingly. Since internal resistance techniques such as pull-ups and sit-ups further reduce the risk of injury in strength training, they are recommended whenever their benefits are sufficient for this purpose.[5,44] The axiom of striving for the optimum in benefits for the minimum of intervention has merit in this arena.

Extrinsic factors

Risk factors external to the host can also greatly increase a young athlete's chances of sustaining an injury. The extrinsic risk factors are, in general, environmental conditions that if identified and controlled could reduce either the incidence or the severity of athletic injuries in children. Environmental conditions can be contributing risk factors that interact with intrinsic factors to cause an injury, or an extrinsic factor might be the exclusive cause of an injury. Environmental factors that have contributed to the risk of injury include (1) the sport, (2) the sports organization, and (3) supervision. Knowledge of the extrinsic factors that account for injuries in young athletes is important, because the resulting injuries are often avoidable.

Sports. Investigations of injury occurrences by sport reveal that all sports do not have an equal risk of injury.* Goldberg et al[34] classified sports according to their impact potential; they found that speed and collision sports have associated higher risks of injury.[34] Football and ice hockey are obviously collision sports, whereas baseball, basketball, soccer, and wrestling have varying degrees of collision.[3] Accordingly, the American Academy of Pediatrics, in its review of competitive sports of elementary school–age children, has warned of the potential hazards of collision and contact activities in this age-group despite many well-intended efforts to control contributing extrinsic risk factors such as poor supervision.[3] Restrictions on a sport may be necessary when the sport puts a population at risk because of its peculiar nature. Since boxing, for instance, seeks injury as a goal, it is therefore an inappropriate activity for children.[3]

In addition to the inherent nature of a sport, are the movement demands or skills that influence the chance of injury. Tackling, for example, is a fundamental skill in football with inherent risks; moreover, mastery of this skill alone may not preclude or diminish the participant's risk of injury. Head and neck injuries are associated with tackling and are a perennial risk in football.[1,53] In lesser contact sports such as tennis, gymnastics, swimming, and running, the determining factors of injury are considerably different. Because a sport incurs limited contact, however, should not suggest that it is safer than a contact sport. In fact, noncontact sports that emphasize repetition, as in swimming or running, may demonstrate greater injury rates related to overuse.[58]

Repetitive loads imparted to musculoskeletal tissues during these activities vary in magnitude, direction, frequency, and duration; further, participants vary in their age, size, and sex. In general, body parts are stressed in disproportionate and varying ways; and as a result athletes incur dissimilar injuries from dissimilar sports.[26] The continued expansion of sports activity in young age-groups necessitates asking critical questions regarding the nature of a sport, the demands of its activities, and the effects on its participants if young athletes are to be expected to fully realize the benefits from sports without incurring undue risk of injury.

Sports organizations. The existence of an organized

*See references 1, 20, 26, 31, 34, 63, 92.

sport program has mixed effects on a young athlete's risks of being injured. Organized children's sports programs have not been shown to unequivocally offer safer athletic environments than free-play situations,[19,34,58] although, within organized programs for youths, responsible administering can prevent the occurrence of certain sports injuries. Comparisons of the reported risks associated with organized versus nonorganized sports reveal conflicting findings. For example, Zaricznyj et al.[99] concluded that nonorganized or free-play sports produce a higher number of injuries than organized sports. However, Goldberg et al.[34] reported that almost half of their observed injury cases occurred under organized or adult-supervised conditions. Micheli[58] concludes that evidence does not currently exist that convincingly answers the question of which condition, organized versus nonorganized, creates a greater threat of injury to the young athlete. Each condition seems to have its own peculiar risks. Micheli,[58] for example, suspects that adult supervision has brought about a higher incidence of repetitive overuse injuries in some organized sports, such as gymnastics, swimming, and running. Since overuse injuries do not appear in free-play situations,[58] they may instead be associated with the presence of competitive adult-supervised programs.

One explanation for the apparent relationship between organized programs and overuse injuries is the emphasis often placed on winning. The risks of injury to young athletes can be no greater than when the fundamental reasons for participation become obscured. For sports programs involving young athletes, winning should remain a contest objective; however, healthy recreation, social learning experiences, and wholesome competition should be the participant objectives.[54] Responsible sports programs for youths have objectives that place the participant first so that if the contest and participant objectives become incompatible, the participants' needs would prevail.

Moreover, when the participant objectives become obscured, the available sports medicine and sports science research has been reported to be underused.[54] Solutions to important questions that have already been systematically determined may not be found when an appraisal of the problem has been based on unclear objectives. Similarly, new research can also become stymied when it is based on invalid assumptions about the purpose of participation.

One way that organized sports appear safer than nonorganized sports has been by reducing the risk of growth plate injuries. Micheli[58] observed that only one third of growth plate injuries in his patients occurred in organized sports, and of those the causative factors were usually macrotrauma injuries resulting from activities such as cross-body blocking in football and sliding in baseball (Fig. 25-10). An organized sports program has a clear advantage over a free-play situation in these instances, because when the cause of an injury is known and the number of incidences seems excessive, an organized program can make appropriate rule changes or require safety equipment.

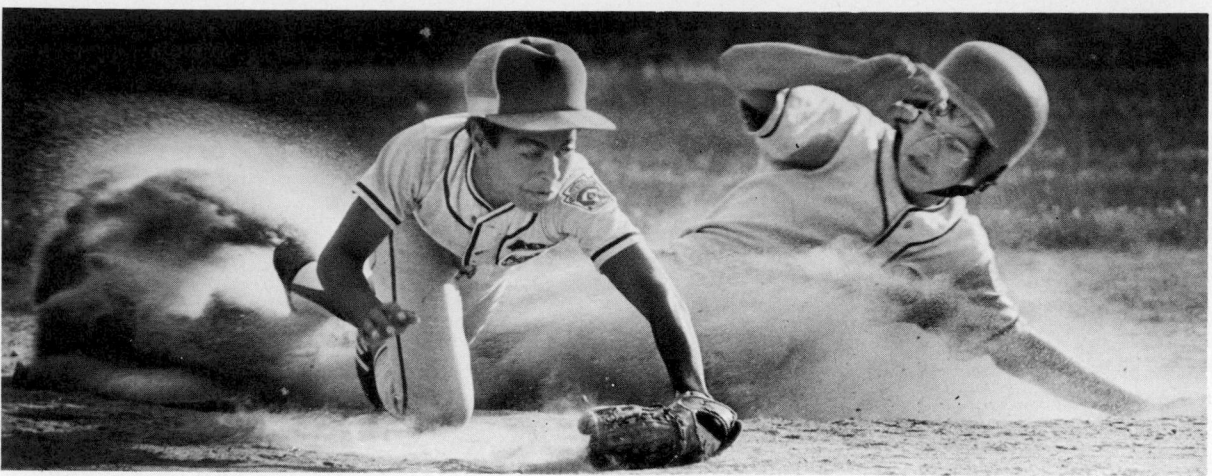

Fig. 25-10. Sliding in baseball increases risk of injury for adolescents.

Rule changes. Within organized sports rule changes have effectively reduced the number of athletic injuries in various sports. In football, for example, some rule changes that have reduced the incidence of injury have included (1) the 1975 blocking and tackling restrictions set by the National Collegiate Athletic Association and the National Federation of High School Athletic Associations in response to improper uses of the helmet[1]; (2) the 1975 ruling to eliminate spearing, which alleviated the prevalence of serious neck injuries; and (3) in 1977 and 1980 rule changes that protected offensive linemen by permitting them the added use of their hands and arms.[1] Further, because cross-body blocking accounts for an excessive number of knee injuries in football, it seems appropriate to consider rule changes to eliminate this activity in games involving growing athletes and to monitor the effects.

Rule changes have also reduced the number of baseball injuries. Little-leaguer's elbow in 8- to 14-year-old children prompted early restrictions, which limited the number of innings pitched to six and required a minimum of 3 days' rest between appearances.[46] Today's sliding injuries might also be avoidable with rule changes, but the popularity of this action may be problematic for those concerned with how this might affect the nature of the game. Organized programs, however, can offer alternative solutions as well, such as using safety equipment (to be discussed).

Regarding gymnastics, rule changes could be an appropriate way to avoid injuries in this sport. For example, since the presence of spotters is not permitted during competition without incurring a point deduction, the use of well-trained spotters to reduce injuries has been recommended.[66] Discriminate use of rule changes should always be a consideration, since it has been shown to effectively reduce or avoid injuries in organized sports. Importantly, when rule changes have been made, the participant has been afforded protection, whereas in most instances the nature of the sport affected has remained unchanged.[99]

Safety equipment. Another advantage of organized programs is the potential for the proper use of equipment. When available protective safety equipment is used either improperly or not at all, the incidence of sports injuries increases.[34,74] Since many young athletes show a disinterest in both the fitting and the care of their safety equipment,[3] properly administered sports programs can reduce injuries by requiring that the athletes wear necessary and appropriate equipment.

Equipment adjustments have effectively reduced the incidence of injuries in young athletes. In young skiers, for example, although the ankle remains a frequently injured region, attention to better-fitting boots, shorter, easily controlled skis, and properly adjusted bindings has substantially reduced the incidence of ankle injuries.[31,32] Nevertheless, across sports, injuries continue to occur that could be avoided by alterations in the available safety equipment.

Soft, thin floor mats are important contributors to the incidence of elbow injuries in young female gymnasts.[66,73] Roy et al.[70] state that with weight bearing by the upper extremity, soft mats exaggerate dorsiflexion of the wrist and contribute to the stress changes of the distal radial epiphysis in gymnasts; they therefore recommend firmer mats. Priest and Weise[66] also conclude that mats add to the incidence of elbow injuries, although they recommend using firmer but thicker mats. Regardless of the mat modification, attention to the type of mat seems key to controlling the growing number of severe elbow injuries that occur when the arm bears weight in gymnastics, since intrinsic structural characteristics of the skeletally immature female gymnast cannot be controlled.

In baseball (including softball) breakaway bases may prove to reduce the high incidence of ankle sprains and hand fractures caused by sliding. Researchers at the University of Michigan reported a sevenfold reduction of sliding injuries when breakaway bases were used.[67] Again, because an extrinsic risk factor was identified and controlled, fewer injuries resulted. Further, this suggests that strategies that use extrinsic-factor interventions may more adequately control macrotrauma injuries.

Finally, equipment interventions may be the best alternative to the problem of baseball-related deaths, since the cause of death is usually a macrotrauma injury and safety equipment protects inexperienced athletes from their own bad decisions. According to a recent study of baseball and softball injuries by the U.S. Consumer Product and Safety Commission, most deaths occur when children are struck by balls.[74] Over a 10-year period 51 baseball-related deaths were reported to have occurred in 5- to 14-year-old children; and in 20 of the cases death was caused by a fatal impact from a ball to the chest. It was determined that deaths occurred because currently available safety equipment was not worn or equipment required for games was not used during practice. Organized programs must enforce the use of available safety equipment and periodically evaluate the need for new equipment, such as chest protectors for young batters, if vulnerable children are to be protected from unpredictable events, which have tragic consequences.

Although some risk factors related to sports organizations have been discussed here, others that may be of greater consequence have been omitted. In general, however, sports organizations have varied risk factors and differ in their ability to ensure safe athletic conditions, because they also vary in their purpose and resources. From well-intended, noncompetitive sports organizations to some exploitive, highly competitive ones, injury risk factors exist. The seriousness of the risks, however, is directly related to the contact nature of the sport, the level of competition, and the vulnerability of the athlete. It would be unrealistic for us to categorically prevent children from competing in a sport, but because of the young athlete's unique vulnerability, careful measures regarding how the sport is organized must be pursued to ensure the athlete's safety.

Supervision. Without responsible supervision a young athlete's risk of injury increases. Supervision becomes responsible when it adapts to the needs and capabilities of growing children. Because we better understand these needs and capabilities as well as the factors that cause the injuries, persons involved in three key supervisory areas— medicine (physicians and health care professionals), coaching, and parenting—should either assume greater responsibility for reducing injuries or accept the responsibility for the consequences.

Medical supervision. Although a growing number of young athletes are sustaining musculoskeletal injuries in competitive sports, growth of medical supervision has not been commensurate. Ironically, youth sports have fewer available trained medical supervisors (physicians, physical therapists, or athletic trainers) than are at the high school and college levels, despite the young athlete's unique predisposition to musculoskeletal injury.[3,13,46,47] Reducing a young athlete's risks of incurring musculoskeletal injuries begins therefore with medical supervision that (1) should minimally include musculoskeletal evaluations and (2) ensures adequate attendance of medical specialists games and practices.

Preparticipation physical examination. Most organized sports involving young athletes require a preparticipation physical examination. Although the content, format, and quality of musculoskeletal examinations vary considerably, the fundamental objectives of every preparticipation musculoskeletal examination should include (1) screening for predisposing structural conditions, (2) assessing the physical maturation, (3) identifying the rehabilitation needs, and (4) determining the physical fitness.[13,47]

Preparticipation examinations are often conducted en masse; that is, large numbers of athletes are screened over a short time. This format offers several advantages, including cost-effectiveness and efficiency, but because of their cursory nature the musculoskeletal physical examinations are not known to provide sufficient information for developing comprehensive rehabilitation plans. Moreover, Blum[13] states that with mass screening, it is typically the history rather than the physical examination that reveals the predisposing factors. This is regrettable because physical examinations offer unique opportunities to assess the status of previously injured musculoskeletal tissues, such as the presence of inflammation; the tissue stage of healing; areas of tenderness; loss of tissue extensibility; and movements that are painful, restricted, or weak. Therefore the trend should be away from mass screening of the neophyte athlete with a previous injury.[46] Comprehensive musculoskeletal evaluation of the previously injured athlete and thoughtful rehabilitation planning if required could prove to be the most effective means for controlling injuries to young athletes.

A last word is individualized examinations irrespective of a previously incurred injury. Mass evaluations also limit dialog and the extent to which the athletes become active in their own health care. Discussion with the young athlete could foster this and could provide the medical supervisor time to consider the child's emotional state. Coddington and Troxell[21] reported that an athlete's mental state affects the risk of sustaining an injury. Individualized evaluations, although more costly and less efficient, could offer young athletes the opportunity to share their feelings and apprehensions with a good listener.

SCREENING. When sports are pursued competitively, the first objective of screening young athletes for musculoskeletal conditions is important because of the risks imposed on immature structures (i.e., articular cartilage, apophyses, and growth plates), postural deviations, and undetected congenital defects. Previous sections on structural conditions have documented the unique and potentially vulnerable musculoskeletal tissues of growing children. Further, postural deviations have been reported to occur frequently in children. For example, because of the high incidence of musculoskeletal deviations in the 4,670 children they screened, Francis and Bryce[29] reported an apparent need for uniform screening examinations for all children. The argument is obviously stronger when the children are engaged in competitive sports.

Effective screening for those musculoskeletal conditions that predispose young athletes to injuries requires qualified medical supervision. Physicians and health care professionals who are qualified are knowledgeable of the musculoskeletal conditions that are unique to young persons. They are familiar with the current epidemiological information that describes by sport, age, and sex the incidence of specific injuries and the areas of the body affected. Further, qualified medical supervisors have sports medicine training and experience with young athletes and their chosen sport. Effective screening therefore has available qualified medical supervisors who, because of their specialized knowledge, are sensitive to the conditions and risk factors of the young athlete.

ASSESSMENT OF PHYSICAL MATURATION. The purpose of assessing physical maturation of young athletes is to primarily allow the physician to determine the likelihood that the child's present stage of physical maturation increases the young athlete's chances of being injured or of injuring others. With this information the physician can recommend to the program supervisors, coach, and parents an appropriate matching with other participants. Occasionally it may be necessary to restrict or disqualify a child whose present physical stature would unreasonably jeopardize the child's safe participation in a contact sport.

REHABILITATION NEEDS. The third objective of identifying the rehabilitation needs of young athletes is perhaps the single most significant way to reduce the athlete's risk of injury. There is strong evidence that many musculoskeletal injuries are caused by inadequate rehabilitation of a previous injury.[13,34,47] Linder et al.[47] screened 1,268 young athletes and reported that about 14% had past joint problems. Goldberg et al.[34] investigated the causes of children's sports injuries and reported that more than 23% resulted from lack of rehabilitation. In his review of adolescent athletes with injuries, Blum[13] reported that rehabilitation was ordered in fewer than half of the cases in which it was needed. Because reinjury is so common in young athletes, it has been said that careful evaluation of previous sites of injury is therefore critical.[13]

Despite the strong need for rehabilitation of previous injuries in young athletes, the youngest are the least likely to benefit from it.[34] Moreover, evidence shows rehabilitation is ordered less often for more severe injuries, which are likely to require more rehabilitation.[34] In one study of 51 sports injuries in children, it was reported that 60% of patients with spine injuries and about 67% of patients with fractures had no rehabilitation.[34]

DETERMINING PHYSICAL FITNESS. The final essential objective of a preparticipation examination is to determine a child's physical fitness for participation and includes such criteria as strength, power, endurance, ability, and flexibility.[13] Rarely, however, do young athletes receive the benefit of qualified athletic trainers, physical educators, physical therapists, or strength coaches with training in these areas.[2] Smilkstein's[84] investigation of preparticipation examinations revealed that the principal deficiency of the physical examination was that it was structured for the nonathlete. If preparticipation examinations are to realize their full potential in preventing injuries, the examination must assess the young athlete's readiness for withstanding the physical demands of a particular sport.

As suggested earlier, evidence shows that deficiencies in musculoskeletal strength, power, and endurance predispose an athlete to injury,[8,44,59,81] and since training gains in young athletes are attainable, it becomes important to determine these deficiencies so that appropriate training can follow. Similarly, flexibility deficiencies have also been attributed to corresponding risks of injury, although findings to support this have been equivocal. For example, Jackson[40] reported no significant relationship between flexibility and joint injuries among 2,300 West Point cadets. Further, it can be argued that flexibility and "maximal" strength are incompatible.[38] This investigator knows of no studies in children that report any meaningful relationship between flexibility and injuries.

There are, however, at least two situations where determining the flexibility of young athletes provides vital information that relates to their risk of injury. The first is when the child has a growth spurt (described earlier). In this situation it is important to recognize that any association with injury could be due to the vulnerability of the tissues rather than the loss of flexibility itself. Moreover, the associated loss of flexibility may actually provide (1) the tissues with some necessary movement restriction, which may be a protective mechanism rather than a risk factor, and (2) a mechanical-compressive stimulus to the articular surfaces and epiphyses that promotes their growth and maturation. Whatever the true purpose, the loss of flexibility occurs at a time when the athlete's involvement in a contact sport may be inappropriate because stresses then become excessive.

The second situation in which determination of the flexibility in a young athlete becomes important is when it is associated with an asymmetry. When asymmetrical flexibility is present, the underlying problem is usually one of alignment. Identification of these asymmetries in flexibility is important, because alignment disorders have been reported to result in overuse injuries.[56]

Flexibility is therefore an important criterion to include in preparticipation examinations of young athletes, because it can be an indicator of growth spurt activity or can serve to alert for alignment disorders. Unlike other fitness criteria, however, flexibility deficiencies do not warrant remedial attention directed at the deficiency. On the contrary, the loss of flexibility should signal a possible need to either restrict a rapidly growing child from activity or assess further the child's alignment. In fact, stretching of the apparently limited tissues would be inappropriate.

Also, most flexibility tests used are generally quick measures of functional capabilities rather than selective procedures that use sound biomechanical or kinesiological approaches to differentiate contractile tissues from noncontractile tissues, or one contractile structure from another. The significance of flexibility as a risk factor of injuries in young athletes will not be known until true flexibility deficiencies are distinguished from apparent deficiencies caused by alignment disorders, and until the tests used are specific.

Medical coverage. In addition to musculoskeletal examinations, young athletes should be provided adequate medical coverage. Since competitive sports increase the chances of injuries occurring, medical supervision must be ready when injuries occur. *Adequate medical coverage* is defined as (1) the availability during games and practices of a medical supervisor who is competent in the care of athletic injuries and (2) a plan to manage the injuries that specifies a procedure for returning the young athlete to participation.[2,46]

Medical coverage for young athletes must address the same details that are the hallmarks of medical supervision for adults. Nevertheless, since children are more vulnerable to injury and depend on adult supervision to ensure their safety, the medical coverage of young athletes should not seek to replicate adult models of medical coverage. After an injury, for example, the onset of swelling in an adult joint might permit an immediate return to participation for this athlete; however, a young athlete with a similar swelling response should be restricted from playing until a growth plate injury has been ruled out. Moreover, a child lacks an adult's experience in determining when an injury is serious. Children therefore should never be encouraged to play when in pain because their judgments related to the severity of their injuries cannot be relied on. Consequently, medical coverage of young athletes is responsible when it acknowledges the vulnerability of children and adapts its coverage with appropriate restrictions and when it pursues conservative management that minimizes the effects of external risk factors.

Unfortunately, most game coverage and first-aid responsibilities provided to young athletes are assumed by coaches or parents with little or no training.[2] It is therefore not surprising that adult-supervised programs are no safer than free-play situations (as reported earlier), since medi-

cal supervision has not been assigned to trained individuals. Further, Goldberg et al.[34] have reported that adult supervision was not associated with prompt referrals for medical care, immediate withdrawal from participation, or a physician's clearance to resume participation despite indications for these.[34] Consequently, experts have agreed that the medical coverage of young athletes would be greatly enhanced by the services of trained medical supervisors such as certified athletic trainers or sports physical therapists.[2,34,46]

Organized youth programs should not begin competitive sports programs unless adequate medical supervision can be provided.[2,68] But because of the growing number of young athletes involved in competitive sports who are at risk of injury from external risk factors, there remains a need for greater support of trained health professionals with knowledge and interest in this undersupervised population.

Coaching. Responsible coaching still plays a vital role in preventing musculoskeletal injuries in young athletes.[2,22] Coaching is responsible when the best interests of the athletes are served, when winning is not at the expense of safety, and when young athletes are recognized for being children, not for being athletes.[44] Most coaches of youth sports are volunteers who lack knowledge of prevention, recognition, or treatment of musculoskeletal injuries.[44] Therefore, as more children compete in sports and are exposed to forces that can place extraordinary stresses on their growing tissues, coaches must be concerned with more than skill and strength development; they must assume a greater responsibility for reducing the young athletes' risks of injury.[96]

Because coaching young athletes does not require a knowledge of the risk factors that predispose these athletes to specific injuries, avoidable risks are often ignored.[44] For example, if all coaches were aware of the number of deaths in children who were struck by a ball, available safety equipment would be used more often. Also, Roy et al.[13] state that if coaches are warned of the incidence of wrist epiphyses injuries and if they establish channels of communications with physicians, then early symptoms of wrist pain can be investigated sooner and the likelihood of the gymnast sustaining a career-threatening stress change (as seen on roentgenograms) can be avoided. Regarding growth plate injuries in general, Jackson[39] has stated that the key to preventing their occurrence in young athletes is through mature, responsible, and reasonable coaching. Moreover, when injuries repeat or increase in incidence, it is a function of responsible coaching to analyze the causes and develop preventative strategies.[46]

When injuries do occur, the coach of a young athlete may need to decide if the child's (or adolescent's) removal from play is warranted. Because of the young athlete's vulnerability, coaches in this situation should restrict the child from further play when the injury initially necessitated the young athlete's removal from play. Further, whenever a youth coach is unsure of the serious nature of musculoskeletal injuries, the athlete should be referred to a physician. Coaching of young athletes therefore is responsible when it relies on competent medical care when an injury occurs (Fig. 25-11).

Skill development. Skill development is necessary in all sports, and when it is lacking in young athletes, it has been shown to be a risk factor that contributes to the incidence of injury.[34,53,58,63] Accordingly, when young athletes have the necessary skills, their chances of being injured are reduced.[46] Because coaching is principally responsible for skill development, it can therefore have its greatest influence on the incidence of injuries in young athletes by selecting and teaching skills that are appropriate.

The selection of appropriate skills for children should be based on knowledge of the sport activities that most often contribute to injuries. For example, because head and neck injuries in football are associated with tackling, and because sliding accounts for many of the injuries that occur in baseball, greater attention to skill development

should be devoted to these activities. Also, with highly skilled noncontact sports, which require repetitive training (such as gymnastics or swimming), the coaching has been reported to be a critical factor in the young athlete's risk of injury.[58] Moreover, the younger the athlete, the more necessary the emphasis on proper skills.

But the selection and teaching of skills must go beyond knowing which activities cause injuries; coaches must then consider the maturational levels of young athletes and adapt their training skills accordingly. Coaches who are more acquainted with the growth characteristics of children will have more reasonable expectations regarding the performance capabilities of young athletes.[83] Modifying the skills to these performance capabilities will foster the learning of the techniques and, perhaps more important, provide maturing musculoskeletal tissues with low-intensity stimuli that would permit them to gradually accommodate the greater demands of the sport for which they were intended.[90]

Strength training. A final contributing risk factor concerning coaching relates to strength training. As stated earlier, it is generally accepted that strength training has been

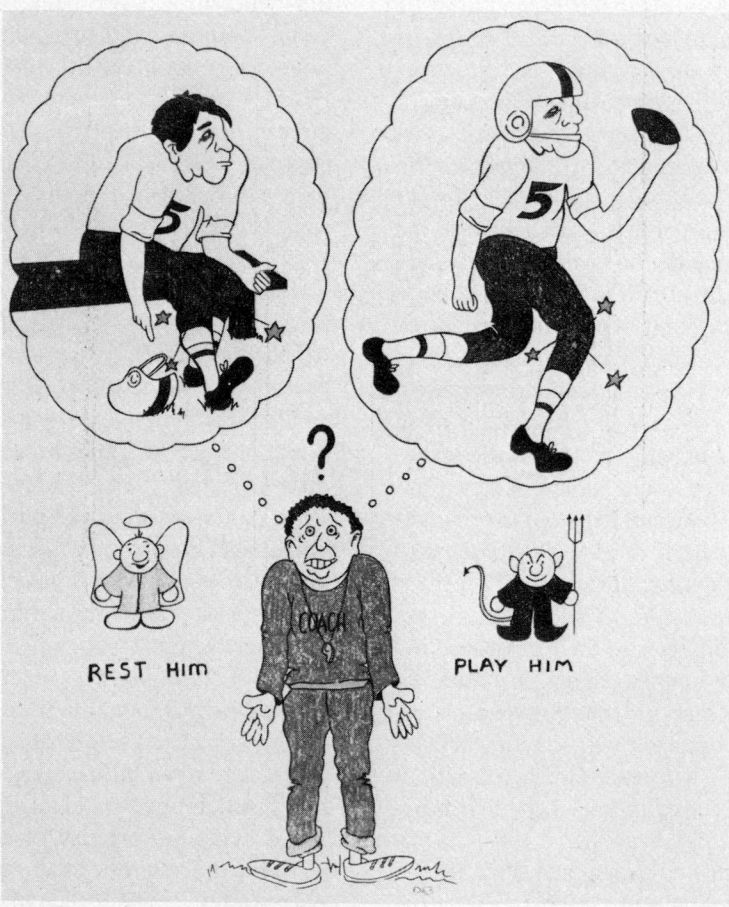

Fig. 25-11. Because of the child athlete's vulnerability, a good coach should restrict playing the injured athlete despite the emotions involved.

shown to reduce injuries in young athletes.[57,59] However, lack of supervision and the limited knowledge of coaches have resulted in injuries to young athletes who are training, ironically, to avoid injuries.[44] Coaching of the young athlete must consider methods of strengthening the athlete's musculoskeletal structure. However, as with teaching skills, responsible coaching requires (1) a knowledge of which injuries are associated with the sport, (2) an understanding of the maturational capabilities of children, and (3) a strategy for modifying the training activities to the needs of the young athlete.

Coaches should know the strength demands of a sport and use training methods that stimulate the movement requirements of the sport.[69] The high incidence of ankle injuries in basketball, soccer, and other sports merits coaching strategies for strengthening this region's musculoskeletal structure.[85] Because these collagen tissues are anisotropic, strengthening activities for preventing ankle sprains should include a variety of mechanical stimuli that would adequately prepare the ankle for the sudden inversion movement that typically produces this injury.

Strengthening ankles of young athletes then might include an activity such as walking on an inverted ankle. This may disturb some readers concerned that this could irreversibly stretch the supporting noncontractile structures on the lateral aspect of the foot. However, since this extreme range is where the injury occurs, it is reasonable to direct gradual stress to the tissues in this position. The eccentric contraction of the peroneal musculature and associated connective tissue hypertrophy could provide these tissues with added capabilities to withstand the stresses of the sport. Variation of the activity, such as rolling in and out to the end of range with gradual amounts of weight bearing, is recommended.

Similar attention should be directed to other sports that demonstrate regional predispositions to injury. Maroon et al.,[53] for example, have stated that strengthening the neck musculature in young athletes before participation in football is essential for preventing catastrophic injuries to this region. Wrist injuries in gymnastics and upper extremity injuries in young children in general require careful consideration of strength-training techniques that would adequately prepare these tissues for the demands of this sport.

Because an effective strength-training program should accomplish its goals without increasing the chance of injury to the individual, it is necessary for coaches, accepting the responsibility of strength training, to understand the maturational capabilities of the young athlete. Decisions regarding appropriate strength-training methods should also be based on a coach's understanding of how subgroups of children differ regarding susceptibility of their structure and the variations of musculoskeletal maturation.

Micheli,[58] for example, reported on the utility of distinguishing between the pubescent (onset of secondary sex characteristics; growth spurt period) and the prepubescent athlete. Because age considerations do affect strength gains, as reported earlier, prepubescent athletes cannot be expected, regardless of their size, to train with heavy resistance. Conversely, pubescent athletes may be more susceptible to growth plate injuries because of their rapidly changing epiphyses. Also, differences in strength between pubescent females and males should be considered, whereas this is not a meaningful consideration in prepubescent athletes. Last, regarding maturational variation, is the need to realize, aside from subgroup considerations, that existing individual maturational variations warrant individualized strength-training approaches.

Finally, strategies for strengthening young athletes to ensure their safety must be modified accordingly. Strength training in young athletes operates on the same principles as those for adults except that it should be adapted to the needs of the child and, above all else, cause no harm. In general, experts recommend that strengthening programs for young athletes emphasize technique and are short, simple, and fun.[12,44,81]

Strength-training activities that are recommended use a low resistance that gradually increases and avoid maximal lifting activities.[12,81] Emphasis on large muscle groups should be considered, with the activity usually designed to complete a full controlled range of motion. Variation of activities provides a variety of musculoskeletal tissue responses and serves to motivate the participant and make the program enjoyable.

Although alternatives to external resistance, such as plyometric training, are recommended, resistance training using external weight, as reported earlier, has been shown to be safe and to reduce injuries in young athletes.[8,17,57,94] Injuries to the wrist and low back, which have been reported in pubescent males training with free weights, could have been avoided if the weight-training activities had been modified to the athlete. Since overhead lifts seem to play a role in these injuries, Micheli[59] has recommended that young athletes training with weights avoid standing lifts and that they do curls and standing lifts from a seated position. Wrist epiphyseal fractures can be avoided if lighter weight is used and the activities are better supervised.[59,76] Coaching supervision of the strength training of athletes cannot expect to maximize the conditions for seeking strength gains unless it first minimizes the unnecessary contributing risk factors.

Parents. The ultimate responsibility for ensuring the safety of a young athlete rests with an athlete's parents. Traditionally, responsible parents have supported the development of competitive sports programs for children perhaps because of their sense that competition promotes physical, psychological, and social maturation of the child.[69] Parents should, however, recognize that the bene-

---

Bill of right for young athletes

1. Right of the opportunity to participate in sports regardless of ability level
2. Right to participate at a level that is commensurate with each child's developmental level
3. Right to have qualified adult leadership
4. Right to participate in safe and healthy environments
5. Right of each child to share in the leadership and decision making of their sport participation
6. Right to play as a child and not as an adult
7. Right to proper preparation for participation in the sport
8. Right to an equal opportunity to strive for success
9. Right to be treated with dignity by all involved
10. Right to have fun through sport

From Singer RN: Different strokes for different folks: teaching skills to kids. In JT Thomas, editor: Youth sports guide for coaches and parents, Washington, DC, 1977, Manufacturers Life Insurance Co.

fits of athletic competition are likely to be offset, sooner or later, by a musculoskeletal injury.

Further, parents should not assume that their child's participation in an organized program ensures high-quality supervision. Since most adult supervision of youth sport programs is provided by well-intended volunteers, parents can best be assured of a safe program by establishing ongoing and frequent dialog with their child, through periodic interaction with the supervisory personnel, and by maintaining an unobtrusive vigilance that assumes nothing.

Because children vary greatly in their physical maturation, there can be no best age to recommend that the child begin a competitive program. This decision begins with establishing the child's interest in playing but requires careful scrutiny of the contributing risks of injury. The accompanying box, Bill of Rights for Young Athletes, offers parents and other adult supervisors a means of appraising the purpose of an athletic program for young athletes and its concern for every child.

SUMMARY

The incidence of injuries to young athletes is growing; different populations of children competing in sports are being injured; the types of injuries incurred by these athletes are changing; more sports of a noncontact nature are accounting for a greater number of injuries; and more factors are contributing to the growing number of injuries to young athletes. Although these findings signify new trends in the arenas of youth sports, higher injury rates have not been reported and so these trends may not suggest a worsening problem. Furthermore, occurrences of injuries in young athletes are no longer viewed as evidence to ex-clude children from competition but have instead resulted in recommendations centered on how to ensure the safety of young athletes.

Sports-related injury in any population will never be eliminated, but investigations can provide valid data that could identify injury trends and the populations at risk.[61] Epidemiological data have shaped our understanding of the existing risk factors, as well as their interactions, and provide insight into the causes of injuries to young athletes. Also, the expanding body of knowledge related to the structure and function of maturing musculoskeletal tissues augments our ability to explain and predict the effects that sport activities have on these tissues.

Recent studies have contributed greatly to our understanding that young athletes are a population at risk. Moreover, despite the constantly changing contributing factors, experts have devised strategies and constructed models that will permit ongoing analysis of youth sport injuries.[16,58] Dissemination of new knowledge must keep pace with this knowledge, and a greater commitment to providing additional resources is needed if unnecessary injuries to young athletes are to be avoided.

REFERENCES

1. Albright JP, et al: Head and neck injuries in college football: An eight-year analysis, Am J Sports Med 13:147-152, 1985.
2. American Academy of Pediatrics: Injuries to young athletes, Physician Sportsmed 9:107-108, 1981.
3. American Academy of Pediatrics: Competitive sports for children of elementary school age, Physician Sportsmed 9:140-142, 1981.
4. American Academy of Pediatrics: Risks in long-distance running for children, Physician Sportsmed 10:82-83, 1982.
5. American Academy of Pediatrics, Committee on Sportsmedicine: Weight training and weight lifting: Information for the pediatrician, Physician Sportsmed 11:157-161, 1983.
6. Antich TJ and Clive EB: Osgood-Schlatter disease: Review of the literature and physical therapy management, J Orthop Sports Phys Ther 7:5-10, 1985.
7. Antich TJ and Lombardo SJ: Clinical presentation of Osgood-Schlatter disease in the adolescent population, J Orthop Sports Phys Ther 7:1-4, 1985.
8. Arheim DD: Modern principles of athletic training, St Louis, 1985, The CV Mosby Co, pp 78-149.
9. Asmussen E: Growth in muscular strength and power. In Rarick GL, editor: Physical activity human growth and development, New York, 1973, Academic Press, pp 60-79.
10. Barnes L: Preadolescent training—How young is too young? Physician Sportsmed 7:114-119, 1979.
11. Benton J: Epiphyseal fracture in sports, Physician Sportsmed 10:63-71, 1982.
12. Bjornaraa BS: Flexibility and strength training considerations for young athletes, National Strength Condition Assoc J 4:62-63, 1982.
13. Blum RW: Preparticipation evaluation of the adolescent athlete, Postgrad Med 78:52-67, 1985.
14. Brady TA, Cahill B, and Bodnar L: Weight training related injuries, Am J Sports Med 10:1-5, 1982.
15. Brighton CT: Structure and function of the growth plate, Clin Orthod Rel Res 136:22-32, 1978.
16. Brown EW: Study of injury mechanisms in youth sports. in Brown EW and Branta CF, editors: Competitive sports for children and youth, Champaign, Ill, 1988, Human Kinetics Books, pp 107-113.

17. Cahill BR and Griffith EH: Effect of preseason conditioning on the incidence and severity of high school knee injures, Am J Sports Med 6:180-184, 1978.
18. Caine DJ and Lindner KJ: Growth plate injury: A threat to young distance runners? Physician Sportsmed 12:118-124, 1984.
19. Caine DJ and Lindner KJ: Overuse injuries of growing bones: The young female gymnast at risk? Physician Sportsmed 13:52-62, 1985.
20. Chambers RB: Orthopedic injuries in athletes (ages 6 to 17), Am J Sports Med 7:195-197, 1979.
21. Coddington RD and Troxell JR: The effect of emotional factors on football injury rates—A pilot study, J Human Stress Dec:3-5, 1980.
22. Collins HR and Evarts CM: Injuries to the adolescent athlete, Postgrad Med 49:72-78, 1971.
23. Costain R and Williams AK: Isokinetic quadriceps and hamstring torque levels of adolescent, female soccer players, J Orthod Sports Phys Ther 5:196-200, 1984.
24. Dehaven KE: Athletic injuries in adolescents, Pediatr Ann 7:96-119, 1978.
25. Dehaven KE, Dolan WA, and Mayer PJ: Chondromalacia patellae and the painful knee, Am Family Phys 21:117-124, 1980.
26. Dehaven DE and Lintner DM: Athletic injuries: Comparison by age, sport, and gender, Am J Sports Med 14:218-224, 1986.
27. Fairbanks LL: Return to sports participation, Physician Sportsmed 7:71-74, 1979.
28. Falkner F and Tanner JM: Human growth—Postnatal growth, New York, 1978, Plenum Press.
29. Francis RS and Bryce GR: Screening for musculoskeletal deviations—A challenge for the physical therapist, Phys Ther 67:1221-1225, 1987.
30. Fulkerson JP: The etiology of patellofemoral pain in young active patients: A prospective study, Clin Orthop Rel Res 179:129-133, 1983.
31. Garrick JG: Symposium on ankle and foot problems in the athlete. Epidemiologic perspective. Clin Sports Med 1:13-18, 1982.
32. Garrick JG and Requa RK: Injury patterns in children and adolescent skiers, Am J Sports Med 7:245-248, 1979.
33. Godshall RW, Hansen CA, and Rising DC: Stress fractures through the distal femoral epiphysis in athletes, Am J Sports Med 9:114-116, 1981.
34. Goldberg B, et al: Children's sports injuries: Are they avoidable? Physician Sportsmed 7:93-101, 1979.
35. Goldberg MJ: Gymnastic injuries, Orthop Clin North Am 2:717-726, 1980.
36. Grana WA and Rashkin A: Pitcher's elbow in adolescents, Am J Sports Med 8:333-336, 1980.
37. Hoshina H: Spondylolysis in young athletes, Physician Sportsmed 8:75-79, 1980.
38. Hettinga DL: Inflammatory responses of synovial joint structures. In Gould JA and Davies GJ, editors: Orthopedic and sports physical therapy, St Louis, 1985, The CV Mosby Co.
39. Jackson DW: Low back pain in young athletes: Evaluation of stress reaction and discogenic problems, Am J Sports Med 7:364-366, 1979.
40. Jackson DW, et al: Injury prediction in the young athlete: A preliminary report, Am J Sports Med 6:6-14, 1978.
41. Jackson DW, et al: Stress reactions involving the pars interarticularis in young athletes, Am J Sports Med 9:304-312, 1981.
42. Kamel M and Rosman M: Disc protrusion in the growing child, Clin Orthod Rel Res 165:46-52, 1984.
43. Kessler RM and Herftling D: Management of common musculoskeletal disorders, Philadelphia, 1983, Harper & Row, pp 107-114.
44. Koz B and Lord RM: Overuse injury in the young athlete, Physician Sportsmed 2:116-122, 1983.
45. Kraemer WJ: The adolescent athlete: Sports performance and specificity of training, Natl Strength Conditioning Assoc J 7:65-66, 1985.
46. Larson RL: Physical activity and the growth and development of bone and joint structures. In Rarick GL, editor: Physical activity human growth and development, New York, 1973, Academic Press, pp 32-59.
47. Linder CW, et al: Preparticipation health screening of young athletes, Am J Sports Med 9:187-193, 1981.
48. Lopez R and Pruett DM: The child runner, J Phys Ed Rec Dance 53:78-81, 1981.
49. Macdougall JD: Morphological changes in human skeletal muscle following strength training and immobilization. In Jones NL and McComas AJ, editors: Human muscle power, Champaign, Ill, 1986, Human Kinetics, Inc, pp 269-285.
50. Malina RM: Exercises as an influence upon growth: Review and critique of current concepts, Clin Pediatr 8:16-26, 1969.
51. Malina RM and Rarick GL: Growth physique and motor performance. In Rarick GL, editor: Physical activity human growth and development, New York, 1973, Academic Press, pp 125-153.
52. Manzione M and Pizzutillo PD: Stress fracture of the schapoid waist: A case report, Am J Sports Med 9:268-269, 1981.
53. Maroon JC, Steele PB, and Berlin A: Football head and neck injuries—An update, Clin Neurosurg 27:414-429, 1980.
54. Martens R: Helping children become independent responsible adults through sports. In Brown EW and Branta CF, editors: Competitive sports for children and youth, Champaign, Ill, 1988, Human Kinetics Books, pp 297-308.
55. Micheli LJ: Low back pain in the adolescent: Differential diagnosis, Am J Sports Med 7:362-364, 1979.
56. Micheli LJ: Overuse injuries in children's sports: The growth factor, Orthod Clin North Am 14:337-360, 1983.
57. Micheli LJ: The prepubescent athlete: Physiological and orthopedic considerations for strengthening the prepubescent athlete, Natl Strength Conditioning Assoc J 7:26-27, 1985.
58. Micheli LJ: The incidence of injuries in children's sports: A medical perspective. In Brown EW and Branta CF, editors: Competitive sports for children and youth, Champaign, Ill, 1988, Human Kinetics Books, pp 279-284.
59. Micheli LJ: Strength training in the young athlete. In Brown EW and Branta CR, editors: Competitive sports for children and youth, Champaign, Ill, 1988, Human Kinetics Books, pp 99-105.
60. Micheli LJ and Santore R: Epiphyseal fractures of the elbow in children, Am Family Physician 22:107-116, 1980.
61. Mueller F and Blyth C: Epidemiology of sports injuries in children, Symposium on Pediatric and Adolescent Sports Medicine 1:343-352, 1982.
62. Murakami S and Nakajima H: Asceptic necrosis of the capitate bone in two gymnasts, Am J Sports Med 12:170-173, 1984.
63. Nilsson S and Rohas A: Soccer injuries in adolescents, Am J Sports Med 6:358-361, 1978.
64. Pappas AM: Epiphyseal injuries in sports, Physician Sportsmed 11:140-148, 1983.
65. Powers JA: Characteristic features of injuries in the knee in women, Clin Orthop Rel Res 143:120-124, 1979.
66. Priest JD and Weise DJ: Elbow injuries in women's gymnastics, Am J Sports Med 9:288-295, 1981.
67. Breakaway bases proposed to avoid softball injuries, PT Bull 3:3, 1988.
68. Rarick GL: Competitive sports in childhood and early adolescence. In Rarick GL, editor: Physical activity human growth and development, New York, 1973, Academic Press, pp 364-385.
69. Rarick GL and Seefeldt V: Characteristics of young athletes. In Thomas JR, editor: Youth sports guide for coaches and parents, Washington, DC, 1973, AAHPER, pp 24-44.
70. Read MT: Stress fractures of the distal radius in adolescent gymnasts, Br J Sports Med 15:272-276, 1981.
71. Reider B, Marshall JL, and Warren RF: Clinical characteristics of patellar disorders in young athletes, Am J Sports Med 9:270-274, 1981.

72. Riegger CL: Mechanical properties of bone. In Gould JA and Davies GJ, editors: Orthopedic and sports physical therapy, St Louis, 1985, The CV Mosby Co, pp 3-49.

73. Roy S, Caine D, and Singer KM: Stress changes of the distal radial epiphysis in young gymnasts, Am J Sports Med 13:301-308, 1985.

74. Rutherford GW, Kennedy J, and McGhee L: Baseball and softball related injuries to children 5-14 years of age, Washington, DC, 1984, US Consumer Product Safety Commission, Epidemiology, Division of Hazard Analysis.

75. Rutherford GW, et al: Overview of sports-related injuries to persons 5-14 years of age, Washington, DC, 1981, US Consumer Product Safety Commission, Divisions of Hazard Analysis and Human Factors.

76. Ryan JR and Salciccioli GG: Fractures of the distal radial epiphysis in adolescent weight lifters, Am J Sports Med 4:26-27, 1976.

77. Salter RB: Textbook of disorders and injuries of the musculoskeletal system, ed 2, Baltimore, 1983, Williams & Wilkins, pp 427-476.

78. Sapega AA and Nicholas JA: The clinical use of musculoskeletal profiling in orthopedic sports medicine, Physician Sportsmed 9:80-88, 1981.

79. Seefeldt V, et al: Physical characteristics of elite young distance runners. In Brown CW and Branta CF, editors: Competitive sports for children and youth, Champaign, Ill, 1988, Human Kinetics Books, pp 247-258.

80. Shaffer TE: The uniqueness of the young athlete: Introductory remarks, Am J Sports Med 8:370-371, 1980.

81. Shankman AG: The adolescent athlete: Special considerations in conditioning the young athlete, Natl Strength Conditioning Assoc J 7:52-53, 1985.

82. Shively RA, Grana WA, and Ellis D: High school sports injuries, Physician Sportsmed 9:46-50, 1981.

83. Singer KM and Roy SP: Osteochondrosis of the humeral capitellum, Am J Sports Med 12:351-360, 1984.

84. Smilkstein G: Health evaluations of high school athletes, Physician Sportsmed 9:73-81, 1981.

85. Smith RW and Reischl S: Treatment of ankle sprains in young athletes, Am J Sports Med 14:465-470, 1986.

86. Snook GA: Injuries in women's gymnastics: A perspective, Med Sci Sports Exerc 16:1-7, 1984.

87. Speer DP and Braun JK: The biomechanical basis of growth plate injuries, Physician Sportsmed 13:72-78, 1985.

88. Stanitski CL: Low back pain in young athletes, Physician Sportsmed 10:77-91, 1982.

89. Tanner JM: Fetus into man. Physical growth from conception to maturity, Cambridge, Mass, 1978, Harvard University Press.

90. Todd TW: Atlas of skeletal maturation, Part I, St Louis, 1937, The CV Mosby Co.

91. Totten L: The prepubescent athlete: Practical considerations in strengthening the prepubescent athlete, Natl Strength Conditioning Assoc J 8:38-39, 1986.

92. US Consumer Product Safety Commission Sports Estimates Reports, National Electronic Injury Surveillance System, 1986.

93. Walsh WM, Hunrman WW, and Shelton GL: Overuse injuries of the knee and spine in girls' gymnastics, Orthod Clin North Am 16:329-350, 1985.

94. Weltman A, et al: The effects of hydraulic resistance strength training in pre-pubertal males, Med Sci Sports Exerc 18:629-638, 1986.

95. Wilkins KE: The uniqueness of the young athlete: Musculoskeletal injuries, Am J Sports Med 8:377-385, 1980.

96. Williams JP: Wear and tear injuries in athletes/and overview, Br J Sports Med 12:211-214, 1979.

97. Wong JC and Gregg JR: Knee, ankle, and foot problems in the preadolescent and adolescent athlete, Clin Pediatr Med Surg 3:731-746, 1984.

98. Worrell RV: The physical development of the young athlete and competitive stress, Ct Med 43:286-288, 1979.

99. Zaricznyj B, et al: Sports-related injuries in school-aged children, Am J Sports Med 8:318, 1980.

Physical therapy in the workplace

Chapter 26

INDUSTRIAL PHYSICAL THERAPY: AN INTRODUCTION

Glenda L. Key

The industrial physical therapist comes to this field of specialization with very little in the literature for definition. Most programs and equipment that have been designed are based on individual experiences and reporting of what has worked and not worked. Because the field is still relatively new, it is difficult for many to recognize what benefits the approach offers. In addition to the specialization being new, very little information is available about the needs in the market that physical therapists are striving to serve.

A growing number of physical therapists are interested in providing services that help companies reach their goals of increasing productivity, returning the injured employees to work quickly and safely, and managing health care costs through programs of prevention.

In a 1988 survey of the membership of the Private Practice Section of the American Physical Therapy Association, 85% reported working more in industry and wellness programs compared with a survey conducted 3 years previously. Ninety-three percent also reported that their involvement in these programs is projected to increase.[16]

Major employers are finding that the use of physical therapists in a variety of functions allows the company to take better control over costs while reducing lost work time. A major brewing company saved $450,000 with its well-back programs, and another saved $154,000 with in-house rehabilitation. A missile company went from a $154,038 annual expenditure for back injuries to $49,911. This represents a 67.5% reduction following back injury prevention training.[22] A communications assembly company saved $1,290,000, representing a 91% decrease in incidence rate the year after upper extremity overuse syndrome prevention training.[10]

Historically, both the number of services available to industry and the therapist's knowledge of how to assist the employer have been limited.

The intent of this chapter is to provide the basic framework of industrial physical therapy, to review terminology, and to assist in program structure.

WORKER CARE SPECTRUM

As represented in Fig. 26-1, the medical community traditionally has become involved with the worker after the trauma has occurred. Therefore the expertise of the medi-

INDUSTRIAL THERAPY
WORKER CARE SPECTRUM

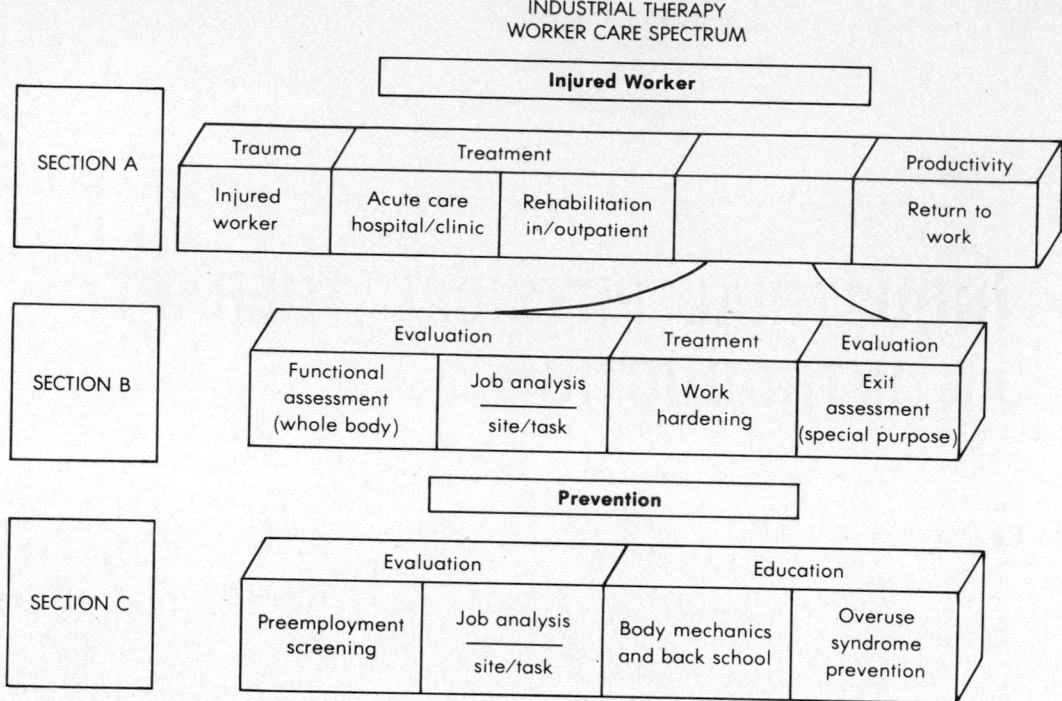

Fig. 26-1. Industrial therapy worker care spectrum. (From Key Functional Assessments, Inc., October 1988.)

cal professional has been primarily postinjury (Fig. 26-1, Section A). Acute care through a hospital or a clinic traditionally has been accepted as the first point of entry into the medical system following injury. If physical therapy treatment was identified as appropriate, it was during or after the acute stage and was provided through rehabilitation at in-patient or out-patient clinics.

The involvement of the medical community therefore has had a very narrow scope, focusing only on postinjury restoration. Rehabilitation has been raised to its highest capability and expressed in terms understood only by the medical community. These terms include *joint range of motion (ROM), muscular strength grades, axial rotations, musculotendinous flexibility, cardiovascular endurance,* and *kinesthetic awareness.* These terms, although understood by the *providers* of the services, were not necessarily understood by the recipients. To the health care providers they represent rates of recovery in impersonal measurable quantities. They do not provide information about what patients can do in relation to the activities of their lives. They do not translate into "functional" activities that are necessary to complete the tasks of work or leisure.

As a provider of patient care, the medical community has filled the need immediately following injury: acute injury treatment. The gap in the system, however, has been with the time between this acute treatment period and the point when the patient is returning to productive employment. This gap is now receiving considerable attention

from the medical community through various programs, including those in Section B of Fig. 26-1. In addition, increasing acceptance by the industrial and labor communities is manifest.

As noted in Fig. 26-1, Section B, functional assessments, job analyses, work hardening, and special purpose assessments are all part of industrial physical therapy and will be reviewed individually.

Section C of Fig. 26-1 represents the services that therapists provide to companies for the purpose of injury prevention. Historically, expertise used for restoration is the same expertise now being brought into use for prevention. Anatomical, physiological, and biomechanical principles must be understood, as well as the organ systems, body tissue responses, and effects of disease and trauma. All these factors are used in the industrial evaluations and training programs for prevention.

In Section C of Fig. 26-1, preemployment screening, job site analysis, job task analysis, and general rules of training programs are indicated as major components of prevention and will be reviewed throughout the chapter.

FUNCTIONAL ASSESSMENTS

Functional assessments (Fig. 26-1, Section B) in the specialization of industrial therapy are also known as *functional capacity assessments, physical capacity evaluations, worker assessments, functional capacity evaluations,* and *work capacity evaluations.* Until consistency of terminology has been reached, it is important that the therapist be very aware that even though the attempted goal may be the same for everyone, all approaches are not equal; nor do the end results always meet the intended goals. The end results, although expressed in similar terms, will not be of equal value.

The easiest way to define functional capacity assessments is to review the individual words.

1. *Functional:* Of or connected with the action for which a person or thing is specially fitted or used or for which a thing exists.[23] Therefore in using *functional* as a guide in assessment means that it must relate to the whole person. The therapist is no longer limiting the assessment to a joint, muscle, or singular body part. The focus is on the entire body and its *ability* level. The specific injury or disorder will have its effect on the ability level of the individual. With *functional* as the focus, one system may compensate for another system's dysfunction or weakness. It is a measure of the whole person's ability that is functional. After all, it is the whole body that goes back to work.

2. *Capacity:* Qualification, competency, power, or fitness; the ability to hold, receive, store, or accommodate. Maximum production or output.[23] The goal of capacity is to assess for maximum safe levels of ability in a number of activities. These activities include, but are not limited to, those of lifting, carrying, pushing, pulling, balancing, squatting, kneeling, crawling, and the tolerances to the time involved in each of these activities. Identifying capability levels has replaced the previous focus of identifying only limitations. As an example, lifting capabilities are now expressed to include details of height, distance, repetition, and posture involved in what one can accomplish. Previously, the recommendations may have been: "30 lb maximal lifting, no bending or stooping." In today's litigious society, that is no longer sufficient or acceptable. Capability information of the individual, of the whole body, is now desired, needed, and expected. The previous focus on limitations has given way to a focus on multiple determinations of *ability*.

3. *Assessment:* To make a valuation; to determine the importance or worth by careful study.[23] Therefore assessment is a valuation or a study of a person's capability level. Measurements must be taken and systematically analyzed against standards that are only now emerging. Assessment indicates a snapshot of how things are—not a pass/fail relationship, as would be reported in a test. Assessment also indicates the need for objectivity. The assessment is strictly one of gathering data, analyzing the data, and reporting this information and what it represents.

A review of the data maintained in the Key Functional Assessments, Inc., Data Back–Data Bank® reveals a comparative analysis of lifting capabilities between injured and uninjured auto mechanics (Fig. 26-2). Other statistics that can be retrieved from the data bank include personal demographics, such as education levels, height, weight, age, sex, and employment status.[7]

The functional capacity assessment is a standardized process that involves participation by the client. A form that can be used in summarizing a portion of the assessment valuation results is represented in Fig. 26-3, *A*.

The functional capacity assessment, as it will be referred to in this chapter, can be divided into four areas: (1) weighted capabilities, (2) tolerances, (3) participation level, and (4) postural examination. Postural examination will also be included secondarily in all loaded or weighted activities and in activities relating to tolerance.

WEIGHTED CAPABILITIES

When conducting a functional capacity assessment, it is essential that a person demonstrate work patterns that include transfer of materials having varying weights or resistance in the act of transfer. Therefore the examination must include what is termed *weight-bearing capabilities*. The weight-bearing or materials-handling activities include:

1. Lifting: Lifting must be assessed in three separate activities. The three standard levels of lifting used in industrial assessment are (1) a lift from the floor, (2) a lift from knee height, and (3) an overhead lift. If unilateral upper extremity weakness is an issue, each height also may be assessed with unilateral techniques. If unilateral testing is done, then nine separate activities are needed in the assessment—three bilateral height activities, three left upper extremity activities, and three right upper extremity activities. NOTE: A contrast to traditional therapy occurs here because the primary focus may now be on the uninvolved extremity. Since the uninvolved extremity usually provides a higher level of ability, it produces a higher functional application in the employee's work. Therefore there are times when the assessment of the uninvolved upper extremity is more critical than assessment of the involved one because it provides the major contribution to the person's *functional* ability level. Therapists must be careful not to fall back to the traditional focus on "disability" rather than "ability," especially when assessing the employee with an upper extremity injury. Therapists must keep in mind that they are assessing the highest functional ability of the person.

Capability Comparison of Injured to Uninjured Auto Mechanics

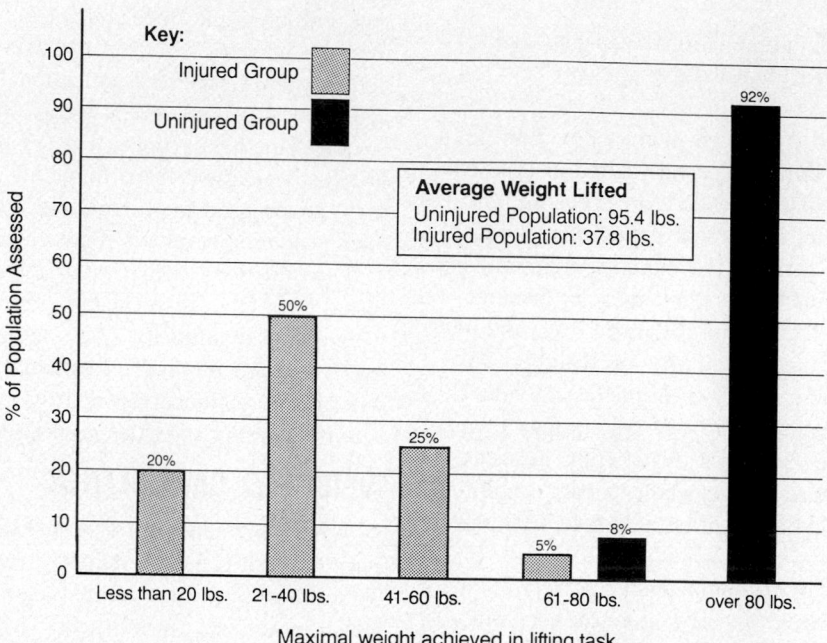

Fig. 26-2. A comparative analysis of lifting capabilities between injured and uninjured auto mechanics.

2. Pushing and Pulling: These need to be recognized as two separate activities performed at a standard height and a given distance. In the case of a back disorder, pushing generally generates higher end values than does pulling. This may not hold true in the upper extremity injury assessment.

Pushing or pulling tests should be designed so that the client stands or walks while performing the task; it is from the standing posture that the employee initiates the movement, and therefore this is when the greatest force is required in an industrial application.

3. Carrying: Two activities are tested in this area: carrying with the right upper extremity and carrying with the left upper extremity. Again, distances are directed by industry standards. A common error made is that of assessing "carry" as a bilateral upper extremity activity. Most materials-handling requir-

ing bilateral activity is actually involved in lifting. If distances are involved, it is a standard requirement that machinery and equipment be provided for mechanical assistance. Therefore what would normally be thought of in the medical model as a bilateral "carry" has been transformed to a lift through mechanical assistance, and the "carry" aspect is relegated to a unilateral activity.

The above components are the basic requirements in testing the weighted activities of a functional capacity assessment. Other materials-handling activities may be added, but attention must be given to the purpose and the need for all tests. Remember that standardization of each test is essential for reporting of results.

Fig. 26-4, *A*, demonstrates a portion of a reporting format for the weighted activities, and Fig. 26-4, *B*, shows a portion of a completed reporting format with assessment

FUNCTIONAL ASSESSMENT OVERVIEW

1. In an 8 hour workday, client can (circle full capacity for each activity):

    a.   Sit: 1-2-3-4-5-6-7-8 hours _____   **A**

    b.   Stand: 1-2-3-4-5-6-7-8 hours _____

    c.   Walk: 1-2-3-4-5-6-7-8 hours _____

2. Client is able to:	Not at all	Occasionally	Frequently	Continuously
a. Bend/stoop				
b. Squat				
c. Crawl				
d. Climb stairs				
e. Reach above shoulder level				
f. Crouch				
g. Kneel				
h. Balance				
i. Push/Pull				

3. Client can carry:	Never	Occasionally	Frequently	Continuously
a. Up to 10 pounds				
b. 11 to 24 pounds				
c. 25 to 34 pounds				
d. 35 to 50 pounds				
e. 51 to 74 pounds				
f. 75 to 100 pounds				

4. Client can lift:	Never	Occasionally	Frequently	Continuously
a. Up to 10 pounds				
b. 11 to 24 pounds				
c. 25 to 34 pounds				
d. 35 to 50 pounds				
e. 51 to 74 pounds				
f. 75 to 100 pounds				

5. Special restrictions, notations, or suggestions:

1. Validity Determination:

2.

3.

_____   _____
Signature of Therapist   Date

Fig. 26-3. A, Functional assessment overview. **B,** Partially filled out assessment.

FUNCTIONAL ASSESSMENT OVERVIEW

1. In an ⓈhourⓈ workday, client can (circle full capacity for each activity):

    a. Sit: 1-2-3-④-5-6-7-8 hours _30 minute durations_

    b. Stand: 1-2-3-④-5-6-7-8 hours _40-50 minute durations_

    B

    c. Walk: 1-2-3-④-⑤-6-7-8 hours _Frequent, long distances_

2. Client is able to:	Not at all	Occasionally	Frequently	Continuously
a. Bend/stoop		X		
b. Squat			X	
c. Crawl			X	
d. Climb stairs			X	
e. Reach above shoulder level			X	
f. Crouch		X		
g. Kneel		X		
h. Balance				
i. Push/Pull		X	X	
		44#	28.5#	

3. Client can carry:	Never	Occasionally	Frequently	Continuously
a. Up to 10 pounds			RIGHT OR LEFT	
b. 11 to 24 pounds		RIGHT OR LEFT	17#	
c. 25 to 34 pounds		32#		
d. 35 to 50 pounds				
e. 51 to 74 pounds				
f. 75 to 100 pounds				

4. Client can lift:	Never	Occasionally	Frequently	Continuously
a. Up to 10 pounds				
b. 11 to 24 pounds	A/S	13.5#	12.5#	
c. 25 to 34 pounds	D/C	28#	17#	
d. 35 to 50 pounds	C/F	23.5#	15#	
e. 51 to 74 pounds				
f. 75 to 100 pounds				

5. Special restrictions, notations, or suggestions:

1. Validity Determination:	
2.	
3.	

_____   _____
Signature of Therapist   Date

Fig. 26-3, cont'd.

A

WEIGHTED ACTIVITES

3. Client can carry:
    (As with a bucket or luggage)
    Right Arm
    Left Arm

0% Never	1-33% Occasionally	34-66% Frequently	67-100% Continuously

4. Client can lift:
    Both Arms:
    Above Shoulders
    Desk to Chair
    Chair to Floor

0% Never	1-33% Occasionally	34-66% Frequently	67-100% Continuously

B

WEIGHTED ACTIVITIES

3. Client can carry:
    (As with a bucket or luggage)
    Right Arm
    Left Arm

0% Never	1-33% Occasionally	34-66% Frequently	67-100% Continuously
	37#	15#	
	37#	15#	

4. Client can lift:
    Both Arms:
    Above Shoulders
    Desk to Chair
    Chair to Floor

0% Never	1-33% Occasionally	34-66% Frequently	67-100% Continuously
	13#	7#	
	28#	14#	
	23#	14#	

Fig. 26-4. A, A portion of a reporting format for the weighted activities and, **B,** demonstrates a portion of a completed reporting format.

values indicated. "Frequency of use" guidelines and principles are provided by engineering resources, human engineering references, anthropometric references, and resources in the area of human factors.

The Minnesota Department of Labor and Industry qualifies frequency of use relating to an 8-hour workday as follows:

Occasionally is equal to 1% to 33% of the workday
Frequently is equal to 34% to 66% of the workday
Continuously is equal to 67% to 100% of the workday

Many state labor departments use this formula or a similar one as a base. The therapist should check with the state forms or the standard forms of industry to identify what is most appropriate for a specific application.

The materials used as weight must be the same with each assessment and must follow the same progression with each assessment. To identify an appropriate weight progression, studies must be performed with test and retest application. The cases are followed into their work activities. It is not sufficient to merely standardize the process. Are the results useful? Are they applicable? Are the amounts of weight lifted too high or too low? The increments of weights must be correlated with the number of repetitions and the speed of the activity performance. A lifting capability assessment that progresses in 10-pound increments, for example, results in an end weight that is higher than that of progressing in 1-kilogram increments, all other factors of speed and height remaining the same. Which is the more accurate? It may be that neither is at the selected speed. The performance pace may need to be adjusted along with the progression of weights. That is why it is necessary to follow a case into application by watching that particular worker and other workers performing the same task and make adjustments accordingly.

Validity discrimination

Valid participation

1. Numbers represent full, safe level of client.

Conditional participation

2. Numbers represent higher than safe level. Client does not have a clear concept of safe end point tolerances and works beyond the level that would be safe over extended periods of time.
3. Numbers represent lower than safe level. Client *perceives* a level as the highest safe level but can physically tolerate more.

Invalid participation

4. Numbers represent lower than safe level. Client is consciously attempting to manipulate the results.

TOLERANCES

Tolerances to a total workday's required demands are determined by a formula based on the results obtained in the assessment itself. These include tolerance of the hours engaged in an activity during a workday, components of those tolerances, and identification of specific durations within the tolerance categories. Fig. 26-5 demonstrates these tolerances in relation to workday hours, sitting, standing, and walking.

PARTICIPATION LEVEL

The usefulness of functional capacity assessment results is dependent on a standardized approach and a scientific basis. The process of determining an individual's participation level has become one of the primary factors in comparing assessments.

BLANK OVERVIEW OF WORKDAY TOLERANCES

1. In an 8 hour workday, client can (circle full capacity for each activity):

Recommendations

a. Sit: 1 - 2 - 3 - 4 - 5 - 6 - 8- hours _____

b. Stand: 1 - 2 - 3 - 4 - 5 - 6 - 8- hours _____

c. Walk: 1 - 2 - 3 - 4 - 5 - 6 - 8- hours _____

COMPLETED OVERVIEW OF WORKDAY TOLERANCES

1. In an [8] hour workday, client can (circle full capacity for each activity):

Recommendations

a. Sit: 1 - 2 - 3 - 4 - 5 - [6] - 8- hours   40-45 minute durations

b. Stand: 1 - 2 - 3 - [4] - 5 - 6 - 8- hours   60 minute durations

c. Walk: 1 - 2 - [3] - 4 - 5 - 6 - 8- hours   Frequent, moderate distances

Fig. 26-5. Tolerance assessment.

It is not enough to simply provide a process by which numbers are reached to indicate a capability level. The assessment must also offer a process for identifying whether those numbers *do* represent the client's capability. This approach must eliminate the concern that they might represent a level higher or lower than the one that would be safe for the worker to perform the activity over an extended time, which rules out single-repetition testing. Previously studied and accepted formulas are used in addition to tests and retests of current methods.

The Key Method of Assessment, developed by physical therapist Glenda L. Key, uses a measure of the participation level during the assessment and categorizes by terms of validity discrimination (see accompanying box on page 660).

Leonard N. Matheson, Ph.D., uses a diagnostic system that analogizes with psychiatric disorders found in the *Diagnostic and Statistical Manual of Mental Disorders (DMS-III)*.[2]

A licensed psychologist, Dr. Matheson uses the term *symptom magnifier* for some clients and further classifies some clients as *refugee, game player,* or *identified patient*. These categories represent learned patterns of behaviors that are used to control the individual's life circumstances.

Industrial therapists must choose the format used for identifying the participation level based on their own expertise and that of their team.

Fig. 26-6 demonstrates the high prevalence of valid participation of the injured workers in the Key Functional Assessment.[1,7]

POSTURAL EXAMINATION

When conducting all parts of the functional capacity assessment, especially the weighted activities, one must always be acutely aware of the posture of the client during the activity. As the load becomes heavier, the client will adapt posturally. This accommodation allows for increased capability.

It is through documentation of the presence or absence of this accommodation that the therapist is able to identify weaknesses in the body that may affect the capability level but may have been missed in traditional screening or evaluation processes. Videotaping a task performance may be helpful to fully analyze the accommodation process. The identified weaknesses can then be addressed in further treatment (e.g., work hardening) or programs of education (e.g., back schools, body mechanics training, and overuse syndrome prevention). These adaptations will also provide valuable information to assist in job modification.

The client's limitations must dictate the assessment termination point. Education for postural changes is not appropriate during the assessment. The posture at the work site is at the discretion of the employee. During the assessment the posture is also at the discretion of the client, not to be controlled by the therapist or the environment. The assessment is designed to be a picture of the client's capability level. If the posture is controlled by the therapist, the capability level would need to be disclaimed or qualified with a statement from the therapist about the changing of the posture, resulting in the increased or changed capability. The therapist needs to remember that this is an assessment—an evaluation. Correction should not be provided to a patient while a gait analysis is being performed. Nor should correction be given in a functional capacities assessment.

An example of the environment controlling the posture is when equipment is used that stabilizes positions of the body. Setting up the assessment station to require or facilitate preferred posture is also an example of controlling the posture through the environment.

Controlling posture and stabilizing portions of the body are appropriate and effective in other parts of the worker care spectrum. Education and treatment for prevention and restoration will be covered later in this chapter.

While fulfilling the needs of the four primary areas, functional capacity assessment design must follow the standards designed into industry. The assessment station for the functional assessment needs to represent standard heights and measures of industry, not measurements associated with the individual's body. The therapist will need to change from the standard movement and posture parameters of the medical community to those of the industrial community. The medical parameters include measurements with direct reference to the individual (e.g., knee height, fingertip level, waist level, and shoulder level). These data vary with each person. An error must not be made by modifying the assessment in relation to the height or the disorder of the client. The workplace design standards do not change. As an example, in following the designs presented by industry, it becomes clear that lifting

PARTICIPATION LEVELS

6,748 Cases of Data Back — Data Bank (TM)

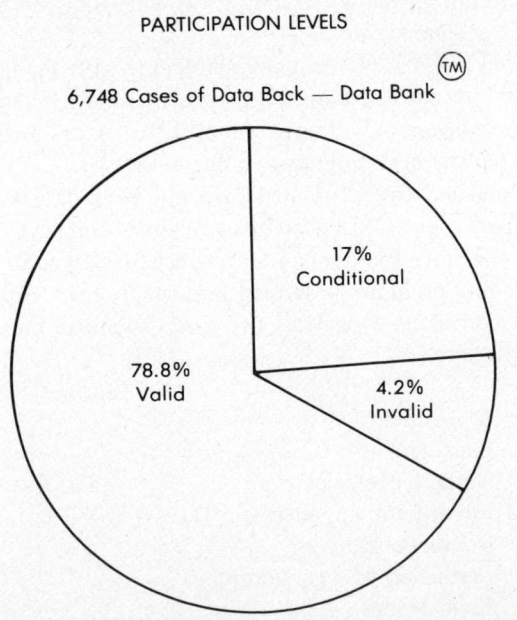

Fig. 26-6. Participation levels, 6,748 cases of Data Back–Data Bank.

usually takes place while turning 90 degrees to place the materials on another surface. To test without including the turning process would invalidate the functional component. Although industry appears quite varied, it should be noted that shelf, table, counter heights, and distances are generally close to standard, as are many applications, such as the angle of the foot when using a foot pedal.

A decision must be made regarding the standard heights that will be used in the functional capacity assessment. Possible sources for this decision are basic human engineering references, architectural references, design engineering references, a qualified human factors task force, or on-site measurements.

Packaged programs available to industrial physical therapists for functional capacity assessment all vary in their depth of initial study with industry. The depth of analysis of industrial sites should be investigated because without this direct information the assessment equipment and protocol may not represent the needs of the industries. Without a standardization of the equipment and the protocol, a new assessment determination area would need to be built for every new job a therapist attempts to evaluate. When there is standardization of the assessment to the *industries,* the same process, protocol, and equipment work for most situations. Standardization of tests not only works but is required for determination of reliability of the assessment.

Neutrality

The therapist, as an assessment specialist, must work to become an independent or neutral observer during the assessment. The specialist must be aware of how much opportunity the therapist has to influence the client. Whenever two human beings interact, an influencing opportunity is present. The therapist must not coach or encourage the client to do more or less than he/she demonstrates after commands are given. One way to assist in the neutral participation of the therapist and eliminate rater bias is to design double-blind techniques into the assessment so that neither the therapist nor the client know the expected results. "Double blind" is an experimental design technique for elimination of preferential (positive or negative) treatment of subjects during particular testing.[26] One of the ways to accomplish this is to have the weights progressed in such a way that neither party is aware of the actual amount being achieved. At the termination of the assessment the amount of weight achieved would then be identified in terms understood by both parties. This can be done simply through the use of conversion charts or basic computer software programs.

The final results of a functional capacity assessment are processed through the specific program's formulas. The report then is presented as a summary of the data and recommendations. An example of a completed report is found in Fig. 26-3, *B*. All programs should provide this information, but there may be differences in how they reach the final assessment numbers. The difference in how the numbers are reached determines the reliability of those numbers and therefore the reliability of the assessment itself.

JOB ANALYSIS

Sections B and C of Fig. 26-1 both include the job analysis. It is the job analysis that provides the critical demands of the work required of an individual. The functional capacity assessment results are matched against the job analysis. The capability of the worker as identified in the functional capacity assessment must equal or exceed the demands of the job as identified in the job analysis. This creates a return-to-work equation for successful and safe job placement.[26] The job task and job site analysis are detailed in this chapter after the section on preemployment screening.

WORK HARDENING

The treatment program that prepares the employee for returning to a specific job or occupation is called *work hardening* (Fig. 26-1, Section B). The term itself does not appear to be very popular. Many programs adopt their own labels but find that they continue to describe it as work hardening. For the sake of simplicity and consistency, *work hardening* is the term used in this chapter.

Fig. 26-1, Section B, identifies work hardening as a treatment program. Functional capabilities are restored through this treatment program, which combines clinical and industrial applications. Baseline capabilities are provided through the results of a functional capacity assessment. The goal is provided through the results of a job description or a job analysis. Both of these include materials-handling information relating to weights required and frequency tolerances.

Two approaches to work hardening are: (1) job task specificity and (2) muscle group conditioning. Many programs concentrate on only one of these factors as their focus, but the best programs combine the two.

Clinical and work-related goals of a work hardening program are found in the accompanying boxes on page 663.

To achieve the clinical and work-related goals, a work hardening program is divided into seven areas. Each area must contribute to at least two goals found in the accompanying boxes.

1. Assessment
2. Education
3. Isotonic exercise
4. Job specific application
5. Isokinetic exercise
6. Cardiovascular conditioning
7. Counseling

Clinical goals of work hardening

1. Increase cardiovascular fitness
2. Improve pain control skills
3. Increase strength
4. Improve safety from reinjury
5. Increase range of motion
6. Increase endurance

Fig. 26-7 is an example of a form used in a work hardening program.[25] Programs are usually standardized by their components or work hardening stations and time elements. The program should be designed primarily by the therapist in conjunction with the client for successful return to work. Others involved may include a representative from the insurance company, a rehabilitation counselor, the physician, or the employer. In the work hardening program's daily schedule the client is responsible for documenting the activities used in tracking the progress. This is reviewed by the therapist, the client, and appropriate members of the team each week during the work hardening treatment program. At the weekly meetings plans are also made for the next week's process and goals are set for progress.

Assessment and evaluation predicate industrial physical therapy, as in traditional therapy, to provide the therapist with the present ability level. End goals are identified and a plan of implementation is agreed on, with intervening goals and methods for attainment developed as progress dictates. The difference is that industrial physical therapists now use applications that relate directly to the work life of the client.

Education is used as a method of improving body mechanics for safety on the job. It can also increase the materials-handling abilities. Videotapes, simulated work tasks, audiotapes, slides, and individual or group sessions with the trainer are acceptable and effective methods used in this education process.

Isotonic exercise is designed to increase range of motion and flexibility. Stretching exercises are commonly employed as methods to promote prevention from reinjury. These exercises may be provided through video programs.

Job specific application combines the greatest number of goals. The clinical goals addressed include those of increasing strength, range of motion, flexibility, and endurance. The work-related goals include items 1 through 4 in the box below: increasing physical strength specific to the demands of a job description, improving body mechanics during the actual work activities, increasing materials-handling levels, and building tolerances to job specific activities.

The equipment used is dependent on the job tasks to which the clients are being returned. Motors, construction framework and tools, electronic assembly models, ladders, electronic and plumbing models, and clerical stations are commonly used in the work hardening simulations. Information from local industry and analysis of the occupational titles of workers referred to the work hardening program dictate the type of equipment purchased or simulations provided. By tracking worker referrals the selection of additional materials and equipment may be accomplished as the job tasks of the referrals changes.

Isokinetic exercise enhances the work hardening program when a specific body part or segment is the focus of the program. The speed and ROM parameters chosen are based on the relationship of the body part to the demands of the job. This addresses the goals of increasing strength, endurance, and conditioning levels to meet the requirements of that job.

Cardiovascular conditioning often involves the use of bicycles, stair machines, or tread mills. This increases endurance and improves the general ability to meet tolerance and endurance requirements of the job.

Counseling is provided to the client to facilitate pain control, address issues of stress, enhance attendance, and develop peer relationships while participating in this work hardening program and at the job site when returning to work.[15] Counseling acts to decrease destructive behavior and increase productivity through positive self-image and better interactional relationships. The primary benefit of counseling is in identifying areas that are causing stress and working with coping mechanisms and developing skills for the management of that stress. It is important that the client establish a positive support system at home and at work. In addition to family members, the closed group atmosphere with the other clients involved in the treatment setting has been identified as effective for the work hardening client.[15] With the multiple issues that evolve around the workers' compensation system, a major injury, or the return-to-work process, it is an important component in any industrial therapy program.

The work hardening facility requires a minimum of

Work-related goals of work hardening

1. Increase physical strength and movement level to match job description
2. Improve body mechanics for safety on the job
3. Increase materials handling level of abilities
4. Improve conditioning level to allow meeting tolerance and endurance requirements of the job
5. Identify responsibilities relating to attendance, following schedules, and ability to work with others
6. Substitute productivity in place of destructive behaviors

WORK CIRCUIT SCHEDULE

NAME: _____   DIAGNOSIS: _____

JOB TITLE: _____   MONTH: _____

WORK CIRCUIT DATE:

TIME IN/OUT										
WARM-UP REPS · SETS										
ISOTONIC ABDOMINAL LBS · SETS										
BACK LBS · SETS										
PULL DOWN LBS · SETS										
PUSH UP LBS · SETS										
BICYCLE RPM · MINUTES										
LIFT ABOVE SHOULDER LBS · SETS										
LIFT_____ LBS · SETS										
LIFT_____ LBS · SETS										
PUSH/PULL LBS · SETS										
CARRY LBS · SETS										
STACKING REPS · MINUTES										
BUILDING UNITS · MINUTES										
LBS · SETS										
LBS · SETS										
LBS · SETS										
LBS · SETS										
LBS · SETS										
LBS · SETS										

Fig. 26-7. Work circuit schedule.

1,000 square feet for basic start-up,[8] but a work hardening facility can be as large as is appropriate for the population number and the economic availability. A program that offers all seven areas of the work hardening process would use approximately 2,500 to 3,000 square feet.[5,8,11,15] This space allottment provides adequate space for 12 clients at one time.[8] As dedicated space, it is separated from the therapy clinic and should offer a nonmedical environment.

Frequency and duration of participation should be daily for 2 to 8 hours. Some programs operate only 3 days a week, but most operate 5 days. The duration of a program is 2 to 8 weeks, with most taking no more than 4 to 6 weeks.[5,8,11,15] An individual's program should be reviewed each week to determine the client's present status and progression to the next step. If the review demonstrates lack of progress or a poor attendance record, the client's program is terminated. Case management must include criteria for admission, discontinuation, and successful completion with discharge. The ultimate goal is productive return to the competitive labor market.

EXIT ASSESSMENT

Exit assessment, a special purpose assessment, is the functional capacity assessment performed on completion of the work hardening program (Fig. 26-1, Section B). The purpose of an exit assessment is to demonstrate elevated or changed capabilities when compared with the assessment on entry into the program. The combination of the two provides the "before" and "after" picture of the individual client. This comparison of ability levels can be used for the following purposes:

1. Identifying the new and current levels of ability for the individual client for return-to-work application
2. Providing documentation of a client's ability to increase his/her capabilities
3. Supporting the viability of a work hardening program to meet the work-related goals identified in the box on page 663.
4. Providing a marketing tool for the work hardening program

When conducting an exit assessment, a full assessment may be repeated; if so, the time element of the exit assessment would be as long as the functional assessment on entry. Another option is that only the critical demands of the job or the assessment are considered. This usually includes primarily the weighted activities. The exit assessment format must follow, exactly, the format of the entry assessment, to allow comparison of the pretest and the posttest. This direct relationship of the "before" and "after" assessments provides valuable information for case management.

PREVENTION

A noninjured workers' spectrum, the prevention spectrum (Fig. 26-1, Section C) frequently includes preemployment screening and job analysis. These services are usually provided on a consultant, contract, or agreement basis.

PREEMPLOYMENT SCREENING

Employers have increased their interest in and pursuit of a selection process to ensure the hiring of employees who meet performance requirements for physically demanding jobs. Ensuring that job performance requirements can be met is certainly not new. Skill tests are a common part of the application process. An example is the speed and accuracy typing test for a clerical position.

Industry is also concerned about an individual's skill level as it relates to the physical demands of the job. The question "Can the perspective employee lift a 32-pound box of paper supplies?" is added to the previous typing skill question. To answer this question a functional capacity assessment is used as a preemployment screening tool. It is an assessment designed specifically to determine the applicant's ability to safely execute select physical tasks, usually weighted tasks. The results of the physical abilities screen is then matched with the results of the job description or the job analysis to make the determination of a performance score.

The Key Job Placement Assessment is one of the physical abilities assessments available to use in the preemployment screening process. This assessment is designed to be a skill or capability assessment, not a tool to predict injury. The measuring or predicting is based on and compared with performance requirements; it is not an attempt to predict injury potential.

The subject of predictability creates great controversy in the academic world. It is understandable that the focus for the medical model has been that of prediction through scientific research process. An industrial physical therapist must ask questions based on the needs from both the medical model and from the viewpoint of the employer. The employer has the primary need of hiring people with the ability to do the work. This can be facilitated and made more successful by a preemployment physical screening assessment. Preemployment screening is gaining increased acceptance as prevention from injury for both the medical and industrial communities.

The design of the preemployment screen or the job placement assessment must be standardized with clear, repeatable guidelines. It must be:

1. Safe to administer; the applicant will not sustain an injury during the assessment
2. Reliable, quantitative, and repeatable
3. Job specific and functional in application
4. Practical in time and cost of administering

5. Independent of user characteristics (e.g., sex, size [height and weight], age, the five senses, etc.)

Cut-off points of acceptable physical abilities must be clearly documented before the assessment or the hiring process. These cut-off points or scores must follow the results of a detailed job analysis. The job analysis is based on functional job-specific activities. This supports the preference of dynamic components in the assessment over isometric or isokinetic components. It is critical for defense in the case of litigation for the industry to (1) have adequate job analysis and (2) use a standardized assessment screen that has functional application.

The industrial therapist should recognize that the physical abilities skill level is but one portion of a hiring process. When matched with the requirements of a job, the relationship should be clear and the decision by the employer can be made objectively.

JOB ANALYSIS

The job analysis is a systematic identification of the components of a job while the worker is performing that job. The therapist may be asked to evaluate a specific job task (job task analysis) or the job site itself (job site analysis), as detailed in the accompanying box. A *job task analysis* provides quantitative data. Materials are weighed, heights and distances are measured, repetitions are counted, and cycle time is clocked. By contrast, a *job site analysis* is the systematic evaluation of the work stations, the tools used, and the relationship between the worker and the work site. Information gathered in the job site analysis is of a qualitative nature.

JOB TASK ANALYSIS

The job task analysis data are used to:

1. Build job descriptions, providing minimal or maximal capacity requirements of a job (also called *critical demands*).
2. Assist in job modification. Comparisons can be made with standards in industry, or acceptable productivity measures and adaptations can be made accordingly.
3. Provide job requirement data by which to compare

Job analysis	
Job task analysis	**Job site analysis**
Quantitative	Qualitative
Weights	Postures
Distances	Positions
Repetitions	Work site standards
Cycle times	Biomechanics

---

functional capacity assessment results or preemployment screening results.

Tools commonly used to do a job task analysis include:

1. Stopwatch
2. Tape measure
3. Video, polaroid, or 35 mm camera
4. Scale for weighing equipment and materials that are handled
5. Resistance dynamometer for push/pull measurements

One of the values of the job task analysis is realized when the information is used to develop job descriptions and the job descriptions are then used in preemployment screening. The screening quantifies the applicant's safe levels of ability. The job task analysis quantifies the critical demands of the job. By using a comparison of job task requirements and safe capabilities, the company is then able to assess the situation and adjust the following factors:

1. Placement of applicants in areas of appropriate capability requirements
2. Transfer of present employees who may be performing tasks beyond their long-term safe levels
3. Modifications of tasks if few applicants are able to demonstrate sufficient ability level
4. Establishment of a standard for entrance into high-risk areas

The job task analysis is intended for use in conjunction with the functional assessment process.

Fig. 26-8 provides a sample job task analysis form.[20] The decision of how detailed the analysis should be is made by both the therapist performing the analysis and the person requesting and paying for it. The decision is based on the expected end use of the data.

If the data will be compared against preemployment screening results, concentration will be placed on the critical demands or the maximal capacity requirements of the job. If a company is considering modifying work stations, or if increasing speed and efficiency is a goal, greater detail will be required. The reporting method will vary according to the initial goals but should be agreed on by both the industrial physical therapist and the employer. An analysis may or may not include recommendations.

JOB SITE ANALYSIS

As contrasted with the job task analysis, a job site analysis can take many forms. A job site analysis is an assessment of the environment and how it fits the worker and the work being done within it.

Within the therapist's area of expertise, the goal of the assessment is to gather the details of the interaction of the

JOB TASK ANALYSIS

Company _____   Video Start _____

Department _____   Stop _____

Job Title _____   Date _____

D.O.T. Number _____   Analyst _____

Tools or Materials	Force Pounds	Verb	Position From	To	Frequency	Other
Move cartons	42#	Lift	18"	31"	5/hr	90° turn

Notes:

Fig. 26-8. Job task analysis.

worker with the job site to draw out the factors that can be changed to allow better synthesis of worker and work site. In the relationship of the worker to the work, the most profound impact that the therapist can have is often one of the simplest of applications; that of working with the employee's posture while he/she completes the job task.

In completing a job site analysis a process is followed that involves moving from the bigger picture of the job itself to the smaller picture of one motion or movement. These units are described in Fig. 26-9, which illustrates a descending order of (1) jobs, (2) tasks, (3) components, and (4) motions and movements. This translates to the fact that each job consists of numerous tasks; each task has multiple components and within each component there are a number of motions and movements. Employers' records

will usually identify the high-risk areas of the work environment that must be analyzed first. Within the high-risk area the jobs in the area must be identified. The tasks involved in completing each job must then be studied with their related components.

An example of this job site analysis scheme follows: When working with a company, the therapist is told by the company representative that from their records the order fulfillment department is an area where they have a higher rate of worker disability problems. When a therapist begins to analyze the problem area, each job category within the department needs to be reviewed. From there the analysis must be made of each task needed to complete each job and the components of each task. Focusing from the big picture down allows the therapist to collect the facts, determine whether the problem is in the worker or in the

JOB SITE ANALYSIS

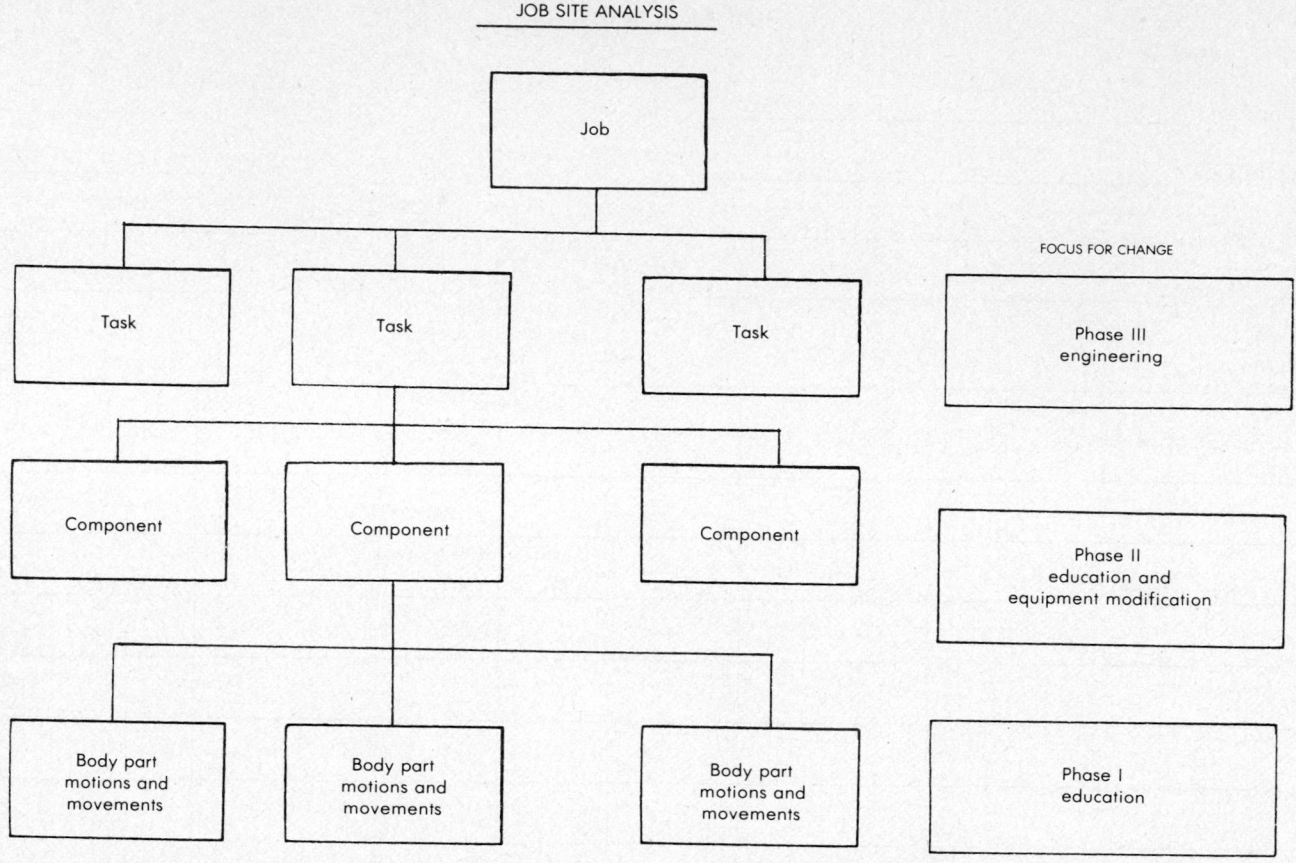

Fig. 26-9. Job site analysis.

environment, and then intervene with solutions to the problems.

Once documented as in Fig. 26-9, the industrial therapist then works through Phase I with the employer. This addresses the smallest unit, the full or partial body movements of the employee while performing the work. This information should be used by the facilitator or trainer to bring about change through education programs. Modification at this level (1) usually has the highest impact in cutting costs, (2) requires participation by the employee, (3) may require participation by the employee's supervisor, (4) can be instructed by the industrial physical therapist to individual employees or in groups, and (5) can be implemented immediately.

This can take the form of changing the movement posture when pulling a lever from that of a primarily isolated wrist action that includes flexion and ulnar deviation to a movement that uses the entire arm or body as the pulling force, which reduces the chance of an overuse syndrome. In job site analysis it is common to see postures that predispose the back or the wrist to injury but can be changed with minimal cost and effort.

Adaptations and modifications may involve total rearrangement of a work space, but others can be as simple as adjusting the angle of the work surface or the angle of the

products. Other simple modifications may be made by placing items closer to the body, placing materials at an angle while working with them, or cutting out large openings in materials (boxes or receptacles) to facilitate proper posture while handling.

Once the analysis is complete and the changes agreed on, these changes are brought about through education programs for the workers, supervisors, and management. Formatting the educational intervention is covered later in this chapter (see section on prevention).

When representatives of industry, including management and on-line workers, are aware of the preferred postures and positions, they are able to carry this information into their own work. If they are the on-line assembly employees, there are modifications that they can make within their areas of responsibility and authority. The industrial engineer, now knowing about the postures and positions necessary to complete a job, has a guide when setting up work stations. The design engineer now can design products and production equipment that avoids inherent faulty postures due to the design of the equipment itself.

When the postures and positions cannot be modified by education and changes of the employee functioning in the work stations, Phase II of the process is to look at the component. The *component* is defined as the tools and equipment used in completion of a task or job. Analysis of components also can lead to modification that will avoid faulty postures and positions.

The component becomes the area of focus when postures and position changes have been initiated and all possibilities have been explored, or when postures and positions cannot be modified without significant changes in the equipment or materials being handled.

The task itself is addressed in Phase III, when Phases I and II have been initiated, and especially if limitations were such that I and II could not be implemented without significant changes to the work station; then concentration must be focused on the structures of the work station itself.

> *Phase I—Postures:* In this phase the therapist is working with people and the physical positions and postures that must be assumed for completion of a task. If a problem is noted, the method of correction is by education of the person to avoid the faulty postures and positions.
>
> *Phase II—Components:* In the component phase an analysis of the equipment used by the person to complete the task takes place to identify modifications that might be made to avoid faulty positions.
>
> *Phase III—Tasks:* In the last phase the work station itself is analyzed for alternatives to the environment where the equipment is used to complete the tasks. Since this is usually the most expensive to adapt or modify, it is addressed only after Phase I and II are without success.

At times it is essential to work with all three components at once or to work in reverse order, but usually a therapist will work in the stated order. The strategy presented in this phased intervention program is to make adaptations or modifications from a simple solution (i.e., change a position in which someone stands) to a complex alteration of the workplace.

The complexity matrix (Fig. 26-10) is used to identify the depth and breadth of the industrial intervention project. Time schedules and changes are built on the development of the matrix. The therapist should also use the matrix to clarify the extent of his/her expected involvement with the company. Each increased level of complexity requires added units of time both on site and in reporting. The schedule of analysis follows from easier (box 1) to more complex (box 4) formats. By following the complexity matrix from the easiest point, the therapist is able to begin with a clearly identified focus and broaden to areas of greater complexity.

A physical therapist has the skills to analyze movement of the body through anatomical, physiological, and biomechanical principles. Organ systems are understood by a therapist, as are tissue responses to disease and trauma. It

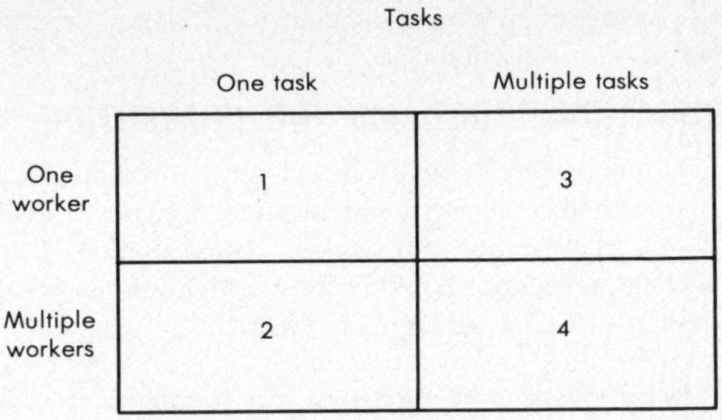

Fig. 26-10. Complexity matrix.

is within this same area of expertise that a therapist must develop the skills necessary to do an analysis of a job site.

Areas that a therapist would not address unless further educated include levels of exposure to chemicals, noise, and VDT radiation. As in traditional ethical practice, the therapist must stay within areas of expertise. Expanding the services into new market areas is acceptable, exciting, and to be encouraged. Expanding into highly sensitive areas beyond one's expertise could be dangerous.

Product-user interfaces that are poorly designed are often a result of a lack of awareness and knowledge of biomechanical and physiological principles by the designer. When understood, general biomechanical standards can be applied by physical therapists in an industrial situation. The industrial therapist needs to apply biomechanical and physiological knowledge to basic ergonomic principles.

The following is a short list of basic principles of positions and movements to observe when performing job analysis activities.*

1. Shoulder abduction angle should be no greater than 30 degrees.
2. Hands should be kept below shoulder level.
3. Reaches over 16 inches should be avoided.
4. Work surfaces should be kept clear of objects at least 3 inches from the edge.
5. Head supports should be used when greater than 30-degree head flexion is sustained.
6. Sharp edges should be avoided or removed.
7. Eye movement should be used for visual scanning; no head movements should be involved.
8. Foot controls should be used only for operation while sitting, not standing.
9. Floor mats should be supplied for standing workers; hard floors should be avoided.

This information, which should be basic to the industrial therapist, may be unknown to an employer and becomes a valuable tool for building a safer environment

*See references 3, 6, 9, 17, 19, and 24.

while saving money in production, medical expenses, and workers' compensation costs.

EDUCATION PROGRAMS FOR PREVENTION

The philosophy of injury prevention is becoming associated with the industrial organization because of rising costs of rehabilitation and workers' compensation. It follows that prevention should become a high priority for the industrial therapist. As stated by Schrich:

Machines used to be fixed only after breakdown. Now we know that machine maintenance is a better approach; it helps prevent breakdown and reduces costs. The human body should be approached with the same philosophy. Instead of waiting for it to break down, or attempting to predict when that will happen, industry is beginning to recognize the importance of a maintenance program. . . .[18]

It is amazing that it has taken the industrial and medical community so long to realize that a philosophy of prevention is a cost-cutting measure in the long run.

As indicated earlier, people problems are corrected through educational programs used as a preventive measure. Implementation of an educational program for prevention follows the progression outlined here:

1. Exploration of the needs within the industry
   Do not assume that you know the problems and needs of the industry with which you propose to do business. There are fact and feeling questions that must be asked and answered before you can determine the real problems and propose answers to those problems. Ronald E. Bates, a marketing consultant, identifies these basic questions to be asked[4]:
   a. How many employees?
   b. How many in management?
   c. How many workers?
   d. Shifts—times and numbers on each?
   e. Hiring cycle?
   f. Areas (divisions, etc.) of incidents?
   g. Number of incidents last year?
   h. Cost of workers' compensation last year?
   i. Programs previously implemented? Examples: smoking cessation, diet programs, back care, safe driving
   j. Organizational structure for implementing programs—who has the final responsibility and authority?
   k. Who signs the check? Are there any budget constrictions?
   l. When implemented, what will be the time and sequence of steps from planning to implementation?
   m. What is their concept of an ideal program?
2. Once this information is gathered, a review of what you, the industrial therapist, have to offer is appro-

priate. It is important to follow the needs as identified through the exploration process.
3. Submission of a proposal for meeting the expressed needs based on the complete analysis
4. On-site activities
   a. Briefing prior to analysis
      Briefings are meetings held with the decision makers. The process that is to occur is reviewed and confirmed. Further exploration is recommended for input by those not having participated in the original exploration processes. The general approach is described, schedules are reviewed, and the debriefing is scheduled.
   b. Analysis-job Site and/or job tasks (as described in detail earlier in this chapter)
   c. Debriefing regarding analysis
      Debriefing is recommended, again with the primary players. This meeting is used to review any significant findings, make recommendations regarding implementation of programs, present an overview of expected price, and identify a schedule for reporting.
5. Report generation

We also recommend that you do some investigation of who the true decision makers are within the given hierarchal structure. Although the president of the company may be the final decision maker, a project can be undermined well before it gets to the president if the true decision makers are not recognized early. Also realize that a union will oftentimes look at a job site analysis as a mechanism to delete a job and feel threatened by it. Early meetings with union officials may be a very wise plan. Initiation of a prevention program is summarized below:

1. Exploration
2. Telling your story
3. Submission of proposal
4. On-site activities
   a. Briefing
   b. Job analysis
   c. Debriefing
5. Report generation

The next step is the delivery of the specific programs of intervention. The two most common programs presently being offered by industrial physical therapists are body mechanics and materials-handling related. The body regions that are most frequently the focus are the back and the upper extremity. Programs for the prevention of back injuries are often in the form of a back school presented to management and hourly employees. Upper extremity injury prevention is usually in the form of overuse syndrome prevention (OSP) programs or cumulative trauma disorder (CTD) prevention. Standard approach in all programs is shown in the box on page 674.

Management and supervisory workshops should be 4 to 6 hours long, highly participatory, and limited in the size of the group. A maximum of 20 participants allows for high levels of participation and interaction between participants, as well as interaction between the participants and the facilitator.[12]

This workshop should include the following: basic anatomy, definitions, economic impact, causes, symptoms, diagnostic procedures, traditional treatment, nontraditional treatment, education as treatment, movements and positions, practical application, exercises, and reinforcement programs.

Employee sessions are usually 1 to 1½ hours in length. Again, a maximum of 20 employees should be encouraged to allow high participation in the session. It is important to teach basic principles in terms that apply to your audience. Use nonmedical terminology, present *their* home and social activities as examples, and use *their* industry's language and work site when giving examples.

Focus on the results you want to see. Do not focus on what will happen if poor posture is used or on the symptoms that are common to back and upper extremity overuse or misuse. Teach participants how to work properly and prevent problems. Do not teach them something that you do not want them to focus on; do not teach them symptoms. Teach what you *want* them to remember.

One-on-one sessions are 1 to 1½ hours in length. The industrial therapist spends this time with an employee who is already demonstrating or reporting symptoms. Basic anatomy of the involved area is reviewed and followed by education for changing postures and/or movements. This includes practice application and concludes with a progressive schedule for integration of the new postures into home and work activities.

ADULT EDUCATION

The process of education for adults has needs and follows principles unlike those associated with children. Adults have established styles of personality, learning, and behavior. Adults also have experiences that can promote or deter learning. The principles of education[12] presented in the accompanying box provide guidelines for carrying out education intervention programs with industrial clients.

As a facilitator, or as a leader, you must consciously include these principles in the interventions as you work with industrial clients.

High participation should be structured to bring out the "aha's" of self-discovery. This occurs for the participant through practice, error, self-evaluation, and accomplishment. When it is well thought out and well structured, this high participation appears to be nonstructured and seems to follow the curiosity and needs of the participants. None of the principles can be taken lightly. The success of the presentation depends on effective use of the three p's—preparation, planning, and participation.

Learning principles for adults

1. People learn when they feel they are actively involved in the learning process. The more the learner can practice and project the information into real life situations, the more learning will take place.
2. People learn when there is a climate of respect for each individual and when the teacher exhibits a sense of caring for each individual.
3. People learn when there is an atmosphere of trust. This trust needs to be established early and is characterized by "unfreezing" of a person's feeling, thinking, and acting. This will happen if the learner can readily perceive the expectation of the present relationship through constructive openness, mutual trust and respect, and honest negotiation and problem solving.
4. People learn when there is a climate of self-discovery, . . .when learners are helped to meet their own needs rather than having their needs dictated to them. Curiosity is natural, built into every person. The skilled leader can bring this natural curiosity out of almost everyone.
5. People learn when there is a nonthreatening teaching-learning situation. People want the opportunity to confront and challenge ideas, but if they fear the consequences of such, learning will be inhibited. The learner needs to see the course leader as supporting and nonthreatening and needs to perceive the climate as nonthreatening and nonjudgmental. People learn when there is a climate of openness, . . .when personal concerns, feelings, ideas and beliefs can be expressed and examined freely.
6. People learn when each participant feels that his/her values, beliefs, feelings, and views are important and significant.
7. People learn when error is accepted as a natural part of the learning process.
8. People learn when differences in people are as acceptable as differences in ideas.
9. People learn when they see themselves as they really are. Self-evaluation is of primary importance in the teaching-learning situation. Evaluation by others is secondary. Every opportunity for self-critique should be undertaken.

From Bates RE: Professional selling skills I, Key Functional Assessments, Inc, Marketing Course (unpublished), 1988.

I. Preparation
  A. You must have a depth of technical knowledge of your material.
  B. Practice your material out loud.
  C. Practice with the audiovisual materials and equipment.
  D. Know your audience.

1. Management level:
   a. Where on the organizational chart; responsibility to the economics; responsibility to the productivity.
   b. Have organizational chart in advance.
   c. Have lists of expected participants.
E. Know the company lingo or industry jargon.
F. Schedule break times around your material.

II. Planning
A. Examples from your own or others' experiences need to be strategically placed. These are necessary to make concepts more concrete and vivid to the participants. Try to make examples fit as closely to the audience as possible.
B. Areas of weakness within the leader need to be self-acknowledged and decisions made relating to extra study to correct those weaknesses.
C. The complexity of the technical material presented needs to be identified. Material should make the participants stretch their knowledge level but not exceed their grasp. Material should be presented in "lay" terminology so that it can be used by the participants.
D. The physical environment needs to be very positive and supportive of a learning experience. Pay attention to details.
   1. Eliminate outside distractions. Arrange for a room with no phone, cool temperature, and good chairs. Tables are to be placed to allow participants to see others easily and to allow ample room for the leader to walk through and up to each participant. A U shape works well. All calls are held until break periods. Be clear in the introduction of the agenda and allow for an appropriate length of breaks and lunch break.
   2. Audiovisual equipment placement should be marked on the floor with tape for easy replacement if it is necessary to move a piece of equipment during the course of the presentation.
   3. Lay out and check the necessary workshop materials against a list.
   4. Have time slotted for each section and follow your plan. If a potential deviation occurs, it is your conscious decision whether to allow that deviation. Another conscious decision needs to be made on where and how the adjustment will take place to include all the material planned.
   5. You are responsible for the physical environment. If the set-up is not as you desire, it is your responsibility to get it corrected *before* you begin. Do not settle for less. The consequences will affect the presentation. Although it may be someone else's responsibility to prepare the room and audiovisuals for you, in the end it is still your responsibility. The physical environment can affect the control you maintain on your group and can thereby reflect on the quality of your presentation.

III. Participation
A. You, the leader, must participate. Communicate interest and enthusiasm in your subject and the sense of being competent. You are the expert. Be clear about what it is that is important to you. That will become important to the participants.
B. The participants must participate. This is one of the most important principles of adult learning. Part of this principle is their responsibility, part of it is yours. You must strategically place challenging questions to enhance the involvement of the group. "Are there any questions?" too easily allows no response. "What do you think about that?" may be too risky for the participant with too much vulnerability in being wrong. Find sentences and situations that work well with you as a participation facilitator. An example might be to say "Let's explore this a little." In the Key Method of Overuse Syndrome Prevention (OSP) program, the tennis racket is one of the "tools" used in the practical application section after a training session on the concepts of prevention. One of the participants demonstrates the typical use of the tennis racket. The demonstration is not necessarily intended to show how that participant would use it, but expected, typical, general use. This allows for a nonthreatening experience, not the "I may do it wrong in front of everyone" fear. The facilitator then works with the group in following the steps previously taught to them in the concept portion. As a group experience, which includes the demonstrator and the facilitator, postures, positions, techniques, and applications are addressed and corrected. This process fulfills nine of the leader-learner principles.

The results include active involvement, respect for the demonstrator and the participants, and an atmosphere of trust, all promoting honest and active problem solving.

The aspect of self-discovery occurs both during a demonstration, with participants revealing concepts during discussion, and when the expert is advising the participant for correction. The self-discovery also comes when participants can actually apply what they have learned—in front of others and especially in front of the expert. This nonthreatening and supportive atmosphere promotes the challenging of ideas and concepts specific to what is being taught. This is an opportunity to call on a participant's previous experiences and beliefs, which allows for further knowledge and understanding.

Using a demonstration in this way takes the burden of error off the individual. It demonstrates that error is a natural part of the learning process. It also shows that people are indeed different in how they use a tool (tennis racket in this case) and how they would problem solve. A demonstration also allows opportunities for self-evaluation: "Do I know the material?" and "Did I learn what I was supposed to learn?"

One of the basic methods used to facilitate early participation is the introduction of each person in a workshop as the first step of the program.

1. The leader learns the names and titles of each participant in that company/group.
2. The leader learns the perceived roles by the participant (this may indicate the role the participant will play during follow-up and implementation of the program).
3. The participant shares expectations.
4. The participant and the leader establish eye contact.
5. The participant is more likely to verbally participate later because of having heard his or her own voice in "this space." This is especially true if the workshop is designed with lecture material first and the participation activities later.

Another highly effective method of teaching is the triad training that is implemented in the training of the Key Method of Assessment.[13] This is a participatory model. The group is divided into teams of three each. Each team is identified as a triad. Learning objectives are clearly identified for a critique process with checklists for the evaluations. Assignments are given based on material previously covered. Each of the three participants rotates through the roles of (1) industrial therapist, (2) client (customer, participant, etc.), and (3) review coach. All have "studied" the same material. This rotating process allows for all nine learning principles to be carried out. The responsibility for learning is on the participant, as is that of coaching. Another benefit of this as a training method is that it allows everyone to assist in his/her own learning while assisting in the learning process of others. Human nature is such that it is important for us to give and contribute. This triad training offers that opportunity in a very true application. The knowledge and capabilities of each person are vital for the training of the others. Error is expected, accepted, and worked on during participatory triad learning. Humor is designed into the roles and facilitated by the personalities of the participants and the leader.

Documentation

Clear documentation is necessary to demonstrate that education is an effective approach for prevention. Information gathered during the exploration stages become the base figures. Tracking occurs on a 3-month, 6-month, and 1-year schedule, as shown in Fig. 26-11.

Fig. 26-12 is a graphic representation of the financial impact that the Key Method of Overuse Syndrome Prevention (OSP) has demonstrated.[10] As identified in the introduction, more and more employers are turning to therapists to assist them in taking better control over their costs and their workers' compensation status.[22]

As an industrial therapist, you can make a significant

Injury type	1 year prior		3 months post		6 months post		1 year post	
	Incidence	Cost	Incidence	Cost	Incidence	Cost	Incidence	Cost
CTS								
Hand								
Wrist								
Elbow								
Shoulder								
Neck								
Back								
TOTAL								

Fig. 26-11. Information gathered during the exploration stages of a 3-month, 6-month, and 1-year schedule.

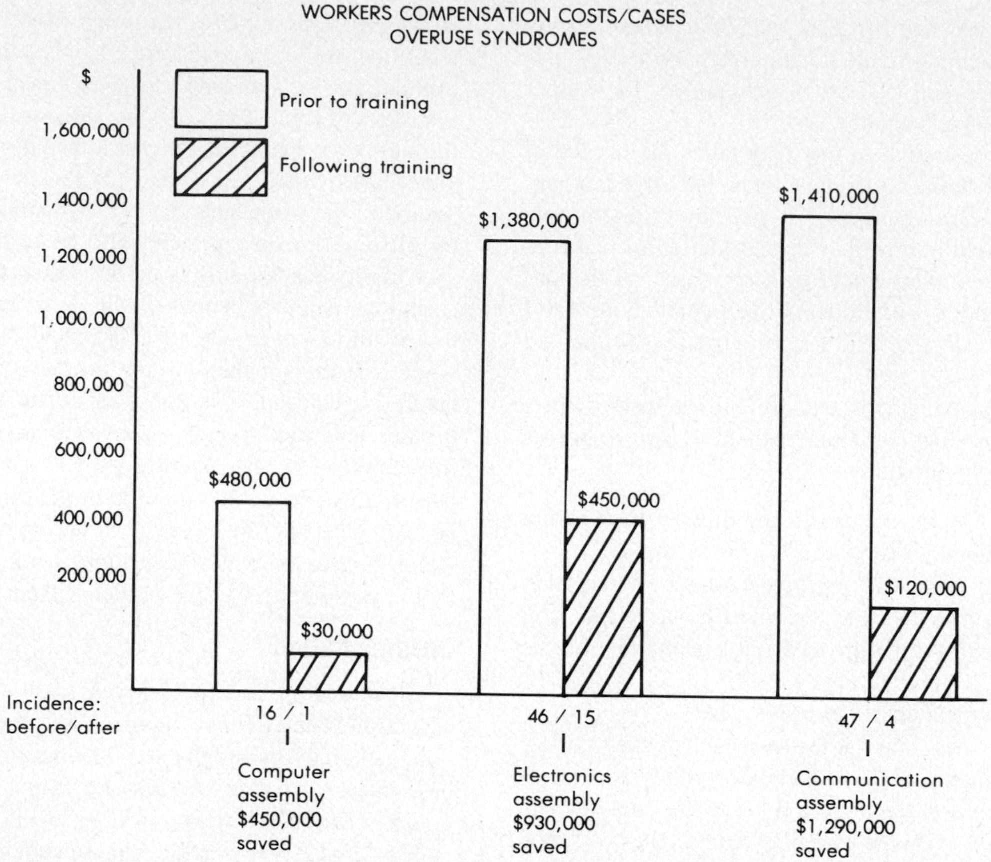

Fig. 26-12. Workers' compensation costs/cases overuse syndrome.

impact on the costs to the employer while reducing pain and suffering (by decreasing injury and incidence rates). Instead of affecting only one individual, as in a traditional treatment, your expertise now works with large numbers of people, having an impact on the improvement of life for many.

A study conducted by the University of Minnesota in 1986 documented the effectiveness of a specific one-on-one education program held with individuals experiencing symptoms of carpal tunnel syndrome (CTS).[21] Their findings identified that 83% of the participants were able to effect modifications at work. Ninety-seven point seven percent (97.7%) reported that they were able to decrease their pain level or stop it from continuing to get worse. Eighty-two percent (82%) were employed at the time of the study, compared to the 36% employed prior to the educational intervention.

SUMMARY

A comprehensive industrial therapy program includes traditional treatment, functional assessments, work-related treatment (work hardening), preemployment assessments, job analysis, and educational interventions for prevention. This chapter has presented an introduction to this new specialization, industrial physical therapy. It is important that the pursuit of this specialization be a conscious decision. It represents a change of traditional process and requires a commitment of energy, resources, and focus. To those of you who choose it, I welcome you. The world of "function" is one where you can have great impact.

Education programs regarding prevention

1. Briefing
2. Management and Supervisory Level Workshops
3. Employee Sessions
4. One-On-One Sessions
5. Organizational Planning for Reinforcement
6. Debriefing
7. Report Generation
8. Follow up

REFERENCES

1. Ahlgren A: Use of statistical information in the physical therapy practice, Key Functional Assessments, Inc, Annual Provider Conference Presentation, Minneapolis, August 1988.
2. American Psychiatric Association: Diagnostic and statistical manual of mental disorders, ed 3, 1980.

3. Ayoub MM: Work place design and posture, Human Factors 15(3):265-268, 1973.
4. Bates RE: Professional selling skills I, Key Functional Assessments, Inc, Marketing Course (unpublished), 1988.
5. Cegelka D: Performance Evaluation and Assessment Center (PEAC), Southbury, Conn, 1988.
6. Chaffin DB: Localized muscle fatigue—definition and Measurement, J Occup Med 15(4):346-354, 1973.
7. Data Back–Data Bank™, Key Functional Assessments, Inc, Minneapolis, 1986.
8. Demers L: How to establish a functional work hardening program, Seminar, Milliken Physical Therapy Center, Scarborough, Me, 1987.
9. Diffrient N, Tilley AR, and Harman D: Humanscale, Cambridge, 1981, Massachusetts Institute of Technology Press.
10. Documented results of the Key Method of Overuse Syndrome Prevention Program: Workers' compensation Cost/incidence reduction, by Key Functional Assessments, Inc, October 1988.
11. Fagan L: New Mexico Occupational Performance Center, Sante Fe, N. Mex.
12. Key GL: Management workshops. In Policies, procedures, and methods for Overuse Syndrome Prevention: industrial applications, 1986.
13. Key GL: Triad training. In Policies and Procedures guide to the Key Method of Functional Assessments, 1986.
14. Key GL: Work capacity analysis. In Physical therapy, Barnes MR and Scully, editors: Philadelphia, 1989, JB Lippincott Co.
15. Miller G: Back to Work Center, Augusta, Me, 1989.
16. Profile of a private practice physical therapist, PT Today, Fall 1988.
17. Roebuck JA, Kroemer KHE, and Thomson WG: Engineering anthropometry methods, New York: John Wiley & Sons, 1975.
18. Schrich LK: Handling carpal tunnel syndrome, Assembly Engineering, November 1988.
19. Tichauer ER: Ergonomic aspects of biomechanics. In the industrial environment—Its evaluation and control, National Institute of Occupational Safety and Health, US Government Printing Office, Washington, DC, 1973.
20. Trainer's guide: Step into industrial therapy, Key Functional Assessments, Inc.
21. University of Minnesota Occupational Therapy Department: Reducing symptoms of carpal tunnel syndrome: A retrospective study of the Key One-on-One Intervention, 1987.
22. Washington Business Group: An employer's guide to obtaining physical therapy services, Healthcare Management and Physical Therapy, March 1988.
23. Webster's New Collegiate Dictionary, 1980.
24. Woodson, WE: Human factors design handbook, McGraw-Hill, Inc, 1981.
25. Work Circuit Schedule. Reprinted with permission of Work Hardening Centers of America, Elkins Park, Pa, 1988.
26. Worth D: CPS National Workshop, CPS Rehab Services, Melbourne, Australia, September 1988.

GLOSSARY

abduction the act of moving away from the midsagittal plane of the body or axis of a joint or limb.

accessory movement manipulation selected arthokinematic movements performed at a joint for the purpose of examination or treatment. Three are commonly noted: distraction, compression, glide. **Distraction:** Separation of joint surfaces perpendicular to the joint plane. **Compression:** The pressing together or approximation of bone, joint surfaces, and/or soft tissue. **Glide:** A sliding or translatoric movement of one joint surface on the other. Therefore a fixed point on the moving surface comes in contact with a new point on the stationary surface.

accessory movements joint movements that are necessary for full range of motion but are not under direct voluntary control of the individual; involving spin and glide.

acute (1) having a short and severe course. (2) Intensification of need, or urgent.

adduction the act of moving toward the midsagittal plane of the body or axis of a joint or limb.

adhesion the result when two or more structures become attached, united, or stuck together.

adjunct rotation osteokinematically, any spin that can occur without any other motion of the bone. This motion can result from gravity, muscle action, other external forces.

analgesia absence of pain sensitivity; patient may experience stimulus, but it is no longer noxious.

anatomical zero joint position the beginning point of a joint range of motion.

anesthesia absence of sensibility to stimuli, with or without loss of consciousness.

angulation (1) the static angle between two anatomical structures, usually bones or body parts. (2) The movement of a rigid body in which all points described circular areas about an axis. See **roll.**

ankylosis stiffening or fixation of a joint secondary to biological tissue.

antalgic pertaining to a compensatory behavior attempting to avoid or lessen pain, usually applied to gait or movement.

anteversion (angle of torsion) the angulation created in the transverse plane between the neck and the shaft of the femur. The normal angle is 15 to 20 degrees; considerably less than this is called *retroversion*.

antiversion turned forward, inclined forward from a plane of reference as a whole without bending; usually applied to the positional relationship between the neck and head of the femur and its shaft.

ARC (1) any line wholly on a curved surface between two chosen points, other than a chord. (2) A portion of a curved surface.

arthro- Greek for joint or articulation.

arthrogram an adjunctive diagnostic procedure that involves injection of a radiopaque dye into a joint with subsequent radiography of the joint.

arthrokinematic movement of the joint surfaces.

arthron the joint composed of bony components, cartilaginous inserts, all the soft tissue structures intervening between the rigid skeletal components, and the adjacent pertinent muscular elements.

arthroscopy an adjunctive diagnostic procedure in which a 2 to 5 mm tube is inserted into a joint to allow direct visualization of the structures within the synovial cavity.

articulation (1) the junction of two or more bones. (2) the process of moving a joint through all or part of its range of motion.

articulatory technique repeated, rhythmic, oscillating joint movements of low velocity and varying amplitude performed within the available range of motion.

assessment to determine the importance, size, or value. Clinically, a judgment or interpretation.

barrier the point or object of restriction of a given movement.

biomechanics (1) an interdisciplinary science that describes, analyzes, and assesses human movement. (2) The study of forces and the effect of those forces on and within the human body.

boundary lubrication coating of a thin layer of molecules on each weight-bearing surface of a joint so that the joint slides on the opposing surface. Effective under low-load situations.

bowstringing spanning the shortest distance between two points.

brittle material a material that has no plastic region and deforms very little before failure.

bruxism clenching and grating of the teeth.

cancellous bone from the Italian word *cancelli*, which are open lattice screens behind which Roman judges sat; bone that is 10% to 70% mineralized tissue.

capsular pattern a characteristic series of limitations of joint motion that are present when the joint capsule is the limiting structure.

cariocas a form of lateral movement in which the side-stepping leg is brought successively behind and then in front of the stance leg.

causalgia burning pain (commonly accompanied by trophic skin changes) that may result from a peripheral nerve injury.

centric occlusion maximal contact of the teeth.

chemotaxis emigration of white blood cells toward the site of injury; dependent on the intensity of the concentration gradient and chemical change.

chord the shortest line (path) between any two points on a surface.

chronic of long duration.

circuit training a method of training involving activities or weight stations that are accomplished in sets during which the participant moves from one activity to another with little rest between sets.

"clearing" tests tests that take the joint to end range and stretch the capsule or other soft tissues in an attempt to reproduce symptoms. If no symptoms are reproduced and the range is within normal limits, the joint is "cleared" from involvement in the problem.

close-packed joint position the point in the range of motion at which the articulating surfaces are the most congruent and the supporting structures are most taut.

cocontraction a simultaneous contraction of agonistic and antagonistic muscle groups about a joint.

component movements see **accessory movements.**

concave-convex rule the principle that expresses the relationship between the osteokinematics and arthrokinematics of a given movement. In the articulating surfaces of a joint, the convex surface is always greater in surface area than that of its adjoining concave surface. Simply stated, when a *concave* joint surface moves on a convex surface, then gliding and bone movement are in the same direction. If a *convex* joint surface moves on a concave surface, then gliding and bone movement occur in the opposite direction. This has been attributed to the axis of motion being in the convex member in either case. A roll is always in the direction of bone movement.

concentric muscle contraction a muscular contraction that results in the origin and insertion of the muscle becoming approximated.

conjunct rotation osteokinematically, the involuntary spin that accompanies all impure (arcuate) swings and diadochal (a succession of two movements at an angle to each other) pure cardinal swings.

contractile unit as defined by Cyriax, those structures that are clinically or functionally related to a muscle regarding diagnosis by provocation. These include the muscle belly, the connective tissue sheaths, the tendons, and the bony insertions.

contraction the development of tension within a muscle or muscle group with or without changes in its overall length.

contracture a shortening of connective tissue that results in decreased range of motion in the corresponding joint.

convex-concave joint relationship the relative shape of each component of a joint's articulating surfaces. One surface is usually convex and the other is concave. The surface being moved determines the direction of the therapeutic procedure.

cortical bone bone in which 70% to 90% is mineralized tissue.

counter nutation the opposite of nutation.

coxa valga the angle of the neck of the femur to the shaft is greater than 120 degrees.

cramp a painful involuntary muscle contraction brought on by use of that muscle or muscle group.

creep a process usually involving metals or viscoelastic materials in which a load applied to an object for a long period of time causes the material to elongate.

crepitation a sense of sound emanating from movement of a joint or fracture site.

crepitus crackling sound or sensation within a synovial-lined cavity produced by movement.

cusps cone-shaped projections of the position teeth that fit into fossae on the tooth they contact.

cyma line a line seen on radiographs formed by the articulation of the talonavicular and calcaneocuboid bones; normally has smooth S shape.

DAPRE (daily adjusted progressive resistance exercise) a program of isotonic exercise that allows for individual differences in the rate at which a person regains strength in an injured area.

degrees of freedom (1) the number of independent coordinates in a coordinate system required to completely specify the position of an object in space. The term is loosely applied to specify the independent motion components involved in the characteristic movements of a given rigid body. The motion of a rigid body in space has six degrees of freedom (three translational and three rotational). When bodies are interconnected in a system, certain constraints are placed on the possible motions, and the number of degrees of freedom decreases (White and Panjabi, 1978). (2) The number of planes of motion through which osteokinematic movement of a joint occurs.

DeLorme technique a widely used method of weight training in which sets of repetitions are repeated with rest between sessions. The technique involves the use of heavier weights and fewer repetitions in successive sets.

derangement (internal derangement) a disturbance of the regular order or arrangement. Clinically, it describes various affections—either intraarticular, extraarticular, or both—that are often caused by trauma or abnormal use, that interfere with the normal function of a joint.

diagnosis see **evaluation.**

diagnosis by selective tension first described by Dr. James Cyriax, a system of diagnostic procedures aimed at localizing a soft tissue lesion based on specific provocation. This includes active movements, passive movements, movements against resistance, and palpation.

diapedesis the process whereby the white blood cell slides through the pore in the vessel wall during the inflammatory process.

disability a medicolegal term denoting a loss of function, either physical or mental (i.e., productivity, earning power, etc.).

dislocation a complete loss of contact of the articular surfaces of a joint.

distraction the surfaces of a joint are pulled apart as in a traction type of pull.

ductile material a material that deforms a great deal before failure and therefore has a long plastic region.

dyesthesia impairment of sensation, usually manifested by unpleasant or painful touch perception.

dysfunction abnormal function.

eburnation the glistening appearance of subchondral bone that appears in osteoarthritic joints where the cartilage has been eroded.

eccentric muscular contraction a muscular contraction that occurs while the origin and insertion of the muscle are moving away from each other.

elastic deformation a deformation of a metal or viscoelastic material caused by a load in which the material will resume its preload form on removal of the load.

electroacupuncture the application of electrical stimulation to acupuncture using a transcutaneous electrical nerve stimulation (TENS) or other electrical stimulator source.

end-feel the sensation imparted to the hands of the clinician at the end point of the available range of movement. This varies according to the limiting structure or tissue.

endurance the ability of a muscle or group of muscles to perform repeated contractions against an immovable object (isometric), against gravity (isotonic), and against a preset speed.

energy the capacity to do work.

enthesitis inflammation of the insertion of muscle with a strong tendency toward fibrosis and calcification. It is painful only when involved muscle is activated.

ergometry the study of work habits or activities.

evaluation an examination and corresponding judgment (diagnosis or assessment).

eversion the movement where the talus moves medially on the calcaneus relative to the neutral position (closed kinetic chain) or the calcaneus moves laterally on the talus relative to the neutral position (open kinetic chain).

examination the act of investigation or collection of data, both subjective and objective.

exit assessment a retest of a person on completion of a rehabilitation program to allow comparison to preadmission testing and/or preinjury tests.

extension a movement that brings two parts of a joint toward a straight position (as in extension of the knee, elbow, etc.). Extension can also be considered as the movement that returns a limb or the trunk from a flexed to a neutral position.

facilitated segment first described by Dr. Irvin Korr; a clinical term denoting the state in which a segment of the spinal cord is hyperresponsive or hyperirritable to impulses coming in from any source. It acts as a "neurological lens," focusing impulses coming in from anywhere to that particular segment. All structures receiving efferent nerve fibers from that segment are potentially exposed to abnormal impulses, including excessive excitation or inhibition.

flexion a movement that brings two parts of a joint or the body into a bent position. Flexion can also be considered as a movement that returns a limb or the trunk from an extended to a neutral position.

force a push or a pull defined as mass times acceleration. If the force on an object produces movement, it is called *dynamics;* if the force does not produce movement, it is called *statics.*

freeway space the gap between occlusal surfaces (teeth) occurring in the normal postural positions; also called *interocclusal distance.*

functional assessment an evaluation of a person's ability levels using task specific tests that involve the whole body versus single joint testing.

glide intrinsic joint movements on a plane parallel to the articulating surface.

grading a scheme or categorization of treatment movements. **Grade I:** A small amplitude movement at the beginning of range. **Grade II:** A large amplitude movement within the range but not to the limit of range. **Grade III:** A large amplitude movement up to the limit of range. **Grade IV:** A small amplitude movement up to the limit of range. **Grade V:** A high-velocity, short-amplitude movement (thrust) at and through the (pathological) limit of range.

herniated nucleus pulposus as defined by the American Academy of Orthopaedic Surgeons, displacement of nuclear material and other disk components beyond the normal confines of the annulus. Various degrees of displacement are recognized. **Protrusion** The displaced material causes a discreet bulge in the annulus, but no material escape through the annular fibers. **Extrusion:** The displaced material present in the spinal canal through disrupted fibers of the annulus; it remains connected to material persisting within the disk. **Sequestration:** Nuclear material escapes into the spinal canal as free fragment(s) that may migrate to other location. NOTE: Discarded term: **prolapse.**

hyperesthesia increased sensitivity, often unpleasant, to cutaneous stimulation.

hypermobile (1) when motion is more than that which would be normally permitted by the structures. (2) Excessive movement in a joint when compared to the normal population.

hyperpathia severely exaggerated subjective painful response to stimuli.

hypesthesia diminished sensitivity to stimuli (hypoesthesia).

hypomobile when motion is less than that which would normally be permitted by the structures.

impairment physical and/or psychological limitation.

inertia a state in which a body remains at rest or in uniform motion until acted on by an outside force.

instability description of a joint that has lost its structural integrity and is overtly hypermobile.

interferential current therapy a form of electrical stimulation technique in which two or three distinctly different currents are passed through an area or tissue, via surface electrodes, and portions of each current are cancelled by the other, resulting in a different net current applied to the target issue.

intrinsic minus hand deformity also called the *ulnar claw hand deformity;* a deformity that results from interruption of innervation of the hand via the ulnar nerve, resulting in metacarpophalangeal joint extensions and interphalangeal joint flexion.

inversion the opposite of eversion.

isokinetic a concentric or eccentric contraction that occurs at a set speed and uses a resistance that accommodates to the force produced at all points in the range of motion.

isometric a concentric muscular contraction of agonistic and antagonistic muscle groups about a joint in which there is no perceptible joint motion.

isotonic concentric or eccentric contractions of variable speed using a set weight or resistance throughout the full range of motion.

job site analysis the measurement of factors at a given location that influence job task performance.

job task analysis an analysis of the components of performing a worker's job through observation and measurement.

joint the junction of two or more bones. (For further definition and description, see *Gray's Anatomy,* ed. 36).

joint play movements see **accessory movements.**

kinematics the study of forces affecting motion.

kinetic chain a complex motor system formed by a series of joints. *Open:* A series of joints in which the terminal one is free. *Closed:* A series of joints in which the terminal one meets sufficient external resistance to prohibit or restrain free movement.

kinetics the study of internal and external forces acting on a body causing motion.

kyphosis a spinal curvature in which the convexity is facing posteriorly.

lateral shift a clinical term denoting an apparent translatoric displacement of the trunk on the lower lumbopelvic region.

lesion the site of an injury, pathological condition, or dysfunction.

loose-pack joint position the point in the range of motion at which the articulating surfaces are the least congruent and the supporting structures are the most lax.

lumbrical plus deformity a situation that often occurs in rheumatoid arthritis in which the lumbricals become contracted and their resultant action results in extension rather than flexion. The action results in metacarpophalangeal joint flexion and interphalangeal joint extension.

luxated joint no contact between articular surfaces of a joint; complete dislocation.

manipulation a therapeutic movement usually of a small amplitude accomplished at the end of the available range of motion but within the anatomical range at a speed over which the client has no control.

margination the accumulation of white blood cells along the margin of the capillary with adherence to the damaged portion of the vessel.

mechanical strain the deformation or change in dimensions that occurs on application of an external load.

mechanical stress the internal reaction to an external load.

mobilization a therapeutic movement of variable amplitude accomplished within the available range of motion at a speed over which the client has control.

muscle guarding/splinting generalized increased muscular tone as a protective response to pain, dysfunction, or stress.

myofascial trigger point a hyperirritable site that is painful on stimulation and gives rise to characteristic referred pain, tenderness, and autonomic phenomena.

neuromodulation altering (inhibiting or facilitating) the transmission of neurological signals, most commonly used regarding nociceptive input.

noncapsular pattern usually a singular, limited movement direction while all other movement directions are relatively unrestricted. This commonly occurs when an extracapsular tissue is the source of joint restriction.

noncontractile unit (inert) as defined by Cyriax, those structures that (1) have no inherent capacity to contract or relax and (2) are not part of the contractile unit. Orthopaedically these include the joint capsule, ligaments, bursa, fascia, dura mater, nerve roots and peripheral nerves, articular cartilage, menisci, disks, and synovial fat pads.

nutation a nodding forward or anteriorly (as in nutation of the sacrum).

open bite existence of vertical space between upper and lower anterior teeth in centric occlusion.

orthopaedic clinical specialist a physical therapist who has successfully met the requirements established by the Orthopaedic Specialty Council of the American Physical Therapy Association.

osteo- bone.

osteokinematic movement of the bones.

ovoid articular surfaces synovial joint surfaces characterized by an egg-shaped articular surface that is either concave or convex in all directions.

ovoid of motion the curved path of motion through which a bone moves. It is always convex away from the joint at which motion occurs.

Oxford technique a method of weight training in which sets of repetitions are repeated with rest between sessions. This technique involves the use of the heaviest weight in the first set with progressively light loads in successive sets.

pain an unpleasant emotional experience that is evoked by activation (mechanical and/or chemical) of the nociceptive afferent system.

pain quality description of the nature, type, or character of pain (i.e., burning, dull, sharp, throbbing, etc.).

painful arc of movement pain is perceived at a central part of a range of movement, with pain ceasing once past that point in either direction, such as when a pain-sensitive structure is impinged between two bony surfaces.

palpation examination by touching and feeling.

parallel force component a nonrotary force that acts to compress or distract a joint (shear).

perpendicular force component a rotary force that acts to rotate a joint (normal).

phagocytosis the process of one cell engulfing another, used by white blood cells to remove foreign materials.

pinocytosis the uptake of extracellular fluid and solutes into membrane-bound vesicles.

plane articular surfaces synovial joint surfaces that are characterized (for functional purposes) as flat, even though anatomically there may be a slight curve.

plastic deformation a permanent deformation in a metal or viscoelastic material created by a sub-yield-point load.

position of maximal joint volume the point in the range of motion at which the capsule has the potential to hold the greatest amount of synovial fluid. This position is usually reflexly assumed by the joint during the time of effusion.

power the rate of doing work or dissipating energy, which is force times linear displacement divided by time. A measure of rotary motion, power is equated to torque times angular displacement divided by time.

pressure force distributed over an area.

pronation (hand or forearm) the act of turning the palm downward, performed by medial rotation of the forearm (radius).

proprioceptive neuromuscular facilitation (PNF) a form of exercise in which accommodating resistance is manually applied to various patterns of movement for the purpose of strengthening and retraining the muscles guiding joint motion.

Q angle the angle of incidence of the quadriceps muscle relative to the patella. The Q angle determines the tracking of the patella through the trochlea of the femur. As the angle increases, the chance of the patellar compression problems increase.

radiating pain a pattern of pain that follows the path of a spinal or peripheral nerve.

recuravatum a curve of a body part opposite to the normal (e.g., genu recurvatum).

referred pain the perception of pain is felt elsewhere than the site of the (tissue) provocation.

resolution a force directed along one line of action.

resolution of force the replacement of a single force by two or more equivalent forces.

rest joint position the position of a joint where the joint surfaces are relatively incongruent and the support structures are relatively lax. This position is used extensively in passive mobilization procedures.

roll intrinsic joint movements on an axis parallel to the articulating surface. The axis can remain stationary or move in a plane parallel to the joint surface.

scar (1) a mark remaining after the healing of a wound or other morbid process. (2) The fibrous tissue replacing the normal tissues destroyed by injury or disease.

sclerotomal pain distribution referral of pain from pain-sensitive tissues covering the axial skeleton.

scoliosis the lateral curvature of the spine.

screening the process of examining a population (usually a high-risk population) for a given state or disease.

sellar articular surfaces synovial joint surfaces characterized by saddle-shaped articular surfaces that are concave in one plane and convex in the plane perpendicular to it. These synovial joint surfaces articulate with corresponding synovial surfaces that are reciprocally concave and convex.

sensation conveyance of an impulse by afferent nerves to the sensorium.

sensibility conscious interpretation of a sensory stimulus.

sign clinically noted as the objective findings associated with an illness or dysfunction.

soft tissue all neuromusculoskeletal tissues except bone and articular cartilage.

spasm an involuntary muscle contraction. Further motion is prevented by vibrant muscular twang (muscle spasm).

spin intrinsic joint movements about an axis perpendicular to the articulating surface.

spinal motion segment described by Junghans, the term denotes those structures and entities that compose the functional unit of the spine. It includes two adjacent vertebrae, the intervertebral disk (except occiput-atlas and atlas-axis), the apophyseal joints, all the interconnecting ligaments, the two intervertebral foramen, and the spinal canal.

sprain an injury to the joint capsule and/or the supporting ligaments resulting from overstress, which causes some degree of damage to the fibers or their attachments. **First degree:** Some disruption of fibers with little or no loss of function. **Second degree:** Some portion of the ligament/capsule is torn with some loss of function. **Third degree:** A complete tear and therefore total loss of function.

squeeze-film lubrication exudation of fluid from the cartilage of joints, forming a film in the transient area of impending contact; termed *squeeze film.*

stenosis a narrowing of any canal (e.g., spinal stenosis denoting a state of decreased diameter of the spinal canal and the intervertebral foramen).

strain an overexertion trauma to a portion of the contractile musculotendinous unit or its attachment to the bone (tendinoperiosteal junction).

strength the ability of a muscle to produce or resist a force.

stretch weakness a clinical term denoting the effect on muscles from prolonged immobilization in a lengthened position, in other words, beyond the neutral or physiological rest position.

subluxated some contact between joint surfaces; partially dislocated.

supination (hand or forearm) the opposite of pronation (i.e., the act of turning the palm upward, performed by lateral rotation of the radius).

supination (subtalar joint) a triplanar motion of the plantar flexion, inversion, and adduction (open kinetic chain).

swing any osteokinematic motion other than a spin. (For further discussion and definition, see *Gray's Anatomy,* ed. 36). **Pure swing** (cardinal swing): When a bone swings without any accompanying spin. The arc of motion created is the shortest distance between two points. **Impure swing** (arcuate swing): When a bone swings and simultaneously undergoes some spin. The arc of motion created is other than the shortest distance between two points.

symptom clinically noted as the subjective findings associated with an illness or dysfunction.

syndrome a group of signs and symptoms that often occur together. Commonly, they characterize a disease or lesion.

synovia also called *synovial fluid;* an ultrafiltrate of blood plasma plus a mucopolysaccharide, hyaluronic acid.

thrust technique a high-velocity, short-amplitude joint motion performed at the end of the available range of motion but within the anatomical ROM.

tibial torsion the rotation occurring inherently in the shaft of the tibia from proximal to distal ends. Normal rotation is approximately 15 degrees.

tidemark a transitional zone, appearing as a wavy line, that marks the junction between calcified and uncalcified cartilage.

tone the tension in a muscle or muscle group resulting from both active (contractile) and passive (inert) mechanisms.

trabeculum the rod portion of cancellous bone.

traction the act of drawing or pulling. Clinically, it is usually along the longitudinal axis of the respective body part.

transcutaneous electrical nerve stimulation (TENS) application of low-intensity, pulsed alternating or direct currents to decrease pain perception.

trigger point see **myofascial trigger point.**

ultimate strain the strain at the point of failure.

ultimate stress the highest load sustained at the point of failure.

valgus an angulation of a body part away from the midline of the body.

varus an angulation of a body part toward the midline of the body.

velocity spectrum rehabilitation a rehabilitation program that uses strength training at multiple speeds of movement, from slow to fast.

weeping lubrication a form of hydrostatic lubrication in which the interstitial fluid of hydrated articular cartilage flows onto its surface when a load is applied.

work hardening a term used to identify a complete program of treatment designed to place an injured worker back into the preinjury job or occupation.

INDEX